Endoscopic Surgery for Gynecologists

Endoscopic Surgery for Gynecologists

Second Edition

Edited by

Chris Sutton

The Royal Surrey County Hospital, Guildford;
Chelsea & Westminster Hospital, London;
Imperial College School of Medicine, University of London, London, UK

and

Michael P. Diamond

Wayne State University School of Medicine, Detroit, USA

Accompanying CD-ROM edited by

Andrew Kent

Senior Registrar, Royal Surrey County Hospital, Guildford, UK

WB SAUNDERS COMPANY LTD

London   Philadelphia   Toronto   Sydney   Tokyo

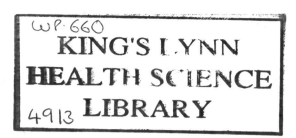
This book is printed on acid free paper

WB Saunders Company Ltd 24–28 Oval Road
London NW1 7DX

The Curtis Center
Independence Square West
Philadelphia, PA 19106–3399

55 Horner Avenue
Toronto, Ontario M8Z 4X6, Canada

Harcourt Brace & Company (Australia) Pty Ltd
30–52 Smidmore St
Marrickville, NSW 2204, Australia

Harcourt Brace Japan Inc.
Ichibancho Central Building, 22–1 Ichibancho
Chiyoda-ku, Tokyo 102, Japan

First published 1993
Second edition 1998

A catalogue record for this book is available from the British Library

ISBN 0-7020-2250-0

CD-ROM produced by Binary Vision, www.binaryvision.com
Cover photograph by Ashley Prytherch, Medical Illustrations Department, Royal Surrey County Hospital

Typeset by Phoenix Photosetting, Chatham, Kent
Printed and bound in Great Britain by Jarrolds, Norwich

Contents

Contributors   xi

Preface   xv

1   History and development of endoscopic surgery   1
A.G. GORDON AND P.J. TAYLOR

2   Medico-legal implications of minimally invasive surgery   9
B.V. LEWIS

LAPAROSCOPIC SURGERY – TECHNIQUES AND EQUIPMENT

3   Setting up a service: instrumentation and administration   19
G.W. PATTON JR

4   Role of the operating room nurse   30
WENDY K. WINER

5   A practical approach to surgical laparoscopy   41
C. SUTTON

6   Advanced laparoscopic techniques   54
H. REICH

7   Lasers in reproductive medicine   68
Y. TADIR AND M.W. BERNS

8   Electrosurgery   83
R.C. ODELL

9   Tissue effects of lasers, electrosurgery and ultrasonic scalpels   93
J. KECKSTEIN AND C. SUTTON

10   Laparoscopic use of the argon beam coagulator   105
J.F. DANIELL AND R.W. DOVER

11   Recent advances in laparoscopic tissue extraction   111
A. POOLEY AND R. STEINER

12 Surgical modalities and clinical results   116
T. TULANDI

LAPAROSCOPIC TUBAL SURGERY

13 Salpingostomy and fimbrioplasty   129
J.-B. DUBUISSON AND C. CHAPRON

14 Laparoscopic fertility-promoting procedures   139
V. GOMEL AND M.G. MUNRO

15 Strategy for treatment of ectopic pregnancy: conservative
treatment   150
J.L. POULY

16 Techniques of mass sterilization   159
S.S. SHETH

17 Laparoscopic female sterilization   167
G.M. FILSHIE

18 Laparoscopic microsurgical tubal anastomosis   176
C.H. KOH

19 Falloposcopy and other tubal cannulation techniques   186
I.W. SCUDAMORE AND I.D. COOKE

LAPAROSCOPIC OVARIAN SURGERY

20 Laparoscopic ovarian surgery: Preoperative diagnosis and
imaging   201
L. DE CRESPIGNY

21 Laparoscopic ovarian surgery and ovarian torsion   212
A.J.M. AUDEBERT

22 Laparoscopic treatment of ovarian endometriomas   221
I. BROSENS AND C. SUTTON

23 Polycystic ovaries, surgical management   233
G.T. KOVACS

24 Laparoscopic treatment of tubo-ovarian abscess   241
D.A. JOHNS

LAPAROSCOPIC UTERINE SURGERY

25 Laparoscopic uterine nerve ablation for intractable
dysmenorrhea   249
C. SUTTON

26 Laparoscopic surgery for pelvic pain   261
E.D. BIGGERSTAFF

27 Laparoscopic myomectomy   272
    J.B. DUBUISSON, C. CHAPRON AND A. FAUCONNIER

28 Laparoscopic leiomyoma coagulation – myolysis   280
    D.R. PHILLIPS

29 Avoidance of complications of laparoscopic hysterectomy   289
    J.H. PHIPPS

30 Laparoscopic assisted vaginal hysterectomy   300
    D.A. JOHNS

31 Laparoscopic supracervical hysterectomy   308
    T.L. LYONS

32 Laparoscopically assisted Doderlein hysterectomy   315
    M.D. WHITTAKER AND R. GARRY

LAPAROSCOPIC PELVIC FLOOR REPAIR AND INCONTINENCE PROCEDURES

33 Laparoscopic colposuspension   325
    A.R.B. SMITH AND T.G. VANCAILLIE

34 Laparoscopic repair of enteroceles and pelvic floor support
    procedures   334
    C.Y. LIU AND S. NAIR

LAPAROSCOPIC SURGERY FOR ENDOMETRIOSIS AND ADHESIONS

35 Diagnosis of endometriosis: laparoscopic appearances   349
    J.A. ROCK AND S. REDDY

36 Rectovaginal septum adenomyotic nodule: A distinct entity.
    A series of 460 cases   357
    J. DONNEZ, M. NISOLLE, M. SMETS, S. BASSIL AND F. CASANAS-ROUX

37 Laser vaporization of endometriosis   363
    J.R. FESTE

38 Monopolar electroexcision of endometriosis   369
    D.B. REDWINE

39 Laparoscopic treatment of advanced endometriosis   380
    D.C. MARTIN

40 Laparoscopic treatment of bowel adhesions (enterolysis)   390
    J.F. DANIELL AND R.W. DOVER

41 Prevention of adhesion development   398
    M.P. DIAMOND AND L.B. SCHWARTZ

LAPAROSCOPIC ONCOLOGIC SURGERY

42 Laparoscopic pelvic lymphadenectomy 407
D. QUERLEU AND E. LEBLANC

43 Laparoscopic aortic lymphadenectomy 417
N. KADAR

44 Laparoscopic vaginal radical hysterectomy 438
D. DARGENT

45 Laparoscopic radical hysterectomy for cervical cancer 447
M. CANIS, A. WATTIEZ, G. MAGE, P. MILLE, J.L. POULY AND M.A. BRUHAT

46 Laparoscopic management of gynecologic malignancy 459
J.M. MONAGHAN

47 Laparoscopic management of ovarian malignancy and
the suspicious adnexal mass 467
L. METTLER

MAJOR COMPLICATIONS OF LAPAROSCOPIC SURGERY – AVOIDANCE AND MANAGEMENT

48 Bowel complications of laparoscopic surgery 481
A. POOLEY AND R. SODERSTROM

49 Major vessel injuries 489
B.S. LEVY

50 Genitourinary complications 494
C.H. NEZHAT, F. NEZHAT, D. SEIDMAN AND C. NEZHAT

HYSTEROSCOPIC SURGERY

51 Initiating a hysteroscopic program and hysteroscopic
instrumentation 501
M.S. BAGGISH

52 Diagnostic hysteroscopy: technique and documentation 511
K. WAMSTEKER AND S. DE BLOK

53 Distension media and fluid systems 525
R. GARRY

54 Laser hysteroscopic resection of fibroids 534
J. DEQUESNE AND N. SCHMIDT

55 Treatment of dysfunctional bleeding by Nd:YAG laser 540
J. DONNEZ, R. POLET, M. SMETS, S. BASSIL, A. BELIARD AND M. NISOLLE

56 Hysteroscopic metroplasty 552
R.F. VALLE

57   Hysteroscopic tubal occlusion   568
F.D. LOFFER

ENDOMETRIAL ABLATION TECHNIQUES

58   Transcervical resection of the endometrium (TCRE)   581
H. O'CONNOR, A.L. MAGOS AND J.A.M. BROADBENT

59   Endometrial electroablation   592
T.G. VANCAILLIE

60   Nd:YAG laser ablation of the endometrium   604
M.H. GOLDRATH AND R. GARRY

61   Endometrial balloon ablation   614
R.W. DOVER

62   Photodynamic therapy   621
Y. TADIR, B. TROMBERG AND M.W. BERNS

63   Microwave endometrial ablation   630
N.C. SHARP, I.B. FELDBERG, D.A. HODGSON, B BUTTERS AND N. CRONIN

MAJOR COMPLICATIONS OF HYSTEROSCOPIC SURGERY – AVOIDANCE AND MANAGEMENT

64   Hazards and dangers of operative hysteroscopy   641
B.J. VAN HERENDAEL

THE FUTURE

65   Fetal surgery   651
J.P. BRUNER

66   Embryoscopy   668
Y. DUMEZ

67   Outpatient local anesthetic laparoscopy   674
E.J. SHAXTED

68   Total laparoscopic hysterectomy using ultrasound energy   679
C.E. MILLER

69   Embolization of myomas   687
B. McLUCAS

Directory of Manufacturers   693

Index   697

Contributors

Dr Alain J.M. Audebert, Institut Robert B Greenblatt, 35 rue Turenne, 33000 Bordeaux, France

Professor Michael S. Baggish, Department of Obstetrics and Gynecology, Good Samaritan Hospital, 375 Dixmyth Street, Cincinnatti, Ohio 45220, USA

Dr Salim Bassil, Catholic University of Louvain, Cliniques Universitaires St Luc, Department of Gynecology, Avenue Hippocrates 10, B-1200 Brussels, Belgium

Dr Aude Beliard, Catholic University of Louvain, Cliniques Universitaires St Luc, Department of Gynecology, Avenue Hippocrate 10, B-1200 Brussels, Belgium

Dr M.W. Berns, Beckman Laser Institute, Department of Surgery, University of California, Irvine, CA 92715, USA

Dr E. Daniel Biggerstaff III, Candler Professional Building, Suite 518, 5354 Reynolds Street, Savannah, Georgia 31405, USA

Dr. J.A. Mark Broadbent, Senior Registrar in Obstetrics and Gynaecology, Elizabeth Garrett Anderson Hospital, Department of Obstetrics and Gynaecology, 144 Euston Road, London NW1 2AP, UK

Professor Ivo Brosens, Leuven Institute for Fertility and Embryology, Tiensevest 168, Leuven B-3000, Belgium

Professor Maurice A. Bruhat, Département de Gynécologie Obstétrique et Reproduction Humaine, Polyclinique de l'Hôtel Dieu, Centre Hospitalier Universitaire, 13 Boulevard Charles de Gaulle, 63033 Clermont-Ferrand, France

Dr Joseph P. Bruner, Vanderbilt Medical Center, Division of Maternal/Fetal Medicine, B1100 Medical Centre North, Nashville, Tennessee 37232-2519, USA.

Dr Brian Butters, Microsulis Ltd, Waterlooville, Hampshire, UK

Dr Michel Canis, Département de Gynécologie Obstétrique et Reproduction Humaine, Polyclinique de l'Hôtel Dieu, Centre Hospitalier Universitaire, 13 Boulevard Charles de Gaulle, 63033 Clermont-Ferrand, France

Dr Francoise Casanas-Roux, Catholic University of Louvain, Cliniques Universitaires St Luc, Department of Obstetrics and Gynecology, Avenue Hippocrate 10, 1200 Brussels, Belgium

Dr Charles Chapron, Clinique Universitaire Baudelocque, Service de Chirurgie Gynecologique, CHU Chochin Port Royal, 123 Boulevarde Port Royal, 75014 Paris, France

Professor Ian D. Cooke, Professor of Obstetrics and Gynaecology, The Jessop Hospital for Women, Leavygreave Road, Sheffield S3 7RE, UK

Dr Nigel Cronin, School of Physics, University of Bath, Bath, UK

Dr James F. Daniell, Women's Health Group, 2222 State Street, Nashville, Tennessee TN 37203, USA

Professor Daniel Dargent, Hôpital Edouard Herriot, Place d'Arsonval, F-69437, Cedex 03, Lyon, France

Dr Sjoerd De Blok, Onze Lieve Vrouwe Gasthuis, 1e Oosterparkstraat 179, Amsterdam 1091 HA, The Netherlands

Dr Lachlan de Crespigny, Associate Professor, Melbourne Ultrasound for Women, Level One, 62 Lygon Street, Carlton, Victoria 3053, Australia

Dr Jacques Dequesne, FMH Gynecologie et Obstetrique, Chemin des Croix Rouges 16, 1007 Lausanne, Switzerland

Professor Michael P. Diamond, Professor of Obstetrics and Gynecology, Wayne State University School of Medicine, Detroit Medical Center, Hutzel Hospital, 4707 St Antoine Boulevard, Detroit MI 48201, USA

Professor Jacques Donnez, Catholic University of Louvain, Department of Gynecology, Cliniques Universitaires St Luc, Avenue Hippocrate 10, Brussels B-1200, Belgium

Dr Richard W. Dover, Research Fellow, Department of Gynaecology, Royal Surrey County Hospital, Egerton Road, Guildford GU2 5XX, UK

Professor Jean-Bernard Dubuisson, Clinique Universitaire Baudelocque, Port-Royal, 123 Boulevard de Port-Royal, Paris F-75014, France

Professor Yves Dumez, Maternité Port Royal, Department of Obstetrics and Gynecology, 123 Boulevard de Port-Royal, Paris F-75014, France

Dr Arnaud Fauconnier, Clinique Universitaire Baudelocque, Service de Chirurgie Gynecologique, CHU Cochin Port-Royal, 123 Boulevard de Port-Royal, Paris F-75014, France

Dr Ian B. Feldberg, School of Physics, University of Bath, Bath, UK

Dr Joseph R. Feste, Ob/Gyn Associates, 7550 Fannin Street, Houston TX 77054-1989, USA

Dr G. Marcus Filshie, Queen's Medical Centre, Department of Obstetrics and Gynaecology, Floor B, East Block, Nottingham NG7 2UH, UK

Dr Ray Garry, Medical Director, Women's Endoscopic Laser Foundation, Gledhow Wing, St James's University Hospital, Leeds LS9 7TF, UK

Professor Milton H. Goldrath, Sinai Hospital – Detroit Medical Center, Department of Obstetrics and Gynecology, 6767 West Outer Drive, Detroit, Michigan 48235, USA

Professor Victor Gomel, University of British Columbia, Department of Obstetrics and Gynecology, 805 West 12th Avenue, Third Floor Willow Pavillion, Vancouver BC V5Z 1M9, Canada

Dr D. Alan G. Gordon, Honorary Consultant Gynaecologist, Princess Royal, BUPA Hospital, Anlaby, Hull HU10 AZ, UK

Dr Bruno J. van Herendael, Jan Palfijn General Hospital, Lange Bremstraat 70, 2170 Merksem, Antwerp, Belgium

Dr David A. Hodgson, Royal United Hospital, Coombe Park, Bath, UK

Dr D. Alan Johns, Richland Medical Center, 3700 Rufe Snow Drive, Fort Worth TX 76180, USA

Dr Grant W. Patton Jr, South Eastern Fertility Center PA, 900 Bowman Road, Suite 108, Mount Pleasant 7SC 29464, USA

Dr Nicholas Kadar, Englewood Hospital and Medical Center, 350 Engle Street, Englewood, New Jersey 07631, USA

Dr Jörg Keckstein, Head of Department, A O Landeskrankenhaus Villach, Department of Obstetrics and Gynecology, 59500 Villach, Nikolaigasse 43, Austria

Dr Andrew Kent, Senior Registrar, Royal Surrey County Hospital, Guildford, GU2 5XX, UK

Dr Charles H. Koh, Reproductive Speciality Centre, Suite 501, Seton Tower, 2315 N. Lake Drive, Milwaukee WI 53211, USA

Professor Gabor T Kovacs, Director/Professor Obstetrics, Monash Medical School, Box Hill Hospital, Nelson Road, Box Hill, Victoria 3128, Australia

Dr Eric Leblanc, Centre Oscar–Lambret, 59000 Lille, France

Dr Barbara S. Levy, University of Washington School of Medicine, Department of Obstetrics and Gynecology, 34509 9th Avenue South, Suite 300, Federal Way, Washington 98003, USA

Dr B. Victor Lewis, Queen's House, 200 Lower High Street, Watford WD1 2EH, UK

Dr C. Y. Liu, Director, Chattanooga Women's Laser Center, 1604 Gunbarrel Road, Chattanooga, Tennessee 37421, USA

Dr Franklin D. Loffer, Department of Obstetrics and Gynecology, University of Arizona School of Medicine, 3410 North 4th Avenue, Phoenix, AZ 85013-3996, USA

Dr Thomas L. Lyons, Center for Women's Care and Reproductive Surgery, 1140 Hammond Drive, Building F, Suite 6230, Atlanta, GA 30327, USA

Professor Gérard Mage, Département de Gynécologie Obstétrique et Reproduction Humaine, Polyclinique de l'Hôtel Dieu, Centre Hospitalier Universitaire, 13 Boulevard Charles de Gaulle, 63033, Clermont Ferrand, France

Dr Adam L. Magos, Consultant Gynaecologist, The Royal Free Hampstead NHS Trust, Minimally Invasive Therapy Clinic, Department of Obstetrics and Gynaecology, Pond Street, London NW 3 2QG, UK

Dr Dan C. Martin, 1717 Kirby Parkway, Suite 100, Memphis, Tennessee 38120-4331, USA

Dr Bruce McLucas, University of California Los Angeles, Medical Plaza, Suite 310, Los Angeles, California 90024-6970, USA

Professor Liselotte Mettler, Universität Kiel, Department of Obstetrics and Gynecology, Michaelisstrasse 16, 24105 Kiel 1, Germany

Sister Diana Miles, Mount Alvernia Hospital, Harvey Road, Guildford, Surrey GU1 3LX, UK

Dr P. Mille, Département de Gynécologie Obstétrique et Reproduction Humaine, Polyclinique de l'Hôtel Dieu, Centre Hospitalier Universitaire, 13 Boulevard de Charles de Gaulle, 63033 Clermont Ferrand, France

Dr Charles E. Miller, Center for Human Reproduction, 750 North Orleans Street, Chicago, Illinois 60610, USA

Dr John M. Monaghan, Senior Lecturer in Gynaecologic Oncology, Queen Elizabeth Hospital, Sheriff Hill, Gateshead, Tyne and Wear NE9 6SX, UK

Professor M. G. Munro, Professor and Associate Chairman, University of California Los Angeles, Department of Obstetrics and Gynecology, 650 Circle Drive South, Los Angeles CA 90095, California, USA

Dr Suresh Nair, Consultant, Kandang Kerbau Hospital, Department of Reproductive Medicine, 2 Hampshire Road, Singapore 219428

Dr Camran Nezhat, Stanford University School of Medicine, 750 Welch Road, Suite 403, Palo Alto, California 94304-1885, USA

Dr Ceana H. Nezhat, Stanford University School of Medicine, Department of Obstetrics and Gynecology, 750 Welch Road, Palo Alto, California 93404-1885, USA

Dr Farr Nezhat, Stanford University School of Medicine, Department of Obstetrics and Gynecology, 750 Welch Road, Palo Alto, California 93404-1885, USA

Professor Michelle Nisolle, Catholic University of Louvain, Cliniques Universitaires St Luc, Department of Gynecology, Avenue Hippocrate 10, B-1200 Brussels, Belgium

Dr Hugh O'Connor, Consultant Obstetrician and Gynecologist, The Coombe Women's Hospital and St James's Hospital, Dublin, Ireland

Mr Roger Odell, Electroscope Inc., 4828 Sterling Drive, Boulder, Colorado 80301, USA

Dr Grant W. Patton Jr, South Eastern Fertility Center, 1376 Hospital Drive, Suite 108, Mount Pleasant, SC 29464, USA

Dr Douglas R. Phillips, Clinical Associate Professor, Department of Obstetrics and Gynecology, School of Medicine, State University of New York at Stony Brook, New York, USA

Dr Jeffrey H. Phipps, George Eliot Hospital NHS Trust, Department of Obstetrics and Gynaecology, College Street, Nuneaton, Warwickshire CV10 7DJ, UK

Dr Roland Polet, Catholic University of Louvain, Department of Gynecology, Cliniques Universitaires St Luc, Avenue Hippocrate 10, B-1200 Brussels, Belgium

Dr Andrew Pooley, Senior Registrar, Mayday University Hospital, Department of Obstetrics and Gynaecology, Mayday Road, Thorton Heath, Surrey CR7 7YE, UK

Professor Jean Luc Pouly, Département de Gynécologie Obstétrique et Reproduction Humaine,

Polyclinique de l'Hôtel Dieu, Centre Hospitalier Universitaire, 13 Boulevard Charles de Gaulle, 63033 Clermont Ferrand, France

Professor Denis Querleu, Hôpital Jeanne de Flandre, CHRU 59037 Lille, France

Dr Sujatha Reddy, Emory University School of Medicine, Woodruff Memorial Research Building, PO Box 21246, 1639 Pierce Drive, Atlanta GA 30322, USA

Dr David B. Redwine, 2190 North East, Professional Court, Bend 97701, Oregon, USA

Dr Harry Reich, Columbia Presbyterian Medical Center, New York, NY 10032, USA

Professor John A. Rock, James Robert McCord Professor and Chairman, Emory University School of Medicine, Department of Obstetrics and Gynecology, PO Box 21246, 1639 Pierce Drive, Atlanta, GA 30322, USA

Dr Norman Schmidt, FMH Gynecologie et Obstetrique, Chemin des Croix Rouges 2, 1007 Lausanne, Switzerland

Dr Lisa Barrie Schwartz, Department of Obstetrics and Gynecology, New York University, New York, New York, USA

Dr Ian W. Scudamore, Leicester General Hospital NHS Trust, Gwendolen Road, Leicester LE5 4PW, UK

Dr Daniel Seidman, Stanford University School of Medicine, Department of Obstetrics and Gynecology, 750 Welch Road, Palo Alto, California 93404-1885, USA

Dr Nicholas C. Sharp, Consultant Obstetrician and Gynaecologist, Royal United Hospital, Combe Park, Bath BA1 3NG, UK

Dr Edward J. Shaxted, Northampton Medical Consultancy Unit, Three Shires Hospital, Cliftonville, Northampton NN1 5DR, UK

Dr Shirish S. Sheth, Breach Candy Hospital, 2/2 Navjivan Society, Lamington Road, Mumbai 400 008, India

Dr Mireille Smets, Catholic University of Louvain, Cliniques Universitaires St Luc, Department of Gynecology, Avenue Hippocrate 10, B-1200 Brussels, Belgium

Dr Anthony R.B. Smith, Consultant Gynaecologist, Saint Mary's Hospital for Women and Children, Whitworth Park, Manchester M13 0JH, UK

Dr Richard Soderstrom, Reproductive Health Specialists PS, 1101 Madison Suite 580, Seattle, Washington 98104, USA

Dr Rolf Steiner, Kantonales Frauenspital Fontana, Lurlibadstrasse 118, 7000 Chur, Switzerland

Dr Chris Sutton, The Royal Surrey County Hospital and Chelsea and Westminster Hospital, 369 Fulham Road, London SW10 9NH, UK

Professor Yona Tadir, Professor of Obstetrics and Gynecology, Beckman Laser Institute, Department of Surgery, 1002 Health Science Road East, University of California, Irvine, CA 92612, USA

Professor Patrick J. Taylor, Professor and Chairman, St Paul's Hospital, Department of Obstetrics and Gynecology, Vancouver, Canada

Dr B. Tromberg, Beckman Laser Institute, Department of Surgery, 1002 Health Science Road East, University of California, Irvine CA 92612, USA

Dr Togas Tulandi, Director, Royal Victoria Hospital, Women's Pavillion, 687 Pine Avenue, West, Montreal, Quebec H3A 1A1, Canada

Professor Rafael F. Valle, Prentice Women's Hospital and Maternity Center, Department of Obstetrics and Gynecology, Northwestern University Medical School, Suite 1552, 333 East Superior Street, Chicago, IL 60611-3095, USA

Professor Thierry G. Vancaillie, Royal Hospital for Women, Barker Street, Randwick, Sydney, NSW 2031, Australia

Dr Kees Wamsteker, Director, Hysteroscopy Training Center, Spaarne Hospital Haarlem, Department of Obstetrics and Gynecology, PO Box 1644, 2003 BRF, Haarlem, The Netherlands

Dr Arnaud Wattiez, Département de Gynécologie Obstetrique et Reproduction Humaine, Polyclinique de l'Hôtel Dieu, Centre Hospitalier Universitaire, 13 Boulevard Charles de Gaulle, 63033 Clermont Ferrand, France

Dr Mark D. Whittaker, Specialist Registrar, Gledhow Wing, St James's University Hospital, Leeds LS9 7TF, UK

Ms Wendy K. Winer, c/o Center for Women's Care and Reproductive Surgery, 1140 Hammond Drive, Suite F-6230, Atlanta, Georgia 30328, USA

Preface

When the first edition of this book was published in 1993 it was a runaway success and very rapidly went into three printings in a relatively short space of time. We were perhaps fortunate, because we were cresting the wave of popularity of laparoscopic surgery and it coincided with the widespread uptake of more advanced procedures, such as laparoscopic hysterectomy and colposuspension.

At that time it was becoming apparent that virtually any operation that could be performed at laparotomy could be tackled using minimal access surgery, with the exception of advanced malignancy. In the first edition the treatment of cancer was hardly mentioned, apart from stern warnings to be careful in the preoperative exclusion of malignancy when dealing with adnexal masses through the laparoscope. In this new edition, one of the largest sections is on laparoscopic oncological surgery and, although the pioneers of laparoscopic surgery were largely reproductive surgeons, it is comforting to note that all of the authors in this section come from reputable oncological subspecialty centers, who have all had considerable experience in treating cancer through a laparotomy incision. In a similar way, the urogynecologists have taken up this new type of surgery and the section on laparoscopic procedures for incontinence and pelvic floor repair reflects a growing trend, that often the best way to obtain a near perfect anatomical result is to perform such surgery laparoscopically rather than by the vaginal approach.

Gynecological endoscopic surgery continues to expand its horizons and continually embraces new technology and we hope that this is reflected in this new edition, because about two thirds of this book has had to be completely rewritten and in many cases completely new chapters have been added. At the time of going to press it is as up-to-date as we can possibly manage to make it and we hope that the addition of CD ROM technology will further increase its appeal.

Since the first edition, the technical virtuosity of some laparoscopic surgeons has ensured that virtually all operations can be performed laparoscopically, although undoubtedly they take considerably more operating time. In certain areas, such as the treatment of ectopic pregnancy and endometriosis, laparoscopic surgery has become the gold standard and is now available in virtually all hospitals, although certainly the very severe cases of endometriosis still require referral to special centers. The question now, is not whether we can do this kind of surgery, but whether it is producing results that are as good as, or even better than, the surgery that it has replaced. It is refreshing in this volume to see that many of the surgical techniques have been subjected to randomized clinical trials, because this is the only way that we can genuinely claim that laparoscopic surgery is not merely better for the patient in terms of reduced postoperative discomfort and morbidity, but also it can be a better way of treating their disease. Such studies must be extended to embrace all aspects of laparoscopic and hysteroscopic surgery, because it is the only way to answer the criticisms of various detractors, usually members of the old guard, who cannot or will not embrace these new surgical techniques.

Chris Sutton
Michael Diamond

1

History and Development of Endoscopic Surgery

ALAN G. GORDON* AND PATRICK J. TAYLOR†

*Princess Royal Hospital and BUPA Hospital, Hull, UK
†Department of Obstetrics and Gynecology, St Pauls Hospital, Vancouver, Canada

Early Endoscopy

'And there is no new thing under the sun' (Ecclesiastes i:8). Nowhere is this more true than in the field of endoscopy. The wish to peer into the body is as old as recorded history. The earliest description of endoscopic examinations were from the Kos school led by Hippocrates (460–375 BC) who described a rectal speculum remarkably similar to the instruments in use today. Clearly recognizable bivalve specula recovered from the ashes of Pompeii, which was buried in 70 AD, can be seen in the Institute Rizzoli in Bologna (Figure 1.1). The Babylonian Talmud (Niddah Treatise), written in 500 AD after 300 years of preparation, described a siphopherot, a tube made of lead with a wooden tip to ease introduction into the vagina, that was used to observe the cervix. Most physicians in the early years used endoscopic techniques to explore the nasal and aural cavities. However, although occasional attempts were made to examine the rectum and vagina, it was not until 1799 that Recamier, who also introduced the curette, reinvented the speculum.

The father of modern endoscopy was Bozzini, who described his technique of examining the interior of the urethra in 1805. He reflected the light from a candle with a mirror directing the rays along a metal tube. One can imagine his chagrin when the august body to whom he reported, the Medical Faculty of Vienna, censured him for 'undue curiosity'. Half a century later Desormeaux (1865) fared rather better. He described a functioning cystoscope that incorporated a lamp burning alcohol and turpentine with a

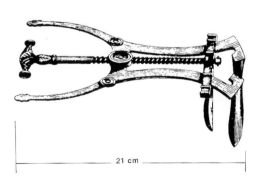

Figure 1.1 Three-bladed vaginal speculum discovered in Pompeii in 70 AD.

21 cm

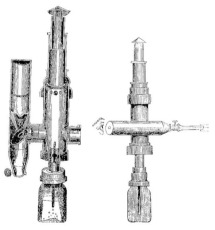

Figure 1.2 The endoscope designed by Desormeaux incorporated a lamp fueled by alcohol and turpentine and a separate viewing channel.

chimney to enhance the flame to the Academie Imperiale de Medicine de Paris, who rewarded him with a share of the Argenteuil prize (Figure 1.2).

Gynecologists were slow to enter the field although Pantaleoni (1869) adapted Desormeaux' telescope for hysteroscopy. He was able to identify an intrauterine polyp in a 60-year-old woman with postmenopausal bleeding and performed the first intrauterine surgery when he cauterized the polyp with silver nitrate. The technique failed to gain the acceptance he had hoped for because most of his students left claiming the only thing they saw through the hysteroscope was an amorphous red blur!

Urologists were more ready to use the new technology, probably because the urethra and bladder were more easy to distend and visualize than the uterus. Maximilian Nitze (1879) in association with a Berlin optician, Reinicke, and a Viennese instrument maker, Leiter, replaced the cumbersome external alcohol-fueled lamp with an incandescent platinum filament sited on the distal tip of the telescope (Figure 1.3). When brought to a white heat it provided reliable illumination, the heat being dissipated by a continuous flow of water.

As is so often the case, medical progress was being driven by technologic advances that were occurring in the wider scientific community. In 1880 Thomas Eddison developed the incandescent light bulb and three years later Newman adapted it for use in a cystoscope. When a separate operating channel was incorporated into the cystoscope, the potential for modern endoscopy and endoscopic surgery was realized.

Hysteroscopy

Diagnostic Hysteroscopy 1900–1950

The early years of the twentieth century saw an increasing interest in endoscopy, but the development of diagnostic hysteroscopy was slow. There were several reasons for this. The uterus was difficult to distend because of the thickness of its walls, and the small size of the cavity and the tendency of the endometrium to bleed on contact provided further obstacles. In addition the illumination from early light sources was poor, the distally situated bulbs caused excessive heat production and were prone to failure, and the lenses available at the time produced poor image quality, even when telescopes with diameters of 12 mm were used. It was little wonder that hysteroscopy did not achieve the popularity it has today.

In spite of all these difficulties, some pioneering clinicians believed in the potential of hysteroscopy and persisted with innovative techniques. In 1907 Charles David described the use of a cystoscope with an internal light and a lens system to examine the uterine cavity. His hysteroscope had a distal bulb, but he improved the design of the original instrument by sealing the end of the telescope to prevent blockage with blood. Rubin (1925) was the first to use carbon dioxide as a distension medium and he also introduced fluid distension to wash away blood that obscured vision. He suggested that visually directed biopsies could be performed and introduced scissors and fulguration loops alongside the telescope to amputate pedunculated fibroids and polyps. Others developed hysteroscopes with multiple channels to allow suction as well as insufflation and channels for introducing operating instruments.

Diagnostic Hysteroscopy 1950–1980

The years after World War II saw an increased interest in hysteroscopy as a result of improved light transmission and lens systems. The first fiberoptic hysteroscopes were designed by Mohri in Japan (1971), who made the first attempts to perform transcervical tuboscopy at about the same time. The quality of the images obtained with flexible endoscopes was, however, poor and it was many years before they produced satisfactory

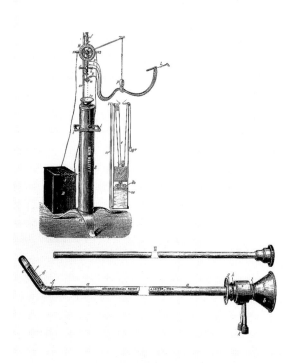

Figure 1.3 The cystoscope designed by Nitze and Leiter.

results. The superior images obtained with the rod lens designed by Professor Hopkins of Reading University in 1953 and the use of cold illumination invented by Fourestiere *et al.* in Paris (1943) have revolutionized endoscopy and allowed the tremendous advances of the past three decades.

Improved distension media were introduced by Edstrom and Fernstrom (1970) who used 32% dextran 70 ('Hyskon'), Levine and Neuwirth (1972) who used 30% dextran, and Lindemann (1973) who demonstrated the safety of carbon dioxide provided the flow rate and intrauterine pressure were kept within specific limits

Further refinements to the hysteroscope were made by Hamou (1980) who developed lens systems with the capability of magnifying up to ×180 that allowed the detection of cellular abnormalities by endoscopy. Modifications have also been made to the irrigation systems to allow a continuous flow of fluid media, which prevents clouding of vision by blood and mucus.

Operative Hysteroscopy 1970–1997

By the early 1970s diagnostic hysteroscopy was becoming accepted even though it was not widely practised. The reluctance of many gynecologists to learn the technique may be attributed to the difficulty the inexperienced clinician finds in obtaining a perfect view every time. However, the realization that hysteroscopy can be used to gain access to the uterine cavity to perform therapeutic procedures has altered opinion and now the popularity of hysteroscopy is increasing.

Initially forceps and scissors were passed alongside the hysteroscope to excise polyps or pedunculated fibroids, to remove misplaced intrauterine contraceptive devices and to divide synechiae. Scissors and forceps of varying strength were later incorporated in the hysteroscope or passed along an operating channel – strong rigid ones for thick adhesions and septa, and semi-rigid or flexible ones for visually directed biopsies.

Robert Neuwirth working in New York has been one of the foremost endoscopists in introducing electrosurgery. He described the use of the urologic resectoscope to remove pedunculated submucous fibroids, either by dividing their pedicles or shaving them off the uterine wall (Neuwirth and Amin, 1976). With increasing experience larger fibroids with a greater intramural component may be excised. Deep-seated myomas may be removed in stages using gonadotropin releasing hormone (GnRH) agonists to reduce the size and vascularity of the fibroid, allowing large deep-seated fibroids to be removed hysteroscopically (Donnez *et al.*, 1989, 1990).

Milton Goldrath of Detroit and colleagues reported the use of the neodymium:yttrium-aluminum-garnet (Nd:YAG) laser to photovaporize the endometrium in 1981. Lasers may also be used for myomectomy and resecting septae as will be discussed in detail later in this book.

In 1983 DeCherney and Polan described the successful use of a resectoscope loop to control intractable uterine bleeding. The concept of removing the endometrium entirely as an alternative to hysterectomy to control abnormal uterine bleeding excited both lay and medical opinion in the late 1980s. More recently electrosurgical ablation with a roller ball has been introduced by Vancaillie (1989). The results appear to be similar to those of resection, and more importantly, the risk of uterine perforation is considerably less (Maresh, 1996). Electrosurgery may also be used to divide uterine septae and synechiae, although the latter procedure is probably safer performed with scissors.

There have been problems with many techniques of endometrial ablation. The prevalence of uterine perforation with the resectoscope loop has been shown in a series of over 10 500 patients to be 3.53% when the loop is used alone and 2.57% when combined with the roller ball. The equivalent figures for laser and roller ball are 0.655% and 0.64%, respectively. The prevalence of hemorrhage or fluid overload is also significantly greater when the loop is used (Maresh, 1996). Clearly simpler and safer alternatives are required. Current developments include the use of a low-power laser, or a laser with photosensitized tissues, thermal destruction using a balloon filled with hot water and the use of intrauterine progestogens. The long-term results of treatment and the ultimate costs of the equipment are eagerly awaited.

Laparoscopy

Diagnostic Laparoscopy 1900–1940

Although the early emphasis of gynecological endoscopy was towards examination of the uterine cavity because of its seemingly easy access, laparoscopy was initially the more popular and potentially the more useful technique. In 1901 von Ott from St Petersburg described the examination of the abdominal cavity of a pregnant woman through a culdoscopic incision using a head mirror to reflect light. In the following year, Georg Kelling, Professor in Dresden, described to the German Biological and Medical Society in Hamburg the examination of the esophagus and stomach of a human and the use of a cystoscope to examine the abdominal cavity of a dog. In this experiment he described one of the key steps in modern laparoscopy, the distension of the peritoneal cavity with gas. He used air filtered through cotton wool to produce a pneumoperitoneum. The credit for the first laparoscopy on a human must go to Jacobaeus of Stockholm (1910) who described inspection of the peritoneal, thoracic and pericardial cavities. Only one month later Kelling reported 45 laparoscopies and described the appearance of the liver, tumors and tuberculosis. Kelling, von Ott and Jacabaeus should be looked upon as the 'fathers' of laparoscopy.

Laparoscopy became popular mainly with general physicians or internists for the diagnosis and treatment of tuberculosis and liver disease, and to them must go much of the credit for the development of laparoscopy over the next 40 years. The first description of laparoscopy in North America was by Bertram M. Bernheim (1911) who used a 10 mm proctoscope with ambient light to inspect the abdominal cavity.

Further developments by internists in the early years of the century include the adoption of Trendelenburg's position to display the pelvic organs by Nordentoeft of Copenhagen (1912), the use of carbon dioxide for insufflation by Zollikoffer in Switzerland (1924), and the invention of the spring-loaded needle by Janos Veress in Budapest (1938), which he devised to introduce a pneumothorax in the treatment of pulmonary tuberculosis.

There was considerable controversy about the nomenclature of these new procedures. Kelling referred to it as 'celioscopy'. Jacobaeus was perhaps less well grounded in the classical languages. He eschewed the terms 'ventroscopy' (Latin: venter, belly) and celioscopy (Greek: koilia, belly) and coined the term 'laparoscopy' (Greek: lapar, flank). The latter term is still widely used, although in France the procedure is still referred to as 'celioscopy'. To confuse matters even further, Steiner (1924) described his experiences with 'abdominoscopy' and Redi (1935) reported several cases of 'splanchnoscopy'.

Operative Laparoscopy 1930–1975

As might be expected, the purely diagnostic application of laparoscopy did not satisfy surgeons for long. In 1929 Kalk began to perform liver biopsies through a second puncture under laparoscopic control and Fervers (1933) designed instruments with which intra-abdominal adhesions could be divided by electrosurgery. He used oxygen as the distension medium and experienced 'great concern' at the audible explosion and

flashes of light produced by the combination of oxygen and a high frequency electric current within the abdominal cavity when he described the first case of laparoscopic adhesiolysis. At about the same time, John C. Ruddock (1934) designed a single-puncture operating laparoscope, which allowed biopsy and coagulation. The first reported use of the laparoscope for the diagnosis of ectopic pregnancy was by Hope (1937), although gynecologists had been using the laparoscope before that time as the first suggestion that female tubal sterilization could be performed by fulguration was by Bosch (1936) in Switzerland and Anderson (1937) in the USA. The first actual sterilization was probably performed in the USA by Power and Barnes (1941). The day of operative gynecological laparoscopy had dawned.

Techniques were developing in parallel in several countries at that time, but because of war, political constraints, language difficulties and the problems in communication produced by distance at that time it is difficult to be certain of the exact sequence of events. In the USA laparoscopy was virtually abandoned from the early 1940s until the late 1960s and was replaced by culdoscopy in most centers (Decker, 1949). In Europe laparoscopy continued to be practised under the influence of Raoul Palmer (1948) in Paris (Figure 1.4), and later, Hans Frangenheim (1959) in Konstanz. Palmer presented his early experiences to the French Society of Obstetrics and Gynecology in 1947. He described the use of a uterine manipulator to display the uterus and tubes and used a Bonney kymograph to control the intraperitoneal gas pressure during laparoscopy under local anesthesia. He also described the optimum site for introducing the spring-loaded needle as 2.5 cm below the left costal margin, a site suggested by Reich nearly 50 years later (Reich, 1991).

Laparoscopic sterilization was developed by Palmer in Paris, but was first described in the English language by Steptoe (1967), who recommended a double-puncture technique with coagulation and division of the tube. Frangenheim (1972) in Europe and Rioux and Cloutier in North America (1974) introduced bipolar electrocoagulation both for sterilization and for controlling bleeding at about the same time as Kurt Semm of Kiel (1972) introduced endotherm coagulation in which no electric current passes through the body (Figure 1.5). Thermal tubal sterilization was largely replaced in the middle 1970s by mechanical methods using spring-loaded clips (Hulka *et al.*, 1975), silastic-lined clips (Filshie *et al.*, 1981) or silastic rings (Yoon and King, 1975).

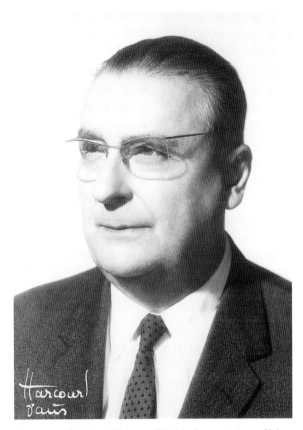

Figure 1.4 Dr Raoul Palmer. (By kind permission of Mme Elizabeth Palmer.)

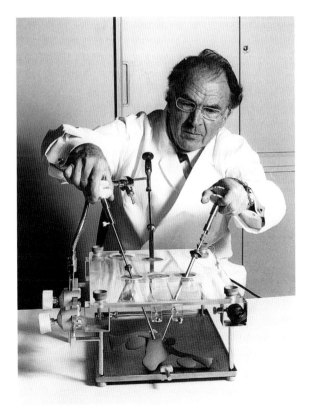

Figure 1.5 Professor Kurt Semm.

Operative Laparoscopy 1975–1988

The first major development in instrumentation after bipolar electrocoagulation and endocoagulation was the introduction of a variety of forms of laser and their application to laparoscopic surgery. Carbon dioxide laser, which is transmitted along a solid lens system, was the first to be used extensively and was introduced to Europe by Maurice Bruhat of Clermont-Ferrand (Bruhat *et al.*, 1979), to the UK by Chris Sutton (1982) and to the USA by James Daniell of Nashville (Daniell and Brown, 1982). Since then lasers transmitted along flexible fiberoptic cables have increased in popularity and include the Nd:YAG, potassium-titanyl-phosphate (KTP) and argon lasers.

Conservative laparoscopic surgery for ectopic pregnancy was first described in France by Bruhat *et al.* (1977) and neosalpingostomy was usually performed by microsurgery in the 1970s and early 1980s. Initially, laparoscopic surgery was confined to those cases where conventional surgery had failed. Soon it was realized that equally good results could be obtained by a laparoscopic approach and some pioneers changed their practise to make laparoscopy the method of choice using electrosurgery (Gomel, 1977; Dubuisson *et al.*, 1985) or laser (Mage and Bruhat, 1983). The use of laparoscopy for the treatment of ovarian cysts was more controversial because of the risk of failing to recognize a borderline or malignant tumor. Careful preoperative assessment by ultrasound (Meire *et al.*, 1978) and intraoperative cystoscopy (Mage *et al.*, 1987) allow a safe laparoscopic approach to ovariotomy. Laparoscopy was accepted as the optimum treatment for minor peritoneal endometriosis, but inevitably, the indications for its use widened until deeply infiltrating endometriomas in the rectovaginal septum came within the purview of expert surgeons (Martin, 1988).

Laparoscopic Surgery 1988–1997

Laparoscopic surgery from 1975–1988 was essentially organ preserving surgery. It was performed by relatively few clinicians and the indications were limited. In 1989 the whole attitude to laparoscopic surgery changed with the publication by Harry Reich of the first case of laparoscopic hysterectomy (Reich *et al.*, 1989). Gynecologists suddenly realized that here was a new operation that could alter the whole practise of their art. The initial disadvantages of prolonged operating times were overcome by adaptations in technique and the introduction of various forms of laparoscopically assisted vaginal hysterectomy (Garry, 1994). Unfortunately some clinicians tried to do too much too soon with the inevitable result of injuries to the ureters and great vessels. Training programs had to be developed and credentialing introduced where they had previously been eschewed.

Once the initial hurdle of performing extirpative surgery using a laparoscope had been crossed, the way was clear for other, even more advanced surgery to be performed using a laparoscopic approach. Almost anything that could be performed by laparotomy was soon to be performed by laparoscopy. The speed with which advances were made was astonishing. Within a few short years gynecologists had progressed from skepticism about endoscopic surgery in general to enthusiasm for adanced procedures such as myomectomy (Dubuisson *et al.*, 1992), treatment of deeply infiltrating endometriosis (Reich *et al.*, 1991), pelvic lymphadenectomy (Querleu, 1989) and para-aortic lymphadenectomy (Childers *et al.*, 1993), presacral neurectomy (Perez, 1990) and pelvic reconstructive surgery (Vancaillie *et al.*, 1991).

The general surgeons, who were the early exponents of laparoscopic surgery, have rediscovered the possibilities presented by the technique to perform cholecystectomy, herniorrhaphy, selective vagotomy and many other procedures. New instruments have been developed to suture and anastomose organs using disposable staples. There has inevitably been controversy about the cost of disposable instruments and this will be addressed in other chapters of this book.

The Future

The development of endoscopy at the end of the nineteenth century was driven by the advances in technology in the field of science – the invention of the electric light and the use of improved lens systems. The end of the millenium will herald a completely new approach to surgical science because of the multiplicity of sophisticated new techniques becoming available.

One of the most radical changes in endoscopic surgery in recent years has been the introduction of microchip video cameras and video monitors in the operating room, which have allowed all of the staff to participate in surgery. Three-dimensional imaging is now becoming available and not only gives the surgeon a much better view of the operative field, but helps to bridge the gap that some surgeons find in changing from three- to two-dimensional vision. The clarity of the images and the potential for accurate record keeping will continue to improve with the development of digital recording technology. Within a few years other technology will further alter practise and training. Computer designed pictures will reproduce anatomic and pathologic images. Virtual reality, which gives both visual and tactile sensation, will allow the trainee to participate in hands-on mock operations before proceeding to live surgery. Computer technology in endoscopic surgery may involve the use of interactive networks. The information highway will enable images to be recorded and transmitted to other terminals to allow intraoperative consultation with colleagues in different centers or, indeed, different continents. A surgeon could be involved in supervising several operations in different hospitals at the same time (DeCherney, 1995).

Other technologic advances include new methods of suturing, allowing microsurgical techniques and materials to be used. New clips, staples, tissue glues and barrier materials will allow organ reconstruction with minimal tissue reaction and adhesion formation. New generation lasers that are more specific in their application, cause less tissue destruction and are easier to control will allow precision beyond today's imagination. Photoactivation of tissues will make them more sensitive to specific laser wavelengths and allow tissue-specific destruction, leaving the normal tissue unaffected. The widespread application of endoscopic surgery to oncology will become a reality.

Tomorrow's surgeon will work in a completely different environment from that we use today. The emphasis on office or outpatient surgery will increase until only a minority of patients will need to stay in hospital after surgery. The operating room will be dominated with electronic equipment and lasers and many procedures will be performed under remote control with robots working to a computerized program.

Today's innovations are tomorrow's history. One can only hope that the surgeon of the twenty-first century will not judge us too harshly and will realize that we are captives of the time in which we practice.

References

Anderson ET (1937) Peritoneoscopy. *American Journal of Surgery* **35**: 136–139.

Bernheim BM (1911) Organoscopy: Cystoscopy of the abdominal cavity. *Annals of Surgery* **53**: 764–767.

Bosch PF (1936) Laparoskopiche sterilization. *Schweizerische Zeitschrift für Krankenhaus und Anstaltswesen.*

Bozzini P (1805) *Der lichtleiter odere beschreibung einer eingachen vorrichtung und ihrer anwendung zur erleuchung innerer hohlen und zwischeraume deslebenden animaleschen korpses.* Landes-Industrie-Comptoi: Weimer.

Bruhat MA, Mage G, Manhes H (1977) Use of CO_2 laser by laparoscopy. In Kaplan I (ed.) *Laser Surgery III. Proceedings of the Third International Congress on Laser Surgery.* Tel Aviv: Jerusalem Press.

Bruhat MA, Manhes H, Choukroun J, Suzanne F (1979). Essai de traitment per coelioscopique de la grossesse extra-uterine. A propos de 26 observations. *Francaise de Gynecologie et d'Obstetrique* **72**: 667–669.

Childers JM, Hatch KD, Surwit EA (1993) Laparoscopic para-aortic lymphadenectomy in gynecologic malignancies. *Obstetrics and Gynecology* **82**: 741–747.

Daniell JF, Brown DH (1982) Carbon dioxide laser laparoscopy: initial experience in experimental animals and humans. *Obstetrics and Gynecology* **59**: 761–764.

David C (1907) De l'endoscopie de l'uterus ares avortement et dans es suites de couches a l'etat pathologique. *Bulletin of Society of Obstetrics, Paris* **December**.

DeCherney AH, Polan ML (1983) Hysteroscopic management of intra-uterine lesions and intractable uterine bleeding. *Obstetrics and Gynecology* **61**: 392–397.

DeCherney AH (1995). The future of endoscopic surgery. In Gordon AG, Lewis BV, DeCherney AH (eds). *Atlas of Gynecologic Endoscopy.* London: Mosby–Wolfe.

Decker A (1949) Culdoscopy: its diagnostic value in pelvic disease. *Journal of the American Medical Association* **140**: 378–385.

Desormeaux AJ (1865) *De l'endoscopie et de ses applications au diagnostic et au traitment des affections de l'uretre et de la vessie.* Paris: Baillière.

Donnez J, Schrurs B, Gillertot S *et al.* (1989) Treatment of uterine fibroids with implants of gonadotrophin releasing hormone agonists: assessment by hysteroscopy. *Fertility and Sterility* **51**: 947–950.

Donnez J, Schrurs B, Gillertot S *et al.* (1990) Neodymium: YAG laser hysteroscopy in large submucous fibroids. *Fertility and Sterility* **54**: 999–1003.

Dubuisson JB, Aubriot FX, Barbot J (1985) Traitment microchirurgical des lesions tubo-peritoneales. Les resultats des plasties distales. *Journal de Gynecologie-Obstetrique et de Biologie de la Reproduction* **14**: 641–645.

Dubuisson JB, Lecuru F, Foulot H *et al.* (1992) Myomectomy by laparoscopy: a preliminary report of 43 cases. *Fertility and Sterility* **56**: 827–830.

Edstrom K, Fernstrom I (1970) The diagnostic possibilities of a modified hysteroscopic technique. *Acta Obstetrica et Gynecologica Scandinavica* **49**: 327–330.

Fervers C (1933) Die laparoskopie mit dem Cystoskope. Ein Beitrag zur Vereinfachung der Technik und zur endoskopichen Strangdurchtrennung in der Bauchole. *Meziniche Klinik* **29**: 1042–1045.

Filshie GM, Casey D, Pogmore JL (1981). The titanium silicone rubber clip for female sterilization. *British Journal of Obstetrics and Gynaecology* **88**: 655–662.

Fourestiere M, Gladu A, Vulmiere J (1943) La peritoneoscopie. *Presse Medicale* **5**: 46–47.

Frangenheim H (1959) *Die Laparoskopie und die Culdoskopie in der Gynaecologie.* Stuttgart: Georg Thieme.

Frangenheim H (1972) *Laparoscopy and Culdoscopy in Gynaecology.* London: Butterworth.

Garry R (1994) Various approaches to laparoscopic hysterectomy. *Current Opinion in Obstetrics and Gynaecology* **6**: 215–222.

Goldrath MH, Fuller TA, Segal S (1981) Laser photovaporization of endometrium for the treatment of menorrhagia. *American Journal of Obstetrics and Gynecology* **140(1)**: 14–19.

Gomel V (1977) Salpingostomy by laparoscopy. *Journal of Reproductive Medicine* **18**: 265–268.

Hamou JE (1980) Hysteroscopie et microhysteroscopie avec un instrument nouveau: le microhysteroscope. *Acta Endoscope* **10**: 415.

Hope R (1937) The differential diagnosis of ectopic pregnancy by peritoneoscopy. *Surgery, Gynecology and Obstetrics* **64**: 229–234.

Hopkins HH (1953) On the diffraction theory of optical images. *Proceedings of the Royal Society* **A217**: 408.

Hulka JF, Omian K, Phillips JM *et al.* (1975) Sterilization by spring clip. *Fertility and Sterility* **26**: 1122–1131.

Jacobaeus HC (1910) Uber due Moglichkeil die Zystoskopie bei Untersuchlung seroser Hohlungen anzerwerden. *Munchener Medizinische Wochenschrift* **57**: 2090–2092.

Kalk H (1929) Erfahrungen mit der Laparoskopie. *Zeitschrift fur Kliniche Medezin* **111**: 303–348.

Kelling G (1902) Uber Oesophagoskopie, Gastroskopie und Koelioskopie. *Munchner Medizinische Wochenschrift* **49** (1): 22–24.

Levine RU, Neuwirth RS (1972) Evaluation of a method of hysteroscopy with the use of 30% dextran. *American Journal of Obstetrics and Gynecology* **113**: 696–703.

Lindemann H-J (1973) Historical aspects of hysteroscopy. *Fertility and Sterility* **24**: 230–243.

Mage G, Bruhat M (1983) Pregnancy following salpingostomy: a comparison between CO_2 laser and electrosurgery procedures. *Fertility and Sterility* **40**: 472–476.

Mage G, Canis M, Manhes H *et al.* (1987). Kysts ovariens et coelioscopie – A propos de 226 observations. *Journal de Gynecologie, Obstetrique et Biologie de la Reproduction* **16**: 1053–1061.

Maresh M (1996) Personal Communication.

Martin DC (1988) Laparoscopic and vaginal colpotomy for the excision of infiltrating cul-de-sac endometriosis. In *Laparoscopic Appearance of Endometriosis*, 2nd edition. vol 1, pp 21–29. Memphis: Resurge Press.

Meire HB, Farrant P, Gutha T (1978) Distinction of benign from malignant ovarian cysts by ultrasound. *British Journal of Obstetrics and Gynaecology* **85**: 893–899.

Mohri T (1971) Demonstration of the Machida hysteroscope. In *Proceedings of the Seventh World Congress on Fertility and Sterility*, Tokyo and Kyoto, October 1971.

Neuwirth RS, Amin JH (1976) Excision of submucous fibroids with hysteroscopic control. *American Journal of Obstetrics and Gynecology* **126**: 95–99.

Nitze M (1879) Beobachtung – und Untersuchungsmethode fur Harnohre, Harnblase und Rectum. *Weiner Medizinische Wochenschrift* **29**: 649–652.

Nordentoeft S (1912) Uber Endoskopie geschlossener Kavitaten mittels meines Trokar-Endoskopes. *Verhandlungen der Deutschen Gesellschaft fur Gynakologie* **41**: 78–81.

Palmer R (1948) La coelioscopie. *Bruxelles Medical* **28**: 305–312.

Pantaleoni DC (1869) On endoscopic examination of the cavity of the womb. *Medical Press Circular* **8**: 26–27.

Perez JJ (1990) Laparoscopic presacral neurectomy. *Journal of Reproductive Medicine* **35**: 625–630.

Power FH, Barnes AC (1941) Sterilization by means of peritoneoscopic fulguration: a preliminary report. *American Journal of Obstetrics and Gynecology* **41**: 1038–1043.

Querleu D (1989) *Lymphadenectomie pelvienne sous controle coelioscopique. Deuxieme Congres Mondial d'Endoscopie Gynecologique.* France: Clermont–Ferrand.

Recamier R (1799) Curette. In *Le Grand Dictionaire Encyclopedique Medical.* Flammarian.

Redi R (1935) Uber ein neues endoskopisches chirurgisches Instrument, das Splannhnoskop. *Zentralblatt fur Chirurgie*: 558.

Reich H, DeCaprio J, McGlynn F (1989). Laparoscopic hysterectomy. *Journal of Gynecologic Surgery* **5**: 213–216.

Reich H (1991) Establishment of pneumoperitoneum through the left ninth intercostal space. *Gynaecological Endoscopy* **4**: 141–144.

Reich H, McGlynn F, Salvat J (1991) Laparoscopic treatment of cul-de-sac obliteration secondary to retrocervical deep fibrotic endometriosis. *Journal of Reproductive Medicine* **36**: 516–522.

Rioux JE, Cloutier D (1974) A new bipolar instrument for laparoscopic tubal sterilization. *American Journal of Obstetrics and Gynecology* **119**: 737–739.

Rubin IC (1925) Uterine endoscopy, endometroscopy with the aid of uterine insufflation. *American Journal of Obstetrics and Gynecology* **10(3)**: 313–327.

Ruddock JC (1934) Peritoneoscopy. *Western Journal of Surgery* **42**: 392–405.

Semm K (1977) *Atlas of Laparoscopy and Hysteroscopy.* Philadelphia: Saunders.

Steiner OP (1924) Abdominoscopy. *Schwizerische Medizinische Wochenschrift* **54**: 84–87.

Steptoe PC (1967) *Laparoscopy in Gynaecology.* Edinburgh, E&S Livingstone.

Sutton CJG (1985) Initial experience with carbon dioxide laser laparoscopy. *Lasers: Medical Science* **1**: 25–31.

Vancaillie TG (1989) Electrocoagulation of the endometrium with the ball-end resectoscope. *Obstetrics and Gynecology* **74**: 425–427.

Vancaillie TG, Schuessler W (1991) Laparoscopic bladderneck suspension. *Journal of Laparoendoscopic Surgery* **1**: 169–173.

Veress J (1938) Neues Instrument sur Ausfuhrung von Brust-oder Bachpunktionen und Pneumothorax-behandlung. *Deutsche Mediziniche Wochenschrift* **64**: 1480–1481.

von Ott D (1901) Ventroscopic illumination of the abdominal cavity in pregnancy. *Zhurnal Akrestierstova I Zhenskikh Boloznei* **15**: 7–8.

Yoon IB, King TM (1975) A preliminary and intermediate report of a new laparoscopic ring procedure. *Journal of Reproductive Medicine* **15**: 54–56.

Zollikofer R (1924) Zur Laparoskopie. *Schwizerische Medizinische Wochenschrift* **15**: 264–265.

2

Medico-legal Implications of Minimally Invasive Surgery

B.V. LEWIS

Watford and Mount Vernon Hospital NHS Trust, UK

Introduction

Complications following minimal access surgery are increasingly resulting in actions for negligence against the surgeon, particularly as more complicated endoscopic surgical techniques are introduced into clinical practice. Although the complication rate will probably continue to increase as the number of surgeons undertaking minimal access surgery increases, the majority of claims follow relatively simple surgery, often performed by unsupervised and untrained junior staff. Alternatively action can follow advanced endoscopic surgery by senior surgeons attempting to teach themselves rather than undergo rigorous training (Royal College of Obstetricians and Gynaecologists, 1994).

Although the Limitation Act 1980 restricts the time for legal action in respect of personal damages to a period of three years from the date on which the cause of action accrued, an action beyond three years is still possible if the plaintiff can demonstrate to the court that they only became aware of a complication at a later date. This applies in English law, but the legislation differs in other countries. In Canada, limitation periods are a provincial matter and vary across the country. Provinces which have a short limitation period (e.g., one year in Alberta) cause a significant barrier to patients seeking compensation for medical injuries (Clements, 1994). All surgeons have a duty of care to their patients, but the responsibilities of duty of care are much wider, involving other specialists involved in treating patients including nursing staff, operating theater attendants, postoperative nursing care and services provided by paramedics and the pathology laboratory (Clements, 1994).

The standard of care applied in medical negligence in English law was laid down in a seminal judgment in Bolam v. Friern Barnet Hospital Management Committee 1957 which states 'The test as to whether there has been negligence or not is not the test of the man on the top of the Clapham omnibus because he has not got this special skill. The test is the standard of the ordinary skilled man exercising and professing to have that special skill. A man need not possess the highest expert skill: it is well established law that it is sufficient if he exercises the ordinary skill of an ordinary competent man exercising that particular art, thus it follows the standard of care for a resident Doctor differs from the standard of care required by the Courts for a Senior Consultant'.

The burden of proof in a civil injury case is not as rigid as required in a criminal case where proof must be beyond all reasonable doubt. In a civil case the standard is 'on the balance of probability'. The Bolam principle is now widely accepted in English law and if it can be demonstrated that a surgeon acted in a way no competent practitioner of the same professional standing would have done, the court will decide in favor of the plaintiff. It also follows that the standard of care need not be the best possible care by the most expert practitioner in the land, but only the standard set by a majority of practitioners (Lewis, 1992).

Courts expect physicians, as in other specialties to be up to date with contemporary literature. Clearly the amount of reading and knowledge required of a primary care physician differs from that required of a hospital specialist; equally the depth of knowledge and experience exercised by a surgeon practicing minimal access surgery on a full time basis differs significantly from that of a general gynecologist practicing endoscopic surgery infrequently. Nevertheless the courts accept that the laparoscope is a standard gynecological instrument and all practitioners should be familiar with its use and dangers.

Surgery without consent is an assault and it follows that informed consent is essential (Table 2.1). However, informed consent need not be in writing and can be oral. Consent implies knowledge, and any surgical operation must be explained to the patient in simple language so that there is no misunderstanding. The extent of information given to patients will vary with the educational background of each patient, but all women should have the operation explained so that they are fully aware what the operation involves and what major complications can occur. Informed consent cannot be given when a patient is under the influence of drugs or has been premedicated, although exceptions are clearly made in an emergency situation.

Many actions occur after a long time interval when staff have changed or the surgeon cannot remember details of the individual patient. The best defense is provided by the clinical records, which should be kept meticulously. All operation notes should be written at the time of surgery in longhand and include as much detail as possible, particularly if untoward or unexpected events have occurred. Under no circumstances should notes or dates be altered unless the alteration is dated and countersigned with a legible signature. Medical notes should always be legible because of the risk of confusion over drug doses or postoperative care (see Table 2.1).

Innovative or unproved surgical techniques present special difficulties. If a patient is included in a clinical trial or a new procedure, she must give informed consent and be fully aware of potential complications. This is especially important when a

new therapy with alleged advantages is compared with established and conventional treatment. A typical example is the introduction of minimal access surgery for the management of ectopic pregnancy. It is now fully established in the literature that laparoscopic salpingostomy or salpingectomy is in many cases the optimum treatment in the management of the tubal pregnancy because series published in the literature show the long-term results. The situation was different five years ago when laparoscopic treatment for ectopics was still a rarity and conventional surgery involved laparotomy. Placebo operations are ethically unacceptable, but surgery with adjunctive drug therapy may involve a group of women taking the active drug and another group of women having placebo. It is incumbent on the surgeon that the highest ethical standards are maintained in all clinical trials and none should be attempted without review and agreement by the hospital ethical committee. The ethical committee's opinion should be available for inspection in writing. While it may be acceptable practise to depart from approved techniques if a patient has not responded to standard therapy and the practitioner is of high reputation within the profession, it is the responsibility of the surgeon to justify any variation from standard practice (Table 2.2). (Garry, 1994).

Table 2.2 Endoscopic cause of action

Failure to recognize trauma
Failure to consult
Inappropriate management of complications

In spite of the above the responsibility always remains on the plaintiff to prove negligence on the balance of probability and in most cases the plaintiff relies upon the information contained in the clinical records. This often presents difficulty for the plaintiff when action is taken against a private practitioner whose clinical records may be poor. An absence of clinical records does not usually impress judges, who are the sole arbiters of negligence in personal injury litigation in the UK. A jury is not involved in the decision either to establish negligence or quantum of damages.

In medical negligence actions, the legal process is prolonged. It begins with a letter before action from the solicitors on behalf of the plaintiff, usually requesting disclosure of all clinical records under the Access to Medical Reports Act (1988) or the Access to Health Records Act 1990. After disclosure of the records the plaintiff employs an expert of high professional standing to review the notes and provide a report, which is reviewed by the solicitor and a barrister at law. A writ of summons and state-

Table 2.1 General cause of action

Delegation to junior staff
Poor communication between staff
No explanation
No consultant input
No consent
Unaware of complications
Poor records

ment of claim are then issued, which is then followed by the defense. On receipt of the defense the plaintiff has an opportunity to serve interrogatories on the defendant, which must be answered and both the defendant and the plaintiff can request further and better particulars to establish the exact source of dispute. If a settlement cannot be reached a date is set for trial. Alternatively when there is no justifiable action a vigorous defense will usually be followed by cessation of action.

The tangled process of English law may be simplified by the reforms that may be introduced following review of civil litigation and the legal aid system by Lord Justice Woolf. However, regrettably the number of actions against doctors is steadily increasing (Table 2.3) and there have been several high profile cases involving minimal access surgery.

Table 2.3 New legal aid certificates for medical negligence (Legal and Annual Reports)

Year	Number
1987	4 761
1988	6 256
1990	6 448
1991	8 879
1992	18 661*
1993	10 857†

* 1992: Easing of legal aid requirements
† 1993: More restrictive legal aid requirements

All operations have complications and the development of a complication does not imply negligence on the part of the surgeon. However, many complications can and should be avoided with good technique. Many actions are started because complications are unrecognized or treated inappropriately. The bowel may be perforated in error, but if the trauma is recognized and closed either laparo-scopically, if the surgeon is experienced, or through a small laparotomy incision, no long-term harm will result. However, failure to recognize bowel trauma inevitably leads to peritonitis, which threatens the patient's life and may end with an ileostomy, colostomy, or permanent sterility (Figure 2.1). In such cases the quantum of damages increases dramatically.

General Accidents in the Operating Room

Many injuries occur when patients are transferred from the anesthetic trolley to the operating table; alternatively injuries can occur during positioning of the patient on the operating table in the lithotomy position or in the steep Trendelenburg's position. Unless the patient is adequately supported, it is possible for the patient to slide off the table, resulting in injuries to the cervical plexus or the cervical vertebrae. Alternatively the brachial plexus can be injured if an arm is hyperextended. The lithotomy poles must be correctly positioned and all screws should be tightened so that the pole does not collapse leading to injuries to the sacral plexus or the lumbar vertebrae. For most minimal access surgery the lithotomy poles can be angled forwards at 45°. The bladder should always be emptied, either by catheterization immediately before surgery or by asking the patient to voluntarily empty her bladder before the induction of anesthesia. The minimum accepted monitoring by the anesthetist is measurement of oxygen saturation using a pulse oximeter, regular recordings of the blood pressure and an ECG. It is advisable, but not essential, for the anesthetist to pass an endotracheal tube.

Electrical safety is paramount (Phipps, 1993). The

Figure 2.1 Medico-legal cases August 1988–February 1995 (571 cases) (Lewis, unpublished). (TOP, termination of pregnancy; B & U, bladder and ureteric).

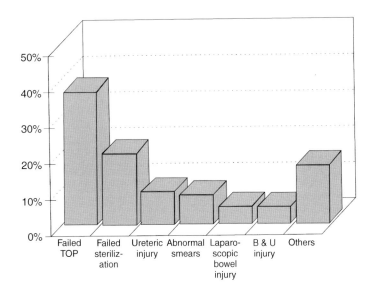

patient should be properly insulated, not touching metal, and the diathermy pad must be accurately applied. Modern electrodiathermy machines will not function if the diathermy pad is misplaced. Simply increasing the current when the machine appears to malfunction without checking on the correct function of the electrical circuit invites disaster, because electrical burns can occur. All instruments should be regularly examined for fractures of the insulating cover. This is particularly likely to occur if instruments are mishandled or subjected to frequent sterilization procedures. The diathermy machine should never be activated unless the surgeon has a clear uninterrupted view of the surgical field and the active electrode is in panoramic view. Laparoscopic instruments attached to the electrical generator must never be left lying on the drapes. Light sources can also generate considerable heat and must not be allowed to rest on the patient's skin where they can cause burns or set the drapes alight. The same precautions apply with the carbon dioxide laser. The outside door of the operating room should have a light indicating that laser surgery is in use, all theater personnel should wear protective glasses if a neodymium:yttrium–aluminum–garnet (Nd:YAG) laser is being used, and the laser must never be activated outside the abdomen because of the risk of injuries to theater staff.

Difficulty with Entry into the Abdomen

Difficulty in establishing a satisfactory pneumoperitoneum can occur, particularly in obese patients (Table 2.4). In order to avoid insufflation of the extraperitoneal fat the abdominal wall should be manually elevated and a long Veress needle inserted at an angle of 45° with its point directed into the pelvis (Lower et al., 1996). The position of the needle point should always be suspect if the initial gas flow rate is low or the pressure is high. If there is doubt about the position of the needle a simple aspiration test using a 10 ml syringe is helpful, and if unsure the needle should be removed and repositioned (Gordon et al., 1995). If a significant volume of carbon dioxide gas is insufflated into the extraperitoneal fat, insertion of the trocar becomes difficult. In these circumstances the surgeon should wait 5–10 minutes for the carbon dioxide to be absorbed and manual pressure on the abdomen will allow most of the carbon dioxide to escape.

Damage to the inferior epigastric artery can occur during insertion of secondary instruments, but should be avoided if the instruments are placed laterally outside the rectus sheath. Alternatively the

Table 2.4 Major complications per 1000 operative laparoscopies (Asch and Studd, 1996).

By instrument	
Veress needle	2.7
Large trocar	2.4–2.7
Accessory trocar	2.5–6.0
Electrocautery	0.5–2.8
Laser	1.2
Pneumoperitoneum	7.4
By site of injury	
Vessels/bleeding	2.6–11.0
Bowel	0.6–2.0
Genitourinary	0.6–1.6
Nerve	6.1
Uterine perforation	3.7
Other indicators	
Death	0.05–0.3
Hospitalization > 72 h	4.2–27.0
Hospital readmission	3.1–5.0
Persistent β-HCG titers	63.2–144.0
Infection	1.4–6.5
Febrile	2.0

secondary instruments should only be inserted after the telescope is in the abdomen with the surgeon visually identifying the course of the artery. The inferior epigastric artery is a major vessel and damage will always cause heavy bleeding. Blood can often be seen dripping from the abdominal incision into the pelvis. Alternatively blood accumulates in the extraperitoneal space causing a hematoma, which can become very large and extend above the umbilicus. Damage to the inferior epigastric artery should be identified and the vessel should be sutured by extending the lateral incision to 2–3 cm and occluding the vessel with mattress sutures. Alternatively a Foley catheter inserted through the lateral port into the abdomen can apply pressure on the vessel when the balloon is distended. If a large hematoma is unrecognized it can be difficult to treat. If the hematoma is left to absorb spontaneously it may take months with pain and discomfort and may eventually require drainage if it becomes infected and forms an abscess. The best treatment is prevention, but alternatively a hematoma should be evacuated through a generous vertical paramedian incision. The wound should then be closed with drainage. Bleeding from the inferior epigastric artery into the abdominal cavity leads to hemoperitoneum and shock. This sequence of events invariably requires an emergency laparotomy and legal action often follows.

Injury to the small or large bowel with either the Veress needle or the trocar should almost always be avoided in a patient without a history of previous surgery (Ward, 1991; Corfman et al., 1993). Patients most at risk of bowel injury are the obese, the thin patient with a small distance between the anterior and posterior abdominal walls, and the patient who has had previous surgery. The stomach can be injured if the anesthetist distends the organ with gas. Women with a history of previous surgery should have a strong indication for laparoscopy and should only be operated upon by experienced surgeons. The patients should be warned of the possibility of laparotomy and the large bowel should be emptied by enemas and a full preoperative bowel preparation instituted. Bowel injury by the Veress needle is usually insignificant and closes spontaneously, but unrecognized injury with the trocar invariably leads to bowel contents leaking into the abdomen and fecal peritonitis. Bowel injuries can be difficult to observe, but should be suspected if extensive intraperitoneal adhesions are present, if the view is restricted, or if there is a fecal smell. Careful inspection of the bowel is mandatory as the telescope is slowly withdrawn at the completion of surgery.

The bowel can also be injured during the division of adhesions, particularly if the sigmoid colon or rectum is adherent to the adnexa by endometriosis or old inflammatory disease. Under these circumstances dissection close to the bowel can be hazardous. Sharp scissors should be used and great care should be taken when hemostasis is obtained with unipolar or bipolar diathermy. If there is any doubt about the integrity of the bowel the pelvis can be filled with saline. The bowel injury will be immediately seen because gas bubbles will appear. This simple precaution can identify even a small hole.

The most important indication of intra-abdominal trauma is excessive postoperative pain. No patient should be discharged from hospital if they are in pain. If a patient returns to the casualty department within a short time of minimal access surgery they should always be seen by a senior doctor who has the records and bowel injury should be assumed until proved otherwise. Many patients have suffered serious injury and had their lives put at risk because they have returned to the hospital with postoperative pain that has been diagnosed as constipation or discomfort due to residual gas in the abdominal cavity. An early laparotomy is much safer than delay.

If the large bowel is injured it must be repaired by laparoscopic suturing or more usually and more safely, by laparotomy. An immediate injury to the large bowel can be closed in two layers. The patient should then be kept in hospital for observation and given broad-spectrum antibiotics and intravenous fluids until fully recovered. Junior surgeons in training asked for emergency help will frequently perform a laparotomy through an unnecessarily large incision and may perform a defunctioning colostomy, which in most cases should be restricted to women where there has been a delay in establishing the diagnosis and there is fecal peritonitis. Such injuries almost always result in a claim for negligence.

Injury to the great vessels on the pelvic sidewall by either the Veress needle or the trocar is a life-threatening complication. If blood is seen in the abdominal cavity or a retroperitoneal hematoma forms, emergency laparotomy with the help of a vascular surgeon is mandatory. Similarly if the anesthetist reports a dramatic fall in blood pressure and decrease in oxygen saturation, a vascular injury should be suspected. These injuries are always avoidable and cannot be justified as a recognized complication.

A different situation arises when there is a trocar or Veress needle injury to a vessel in the mesentery or omentum. The bleeding often stops spontaneously and the surgeon should merely observe to see if a large hematoma is developing. An early laparotomy through a small incision may be appropriate. In contrast to laparotomy for vessels on the posterior abdominal wall, a laparotomy may not be needed for injury to a mesenteric vessel and a laparotomy is only indicated if the hematoma enlarges. Injuries to the stomach should always be closed. They usually occur if the stomach is distended by the anesthetist.

Bladder injuries cannot occur if the bladder is empty. If the bladder is perforated it should either be closed by laparoscopic suturing or laparotomy. A small injury will close spontaneously if an indwelling catheter is inserted for five days.

There have been several reported cases of a volvulus with a strangulated loop of small bowel appearing through the entry ports. This is likely to occur when 10 mm or 12 mm instruments are used and all the larger secondary incisions must be sutured, closing the peritoneum. Simple instruments are now available to close the peritoneum with a catgut or a silk mattress stitch.

Sterilization

In spite of the advances in minimal access surgery the single most frequent operation giving rise to litigation is laparoscopic sterilization. Although it is almost universal to advise patients of the risk of pregnancy, such a disclaimer does not prevent legal action because the surgeon owes a duty of care to the patient and inappropriate or unacceptable surgery will therefore result in litigation. A menstrual history is essential before sterilization.

If a patient is overdue, β-human chorionic gonadotropin (β-HCG) estimation is mandatory and the operation should be delayed until pregnancy has been excluded. Even if a β-HCG test is negative patients should be warned to report to their doctors if they do not have a period.

It is probably best if unipolar electrodiathermy is avoided. This is an effective method of sterilization, but destroys the whole fallopian tube and makes reversal impossible. There is also an increased risk of electrical injury to the bowel unless the surgeon always has a panoramic view of the pelvis to ensure that the bowel is well away from the surgical field. Bipolar diathermy is not sufficient to cause permanent sterilization because the electrical current may destroy only the muscle and peritoneal layer of the tube leaving the endothelium intact (Soderstrom, 1984, 1993). However, bipolar diathermy is acceptable if the surgeon applies the electric current in two areas separated by 1–2 cm of tube and then divides the tube with scissors to separate both ends. Electrodiathermy should be applied at the narrowest part of the tube in the isthmic area. Most surgeons use mechanical clips or plastic rings. The Yoon ring may be ineffective if it is applied to the wide ampullary end of the tube, but is highly effective if it is placed on the isthmic area. Care must be taken to avoid tearing of the mesentery with bleeding.

The usual mechanical devices are the Hulka Clemens clip and the Filshie clip, which is more popular in the UK and is now available in the US. Both clips are effective so long as they are placed on the narrow isthmic length of tube, are correctly locked, and care is taken to ensure that the whole diameter of the tube is included in the clip. This can sometimes be difficult because the surgeon is viewing in two rather than three dimensions. It is a good practise to insert the telescope deeper into the pelvis for a close-up view after the tubes have been clipped to ensure that the clips are accurately applied. Ideally the operation should be performed on a television monitor so that other members of the team can see what is happening, and if possible, polaroid photographs should be taken and placed in the notes. The faulty application of a clip to the round ligament or the superficial area of the tube is indefensible in law and can always be avoided by positively identifying the tube by viewing the fimbria. If a clip falls out of the applicator into the pelvis it should be recovered, but if it disappears into loops of bowel a laparotomy is not necessary. The patient and her family practitioner should be told of the mishap, which should be fully documented. If a patient becomes pregnant within a year of laparoscopic sterilization it is probable that the clips or rings have been negligently applied (Clements, 1994). Pregnancy after 15 months is more likely to be caused by recanalization following correct application of rings or clips and constitutes a valid defense to a negligence claim. The longer the interval between pregnancy and sterilization the more likely it is that recanalization has occurred. At least 35% of pregnancies that occur after sterilization are ectopic and patients should be warned of this risk.

If a surgeon has difficulty applying the clips because of adhesions due to previous endometriosis, pelvic inflammatory disease or a cesarean section, this should be fully documented and a hysterosalpingogram should be performed to confirm tubal blockage. In the interim patients should be warned of the risk of pregnancy and advised to use mechanical birth control. Hysterosalpingograms provide good confirmatory evidence of sterilization providing adequate pressure can be obtained to fill the uterine cavity and the proximal part of each tube. Failure of dye to enter the tubes because of leakage around the cervix can lead to a mistaken diagnosis of sterility.

Following failed sterilization many women are resterilized either at cesarean section, by laparotomy or by repeat laparoscopic sterilization. It is imperative that the surgeon performing the second operation is aware of the failed sterilization and documentation should be meticulous. The surgeon must try and explain why the patient has become pregnant, acknowledging the fact that the tube must be patent for pregnancy to occur, and must identify the precise site of the rings or clips and describe the anatomy. If salpingectomy is performed the role of the pathologist is critical; the pathologist must be aware of the previous sterilization and should discuss the clinical problem with the clinician. It is insufficient for either the surgeon or the pathologist to state that the clip is not on the tube. The natural history of a correctly applied clip is that the tissues between the jaws necrose, and in a high proportion of women, perhaps as many as 35%, the clip will then fall off within a few weeks, leaving the two separate ends. If recanalization occurs the ends grow together to become continuous, but the clip may be several centimeters away or in the pouch of Douglas. It follows that a clip in the pouch of Douglas does not imply misapplication. It is also essential that the pathologist looks for histopathologic evidence of tubal injury. If the pathologist can demonstrate inflammatory cells or histologic evidence of old trauma the court might accept this as evidence of recanalization. Unfortunately it is only too common for a pathologist to report that a section of tube is 'patent', but this result depends on whether the section is taken from the site of injury, which the pathologist often fails to identify. There have been many cases when settlement of a claim has been necessary because the pathologist failed to describe the accurate anatomic findings. These cases often come to court many years later and the specimen is not available for further histopathologic examination.

Ectopic Pregnancy

It is now accepted that minimal access surgery provides the best and most efficient method of treating ectopic pregnancies unless there is a massive hemoperitoneum with hypovolemic shock. Laparoscopic salpingectomy is a simple operation with minimal complications. The tube can be removed using electrodiathermy or ready-tied loops for hemostasis (Roeder-loop, Ethicon, autosuture). The whole length of the tube is then available for pathologic analysis. It is important that the contralateral tube is examined, and confirmed to be normal and that this information is documented before the ectopic pregnancy is removed. Salpingotomy with conservation of the tube is also an acceptable technique. However, it is essential that the tubal lumen is thoroughly washed to ensure all residual trophoblast is removed and that the patient is followed up with serial β-HCG estimations. If the β-HCG rises it is probable that there is residual trophoblast, which will cause symptoms. The patient should also be warned of the risk of a recurrent ectopic pregnancy in a conserved tube.

Injury to the Ureter

The ureter can be injured during laparoscopic oophorectomy (Bruhat, 1994), laparoscopically assisted vaginal hysterectomy, laparoscopic adhesiolysis for endometriosis, pelvic inflammatory disease or the residual ovarian syndrome, laparoscopic uterine nerve ablation and laparoscopic colposuspension (Bassil *et al.*, 1993; Grainger *et al.*, 1990). The ureter must therefore be identified in all cases where it is at risk. This is usually best done by identifying the ureter at the pelvic brim where it can be seen to vermiculate behind the peritoneum. Clamps around the ovarian pedicle or the uterine artery should never be applied until the ureter has been identified. The endo-GIA stapler is a frequent cause of ureteric injury when the clips are placed on the uterine artery, especially if the anatomy is distorted by endometriosis (Garry and Reich, 1993; Phipps,

1993). The 12 mm device is capable of clamping and dividing tissue over a length of up to 30 mm, simultaneously securing hemostasis. When fired, the stapler delivers two triple staggered rows of titanium staples into the tissues, then drives a knife blade between the rows to divide them. Identification of the ureter with illuminated stents inserted through a cystoscope has been advocated. The light can be seen through the laparoscope as the dissection is near the ureter and traction on the stent from below will show movement, which is proof that the ureter is intact after the endo-GIA stapler has been locked. However, there has been some criticism of illuminated stents because they can cause transient hematuria and may themselves damage the delicate endothelium of the ureter.

Hysteroscopic Surgery

The main complications of the hysteroscope are perforation of the uterus with bowel damage, absorption of irrigating fluid into the circulation causing cerebral and pulmonary edema, and post-ablation infection (Gordon, 1995). The Nd:YAG laser or electrodiathermy should never be activated until the surgeon has a clear view of the endometrium and only when the electrode or quartz fiber is withdrawn towards the surgeon. All fluid should be measured and tissue should always be sent to the laboratory for histology following endometrial resection.

Summary

Most documented complications of minimal access surgery can be avoided with good technique (Ward, 1991). Where patients are known to be at risk they must be fully informed of possible and potential complications and the operation should be carried out by a senior, fully trained practitioner. Care should be taken with entry and the introduction of the pneumoperitoneum. If there is a history of previous surgery with likely adhesions, insertion of the Veress needle in the left hypochondrium may be helpful because there is almost always a free space, but care must be taken to avoid inserting the needle into the chest cavity. When an injury occurs this should be fully documented. Trauma should be identified as early as possible and remedial surgery instituted without delay. Delaying surgery almost always makes matters worse and can lead to larger incisions, pelvic sepsis, more complicated surgery and a possible colostomy or ileostomy. Ureteric damage can usually be treated by stenting if it is recognized early. However, if an injury to the ureter is unrecognized, laparotomy and reimplantation of the ureter may be the only alternative and will result in a much longer convalescence. It must always be remembered that legal action can often be avoided by offering the patient a full explanation, apologies if necessary and careful follow-up maintaining a good doctor–patient relationship. Above all surgeons should only attempt operations for which they have been adequately trained.

References

Asch R, Studd J (1996) In Nezhat CR, Nezhat F and Nezhat CH (eds). *Progress in Reproductive Medicine*. New York: Parthenon Publishing.

Bassil S, Nisolle M, Donnez J (1993) Complications of endoscopic surgery in gynaecology. *Gynaecological Endoscopy* **2**: 199–209.

Bruhat MA (1994) *Management of Adnexal Cysts*. Oxford: Blackwell Scientific Publications.

Clements RV (1994) *Safe Practice in Obstetrics and Gynaecology*. Edinburgh: Churchill Livingstone.

Corfman RS, Diamond MP, De Cherney A (1993) *Complications of Laparoscopy and Hysteroscopy*. Oxford: Blackwell Scientific Publications.

Garry R (1994) The Achilles heel of minimal access surgery. *Gynaecological Endoscopy* **3**: 201–202.

Garry R, Reich H (1993) *Laparoscopic Hysterectomy*. Oxford: Blackwell Scientific Publications.

Gordon AG (1995) *Endometrial Ablation. Clinical Obstetrics and Gynaecology*. London: Baillière Tindall.

Gordon AG, Lewis BV, De Cherney AH (1995) *Atlas of Gynecologic Endoscopy*, 2nd edn. London: Mosby–Wolfe.

Grainger DA, Soderstrom RM, Sciff SF, Glickman G, De Cherney AH, Diamond MP (1990) Ureteral injuries at laparoscopy. *Obstetrics and Gynaecology* **75**: 840–843.

Lewis CJ (1992) *Medical Negligence*, 2nd edition. Tolley Publishing.

Lower A, Sutton C, Grudzinskas G (1996) *Introduction to Gynaecological Endoscopy*. Oxford: Isis Medical.

Phipps JH (1993) *Laparoscopic Hysterectomy and Oophorectomy*. Edinburgh: Churchill Livingstone.

Royal College of Obstetricians and Gynaecologists (1994) *Training in Gynaecological Endoscopic Surgery*. London: Chameleon Press.

Soderstrom RM (1984) Sterilisation failures and their causes. *American Journal of Obstetrics and Gynecology* **152**: 395–403.

Soderstrom RM (1993) Bowel injury litigation after laparoscopy. *Journal of the American Association of Gynecological Laparoscopists* **I**: 74–77.

Ward CJ (1991) An Analysis of 500 Obstetric and Gynecologic Malpractice Claims. *American Journal of Obstetrics and Gynecology* **165**: 298–306.

Laparoscopic Surgery –
Techniques and Equipment

3

Setting up a Service: Instrumentation and Administration

GRANT W. PATTON, Jr

Southeastern Fertility Center, Mt Pleasant, South Carolina, USA

Introduction

Gynecologic endoscopic surgery has changed and continues to evolve rapidly. This text discusses operative laparoscopic and hysteroscopic techniques that are generations away from laparoscopic tubal ligation. The magnitude of change is reflected in the rapidity with which general surgeons embraced laparoscopic cholecystectomy, herniorrhaphy and limited bowel resection. Certainly laparoscopic hysterectomy has become common, as has the resection of severe endometriosis and rectosigmoid resection. The sense of change is critical when evaluating operating room design since this area has also changed dramatically and will continue to change in the years ahead.

Operating Room Arrangement

Operating room (OR) arrangement may include a number of luxuries, but must include certain basic equipment, since the setup will have a significant impact on surgical technique. Nowhere is this more apparent than the standard that operative laparoscopy should be performed by viewing the monitor rather than peering down the telescope. In many respects a well designed and equipped operating room leads the surgeon to a higher level of surgical expertise.

It is our goal in this chapter to describe a fundamental approach to OR layout and equipment that permits the endoscopic surgeon to function comfortably at various levels of surgical expertise. The design for the surgeon who performs occasional operative laparoscopic surgery will not differ from that used for the most complicated endoscopic procedures. Obviously the number of instruments will vary, but the OR layout will not, thus permitting the surgeon to move with ease from the simple vaporization of endometriosis to the excision of severe endometriosis with bowel resection with minimal change in layout or staffing. Combined operative hysteroscopic and laparoscopic procedures would be easily performed in this setting, as would laparoscopic hysterectomy and cholecystectomy.

A new development since the first edition of this text has been the use of 'office or emergency room' laparoscopy. This approach has reduced laparoscopy to its diagnostic function and simple operative procedures including tubal ligation, gamete intrafallopian transfer (GIFT) and second-look. The set-up for this technique will be discussed.

Overall Concept

Successful operative laparoscopy requires three essential ingredients:

1. surgical skill;
2. a well designed and equipped OR;
3. a surgical team.

The discussion that follows will assume that the surgeon is aware of his level of surgical expertise and operates comfortably at that level. That different levels of skill exist among various gynecological surgeons is obvious to the OR staff, as well as to fellow surgeons. Operative gynecologic endoscopy permits the surgeon to 'get in over his or her head' and requires discipline on the part of the surgeon to know when to stop.

This chapter will discuss a concept of OR design for operative laparoscopy that integrates the surgical team into this design much as an architect must consider function when designing a building. It is the author's opinion that operative laparoscopy hinges on the ability of the surgeon to use the team members successfully.

Technique and Team

Surgical Assistant

The right-handed surgeon stands on the patient's left side, while the left-handed surgeon usually stands on the opposite side of the patient. The need for a high degree of hand–eye coordination during these procedures means that moving from one side of the table to the other during operative laparoscopy is difficult. A second surgeon often makes a poor assistant because of this orientation. In most cases, a well trained nursing assistant familiar with the surgeon's technique and comfortable working across the table will complement the surgeon's approach as experience teaches this individual to anticipate surgical moves and equipment changes.

Practise and experience are invaluable aids and should be emphasized during the training of a surgical assistant. This is a highly specialized job and certainly not suitable for the untrained technician who is unfamiliar with the case at hand. The author has had the same surgical assistant for many years and feels that it is a luxury that significantly improves the quality of surgery.

The author would counsel residents and fellows against operating on the opposite side of the table while working with an attending physician, a point that also applies to physicians attending a surgical training program.

Scrub Nurse

The scrub nurse should play an active role. In the author's OR, the scrub nurse stands at the foot of the table between the patient's legs. He or she hands equipment to the surgeon from either the surgeon's side table or the back instrument table, holds the uterine manipulator and manipulates second puncture instruments when necessary. Naturally he or she checks to see that various instruments, suction, cautery, etc. are properly attached. Most importantly, the scrub nurse cleans and cares for the equipment, which in view of the delicate instrumentation is a major role. The scrub nurse is also responsible for sending instruments to be repaired and for recommending that new instruments be ordered when necessary.

Biomedical Technician

This new position is critical to the success of a high-technology OR. This individual may not be assigned to a specific OR, but rather functions to oversee the equipment in a number of ORs, and is able to step into an operating procedure and adjust the video, light source or laser, or correct other potential trouble spots. This individual should be trained in electronic, digital and analog equipment, with specific training in the video and laser instrumentation specifically used. He or she must also develop OR expertise and assume a clinical role to some degree, thereby developing a sensitivity to the equipment needs of specific surgeons and procedures. The primary goal of this individual is to avoid crisis management by keeping all equipment in good working order and by teaching team members to use all instruments comfortably. The biomedical technician should also function as the laser nurse and assume responsibility for in-service instruction for those individuals who will be running the specific lasers in the OR. In a large OR suite, it is essential to train a number of nurses and OR technicians to act in the role of the biomedical technician. This training should include laser operation and is designed to provide personnel to assume this role when necessary during operative laparoscopic procedures in a number of ORs.

Circulating Nurse

The circulating nurse is the 'captain of the team', knowledgeable in the roles of other team members, able to help each when necessary, and able to relate to the surgeon. Communication with the surgeon is most critical to successful operative laparoscopy, particularly when a procedure goes poorly. There is an element of tension present during operative laparoscopic surgery that does not exist during a microsurgical procedure. Perhaps it is the threat of bleeding, the possibility of a bowel or bladder injury, the fear of fatigue during prolonged procedures. Whatever the problem, the circulator should help everyone deal with the situation and provide support when and where it is needed. He or she may check the light source, call the biomedical technician, find a lost instrument, adjust the suction, turn up the stereo, and in general maintain the rhythm. The circulating nurse is specifically responsible for the operation of the bipolar and monopolar electrosurgical generators, and also adjusts the wall suction and laser and electrosurgical pedals for appropriate use during an operative procedure. It is expected that this individual will be familiar with all laser units and be able to operate them when necessary; however, during an operative procedure the biomedical technician (laser nurse) in attendance should be primarily responsible for this equipment.

In many ways the circulating nurse orchestrates the procedure as much as the surgeon. During endoscopic procedures by a young or inexperienced surgeon, he or she must hold the procedure together. This is obviously an important role beyond the scope of the traditional circulating nurse.

Summary

These four individuals must be able to function comfortably within the OR designed for operative laparoscopy (Figure 3.1). It is clear that all hospital OR services will not be able to maintain identical team members for all surgeons. The principle that these four roles are essential to successful operative laparoscopy is critical, however.

Instrumentation for Endoscopic Surgery

Video

Perhaps the most difficult area to maintain at a high level is the quality of the video picture. A high quality camera with both focus and zoom adjustments is essential. This camera is attached to the telescope lens before placing the telescope into the abdominal cavity. The camera is white balanced when necessary and the camera–telescope unit inserted through the trocar sleeve. A beam splitter is not used since it reduces light to the video picture, and secondly, after adequate surgical experience, produces no improvement in surgical technique. The surgeon must learn to work from the monitor and break the old habit of looking through the telescope. This has been easier for general surgeons who learned laparoscopic surgery by working from the monitor, and most difficult for those gynecological surgeons accustomed to keeping the field of view to themselves.

Two monitors are the gold standard, providing ease of viewing for both surgeon and assistant. A single video screen placed at the foot of the table

Figure 3.1 Photograph of the operating team that is essential for operative laparoscopy. The team includes a circulating nurse, surgeon, scrub nurse, surgical assistant and biomedical technician.

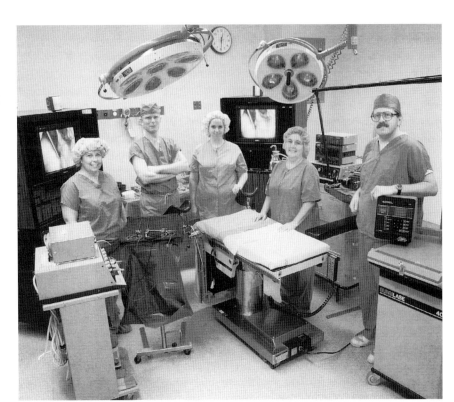

will work, but limits the role of the scrub nurse and is inconvenient for the assistant and occasionally for the surgeon. One video screen works, but two improve the quality and ease of surgery.

The author uses two Storz cameras and two 20-inch high resolution Sony monitors placed on floor stands that move easily. The monitors are wired above through the ceiling with flexible cables that permit adequate mobility.

Ceiling-mounted monitors have been replaced by a new design marketed by Berchtold Corporation, termed the Berchtold Teletom Power Boom. This ceiling-mounted unit holds the monitor, CO_2 insufflator, light and camera box and is easily positioned for the surgeon's convenience. It is the author's opinion that placement of these ceiling units on either side of the endoscopic operating table is the state-of-the-art. One caveat, however, is the need

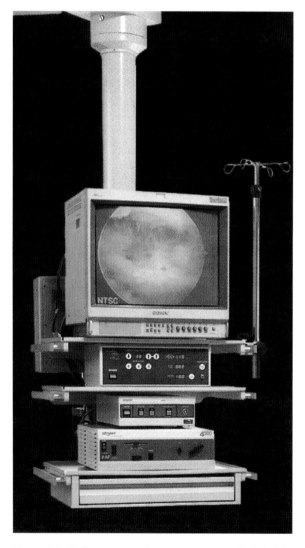

Figure 3.2 Ceiling-mounted 'power boom' which holds the complete laparoscopic setup including the monitor. All electrical connections pass through the ceiling attachment.

for an adequately sized operating suite to permit comfortable movement during surgery (Figure 3.2).

Light Source

The old 150 W light source has been superseded; at least it is not useful during operative laparoscopy. The xenon light is extremely useful; however, the automatic adjustment used on early models that permitted the light source to adjust the light requirement is no longer of value since the new video cameras perform this function more successfully. The xenon units are reliable, the bulb lasts many hours (warranty covers 400–500 hours of operating time), and in general, are a major advance over earlier light sources. A 150 W halogen light sold by Stryker is promising, but requires a complete surgical setup including camera, cable, light source and video monitor.

The new generation three-chip cameras provide 25–50 mm parafocal zoom, which permits the surgeon to adjust the image size and provides a highly magnified image. Image quality has improved greatly.

Electrosurgical Generator

A surgical technique that combines sharp incision with scissors and coagulation of specific vessels with bipolar current has become a standard approach of laparoscopic surgeons dealing with extensive pelvic adhesions and fimbrial occlusion. A fine tip monopolar electrode has also been employed when necessary in an effort to mimic microsurgical technique.

The standard Wolfe bipolar coagulating instrument is of value when used with the Kleppinger bipolar forceps to coagulate significant bleeding vessels. The tip of the instrument remains hot for short intervals following coagulation and should be used as a probe or grasping forceps with care.

Storz Instrument Co. recently introduced a series of bipolar forceps that vary in size from micro to a macro size equivalent to the Kleppinger. An advantage of this new design is the ability of the forceps blades to close smoothly on an object rather than retract during closure, as occurs with the Kleppinger forceps. The new bipolar forceps has been a pleasure to use. Extensive bipolar coagulation during laparoscopic hysterectomy procedures may require the Kleppinger forceps, however. A fine-tip monopolar electrode can be passed through a hollow cannula, permitting suction and irrigation as needed during the cutting procedure. The Bard,

Valley Lab or Bircher electrosurgical generators provide monopolar and bipolar current and are useful with macro and micro bipolar forceps as well as a microelectrode when necessary. Recently the argon beam coagulator has been used for hemostasis with good results. Reintroduction of the technique by Bircher includes a long 10 mm tip, which is useful as a second-puncture instrument during operative laparoscopy. A smaller 5 mm tip will soon be available. This instrument provides both coagulation and monopolar current. The ability to provide both bipolar and argon beam coagulation, as well as monopolar cutting is essential during operative laparoscopy. Again, this is an area in which availability is essential, since coagulation may be required at short notice if bleeding occurs. Monopolar cutting and coagulation may be used by individual surgeons and should be discussed before a surgical procedure, as should the use of the argon beam coagulator. In the author's OR, these instruments are assembled and placed on the surgeon's small instrument table for easy access.

Laser

A CO_2 laser technique using a third generation sealed tube CO_2 laser is used for lysis of adhesions, excision of endometriosis and other operative laparoscopic procedures. The potassium–titanyl phosphate (KTP) and neodymium: yttrium-aluminum garnet (Nd:YAG) fiber lasers can serve this purpose, but have been found most effective when significant coagulation is required (i.e. during a myomectomy procedure). The surgeon must discuss his surgical technique with the OR staff before the actual procedure in order to permit adequate preparation of instruments and placement of individual lasers. As discussed earlier, the operating endoscopic OR staff must be well trained in both electrosurgical and laser techniques and be comfortable moving from one to the other. When the CO_2 laser is used during operative laparoscopy, the articulating arm of the laser is attached to the operating laparoscope (12 mm, 6° operating telescope with a 6 mm operating channel), and the telescope is placed in the warming unit for later use. The arm is usually covered with a sterile drape.

A word should be said concerning the articulation of the CO_2 laser with the endoscope. This articulation usually involves a fixed focus lens, which differs from a variable focus lens used to produce variable degrees of a defocused beam. Misalignment of the laser beam in this situation is caused by either a loose attachment of the coupler or misalignment of the beam through the articulating arm due to improper mirror adjustment, which might have occurred by bumping the arm or hitting it against a stationary object. This is easily detected by the biomedical technician and should be corrected. In this regard, the biomedical technician or a substitute should be able to monitor beam alignment during the procedure and advise the surgeon and staff regarding problems with alignment, suggesting simple solutions such as condensation inside the telescope channel. With adequate training the circulating nurse will also be able to fill this role.

CO_2 Insufflation and Smoke Evacuation

The ability to visualize the pelvis clearly while using cautery or laser hinges on rapid flow of CO_2 in and out of the pelvis. Smoke and plume evacuation can only keep pace with CO_2 insufflation, which fortunately has improved recently. The original 1–3 l min^{-1} instrument gave way to the second generation, which delivered 7–9 l min^{-1}. Recently Storz and others have introduced a third generation insufflation device that will deliver up to 20 l min^{-1}, a huge asset in selected circumstances. The new Storz instrument offers adjustable pressure and gas flow.

Most OR assistants control insufflation by varying the rate of smoke evacuation. Exit pressure can be varied most conveniently by use of an in-line filter attached to the hospital OR suction line. These disposable in-line filters have been found to be completely satisfactory and do not appear to permit contamination of the main hospital system. Free-standing smoke exhaust units are available from most laser companies and prevent smoke and plume from contaminating the OR environment and hospital suction.

Telescope and Instruments

The author performs an operative laparoscopic procedure using a 0° 10 mm panoview diagnostic telescope, which produces an excellent picture and permits careful exploration of the pelvic area. Once the operative approach has begun, he changes to a 12 mm, 6° operating laparoscope, although one could use the operating telescope throughout. An angled 30° lens on a diagnostic telescope will assist in evaluating the anterior abdominal wall and is used by general surgeons in inguinal hernia repair. The smaller lens and lower number of fiber bundles contained in the 5 mm operating telescope reduce light and the quality of the video picture. Successful use of this telescope requires high intensity light and a high quality camera. A good quality video picture will often deteriorate during a difficult operative procedure when the early contrast of tissues is blunted by the colors red (blood) and dark blue (methylene blue), yet the quality of the video image must be maintained throughout.

Individual Operating Instruments

A selection of operating instruments (Table 3.1) should be available and, if possible, the surgeon should discuss these with the scrub nurse before the surgical procedure. At least three 5.0 mm puncture trocars and sleeves are of value, one containing a stopcock and vent for smoke exhaust. The need for both 5 mm and 5.5 mm sleeves has been eliminated since the new Nezhat–Dorsey suction irrigation cannula has been reduced to 5.0 mm. The pyramidal trocar tip is safer to use. The author prefers reusable metal trocar and sleeves, but has found that a combination of metal and disposable trocars is a great convenience. Disposable trocars have gained popularity in general surgery, and permit flexibility when the number of second punctures and instrument sizes vary. A metal trocar and sleeve pass through the fascia and peritoneum with little resistance under better control than the older model Teflon sleeve. The 12 mm disposable trocars are also easy to use and permit removal of tissue and elements hung up on the flap valve. In an effort to reduce cost, the author primarily uses the metal trocar and sleeves, and uses disposable units when necessary.

Each surgeon will express his preference for second-puncture accessory instruments. A selection of these instruments is important, however, in order to deal with surgical emergencies.

Equipment Summary

Obviously, laparoscopic equipment used for diagnostic procedures as well as tubal ligation will not suffice for modern operative laparoscopic procedures. Neither will the early CO_2 insufflator, telescope, or early model beam-splitting cameras be adequate. The hospital must therefore purchase new equipment suitable for individual procedures. Successful operative gynecological laparoscopy requires the instruments mentioned earlier. These instruments, the team and the OR layout to be noted later will suffice for virtually all laparoscopic procedures, including those now being performed by many general surgeons.

Table 3.1 Basic instruments.

1. Grasping forceps
   5 mm Platapus style grasper
   3 mm alligator
   Flat pancake forceps
   3, 5 mm needle drivers

2. Scissors – 55 mm
   Semm microdissecting scissors
   Semm Hook scissors
   Sharp cutting scissors
   'Scissors must cut, not cauterize or tear'

3. Bipolar cautery
   Kleppinger, bipolar microforceps
   Storz bipolar instruments (Manhes instrument style)

4. Monopolar current
   2 mm micro tip
   Corson suction irrigation unit
   5 mm suction cannula
   Scissors
   Forceps

5. Other
   Angled backstop (deflecting)
   Oviduct forceps
   Grasping forceps for suturing
   Deflecting mechanism for laser fiber

6. Suction, irrigation
   Single instrument with dual function control, permitting easy digital control of both suction and irrigation
   Nezhat (Cooper): Updated Nezhat–Dorsey (Storz). The Nezhat–Dorsey suction irrigation system has replaced the older stage Aqua-Purator. The basic components of this system are adjustable pressure unit, reusable variable-tip cannulas, and disposable trumpet valve and tubing. The hospital wall suction is attached to this unit as well. The technique of aquadissection discussed in later chapters uses the Nezhat–Dorsey instrument to force fluid into peritoneal spaces, thereby permitting safe excision. The single lumen cannula should have a non-perforated tip of decreasing size to achieve maximum pressure.

7. Suturing
   Intracorporeal knot tying is the state-of-the-art in operative laparoscopy. A microsurgical laparoscopic approach to suturing has been discussed by the author (Szabo and Patton, 1994). At present, knot tying within the abdominal cavity can be accomplished by three techniques:
   a. traditional suture forceps or groping forceps;
   b. Szabo–Berci suturing instruments: flamingo assistant's grasper and parrot needle holder
   c. Endo stitch instrument sold by US Surgical, which passes the needle between two toggle levers and is a great convenience when suturing.

OR Design

The basic OR design permits easy adaptation to various gynecological endoscopic surgical procedures. Figure 3.3 is a diagram of the author's OR arrangement, arranged for a typical laparoscopic procedure. A photograph of this arrangement is shown in Figure 3.1. It is apparent that the staff have also anticipated the possibility that the surgeon may wish to use an operative laparoscopic technique. This typical arrangement, permitting transition from a diagnostic to an operative approach, is accomplished with minimal confusion. Single-use equipment such as the suction irrigation handle, tubing and trocars can be opened once the surgeon decides to proceed with operative laparoscopy.

The primary (back) instrument table (Figure 3.4) used primarily by the scrub nurse, contains all of the laparoscopic instruments for diagnostic laparoscopy as well as those instruments the surgeon prefers during an operative approach. The selection of operative instruments should be made before surgery since individual surgeons will have different preferences. Extra instruments such as needle holders should be kept in sterile packages in a drawer of the laparoscopy cart (Figure 3.5).

The surgeon's instrument table is usually a draped jumbo Mayo stand containing electrosurgical instrumentation, including the macro and micro bipolar forceps, a monopolar needle instrument and the argon beam coagulator. These instruments should be available at all times in case unexpected bleeding occurs. Additional selected instruments such as a favorite forceps or grasping instrument can also be placed here for easy access. This table can also act as an interchange between the surgeon and scrub nurse, with placement of instruments on this table either for anticipated use by the surgeon or anticipated removal by the scrub nurse.

Figure 3.3 Diagram of operating room layout. 1, KTP/YAG laser; 2, video display monitor; 3, operating instrument table; 4, video supply cart; 5, patient table with stirrups; 6a, surgeon; 6b, scrub nurse; 6c, operating room technician; 6d, biomedical technologist; 6e, circulating nurse; 7, endoscopic supply cart with CO_2 insufflator and suction machine; 8, surgeon's instrument table; 9, electrosurgical cart; 10, CO_2 laser; 11, warming tray for endoscopes; 12, VCR power source and cassette storage; 13, stereo.

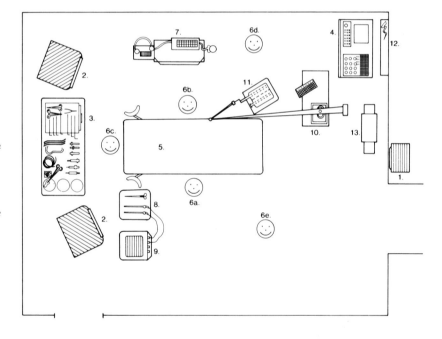

Figure 3.4 Back instrument table.

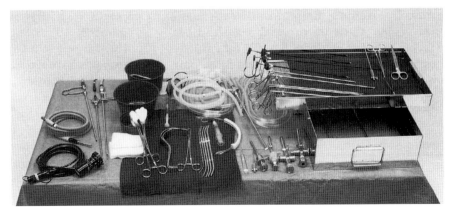

Figure 3.5 Photograph of laparoscopy cart consisting of mobile cart with drawers, endoscopic light source, CO_2 insufflator, camera, power source and irrigation system.

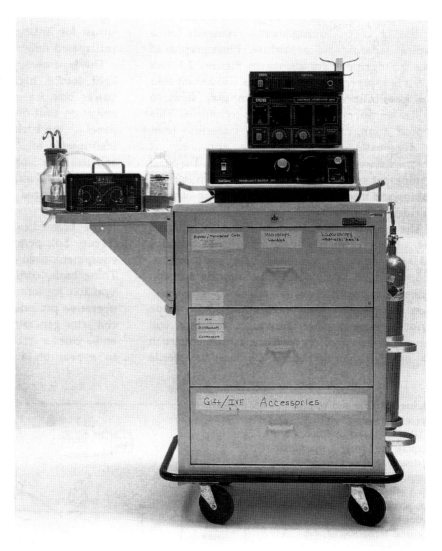

The laparoscopy cart or ceiling-mounted unit each have a compact organization. The light source, high flow insufflator and camera power box are stacked on top with a suction irrigation unit on the side platform. An electric panel permits all of these instruments to be plugged into a single source and use of a single electrical cord from the cart or ceiling unit to an electrical outlet. Additional instruments that may be required during laparoscopy are kept in drawers.

The biomedical cart is used to store instruments and equipment used by the biomedical technician. These tools, cords, instruments, bulbs, etc. are available for immediate use as needed during an operative procedure. On top of the cart are the character generator used with the video system and a video mixer that permits two camera images to appear on a single video monitor screen. Behind this cart is the wall cabinet that contains the camera power source for both the laparoscope and operating microscope camera, as well as a VCR.

Video monitors mounted on large mobile carts are easily moved to accommodate comfortable viewing by the surgeon and assistant. This system permits adaptation to operative hysteroscopy as well as both laparoscopic hysterectomy and laparoscopic cholecystectomy.

Electrosurgical generators are placed on the patient's left side just behind the surgeon's instrument table. This will include the argon beam coagulator when it is used.

The CO_2 laser is placed to the right of the patient's shoulder, a little behind the anesthesia machine, and is moved into the surgical field when needed. The operating laparoscope is usually attached to the CO_2 articulating arm and placed in a warmer during initial setup. In this design, a single weakness is the need to move the telescope warmer table and tray out of the field when using the CO_2 laser.

The KTP and YAG lasers used during operative laparoscopy and hysteroscopy are placed to the left of the patient at shoulder level when needed. The fiber may be positioned on either side of the surgeon for his comfort.

Office or Emergency Room Laparoscopy

A simplified laparoscopic technique has evolved recently in response to a new technology in which fiberoptic cables replace the rod lens in a 2 mm telescope. Although this approach appears reminiscent of outpatient laparoscopy during 1971, it is in fact a high tech procedure that permits the reproductive surgeon to perform diagnostic laparoscopy, GIFT and tubal ligation in an office setting. It may also hold promise as a second-look option in patients following treatment for endometriosis or ovarian cancer.

It appears that office or emergency room laparoscopy presents a challenge to skilled endoscopists, demanding the same high quality video images and exposure achieved in the formal OR. This technique is not a return to 1971, but an advance for the 1990s. The OR setup used for simplified laparoscopy shown in Figure 3.6 should include the following:

1. electric table with arm boards and leg-holding stirrups;
2. simplified anesthesia machine, including pulse oximeter, automatic blood pressure cuff and ECG monitor;
3. crash cart with cardioversion set;
4. laparoscopic cart;
5. instrument table.

The laparoscopy cart shown in Figure 3.6 looks much like the equipment discussed earlier. The author has used the Storz equipment shown in this figure, which includes a CO_2 monitor, light source, video camera and VCR. An electrosurgical generator would permit monopolar cautery with lysis of adhesions, and a bipolar unit would permit coagulation of vessels during manipulation in an emergency situation.

The author has used three telescopes, including Storz 2 mm and 4 mm, as well as the fiberoptic telescope now marketed by US Surgical. The 4 mm telescope, which is really the same telescope used in

Figure 3.6 OR setup for 'office laparoscopy'. Not shown in this photograph are the anesthesia machine at the head of the table and the emergency cart. The automatic blood pressure cuff, pulse oximeter and ECG monitor are placed on the anesthesia machine.

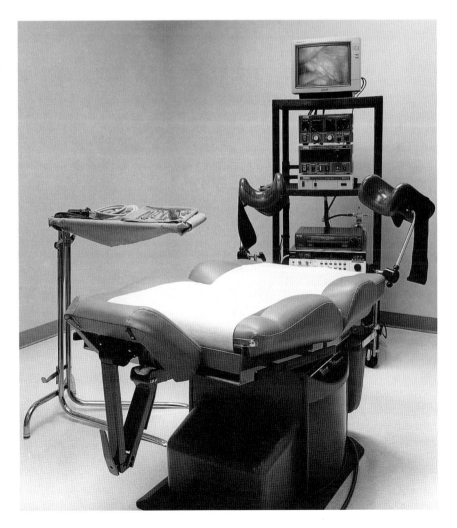

hysteroscopy, provides a superior picture during the introduction of this technique. The smaller telescope provides an excellent picture in the hands of an experienced surgeon.

Personnel

Office and emergency room laparoscopy requires high levels of experience and preparation to be carried out successfully. The scrub nurse and surgical assistant are moulded into a single individual who sets up the case, handles instruments and assists at surgery. A circulating registered nurse may not be required; although such an individual could provide assistance during the procedure, he or she would also crowd a small operating room area. The surgeon must become a more active member of the team, however, and is certainly capable of turning on the video camera, white balancing the video, and connecting tubes, as well as performing the surgery. In a sense, the surgeon assumes many of the circulating nurse's functions.

Anesthesia

This simplified laparoscopic approach is greatly aided by the use of anesthesia provided by a nurse anesthetist using propofol. Combined with the use of local anesthesia (bupivacaine) at three puncture site locations, a high quality procedure is possible and very comfortable. Certainly the combination of meperidine and midazolam with local anesthesia is a second excellent option.

Operative Hysteroscopy

Hysteroscopy is frequently used during the evaluation of patients who may also require diagnostic laparoscopy as well as an operative endoscopic procedure.

Most diagnostic procedures are performed in an office setting, as discussed earlier for office laparoscopy. Operative hysteroscopy is therefore the procedure most frequently performed in the hospital.

The ability to incorporate operative hysteroscopy easily into the OR setup is essential. This is accomplished by using a small Mayo size stand for hysteroscopic instruments placed next to the main instrument table, and a second stand on which is placed a high intensity light source and video camera power source. Both are easily incorporated into the OR design as discussed below.

OR Team

The OR team used for operative laparoscopy remains the same for operative hysteroscopy. These individuals must be trained in basic hysteroscopic technique and become familiar with types of operative hysteroscopy, and of course, safety procedures involving the use of equipment, particularly the YAG and KTP lasers.

Equipment

The telescope used during operative hysteroscopy is a 4 mm 30° telescope, which is usually inserted through a double operating channel. Recently Baggish has designed a hysteroscope sleeve that includes three channels, permitting insertion of a flexible instrument or laser fiber through one, and fluid or suction exhaust through a second accessory channel. Urological instrumentation, including the Olympus Ignasius resectoscope, typically employed during transurethral prostatectomy, has been of great value during operative hysteroscopy for resection of submucous uterine myomas and endometrial polyps. Distension of the uterine cavity with dextran 70 (Hyskon) although of some use during a diagnostic procedure has been replaced by the use of glycine and 3% sorbital used under pressure to increase distension of the uterine cavity and improve the ability to use the resectoscope for a prolonged interval without fear of overloading the patient with excessive fluid. These subjects are discussed in Chapter 52 on operative hysteroscopy.

Light Source

Adequate light is necessary during operative hysteroscopy performed in a fashion similar to operative laparoscopy: the video camera is attached to the telescope, and the surgeon views the procedure by observing the video monitor. A xenon light source similar to that for operative laparoscopy and the video camera used during laparoscopy can be used.

Dual Image Video Hysteroscopy/Laparoscopy

Many operative hysteroscopic procedures are facilitated by the ability to visualize the laparoscopic view of the uterus and tubes during the procedure by having both video images on the same monitor. This is particularly useful during tubal cannulation as while inserting the cannula through the tubal ostia, the surgeon can view the fallopian tube and

Figure 3.7 Photograph of video mixer with two telescopes and cameras. This unit permits synthesis of images from two cameras with display of both on a single monitor as shown. This is of great value during hysteroscopic tubal cannulation to avoid tubal perforation.

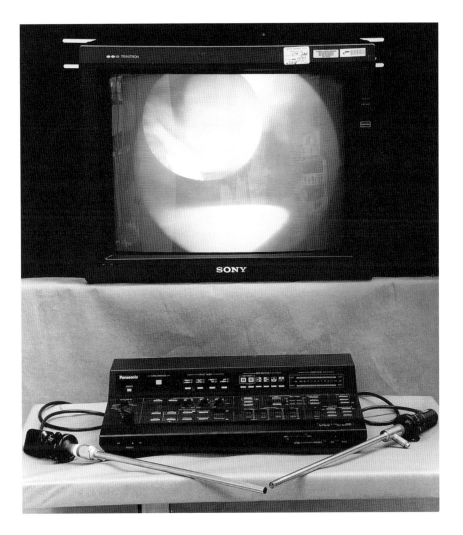

passage of the catheter through it. This greatly diminishes the incidence of tubal perforation. Additional uses include concurrent laparoscopy and falloposcopy as well as exploration of the common bile duct during laparoscopic cholecystectomy. A video mixer is used to project images from two cameras on the monitor at the same time (Figure 3.7). Two high quality cameras are therefore necessary and two xenon light sources are also used to carry out concurrent laparoscopy and hysteroscopy.

Two monitors are not absolutely necessary during operative hysteroscopy since both assistant and surgeon may view a single monitor. However, concurrent laparoscopy can make a second monitor necessary and clearly two monitors are obviously helpful.

Reference

Szabo Z, Patton GW (1994) Microsurgical laparoscopy. In Behrman SJ, Patton GW, Holtz G (eds). *Progress in Infertility*, 4th Edition. Boston: Little, Brown & Co.

4

Role of the Operating Room Nurse

WENDY K. WINER

Center for Women's Care and Reproductive Surgery, Atlanta, Georgia 30327
and Emory University School of Nursing, Atlanta, Georgia, USA

Introduction

Many things in surgery have changed over the past two decades (Semm, 1987; Kelly, 1988; Thompson and Rock, 1992). One of the most remarkable changes has to do with the role of the operating room (OR) nurse during endoscopic procedures in gynecology (Gomel, 1989; Gomel and Taylor, 1995). Previously the nurses had a more peripheral role. This is no longer the case when the surgery is carried out using the videocamera in conjunction with the endoscope (Yuzpe, 1977). As a result of the advances in the area of gynecologic endoscopy and the adaptation of the videocamera to the laparoscope and hysteroscope (Winer, 1996a), nurses can now play an active role during these surgical procedures (Winer, 1993a, 1995a).

The Endoscopy Team

The camera is attached to the eyepiece of the scope enabling everyone in the OR suite to be a part of the procedure, thus, the development of endoscopic teams (Figure 4.1). These teams are generally made up of the surgeon, surgical assistant, scrub nurse or surgical technologist, anesthesiologist, circulating nurse and laser nurse (if laser is used). Everyone in the room can follow the procedure by looking at the videomonitors; this is made easier when two monitors are used. This enables the nurses to play a more

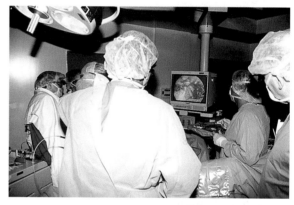

Figure 4.1 Videocamera with the laparoscope enables everyone in the OR to follow the procedure on the videomonitor.

integral role in the procedure since not only can they observe what the surgeon sees, but they can also offer better assistance and anticipation as a result of being able to follow the procedure on the videomonitor (Winer, 1994a). In this chapter we focus on the role of the OR nurse as part of the endoscopy team in operative gynecologic endoscopy (Gomel and Taylor, 1995).

There are some different pieces of instrumentation and equipment with which nurses must familiarize themselves (Winer, 1991, 1995b). These include videocameras, videomonitors, videorecorders, printers, high intensity light sources, electrosurgery generators, lasers, harmonic scalpel, suction and irrigation devices, and high flow insufflators (Winer, 1993b, 1994b). In addition to knowing how to operate these items there is the challenge of finding the most efficient way to lay out the equipment and instrumentation. This also includes the most efficient placement of the nurses as well as their individual responsibilities. Ultimately, the goal, as with any surgery, is to have the most efficient layout of instrumentation and equipment with a team of nurses who position themselves in roles that will aid this or so that the surgeon and ultimately the patient can benefit from the many advances and advantages of the new high tech endoscopic surgery (Soderstrom, 1993) (Figure 4.2).

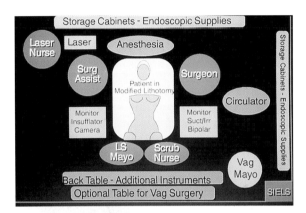

Figure 4.2 A suggested placement of the endoscopy team and equipment for gynecologic endoscopy.

Preoperative Nurses

The role of the OR nurse begins before the patient enters the OR itself. In the preoperative area the nurse begins by preparing the patient mentally and physically. An assessment of the patient and family is also completed at this time (Association of Operating Room Nurses, 1996). The assessment includes checking with the patient to see what her understanding of the surgery is. This is one of the most important roles nurses play as they provide 'patient and family education'. This includes preoperative assessment and follow-through, educating the patient and family about the procedure, helping to decrease their anxiety level, reassurance, answering all questions and when necessary arranging for the surgeon to answer questions. At this time, postoperative instructions are briefly covered verbally and reiterated in more detail postoperatively in conjunction with written going-home instructions as well as follow-up phone calls after the patient is discharged home.

During the assessment not only is the patient's level of education examined, but her chart is also reviewed. Laboratory investigations are checked to

be sure that the appropriate laboratory tests have been done and the results are within normal limits. The history and physical are reviewed with special emphasis on the patient's surgical history and any medical problems. The consent form is reviewed to verify it has been signed for the planned procedure or procedures and that the patient is comfortable with the planned treatment. Reassuring the patient and family is very important during this time to help reduce everyone's anxiety level.

Preparation of the OR by the Endoscopy Team

While the patient is prepared by the nurse and anesthesiologist in the preoperative area, the nurses and surgical technologist prepare the OR. All necessary sterile instrumentation is opened and the surgical technician sets up and organizes the instrumentation. The setup may vary from one institution to another. In general, two Mayo stands are used: one for laparoscopic instruments and one for vaginal instruments. In addition, a back table for additional laparoscopic instrumentation is used (Figure 4.3) as well as a secondary back table for additional vaginal instrumentation that may be used in more extensive vaginal procedures (e.g. operative hysteroscopy, total laparoscopic-assisted vaginal hysterectomy or perineorrhaphy). An optional ring stand with one or two large basins may be used for rinsing, separating cords and tubing during setup or placing items after they have been used to simplify cleaning.

Initially the items on the laparoscopic Mayo consist of trocars. After the trocars are placed the commonly used laparoscopic instruments (i.e. atraumatic graspers, needle driver, knot pusher, scissors and a cotton tip endoscopic dissector or kittner) are transferred from the back table to the

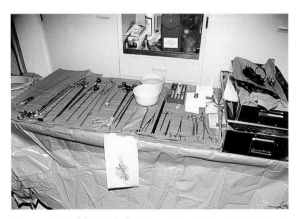

Figure 4.3 Additional laparoscopic instrumentation is placed on the back table.

Mayo while used trocars are placed on the back table. Additional laparoscopic instrumentation is kept on the back table (i.e. instruments for tissue removal and additional types of graspers) until they are needed (Carter, 1994).

The circulating nurse assists in opening the appropriate sterile items, which may include table covers and a laparoscopy pack. The circulator and laser nurse (if laser is used) are busy testing equipment and organizing it in an efficient manner. In addition, all other equipment should be checked out at this time (i.e. video equipment, light cable, light source and bulb, insufflator and gas tank level, irrigation pump and tank level, suction, electrosurgery unit and laser). If the surgeon has a surgical assistant, such as a registered nurse first assistant, this individual may also help assess the patient (Figure 4.4), educate the patient and family preoperatively and help with opening up instrumentation and organizing the equipment according to the preference of the particular surgeon (Nezhat F *et al.*, 1988a; Nezhat C *et al.*, 1989; Nezhat F *et al.*, 1990; Nezhat F *et al.*, 1991). A preference card on each surgeon's preference for each procedure is strongly

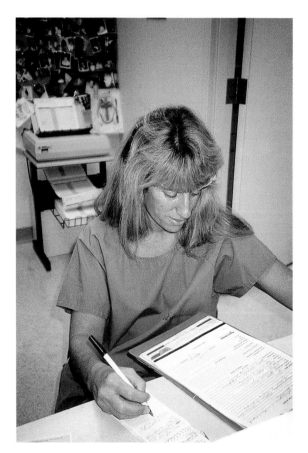

Figure 4.4 The registered nurse first assistant looks at the chart preoperatively to review the patient's history, consent form and laboratory investigations.

recommended so any OR nurses can come in and set up the case even if they do not routinely work with that surgeon. As cost containment is so important it is strongly recommended that nurses take care not to open sterile items unless it is quite probable that they will be used. This is another benefit of having an accurate preference card and if there is any doubt it is better to wait and confer with the surgical assistant or surgeon who is more familiar with the procedure to be carried out on that specific patient (Lyons, 1994; Lyons and Winer, 1995a,b; Lyons, 1996). One of the benefits of operative endoscopy is that individual procedures can be specifically tailored to each patient giving them the best possible surgical outcome; however, keep in mind that this may require some flexibility on the team's part as well as influencing what items are necessary for that patient's procedure. The assistant will then scrub and help the scrub technician to check the instrumentation to ensure it is all in good condition and operating properly as well as review the layout of these items on the back table and Mayo stands.

While the final checks are being carried out the circulating nurse goes to the preoperative area. He or she will review the patient's history and chart with the preoperative nurse, verifying that the laboratory work and consent form are complete and what procedures are to be done. She will briefly visit the patient and family. Many patients come to the OR with no preoperative medication, thus it is vital that the nurse projects a warm, caring and reassuring tone to the patient and family to help decrease normal preoperative anxiety. The patient is then accompanied by the circulator and anesthesiologist back to the OR.

It is particularly important that the patient is in a relaxed quiet environment as she is anesthetized. All noise and chatter should be kept to a minimum. Keep in mind that anesthesia is generally one of the things patients fear most. It is important that the number of people in the OR is limited to all who need to be there. Any invited guests should not be permitted to enter until the patient is asleep and draped.

When the surgeon enters the room he or she may assist the nurse and carefully position the patient's legs in padded stirrups before the patient is draped (Schmaus *et al.*, 1986; AMSCO, 1987). Generally, the surgical assistant and scrub technician will drape the patient, place the Foley catheter, and hook up and connect all of the cords to the appropriate instruments in preparation for the beginning of the procedure. The cords are organized and carefully secured to the drape and then passed off to the circulator and laser nurses so that they can be connected. Generally two video carts or hanging orbiters are used. The primary cart or orbiter houses the surgeon's monitor, insufflator, light source, camera box, video cassette recorder (VCR), and (optional) printer. The secondary cart or orbiter, opposite the assistant, houses a second monitor and the electrosurgery generator. The suction and irrigation are also kept on that side with the laser on the opposite side. Some of the placement of these items is dependent upon each room's particular hook-up locations. The key is to use the most efficient setup and layout conducive to your setting. The light cord is not placed on the drape until it is safely secured to the laparoscope. It is helpful to use an endoscopic organizing pouch to secure and house the bipolar forceps and suction and irrigation probe until they are to be used. After everything has been prepared the surgeon scrubs and the procedure is ready to begin.

Whatever protocol is followed and however this works best in your setting, it is paramount that everyone works together as a team, never losing sight of the primary goal – providing optimal care for the patient who is undergoing surgery (Meeker and Rothrock, 1995). A good team can enable the surgeon to focus on his or her work and perform surgery at an optimal level without having to be concerned with instrumentation and equipment as well.

Intraoperative Nurse Circulator Responsibilities

During the gynecologic endoscopic procedure the circulating nurse runs the equipment and monitors it. His or her responsibilities may include changing gas tanks when low, replacing irrigation bags (Figure 4.5), changing suction canisters, collecting specimens, recording input and output of fluid,

monitoring the VCRs, making any adjustments on cameras and or light sources, adjusting electrosurgery units and opening additional sterile instrumentation as necessary.

Laser Nurse Responsibilities

The laser nurse should be thoroughly trained in appropriate laser safety guidelines as established by the laser committee of the hospital (Martin and Diamond, 1986; Nezhat C et al., 1987; Nezhat F et al., 1988b). These guidelines will vary depending upon the specific laser and wavelength being used. (Absten, 1992). The guidelines should include information regarding appropriate eye protection for the patient, the endoscopy team and anyone else who may be present during the case. In addition to protective eyewear in the room, there should be a sign on the door alerting anyone who may enter during the procedure (i.e. 'laser in use' and 'protective eyewear required'). Goggles should be kept just outside the door. A fire extinguisher should be located just outside the room. The laser nurse stays with the laser throughout the case to be sure it is running appropriately and to adjust the laser control board during the procedure (Figure 4.6). The laser should be placed on 'ready' only when the surgeon is ready to activate it. The power setting is determined by the surgeon and the laser then set accordingly. The foot pedal is placed in a convenient location for the surgeon and safely separated from any other power source pedal such as the electrosurgery unit so that the surgeon does not inadvertently press the wrong foot pedal. The laser nurse should follow the procedure on the monitor to be ready to place the laser on 'standby' when it is not being used and also prepared to place it on 'ready' so that the surgeon does not have to be

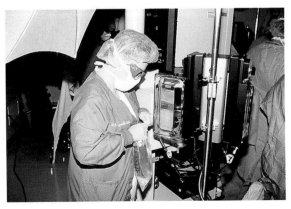

Figure 4.5 The circulating nurse changes irrigation bags as necessary during the procedure.

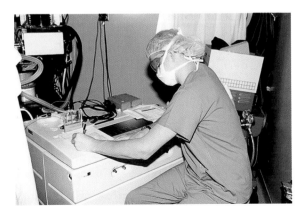

Figure 4.6 The laser nurse stays with the laser throughout the procedure.

delayed when he or she is ready to use it. The laser nurse or anyone using the laser should be trained on that particular laser unit. Initial training may be provided by the manufacturer upon installation with periodic updating. The laser nurse should organize and provide in-service training for all OR personnel. Anyone who operates the laser should have appropriate credentials from the laser committee of the hospital. This committee is generally comprised of physicians and nurses. If at any time proper guidelines are not followed the chairman of the laser committee should be notified immediately, preferably verbally as well as in writing (Winer, 1994c).

Registered Nurse First Assistant

To enhance the surgeon's ability to carry out optimal surgery and for the patient to get the best possible care and surgical result the team must be 'together'. A registered nurse surgical assistant can be a great asset to patients and their families, the surgeon and the rest of the team. He or she can help orient the staff to the surgeon's particular preferences, help the staff set the OR up accordingly and will know the surgeon's routine if he or she operates with the surgeon all the time. This person can be an invaluable team member, not just for the physician, but also for the rest of the team or staff and for the patients and their families.

A well trained assistant should be able to handle the laparoscope with ease so that someone watching the monitor will be unable to detect whether the surgeon or assistant is holding the instrument. The assistant should use two hands and not be just a camera holder. He or she holds the laparoscope

with the left hand and uses the right hand to dissect, grasp tissue, retract tissue and suction or irrigate throughout the procedure (Figure 4.7).

Positioning of OR Personnel

Positioning of OR personnel during operative endoscopy is paramount in providing optimal efficiency. The surgeon usually stands on the patient's left side with the surgical assistant directly across from the surgeon. The surgical technician stands between the patient's legs with the laparoscopic Mayo table elevated safely over the patient's right leg and close enough to the operating field that the surgeon and/or assistant can easily reach instruments on that stand (Figure 4.8). The back table is placed directly behind the scrub technician with additional items that may be needed during the procedure. Off to the side is the vaginal Mayo stand, with any vaginal instrumentation to be used which is kept sterile throughout the procedure. During the procedure the laser nurse is positioned adjacent to the laser and also positioned so that he or she may follow the entire procedure on the monitor. Initially, the circulating nurse is busy adjusting the camera, light source, videomonitor, VCR, and insufflator on the primary video cart or orbiter placed on the right side of the room and opposite the surgeon. The laser nurse may conveniently sit between the laser and the primary cart adjacent to these items in case any adjustments are needed during the procedure. The circulator stays primarily on the left side of the room opposite the assistant after he or she has positioned the secondary cart with monitor, adjusted the electrosurgery generator, and set up the irrigation and suction.

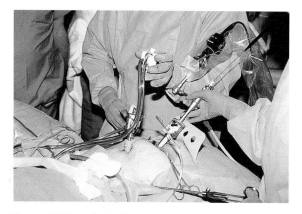

Figure 4.7 The surgical assistant guides the scope with the left hand and uses the right hand to assist; in this way, the surgeon has two hands free to operate.

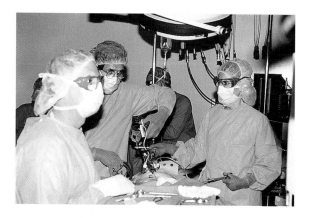

Figure 4.8 Instrumentation on the laparoscopic Mayo can be reached by the surgeon and assistant in addition to the scrub technician.

Once all of the video and laparoscopic equipment is functioning properly and the case is under way most of the adjustments are on the left side of the room. These most frequently include changing irrigation bags of fluid, switching suction canisters and possibly adjusting the electrosurgery settings. In addition, the circulator may have a small stand to document input and output of fluid and to carry out other documentation that may be necessary during the procedure (Nezhat F *et al.*, 1989) (Figure 4.9). In addition, the circulator will be responsible for collecting and labeling any specimens for pathology. It

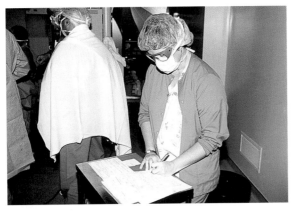

Figure 4.9 Nurses carry out necessary documentation throughout the procedure.

is imperative that all members of the team maximize the benefit of the videocamera by following the procedure on the monitor. If the surgeon needs an additional instrument, piece of equipment or particular suture a nurse can often anticipate this and have it ready before the surgeon asks for it. It is helpful if the items most frequently needed, such as an additional trocar, instrument or suture are conveniently kept in that room in clearly labeled cabinets or drawers. A team that works together on a regular basis can prove to be extremely efficient and save operating time by accurate anticipation. This may decrease surgeon frustration resulting from time delays waiting for any equipment or instrumentation or any malfunctions of these items.

Surgeon, Surgical Assistant and Surgical Technician

A team within a team can also be an integral part to the success of the procedure. This may include the immediate surgical team consisting of the surgeon, surgical assistant and scrub technician. When the surgeon and assistant work together regularly they

may function almost as one operator with four hands by working in concert (Figure 4.10). A three chip videocamera with high intensity light provides such an excellent panoramic view that the surgeon and assistant can function optimally provided they have had proper training and experience in conjunction with the benefits of the latest in new technology. When a surgeon's regular assistant holds the laparoscope and anticipates appropriately the surgeon can operate with two hands just as in traditional open surgery and the assistant still has his or her right hand free to assist. In addition, by carefully following the procedure the scrub technician can have instruments readily available on the laparoscopic Mayo table as well as assist in manipulation of the uterus.

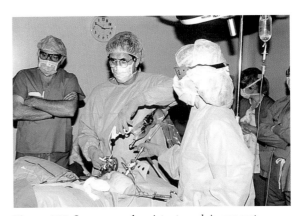

Figure 4.10 Surgeon and assistant work in concert together using four hands.

Nursing Responsibilities Specific to Operative Hysteroscopy

The nursing roles are similar for operative hysteroscopy as for operative laparoscopy. Accurate measurement of intake and output of fluid is crucial and needs to be documented and reported to the surgeon regularly (at least every 15–30 minutes) throughout the procedure. Generally glycine or sorbitol solution in 3 l bags is used for operative hysteroscopy. These bags are hung on elevated intravenous infusion poles. Specific guidelines should be established at each institution and then closely followed for the safety of the patient. It is important with operative hysteroscopy, as with operative laparoscopy, that the nursing staff are properly trained initially and continually updated, as this is also a rapidly advancing area in gynecologic endoscopy. A drainage bag attached to the sterile drape or a bag placed under the buttocks is attached so that all hysteroscopic outflow drains into the bag to aid accurate calculation of outflow.

DATA FOLLOW-UP SHEET

PATIENT'S NAME: _____

HOSPITAL #: _____

CHARGES: HOSPITAL: _____   PHYSICIAN: _____

FOLLOW-UP: _____3 MONTHS _____6 MONTHS_____12 MONTHS

IF STRESS INCONTINENCE:

1. _____MILD   2. _____MODERATE   3. _____SEVERE

PAIN? IF SO WHERE? _____

HOW IS IT COMPARED TO BEFORE SURGERY?:

1. _____WORSE   2. _____SAME   3. _____BETTER

DID YOU REQUIRE PAIN MED.? _____   & FOR HOW LONG?   _____

ARE YOU TAKING PAIN MEDICATIONS NOW?

LENGTH OF POST-OP UNTIL NORMAL ACTIVITIES RESUMED?

1. _____3–5 DAYS   2. _____5–8 DAYS   3. _____8–10 DAYS

4. _____10–14 DAYS

ANYTHING OF SIGNIFICANCE?:_____

3 MONTHS POST-OP: HOW DO YOU FEEL COMPARED TO BEFORE SURGERY?

1. _____WORSE   2. _____SAME   3. _____BETTER

BURCH LAPAROSCOPIC COLPOSUSPENSION

1. ARE YOU DRY? Yes_____   No _____

2. IF NO, HOW MANY PADS ARE REQUIRED PER DAY? _____

3. DO YOU HAVE ANY RECURRENT PROLAPSE? _____

4. DO YOU HAVE DIFFICULTY INITIATING A STREAM OF URINE? _____

5. ANY COMMENTS? _____

Figure 4.11 Sample follow-up questionnaire.

LAPAROSCOPIC SUPRACERVICAL HYSTERECTOMY (LSH)

1. HAVE THE SYMPTOMS WHICH NECESSITATED YOUR SURGERY SUBSIDED?_____

2. ARE YOU HAVING CYCLIC BLEEDING? _____

3. COMPARED TO BEFORE SURGERY, DO YOU FEEL THAT SEXUAL RELATIONS ARE . . .

_____THE SAME _____BETTER _____WORSE

4. DO YOU HAVE PAIN WITH INTERCOURSE? _____

5. ANY COMMENTS? _____

SACRAL CULPOPEXY

1. IS THE PROBLEM CORRECTED? _____

2. ARE YOU HAVING PROBLEMS WITH VOIDING? _____

3. ANY COMMENTS? _____

OTHER SURGERIES

1. HAVE THE SYMPTOMS BEEN RELIEVED? _____

PAIN?_____Yes _____No   BLEEDING?_____Yes _____No

2. ARE YOU TAKING ANY MEDICINE NOW FOR YOUR SYMPTOMS?

LUPRON? _____Yes _____No

BIRTH CONTROL PILLS (BCPS)? ____Yes ____No

ANTIPROSTAGLANDINS?   _____Yes ____No

3. ANY COMMENTS? _____

Figure 4.11 (*cont.*)

This fluid is then drained by suction connected to a suction canister and in turn to the wall suction. If at all possible it is helpful to have an additional circulator who solely measures input and output while the other circulator makes sure that all equipment is operating properly and keeps the inflow solution running, reducing unwanted delays (Winer, 1996a).

Care of Instrumentation and Equipment

Upon conclusion of the procedure it is paramount that all instrumentation and equipment are carefully cleaned and cared for as this is frequently the time when items are damaged due to careless handling (Hulka and Reich, 1994). The scrub technician carefully organizes and handles the instrumentation as it is disconnected from cords and disassembled; it is vital that only items meant to be disposable are discarded at this time. In addition, endoscopes, cameras, and light cords should be separated to help prevent endoscopes from being inadvertently autoclaved unless they are designed for autoclaving (Association of Operating Room Nurses, 1995). The instrumentation needs to be carefully cleaned by a designated person who knows how to disassemble the instrumentation properly for thorough cleaning. It may be helpful to package small items separately so they are not lost. Small adapters can be costly and can prevent a procedure from being performed if they are not in their proper place. It is recommended that the same personnel do this regularly so that they are familiar with the endoscopic instrumentation. Knowing the proper care and cleaning of instrumentation is a 'behind the scenes role' that is an integral part of maintaining the vital tools that the surgeon uses.

After the patient has been thoroughly cleaned of any betadine and blood, the bandages have been secured, the legs are lowered gently together from the stirrups, warm blankets are placed, wet gowns or sheets are replaced and the usual safety precautions are taken as the patient is carefully transferred from the OR table to a bed. It expedites this transfer if additional OR personnel are available to help during this time. The safe transfer and care of the patient is always the primary concern and must never be overlooked. The patient is moved to the recovery area by the circulating nurse and anesthesiologist.

Postoperative Nurse

The nurses in the recovery room receive the report from the circulating nurse regarding the procedure,

incision sites and any special instructions for that particular patient. The recovery room nurses need to be aware of the unique features to check for in patients who have undergone gynecologic laparoscopy. The patient's temperature is often a concern in the immediate postoperative area. This can often be regulated with the help of a patient warming device intraoperatively and in the recovery room. Some drainage from the incision sites is normal as a result of irrigation during the procedure. Comprehensive postoperative care instructions are given to the patient and/or her family verbally and instructions should also be given in writing so that the patient can review them when she gets home and is more alert.

Postoperative Written Instructions

Education of the patient and the person who will be helping care for her for the first few days postoperatively is crucial as these patients generally go home within 23 hours, so they can be considered as 23 hour stay for insurance purposes. One of the benefits of gynecologic laparoscopy is significantly decreased patient morbidity, but patients still need to have comprehensive going-home instructions (Winer 1995b). These may include what to expect such as possible shoulder pain due to gas insufflation, acceptable activities, diet, keeping track of temperature and reporting anything out of the ordinary such as a temperature of 101°F or higher, bleeding that is heavier than a period, inability to void, severe abdominal pain and excessive nausea or vomiting. The patient also needs to know when to return for a follow-up appointment. These instructions should be coordinated between the physician and the surgical care facility with a 24-hour phone number patients can call if they encounter any of these problems or have any additional questions.

Short- and Long-Term Follow-up

Follow-up of these patients short term as well as long term for at least a five-year period is recommended to be able to provide adequate evaluation of laparoscopic surgical outcomes short term and long term (two weeks, three months, six months, and annually) (Kadar, 1994) (Figure 4.11). This is an area where a well trained endoscopic nurse can be very active as it is so important to collect data on these procedures to enable physicians to evaluate their surgical techniques and whether positive patient outcomes have been attained (Winer 1996b).

For decades nurses have played an important role in the surgical area. Advanced operative laparoscopy in the area of gynecology presents nurses with exciting opportunities that include challenging and key roles not only intraoperatively, but also preoperatively and postoperatively. The role of the 'endoscopy team' is to improve patient care while taking advantage of today's high level of technology in the OR.

The Importance of Training for Nurses

Due to the rapidly advancing field of advanced operative laparoscopy it is critical that nurses are adequately trained in these new techniques and maintain excellent continued learning. The endoscope in conjunction with the video camera has totally changed the procedure for OR nurses. Nurses have an enhanced opportunity to play an active role in the procedures and to participate in the team concept. The recommendations in this chapter are designed as a helpful guide, as each setting varies and some flexibility may be necessary to provide the most organized efficient setup for a particular institution. The importance of adequate training of the team must be emphasized for the safety and optimal care of the patient. This may be best achieved by participating in frequent continuing education programs at the surgery facility, attending local and national meetings pertaining to surgery as well as specific to endoscopy, reading key laparoscopic journals, attending preceptorship programs (where a nurse who may have expertise in laparoscopic surgery can be observed first hand) and videoconferencing. Nurses should attend regular training courses, perhaps ideally with the surgeon, to receive hands-on practice along with the surgeon. Courses are being taught with hands-on laboratory sessions where nurses and surgeons can work together, each learning their role, to better simulate 'real surgery'. Learning the procedures, anatomy and instrumentation, troubleshooting the equipment, and following proper intake and outflow guidelines are key ingredients for a successful endoscopic program. The learning process never ends as techniques are refined, new products developed and continued advances are made in this field. In this way, the field of endoscopy (Winer, 1995b; Winer, 1996a; Winer, 1996c) will continue to advance and provide benefits to patients if team members maintain an active and dedicated role as

they continue to learn and stay on the cutting edge of today's high tech surgical arena.

References

Absten GT (1992) The physics of light and lasers. In Sutton CJG (ed.) *Lasers in Gynaecology*, Ch 1, pp 1–23. London: Chapman Hall.

AMSCO (1987). *Positioning Patients for Surgery*. AMSCO Education Services.

Association of Operating Room Nurses (1995) New sterilization technology. *Surgical Services Management* **2**: 4–44.

Association of Operating Room Nurses (1996) *1996 Standards and Recommended Practices*. pp. 95–125, 163–9, 191–211, 233. AORN.

Carter J (1994) A new technique of fascial closure for laparoscopic incisions. *Journal of Laparoendoscopic Surgery* **4(2)**: 143–148.

Gomel V (1989) Operative laparoscopy: Time for acceptance. *Fertility and Sterility* **52**: 1–11.

Gomel V, Taylor PJ (1995) Diagnostic and operative gynecologic laparoscopy. St. Louis: Mosby Year Book.

Hulka JF, Reich H (eds) (1994) *Textbook of Laparoscopy*, 2nd edition. Philadelphia: W.B. Saunders.

Kadar N (1994) Randomized trials involving laparoscopic surgery: Valid research strategy or academic gimmick? *Journal of Gynecologic Endoscopy* **3(2)**: 69–73.

Kelly HA (1988) *Operative Gynecology*. New York: Appleton.

Lyons TL (1994) Laparoscopic treatment of urinary stress incontinence. Tulandi T (ed.) *Atlas of Laparoscopic Technique for Gynecologists*. pp. 131–136 London: WB Saunders.

Lyons TL, Winer WK (1995a) The Nolan–Lyons modification of the Burch procedure. *Journal of the American Association of Gynecologic Laparoscopists* **2(2)**: 95–99.

Lyons TL, Winer WK (1995b) Vaginal vault suspension. *Endoscopic Surgery* **3**: 88–92.

Lyons TL (1996) Laparoscopic resection of rectovaginal endometriosis using the contact Nd:YAG laser and primary closure with suturing techniques. *Journal of Pelvic Surgery* **2(1)**: 8–11.

Martin DC, Diamond MP (1986) Operative laparoscopy: comparison of lasers with other techniques. *Current Problems in Obstetrics, Gynaecology and Fertility* **9**: 656–658.

Meeker M, Rothrock J (1995) *Alexander's Care of the Patient in Surgery*, 10th edition. St Louis: Mosby Year Book.

Nezhat C, Winer WK, Crowgey S (1987). Videolaseroscopy for treatment of endometriosis and other diseases of the reproductive organs. *Obstetrics and Gynecologic Forum* **1**: 2–5.

Nezhat C, Winer WK, Cooper JD *et al.* (1989) Endoscopic infertility surgery. *Journal of Reproductive Medicine* **34**: 127–134.

Nezhat F, Winer WK, Nezhat C (1988a) Videolaparoscopy and videolaseroscopy: Alternatives to major surgery? *Female Patient* **13**: 46–53.

Nezhat F, Winer WK, Nezhat C (1988b) Is endoscopic treatment of endometriosis and endometrioma associated with better results than laparotomy? *American Journal of Gynecologic Health* **2**: 10–16.

Nezhat F, Winer WK, Nezhat C (1989) Laparoscopic removal of dermoid cysts. *Obstetrics and Gynecology* **73**: 278–281.

Nezhat F, Winer WK, Nezhat C (1990) Fimbrioscopy and salpingoscopy in patients with minimal to moderate pelvic endometriosis. *Obstetrics and Gynecology* **75**: 15–17.

Nezhat F, Winer WK, Nezhat C (1991) Salpingectomy via laparoscopy: A new surgical approach. *Journal of Laparoendoscopic Surgery* **1**: 91–95.

Schmaus D, Nelson S, Davis D (1986) *Association of Operating Room Nurses, Positioning the Surgical Patient,* pp 1–6, 40–44.

Semm K (1987) Instruments and equipment for endoscopic abdominal surgery. In Semm K (ed.) *Operative Manual for Endoscopic Abdominal Surgery.* pp. 46–123. Chicago: Year Book.

Soderstrom R (1993) *Operative Laparoscopy, The Master's Techniques.* pp 1–15, 47–86. New York: Raven Press, Ltd.

Thompson JD, Rock JA (1992) *Te Linde's Operative Gynecology.* pp 1–12, Philadelphia: JB Lippincott.

Winer WK (1991) The set-up for operative endoscopy. *Laser Nursing* **5**: 139–145.

Winer WK (1993a) The role of the operating room staff in operative laparoscopy. *Journal of the American Association of Gynecological Laparoscopists* **1**: 86–88.

Winer WK (1993b) A comparison of the CO_2 laser and the harmonic scalpel. *Minimally Invasive Surgical Nursing* **7**: 54–56.

Winer WK (1994a) Minimal access surgery for nurses and technicians. In Hall FA (ed.) *Gynaecology.* pp 94–109. Oxford: Radcliffe Medical Press.

Winer WK (1994b) Harmonic scalpel. What it is, is it better than laser, electrosurgery or scissors for advanced operative laparoscopic procedures? *Lasers and Advanced Technology Specialty Assembly Newsletter for AORN* **2**: 2.

Winer WK (1994c) Why the use of lasers in gynecological laparoscopy has declined. *Minimally Invasive Surgical Nursing* **8**: 136–139.

Winer WK (1995a) Nursing aspects of gynecologic endoscopy. In *Endoscopic Surgery* **3**: 109–111. New York: Georg Thieme Verlag.

Winer WK (1995b) New procedures for women that are being done endoscopically. *Minimally Invasive Surgical Nursing* **9(2)**: 87–89.

Winer WK (1996a) Operating room personnel. In Sanfilippo JS, Levine RL (eds) *Operative Gynecologic Endoscopy,* 2nd edition. pp 412–422. New York: Springer-Verlag.

Winer WK (1996b) Thorough patient follow up encouraged for all cases, not just research and booklets help prepare patients for laparoscopy, ensure informed consent. *Laparoscopic Surgery Update* **4(3)**: 28–31.

Winer WK (1996c) A laparoscopic approach to rectocele repair. *Today's Surgical Nurse,* **18(3)**: 37–40.

Yuzpe AA (1977) Television in laparoscopy. In Phillips JM, Corson SL, Keith L, *et al.* (eds) *Laparoscopy.* pp 306–325. Baltimore: Williams & Wilkins.

5

A Practical Approach to Surgical Laparoscopy

CHRIS SUTTON

The Royal Surrey County Hospital, Guildford, The Chelsea and Westminster Hospital, London
and Imperial College School of Medicine, University of London, UK

Introduction

During the past few years laparoscopy has become one of the most frequently performed operations in gynecological departments. Initially it was used for occlusion of the fallopian tube as a simple method of female sterilization and for the diagnosis of pelvic pain and infertility, but increasingly it is being used for operative procedures, which are described in detail in different sections of this book. Before embarking on such procedures it is essential that each surgeon develops a safe technique for insufflating the abdomen and inserting the laparoscope and various ancillary probes and instruments.

Complications and Consenting the Patient

Modern laparoscopy is essentially a safe procedure and serious complications are rare. One of the pioneering examples of detailed surgical audit was the *Confidential Enquiry into Gynaecological Laparoscopy* conducted on behalf of the Royal College of Obstetricians and Gynaecologists (RCOG) by Professor GVP Chamberlain, which revealed an overall complication rate of 34/1000 and a mortality rate of 0.08/1000 (Chamberlain and Brown, 1978). A much larger survey from West Germany, reporting operative laparoscopies as well, drew attention to the relative safety of laparoscopic surgery in the hands of experienced operators. Major complications, requiring laparotomy or re-laparoscopy were four times greater with operative procedures than with diagnostic procedures, but the rate was only 3.8/1000 with an overall mortality for all procedures of 0.05/1000 (Riedel *et al.*, 1986).

A more recent study, which was partly retrospective but then prospective, was performed by Denis Querleu and colleagues, who reported the complications from 17 French centers performing extensive and advanced laparoscopic surgery. Of a total of 17 500 cases, there was only one death, which was due to a great vessel injury, and not surprisingly they came to the conclusion that the more advanced the surgery the greater the likelihood of complication (Querleu *et al.*, 1993).

The most dangerous time for direct trauma is when the Veress needle and the first trocar cannula are being introduced blindly (closed laparoscopy), especially in a patient who has had previous surgery. Another group at increased risk are very thin athletic women in whom the typical feel of traversing different layers of the abdominal wall is lost. The great vessels, which lie only 2.5 cm below the skin at the umbilicus, can be impaled unless great care is taken. Another group with an increased risk of complication are the morbidly obese in whom there is an increased risk of visceral injury because the thick fat-laden peritoneum is often unyielding, increasing the chance of surgical emphysema, making subsequent attempts at entry more difficult and often requiring much longer instruments.

Major direct trauma injuries and diathermy

Picolax Information Sheet for Patients

Picolax has been prescribed to clear the bowel before your operation. Two sachets are to be taken the day before according to the schedule below. It is important that you follow the instructions carefully.

The success of your laparoscopic surgery depends on the bowel being as clear as possible.

Directions for the Preparation of Picolax
Dissolve the contents of ONE sachet in a cup of water. Stir for 2–3 minutes and drink the mixture.

Be prepared for frequent bowel movements starting within three hours of the first dose.

Suggested Treatment Plan the Day Before Your Laparoscopic Surgery
Drink plenty of clear fluids throughout the treatment with Picolax. Try to drink at least a tumblerful every hour during the treatment day. Water, fizzy drinks, clear soups or meat extract drinks can be taken at any time. Tea or coffee should not be taken later than mid-afternoon.

BREAKFAST (8.00–9.00 a.m.)
Breakfast, if taken, should be limited to a boiled or poached egg and/or white bread; a scraping of butter or margarine is allowed, but no jam or marmalade.

1st sachet of Picolax dissolved in water as described above – *To be taken at 12 noon*

LUNCH (12.30–1.30 p.m.)
A small portion of steamed, poached or grilled white fish or chicken can be taken with a very small portion of boiled potato OR white bread. Clear jelly can be taken for dessert.

Second sachet of Picolax dissolved in water as described above – *To be taken at 5 p.m.*

SUPPER (7.00–9.00 p.m.)
No solid food is allowed.
Clear soup or a meat extract drink can be taken followed by clear jelly for dessert.

No Further Food is Allowed Until After the Operation. Continue to Take Fluids Until the Bowel Movements Have Ceased. Drink as Much as is Required to Satisfy Thirst.

On The Day of Surgery You Must Have Nothing to Drink or Eat for Six hours Before the Procedure.

Figure 5.1 Bowel preparation before laparoscopic surgery.

accidents to the bowel are one of the most serious complications of operative laparoscopy, and are associated with a high mortality and a high rate of surgical intervention, often associated with a temporary defunctioning colostomy, particularly if unrecognized at the time of surgery. In view of the fact that these surgical accidents can occur even in patients with no predisposing factors, all patients should be warned of the possibility of proceeding to laparotomy in the event of major hemorrhage or perforation or laceration of the bowel or urinary tract. The risk of having to perform a colostomy is considerably reduced if the bowel is thoroughly prepared, and all patients having laparoscopic surgery involving the bowel should undergo a thorough bowel preparation one day beforehand. The regimen used is shown in Figure 5.1.

The various complications of laparoscopic surgery and tips for avoiding them are dealt with in detail in the section on major complications (see Chapters 48–50).

Injuries to the bowel, urinary tract and pelvic organs contributed 1.8/1000, 0.2/1000 and 3.4/1000 complications in the RCOG series, respectively. In order to avoid these injuries with the primary trocar many laparoscopists, particularly our surgical colleagues, have advocated the open approach with the Hasson cannula (Hasson, 1978). In this technique the abdominal wall is elevated by two sutures or skin graspers and the layers of the abdominal wall are opened by a scalpel under direct vision. Once the peritoneum has been opened, the blunt ended Hasson trocar is inserted and the cone sutured in place to produce an airtight seal. Although bowel laceration can occur with open laparoscopy and occurred in 6 of 11 000 cases reported by Penfield (1985), the major advantage of this method is that accidental perforation is usually recognized and can be repaired at the time of the operation – nevertheless the diagnosis was missed in two of the six perforations that occurred.

Contraindications

This subject has been well reviewed by Gordon and Magos (1989) and the absolute and relative contraindications are listed in Table 5.1.

Abdominal distension secondary to bowel obstruction is an absolute contraindication because of the dangers of bowel trauma and perforation. An irreducible hernia is likely to be exacerbated and possibly made ischemic by the added pressure of the pneumoperitoneum. Similarly intraperitoneal gases under pressure are also likely to aggravate the

Table 5.1 Contraindications to laparoscopic surgery

Absolute
   Mechanical and paralytic ileus
   Large abdominal mass
   Generalized peritonitis
   Irreducible external hernia
   Cardiac failure
   Recent myocardial infarction
   Cardiac conduction defects
   Respiratory failure
   Severe obstructive airways disease
   Shock

Relative
   Multiple abdominal incisions
   Abdominal wall sepsis
   Gross obesity
   Hiatus hernia
   Ischaemic heart disease
   Blood dyscrasias and coagulopathies

anesthetic risks associated with severe respiratory and cardiac disease due to the effects on acid–base balance, myocardial contractility, venous return and blood pressure.

Patients should be hemodynamically stable and clinical shock is therefore a contraindication and if due to a ruptured ectopic pregnancy, is a reason for immediate laparotomy to stem the hemorrhage rather than subjecting the patient to the further delay implicit in setting up for a laparoscopy.

Relative contraindications depend upon the experience of the laparoscopic surgeon and the anesthesiologist. Previous abdominal scars require special skill in introducing instruments and employing techniques such as entering at Palmer's point in the left upper quadrant or the Z-introduction of Semm (see below). Alternatively CO_2 insufflation can be achieved through the posterior fornix or even through the uterine fundus.

Patients with hiatus hernias pose a special problem and the Trendelenburg position should be limited to 15° of downward tilt and the intra-abdominal pressure should not exceed 10 mm Hg. Some authorities have advocated direct insertion of the laparoscopic trocar without prior pneumoperitoneum as a safer approach in patients with this condition (Dingfelder, 1978).

Laparoscopic surgery should be kept to the minimal possible time in patients with ischemic heart disease, while bleeding disorders should be corrected before laparoscopic surgery in the same way as they would be before conventional surgery. The same protocol for prophylactic anticoagulants as advised for conventional surgery should be adhered to and should be used for those patients with a previous history of thromboembolism, obese women over 40 years of age, when carcinoma is

Table 5.2 Anticoagulant prophylaxis against thromboembolism for gynecological surgery (Thrift Consensus Group, 1992).

	High risk	Moderate risk	Low risk
Criteria	Three or more moderate risk factors	Age > 40 and surgery > 30 min	Age < 40 or surgery < 30 min
	Major pelvic or abdominal surgery for malignancy	Minor surgery < 30 min in patient with previous history of DVT/PE or thrombophilia	Age > 40 and no other risk factors
	Major surgery or trauma in patient with previous history of DVT/PE or thrombophilia	Obesity	
	Paralysis or immobilization of legs	Emergency surgery	Note: HRT and the oral contraceptive are not considered risk factors in the absence of other risk factors
		Gross varicose veins	
		Immobility > four days	
		Major concurrent illness (e.g. heart/lung disease, malignancy)	
Prophylaxis	Heparin† 5000 iu 8 hrly sc + TEDS	Heparin† 5000 iu 12 hrly + TEDS	Early mobilization

DVT, deep vein thrombosis; HRT, hormone replacement therapy; PE, pulmonary embolism; TEDS, thromboembolic disease stocking. †Heparin prescribed preoperatively (1st dose timed 1–3 h preoperatively), but with the instruction 'to start postoperatively' if an epidural or spinal is planned. The combination of epidural catheter, non-steroidal anti-inflammatory drug and heparin should be avoided at all times. Heparin should only be withheld on specific surgical instruction for a particular case. Pneumatic calf compression may be added to any of the above groups where feasible, especially when heparin has been withheld.

suspected and when the operation is expected to last more than 30 minutes (Table 5.2).

Anesthetic Considerations (Contributed by Dr Gareth Jenkins, Royal Surrey County Hospital, Guildford, UK)

In our unit patients are usually admitted on the day of operation and are not usually given a premedication, though if particularly anxious, they are given oral benzodiazepine. Intravenous induction of anesthesia is achieved with propofol and muscle relaxation with atracurium. Endotracheal intubation is used for all patients since we believe that a laryngeal mask is inherently unsafe, particularly for prolonged procedures. We do not use a gastric tube to empty stomach contents since all our patients are starved for at least six hours before operation. The operation is conducted under intermittent positive pressure ventilation with oxygen, nitrous oxide and enflurane or isoflurane. Analgesia is achieved with fentanyl and metoclopramide is employed as an antiemetic.

At the end of the procedure residual paralysis is rapidly reversed with neostigmine 2.5 mg and glycopyrrolate 0.5 mg, and diclofenac 100 mg is inserted rectally as a suppository for postoperative analgesia. After that most patients only need oral analgesics and can go home with a responsible adult accompanying them four hours later. However, after lengthy procedures most patients benefit from an overnight stay in hospital and can then be safely discharged the following day; the nursing staff and many of the patients seem to prefer this and the patients are much more likely to retain information concerning their operation when it is imparted to them the following day.

Preparation and Positioning the Patient

Our patients are routinely catheterized before laparoscopy unless we can be absolutely sure that they have voided just before their arrival in the operating suite. If the procedure is likely to be prolonged, an indwelling catheter should be inserted. If extensive surgery is likely in the vicinity of the large bowel, as occurs with complete obliteration of the cul-de-sac with endometriosis, it is advisable to administer a mechanical bowel preparation such as the polyethylene glycol-based iso-osmotic solution

---

Patient Preparation

- Patient should be fasted and the bladder emptied.
- Shaving is rarely necessary, but if it is it should be done immediately before the operation.
- Bowel preparation is necessary if the surgery is close to or involving large bowel.
- Antibiotic prophylaxis if vagina is opened or there are fluid instillations via the cervix.
- Thromboembolism prophylaxis if indicated.

GoLytely (Braintree, Braintree, MA, USA), or sodium picosulfate 10 mg and magnesium citrate 13.1 g (Picolax; Ferring, Feltham, UK) (see Figure 5.1). Prophylactic antibiotics are not used routinely, but can be administered in prolonged cases. They are *always* used if the vagina is opened for tissue extraction and after dye hydrotubation, and whenever there is an increased risk of infection.

The patient is placed in a modified lithotomy position once she has been anesthetized and care is taken to abduct the thighs slowly and symmetrically. Pads are placed between the poles and the calf muscles and diathermy pads are carefully attached to ensure wide and uniform application to the skin. Lower abdominal, pubic and perineal hair is not shaved, and if this is deemed necessary by overzealous operating room staff any shaving should be performed in the anesthetic room immediately before surgery. Shaving of patients on the wards several hours beforehand with the inevitable serosanguineous discharge from cut hair follicles produces a perfect culture medium for *Staphylococcus aureus*. This is an ideal way to ensure wound infections and introduces a totally avoidable risk factor into laparoscopic surgery.

The patient is supine until after the initial insertion of the primary trocars and is then placed in a steep Trendelenburg position of about 30°. It is therefore essential to have a non-slip mattress or shoulder braces, otherwise the assistant is unable to antevert the uterus. Some laparoscopic surgeons employ Trendelenburg positions as steep as 40° and have reported no adverse effects (Reich, 1993a), although there are likely to be some protestations from the anesthesiologist until he or she becomes familiar with the ventilation pressure changes induced by this degree of tilt.

Insufflation of the Abdominal Cavity with CO_2

A vertical incision is usually made deep inside the inferior aspect of the umbilicus, as the scar resulting from the sloughing of the umbilical cord overlies the area where skin, deep fascia and parietal peritoneum meet. The Veress needle is inserted, initially almost at right angles (Figure 5.2), and advanced through the layers of the abdominal wall, feeling each layer as it is penetrated, for about 1 cm before angling it forwards towards the anterior pelvis. Although a vertical incision is the most popular, other incisions, such as an elliptical one beneath the rim, can be made, depending upon the actual configuration of the navel, to produce a better cosmetic result. Nevertheless the incision should still be within the umbilicus since this minimizes the chance of the peritoneum tenting away from the end of the needle and producing surgical emphysema of the anterior abdominal wall.

The Veress needle should be tested before insertion and the resting insufflation pressure noted. During insertion the tap should be open and the gas tubing unconnected so that once the negative pressure inside the peritoneal cavity is encountered room air enters and bowel and omentum fall away from the needle tip.

After insertion the needle is connected to a CO_2 insufflator flowing at 1 l min^{-1} with a pressure only slightly above that registered when the needle was tested before insertion. The abdomen is percussed for the characteristic uniform tympanitic sound that signifies that the gas is flowing into the abdominal cavity. Once liver dullness is lost, the controls are switched to deliver a fast flow of gas until at least 3 l of CO_2 have been introduced to distend the peritoneal cavity.

Reich (1993) believes that intra-abdominal pressure is more important than volume, and deliberately increases the pressure to 25 mm Hg, which will thin the abdominal wall, the increased tension making it easier to introduce the trocar. More importantly it significantly increases the distance between the anterior abdominal wall and the great vessels, the aorta and the inferior vena cava, thus reducing the chance of lacerating them – the most feared complication of laparoscopy. Once the main trocar is inserted, the pressure should be reduced to 15–18 mm Hg. Although Reich's technique has much to recommend it the volume of gas required and the time taken to reach this pressure are greatly increased and we tend to insert the primary trocar when the intraperitoneal pressure has reached 18 mm Hg. This often requires 5–6 l of insufflated gas.

A muffled sound on percussion or asymmetric swelling of the abdomen suggests failure to perforate the peritoneum, which can be very thick and elastic, especially in obese patients, resulting in surgical emphysema. If the surgeon is uncertain that insufflation is intraperitoneal, the Veress needle should be removed and reinserted before too much surgical emphysema has developed. If a second attempt at insertion is unsuccessful, insufflation should be attempted elsewhere – either through a suprapubic incision into the uterovesical pouch, by a colpotomy into the cul-de-sac, or transfundally. This latter approach is used almost exclusively by some gynecologists and requires strict aseptic preparation of the lower genital tract and careful uterine sounding to measure the distance from the cervix to the internal surface of the fundus. The Veress needle is pushed through the myometrium with the patient in a steep Trendelenburg position until a loss of resistance signifies fundal perforation.

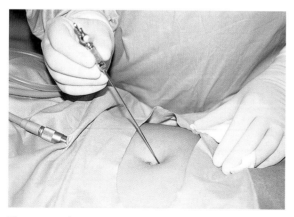

Figure 5.2 The Veress needle is inserted intraumbilically almost vertically then, when the peritoneum is pierced, it is angled towards the anterior pelvis.

Entry Technique

- Intraumbilical incision. Veress needle inserted vertically until peritoneum pierced and then angled towards the anterior pelvis.
- Confirm peritoneal position of needle.
- Insufflate until pressure of 18 mm Hg.
- Insert primary trocar, withdrawing sharp point when peritoneum is pierced.
- Steep Trendelenburg position once primary trocar has been correctly positioned.
- Check all around umbilical area for any sign of damage to bowel.
- If bowel has been damaged by the trocar it should be repaired immediately by a laparotomy.

There is considerable risk if the bowel is adherent to the uterus from previous surgery or severe endometriosis.

The induction of a pneumoperitoneum can be particularly difficult in very obese patients, often due to the thickness and elasticity of a peritoneum densely infiltrated with adipose tissue. For some patients weighing 120 kg or more we use longer trocars and needles, but these instruments must never be used for women with a normal habitus since they would pose a very real risk of penetrating pelvic organs, particularly the fundus of the uterus, or more seriously, the great vessels. The correct siting of the Veress needle can also be very difficult, paradoxically, in the very thin, when the tactile recognition of the separate layers is often absent.

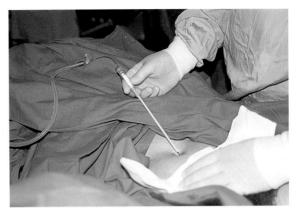

Figure 5.3 An optical catheter is probably the safest way to enter the peritoneal cavity, but at the moment these devices are expensive and relatively fragile.

Confirmation of Peritoneal Entry

Several of the disposable Veress needles are fitted with a hollow chamber containing a small ball just above the spring mechanism and the characteristic double click, which is clearly heard when the needle tip pierces the rectus sheath and then the peritoneum, is satisfactory confirmation of the intraperitoneal position of the needle tip when in the hands of an experienced laparoscopist. A number of tests can be used to confirm peritoneal entry, such as the syringe test, where a 10 ml syringe filled with saline is attached to the Veress needle and 5 ml are injected into the peritoneal cavity and the plunger is then withdrawn. No aspirate should be obtained if the needle is correctly positioned as the fluid will have dispersed between the loops of bowel. If the needle lies in the abdominal wall, clear fluid will be obtained, but if the aspirate is stained red or brown, perforation of bowel or a blood vessel has probably occurred. A variation of this test is to put a droplet of saline on the Veress needle during insertion and watch it disappear once the negative intraperitoneal pressure is encountered. Another test of intraperitoneal position is the swinging needle test to confirm that the tip of the needle is lying free, but the disadvantage of this test is that if bowel has been perforated this will merely increase the damage.

Probably the safest way to be certain of correct Veress needle placement is with an optical catheter (Figure 5.3), which will fit inside the Veress needle or replace the Veress needle (Storz, Tuttlingen, Germany) and allow the surgeon to directly visualize entry into the abdominal cavity. At the moment these catheters are expensive and relatively fragile, but it is likely that in the future they will be the entry mechanism of choice and will provide added safety, taking away the blind nature of the present procedure.

If the Veress needle punctures the bowel, it is probably acceptable to treat the patient with metronidazole and a broad-spectrum antibiotic, to observe carefully over a period of 72 hours in hospital, and to give the patient strict instructions to take her temperature when she returns home and to report back if she feels any increasing pain or malaise. If, however, the injury is caused by the main trocar, exploration is mandatory. Normally it should be performed by laparotomy by an experienced gastrointestinal surgeon, but occasionally a minimal access approach can be used to resolve the problem. Figure 5.4 shows a case treated in this manner. The patient had previously had a laparoscopy, but no other surgery, and the

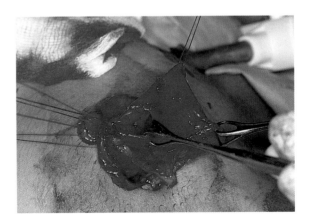

Figure 5.4 Perforation of transverse colon stuck to previous laparoscopy scar repaired by minimally invasive surgical technique employing minimal extension of umbilical scar.

transverse colon was stuck to the umbilical scar from her previous laparoscopy. When the laparoscope was inserted, it was clear that the trocar was in the bowel. The trocar was not removed, a small incision was made laterally in the right iliac fossa and the site of the perforation was visualized through a 5 mm laparoscope. There was no fecal contamination and a general surgeon with considerable experience in laparoscopic surgery was called. A small incision was made circumferentially around the umbilicus and a grasping forceps was inserted through the primary trocar to exteriorize the bowel, which was then repaired in the usual manner. After reinsertion the peritoneal cavity was cleansed with copious irrigation and the patient was given antibiotics. The laparoscopic surgery was then continued to remove the patient's endometriosis by the CO_2 laser. The patient stayed in hospital for two days and was discharged well, with an almost unnoticeable incision around the inner rim of the umbilicus. A minimal access surgical accident was thus repaired by minimal access surgical techniques, but this could only be achieved in this particular case because the trocar had not been removed once the accident had been recognized and there was no fecal contamination.

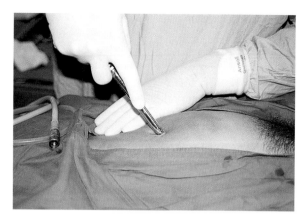

Figure 5.5 At 18 mm Hg intra-abdominal pressure, gas can be forced into the lower abdomen by pressure with the left hand increasing the volume of pneumoperitoneum and allowing safer entry of the main trocar.

Other organs at risk of damage by the trocar are the full bladder, and rarely, the transverse colon, a low slung stomach or pelvic kidney, either naturally occurring or following renal transplantation.

Insertion of the Umbilical Trocar and Laparoscope

If the abdominal cavity is well distended it is not necessary to lift up the anterior abdominal wall during insertion of the trocar because this can give rise to unpleasant bruising. The gas can be forced into the lower abdomen by simply pressing on the upper abdomen with the left hand while the trocar is inserted in the palm of the right hand with the index finger acting as a guard to allow only a few centimetres of the sharp end to penetrate the peritoneum (Figure 5.5). Once inserted, the trocar is angled almost horizontally and pushed forwards towards the anterior pelvis, taking care to avoid the major vessels as they course over the sacral promontory. This is particularly important on the rare occasion when laparoscopy is performed on an achondroplastic dwarf since the true conjugate of the pelvis is considerably reduced, thus exposing the aorta and inferior vena cava to serious risk of laceration and the inevitable catastrophic hemorrhage that ensues.

The patient should not be placed in the steep Trendelenburg position before the trocar has been inserted because this angle of tilt increases the risk of retroperitoneal injury by rotating the sacral promontory into a position closer to the umbilicus (Lynn *et al.*, 1982).

Patients with Previous Laparotomy Scars

Previous abdominal surgery used to be considered a contraindication to laparoscopy. Certainly loops of bowel adherent to a midline scar are at risk of perforation and such patients should have a bowel preparation such as GoLytely, or Picolax. The Veress needle and the trocar should be angled at 45° away from the scar, but great care must be taken to introduce only the sharp tip of the trocar just inside the peritoneum before checking the site visually with the laparoscope. An alternative technique in these patients is the Z-puncture technique of Semm and O'Neill-Freys (1989) where a 10 mm trocar is inserted proximal to the peritoneum and penetration of a thin translucent sheet of peritoneum is selected visually, thus avoiding adherent bowel or omentum. Unfortunately this technique will not work in obese women with a fatty peritoneum since the intra-abdominal contents will not be seen clearly if at all.

Reich (1993b) has described entry through the left ninth intercostal space in the anterior axillary line (Figure 5.6). A 5 mm trocar is inserted at the left costal margin in the midclavicular line (Palmer's point) and a small 5 mm laparoscope is inserted to give a panoramic view of the entire abdominal cavity. Any adhesions around the

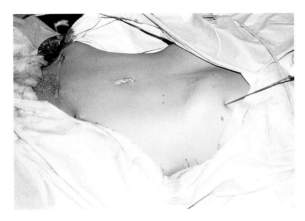

Figure 5.6 Reich's technique of insufflation in patients with midline scars. The Veress needle is introduced through the left ninth intercostal space in the anterior axillary line and then the 5 mm trochar is inserted beneath the lowest rib at Palmer's point.

umbilicus can be divided by scissors before inserting the laparoscope intraumbilically under direct vision. The left upper quadrant is rarely involved in adhesive disease, but care should be exercised in patients with splenomegaly and in malarious areas. Personally I have never dared to insert the Veress needle between the ribs and have modified this technique by inserting both the insufflating needle and the 5 mm trocar at Palmer's point with good results.

Initial Inspection

Following insertion of the laparoscope the surgeon should consciously perform an anatomic tour of the pelvis to identify any structures that could be harmed if inadvertently hit with the laser beam or electrodiathermy. This first step is vital to ensure the safety of operative laparoscopy and should never be omitted since no two pelvises are identical and anatomic variations, particularly concerning the course of the ureter, are not unusual.

The pelvic sidewall is inspected to determine the position of the ureters, which can occasionally lie close to the uterosacral ligaments, but usually run 1–2 cm laterally. They can be 'palpated' with a blunt probe and often the characteristic peristaltic movements can be recognized beneath the peritoneal surface. In extreme cases they can be dissected out with the CO_2 laser, scissors and aquadissection (Reich, 1990) or illuminated by special ureteric catheters (Rocket, London, UK), but although such measures

may be justified during laparoscopic hysterectomy or a difficult dissection of an ovary plastered onto the pelvic sidewall by endometriosis they should not be necessary for most operative laparoscopic procedures. Once the anatomic landmarks have been established the surgeon should carefully inspect the pelvis for evidence of any pathology, particularly endometriosis. The laparoscope when held close to the peritoneal surface can provide $\times 8$ magnification and close inspection may reveal subtle or atypical appearances (Jansen and Russel, 1986), which are described in detail in Chapters 35 and 37. Figure 5.7 shows some of these changes with vesicles (sago grains), white scarring (powder puff burns) and abnormal vessels radiating from an endometriotic lesion lying perilously close to the ureter. The ovarian fossa and posterior surface of the ovary must also be inspected for evidence of endometriosis and sub-ovarian adhesions, and in the absence of ovarian ultrasound or nuclear magnetic resonance imaging (MRI) techniques, the ovaries may have to be 'needled' for the presence of hemosiderin to avoid missing ovarian endometriomas.

It is impossible to perform an adequate diagnostic laparoscopy with a single puncture technique and nearly all operative procedures require additional punctures in the suprapubic area or in one or other iliac fossae.

Insertion of the Suprapubic Probe

This probe is inserted through a 5 mm trocar introduced via a small incision placed centrally

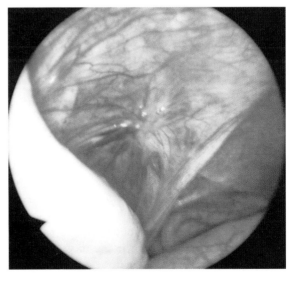

Figure 5.7 Atypical endometriosis on the back of the broad ligament close to the ureter.

just above the pubic bone in the hair-bearing area of the mons veneris so that no visible scar remains following the procedure. Since a full bladder would be punctured by a stab at this site it is imperative that the bladder is emptied before the start of the operation by catheterization using a sterile technique. An alternative to a rigid metal probe is to use a suction–irrigation instrument to wash off residual carbon deposits and cool the tissues if laser or electrosurgery is being used. Some of these devices are not as strong as the rigid stainless steel probes and since they are expensive great care must be taken not to distort them while applying pressure to the posterior aspect of the cervix to delineate the uterosacral ligaments before a laparoscopic uterine neurectomy. Some surgeons prefer to use flexible fiber lasers, in which case the suction–irrigation probe is inserted in the right iliac fossa as described below and the central channel of the probe is used to conduct the silicone quartz fiber, which transmits the laser energy.

Insertion of the Second and Third Operative Trocars

An incision is made either at the right-hand end of an imaginary Pfannenstiel incision just above the pubic hairline or higher in the right iliac fossa just lateral to the deep inferior epigastric vessels. These vessels – an artery flanked by two veins (venae comitantes) – can bleed profusely if accidentally punctured and this is an accepted and unfortunate

---

Placement of Lateral Trocars

- Positively identify the deep epigastric arteries lateral to the umbilical ligament, which are visualized from underneath the peritoneal surface
- Insert lateral trocar under direct vision, vertically at first and then guiding it towards the anterior pelvic compartment.
- Avoid hybrid trocars and ensure that all elements of the trocar are made of the same material.
- Close all incisions 10 mm or more in length, with non-absorbable sutures placed under laparoscopic vision before removing the laparoscope.

hazard of operative laparoscopy. Transillumination of the abdominal wall will often pick out the superficial vessels, but cannot be relied upon to locate the deeper vessels, especially in a 'well covered' woman. These must routinely be located by direct vision of the peritoneal surface of the anterior abdominal wall where they run just lateral to the umbilical ligaments – the obliterated umbilical artery (Figure 5.8). A finger tapping the skin lightly from above can be identified and it is moved to an avascular area lateral to these vessels and the incision made at this site. The 5 mm trocar is inserted there, preferably with a self-retaining thread to prevent it sliding during instrument movements. Please note that the trocar, when introduced lateral

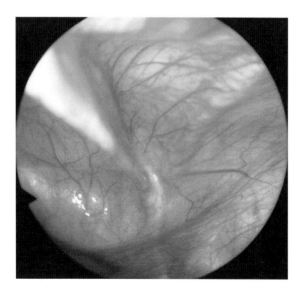

Figure 5.8 Obliterated umbilical artery and inferior epigastric vessels running parallel and to the left.

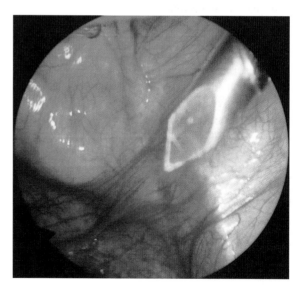

Figure 5.9 Second portal trocar inserted under direct vision to avoid damage to external iliac vessels.

to the rectus sheath, is very close to the external iliac vessels and the forefinger should always act as a guard to prevent deep insertion. Penetration of the peritoneum by the sharp trocar should always be conducted under direct vision and as soon as the sharp point perforates the peritoneum it must be angled more horizontally towards the uterus so that perforation of the external iliac vessels can be avoided (Figure 5.9).

Most operative laparoscopies can be performed through these three trocars, but it is occasionally necessary to employ a fourth 12 mm port, which is usually placed just beneath the umbilicus in the right or left flank. This is needed to introduce larger instruments such as the Semm or Steiner morcellator and tissue extractor or large stapling devices. In practise they are used for only a relatively short time during complicated procedures such as hysterectomy and oophorectomy or for removing large ectopic pregnancies or myomas. The development of reducing sleeves to enable smaller diameter instruments to be introduced through the large trocars without loss of pneumoperitoneum represents a very real advance and is a classic example of how complex problems can be solved by simple solutions. Care must be taken to keep the incisions well apart to avoid interference with other instruments – the so-called 'clashing swords' effect, which can be annoying and frustrating for both the surgeon and the assistant. The laparoscopic surgeon should try to adopt a situation where the positioning of the trocars is constant for specific procedures to allow the surgeon and assistants to gain a certain familiarity with the technique (Figure 5.10). Incisions should be kept to the minimum necessary because multiple scars, albeit small, are unsightly and can be the site of implantation endometriosis. (Figure 5.11).

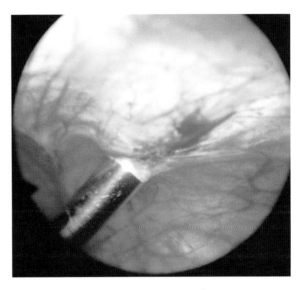

Figure 5.11 Endometriosis in previous laparoscopy scar.

It is important to avoid the use of hybrid trocars (i.e. a metal trocar and plastic retaining thread) because this increases the risk of capacitive coupling. Use only trocars made of the same material – metal and metal or plastic and plastic.

Management of Profuse Bleeding during Trocar Introduction

The procedure outlined above to avoid puncturing the inferior epigastric vessels should always be followed, but sometimes, regardless of the preventive measures taken, a large vessel is pierced and deep suture equipment should be immediately available. The bleeding can sometimes be very dramatic and if this occurs DO NOT REMOVE THE TROCAR because it is marking the track of insertion along which the bleeding vessel must be located. A strong suture on a straight needle should be passed directly beside the trocar and retrieved inside the abdomen with a needle holder and passed up on the other side of the trocar and extracted through the skin using a conventional needle holder. The procedure is then repeated to embrace the tissue occupied by the trocar in a Z-fashion. The trocar is then removed and a knot carefully tied to achieve hemostasis. Unfortunately this often results in an untidy scar, but if the trocar is removed and the excision extended it can be almost impossible to locate the bleeding point.

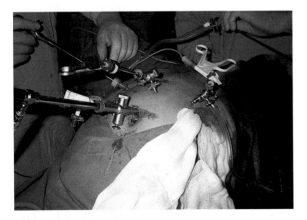

Figure 5.10 The placement of trocars for advanced laparoscopic surgery.

Closure

The umbilical incision is closed with a 4.0 Vicryl suture opposing deep fascia and skin dermis. The other incisions can be closed with plain catgut for day cases or Michelle clips, which are removed the following morning before the patient goes home. If large incisions are made for the removal of ovarian tumors or myomas it is important to close the rectus sheath with a non-absorbable suture, otherwise there is a risk of incisional hernia (Richter's hernia) and occasional fatalities have been reported when loops of small bowel have been incarcerated in the abdominal wall. Various J needles are available to close all layers under laparoscopic vision and even the old-fashioned Bonney–Reverden needle holder can be used to good effect.

Postoperative Care

If the laparoscopic surgery is on a morning list, the patient is usually able to go home accompanied by a responsible adult the same evening. Although the incisions are only small many of the patients have had a lot of surgery performed inside and should be warned to expect some soreness over the following week. Temperature elevation is unusual beyond the first day and they should be told to report any other temperature rise. They should also be warned to expect some vaginal bleeding due to the intrauterine manipulator.

As a general rule, patients get better with each passing hour following laparoscopic surgery. Patients with increasing pain and malaise should be told to report back to the ward so that they can be reassessed to make sure that they do not have peritonitis due to an unrecognized bowel injury. The family physicians and accident and emergency doctors are often unfamiliar with the complications of laparoscopic procedures and may give misplaced reassurance or adopt a 'wait and see' policy, often accompanied by antibiotics, when the patient urgently requires laparotomy and repair of any bowel damage by a gastrointestinal surgeon (Thompson and Wheeless, 1973). This is the 'Achilles heel' of laparoscopic surgery (Garry, 1994), and delay in recognizing intestinal and ureteric injuries are the leading reason for litigation. This subject is covered comprehensively in Chapter 48.

Complications of laparoscopy

General Complications

- Peri-operative – pulmonary, thrombo-embolic, urinary
- Anesthetic – particularly associated with long procedures and patients classed as poor anesthetic risk

Laparoscopy-specific Complications

- Entering the peritoneal cavity – various needle injuries, trocar injuries
- All viscera and blood vessels potentially at risk, particularly the bowel, urinary tract and great vessels
- Insertion of lateral ports – injury to epigastric vessels should largely be avoided by direct visualization internally, and lateral ports should be inserted carefully under direct vision
- Electrosurgical injuries – transmitted heat, open circuit, faulty insulation, capacitative coupling; these should be avoided partially by not using hybrid ports and completely by using electronic devices which will switch off the current if this occurs
- Laser injuries (transmitted heat, overshooting of target) – failure to use back stops appropriately, failure to appreciate the greater depth of penetration of fiber lasers
- Port site complications (hematoma, infection and hernia). All ports more than 7 mm must be closed with a suture that involves the rectus sheath and peritoneum

Key Points

- Patients get better and experience less pain with each passing hour following laparoscopic surgery.
- Patients with increasing pain, malaise and fever must return to the hospital to be carefully assessed. Unsuspected bowel injury is the most likely diagnosis and further morbidity and mortality can be avoided by early laparotomy and bowel repair performed by a gastrointestinal surgeon.

References

Chamberlain GVP, Brown JC (1978) *Gynaecological Laparoscopy – The Report of the Working Party of the Confidential Enquiry into Gynaecological Laparoscopy*. London: Royal College of Obstetricians and Gynaecologists.

Dingfelder JR (1978) Direct laparoscopic trocar insertion without prior pneumoperitoneum. *Journal of Reproductive Medicine* **21**: 45–47.

Garry R (1994) The Achilles heel of minimal access surgery. *Gynaecological Endoscopy* **3(4)**: 201–202.

Gordon AG, Magos AL (1989) The development of laparoscopic surgery. In Sutton CJG (ed.) *Laparoscopic Surgery. Ballière's Clinical Obstetrics and Gynaecology* **3(3)**: 429–449.

Hasson HM (1978) Open laparoscopy versus closed laparoscopy: a comparison of complication rates. *Advanced Planned Parenthood* **13**: 41–51.

Jansen R, Russel P (1986) Non-pigmented endometriosis: Clinical, laparoscopic and pathological definition. *American Journal of Obstetrics and Gynecology* **3(3)**: 655–681.

Lynn SC, Katz AR, Ross PJ (1982) Aortic perforation sustained at laparoscopy. *Journal of Reproductive Medicine* **27(2)**: 17–19.

Penfield AJ (1985) How to prevent complications of open laparoscopy. *Journal of Reproductive Medicine* **30**: 660–663.

Querleu D, Chevallier L, Chapron C, Bruhat MA (1993) Complications of gynaecological laparoscopic surgery. A French multicentre collaborative study. *Gynaecological Endoscopy* **2**: 3–6.

Reich H (1990) Aquadissection. In Baggish M (ed.) *Laser Endoscopy. The Clinical Practice of Gynaecology Series.* pp. 159–185. New York: Elsevier.

Reich H (1993a) Advanced laparoscopic surgery. In Garry R, Reich H (eds) *Laparoscopic Hysterectomy.* Ch 4, p. 51. Oxford: Blackwell Science.

Reich H (1993b) New laparoscopic techniques. In Sutton C, Diamond M (eds) *Endoscopic Surgery for Gynaecologists.* Ch. 4, p. 31. London: W B Saunders.

Riedel HH, Lehmann-Willenbrock E, Conrad P, Semm K (1986) German pelviscopic statistics for the years 1978–1982. *Endoscopy* **18**: 219–222.

Semm K, O'Neill-Freys I (1989) Conventional operative laparoscopy (pelviscopy). In Sutton CJG (ed.) *Laparoscopic Surgery. Ballière's Clinical Obstetrics and Gynaecology* **3(3)**. 451–485.

Thompson BH, Wheeless CR Jr (1973) Gastrointestinal complications of laparoscopic sterilisation. *Obstetrics and Gynecology* **41**: 669.

Thrift Consensus Group (1992) Report of the RCOG Working Party on prophylaxis against thromboembolism in gynaecology and obstetrics. *British Medical Journal* **305**: 567–574.

6

Advanced Laparoscopic Techniques

HARRY REICH

Columbia Presbyterian Medical Center and Columbia University College of Physicians and Surgeons, New York, USA

Introduction

Operative laparoscopy requires a level of skill, facilities, and equipment far beyond the standard diagnostic and sterilization procedures of the 1970s and 1980s. Advanced laparoscopic surgery uses special techniques, some new and others similar to traditional techniques, to perform procedures with better visualization. Most laparoscopic procedures are not new, but are minimally invasive versions of traditional operations. I have no doubt that 25 years from now, surgical students will be amazed to learn that laparoscopic gynecological operations had such a difficult beginning. Kurt Semm's fame will grow, and we will all appreciate the wonders of the team that Maurice Bruhat assembled in Clermont–Ferrand and their formidable research in establishing laparoscopic surgery as the standard.

This chapter will concentrate on laparoscopic techniques that are new to many surgeons, though some of these techniques have been known for over 20 years. Ideas and techniques are not listed in any particular order of importance and only reflect this author's preferences.

Pre-operative Evaluation

Endovaginal ultrasound is carried out to evaluate the pelvis in cases involving a pelvic mass, retrocervical nodules or fibroids. A CA-125 assay, which uses a monoclonal antibody that reacts to an antigen found in most non-mucinous ovarian cancers, is obtained when a mass is present, but is rarely useful as it is elevated in many cases of extensive endometriosis. Intravenous pyelograms are rarely carried our preoperatively, but should be obtained when abdominal pain persists after surgery on or near the ureter. Before laparoscopic surgery, there are few indications for CT scanning or MRI that justify their expense. This author has little experience with these procedures and believes that laparoscopy is better for diagnosis.

Pre-operative Preparation

Patients are encouraged to drink and eat lightly for 24 hours before admission. When extensive cul-de-sac involvement with endometriosis is suspected, either clinically or from another doctor's operative record, a mechanical bowel preparation is advised (polyethylene glycol-based isosmotic solution: Golytely or Colyte). Lower abdominal, pubic, and perineal hair is not shaved. Patients are encouraged to void on the way to the OR, and a Foley catheter is inserted only if the bladder is distended, a long operation anticipated, or recovery room personnel feel uncomfortable with the early discontinuation of intravenous fluids. (Postoperative urinary retention is usually secondary to overhydration.) Antibiotics (usually cefoxitin or cefotetan) are administered at the start of all cases.

Leuprolide acetate for depot suspension (Lupron Depot, TAP Pharmaceutical, Deerfield, IL, USA), 3.75 mg IM, is often administered after ovulation in the cycle preceding surgery to avoid operating on ovaries containing a corpus luteum; it is not used to treat endometriosis or fibroids as it is ineffective. The preoperative use of gonadotropin-releasing hormone (GnRH) analogues for more than two months before myomectomy or hysterectomy for large myomas is discouraged. GnRH analogs rarely reduce the total uterine and leiomyoma volumes enough to make laparoscopic or vaginal hysterectomy easier, though anemia secondary to hypermenorrhea should resolve. Preoperative treatment with GnRH analogs for longer than two months may result in degeneration of the myoma, making the dissection planes between the myoma and its myometrial pseudocapsule difficult to distinguish during surgery. In addition, the myoma may be made so soft that it cannot be grasped with a tenaculum or corkscrew for adequate traction. Autologous blood donation can be considered before laparoscopic hysterectomy, but most blood obtained for this purpose is discarded; packed red blood cells have a shelf life of 35 days if stored at 1–6° C.

Recently, techniques have been developed to denature myomas to cause their regression. Specially designed bipolar or monopolar probes and cryoprobes are used to puncture the myoma capsule and desiccate the tissue inside it. Small myomas are desiccated until they turn white (Gallinat, 1992). This surgeon (HR) has experience with a patient return electrode burn when using low voltage cutting current above 200 W power for a long duty cycle.

Equipment

High Flow CO_2 Insufflators

High flow CO_2 insufflation is necessary to compensate for the rapid loss of CO_2 during suctioning. Models to filter smoke produced by electrosurgery or laser from the CO_2 gas are available (ICM 350D, I.C. Medical, Phoenix, AZ, USA), and should decrease operative time spent suctioning smoke and smoke products absorbed by the patient and operating room personnel. The ability to maintain a relatively constant intra-abdominal pressure of 10–15 mm Hg during long laparoscopic procedures is essential. Higher pressure settings are used during initial insertion of the trocar (25 mm Hg), with the setting lowered thereafter in order to diminish the development of subcutaneous emphysema. High pressure settings can be used to control venous bleeding, but only for short periods to avoid the possibility of CO_2 embolism and delayed bleeding.

30° Tiltable Operating Room Table

Operating room tables capable of a 30° Trendelenburg position are extremely valuable for advanced laparoscopic surgical procedures, especially when the deep pelvis is involved. Unfortunately these tables are rare, and this author has great difficulty when operating in other institutions where a limited degree of body tilt can be obtained.

For the past 20 years this author has used a steep Trendelenburg position (20–40°), with shoulder braces and the arms at the patient's sides (Romanowski et al., 1993). Presently, the hand-controlled Champagne model 600 (Affiliated Table Company, Rochester, NY, USA) is used; electronically controlled tables capable of this degree of body tilt are rarely available. This author's patients have experienced no adverse effects from the steep Trendelenburg position.

Uterine Manipulators

A Valtchev uterine mobilizer (Conkin Surgical Instruments, Toronto, ON, Canada) is the best available single instrument to antevert the uterus and delineate the posterior vagina throughout complicated cases. The uterus can be anteverted to about 120° and moved in an arc about 45° to the left or right by turning the mobilizer around its longitudinal axis. Four interchangeable detachable uterine obturators of various lengths and diameter ranging from 3 mm thickness and 45 mm length to 10 mm thickness and 100 mm length, and two cannulas for injection of dye measuring 3 mm thick by 35 or 50 mm length, are also available. With this device in the anteflexed position, the cervix sits on a wide acorn, which is readily visible between the uterosacral ligaments when the cul-de-sac is inspected laparoscopically. The 80 mm long, 80 mm thick obturator is used for uterine manipulation during hysterectomy. The 50 mm long, 3 mm thick acorn cannula is used for most other procedures, including cul-de-sac dissections and as a backstop during laser culdotomies.

Rectal and Vaginal Probes

If a Valtchev uterine mobilizer is not available, a sponge on a ring forceps is inserted into the posterior vaginal fornix and a #81 French rectal probe (Reznik Instruments, Skokie, IL, USA) is placed in the rectum. This is used to define the rectum and posterior vagina in endometriosis and adhesion cases with some degree of cul-de-sac obliteration and to open the posterior vagina (culdotomy). In addition, a #3 or 4 Sims curette or Hulka uterine elevator is placed in the endometrial cavity to antevert the uterus markedly and stretch out the cul-de-sac. The rectal probe and intraoperative rectovaginal examinations remain important techniques even when the Valtchev is available. Whenever rectal location is in doubt, it is identified by placing a probe.

Trocar Sleeves

Trocar sleeves are available in many sizes and shapes. This author uses a 10 mm Apple trocar sleeve in the umbilicus in all cases as it does not slip when moving the laparoscope in and out. For lower quadrant incisions, 5.5 mm cannulas are adequate. Short trapless 5 mm trocar sleeves with a retention screw grid around the external surface are used (Richard Wolf, Vernon Hills, IL, USA; Apple Medical, Bolton, MA, USA) as they facilitate efficient instrument exchanges and evacuation of tissue while allowing unlimited freedom during extracorporeal suture tying. With practice, a good laparoscopic surgical team makes instrument exchanges so fast that little pneumoperitoneum is lost. Once placed, the portal of exit stays fixed at the level of the anterior abdominal wall parietal peritoneum, permitting more room for instrument manipulation (Reich and McGlynn, 1990).

Positioning of Patient

All laparoscopic surgical procedures are done under general anesthesia with endotracheal intubation and an orogastric tube. The routine use of an orogastric tube is recommended to diminish the possibility of a trocar injury to the stomach and to reduce small bowel distension. The patient is flat ($0°$) until after the umbilical trocar sleeve has been inserted and then placed in a steep Trendelenburg position ($20-30°$). The lithotomy position with the hip extended (thigh parallel to abdomen) is obtained with Allen stirrups (Edgewater Medical Systems, Mayfield Heights, OH, USA) or knee braces, which are adjusted to each individual patient before she is anesthetized. Examination under anesthesia is always performed before prepping the patient for surgery.

Positioning of Video Equipment and Assistants

The videomonitor is placed opposite the surgeon if only one is available. The monitor is on the patient's right, the surgeon on her left, and a specially trained assistant between the patient's legs. The circulating nurse tends the video recorder (two tapes: one for the patient and the other for the surgeon), irrigation supply, laser and surgical specimens. This arrangement requires some hand–eye adjustment for the surgeon since the monitor is rotated $90°$ from the plane of surgery. However, it avoids neck and back strain from twisting to see a monitor placed between the patient's legs, especially if the surgeon operates with instruments in the left hand and laparoscope in the right. Hand–eye coordination (almost mirror-image) is extremely difficult for the assistant, who often assumes a passive role of maintaining retraction or grasper positions achieved by the surgeon. Mirror-image operating skills are attainable after extensive training and greatly increase the efficiency of the surgical team.

The importance of the assistant who holds and manipulates the uterus cannot be emphasized enough. Unfortunately most medical doctor assistants try to position themselves opposite the surgeon where they obstruct the surgeon's video monitor view and hold the camera with their non-dominant left hand, which can rarely focus, center, and give alternate panoramic and close-up views.

Scrubbing and Masking

Laparoscopy was never thought of as a sterile procedure before the incorporation of video with the laparoscope as the surgeon operated with his head in the surgical field, attached to the laparoscopic optic. Since 1983, this author has maintained a policy of not scrubbing for laparoscopy and not sterilizing or draping the camera or laser arm. Infection has been rare: less than 1/200 cases. This author attributes this to his policy of absolute hemostasis by underwater examination, copious irrigation and clot evacuation, and leaving 2–4 l of Ringer's lactate in the peritoneal cavity at the end of each operation. Bacteria grow poorly in Ringer's lactate solution, especially if all blood clot is evacuated from the peritoneal cavity. The umbilical incision is closed with a single 4–0 Polyglectin 910 suture, opposing deep fascia and skin dermis, with the knot buried beneath the fascia to prevent the suture from acting like a wick to transmit bacteria into the soft tissue or peritoneal cavity.

Masking by the whole operating room team for laparoscopy is a primitive practise with no redeeming features for the patient. I am glad to see that masks are not used for laparoscopic surgery in some localities.

Hysteroscopy

CO_2 hysteroscopy is carried out on all laparoscopic surgical patients with a uterus while the pneumoperitoneum is being developed to 20–25 mm Hg for safe trocar insertion. All indicated hysteroscopic surgery is done after the laparoscopic portion of the case using the resectoscope attached to a continuous flow controlled distension irrigation system (CDIS, Zimmer, Warsaw, IN, USA), which pumps sorbitol into the uterus for distension at a constant intrauterine pressure of 80 mm Hg. Two new techniques have recently been introduced to increase safety during high voltage resectoscope surgery (Reich et al., 1993).

Bulldog Clamps

Before resectoscope myomectomy procedures, tubal lavage is carried out with indigo carmine dye. Visualization of blue dye in the infundibulopelvic ligament vessels during tubal lavage signifies direct communication to the venous system, making fluid overload likely. When this dye is seen coursing through the infundibulopelvic ligament vessels, bulldog clamps inserted through the 10 mm umbilical cannula are applied to the infundibulopelvic ligaments to decrease the risk of fluid overload in these high risk women.

Underwater Resectoscope Surgery

The uterus is submerged in a 2000 ml isotonic electrolyte solution instilled laparoscopically to prevent thermal burns of intraperitoneal organs by dispersing current near the uterine serosa. For fibroids, 100–140 W cutting current is used through a wire loop electrode for cutting and 60–80 W coagulation current for fulguration of bleeding vessels. For endometrial ablation, high voltage electrosurgery is used: 80 W of coagulation current (5000 V peak) through a resectoscope roller cylinder (Wolf). Amenorrhea is the goal, not hypomenorrhea!

Incisions

For most pelvic procedures, the operative incisions are limited to three: 10 mm umbilical, 5 mm right, and 5 mm left lower quadrant. I stand on the left side of the patient and use my dominant right hand to hold, manipulate, and focus the camera. My laparoscopic puncture sites have not evolved over the past 21 years as I do not feel that more and larger trocar sleeve incisions, used by many surgeons today, represent progress. Most women prefer the cosmetic appearance of a 15 cm Pfannenstiel incision to multiple 12 mm incisions required for stapling devices (Currie et al., 1996).

The left lower quadrant puncture is the major portal for operative manipulation. The right trocar sleeve is used for retraction with atraumatic grasping forceps. Large masses are removed through the upper posterior vagina. Large puncture sites or incisions bordering on minilaparotomies for tissue extraction should be replaced by an umbilical extension or a laparoscopic culdotomy approach.

Lower Quadrant Lateral to the Deep Epigastric Vessels

Placement of the lower quadrant trocar sleeves lateral to the deep epigastric vessels is preferred as it avoids the rectus muscle while making a tract through the external oblique, internal oblique, and transversalis fascia, which is easily identifiable for replacement of the trocar sleeve during suturing and specimen excision. These vessels, an artery flanked by two veins (vena comitantes), are located by direct inner laparoscopic inspection of the anterior abdominal wall. They are found lateral to the lateral umbilical ligament (obliterated umbilical artery) and cannot be consistently found by traditional transillumination.

Ninth Intercostal Space (Reich et al., 1995)

Special entry techniques are used in patients who have undergone multiple laparotomies or who may have extensive adhesions, either clinically or from another doctor's operative record. If CO_2 insufflation is not obtainable through the umbilicus, Veress needle puncture is carried out in the left ninth intercostal space, anterior axillary line. The trocar is then inserted below the left costal margin in the midclavicular line, giving a panoramic view of the entire peritoneal cavity. Likewise when extensive adhesions are encountered initially surrounding the umbilical puncture, the surgeon should leave the trocar in place and immediately seek a higher site. Thereafter, the adhesions can be freed down to and just beneath the umbilicus, at which time it becomes possible to reestablish the umbilical portal for further work.

Operative Techniques

The advanced laparoscopic surgical techniques used by this author include aquadissection, scissors dissection, electrosurgery, laser and suturing. Aquadissection and scissors dissection are used in preference to thermal energy sources.

Aquadissection

Aquadissection is broadly defined as the use of hydraulic energy from pressurized fluid to aid in the performance of surgical procedures. It differs from mechanical energy applied with a blunt probe, which is a unidirectional force, the direct prolongation of the surgeon's hand. The force vector with hydraulic energy is multidirectional within the volume of expansion of the non-compressible fluid. Installation of fluid under pressure displaces tissue, often resulting in the fluid creating cleavage planes in the least resistant spaces. In addition, the installation of fluid under pressure into closed spaces or behind enclosed areas of adhesions produces edematous, distended tissue and with loss of elasticity, making further division easy and safe using blunt dissection, scissors dissection, laser or electrosurgery.

Aquadissectors (suction–irrigators with the ability to dissect using pressurized fluid) should have a single channel to maximize suctioning and irrigating capacity. An aquadissector with a solid (not perforated) distal tip is necessary to perform atraumatic suction–traction–retraction, irrigate directly and develop surgical planes (aquadissection). Small holes at the tip impede these actions and serve no purpose. Likewise, systems with tubing entering the handpiece at right angles cannot generate the power of in-line entry devices.

The Aqua-Purator (WISAP, Tomball, TX, USA) was the first of the aquadissection devices. It delivers fluid under 200 mm Hg pressure at a rate of 250 ml every 10 seconds. 1 l can be instilled in 35 seconds. The handle of the Aqua-Purator uses large staples to occlude separate suction and irrigation tubing, each of which funnels into a single-channeled tube. Aquadissection has not changed except for the incorporation of warmed fluids in the past 15 years (Reich, 1990), though the market is crowded with other aquadissection devices. This author uses much less aquadissection today as his ability to dissect with scissors has improved.

Scissors that Cut

Scissors that actually cut most of the time are truly a new laparoscopic technique. Sharp dissection is the primary technique used for adhesiolysis to diminish the potential for adhesion formation; electrosurgery and laser are usually reserved for hemostasis. Straight scissors, 5 mm, with blunt, rounded or sharp tips, are used to lyse thin and thick bowel adhesions. Since scissors notoriously become dull after processing between cases, a large number and variety should be available to ensure that some will cut. Blunt tipped, sawtooth scissors (Wolf), Manhes scissors (Storz, Culver City, CA, USA), and in-line curved scissors (Olympus, Melville, New York, USA) all cut. Most disposable scissors depend too much on electricity to cut. Hook scissors are used when the surgeon can get completely around the structure being divided (e.g. suture), but rarely maintain their sharpness.

Electrosurgery

Electrosurgical knowledge and skill are essential (Odell, 1987). The terms 'cautery' and 'diathermy', when referring to electrosurgery, should be abandoned. Unipolar cutting current has been used by this author for 20 years with minimal complications from this energy source. More effective surgery can be done with electrosurgery than with most lasers. Electrosurgery at laparoscopy is safer than at laparotomy as it takes 30% more power to spark or arc in CO_2 than in room air; at the same electrosurgical power setting, less arcing occurs at laparoscopy. Newer electrosurgical electrodes that eliminate capacitance and insulation failure (Electroshield from Electroscope, Boulder, CO, USA) are available.

Cutting current is used to both cut or coagulate, depending upon the configuration of the electrode in contact with the tissue. The tip cuts, while the wide body coagulates. Unipolar coagulation current is set at 0; it is rarely used and then only to fulgurate (i.e. in close proximity to tissue, but not in contact). This waveform uses voltages over ten times that of cutting current and should not be used in contact with tissue. The high voltage allows it to arc or spark for 1–2 mm, producing hemostasis with diffuse venous and arteriolar bleeding, but excessive tissue destruction and charring.

Bipolar desiccation for large vessel hemostasis of uterine and ovarian vessels has been carried out since 1980 (Reich and McGlynn, 1986; Reich, 1987). A more uniform bipolar desiccation process is obtained using a cutting current. Coagulating current is not used as it quickly desiccates the outer layers of the tissue, producing superficial resistance, which may prevent deeper penetration. Large blood vessels are compressed and bipolar cutting current passed until complete desiccation is achieved (i.e., the current depletes tissue fluid and electrolytes until it ceases to flow between the forceps as determined by an ammeter or current flow meter – end point monitor, Electroscope EPM-1). In most cases, three contiguous areas are desiccated. Complete endpoint desiccation results in full thickness coagulation (Soderstrom and Levy, 1987; Soderstrom et al., 1989), fusion of collagen and elastic fibers (Sigel and Dunn, 1965) and vessel weld strength (Harrison and Morris, 1991). The ammeter provides a scientific measurement of complete coaptive desiccation, allowing the surgeon to make an objective decision of how much current is enough and when it is safest to divide. This author uses his right foot to activate the CO_2 laser, his left foot for the bipolar electrosurgical pedal, and hand controls for unipolar electrodes.

Argon Beam Coagulation

Argon beam coagulation is rarely used for laparoscopic surgery today. Uses include intraovarian bleeding after cystectomy, uterine hemostasis after myomectomy, and pelvic hemostasis after hysterectomy and endometriosis surgery.

Beacon Labs (Boulder) made the first argon beam coagulator for laparoscopic use at this author's request in April, 1990. It uses argon gas at $2\,l\,min^{-1}$ and high voltage coagulation current to increase the spark or arc possible with conventional fulguration while penetrating the tissue very superficially. Advantages of the argon beam coagulator include the ability to clear the operative site of surface blood and fluids making the bleeding vessel or rent in that vessel visible by the gentle flow of argon gas as it moves towards the tissue, but before it is close enough to activate current. Conventional spray coagulation current at 80 W will arc approximately 1 cm through the argon gas with resultant superficial charring and hemostasis. As argon is cooler than CO_2, there is less smoke generated than with a conventional electrode.

Laser

Laser is required by most surgeons who undertake extensive endometriosis surgery. Laser to this author means CO_2 laser. The physics are not appropriate with the fiber lasers as they coagulate before they cut and lack the precision and the ability to operate across space that CO_2 laser possesses. The ability to align the CO_2 laser beam has improved, though an ice-pack is still sometimes necessary between the laserscope coupler and the surgeon's hand to prevent skin burns when using lasers with large raw beams and beam-coupler mismatches. The newer CO_2 lasers from Sharplan (Tel Aviv, Israel), Coherent Laser (Palo Alto, CA, USA), and Laserscope (formerly Heraeus LaserSonics, Milpitas, CA, USA) are highly sophisticated instruments that do very fine work in an uncluttered field with a collimated (parallel) beam traveling through the operating channel of the laparoscope.

The passage of CO_2 gas through the laparoscope lumen, presently a necessity to purge this channel of debris, results in a decrease in both power delivered to the tissue and power density at the tissue because the $10.6\,\mu m$ wavelength of the laser beam is the same as that of the purge gas. Power to tissue is reduced by 30–50% with a 7.2 mm laparoscopic operating channel (12 mm scope) and by 60% with a 5 mm operating channel (10 mm scope) (Reich et al., 1991a). While it is desirable to operate at high power density for a short time to minimize damage to surrounding tissue, the passage of CO_2 gas through the laparoscope lumen results in an increase in spot size and thus a reduction in power density (the concentration of laser energy on the tissue) at higher power settings. At high power settings with the CO_2 laser (80–100 W), a very large spot size, 3–4 mm, is obtained, which is extremely coagulative and provides very good hemostatic cutting. Considering these limitations with a Sharplan 1100 laser through a 10 mm laparoscope with a 5 mm operating channel, a setting of 20–35 W in superpulse mode is used for most procedures ($<1000\,W\,cm^{-2}$ at the tissue) and at 80–100 W continuous mode to obtain a diffuse hemostatic effect for myomectomy and culdotomy.

Coherent laser has advanced CO_2 laser technology by modifying the $10.6\,\mu m$ wavelength to $11.1\,\mu m$ (Ultrapulse 5000 L), resulting in little interference in power transmission from the purge gas (Adamson et al., 1994). With this modification, settings of 10–20 W Ultrapulse are used for precise cutting and 50–80 W for extirpative procedures. Also little power is lost in the Coherent coupler from the 6 mm raw beam. Laserscope (Heraeus LaserSonics, Malpitas, California) maintains a small spot size by performing rapid exchanges of gas through the operating channel of the operating laparoscope using the ICM 350 smoke evacuator from IC Medical, Phoenix, AZ, USA. This gas is exchanged faster than it can be heated up, a technique that also minimizes smoke in the peritoneal cavity, while actively using the laser. Argon gas can be added to the CO_2 purge gas to produce a high power density beam with little interference in power transmission.

Average power is measured in W; average energy per pulse is measured in mJ per pulse. I usually like to work at 25 W average power with 200 mJ energy pulses. Superpulse mode implies very high power (500 W) low energy (<50 mJ) pulses for brief surges, theoretically allowing tissue to cool between spikes to reduce the surrounding thermal effect. Surgipulse and Ultrapulse deliver short duration high energy pulses (>200 mJ) at the same high power (500 W), allowing longer cooling intervals between pulses with resultant reduced heat conduction and char-free vaporization. At the same average power, the superpulsed laser must produce five pulses to deliver as much energy as one Ultrapulse.

Suturing

Suturing is not as new as some like to think it is. A knot-pusher (Marlow Surgical, Willoughby, OH, USA) is used to tie in a manner very similar to the way one would hand-tie sutures at open laparotomy. This technique was developed in 1970 by Dr H Courtenay Clarke, presently residing in Windsor, Ontario. It was published in 1972 in *Fertility and Sterility* and promptly forgotten. H. Courtenay Clarke should be recognized as the first to suture well laparoscopically. His device is just like an extension of the surgeon's fingers (Clarke, 1972).

To suture with a straight needle (Fig. 6.1), the surgeon applies the suture to the tissue, pulls the needle outside, and then, while holding both strands, makes a simple half-hitch, but not a surgeon's knot, which will not slip as well. The Clarke knot-pusher (Marlow Surgical) is put on the suture, held firm across the index finger and the throw is pushed down to the tissue. A square knot is made by pushing another half-hitch down to the knot to secure it while exerting tension from above. Suture tying outside the peritoneal cavity is made easy by using trocar sleeves without traps, as traps make it very hard to slip knots down from outside the peritoneal cavity.

The Endoloop (Ethicon, Somerville, NJ, USA) is a preformed knotted loop designed to fit over vascular pedicles and then be tightened. Over the last 15 years, this author has used it for appendectomies and omentectomies, but never for oophorectomy. Bipolar desiccation or free ligatures work better and eliminate any chance of slippage. Postoperative pelvic pain is less in desiccated pedicles; an endolooped pedicle leaves living cells distal to the loop to necrose, releasing lysozymes.

A special technique is used to put any sized curved needle into the peritoneal cavity through a 5 mm lower quadrant incision (Reich *et al.*, 1992). To do it, the lower abdominal incisions are placed lateral to the deep epigastric vessels, and thus lateral to the rectus muscle, as previously described. Upon removing the trocar sleeve, a tract is obvious and is easy to get back into. To suture with a

Figure 6.1 (A) Clarke knot-pusher. (B) Application to a single tie. (C) The first throw of the knot is passed through the trapless trocar sleeve. (D) The second throw is passed through the trocar sleeve to secure the first. Reprinted with permission from The American College of Obstetricians and Gynecologists (*Obstetrics and Gynecology*, 1992, **79**: 143–147.)

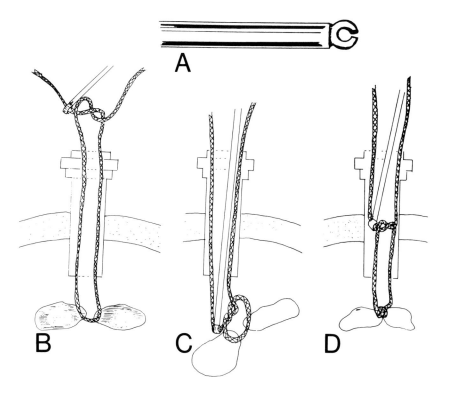

Figure 6.2 (A) Short trocar sleeve in place. (B) Distal suture is loaded into the sleeve removed from the peritoneal cavity. (C) The suture is grasped 3 cm from the curved needle. Reprinted with permission from the American College of Obstetricians and Gynecologists (*Obstetrics and Gynecology* 1992, **79**: 143–147.)

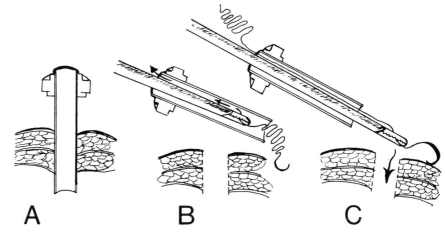

Figure 6.3 (A) Needle holder is directed back through the original incision. (B) The sleeve is replaced over the needle holder. (C) Suture is applied with the curved needle holder. Reprinted with permission from The American College of Obstetricians and Gynecologists (*Obstetrics and Gynecology* 1992, **79**: 143–147.)

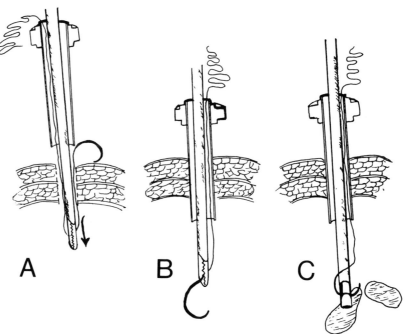

CT-1 needle, the trocar sleeve is taken out of the abdomen and loaded by grasping the end of the suture with a needle holder, pulling it through the trocar sleeve, reinserting the instrument into the sleeve, and grasping the suture about 2–3 cm from the needle (Fig. 6.2). The needle driver is inserted into the peritoneal cavity through the original tract, as visualized on the monitor and the needle follows. Even large needles can be pulled into the peritoneal cavity in this manner. At this stage, the Semm straight needle holder is replaced with a Cook curved needle driver (Cook OB/GYN, Cook Urological Inc., Spencer, IN, USA), and the needle is driven through the tissue (Fig. 6.3). Afterwards the needle is stored in the anterior abdominal wall parietal peritoneum (like in a pin cushion) for later removal after the suture has been tied (Fig. 6.4). The needle is cut, the cut end of the suture is pulled out of the peritoneal cavity, and the knot is tied with the Clarke

knot-pusher. To retrieve the needle, the trocar sleeve is unscrewed, after which the needle holder inside it pulls the needle through the soft tissue (Fig. 6.5). The trocar sleeve is replaced with or without another suture.

Staples

Disposable stapling instrumentation for laparoscopic surgery are used for large vessel hemostasis during cholecystectomy, oophorectomy and hysterectomy. This author worked with US Surgical in 1988 developing clips and staples for laparoscopic gynecological work. Unfortunately, the randomized studies planned for these products were never carried out because the general surgeons entered the laparoscopic cholecystectomy market. US Surgical had clips available when laparoscopic

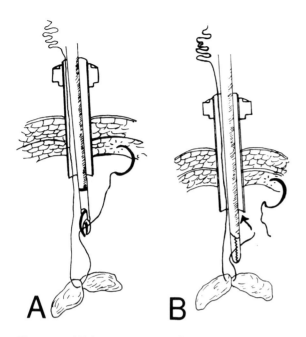

Figure 6.4 (A) Suture is cut 3 cm from the needle. (B) The cut end is pulled through the trocar sleeve and the needle is placed in the parietal peritoneum. Reprinted with permission from The American College of Obstetricians and Gynecologists (*Obstetrics and Gynecology* 1992, **79**: 143–147.)

cholecystectomy was first performed because they had developed them for gynecology.

An automatic clip applier (Auto Suture Endo Clip Applier) stacks 20 clips of medium to large size (9 mm long when closed), which are made of titanium, an inert, nonreactive metal. The disposable loaded unit is designed for introduction through a 12 mm trocar sleeve (Surgiport). Skeletonization of vessels is necessary before application of this staple. When applied to vessels with overlying peritoneum, the staple will frequently slip off during further manipulation of the tissue. The Endo Clip may be used to ligate the uterine artery after both it and the ureter have been skeletonized.

A laparoscopic stapler (Multi-Fire Endo GIA 30) places six rows of titanium staples, 3 cm in length, and simultaneously divides the clamped tissue. It consists of a disposable handle and shaft, the end of which contains a replaceable single-use stapling cartridge. The standard staple compresses on firing to 1.5 mm, while the vascular cartridge compresses to 1 mm. The disposable handle is designed to fire up to four staple cartridges through a 12 mm cannula before being discarded. This instrument functions similarly to the gastrointestinal anastomosis stapler (GIA) that thoracic and general surgeons have used for the past 25 years. The Multi-Fire Endo GIA 30 is useful in gynecology for hysterectomy with ovarian preservation to divide the pedicle next to the uterus (the utero-ovarian ligament, round ligament and fallopian tube); it was first used in laparoscopy by this author for appendectomy and two hysterectomies in August 1990.

Figure 6.5 (A) Knot placement. (B) The needle end is retrieved. (C) The needle is removed from the peritoneal cavity after withdrawing the trocar sleeve, which is then replaced. Reprinted with permission from The American College of Obstetricians and Gynecologists (*Obstetrics and Gynecology* 1992, **79**: 143–147.)

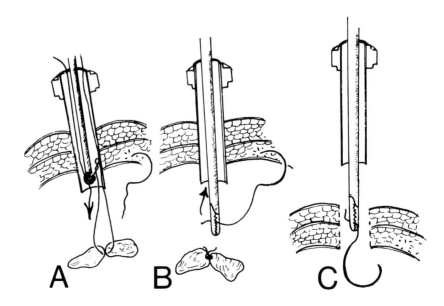

A multiple staple applicator in a circular design – Proximate ILS Curved Intraluminal Stapler (Ethicon, Somerville, NJ, USA) or EEA (US Surgical) – is intended for rapid end-to-end anastomosis of the rectosigmoid colon. Introduced through the rectum, this large device fires off a circle of staples into aligned proximal and distal stumps of a rectosigmoid resection. This procedure can be done during laparoscopic resection of cul-de-sac endometriosis if there is a bowel stricture.

Culdotomy (Reich, 1989)

A posterior culdotomy incision using CO_2 laser or electrosurgery through the cul-de-sac of Douglas into the vagina is preferable to a colpotomy incision using scissors through the vagina and overlying peritoneum because complete hemostasis can be obtained while making the culdotomy incision. Vaginal bleeding greater than 100 ml is usual before all cuff bleeding is stopped after scissors colpotomy.

Infection after culdotomy incision using a relatively non-sterile technique is so rare that it should be a reportable event. The culdotomy incision is closed laparoscopically with interrupted or running 0-Polyglectin 910 suture. Vaginal suturing can be difficult if the vaginal incision becomes edematous during the procedure making exposure inadequate. Thus, the surgeon should elect to close the culdotomy incision from above using 1–3 curved needle sutures (Polyglectin 910 on a CT-2) tied extracorporeally with the Clarke knot-pusher.

Tissue Removal

Specimens slightly larger than the 5 mm trocar channel are often removed by slipping the trocar sleeve upward on the biopsy forceps shaft out of the peritoneal cavity and then pulling the biopsy forceps with the specimen out in one motion through the soft tissue of the anterior abdominal wall. The biopsy forceps are then reinserted through their exit tract and the trocar sleeve pushed back into the peritoneal cavity over the forceps.

Larger masses are removed through a cul-de-sac culdotomy. My technique for unruptured ovaries or cysts is to insert an impermeable sac (LapSac: Cook OB/GYN) intraperitoneally through the culdotomy incision. This 5″ × 8″ nylon bag has a polyurethane inner coating and a nylon drawstring. It is impermeable to water and dye. The ovary with intact cyst is placed in the bag, which is closed by pulling its drawstring. The sac is delivered by the drawstring through the posterior vagina, the bag opened and the intact specimen visually identified, decompressed and removed.

For fibroids (or a large fibroid uterus), an 11 mm corkscrew device is screwed into the myoma vaginally through the culdotomy incision. The myoma is put on traction and further morcellated vaginally with scissors or scalpel if necessary until removal is completed. This can be a particularly time-consuming portion of the procedure. It is wise to change from laparoscopic stirrups (Allan stirrups or knee supports) to candy cane stirrups to obtain better hip flexion to permit assistance with vaginal sidewall retractors during long procedures. Self-retaining lateral vaginal wall retractors or Vienna retractors (Breisky–Navatril, Baxter Health Care Corp., McGaw Park, IL, USA) are considered for shorter procedures.

Morcellation of fibroids through anterior abdominal wall puncture sites is now practical with presently available instruments. Kurt Semm (WISAP) has developed a manual circular saw to core out 2 cm cylinders of fibromyomatous tissue while the fibroid is still in or attached to the uterus. This device is inserted through a 2 cm lower abdominal trocar sleeve and depends upon a corkscrew inside it to fixate the fibroid before twisting the circular saw into it. Loss of resistance during the twisting indicates the base of the fibroid, after which the cylindrical specimen is pulled free by traction, the specimen removed, and the instrument reinserted. After the bulk of the lesion has been removed in this fashion, a claw forceps is substituted for the corkscrew in the device for traction, and the compressible, fenestrated, remaining tissue is removed from the uterus through the 2 cm cannula. Professor Semm accomplishes supracervical hysterectomy using this same device after coring out the endocervical canal with a 1 cm circular saw. These 2 cm puncture sites require direct peritoneal and/or fascial closure with skin hooks to prevent hernias.

Cook Urological has developed a 1 cm motorized circular saw with suction for laparoscopic nephrectomy. After placement of the kidney into the LapSac, it is morcellated into small soft pieces, which are sucked into the device until the LapSac is small enough to be pulled out of the umbilicus. This author has used this instrument for myoma morcellation during laparoscopic hysterectomy and myomectomy, and for fibroma oophorectomy. We are currently working on 2 and 3 cm versions for culdotomy morcellation.

The Steiner Electromechanic Morcellator (Karl Storz, Tuttlingen, Germany) is a 10 mm diameter motorized circular saw that uses claw forceps or a tenaculum to grasp the fibroid and pull it into contact with the fibroid. Large pieces of myomatous tissue are removed piecemeal until the myoma can be pulled out through the trocar incision. With practice this instrument can often be inserted through a stretched 5 mm incision without an accompanying trocar.

I have developed the poor man's morcellator, a #10 blade on a long handle introduced gently through the left 5 mm trocar incision after removing the trocar. With care the myoma can be bivalved with the blade. The surgeon's fingers in contact with the skin prevent loss of pneumoperitoneum. Multiple blades may be necessary.

In addition, there are now numerous organ and cyst retrieval systems available commercially that allow for specimen removal through the trocar sites without enlarging the incision. These systems allow for entrapment, fragmentation and retrieval of resected tissue. They are available in various sizes ranging from 200–800 ml with special introducers that mostly fit through a 10 mm trocar sleeve. The retrieval bags are made of different materials including:

1. Polyurethane (PU) foil: Endobag™ (Dexide Co., Forthworth, Texas, USA), Endo Catch™ (US Surgical, Norwalk, Connecticut, USA), Extraction Bag™ (Karl Storz Co., Tuttlingen, Germany). These are gas and liquid impermeable, but have limited tensile strength and mechanical resistance. The risk of perforation with morcellation of pathologic tissue (cancer, infected tissue) and consequent peritoneal contamination limit their use to extraction of tissue without morcellation.
2. Special plastic foil: Endopouch™ (Ethicon Co., Somerville, New Jersey, USA). Main use is retrieval of small tissue that does not require morcellation. The material has a potential for instrument perforation, which makes tissue morcellation potentially dangerous.
3. Polyamide textile and PU coating: LapSac™ (Cook Co., Spencer, Indiana, USA), Espiner Bag™ (Espiner Co.), Lap Bag™ (Angiomed Co.). Polyamide is a plastic material manufactured with nylon fibers of appropriate diameter that provides high tensile strength and mechanical resistance to perforation. Also tears in the material do not widen further. This combined with PU coating for waterproofness makes them safer for tissue morcellation.

For deployment, most devices have an introducer or tube with the sack packaged inside. This arrangement allows its placement in a 10 mm trocar without loss of pneumoperitoneum. In addition, they are also designed to stabilize the sack and to maintain contact in order to prevent its loss in the abdominal cavity. While some systems require the use of endoscopic forceps or dissectors to open the mouth of the bag, other designs use springs, wires and rubber rings that allow for spontaneous opening once deployed in the abdominal cavity, and some have designs that allow for easier capture of specimen. Others allow the use of instruments while the sac remains open. This is particularly useful when performing cystectomy with the ovary in the sac to avoid spillage in case of cyst perforation (if one chooses not to drain the cyst). All these features increase sack bulk and limit its potential size.

For specimen removal, some sacks have incorporated a drawstring to close its mouth before extraction while others have a long extended tail so that it can be drawn into the mouth of the trocar. Extraction of specimen from the abdomen (after the mouth of the bag has been secured) requires the removal of the trocar from the body wall along with the device. At this point, the mouth of the bag should be outside the body wall where it can be grasped with fingers and removed entirely by pulling. If the specimen is larger than the 10 mm incision, the incision can be extended or the specimen can be morcellated with fingers, forceps, scissors or morcellators within the bag. Smaller pieces of tissue are then removed until the entire specimen within the sack can be extracted through the 10 mm incision. Again, for morcellation of pathologic specimens, one should use a system made of polyamide textile in order to prevent perforation and spillage into the abdominal cavity. Additionally, for endoscopic morcellation or dissection (e.g. cystectomy), it is advantageous to use a system that has an endoscopically visible transparent sack. Moreover, these organ retrieval systems also afford protection of the exit wound from contamination by an infected or cancerous specimen.

As one can see, numerous options are now available for laparoscopic retrieval of specimens. In closing, the optimal device should be easy to deploy, endoscopically visible for manipulation and dissection, and easy and safe to extract, with a sac that is strong, liquid impermeable, resistant to tear and of sufficient size to capture the specimen.

Underwater Surgery at the End of Each Procedure (Reich, 1989)

At the close of each operation, an underwater examination is used to document complete intraperitoneal hemostasis in stages; this detects bleeding from vessels and viscera tamponaded during the procedure by the increased intraperitoneal pressure of the CO_2 pneumoperitoneum. The CO_2 pneumoperitoneum is displaced with 2–4 l of Ringer's lactate solution, and the peritoneal cavity is vigorously irrigated and suctioned with this solution until the effluent is clear of blood products, usually after 10–15 l. Underwater inspection of the pelvis is performed to detect any further bleeding, which is controlled using specially insulated microbipolar forceps containing a channel for irrigation and a fixed distance between the electrodes to coagulate through the electrolyte solution. The bleeding sites are irrigated with irrigant pushed through the microbipolar forceps by the Marlow Pump Vac Plus for vessel identification before coagulation and to prevent formation of an eschar that can stick to the electrode.

First, complete hemostasis is established with the patient in the Trendelenburg position. Next, complete hemostasis is secured by underwater examination with the patient supine and in reverse Trendelenburg position using underwater microbipolar coagulation. Finally, complete hemostasis is documented with all instruments removed, including the uterine manipulator.

To visualize the pelvis with the patient supine, the 10 mm straight laparoscope and the aquadissector are manipulated together into the deep cul-de-sac beneath floating bowel and omentum, and this area is alternately irrigated and suctioned until the effluent is clear, both in the pelvis and the upper abdomen. During this copious irrigation procedure, clear fluid is deposited into the pelvis and circulates into the upper abdomen, displacing upper abdominal bloody fluid, which is suctioned after flowing back into the pelvis. An 'underwater' examination is then performed to observe the completely separated tubes and ovaries and to confirm complete hemostasis.

The 'chopstick' maneuver refers to the synchronized moving of the actively irrigating aquadissector tip just in front of the laparoscope tip to maintain a clear underwater view in a bloody field deep in the pelvis. Bloody fluid is diluted, circulated and aspirated. Individual blood clots are isolated, usually in the pararectosigmoid gutters, and aspirated.

A final copious lavage with Ringer's lactate solution is undertaken and all clot directly aspirated; at least 2 l of lactated Ringer's solution are left in the peritoneal cavity to eliminate the pneumoperitoneum, prevent fibrin adherences from forming by separating raw operated-upon surfaces during the initial stages of reperitonealization, and dilute the peritoneal cavity bacterial count, especially after hysterectomy or bowel resection; this may decrease postoperative infection, further reducing postoperative hospitalization and recovery time. No other anti-adhesive agents are employed. No drains, antibiotic solutions or heparin are used.

Adhesion Prevention

Dr Jaroslav Hulka said in 1988 that 'Reich's solution to pollution is dilution', and that opinion has not changed. This author currently believes that the following will reduce adhesions: a reduction of thermal damage to tissue, absolute hemostasis, clot evacuation, copious irrigation to dilute fibrin and prostaglandins arising from operated surfaces and bacteria, and leaving 2–4 l of Ringer's lactate in the peritoneal cavity at the end of each operation to physically separate normal and compromised structures. Currently, lactated Ringer's solution (1–2 l) postoperatively is widely used, but has rarely been prospectively studied. Rose determined that lactated Ringer's solution is absorbed over 2–3 days by weighing patients (Rose et al., 1991).

The Gore-Tex Surgical Membrane (WL Gore, Flagstaff, AZ, USA) is probably the best of the presently available surgical barriers. It is a non-absorbable inert membrane with pore size less than 1 μm. It is used after division of severe adhesions (e.g. retroperitoneal ovary) and is sutured in place. It is this author's belief that Interceed (TC7) (Johnson & Johnson, New Brunswick, NJ, USA) is impossible to use successfully laparoscopically as it requires absolute hemostasis at the applied site and no fluid. Bleeding from vessels and viscera tamponaded during the procedure by the increased intraperitoneal pressure of the CO_2 pneumoperitoneum cannot be detected without an underwater examination. This author suspects that bleeding from a raw site after the pneumoperitoneum is expelled results in the filling of the Interceed with blood, making it adhesiogenic. The use of Interceed as a carrier to deliver heparin to traumatized surfaces looks promising (Diamond et al., 1991). Seprafilm Bioresorbable Membrane (Genzyme, Cambridge, MA, USA), a hyaluronic acid derivative, remains untested at laparoscopic surgery.

Surgicel (oxidized regenerated cellulose) application is a very useful, time-saving technique for hemostasis and adhesion prevention in most myomectomy procedures. A piece is packed into the myomectomy defect, which is then repaired with 0-Polyglectin 910 suture on CT-1 curved needles to compress the full thickness of exposed myometrium. Swelling of the material applies pressure to the myoma bed bleeding. The clotting process is initiated by physical means instead of alteration of the clotting mechanism itself. After the products are saturated with blood, a dark, gelatinous mass forms that aids in clot formation and absorbs seven to eight times its weight in blood. This gelatinous mass also exerts pressure, which further enhances hemostatic activity. Surgicel does not interfere with epithelialization and is bacteriostatic against a wide range of gram-positive and gram-negative organisms due to its low pH.

Bowel Injury

Gastrointestinal injuries may occur during laparoscopic surgery and the surgeon should be familiar with their management; in many cases laparotomy can be avoided, regardless of specialty training. Treatment of gynecologic conditions like rectal endometriosis requires special understanding. This author did the first laparoscopic repair of a small bowel trocar perforation in July, 1988, and a planned full-thickness resection of deep fibrotic rectal endometriosis in August, 1989 (Reich *et al.*, 1991b).

Small bowel perforation occurs at laparoscopic surgery in cases involving extensive small bowel adhesions while inserting umbilical or lower quadrant trocars or during the division of adhesions. Small bowel perforation during small bowel adhesiolysis surgery for pain secondary to adhesions from multiple previous surgeries is common, occurring in over 25% of these procedures. Despite the application of traction and countertraction to each adhesion, bowel punctures are inevitable as these adhesions are carefully cut.

Following recognition of a small bowel perforation, it can be repaired transversely with interrupted 3–0 Polyglectin 910, silk, or Polydioxarone suture on a taper gastrointestinal needle tied either externally by pulling the affected bowel out through the umbilicus or with intracorporeal instruments. Sterile milk is instilled into the bowel lumen before closing the last suture to detect leakage from the laceration and occult perforations near the small bowel mesentery.

In the bowel-prepared patient, injury to the anterior rectum can usually be repaired laparoscopically. These injuries usually occur during excision of nodules in the muscularis of the anterior or lateral rectum (Reich *et al.*, 1991c). Full-thickness penetration of the rectum may occur during this surgery. After excision of the nodule and identification of the rent in the rectum, usually surrounded by fibrotic endometriosis, a closed circular stapler – Proximate ILS Curved Intraluminal Stapler (Ethicon, Stealth) – is inserted into the lumen just past the hole, opened 1–2 cm, and held high to avoid the posterior rectal wall. The proximal anvil is positioned just beyond the hole, which is invaginated into the opening and the device is closed. Circumferential inspection is made to ensure the absence of encroachment of nearby organs and posterior rectum in the staple line and the lack of tension in the anastomosis. The instrument is fired and then removed through the

anus. The surgeon inspects the donut of tissue representing the excised hole contained in the circular stapler. After closure, anastomotic inspection is carried out laparoscopically underwater after filling the rectum with indigo carmine solution through a #26 F Foley catheter with a 30 ml balloon. This author has had no late sequelae following 40 such procedures.

Concerning the unprepared bowel, the decision whether to repair laparoscopically depends upon the amount of fecal spillage present. Should a large amount of fecal contamination occur, laparotomy followed by repair should be considered. Laparoscopic suture closure followed by copious irrigation until the effluent clears may be satisfactory. I have found no indication for colostomy during the repair of bowel injuries noted during the course of a laparoscopic procedure.

The practice of performing a colostomy during treatment of bowel injury began following the report of Ogilvie who noted significant reductions in mortality following treatment of colon injuries during World War II (Ogilvie, 1944). In fact in 1943, the Surgeon General of the United States issued an order that all colon injuries sustained in battle should be treated by performing a colostomy (Office of the Surgeon General, 1943). In 1951, Woodhall and Ochsner reported their experience with primary repair without colostomy: their mortality rate fell from 23% to 9% with primary repair (Woodhall and Ochsner, 1951). In 1979, Stone and Fabian reported the first well controlled prospective randomized study on primary closure of traumatic colon perforations. Morbidity for the randomized colostomy group was 10-fold higher and average hospital stay six days longer (Stone and Fabian, 1979). Similar results were obtained by George *et al.* (1989) and Burch *et al.* (1986). Thus, this author finds little indication for colostomy at the time of repair of bowel injuries noted during the course of a laparoscopic procedure.

References

Adamson GD, Reich H, Trost D (1994) CO$_2$ isotopic laser (Ultrapulse 5000 L) used through the operating channel of laser laparoscopes: A comparative study of power and energy density losses. *Obstetrics and Gynecology* **83**: 717–724.

Burch JM, Brock JC, Gevirtzman L *et al.* (1986) The injured colon. *Annals of Surgery* **203(6)**: 701.

Clarke HC (1972) Laparoscopy – new instruments for suturing and ligation. *Fertility and Sterility* **23**: 274–277.

Currie I, Onwude JL, Jarvis GJ (1996) A comparative study of the cosmetic appeal of abdominal incisions used for hysterectomy. *British Journal of Obstetrics and Gynaecology* **103**: 252–254.

Diamond MP, Linsky CB, Cunningham T, Kamp L, Pines E, DeCherney AH, diZerega GS (1991) Synergistic effects of INTERCEED (TC7) and heparin in reducing adhesion formation in the rabbit uterine horn model. *Fertility and Sterility* **55**: 389–394.

Gallinat A (1992) Current trends in the therapy of myomata. In Lueken RP, Gallinat A. (eds) *Endoscopic Surgery in Gynecology.* pp. 69–71 Demeter.

George SM Jr, Fabian TC, Voeller GR *et al.* (1989) Primary repair of colon wounds. *Annals of Surgery* **209(6)**: 728.

Harrison JD, Morris DL (1991) Does bipolar electrocoagulation time affect vessel weld strength? *Gut* **32(2)**: 188–190.

Odell R (1987) Principles of Electrosurgery. In Sivak M (ed.) *Gastroenterologic Endoscopy.* pp. 128–142. Philadelphia: W.B. Saunders Company.

Office of the Surgeon General (1943) Circulation Letter, no. 178.

Ogilvie WH (1944) Abdominal wounds in the Western Desert. *Surgery, Gynecology and Obstetrics* **78**: 225.

Reich H (1987) Laparoscopic oophorectomy and salpingo-oophorectomy in the treatment of benign tubo-ovarian disease. *International Journal of Fertility* **32**: 233–236.

Reich H (1989) New techniques in advanced laparoscopic surgery. In Sutton C (ed.) *Baillière's Clinical Obstetrics and Gynaecology,* pp. 655–81. New York: Harcourt Brace–Jovanovich.

Reich H (1990) Aquadissection. In Baggish M (ed.) *Laser Endoscopy, The Clinical Practice of Gynecology Series.* pp 159–185. New York: Elsevier.

Reich H, McGlynn F (1986) Laparoscopic oophorectomy and salpingo-oophorectomy in the treatment of benign tuboovarian disease. *Journal of Reproductive Medicine* **31**: 609.

Reich H, McGlynn F (1990) Short self-retaining trocar sleeves for laparoscopic surgery. *American Journal of Obstetrics and Gynecology* **162(2)**: 453.

Reich H, MacGregor TS, Vancaillie TG (1991a) CO_2 laser used through the operating channel of laser laparoscopes: *In vitro* study of power and power density losses. *Obstetrics and Gynecology* **77**: 40–47.

Reich H, McGlynn F, Budin R (1991b) Laparoscopic repair of full-thickness bowel injury. *Journal of Laparoendoscopic Surgery* **1**: 119.

Reich H, McGlynn F, Salvat J (1991c) Laparoscopic treatment of cul-de-sac obliteration secondary to retrocervical deep fibrotic endometriosis. *Journal of Reproductive Medicine* **36**: 516–522.

Reich H, Clarke HC, Sekel L (1992) A simple method for ligating in operative laparoscopy with straight and curved needles. *Obstetrics and Gynecology* **79**: 143–147.

Reich H, DeCaprio J, Polin M, Sekel L, McGlynn F (1993) High-voltage resectoscope surgery: safety measures. *Endoscopy in Gynecology/AAGL 20th Annual Meeting Proceedings.* Baltimore, MD: Port City Press.

Reich H, Levie M, McGlynn F, Sekel L. (1995) Establishment of pneumoperitoneum through the left ninth intercostal space. *Gynaecological Endoscopy* **4**: 141–143.

Romanowski L, Reich H, Adelson MD, McGlynn F, Taylor PT (1993). Brachial plexus neuropathies after advanced laparoscopic surgery. *Fertility and Sterility* **60(4)**: 729–732.

Rose BI, MacNeill C, Larrain R, Kopreski MM (1991) Abdominal instillation of high-molecular-weight dextran or lactated Ringer's solution after laparoscopic surgery: a randomized comparison of the effect on weight change. *Journal of Reproductive Medicine* **36**: 537–539.

Sigel B, Dunn MR (1965) The mechanism of blood vessel closure by high frequency electrocoagulation. *Surgery, Gynecology and Obstetrics* **10**: 823–831.

Soderstrom RM, Levy BS (1987) Bipolar systems – do they perform? *Obstetrics and Gynecology* **69**: 425–426.

Soderstrom RM, Levy BS, Engel T (1989) Reducing bipolar sterilization failures. *Obstetrics and Gynecology* **74(60)**: 60–63.

Stone HH, Fabian TC (1979) Management of perforating colon trauma. *Annals of Surgery* **190(4)**: 430.

Woodhall JP, Ochsner A (1951) The management of perforating injuries of the colon and rectum in civilian practice. *Surgery* **29**: 305.

7

Lasers in Reproductive Medicine

YONA TADIR AND MICHAEL W. BERNS

Beckman Laser Institute and Medical Clinic, University of California, Irvine, USA

Introduction

Lasers were introduced into gynecologic practise in 1972, and for several years were considered as an experimental tool (Kaplan and Goldman, 1973). With the ongoing development of instruments and applications for minimally invasive therapy (MIT) and assisted reproduction technologies (ART) the range of laser treatments for female infertility now spans a broad spectrum of applications. This chapter briefly describes the basic physics underlying lasers and laser–tissue interactions.

Current applications of lasers in pelvic reconstructive surgery and assisted reproduction will be reviewed. The potential use of light in photodynamic therapy (PDT) is reviewed in Chapter 62.

Physical Principles of Lasers

Light is composed of packets of energy known as photons. Laser is an acronym for 'light amplification by the stimulated emission of radiation'. Amplification by the stimulated emission of radiation is the physical process that occurs within the laser tube. This physical process will be discussed in more detail in the following section.

Light is an electromagnetic wave generated by atomic processes. The ground state for atoms also represents their lowest state of energy, but atoms can be raised from this resting state to a higher energy level by exciting them with chemical, optical or electrical energy. The excited atom quickly returns to its ground state and gives up its excess energy. This excess energy occurs in the form of a light particle called the photon – a process called 'spontaneous emission of light'.

Laser Light is Coherent (Parallel)

Light from a light bulb radiates in all directions. As an observer walks away from it, the light gets dimmer and dimmer; there is a direct mathematical relationship between loss of light intensity and the distance of the observer from the source. In the laser, however, photons are emitted in parallel and in phase with each other – a property known as 'coherence'.

Laser Light is Monochromatic (One Wavelength, One Color)

Light emitted by the light bulb is white or yellowish-white in color and contains all colors and wavelengths in the visual portion of the electromagnetic spectrum and is therefore polychromatic. Laser light contains light of only one wavelength or color and is therefore monochromatic. In most cases, the number of photons in a laser beam is greater per unit area of emission than any other light source.

The Four Basic Qualities of Light

All light, regardless of its source, has four basic qualities: wavelength, frequency, velocity and amplitude.

- Wavelength, the distance between two successive crests, determines the color of the light. By convention, a medical laser is referred to in terms of its wavelength in either nanometers (nm), micrometers (μm), or millimeters (mm).
- Frequency, expressed as cycles per second or hertz (Hz), is the number of waves passing a given point per second. Wavelength and frequency are inversely related. As wavelength increases or decreases, frequency decreases or increases, respectively. Higher frequencies (short wavelengths), such as cosmic, gamma and X-rays, are high energy waves. As such, they are the most dangerous because unlike laser light they emit ionizing radiation, which disrupts molecular structure.
- Velocity is the speed of light which is a constant.
- Amplitude is the height of the wave. The higher the wave, the greater the power.

Laser Design

Although the details and purposes for lasers may vary greatly, their designs are similar. When discussing different kinds of lasers, identification is made by the type of material inside the device going through the 'lasing process', for example ruby lasers, argon lasers, and carbon dioxide (CO_2) lasers. The lasing medium (gas, solid or liquid) is contained in an optical cavity or resonator, which is closed at both ends by mirrors. The optical axis of both mirrors coincides with the axis of the resonator. One end of the resonator has a pinhole through which the light produced exits as laser light. An exciting source (electrical, chemical or mechanical) is applied to the atoms of the medium. The atoms are excited and spontaneously emit their photons in various directions. Many of these photons will pass back and forth between the mirrors, hitting other excited atoms and stimulating them to release more photons – all having the same wavelength. Solid state diode pumped lasers represent the latest developments in semiconductor technology. The diode laser is formed from a minute chip of gallium arsenide semiconductor material. It converts electricity to laser light with no mirrors.

The photons exit from the pinhole as a beam of laser light, which can then be focused by a lens or a laser fiber to a finite spot. The spot size of the laser beam and its capability for adjustment are crucial to the application for which the laser is being used. Accordingly, when combined with other factors, it produces different types of tissue interaction.

Effects of Lasers in Surgery

The three primary results of tissue interaction with lasers used for surgical applications are vaporization, excision and coagulation. Thus, the power density of the laser beam determines the effects of the laser on tissue, as will be discussed later. Understanding the power density of the laser beam is the most important factor in effectively using any laser. The laser lens directs the energy of the laser beam to a small spot. The concentration of energy per surface area of the spot is called its power density (or irradiance) expressed in W/cm^2. To determine approximate power density, clinicians use the following formula:

$$\text{Power density (PD)} = \frac{(\text{Power in watts}) \times 100}{(\text{Spot diameter in mm})^2} = W\,cm^{-2}$$

With an equal distribution of energy, the smaller spot size of the beam will produce a greater concentration of energy per surface area and thus a greater power density than a larger spot size. Higher power densities (smaller spot sizes) will vaporize tissue layer by layer; however, if too high, the depth of destruction is difficult to control. Lower power densities (larger spot sizes) are used to produce tissue coagulation. The energy fluence of a laser beam consists of both power density and exposure time and is expressed as joules (J) per unit surface area ($1\,J = 1\,W \times 1\,s$).

Lasers are generally operated in one of the following modes:

- Continuous wave (CW).
- Pulsed.
- Q-switched.
- Mode-locked.

In pelvic surgery, a CW beam of constant power is usually practiced. In a pulsed operation, pulsed pumping of the active medium results in relatively high-energy pulses at repetition rates from one to hundreds of pulses per second. The techniques of Q-switching and mode-locking are often employed when pulses of extremely short duration are required. More information on basic laser physics are provided by Bellina and Bandieramonte (1984) and Gardner (1985).

Laser–Tissue Interactions

The interaction of light with tissue can be described according to properties such as absorption, reflection, scattering and transmission (American

National Standards Institute, 1991). For a laser to produce an effect on tissue, its beam must first be absorbed by the tissue. If it is transmitted through or reflected from tissue, the beam will not accomplish its intended purpose. When light is scattered, it is absorbed over a broader area, thus diffusing its effects and possibly scattering light to places where it is not wanted. Other important considerations regarding laser tissue interactions include heat formation, photochemistry, photoablation, fluorescence, ionization, and plasma formation (Figure 7.1).

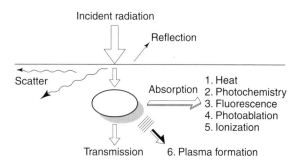

Figure 7.1 Laser–tissue interactions.

Laser Absorption

The tissue molecules that absorb the light are usually referred to as pigments. Hemoglobin and water are two common body constituents that can function as pigments. Hemoglobin has a very high absorption in the violet and blue/green portions of the visible spectrum. Absorption declines in the red region of the spectrum, which is why hemoglobin is red – it does not absorb red light. This is the rationale for using an argon laser, which emits blue/green light for treating hemoglobin and hemosiderin-containing lesions, such as endometriosis. Water, however, is absorbed maximally in the far infrared (IR) regions of the spectrum. Thus, a CO_2 laser has a direct effect on any tissue in the body. The CO_2 laser removes cell layer by cell layer by volatilizing the water. The selection of the correct laser for a particular clinical procedure requires an understanding of the absorptive as well as the reflective, scattering and transmissive properties of the target tissue.

Heat

Laser light works primarily by causing molecular vibration, which in turn produces heat. Controlling tissue heating is an important consideration for the

laser surgeon. At 37–60°C, tissue retracts; above 60°C, there is protein denaturation and coagulation; from 90–100°C, carbonization and tissue burning occur. Above 100°C, the tissue is vaporized and ablated. The physician should be able to stop the heating process at any one of these thermal ranges to produce the desired clinical result. Moreover, for certain applications, such as assisted reproduction, heat formation may be detrimental to gametes (*in vivo* or *in vitro*) and to sensitive organs, such as the fallopian tubes.

Photochemistry

Certain molecules can function as photosensitizers. The presence of these photosensitizers in certain cells makes the cells vulnerable to light of an appropriate wavelength and intensity. The photosensitizers absorb the photons and are thereby elevated to an excited atomic state, subsequently reacting with a molecular substrate, such as oxygen, producing singlet oxygen and causing irreversible oxidation of selected cellular components. This entire process occurs without the generation of heat. Currently, the most common clinical use of this process has been in the treatment of cancer and precancerous tissue; however, preliminary data suggest that dysfunctional endometrial bleeding and endometriosis may be treated as well. PDT is accomplished in a two-step procedure. The physician administers a photosensitizing agent either topically or intravenously. Once an optimal level is reached in the target tissue, the organ is illuminated with visible light tuned to 630–690 nm (depending upon the photosensitizing agent). Photochemical changes induce cell necrosis within a few days through the generation of highly reactive oxygen intermediates.

Fluorescence

Photon energy may be dissipated as the re-emission of light. If this happens within 10^{-6} seconds after absorption, it is called fluorescence. Many of the photosensitizing dyes used to induce photochemistry are also fluorescent. This makes it possible for the physician to detect the cells containing the photosensitizer and, if needed, selectively damage these cells.

Photoablation

This tissue–laser light interaction can be described as breaking intermolecular bonds in polymeric chains. In this interaction, the tissue absorbs the high energy ultraviolet photons that are produced by the excimer laser. The lasing material of the excimer laser are excited dimers of unstable gases, usually a halogen and some rare elements. The ultraviolet (UV) photons generated by these lasers possess so much energy that they break apart molecular bonds before their energy can be dissipated as heat. The lased tissue is reduced to its atomic constituents. Because UV radiation from 200–360 nm is well absorbed by most biological tissue, the penetration depths are only a few micrometers with minimal thermal damage to adjacent tissue. Thus, minimal thermal damage is combined with the ability of excimer lasers to produce well defined non-thermal cuts. These effects can be used in assisted hatching as will be discussed later (see p. 78).

Ionization

Ionization is the ejection of an electron from an atom. It is generally believed that the individual photons generated from existing lasers do not have enough energy to cause the absorbing molecule to lose an electron; however, it is possible to have absorption of more than one photon simultaneously in a multiphoton process.

Plasma Formation

This is an effect that does not obey the basic laws of photobiology. With Q-switched (nanosecond) and short-pulsed (picosecond) lasers, it is possible to generate very high power densities (gigaW cm^{-2}) in focal spots of 25–50 µm. When these lasers are focused on a small spot of tissue, it is possible to generate a plasma, which is sometimes referred to as the 'fourth state of matter' because the properties of its gaseous cloud of free electrons are very different from those of solids, liquids or gases. Due to the sudden production of an electrical field in 10^{-9} to 10^{-12} seconds, an intense acoustical shock wave is generated in the medium. At present, there are no clinical applications in reproductive medicine in which these effects are used.

Laser Safety

Unlike most standard surgical devices, the laser can harm surgeons and operating personnel as well as patients. Appropriate eye wear, such as goggles with filters capable of protecting against the wavelength in use, must be worn at all times. Operating room access must be controlled so that individuals without appropriate eye wear do not enter. Surgical instruments in the field must be nonreflective and operating room drapes must also be nonflammable. Endotracheal tubes must be either metal or wrapped with reflective tape to prevent ignition or melting.

Installation of a laser plume management system is also a critical precaution. The system should be appropriate to the laser wavelength and clinical application, and it should always be employed when the laser is in use. These systems are most typically referred to as smoke evacuators and recirculation units. They are designed to remove laser plume contaminants from the laser impact site in order to reduce the risks of transmission of potentially hazardous particles to personnel in the room (American Standards Institute, 1991).

Lasers in Pelvic Reconstruction

The incorporation of the laser into reconstructive surgery is appealing because of its potential accuracy and high versatility. It was first introduced into pelvic reconstructive surgery in the late 1970s and early 1980s when the CO_2 laser (operating at 10 600 nm wavelength) was coupled to operative microscopes (Bellina, 1983) and laparoscopes (Bruhat et al., 1979; Tadir et al., 1981). Later on, specially designed rigid (Tadir et al., 1984) and flexible (Baggish and ElBakrey, 1986) delivery systems for this laser, as well as other lasers – argon, operating at 540 nm (Keye and Dixon, 1983), neodymium: yttrium–aluminum–garnet (Nd:YAG) 1 064 nm (Lomano, 1985) and frequency doubled potassium titanyl phosphate (KTP) crystal YAG at 532 nm (Daniell et al., 1986) – were developed and clinically evaluated. Further advances in laser technology have introduced a large variety of other lasers in the UV, visible, IR range of the electromagnetic spectrum. These lasers are being assessed clinically and scientifically for various applications in reproductive medicine (Figure 7.2).

Numerous publications describe conflicting data following the application of lasers in endoscopic surgery and, thus, critical questions on the potential superiority of each of these lasers over conventional approaches are being raised (McDonough, 1992; Pitkin, 1992). Different criteria for patient selection as well as surgical skill and personal bias could affect these data. There is no doubt that for certain applications, laser light may selectively interact with tissue (i.e. pigmented endometriotic implants), cause minimal effect to surrounding tissue and,

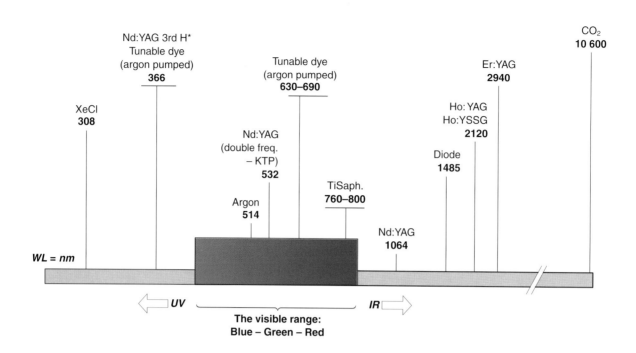

Figure 7.2 Lasers in clinical and experimental use in clinical medicine. (Er, erbium; Ho, holmium; TiSaph, titanium sapphire; WL, wavelength; YSSG, yttrium scandium gallium garnet) *Harmonic.

thus, offer significant advantages over other techniques. However, most indications for operative laparoscopy can be handled without the use of the laser. The experienced endoscopist can take advantage of the laser's special effects (i.e. alternate quickly between a small spot size cutting beam to superficial vaporization) by using a large spot or an electronically controlled laser beam scanner (Donnez *et al.*, 1994). Some procedures can be performed by combining maneuvers of cutting and coagulation. This can be achieved by using contact fibers with different tip profiles or as a result of different tissue colors (Tadir *et al.*, 1994).

Controversies on the place of the laser in operative laparoscopy are anticipated, and its existence has to be viewed as an additional tool. In experienced hands, it can offer significant advantages for properly selected indications (Gant, 1992).

The incorporation of video equipment to endoscopic surgery contributed significantly to the increased interest in minimally invasive therapy (Nezhat, 1986). The consequent improvement in resolution dramatically enhanced the accuracy and therefore the safety of this approach. The bright illuminating light used in endoscopic surgery required upgrading the helium–neon (He–Ne) aiming beam used with non-visible lasers, such as CO_2 and the Nd:YAG. Concomitantly, the accuracy of the CO_2

laser beam alignment, being delivered through long rigid tubes, enabled a reduction in the laparoscope's laser port from the initial size of 8 mm to the currently available 5 mm channels (Tadir *et al.*, 1986). Efficient use of the operative laser laparoscope requires direct coupling to the entire video-endoscopy unit in a way that allows fast interchange from conventional accessories to the laser set-up without requiring significant maneuvers and time wastage.

Delivery Systems

The CO_2 laser, which is an ideal cutting and vaporization beam, is still the most commonly used laser in operative laparoscopy (Tadir *et al.*, 1993b). The beam is reflected by mirrors and is mainly delivered through a rigid set of tubes. Flexible hollow wave guides for CO_2 laser laparoscopy are also available; however, for most indications, pelvic anatomy and surgical needs do not require flexible instruments. Other lasers, such as Nd:YAG, argon and KTP, are also available for laparoscopic surgery. Various technical aspects that influence the development and the handling of these devices for laser endoscopy will be described.

CO_2 Laser

Laparoscopic application of the CO_2 laser through long and rigid channels requires lenses with 200–300 mm back focal length (BFL), which means a long focal depth. For example, if the beam's minimum spot size (at the focal point) after passing through the lens is about 1 mm in diameter, the beam will remain relatively collimated 2 cm before and 2 cm behind the focal point with a diameter of approximately 1.1 mm. This means that PDs within the long range of the focal plane, which in turn, determine the effects of the laser beam on tissue, remain similar to those at the focal point.

In order to increase laser effectiveness as a cutting and coagulating tool, special lenses with different focal lengths are used. The distance between the lens and the focal point (the point where idealized light rays will converge after passing through the lens) is termed the BFL (Baggish et al., 1988). The shorter the BFL of a given lens, the smaller the spot size (or 'waist') of a laser beam that passes through the lens, and the smaller the depth of focus. Depth of focus is defined as length along the beam direction of propagation where the laser beam possesses its smallest waist (for a given lens) and the beam is most collimated (i.e. the beam of light in this region is neither diverging nor converging).

Indeed, one of the main advantages of the CO_2 laser is that varying the PD yields different effects on tissue. This is especially relevant in reproductive surgery where minimizing heating and heat conductance will prevent unwanted damage to adjacent tissues. Long focal length lenses used in the rigid laser laparoscopes limit the achievable minimum spot size of the beam at the waist and thus result in lower PDs. In turn, using very low PDs can superficially ablate endometrial implants or cause serosal shrinkage needed for fimbrial eversion during salpingostomy.

Changes of PD can offer versatile tissue effects to this surgical modality. Minimal PD changes can be obtained by sliding the lens in the endoscopic coupler – termed as continuous variable defocus (CVD) coupler. However, in view of the long BFL and the wide focal plane, these changes are minimal. A simple way to reduce PD is to reduce the power output of the laser source or to move the joystick and reflect the beam on the inner cannula surface. The emerging beam profile will be crescent-shaped instead of round, but the effects on tissue may be superficial as needed. Another innovative modality for superficial tissue ablation on relatively large areas (5–6 mm) with minimal thermal damage to the underlying layers may be obtained with an electronic scanner (Donnez et al., 1994). By reducing the power output, superficial effects can be safely performed. This might be useful for procedures, such as salpingostomy (Bruhat manoevre), ablating endometriotic implants and superficial ablation of the peritoneum over vital organs.

The CO_2 laser, unlike any other cutting tool, acts in the non-contact mode. The lack of tactile feeling is unfamiliar to most surgeons and it takes some time to get used to. The collimated beam of light may cause damage to organs located behind the 'lased' area. Several instruments and maneuvers protect against such damage. In general, these can be divided into mechanical and optical methods. Various types of rigid cannulas inserted at the suprapubic region usually contain a metal tongue at the distal end. This part is located behind the cutting area and prevents further delivery of the beam. Adding such a tongue to the single puncture operative laparoscope is impossible since it may obstruct visibility. Several types of metal probes and hooks can be used as backstops when the beam is delivered through the operative laparoscope. Different tip profiles assist during tissue handling, and a channel for smoke evacuation is built into the device. It is important to note that in the single puncture operative laparoscope, the laser port and the viewing lens are parallel to each other. When the target area is too close to the tip of the laser laparoscope, the He–Ne aiming beam is invisible and activating the laser might cause damage to hidden organs.

Another way to protect deep pelvic organs from unwanted damage by the CO_2 laser beam is by using fluid that absorbs the light and acts as a backstop. This can be achieved as part of the ongoing process of tissue irrigation or by simply applying the fluid to the lower pelvis, in the event that this is the area behind the dissected region.

One of the problems encountered during laser endoscopy is evacuating the smoke produced during tissue vaporization without compromising visibility and peritoneal cavity distention. Several methods can be used to allow smoke evacuation during laser laparoscopy:

- High flow CO_2 gas insufflation.
- Synchronized laser suction unit activated by the laser apparatus with preset suction delay.
- Pressure valves designed to prevent the occurrence of overpressure during high gas inflow.
- A closed circuit of pumped plastic tubing and filters allowing continuous filtration at high flow under constant gas pressure.
- Ports for smoke evacuation are:
- The suction–irrigation probe, which can be used as a backstop as well as smoke evacuator.
- The double channel in the second puncture probe.

Optical fibers made of silver halide crystals are capable of transmitting CO_2 laser energy (Katzir and Arieli, 1982). Although the transmission losses at low power levels are minimal, some limitations, such as low flexibility, low cutting effects and high cost, have prevented its clinical use in gynecologic endoscopy. When CO_2 gas is used for pneumoperitoneum, higher powers of the CO_2 laser induce high gas temperatures, which in turn create a larger spot size by an effect defined as 'blooming'. This effect of the laser beam reduces PD at the tissue and eliminates the pinpoint spot size needed for microdissection (Tadir *et al.*, 1986; Reich *et al.*, 1991). Clinically, this effect results in optimal cutting (vaporization) at low power settings and coagulation accompanying cutting at higher settings.

Flexible hollow wave guides for CO_2 laser laparoscopy are also available (Gannot *et al.*, 1992). However, pelvic anatomy and satisfactory organ visibility allows workable laser transmission through rigid wave guides (Baggish *et al.*, 1988). Such probes allow the passage of the CO_2 laser beam via standard laparoscopes.

The principles of reconstructive pelvic microsurgery – careful tissue handling and continuous irrigation – are relevant to laparoscopic surgery as well. Suction irrigation probes were available before the era of laser laparoscopy. However, the increased need for fluid and smoke evacuation during laser surgery call for instrument modifications, such as surface abrasion (to prevent laser reflection), a variety of probe diameters, easy valve manipulation and a dedicated port for fiber insertion (for visible and near IR lasers). The correct handling of these multipurpose devices is very important during laser laparoscopy particularly since they may also serve as backstops.

Nd:YAG, KTP and Argon Lasers

Delivery of these laser beams (and others, such as holmium:YAG, argon pumped dye, flashlamp pumped dye, and more) via optical fibers makes them potentially ideal energy sources for flexible endoscopy. Current technology in laser laparoscopy is based mainly on direct thermal effects on the target area. Some differences between such thermal systems still exist: Nd:YAG laser, which is in the near IR range, is poorly absorbed by water and thus results in deep coagulating effects. However, by using conical sculpted tips in a contact mode, cutting effects can become predominant. The KTP laser – in which the Nd:YAG frequency is doubled by a potassium titanyl phosphate (KTP) crystal emitting at 532 nm – as well as the argon laser (wavelengths 488–514 nm) fall in the visible range

of the spectrum. Their absorption in water is poor, and tissue penetration is relatively high. However, because of their strong interaction with absorption centers embedded in the tissue, such as small pigmented endometrial implants, the CW argon laser is useful in applications where selective ablation is required. The KTP laser, operating at a similar wavelength but with higher power and in the pulsed mode, is a more efficient cutting tool.

For certain procedures, advantages of the Nd:YAG over the CO_2 laser include deeper penetration, improved hemostasis and decreased plume formation. Effective transmission through fluids may be an advantage or a disadvantage depending upon the type of procedure performed. The main disadvantages of the Nd:YAG systems compared to the CO_2 laser are:

- Extent of tissue damage (similar to electrocautery) which may be critical in some areas (such as damage to the fallopian tube during reconstructive surgery).
- The need for disposable fibers.

Other lasers in the UV range (such as XeCl (308 nm) or nitrogen (337 nm)), visible range (such as the flash lamp dye (504/590 nm)), IR range (such as Ho:YSSG (2120 nm) or Er:YAG (2940 nm)) and the diode laser in the visible and IR range are also available for clinical evaluation. Each of these lasers have different effects on tissue and may offer some advantages for specific applications as will be discussed later. It is beyond the scope of this chapter to compare or evaluate all of these new devices; however, it is expected that some of them will be used in the future when appropriate delivery systems have been developed.

Laser Laparoscopy: Surgical Techniques and Clinical Applications

Almost all pelvic reconstructive procedures previously performed conventionally or microsurgically can be performed similarly through the laparoscope. However, pregnancy rates may vary and appropriate patient selection is still the most important factor in predicting the outcome. If laser laparoscopy is performed, it should be connected to a video system. The final decision about whether to use electrosurgery or laser is dependent upon the type and location of the diagnosed pathology and the surgeon's expertise. Experienced surgeons are using laser equipment in combination with other techniques, such as electrosurgery and stapling devices. The continuous use of standard grasping forceps for stabilizing the area selected for 'lasing' and suction and irrigation cannula (also serving as a backstop) is mandatory. Several sources of information describe the combined use of these technologies on a step by step basis (Hulka and Reich, 1994; Nezhat *et al.*, 1995).

Pelvic Adhesiolysis

Salpingolysis and ovariolysis can easily be dissected without the need of the laser. However, vascular adhesiolysis (blood vessels are usually less than 0.5–1 mm in diameter) is carried out with the CO_2 laser laparoscope or with electrocautery (Donnez *et al.*, 1994). Most surgeons prefer the single puncture laparoscope. The double puncture tube with the backstop or the laparoscopic probes are also suitable for lysis of vascular or avascular adhesions. The ovary, uterus and cul-de-sac fluid may serve as a backstop (Nezhat *et al.*, 1995).

Vaporization of Endometriosis

A large meta-analysis study suggested that laparoscopic surgery with laser techniques may be superior to laparotomy in the management of infertility resulting from moderate and severe endometriosis (Gant, 1992). Laparoscopic laser surgery has been subjected to a randomized prospective double-blind controlled study and has been shown to be effective for pain relief in patients with stage I–III endometriosis compared with the sham arm of the study who had laparoscopy alone (Sutton *et al.*, 1994). Peritoneal endometriotic implants can be removed by CO_2 (Kelly and Roberts, 1983; Martin, 1985), argon (Keye and Dixon, 1983), Nd:YAG (Lomano, 1985) and the KTP (Daniell *et al.*, 1986) lasers. The tissue effect is different for each of these lasers and the superiority of one over the other has not been demonstrated. However, most surgeons prefer the CO_2 laser via the operative single puncture probe. Separate incisions allow the insertion of other accessories, such as grasping forceps and suction irrigator probe. This device is particularly important in draining the contents of endometriotic cysts. A focused beam (0.6–0.8 mm spot size at 15–30 W PD: 5000–12 000 W cm^{-2} is employed to vaporize endometriotic implants from the ovary, uterosacral ligaments, bladder, tubes and pelvic sidewall.

The argon laser may offer some advantages for small endometriotic implants due to its selective absorption by the red pigmented lesions. This causes less damage to the overlying peritoneum. However, since the argon laser is not an ideal cutting tool, its use is limited to the small implants where adhesiolysis is not required. A combined approach of medical treatment – gonadotropin releasing hormone (GnRH) analog – and CO_2 laser laparoscopy is recommended for large endometriotic cysts (Donnez and Nisolle-Pochet, 1992).

Terminal Salpingostomy

The correlation between tubal damage and predictive prognostic criteria for intrauterine pregnancy following salpingostomy performed microsurgically for the treatment of hydrosalpinx are well known (Boer-Meisel *et al.*, 1986). Salpingostomy on a thin wall hydrosalpinx with minimal adhesions can offer a 77% chance of intrauterine pregnancy. The same operation carried out on moderately damaged tubes may yield a 21% pregnancy rate, whereas only 3% of those operated on for thick wall hydrosalpinx with dense adhesions ever conceive spontaneously. Thus, although meticulous tissue handling and minimal thermal damage can influence the outcome of the operation, patient selection still appears to be the dominant factor affecting the success rate.

The improved success rate in *in vitro* fertilization may even justify laparoscopic removal of severely damaged tubes. This approach may reduce the risk of tubal pregnancy following *in vitro* fertilization and embryo transfer (IVF–ET) (Zouves *et al.*, 1991).

Terminal salpingostomy can be performed with various laser types (Daniell and Herbert, 1984; Daniell, 1989); however, the CO_2 laser is probably the ideal tool for thin wall hydrosalpinx (Tadir and Fisch, 1993). The routine steps preceding laparoscopic salpingostomy must include cervical cannulation to provide a route for the intraoperative injection of dye to distend the tubes and two grasping forceps which are introduced for traction and manipulation at the ampullary–fimbrial segment. The blocked tube is held so that the focused laser beam can be aligned at a 90° angle to the 'dimple'. The laser is set on continuous mode and a linear incision is made, cutting at the dimple along blood vessels. As soon as the lumen is entered, the tube collapses and continuous dye injection keeps it distended. At this point, the grasping forceps gently hold the incision edges and a reduced power (4–7 W, 150–300 W cm^{-2}) defocused beam is used to contract and evert the serosal aspect of the incised edge (Bruhat manoeuvre) (Mage *et al.*, 1985). A similar procedure can be performed with the laparoscopic scanner (Donnez *et al.*, 1994).

Uterosacral Ligament Ablation

In patients with dysmenorrhea not responsive to medical treatment, the uterosacral ligaments can be vaporized using the laser (Feste, 1984). The nerve fibers passing into the uterus are damaged by a shallow crater at the ligament's insertion on the posterior wall. The close proximity to the ureters requires precise tools and the CO_2 laser may be the safest. This procedure, also known as the 'modified Doyle procedure' (though originally described by Fraenkl in 1909), is still open to the surgeon's judgment and should be based on subjective criteria such as magnitude of pain. Technical details of this procedure are discussed in detail in Chapter 25 (Nezhat et al., 1995).

Tubal Pregnancy

Early detection of unruptured tubal pregnancy has changed the surgical approach and introduced medical treatments as well (Slaughter and Grimes, 1995). Laparoscopic salpingostomy using scissors, electrocautery or laser has replaced the conventional approach of salpingotomy via laparotomy. If a laser is used, a longitudinal incision is made at the antimesenteric aspect of the tube over the bulging area of the implantation site using a focused beam. The CO_2 laser is preferred since minimal thermal damage prevents additional damage to the tube. Some surgeons prefer using a vasopressin agent to prevent bleeding from the implantation site. Removal of conception debris is performed with a suction cannula or with an ovum forceps introduced suprapubically. If bleeding occurs following aspiration, hemostasis is achieved by compression with atraumatic forceps or by application of bipolar coagulator. The tube is usually left open for secondary healing. Segmental resection or salpingectomy can also be performed laparoscopically. In this case, the CO_2 laser or other non-laser resection means is combined with hemostatic methods, such as bipolar coagulation, loop ligation or laparoscopic staples.

Myomectomy

Patients with indications for laparoscopic myomectomy can be managed preoperatively with GnRH analogs for up to three months in order to reduce tumor size and blood loss. Laparoscopic myomectomy has two stages.

- First, removing the fibroid from the uterus.
- Second, removal from the abdominal cavity.

A pedunculated myoma is simply excised at the stalk using high power (> 40 W) CO_2 laser, scissors or electrocoagulation, and bleeding is best controlled with a bipolar electrocoagulator. For a subserosal or intramural myoma, vasopressin is injected under the capsule, which is then excised with a CO_2 laser and gradually dissected using a combination of forceps and suction irrigation probe (Donnez et al., 1994).

Intraligamentary fibroids are approached by incising the anterior or posterior leaf of the broad ligament with the laser after identifying the location of the large vessels, ureter and bladder. Extraction of the tumor from the abdominal cavity is sometimes difficult. Posterior colpotomy or morcellation are some of the options available (Steiner et al., 1993).

Patients approaching menopause who wish to avoid abdominal myomectomy or hysterectomy can be treated with Nd:YAG laser which is coagulating and blocking the blood supply to the fibroid. The Nd:YAG laser dispersion effect, 2–5 mm in diameter, can be used to coagulate and reduce symptomatic serosal and intramural myomas of moderate size (less than or equal to 10 cm) (Donnez et al., 1990; Goldfarb, 1992). Small fibroids accidentally found during laparoscopy can be easily vaporized with the laser beam; however, the indication for their removal is doubtful.

Hysteroscopic Laser Applications

Hysteroscopic laser applications may hold several advantages and disadvantages compared to those of conventional techniques. In order to perform safe and effective hysteroscopic procedures, special equipment must be used. The instrumentation is similar to the urologic cystoscope; however, anatomic dissimilarity between the urinary bladder and the uterus require several modifications to accommodate different flow and pressure mechanisms (Baggish, 1988). A double lumen set for irrigation maintains intrauterine pressure around 100 mm Hg. Uterine distention is a prerequisite condition for a safe and effective procedure; however, the preferred distention medium is still a controversial issue. While all media – CO_2 gas or liquid media – can be used for diagnostic hysteroscopy, there are special indications and limitations for operative hysteroscopy. CO_2 gas offers an optimal view; its safety for operative procedures has been demonstrated by Lindemann et al. (1976) and it is the most cost-effective distending medium. However, the risk of gas embolism is higher during laser hysteroscopy, which is performed under high flow and pressure to maintain uterine distention and fiber cooling. Several cases of gas embolism have been reported in the USA and, thus, only liquid medium is allowed in the USA for laser hysteroscopy (Baggish and Daniell, 1989). The optimal laser for hysteroscopic application is the Nd:YAG. It operates through water and the uterine wall thickness offers good protection for its depth of penetration.

Dysfunctional uterine bleeding that in many cases leads to hysterectomy is a common gynecologic complaint. The standard management requires exclusion of any malignant or premalignant conditions, and if hormonal treatment has failed or is contraindicated, endometrial ablation with Nd:YAG laser is beneficial (Goldrath et al., 1981). High frequency electrocautery using the rollerball or a modified resectoscope may offer several advantages and disadvantages over Nd:YAG laser ablation (Wamsterker and De Block, 1992). Pretreatment with danazol or GnRH analogs is recommended to render endometrial atrophy. The endometrial cavity is inspected with an operative hysteroscope. Constant irrigation allows clear viewing by removing blood and tissue debris. Inflow and outflow of fluid are precisely measured. A 600–800 µm fiber is inserted through the operating channel of the hysteroscope and the procedure is monitored by the closed circuit TV system. In cases with direct vision, a protective filter is placed over the eyepiece to prevent injury. The power output selected for photocoagulating the endometrial surface is ±50 W. The fiber tip is longitudinally moved in close approximation to the surface until the whole cavity is ablated. The success rate for endometrial ablation with either technique ranges between 65–85% (Daniell et al., 1992; Garry et al., 1995); however, these procedures are not risk free. In 1991, a large survey – 630 surgeons who performed 17 298 operative hysteroscopies – revealed that the most frequent complication was uterine perforation (11/1000 procedures). The rate of water intoxication or pulmonary edema was 1.4/1000 procedures, and some serious complications (eight laparotomies for bowel injury, three CO_2 embolisms and three deaths) were reported (Hulka et al., 1993). An alternative approach for selective endometrial destruction will be discussed in the PDT section.

The septate uterus is amenable to hysteroscopic metroplasty. The technique was first proposed by Edstrom in 1974 but was not widely employed until appropriate instruments were developed (Chervenak and Neuwirth, 1981). The use of high frequency cutting current is hemostatic in this situation, but it does have some risks in that it is impossible to determine the degree of electric spread.

This operation can be performed with the Nd:YAG (Goldrath, 1985) and KTP laser (Daniell et al., 1987). It is important that laparoscopy is performed before or during the laser metroplasty to make sure that the uterus is not bicornuate. The procedure should be scheduled in the first half of the menstrual cycle when the endometrium is thin or following hormonal suppression. Other treatment modalities for menorrhagia, such as thermal energy (Singer et al., 1994; Baggish et al., 1995) and PDT (Wyss et al., 1995), may replace existing methods with a less invasive approach.

Lasers in Micromanipulation of Pre-Implantation Embryos and Gametes

The introduction of IVF into clinical practise has changed the approach towards the infertile couple. Two main areas have received special attention in the last few years:

- The use of IVF for the treatment of severe male factor infertility.
- Improvement of the implantation rate.

Several methods have been studied in these areas and recent studies suggest that gamete manipulation may play a major role in solving both problems. Meticulous handling of gametes during such manipulations requires special tools and laboratory expertise. Mechanical methods of sperm injection and zona manipulations have been studied by several groups and will be discussed in other chapters. Laser microbeams offer some advantages as accurate manipulating tools for cellular and subcellular organelles (Berns et al., 1969) and as such were tested for gamete manipulations (Tadir et al., 1989a, 1989b).

The high precision of laser beams and the possibility of narrowing beam spot size from 500–800 µm used for tissue microsurgery to the 0.5–3 µm needed for cellular microsurgery suggested its adaptability for IVF.

A CW laser at very low power can be used as an optical tweezer if focused above a single cell and pulsed lasers have been applied to drill oocytes. As previously mentioned, several parameters determine the laser effect on the target: these are wavelength, pulse duration, energy per pulse, pulse repetition rate, total time of radiation exposure, beam spot size and the focal plane. The water content of the manipulated object, and the surrounding environment (i.e. gas or liquid, water or oil) may also influence the laser effect (Tadir et al., 1993a; Neev et al., 1995).

Since the introduction of laser to the IVF laboratory, it has been tested for the following applications:

- Optical trapping to manipulate sperm and study new physiologic aspects of sperm motility.
- Laser zona drilling (LZD) to improve fertilization in the presence of abnormal sperm.
- Laser assisted hatching (LAH) to improve implantation.
- Interactions with the zona pellucida (ZP) to study potential effects of the beam on the oocyte and investigate unique properties of the ZP.

Several commercial systems dedicated to gamete manipulations have been developed. Some are based on a contact fiber delivery system and others are contact-free units that take advantage of the laser as a 'light scalpel'.

Sperm Manipulations with Optical Trapping

Optical trapping to manipulate single cells was initially described by Ashkin and Dziedzic (1987). The mechanical force exerted on a microscopic particle by light is a result of momentum carried by the electromagnetic wave. A single beam gradient force trap consists of a laser beam with a Gaussian intensity profile, focused to a spot smaller than the particle being trapped. This trap confines the particle to a location just below the focal point of the laser beam in the axial direction and centered in the beam in the transverse direction. The force generated by the light is greater than all other forces acting on the particle and as such creates a trapping effect.

Using these principles, a laser generated optical tweezer was applied to manipulate sperm. Initially, the Nd:YAG laser was used to determine relative force generated by single spermatozoa compared to velocity and motility patterns (Tadir *et al.*, 1990). Zig-zag motile sperm produced swim with more force than straight motile sperm. Other experiments revealed that similar effects could be achieved with a tunable TiSaph laser (700–800 nm wavelength) (Araujo *et al.*, 1994). Several studies were performed to explore new physiologic parameters of sperm exposed to the trapping system. Measurements of the relative sperm force before and after exposure to cumulus cell mass determined a significant increase following interaction with the cumulus mass (Westphal *et al.*, 1993). The relative force of human sperm before and after cryopreservation demonstrated that there was no significant difference when a yolk buffer freezing media was used as cryoprotectant (Zoentania *et al.*, 1995). In a recent study (Patrizio *et al.*, 1996) using the same system, it was determined that *in vitro* exposure of human sperm to pentoxifylline significantly increases sperm intrinsic relative forces in normospermic and asthenospermic samples. This experiment confirmed that optical tweezers can provide an accurate determination of sperm force in experimental *in vitro* conditions.

Embryo Manipulation: LAH

Micromanipulation of embryos before transfer into the uterus has been suggested to enhance implantation following IVF. This was based on observations in selected groups of patients that an artificial opening of the ZP (assisted hatching) promoted implantation rate (Cohen, 1991) and accelerated the process of implantation as indicated by the early rise of hormonal markers such as luteal estradiol, progesterone and human chorionic gonadotropin (hCG) (Liu *et al.*, 1993). Thickness and hardness of the ZP are probably some of the factors playing a role in this complex process. The accuracy and simplicity with which lasers can be used to open the ZP without causing visible damage to the ooplasm membrane increased the interest of this approach.

Effects on embryonic development were evaluated following use of the XeCl excimer laser (Neev *et al.*, 1993). Zonae of 8–16-cell mouse embryos were either lased ($n=189$), zona drilled with acidified Tyrode's solution ($n=183$), or left intact ($n=188$). Blastocyst formation (99–100%) was similar in the three groups. Hatching occurred earlier in the lased embryos than for those of the control groups. These embryos hatched through the laser ablated area. Significantly more embryos were hatching on days 4 and 7 in the conventionally drilled group compared to those in the laser treated group. However, implantation rates of morphologically normal laser ablated embryos were not impaired compared to those of the control embryos. As mentioned earlier, even though the 308 nm laser is safe, the sensitivity of gamete manipulation justifies staying away from the UV range. As such, most of the research in this area has been shifted to various lasers in the IR range.

The Ho:YAG laser operating in the IR range (2100 nm) and delivered through a silicon fiber was applied on the ZP of 2–8-cell stage mouse embryos in order to assist hatching (Reshef *et al.*, 1993). The rate of development to blastocyst stage or beyond and the rate of hatching between the laser treated and control embryos were compared. Embryos were placed during lasing in phosphate-buffered saline under oil and assessed 72 hours later. Of 49, 33 laser drilled embryos (67%) progressed to hatching compared to 36 of 82 (44%) untreated controls ($P<0.01$).

Schiewe *et al.* (1995) assessed the efficacy of the same wavelength generated from a Ho:YSGG laser operating at 2100 nm in a pipette-free non-contact mode to assist hatching and sustain normal embryonic development. They tested the unit with a pulse duration of 250 µs and pulse repetition rates at 10 Hz. Incisions in the zona were obtained by using the laser at 10 mJ per pulse. Two-cell mouse embryos were recovered and assigned to LAH or control culture. The laser beam was directed through a mechanical shutter into an input port of a Zeiss Axiomat (Carl Zeiss, Inc.) inverted microscope. Fewer (*P*<0.05) embryos developed to the blastocyst stage in the control group (81%) in contrast to the LAH group (90%), and the procedure was simple and accurate.

Feichtinger *et al.* (1992) applied the Er:YAG contact laser to mouse embryos and subsequently to human embryos. Groups of 10–15 mouse embryos were placed under oil on two slides. A control slide was maintained on a warming stage while embryos on the other slide were subjected to the laser to produce holes in the ZP. Subsequently, the embryos were assessed for the number developing to the blastocyst stage. There was no difference between the laser treated mouse embryos and the untreated controls on day 1 and 2 of culture. On day 3, however, complete hatching was significantly enhanced in the laser treated group – 44/55 (80%) in the laser group, 17/58 (29.3%) for controls (*P*=0.0001).

The same laser was used in a multicenter study for human application (Oburca *et al.*, 1994). Embryos obtained from 129 patients who had previously experienced repeated implantation failures following IVF and ET were exposed to similar laser treatment for assisted hatching. During the procedure, embryos were held by negative pressure using a glass holding pipette, and ZP ablation performed by depositing approximately 10 µJ in the contact mode; 5–8 pulses were employed to penetrate the ZP creating a 20–30 µm opening. Ongoing pregnancy rates of 36% (30/84 patients) and 29% (13/45 patients) were achieved, in the two centers. Considering the patient group studied these results were encouraging. Preliminary results of an ongoing prospective randomized study in patients with an initial IVF attempt exhibited a 50% pregnancy rate (10/20 patients) in the LAH group in contrast to 44% (10/23 patients) without assisted hatching. The implantation rate per embryo in this preliminary study was also not significant (23.8% versus 21%, LAH versus control). This demonstrates that the laser has no detrimental effect on embryo survival and implantation.

An alternative IR diode laser operating in the contact free mode at 1485 nm was introduced to the IVF laboratory in 1994 (Rink *et al.*, 1994). In a set of several studies, the beam was delivered through a 45× objective of an inverted microscope (2–4 µm spot diameter, 10–40 ms pulse, 0.5–1.2 mJ) to produce laser ZP dissection in mouse zygotes (Germond *et al.*, 1995a; Rink *et al.*, 1996). One discharge was sufficient to drill openings in the ZP ranging from 5–20 µm depending upon laser power and exposure time and 70% of the drilled zygotes developed to the blastocyst stage, which was comparable with the control group, and there was no evidence of thermal damage. The same group further explored the effects of the same diode laser in a set of studies. Germond *et al.* (1995b) demonstrated that the energy needed to drill a hole of a given diameter is greater for mouse and human zygotes than for oocytes by using this accurate non-touch technique. Safety of the drilling procedure was demonstrated by the observation that 42 normal mice were born following the procedure, and 33 normal second generation newborns were produced by four males and four laser treated females that were cross-mated. Various laser parameters were tested (irradiation time of 3–100 ms, and laser power 22–55 mW) in order to determine potential thermal damage. The authors concluded that the microdrilling procedure can generate standardized holes in mouse ZP without any visible side effects. Human studies using the same diode laser demonstrated improved pregnancy rate following assisted hatching of cryopreserved embryos (Germond *et al.*, 1995b).

Conclusion

This chapter covers a large variety of procedures in reproductive medicine, some of which are still experimental. Further developments in laser and other technologies are underway and new products are being evaluated in clinical settings.

Supported by grants:
NIH: #2RO1 CA32248, #5P41 RR01192, #R29GM50958;
DOE: #DE-FG03-91ER61227;
ONR: #N00014-91-C-0134;

References

American National Standards Institute (1991) *American National Standards for the Safe Use of Lasers in Health Care Facilities.* Orlando, FL: American National Standards Institute.

Araujo E, Tadir Y, Patrizio P, Ord T, Silber S, Berns MW, Asch R (1994) Relative force of human epididymal sperm correlated to the fertilizing capacity *in vitro*. *Fertility and Sterility* **62**: 585–590.

Ashkin A, Dziedzic JM (1987) Optical trapping and manipulation of viruses and bacteria. *Science* 235: 1517.

Baggish MS (1988) New laser hysteroscope for neodymium-YAG endometrial ablation. *Lasers in Surgery and Medicine* 8: 99–103.

Baggish MS, Daniell JF (1989) Catastrophic injury secondary to the use of coaxial gas-cooled fiber and artificial sapphire tips for intra uterine surgery. *Lasers in Surgery and Medicine* 9: 581–584.

Baggish MS, ElBakrey MM (1986) A flexible CO_2 laser fiber for operative laparoscopy. *Fertility and Sterility* 46: 16.

Baggish MS, Sze E, Badawy S, Choe J (1988) Carbon dioxide laser laparoscopy by means of 3.0-mm diameter rigid wave guide. *Fertility and Sterility* 50: 419.

Baggish M, Paraiso M, Breznock EM, Griffey S (1995) A computer-controlled, continuously circulating, hot irrigating system for endometrial ablation. *American Journal of Obstetrics and Gynecology* 173(6): 1842–1848.

Bellina JH (1983) Microsurgery of the fallopian tube with the carbon dioxide laser: Analysis of 230 cases with a two year follow up. *Lasers in Surgery and Medicine* 3: 255–259.

Bellina J, Bandieramonte G (1984) An introduction to lasers. In Bellina J, Bandieramonte G (eds) *Principles and Practice of Gynecologic Laser Surgery*, pp. 1–26. New York: Plenum Medical Book Company.

Berns MW, Rounds DE, Olson RS (1969) Effects of laser microirradiation on chromosomes. *Experimental Cell Research* 56: 292–298.

Boer-Meisel ME, te Velde ER, Habbema JDF, Kardaun JWPF (1986) Predicting the pregnancy outcome in patients treated for hydrosalpinx: a prospective study. *Fertility and Sterility* 45: 23–29.

Bruhat M, Mage C, Manhes M (1979) Use of the CO_2 laser via laparoscopy. In Kaplan I (ed.) *Laser Surgery III, Proceedings of the Third International Society for Laser Surgery*, pp. 274–276. Tel-Aviv: Ot-Paz.

Chervenak FA, Neuwirth RS (1981) Hysteroscopic resection of the uterine septum. *American Journal of Obstetrics and Gynecology* 141: 351.

Cohen J (1991) Assisted hatching of human embryos. *Journal of In Vitro Fertilization and Embryo Transfer* 8: 179–190.

Daniell JF (1989) Fiberoptic laser laparoscopy. *Clinical Obstetrics and Gynecology*. 3: 545–562.

Daniell JF, Herbert CM (1984) Laparoscopic salpingostomy utilizing the CO_2 laser. *Fertility and Sterility* 41: 558.

Daniell JF, Miller W, Tosh R (1986) Initial evaluation of the use of potassium-titanyl-phosphate (KTP/532) laser in gynecologic laparoscopy. *Fertility and Sterility* 46: 373–377.

Daniell FJ, Osher S, Miller W (1987) Hysteroscopic resection of uterine septa with visible light laser energy. *Colposcopy and Gynecologic Laser Surgery* 3: 217.

Daniell JF, Kurtz BR, Ke RW (1992) Hysteroscopic endometrial ablation using the rollerball electrode. *Obstetrics and Gynecology* 80(3)(Pt 1): 329–332.

Donnez J, Nisolle-Pochet M (1992) Endometriosis associated with infertility: Therapeutic approaches to endometriosis. In Bastert G, Walwiener D (eds) *Lasers in Gynecology* pp. 135–141. Berlin: Springer Verlag.

Donnez J, Gillerot S, Bourgonjon D, Clerckx F, Nisolle M (1990) Neodymium:YAG laser hysteroscopy in large submucous fibroids. *Fertility and Sterility* 54: 999–1003.

Donnez J, Nisolle M, Casanas-Roux F, Anaf V, Bassil S (1994) CO_2 laser laparoscopic surgery: adhesiolysis, salpingostomy and fimbrioplasty. In Donnez J, Nisolle M (eds) *Atlas of Laser Operative Laparoscopy and Hysteroscopy*, p. 97 Pearl River, NY: Parthenon Publishing Group.

Edstrom K (1974) Intrauterine surgical procedures during hysteroscopy. *Endoscopy*, 6: 175.

Feste JR (1984) CO_2 laser neurectomy for dysmenorrhea. *Lasers in Surgery and Medicine* 3: 327.

Feichtinger W, Strohmer H, Fuhrberg P, Radivojevic K, Antoniori S, Pepe G, Versaci C (1992) Photoablation of oocyte zona pellucida by erbium:YAG laser for in-vitro fertilization in severe male infertility. *Lancet* 339: 811.

Fraenkl L (1909) Anatomische und klinische beitrage zur parametritis posterior chronica. *Deutsche Medizinische Wochenschrift* 47: 258.

Gannot I, Dror R, Dahan N, Croitoru N (1992) Improved plastic hollow fibers for CO_2 laser radiation transmission for possible endoscopic use. *The International Society for Optical Engineering, Proceedings* 1649.

Gant NF (1992) Infertility and endometriosis: Comparison of pregnancy outcome with laparotomy versus laparoscopic techniques. *American Journal of Obstetrics and Gynecology* 166: 1072–1081.

Gardner MF (1985) Laser physics. In Baggish MS (ed.) *Basic and Advanced Laser Surgery in Gynecology*, pp. 23–35. Norwalk, CT: Appleton-Century-Crofts.

Garry R, Shelley-Jones D, Mooney P, Phillips G (1995) Six hundred endometrial laser ablations. *Obstetrics and Gynecology* 85(1): 24–29.

Germond M, Nocera D, Senn A, Rink K, Delacretaz G, Fakan S (1995a) Microdissection of mouse and human zona pellucida using a 1.48 μm diode laser beam: efficacy and safety of the procedure. *Fertility and Sterility* 64: 604–611.

Germond M, Senn A, Rink K, Delacretaz G, De Grandi P (1995b) Is assisted hatching of frozen-thawed embryos enhancing pregnancy outcome in patients who have several previous nidation failures? (abstract) Presented at the Three Country Fertility and Sterility Meeting. Innsbruck, Austria, Oct. 12–14: *J fur Fertilitat und Reproduktion* 3: 41.

Goldfarb HA (1992) Nd:YAG laser laparoscopic coagulation of symptomatic myomas. *Journal of Reproductive Medicine* 37: 636–638.

Goldrath M, Fuller T, Segal S (1981) Laser photovaporization of endometrium for the treatment of menorrhagia. *American Journal of Obstetrics and Gynecology* 140: 14–19.

Goldrath M (1985) Hysteroscopic laser surgery. In Baggish MS (ed.) *Basic and Advanced Laser Surgery in Gynecology*. pp. 357–372. Norwalk, CT: Appleton-Century-Crofts.

Hulka J, Reich H (1994) *Textbook of Laparoscopy*. Philadelphia, PA: Saunders.

Hulka JF, Peterson HB, Phillips JM, Surrey MW (1993) Operative hysteroscopy. American Association of Gynecologic Laparoscopists 1991 membership survey. *Journal of Reproductive Medicine* 38: 572–573.

Kaplan I, Goldman J (1973) The treatment of erosion of the

uterine cervix by means of CO_2 laser. *Obstetrics and Gynecology* **4:** 795–796.

Katzir A, Arieli A (1982) Long wavelength infrared optical fibers. *Journal of Non-Crystalline Solids* **47:** 149–158.

Kelly RW, Roberts DK (1983) CO_2 laser laparoscopy: a potential alternative to danazol in the treatment of stage I and II endometriosis. *Journal of Reproductive Medicine* **28:** 638–640.

Keye WR, Dixon J (1983) Photocoagulation of endometriosis by the argon laser through the laparoscope. *Obstetrics and Gynecology* **62:** 383–386.

Lomano JM (1985) Nd:YAG laser applications in gynecology. In: Joffe SN, Ogurs Y (eds) *Advances of Nd:YAG Laser Surgery* pp. 201–207. Berlin: Springer Verlag.

Lindeman HJ, Mohr J, Gallinat A, Buros M (1976) Der einfluss von CO_2 gas wahrend der hysteroskopie. *Geburtshifle Frauenheilkunde* **36:** 153.

Liu HC, Noyse N, Cohen J, Rosenwaks Z, Alikani M (1993) Assisted hatching facilitates earlier implantation. *Fertility and Sterility* **60:** 871–875.

McDonough PG (1992) The need for technology assessment in the reproductive sciences. *American Journal of Obstetrics and Gynecology* **166:** 1082–1090.

Mage G, Pouly JL, Bruhat MA (1985) Laser microsurgery of the oviducts. In *Basic and Advanced Laser Surgery in Gynecology*, pp. 299–322. Norwalk, CT: Appleton-Century-Crofts.

Martin DC (1985) CO_2 laser laparoscopy for the treatment of endometriosis associated with infertility. *Journal of Reproductive Medicine* **30:** 409–411.

Neev J, Gonzales A, Licciardi F, Alikani M, Tadir Y, Berns MW, Cohen J (1993) A contact-free microscope delivered laser ablation system for assisted hatching of the mouse embryo without the use of a micromanipulator. *Human Reproduction* **8:** 939–944.

Neev Y, Schiewe MC, Sung WV, Kang D, Berns MW, Tadir Y (1995) Use of Ho:YSSG laser system delivered in a non-contact mode for zona pellucida dissection. *Journal of Assisted Reproduction and Genetics* **12,** 228–293.

Nezhat C (1986) Videolaseroscopy: A new modality for the treatment of diseases of the reproductive organs. *Colposcoscopy and Gynecologic Laser Surgery* **2:** 221–224.

Nezhat CR, Nezhat FR, Luciano AA, Siegler AM, Metzger DA, Nezhat CH (1995) *Operative Gynecologic Laparoscopy: Principles and Techniques.* New York: McGraw-Hill.

Oburca A, Strohmer H, Sakkas D, Menezo Y, Kogosowski A, Barak Y, Feichtinger W (1994) Use of laser in assisted fertilization and hatching. *Human Reproduction* **9:** 1723–1726.

Patrizio P, Liu Y, Sonek G, Berns MW, Tadir Y (1996) Effect of pentoxifylline on the intrinsic force of human sperm. Presented at the American Academy of Andrology, Minneapolis, MN, April 25–29.

Pitkin RM (1992) Operative laparoscopy: surgical advance or technical gimmik? *Obstetrics and Gynecology* **79:** 441–442.

Reich H, MacGregor TS, Vancaillie TG (1991) CO_2 laser used through the operating channel of laser laparoscopes: *in vitro* study of power and power density losses. *Obstetrics and Gynecology* **77:** 40–47.

Reshef E, Haaksma CJ, Bettinger TL, Haas GG, Schafer SA, Zavy MT (1993) Gamete and embryo micromanipulation using the holmium:YAG laser. Presented at the 49th American Fertility Society, Montreal, Canada, Oct. 11–14. *Fertility Sterility Program* supplement P-016, S88.

Rink K, Delacretaz G, Salathe RP, Senn A, Nocera D, Germond M, Faken S (1994) 1.5 μm diode laser microdissection of the zona pellucida of mouse oocytes. Biomedical Optics. The International Society for Optical Engineering. *Proceedings from the Biomedical Optics Program.* 2134A–53.

Rink K, Delacretaz G, Salathe RP, Senn A, Nocera D, Germond M, De Garnadi P, Fakan S (1996) Non contact microdrilling of mouse zona pellucida with an objective delivered 1.48 μm diode laser. *Lasers in Surgery and Medicine* **18:** 52–62.

Schiewe MC, Neev Y, Hazeleger NL, Balmaceda JP, Berns MW, Tadir Y (1995) Developmental competence of mouse embryos following zona drilling using a non-contact Ho:YSSG laser system. *Human Reproduction* **10:** 1821–1824.

Singer A, Almanza R, Gutierrez A, Haber G, Bolduc LR, Neuwirth R (1994) Preliminary clinical experience with a thermal balloon endometrial ablation method to treat menorrhagia. *Obstetrics and Gynecology* **83:** 732–734.

Slaughter JL, Grimes DA (1995) Methotrexate therapy. Nonsurgical management of ectopic pregnancy (meta-analysis). *Western Journal of Medicine* **162:** 225–228.

Steiner R, Wight E, Tadir Y, Haller U (1993) Electrical cutting device for laparoscopic removal of tissue from the abdominal cavity. *Obstetrics and Gynecology* **81:** 471–493.

Sutton CJG, Ewen SP, Whitelaw N, Haines P (1994) Prospective, randomized, double-blind controlled trial of laser laparoscopy in the treatment of pelvic pain associated with minimal, mild, and moderate endometriosis. *Fertility and Sterility* **62:** 696–700.

Tadir Y, Fisch B (1993) Operative laparoscopy: a challenge for general gynecology. *American Journal of Obstetrics and Gynecology* **169:** 7–12.

Tadir Y, Ovadia J, Zukerman Z et al. (1981) Laparoscopic application of CO_2 laser. In Atsumi K, Nimsakul N (eds) *Laser Tokyo 81.* pp. 13–27. Tokyo: Inter Group Corp.

Tadir Y, Kaplan I, Zukerman Z et al. (1984) New instrumentation and technique for laparoscopic carbon dioxide laser operations: a preliminary report. *Obstetrics and Gynecology* **63:** 582–585.

Tadir Y, Kaplan I, Zukerman Z, Ovadia J (1986) Effective CO_2 laser power on tissue in endoscopic surgery. *Fertility and Sterility* **45:** 492–495.

Tadir Y, Wright WH, Berns MW (1989a) Cell micromanipulation with laser beams. In Capitanio GL, Asch RH, De Cecco L, Croce S (eds) *G.I.F.T.: From Basics to Clinics.* pp. 359–368, New York: Raven Press.

Tadir Y, Wright WH, Vafa O, Ord T, Asch R, Berns MW (1989b) Micromanipulation of sperm by a laser generated optical trap. *Fertility and Sterility* **52:** 870–873.

Tadir Y, Wright WH, Vafa O et al. (1990) Force generated by human sperm correlated to velocity and determined using a laser trap. *Fertility and Sterility* **53:** 944–947.

Tadir Y, Neev J, Berns MW (1993a) Delivery systems for laser laparoscopy. In Sutton C, Diamond M (eds) *Practical Manual of Gynecologic Endoscopy,* pp. 40–50. London: WB Saunders Ltd.

Tadir Y, Neev J, Ho P, Berns MW (1993b) Lasers for gamete micromanipulation: basic concepts. *Journal of Assisted Reproduction and Genetics* **10**: 121–125.

Tadir Y, Rosenberg K, Rozenberg Z, Fisch B, Ovadia J (1994) Safety characteristics of the conically sculpted Nd:YAG laser fiber for operative laparoscopy. *Journal of Gynecological Surgery* **10**: 71–77.

Wamsterker K, De Block S (1992) HF electrosurgery versus laser hysteroscopy. In Bastert G, Wallwiener D (eds) *Lasers in Gynecology*. pp. 211–213. Berlin: Springer Verlag.

Westphal L, El-Danasouri IE, Shimizu S, Tadir Y, Berns MW (1993) Exposure of human sperm to the cumulus oophorus results in increased relative force as measured by a 760 nm laser optical tram. *Human Reproduction* **8(7)**: 1083–1086.

Wyss P, Svaasand L, Tadir Y, Haller U, Berns MW, Wyss MT, Tromberg B (1995) Photomedicine of the endometrium: experimental concepts. *Human Reproduction* **10**: 221–226.

Zoentania ND, Araujo E, Berns MW, Tadir Y, Schell MW, Stone SC (1995) Effect of freezing on the relative escape force of sperm as measured by laser optical trap. *Fertility and Sterility* **63**: 185–188.

Zouves C, Erenus M, Gomel V (1991) Tubal ectopic pregnancy after *in vitro* fertilization and embryo transfer: a role for proximal occlusion or salpingectomy after failed distal tubal surgery? *Fertility and Sterility* **56**: 691–695.

8

Electrosurgery

ROGER C. ODELL

Electroscope, Inc., Boulder Colorado, USA

With the increased acceptance of laparoscopic access for major surgical procedures it is clear that the fundamental therapeutic modalities of electrosurgical energy must be understood to enhance the art of delivery in practice. It is equally important to maximize the safe delivery of this most commonly used energy source. The intention of this chapter is to introduce the fundamental therapeutic modalities and discuss the inherent risks of electrosurgical energy during laparoscopy and methods available which allow the surgeon to deliver electrosurgical energy with the same level of patient safety as in open laparotomy.

Unfortunately most clinicians learn the application of electrosurgical energy on the job (i.e. observing one's mentor across the operative table). In open surgery this may have been sufficient considering the vantage point and additional options available to the clinician that laparoscopy does not offer (see Figure 8.1). In minimally invasive surgery (MIS) the surgeon must operate from outside the patient's

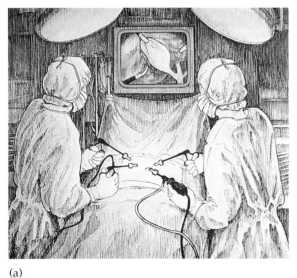

(a)

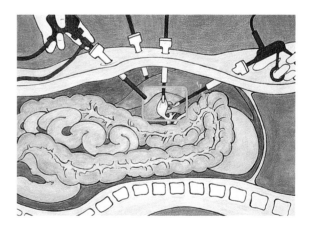

(b)

Figure 8.1 (a) In minimally invasive surgery (MIS), the surgeon must operate from outside the patient's body. The elimination of a major incision for access substantially reduces patient trauma, postoperative recovery times and the cost of the procedure. MIS does, however, require the surgeon to operate remotely, with long instruments, viewing the surgical site by way of a small camera and TV monitor. (b) The camera system views only a 1–2″ diameter portion of the surgical site, showing only the operating tips of the surgical instruments. In fact, over 90% of the instrument shaft length is outside the surgeon's view. Radiofrequency (RF) energy is used for cutting and coagulating tissue in MIS surgery. The electrical characteristics of this energy make it possible for stray energy to cause patient injury in the form of unintended, and unobserved electrosurgical burns along the instrument shaft outside the surgeon's view.

body. This change from open surgery sets the stage for the laparoscopist to work remotely (outside the patient) which, logistically, does not have the advantages offered in open surgery when it comes to controlling bleeding. Bleeding and other surgical misadventures are avoided by good surgical technique, but when misadventures are encountered the full complement of tools is needed to insure the best outcome for the patient. This chapter is intended to introduce the reader to the fundamental applications of electrosurgical energy with in-depth discussion on the biophysics of each. It will also introduce the reader to the hidden risks of the application of electrosurgical energy during laparoscopy and the preventive options offered to allow the surgeon to apply this form of energy with the same safety as with open surgical access procedures.

The use of high-frequency electrical energy for surgical application dates back nearly a century. Electrosurgery is the generation and delivery of RF current between an active electrode and a dispersive electrode in order to elevate the tissue temperature for the purpose of cutting, fulguration and desiccation. In contrast to electrocautery, the electric current actually passes through the tissue. Harvey W Cushing with the assistance of William T Bovie was the first surgeon to document the principles in depth regarding both the art as well as the biophysics of electrosurgery. These early documents detailed his appreciation of Dr. Bovie's device and his encouragement regarding the versatility of this energy source. It truly changed the course of neurosurgery and other surgeons' views during his practising years for the potential uses of electrosurgical energy. The intent of this chapter is to highlight the practical application of the three modalities and how to maximize their intended uses. With the rapid shift to MIS technique, there is a detailed discussion about how electrosurgical energy is delivered. The pitfalls associated with laparoscopy are also covered.

Temperature and Tissue

Energy cannot be created or destroyed, but it can be converted from one form to another. In electrosurgery electrosurgical current is converted to heat in the tissue for the purpose of vaporizing/cutting and coagulation. The principles are quite similar to those of laser energy when converted to heat within the tissue:

- At or above 44°C tissue necrosis starts.
- At or above 70°C coagulation begins when collagen is denatured and the clotting mechanism is activated.
- At or above 90°C tissue desiccation begins when the tissue is dehydrated.
- At or above 100°C vaporization occurs when the tissue is converted into a vapor.
- At or above 200°C carbonization starts; this black eschar can only result from fulguration (Table 8.1).

How Electrical Energy Affects Tissue Temperature

The three electrical properties that cause temperature rise are:

- Current (I).
- Voltage (V).
- Resistance (impedance) (R).

To help understand the terms and meanings for electrical energy a direct analogy to water or hydraulics energy source will be made. The water tower in Figure 8.2a presents a hydraulic energy source for the purpose of performing work. Figure 8.2b shows an equivalent electrosurgical tower with the electrical terms, current, voltage, and resistance

Table 8.1 Tissue effects of electrosurgery at different temperatures.

	Temperature (°C)					
	34–44	44–50	50–80	80–100	100–200	>200
Visible effect	None	None	Blanching	Shrinkage	Steam 'popcorn'	Carbonization cratering
Delayed effect	Edema	Necrosis	Sloughing	Sloughing	Ulceration	Larger crater
Mechanism	Vasodilation Inflammation	Disruption of cell metabolism	Collagen denaturation	Desiccation	Vaporization	Combustion of tissue hydrocarbons

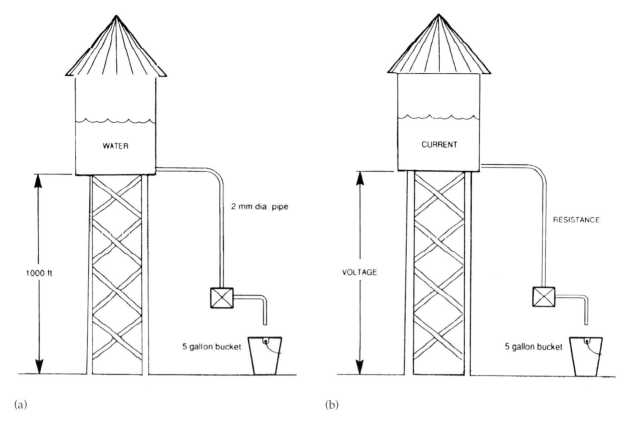

Figure 8.2 (a) Hydraulic energy source. (b) An equivalent electrosurgical tower.

inserted. This direct relationship is important in overcoming the mystique of electrosurgical unit (ESU) modalities.

Ohm's law, I = V/R shows the relationship between the properties of electrosurgical energy.

Power Formula

The energy the surgeon induces into tissue creating a rise in temperature is equal to wattage multiplied by time, where watts (W) = V × I. The ratio of V:I of the electrosurgical waveforms is what is primarily responsible for the observed effects on the tissue when time and electrode size are kept equal.

Power Density

Power density = (I density)^2 × resistivity. Power density is the relationship of the size of the active electrode in contact with the tissue and the effect on the tissue at a given energy setting. In non-contact modalities (i.e. cutting and fulgurating) this would be equivalent to the sparking area between the active electrode and the tissue. The exact surface area of the electrode in contact with the tissue is important when calculating power density only

when desiccating. During fulguration and cutting the electrode is not in contact, therefore the power density can only be approximated.

In general, the larger the electrode surface area the lower the power density, the smaller the electrode surface area the higher the power density.

Time

The time element is the primary component determining the depth and degree of tissue necrosis at a given energy setting. Many other components contribute to this discussion, but time is important as will be demonstrated in the following sections.

Cut – Fulgurate – Desiccate

Cutting, fulguration and desiccation are the three distinct therapeutic effects to tissue that electrosurgical energy has been reduced to in practise. Unfortunately most electrosurgical units are labeled simply by two modes, 'cut' and 'coag'. These terms do not help in the present confusion pertaining to the optimal use of the energy.

Cut

A high current, low voltage (continuous) waveform elevates the tissue's temperature, rapidly producing vaporization or division of tissue with the least effect on coagulation (hemostasis) to the walls of the incision (Figure 8.3a, cutting waveform with electrosurgical unit (ESU) set at 50 W). During optimal electrosurgical cutting the current travels through a steam bubble (Figure 8.3b) between the active electrode and the tissue. Therefore it is important to recognize that electrosurgical cutting is a non-contact means of dissection. The electrode floats through the tissue and there is very little tactile response transmitted to the surgeon's hand. The continuous waveform is analogous to the garden valve shown in Figure 8.2a with a constant even flow of water. Due to the constant flow of current and the lowest possible voltage to dissect, the width and depth of necrosis to the walls of the incision are minimal. Therefore the ratio of high current to low voltage within the waveform produces less necrosis. If the electrode is allowed to remain stationary or is slowed, the maximum temperature attained is increased as well as the width of thermal damage to the tissue.

Blend 1, 2 and 3

With a ratio modification of the cutting waveform (i.e. changing the current, voltage product) by interrupting current and increasing the voltage, the waveform becomes non-continuous with a series of energy packets consisting of higher voltage and reduced current per time. Total energy remains the same, but the ratio of voltage and current are modified to increase hemostasis during dissection with electrosurgical current (Figure 8.4).

This would be analogous to the garden valve pulsing the water, with an increased height to the water tower to make up for the reduction of hydraulic energy as a result of reducing the time that the water is allowed to flow. In using the blend modes as well the electrode should float through the tissue. The blend waveforms will require a longer period of time to dissect the same length of incision than the cutting waveform due to the interrupted delivery of current at the same power setting. With this increased time comes an increase in thermal spread from the voltage component of the blend waveform. This increased thermal spread improves coagulation of small vessels while dissecting. When needed these blend modes can be a very valuable option in controlling bleeding, as needed when dissecting.

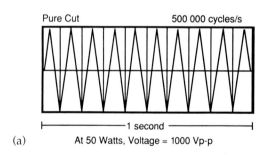

(a)   At 50 Watts, Voltage = 1000 Vp-p

ELECTROSURGICAL CUTTING

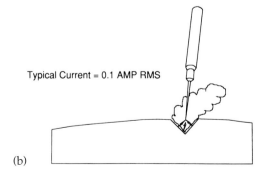

Typical Current = 0.1 AMP RMS

(b)

Figure 8.3 (a) Electrosurgical cutting waveform. (b) The electrode is not in contact with the tissue.

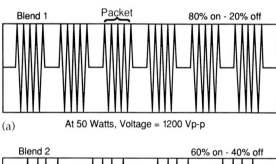

(a)   At 50 Watts, Voltage = 1200 Vp-p

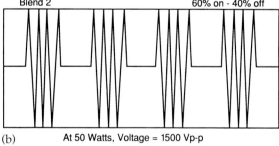

(b)   At 50 Watts, Voltage = 1500 Vp-p

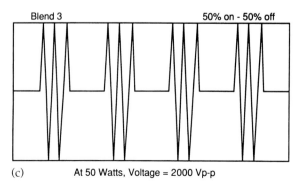

(c)   At 50 Watts, Voltage = 2000 Vp-p

Figure 8.4 (a) Blend 1 waveform. (b) Blend 2 waveform. (c) Blend 3 waveform. Vp-p, voltage peak to peak.

On the other hand, if used and not needed the increase in the width of necrosis may result in a higher postoperative infection level as a direct result of the increased amount of tissue necrosis. Also the amount of smoke plume will be increased at laparoscopy using high blend or coagulation modes. Blend 1 causes slightly increased hemostasis, blend 2 moderately increased hemostasis with blend 3 showing a marked increase in hemostasis while dissecting.

When dissecting tissue with a cut or blended mode the ESU should be activated first before the electrode touches the tissue. A feathering or light stroking similar to when painting with a two bristle paint brush for touch-up or fine detail work needs to be simulated. This will allow for the maximum power density as the electrode approaches the tissue just before contact. This will help initialize vaporization or dissection of tissue. In theory and in practise with optimum technique and control setting the force required to dissect tissue would be 0 g of pressure between the electrode and the tissue.

Fulgurate

A high-voltage, low-current non-continuous waveform (highly damped) is designed to coagulate by means of spraying long electrical sparks to the tissue (Figure 8.5a – coagulation (fulguration) waveform set at 50 W). The most common use of fulguration is when coagulation is needed in an area that is oozing such as in a capillary or arteriole bed where a discrete bleeder cannot be identified. The benefit of fulguration is its ability to arrest oozing emanating from a large area in a most efficient manner. Cardiovascular, urological and general surgeons have relied on fulguration for their most demanding applications (i.e., hepatic resections, bleeding from a bladder tumor resection and surface bleeding on the heart). With fulguration a very superficial eschar is produced, therefore the depth of necrosis is minimal as a result of the defocusing of the power density. By drawing the electrode away from the tissue, the power density goes down. A great deal of the energy is lost in the air that the current passes through. Fulguration like electrosurgical cutting is a non-contact modality.

Fulguration can be initiated in two ways:

- By very slowly approaching the tissue until a spark jumps to the tissue whereupon a raining effect of sparks will be maintained until the electrode is withdrawn or the tissue is carbonized to the point where the sparks cease.
- Bouncing the electrode off the tissue will result in a raining effect of sparks to the tissue without the painstaking effort of approaching the tissue until a spark jumps without touching.

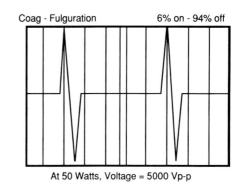

(a) Coag - Fulguration   6% on - 94% off

At 50 Watts, Voltage = 5000 Vp-p

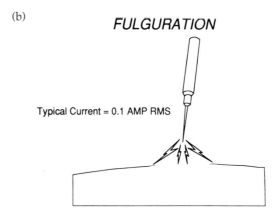

(b) *FULGURATION*

Typical Current = 0.1 AMP RMS

Figure 8.5 (a) Fulguration waveform. (b) Electrode not in contact with tissue.

Electrosurgical fulguration is the most effective means of arresting this form of bleeding.

Desiccation

Any waveform will desiccate due to the electrode being in contact with the tissue for the first time (Figure 8.6). Regardless of the current voltage ratio with the electrode in contact with the tissue, the magnitude of energy in watts is of the greatest importance. Desiccation is another form of coagulation. Most surgeons do not make a distinction between fulguration and desiccation, but refer to both as coagulation. The application of electrosurgical current by means of direct contact with the tissue will now result in all of the energy set on the ESU being converted into heat within the tissue. By contrast, in both cutting and fulguration mode a significant amount of the electrical energy converted to heat went into heating up the atmosphere or air/carbon dioxide between the electrode and the tissue. Therefore with contact coagulation/desiccation the increased energy delivered into the tissue results in deep necrosis, as deep as it is wide, as observed on the surface where the electrode makes contact (see Figure 8.6).

DESICCATION

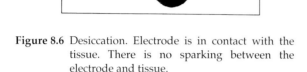

Typical Current
= 0.5 AMP RMS

Figure 8.6 Desiccation. Electrode is in contact with the tissue. There is no sparking between the electrode and tissue.

The most common application of desiccation is when a discrete bleeding vessel is encountered and a hemostat is introduced to occlude the vessel first by mechanical pressure, then the electrosurgical energy is applied to the body of the hemostat. In this way the current must pass through the hemostat into the tissue grasped by the jaws and back to the patient return electrode. The coaptation of vessels was documented as producing a collagen chain reaction resulting in a fibrous bonding of the dehydrated denatured cells of the endothelium (Sigel and Dunn, 1965). Because the electrode is in good electrical contact with the tissue the voltage current ratio is not nearly as important as in cutting and fulgurating. In practical terms the cut/blend waveforms are superior for this application over the fulguration waveform when desiccation is desired. The primary reason is that the fulguration waveform will tend to spark through the coagulated tissue, resulting in voids in the bonding to the end of the vessel. Also when sparks occur at the electrode point of contact with tissue, the metal in the electrode will heat up rapidly, causing the tissue to adhere to the electrode when drawn off the target site. Bleeding will continue each time the tissue is pulled off due to adhesion from heat within the electrode.

In bipolar desiccation, the waveform plays a far more important role. Today, for the most part, the manufacturers have incorporated a continuous low-voltage, high-current waveform in the bipolar output to maximize the effect on desiccation. With the older models, the manufacturers allowed the surgeon to select either a continuous cut, blend or fulguration waveform when desiccating in bipolar. The lack of understanding on the physician's part, in combination with the literature not being clear on the tissue effect when bipolar desiccation is performed with these waveforms, led to a number of documented associated problems (Soderstrom, 1982). Therefore

at this time the generally accepted waveform for bipolar desiccation is a continuous low-voltage, high-current waveform. The author recommends that when bipolar desiccation is critical a newer model ESU with a dedicated continuous bipolar waveform is used. If one must use an ESU that allows you to select cut/blend, fulguration and bipolar currents, it is best to start with the pure cut (continuous) waveform for best results. When performing desiccation, patience is the key to good results. Typically the power density is much lower when desiccating. The physical size of the active electrodes is therefore larger. The larger electrode or contact area relative to tissue will require longer activation times to attain the desired therapeutic effect. If higher energy is introduced to speed up the desiccation process, this will most likely be counterproductive. Higher energy levels will increase the temperature to the tissue adjacent to the electrode/s, potentially forcing the current to spark through the necrosis, resulting in fulguration rather than desiccation. Fulguration or sparking immediately stops the deep heating process and starts to carbonize the surface of the tissue only. Therefore when sparking is observed during desiccation, it is wise to stop and reduce the power or pulse the current by keying on and off the ESU to overcome this natural tendency of the electrosurgical energy. Sparking is not needed or wanted when desiccating. It causes tissue sticking and creates uneven necrosis and may compromise the intent to coapt the vessel. To assist the surgeon when desiccating, an ammeter (Model EM-2+ ammeter, Electroscope, Inc., Boulder, CO, USA) may be used to control the amount of current as well as to determine end-point coagulation/desiccation. This will help confirm the visual effect seen by the surgeon. The ammeter will only show current flow when the tissue still contains electrolytic fluid. Total or complete desiccation occurs after dehydration has taken place.

Inherent Risks

Since the inception of monopolar electrosurgery, there have been three potential sites for patient burns due to the presence of electrosurgical current – one intended, two unintended. The intended site is at the active electrode where the unit is used to cut, fulgurate or desiccate the tissue in surgery. Due to its design, the active electrode has a high power density to heat tissue rapidly. This electrode can burn the patient severely if not kept in control at all times. Therefore the author strongly recommends that the active electrode is stored in an insulated holster or tray when not in use.

There are two unintended sites:

- The first is a consequence of current division. Current division to alternate ground points to the patient can only occur on ground referenced ESUs.
- Second, the patient may be burned due to a fault condition at the site of the patient return electrode, i.e. partial detachment or a manufacturing defect that forces the current returning to the ESU via a high current density.

The patient return electrode (ground plate) has an approximate surface area of 20 square inches or larger when properly applied. Therefore very little temperature rise occurs at this site under normal conditions.

Both of the potential burn sites have been overcome by improved design within the newer ESUs developed in the last two decades. These safety circuits or features are available on most ESUs sold within the past ten years. The two major advancements in overcoming these risks are isolated electrosurgical outputs and contact quality monitors (see below). These two technological advances have reduced the potential for patient burns while performing classic open electrosurgical procedures. These features are now found on equipment supplied by the major manufacturers of ESUs such as Aspen (Denver, CO, USA), ERBE (Germany), Eschmann (UK) and Valleylab (Boulder, CO, USA).

Isolated Electrosurgical Outputs

Isolated ESUs were introduced in the early 1970s. The primary purpose of their introduction was to prevent alternate ground site burns due to current division. Today the number of alternate site burns as a direct result of current division is essentially zero with the introduction of isolated ESUs. As a small percentage of hospitals use ground reference ESUs it is therefore wise to qualify the type of ESU in service at your hospital regarding the type of output.

Contact Quality Monitors

Contact quality monitoring circuits were introduced in the early 1980s. The primary purpose of their introduction was to prevent burns at the patient return electrode site. The contact quality monitor incorporated a dual section patient return electrode and circuit for the purpose of evaluating the total impedance of the patient return electrode during surgery. Therefore during the course of surgery if the patient return electrode became compromised the contact quality circuit would inhibit the electrosurgical generator output based on this dual section patient return electrode and circuit combination. This feature has essentially eliminated the secondary unintended patient burns (i.e. those that appear at the site of the patient return electrode).

Laparoscopic Issues

Electrosurgery has been used in laparoscopic surgery by gynecologists for the past two and a half decades (Rioux, 1973). With the major shift since 1990 by general, urologic, thoracic surgeons and gynecologists performing advanced minimal access laparoscopic techniques, greater attention to the safe delivery of electrosurgical energy needs to be discussed. The purpose of this section is to address the real issues pertaining to its safe use in laparoscopy, in a similar detailed manner as the potential hazards discussed previously regarding the general use of electrosurgery in open surgery. Additionally, options available to help minimize or eliminate the potential of unintended burns within the peritoneal cavity during laparoscopic surgery will be described.

There are two potential hazards in the use of electrosurgical energy during laparoscopy (Voyles and Tucker, 1992). They are a direct result of two factors:

- How access is obtained to the peritoneal cavity through the trocar cannulas;
- The laparoscope views less than 10% of the total electrosurgical probe.

In passing the electrosurgical active electrode through the access channels there is potential for unintended burns.

Most laparoscopic accessories are approximately 35 cm long. The laparoscopic images viewed on the monitor show a small portion, typically less than 5 cm of the distal end of the device. Therefore, the active electrode used for the delivery of the electrosurgical energy has insulation covering most of the electrode. Unfortunately 90% or more of this insulated portion of the electrode is out of the viewing image seen on the monitor. Therefore, if a breakdown of the insulation occurs on the shaft of the electrode out of view from the operator, a severe burn may occur on the bowel or other organs near or touching the electrode at this site (Figure 8.7). These burns may not be noticed during the course of surgery and may result in severe postoperative complications. It is most important to examine or have biomedical staff set up a routine inspection of these electrodes periodically.

The second hazard that exists is one of capacitively coupled energy into other metal

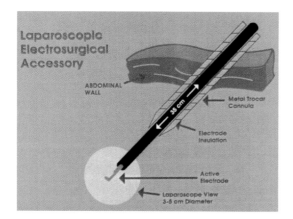

(a)

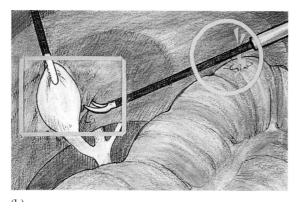

(b)

Figure 8.7 (a) Full view of electrosurgical accessory in the peritoneal cavity. (b) Full view of electrosurgical accessory with insulation failure.

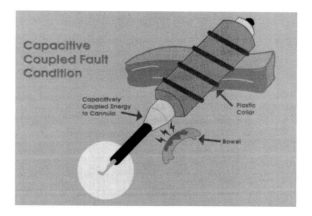

(a)

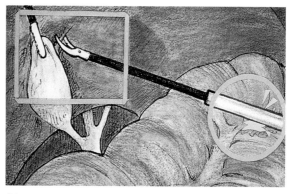

(b)

Figure 8.8 (a) Hybrid trocar cannula that blocks the capacitive current from the abdominal wall. (b) Capacitive coupling with dangerous stray pathway back to patient return electrode.

laparoscopic instruments or trocar cannulae. The principle of how capacitance occurs requires a degree of understanding of electrical physics beyond the scope of this chapter. The bottom line is that 5–40% of the power level that the ESU is set to deliver, can be coupled or transferred into the (10 cm) trocar cannula. This energy in itself may not be dangerous providing it is allowed to pass through a low power density pathway such as the all metal (conductive) trocar cannula inserted into the abdominal wall and returned to the patient return electrode. The problem arises when this energy is allowed or made to pass through a high power density pathway (Figure 8.8). This can happen for example with the part-plastic (non-conductive) and part-metal (conductive) trocar cannulas on the market. Some trocar manufacturers supply a plastic thread to the metal cannula tube to help hold the cannula in the abdominal wall when the laparoscopic electrode is positioned in and out of the cannula port (see Figure 8.8). To avoid this hazard the author strongly recommends that the electrosurgical active laparoscopic electrode is passed through an all-metal or all-plastic trocar cannula.

Capacitive coupling can occur to a lesser degree by crossing another laparoscopic instrument with the electrosurgical laparoscopic electrode within the peritoneal cavity (e.g. atraumatic grasper). The energy transfer to these instruments can range from 1–10% of the power set on the ESU. Some caution should be taken under these conditions, especially during long activation times.

The issue of capacitive coupling was first detected when performing operative single-puncture laparascopic procedures (Corson, 1974; Engel, 1975). The laparoscope has an operating channel (30–40 cm long) to pass various instruments through. It was observed that when a plastic 10/12 mm cannula was used to pass the operating laparoscope through that the distal end of the metal laparoscope could deliver a portion of the power (40–80%) set on the ESU, and burns to adjacent tissue were documented. Therefore during single-puncture operative laparoscopy where electrosurgery may be used, only all-metal trocar cannulae should be used to pass both the laparoscope and electrosurgical electrode into the peritoneal cavity.

There was a strong recommendation made to this effect by the FDA in the late 1970s.

The all-metal trocar cannula is also beneficial in multiple-puncture laparoscopic procedures in the event of the active electrode accidentally touching the end of the metal laparoscope during activation. The metal trocar cannula will allow this energy to pass safely into the abdominal wall via a low power density pathway. If a plastic cannula were used, the current may exit to the bowel or other organs touching the laparoscope (Figure 8.9), out of view of the

monitor. This is due to the plastic cannula blocking the directly coupled energy from being safely passed into the abdominal wall and back to the patient return electrode.

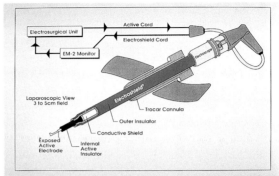

5mm Integrated Electroshield® Electrode Diagram

(a)

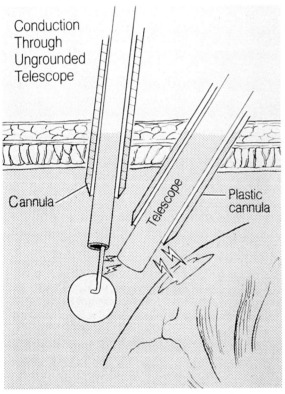

Figure 8.9 Full view showing how direct coupling may prove hazardous when a plastic cannula is used.

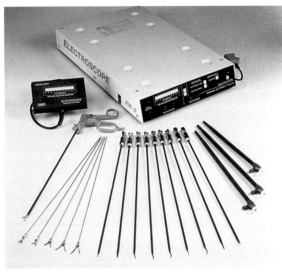

(b)

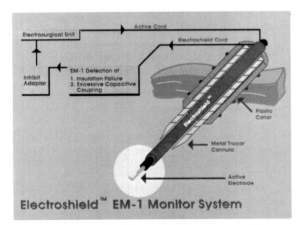

Figure 8.10 Electroshield monitoring system (Electroscope) dynamically detects any insulation faults and shields against capacitive coupling.

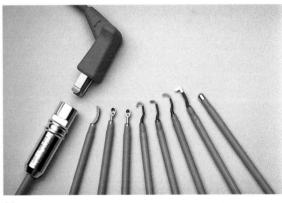

(c)

Figure 8.11 The Electroshield system for use in laparoscopy. (a) Cut-away view showing the conductive shield that diverts stray current to the EM-2+ monitor. (b) EM-2 Electroshield monitor and related shielded reusable electrodes. (c) Electroshield cord which connects the active electrode to the ESU and AEM.

There are increasing reports of bowel perforation and the delayed presentation of peritonitis (Willson *et al.*, 1994). The need to address stray electrosurgical energy (capacitive coupling and insulation failure) out of the view of the laparoscope and therefore out of the control of the surgeon is essential to maintain the same level of safety as with the open surgical technique.

Recently an integrated shielded 5 mm reusable (fixed and hinged) array of instruments that are dynamically monitored for stray energy in the form of capacitive coupling and insulation failure have been released on the market (Emergency Care Research Institute, 1995). Electroscope, Inc of Boulder, CO, USA has released Electroshield-R, Model EM-2+ Monitoring System, which protects against both these primary hazards while performing laparoscopic application of electrosurgical energy. The Electroshield system features a reusable shield (Figure 8.10) that surrounds 'existing' dissecting and coagulating laparoscopic electrodes as well as a totally integrated 5 mm (fixed and hinged) array of reusable instruments (Figure 8.11). Electroshield Monitor (EM-2+) dynamically detects insulation faults and shields against capacitive coupling out of the view of the surgeon. If an unsafe condition exists, the Electroshield system (see Figure 8.11a) automatically deactivates the generator before a burn can occur. The EM-2+ provides the surgeon with continous active electrode monitoring (AEM). AEM was developed for the same reason as contact quality monitoring circuits: 'to protect the patient from being exposed to a hidden risk of the surgical staff' (Kirshenbaum and Temple, 1996).

The use of ESUs with contact quality monitoring, isolated outputs and AEM optimizes patient safety when performing laparoscopy.

With this technological advancement, electrosurgical energy can be used in laparoscopy with the same efficacy and safety as in classical open surgical procedures.

Summary

Compared with other energy sources electrosurgical energy has by far the most diverse capabilities. The technological advances in performance and safety have positioned this device as one of the more useful tools in a surgeon's armamentarium. As with any surgical tool or energy source, education and skill are required. This introduction to the principles of the biophysics of electrical energy on tissue and the safety considerations should help further the clinician's understanding of this powerful surgical tool.

References

Corson SL (1974) Electrosurgical hazards in laparoscopy. *Journal of the American Medical Association* **227(11)**: 1261.

Emergency Care Research Institute (1995) Focus on laparoscopy. *Health Devices* **24(1)**: 4–38.

Engel T (1975) Electrosurgical dynamics of laparoscopic sterilization. *Journal of Reproductive Medicine* **15** (1).

Kirshenbaum G, Temple DR (1996) Active electrode monitoring in laparoscopy: the surgeon's perspective. *Surgical Services Management* **2(2)**: 46–49.

Sigel B, Dunn MR (1965) The mechanism of blood vessel closure by high frequency electrocoagulation. *Surgery, Gynecology and Obstetrics* **121**: 823–831.

Rioux JE (1973) Laparoscopic tubal sterilization; sparking and its control. *La Vie Medicale au Canada Fransçais* **2**: 760–766.

Soderstrom NM (1982) Hazards of laparoscopic sterilization. *Gynecology and Obstetrics*, Ch. 24, pp. 1–6. Harper & Row.

Voyles CR, Tucker RD (1992) Education and engineering solutions for potential problems with laparoscopic monopolar electrosurgery. *American Journal of Surgery* **164**: 57–62.

Willson PD, McAnena OJ, Peters EE (1994) A fatal complication of diathermy in laparoscopic surgery. *Minimally Invasive Therapy* **3(1)**: 19–20.

9

Tissue Effects of Lasers, Electrosurgery and Ultrasonic Scalpels

JORG KECKSTEIN* AND CHRIS SUTTON†

*Department of Obstetrics and Gynecology, Landeskrankenhaus, Villach, Austria
†Royal Surrey County Hospital, Guildford, The Chelsea and Westminster Hospital, London, and Imperial College School of Medicine, University of London, UK

Introduction

In surgery great importance has always been attached to the techniques of incision, preparation and hemostasis. With the advent of endoscopic operations most surgical techniques required either modification or complete change. A profound knowledge of the interaction between biologic tissue and implements used is of vital importance for achieving optimal results.

The method most commonly practiced in surgical medicine is that using operative therapeutic heat to destroy or coagulate tissue. Table 9.1 shows the various incision and coagulation procedures available for biologic tissue. Although the scalpel is still the most inexpensive and most commonly used instrument for the separation of tissue, its use in conjunction with endoscopic instruments is rather limited.

Bleeding control during cutting affords a good overall view of the operational site and consequently reduces operating time. Here the laser

Table 9.1 Different instruments for incision used in endoscopic surgery.

Scalpel
Electric blade – high-frequency (HF) surgery
Laser
Ultrasound dissector
Jet of liquid
Plasma scalpel
Microwave scalpel
HF-controlled rare gas jet

systems and HF surgery come into their own. The tissue changes brought about by these instruments are chiefly due to thermal effects. In Table 9.2, the correlation between tissue effect and temperature is demonstrated.

Electrosurgery

The term 'diathermy' is often used in connection with HF surgery and is in this context a regrettable misnomer. In actual fact, diathermy stands for the application of extremely HF alternating current (>1 GHz) to yield heating of entire body parts. In contrast, the term 'HF surgery' applies to alternating current with a frequency range starting at 300 kHz and used for incision and coagulation.

Table 9.2 Thermal tissue effect of different temperatures.

Temperature (°C)	Tissue effect
37–43	Heating
43–45	Retraction
>50	Reduction of enzyme activity
45–60	Denaturation of protein coagulation
90–100	Drying
>100	Boiling point of water, destruction of cell membrane
>150	Carbonization
>300	Vaporization
>500	Burning

Electric current renders living tissue electrically conductive, the degree of conductivity depending upon the electrolyte content. When electrical current passes through living tissue, three qualitatively different endogenous effects can be observed:

- Electrolytic effect.
- Stimulation of nerves and muscles.
- Thermic effect.

Cutting with HF surgical instruments requires the presence of a high voltage (peak voltage of approximately 200 V) between the electrode and the tissue. Such HF excludes stimulation of nerves and muscles likely to interfere with the surgical procedure. It is produced by a small active electrode whose outgoing current is highly concentrated on tissue contact, but is then dispersed in the body, eventually rendering the electrode quasineutral. This means that an effect is only produced at the point of entry. The resulting electric arcs (Figure 9.1) are like microscopic flashes and appear when the electrode and tissue are within close proximity of each other. If the voltage is below 200 V the tissue cannot be cut.

In addition to the cutting effect, a variable coagulation effect (see Figure 9.1) is produced along the incision line. Both these effects depend upon parameters such as peak voltage, frequency, modulation, cutting and coagulation speed, shape of electrode, and tissue.

Experimental studies show a close association between 'peak voltage' and coagulation zone. The correlation between the depth of coagulation and voltage is demonstrated in Figure 9.2. Low voltage current produces incisions with little coagulation effect, while high voltages create incisions with broader coagulation zones (see Figure 9.2).

The 'frequency' of HF current ranges between 400–40 000 kHz and is produced by a tube generator and a spark generator. For cutting, unmodu-

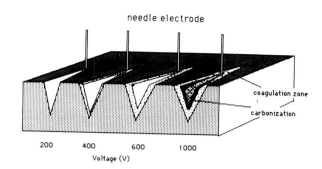

Figure 9.2 Tissue effect of HF surgery. Correlation between intensity of voltage and coagulation effect. A relatively low peak voltage of 200 V is used to produce cuts with small necrosis zones.

lated HF current (Figure 9.3) is produced by the tube generator. The spark generator provides amplitude-modulated HF voltages yielding a greater coagulation effect (see Figure 9.3). A combination of the different HF 'voltage modulations' permits tissue effects to be varied.

Another factor influencing tissue effect is the 'cutting speed' of the electrode. When the electrode is moved at high speed, there is little coagulation effect (Figure 9.4). Slowing down the rate increases the coagulation effect.

The 'shape' of the cutting electrodes is of decisive influence on tissue effect. The thicker the electrode, the deeper the coagulation zone. Thin needle electrodes used in microsurgery or wire loops have

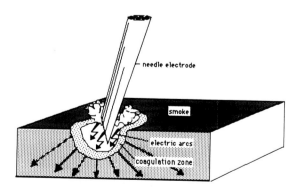

Figure 9.1 Incision with HF current. A cut is produced when a peak voltage of over 200 V is reached between the electrode and the tissue, resulting in vaporization of the tissue.

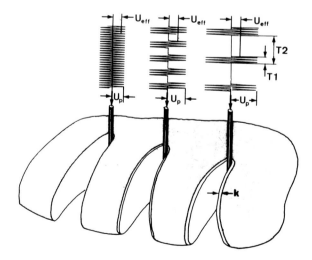

Figure 9.3 Different tissue effects depending upon different voltages and modulation. The depth of the coagulation effect increases with increasing peak value U_p. Some HF surgical equipment offers the option to modulate electric current, enabling the surgeon to determine the quality of the cut. (Published by kind permission of G. Farin, Erbe, Tübingen.)

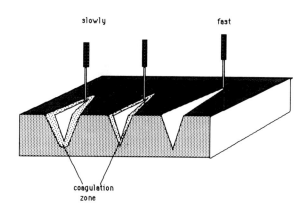

Figure 9.4 Tissue effect of HF surgery in relation to the cutting rate.

poorer coagulation properties than knife- or ball-shaped electrodes (Figure 9.5). Knife-shaped electrodes permit very smooth incisions, but create a larger coagulation border. When the electrode is used to aid coagulation its broad end is pressed against the incision surface.

Coagulation

Biologic tissue to be coagulated requires a temperature build-up of 70°C. Table 9.2 shows the different tissue effects in relation to temperature.

With HF electric alternating current used for heating biologic tissue, tissue temperature rises in proportion to tissue resistance. A temperature increase beyond 70°C may trigger additional problems. Dehydration, vaporization, or carbonization may interfere with the coagulation effect and thus hamper the determination of the size of the coagulation zone.

The lack of homogeneity of the tissue's electrical and thermal properties causes the temperature to rise at varying rates, rendering control of the coagulation effect quite difficult. The coagulation of tissue is a dynamic process and presents the surgeon attempting to obtain a specific tissue effect with a variety of complex problems.

The size of the coagulation zone can be determined by the type of technique applied and by the rate of coagulation. There are three different coagulation modes (Figure 9.6):

- Soft coagulation.
- Forced coagulation.
- Spray coagulation.

SOFT COAGULATION (SEE FIGURE 9.6a)

This refers to voltages below 200 V. The electrodes are brought into direct contact with the tissue.

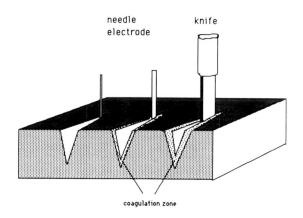

Figure 9.5 Tissue effect of HF surgery with different shapes of electrode: small coagulation zone with needle electrode; large coagulation zone with thick blades.

Figure 9.6 Coagulation modes with different techniques and electrodes. Each technique has a different peak voltage and modulation of the HF current. (a) Soft coagulation. (b) Forced coagulation. (c) Spray coagulation. (Published by kind permission of G. Farin, Erbe, Tübingen.)

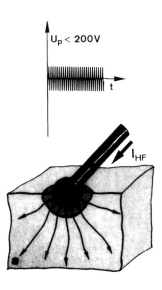

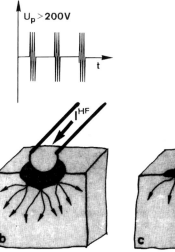

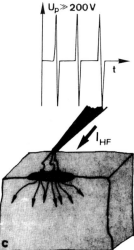

Unmodulated HF voltages with an absence of electric arcs exclude tissue vaporization or carbonization. The tissue is heated gradually according to coagulation time and electric resistance of the tissue. Because of the low voltage the tissue does not become carbonized.

FORCED COAGULATION (SEE FIGURE 9.6b)

This uses small electrodes and is characterized by electric arcs generated between the coagulation electrode and tissue to obtain deeper coagulation. This specific mode requires voltages of over 500 V. HF current needs to be modulated and voltages must not be too high as this creates a cutting effect.

SPRAY COAGULATION (SEE FIGURE 9.6c)

HF voltages with peak values of a few kV are recommended for 'spray coagulation'. With this technique, which is particularly used for surface coagulation, long electric arcs produced between the electrode and tissue make direct contact superfluous.

Monopolar versus Bipolar HF Surgery

Density distribution of the HF current is chiefly determined by the technique applied. Totally different results are achieved when using monopolar as opposed to bipolar HF current.

The size of a coagulum produced by the monopolar and bipolar technique is depicted in Figure 9.7.

Laser

In the field of medicine the carbon dioxide (CO_2), neodymium:yttrium-aluminum-garnet (Nd:YAG), argon, potassium titanyl phosphate (KTP), and dye lasers have been in use for some time now and have proved worthwhile, whereas the excimer laser, so far chiefly used in research, is only just beginning to gain ground in the medical field.

Table 9.3 shows the emission wavelengths of lasers used in medicine. The aiming beam of the individual types of invisible lasers is the helium–neon (He–Ne) laser. Each of these lasers has distinctive properties, which yield different tissue effects and thus allow specific applications (Figure 9.8).

We carried out a number of experimental *in vitro* studies to assess and compare CO_2, argon, and Nd:YAG laser performance, testing the cutting and coagulation effects on the extirpated uteri of pigs. Fibers of 600 µm diameter were chosen. To ensure uniform experimental conditions with regard to tissue tension and cutting velocity, equal-length strips of material were stretched on a portable cart and secured by weights. The laser guide was fixed on a

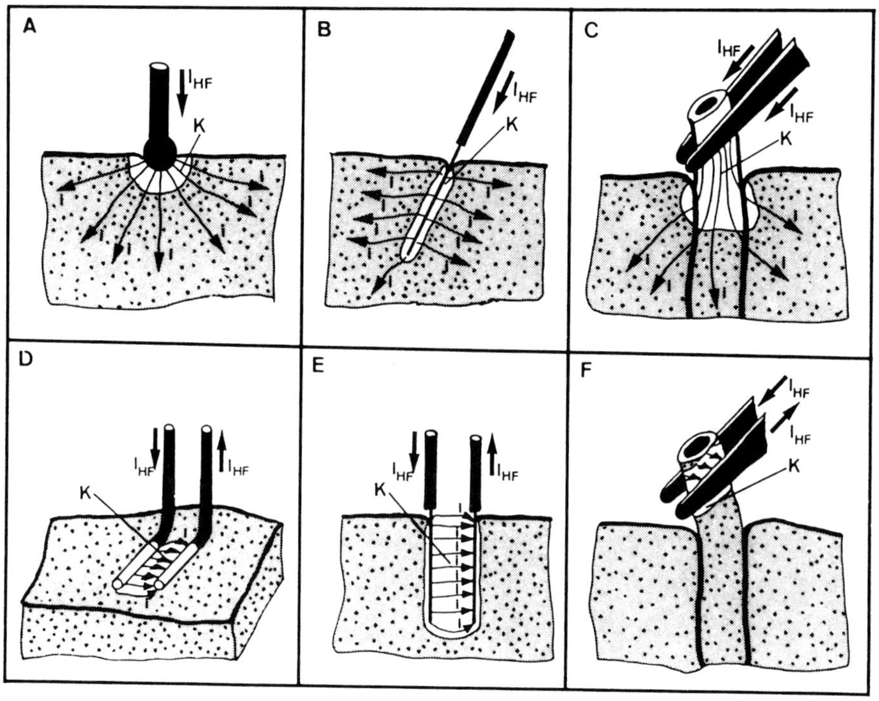

Figure 9.7 Tissue effect of monopolar and bipolar HF coagulation with different application techniques. (A–C) These depict monopolar coagulation with a ball electrode and a thin needle electrode for interstitial coagulation, and coagulation of a vessel by forceps. (D–F) In bipolar coagulation the current flow between the two electrodes affords better control of the coagulation effect. (K, coagulation zone, I, current.) (Published by kind permission of G. Farin, Erbe, Tübingen.)

Table 9.3 Different wavelengths of laser systems used in endoscopic surgery.

System	Wavelength
CO_2 laser	10.60 μm
Nd:YAG laser	1.06 μm or
	1.32 μm
Argon laser	488/514 nm
KTP laser	530 nm

support and the tissue moved with a speed of 2.5 cm s⁻¹ (Figure 9.9).

Criteria for effect evaluation were vaporization depth and coagulation of the cut borders. Results are shown in Figures 9.13–9.17 (see later).

Laser systems

CO_2 LASER

The coherent monochromatic CO_2 laser beam can be accurately focused through an optical lens system. The high-energy laser beam passes through air and is absorbed as it hits liquid or solid objects. It can thus be used for precise surgical work such as tissue incision, vaporization and coagulation. Body tissue with a water content of 80–90% absorbs the laser energy very rapidly.

The tissue is incised by heating intracellular and extracellular water to boiling point, resulting in the formation of steam. The energy of a continuously emitted CO_2 laser beam creates an incision by tissue vaporization. This makes the laser eminently suitable for surgery. Some of the debris is carbonized as it passes through the beam, some ignites and burns, thus creating the 'laser plume'.

The defocused laser beam has low energy density and causes a rapid rise of tissue temperature, with gradual fluid vaporization, dehydration and carbonization.

Histologic examination of sections derived from laser wounds of various organs (Figure 9.10) has shown that cellular damage occurs within a range of 500 μm from laser impact. The depth of thermal necrosis is, however, generally below 100 μm. With normal blood flow, veins and arteries up to 0.5 mm vascular diameter can be sealed by laser. The CO_2 laser has been the subject of many studies investigating the tissue effects of the laser beam (Bellina *et al.*, 1984; Badaway *et al.*, 1986; Baggish and ElBakry, 1986; Filmar *et al.*, 1986; McKenzie, 1986; Barbot *et al.*, 1987; Luciano *et al.*, 1987; Puolakkainen *et al.*, 1987; Keckstein, 1990).

Our experiments showed that with increasing power the vaporization effect intensified whereas the coagulation effect weakened (Keckstein, 1990). Various authors report a reduced rate of tissue necrosis when using the CO_2 laser in superpulse mode (Badaway *et al.*, 1986; Baggish and ElBakry, 1986; Luciano *et al.*, 1987; Keckstein, 1990). This is attributable to the interval between each laser pulse, which eliminates the constant tissue heating experienced with the continuous mode.

A recent development in CO_2 laser technology is the 'ultrapulse' closed facility. In this mode the laser beam is delivered as very high pulse energy bursts of up to 250 mJ and average powers of 950 mW. The advantage of this mode is char-free extremely precise cutting with minimal thermal damage to surrounding tissue, even at spot sizes up to 3 mm in diameter.

Figure 9.8 Different tissue effects of CO_2, Nd:YAG and argon lasers.

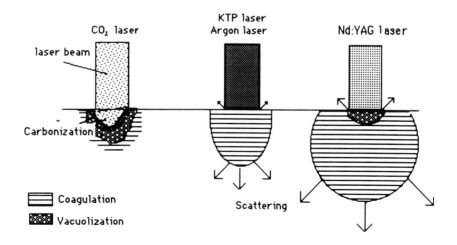

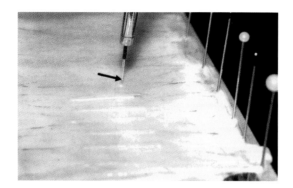

Figure 9.9 Experimental study of tissue effect with different laser systems. The picture shows a bare fiber (arrow) for the use of Nd:YAG laser in non-contact technique.

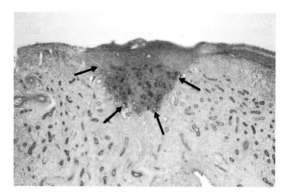

Figure 9.11 Tissue effect of Nd:YAG laser. The section demonstrates a deep coagulation effect (arrows) without any vaporization effect.

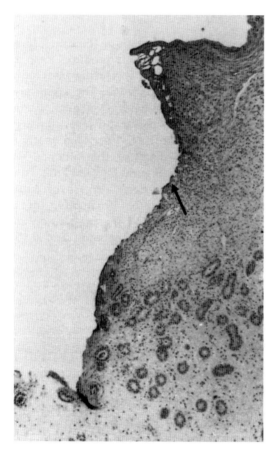

Figure 9.10 Incision with the CO_2 laser. The depth of thermal necrosis is less than 100 µm (arrow).

THE ND:YAG LASER

In contrast to the CO_2 laser, the beam of the Nd:YAG laser has a greater depth of tissue penetration, yielding totally different tissue effects (Figures 9.8, 9.11). The amount of energy available does not usually suffice for instant tissue vaporization. Thus,

brief laser application only produces coagulation (see Figure 9.11). With increasing time of application, tissue temperature rises to approximately 100 °C. The ensuing tissue dehydration impairs heat conduction, causing a further rise in temperature. Once the laser-treated surface is dry and begins to carbonize, the absorption properties of the tissue change. The result is a vaporization effect.

Due to its great depth of tissue penetration the Nd:YAG laser beam is capable of coagulating, shrinking, and hence sealing blood vessels of up to 5 mm diameter.

ARGON LASER/KTP LASER

The depth of penetration of the argon laser lies between 0.5–2.5 mm. Its applicability ranges between that of the CO_2 laser and the Nd:YAG laser. The KTP laser has a wavelengths similar to the argon laser and is equivalent to the argon laser in terms of practicability.

The argon laser produces a blue light and is a mixture of different wavelengths between 488–515 nm. The KTP 532 laser is essentially Nd:YAG laser energy passed through a potassium titanyl phosphate crystal, effectively halving the wavelength so that emerald green light at 532 nm emerges from the laser generator. One advantage of this laser is that at a flick of a switch a mirror is interposed, which stops the Nd:YAG laser energy from hitting the crystal and allows it to come out as pure Nd:YAG energy, effectively giving two lasers for the price of one.

Although these lasers have very similar wavelengths, it is obvious on using them clinically that the argon laser is more effective as a photocoagulating laser, whereas the KTP laser is a very effective cutting instrument, especially using a 300 µm fiber, and if the fiber is withdrawn from the tissue it acts as a very effective coagulator. The argon laser seems to be less effective at cutting, possibly because of the lower power at which it works, but also because the end of the fiber burns off during cutting. Continuous measurements of the loss of laser power at the fiber tip during cutting show a nearly exponential decrease of power output with length of cut; after 50 cm only 10% of the laser power exits from the fiber tip. Correspondingly the cutting efficiency is reduced to 30%, but without any influence on the coagulation zone (Keckstein *et al.*, 1988). The KTP 532 laser is particularly suitable for dealing with advanced endometriosis, especially ovarian endometriomas, and is also useful for dealing with hemorrhagic ovarian cysts and ectopic pregnancies.

Laser Techniques

LASER APPLICATION IN CONTACT AND NON-CONTACT TECHNIQUE – ARGON VERSUS Nd:YAG LASER

The use of Nd:YAG (Keckstein *et al.*, 1987; Wallwiener *et al.*, 1987; Grochmal, 1988; Kojiama *et al.*, 1988; Daniell, 1989; Keckstein, 1990) and argon lasers (Bellina *et al.*, 1983; Keye and Dixon, 1983; Keckstein *et al.*, 1988; Keckstein, 1990) for endoscopic operations has been described by a number of authors. The poor cutting properties of the Nd:YAG laser were overcome by using sapphire tips or by adapting the bare fiber technique.

We carried out *in vitro* studies to examine the tissue effects produced by Nd:YAG and argon lasers both in contact and non-contact technique (Figure 9.12). Measurements obtained for the individual lasers and techniques showed that cutting depth and coagulation were a function of laser power and energy density (Figures 9.13–9.17).

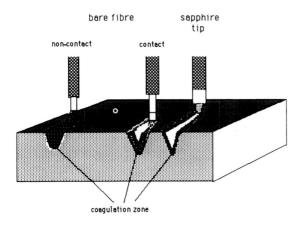

Figure 9.12 Application modes of 'fiber lasers': bare fiber technique in non-contact mode, bare fiber in contact mode, sapphire tips.

Non-contact Technique

With the non-contact technique (see Figures 9.13, 9.14), the Nd:YAG laser only produces deep and wide tissue coagulation. Increasing laser power enlarges the coagulation zone. The argon laser, too, at low power produces a coagulation effect only. With increased power, however, the argon laser, unlike the Nd:YAG laser, can reach the same vaporization depth as that attained with the contact technique (see Figures 9.15, 9.16). Power increase results in a clear increase of cutting depth, with only minor broadening of the coagulation zone. At 10 W the coagulation zone is 70% of the cutting depth, and at 15 W it is 50% of the cutting depth.

Contact Techniques – Nd:YAG

Sapphire Tips versus 'Bare Fiber'
With both contact and non-contact techniques (see Figures 9.13–9.16), the Nd:YAG laser produces tissue vaporization. Histologic tissue preparation and measurement of the cuts showed that, on average, the use of the bare fiber technique (see Figure 9.13) produced a 30% deeper cut than sapphire tips (Figure 9.16). With either technique cutting depth and coagulation increased with increasing power.

Sapphire Tips
Sapphire tips (see Figure 9.17) have been widely used and their specifications and limitations are well known. The role of the laser light in connection with such probes is still a point of debate. It is obvious that heating the tip enhances cutting efficacy. A new tip with an optically clean surface does not cut at all, it must first be immersed in blood or other biologic matter to absorb enough laser light. Heat will therefore not only be generated at the end of the tip, but also in part of the probe. The heat absorbed by the tissue in the cutting process must be regenerated by the laser light. Only a small amount of laser light is transmitted directly to the tissue, contributing to coagulation.

Any cutting and coagulation achieved with sapphire tips is thus chiefly attributable to a heating effect.

Bare Fiber
This technique presents totally different results. Histologic tissue preparation and measurement of the cuts generally showed greater depth of incision compared with that realized with sapphire tips (see Figures 9.15, 9.16). Moreover, the depth of necrosis exceeded incision depth. This is due to the fact that a far higher proportion of laser light penetrates into the tissue with the bare fiber technique, than with the conically shaped contact probes.

Figure 9.13 Coagulation versus vaporization. Argon laser radiation with bare fiber in non-contact technique.

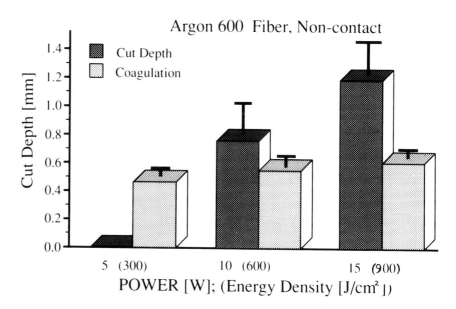

Figure 9.14 Coagulation versus vaporization. Nd:YAG laser radiation with bare fiber in non-contact technique.

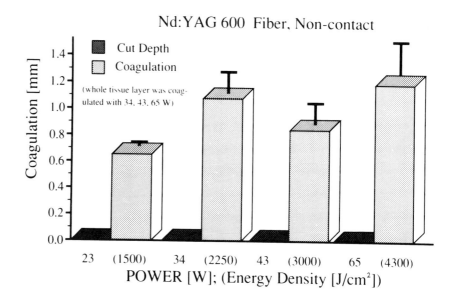

Figure 9.15 Coagulation versus vaporization. Argon and Nd:YAG laser application with the bare fiber (0.6 mm) in contact technique.

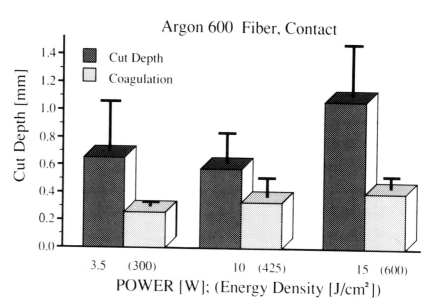

Figure 9.16 Coagulation versus vaporization. Argon and Nd:YAG laser application with the bare fiber (0.6 mm) in contact technique.

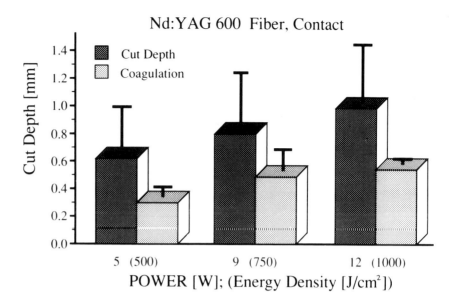

Figure 9.17 Coagulation versus vaporization. Use of sapphire tips with the Nd:YAG laser.

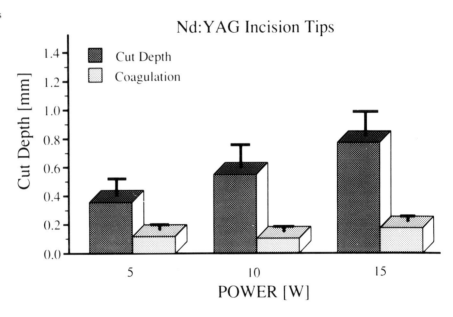

The use of the bare fiber technique may cause various technical problems. High power densities on the very end of the quartz fibers produce high temperatures, which result in a good vaporization effect. During the vaporization process, tissue debris may stick to the fiber surface causing a change in transmission properties. The high absorption rate of the laser light within the fiber or on the surface then leads to a rapid temperature increase of up to 800 or 1000°C. Although this may diminish the laser light transmission rate into the tissue and thus enhance the thermal tissue effect, the laser fiber may be damaged by such a high temperature and by the change in transmission characteristics. A highly contami-

nated or destroyed fiber surface, however, rules out any subsequent non-contact procedure.

Using a constant temperature control at the fiber tissue interface, the Fibertom (MBB) protects the laser fiber against rapid destruction. During vaporization, visible light is produced, which correlates with the temperatures at the fiber end. This allows temperature control by way of a feedback system with integrated microprocessors, regulating laser output in accordance with the visible light (temperatures) produced during laser application. The visible light is kept at a constant intensity according to the control parameters (power and reference values). Alteration of these parameters leads to varying tissue effects. The system's advantages are:

- Protection of the optical fiber through temperature control.
- Possibility of combined procedures (non-contact/contact).
- No need for a cooling system (saline, gas) for fiber protection.
- Controllable coagulation and vaporization effect.

Our experimental studies on uteri showed vaporization depths of 0.4–0.9 mm and coagulation zones of 0.2–0.6 mm. The fiber surface was controlled by alternating non-contact with contact mode laser use. Due to the feedback control system the laser fiber can be used 2–3 times longer than conventional Nd:YAG laser systems. The fibers are, however, not totally invulnerable to surface destruction.

In summary, it can be said that the Nd:YAG laser is well suited as a cutting instrument in contact technique, using either sapphire tips or bare fibers. Sapphire tips yield a smaller coagulation zone. Comparing argon with Nd:YAG lasers using the bare fiber technique, the argon laser produces a 10% greater depth of vaporization, which is not significant. This effect is not dependent upon energy density. Coagulation zone width follows the same pattern as cutting depth in that it is only power dependent at a certain cutting speed and unaffected by fiber diameter. Comparing the contact versus non-contact mode of the different laser systems, the former produces a smaller coagulation zone in the incisions.

Ultrasonic Scalpel

Although both lasers and electrosurgery have been used extensively for laparoscopic surgery, they are not without considerable disadvantages. They both generate a great deal of smoke and char, which can obscure the operative field and necessitate removal by pressurized irrigation fluid. Electrosurgery has been implicated in 'off screen' tissue injury due to capacitative coupling and faulty insulation. There is always a risk that tissue may be inadvertently damaged unless lasers are used very carefully and the energy is only activated when the aiming beam can be clearly seen. In addition, if backstops are not correctly used the beam can cause damage beyond the intended target. Most laser injuries have been due to operator error and if the surgeon is fastidious in laser safety, then it is an extremely safe energy source. Nevertheless laser equipment is very expen-

sive compared with other energy sources, electrosurgical equipment tends to be more unreliable, and there is a much greater tendency for the equipment to stick to tissue and to generate bleeding when the eschar is removed.

For some years ultrasonic scalpels have been proposed as an alternative energy source, but the initial devices seemed to generate a large quantity of fatty droplets, which obscured vision almost as much as smoke, and were relatively expensive, because there was a need for disposable equipment. Although the latter criticism still applies, the newer devices appear to be much more effective with the improved design of the newer ultrasonic scalpels (Harmonic scalpel, Ultracision Inc, Smithfield, Rhode Island; Ethicon Endosurgery, Edinburgh, UK) and the instrument operates by means of a blade that vibrates longitudinally at a frequency of 55.5 kHz (Hambley *et al.*, 1988) The end of the device oscillates at about 50 000 cycles s^{-1}, which results in precise cutting, generating neither smoke nor char (Figures 9.18, 9.19) (Amaral, 1994). The

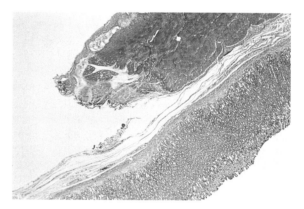

Figure 9.18 Seromyotomy performed using the Harmonic scalpel, showing sealed serosa and no damage to the mucosal layer.

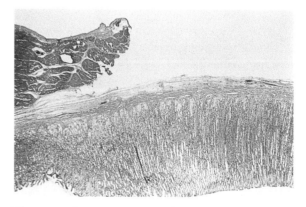

Figure 9.19 Seromyotomy performed using electrosurgery, again showing sealed serosa, but with extensive thermal damage seen in the mucosal layer beneath.

newer devices have a sharp blade that can be rotated at 90° to expose a blunt blade, which will result in a degree of coagulation and will achieve hemostasis without tissue adherence. The device is excellent for laparoscopic myomectomy (Stringer, 1994) and is also useful for hysterectomy as described by Charles Miller in Chapter 67.

It is noteworthy that clinical experience with these new devices is often published before experimental studies on the animal model. Recently Schemmel et al. (1997) published their studies on 16 mature female New Zealand white rabbits and compared the effects of steel scalpel, the ultrasonic scalpel at power level 3 (blade excursion: 60 µm) and power level 5 (blade excursion 80 µm) with the CO_2 laser at 30 W on continuous power and the needle tip electrosurgery device at 30 W cutting power. They were used to perform an ovarian wedge resection and to remove a distal uterine horn and during the procedure a 3 cm longitudinal incision was also made in the contralateral uterine horn. As their main outcome measures they looked at the number of 1 s bursts of needle tip electrosurgery required for hemostasis, the depth and degree of coagulation necrosis, the degree of fibrin deposition and postoperative adhesion formation. This was a prospective randomized animal study and they found that the amount of electrosurgery needed to achieve hemostasis was less for any of the four power techniques than for the steel scalpel, with the exception of the ultrasonic scalpel at level 5 when used on the ovary. The depth (range: 0.30–0.38 mm) and the degree of coagulation necrosis did not differ for any of the power techniques. The fibrin score was greatest with the ultrasonic scalpel at level 5 in both the ovarian tissue and the uterine tissue. There was no difference in adhesion scores for the power techniques and the steel scalpel. From this study they concluded that the ultrasonic scalpel at level 3 does not differ from either CO_2 laser or electrosurgery in terms of hemostatic properties, coagulation necrosis or adhesion formation in the rabbit model.

Thus the ultrasonic scalpel with the advantage of producing neither smoke nor char appears to be a reasonable alternative when the precision, control and hemostatic properties of a power instrument are desired for reproductive surgery. It does, however, have the disadvantage that the ultrasonic tip has a very limited life span, and in some cases is even disposable, making the cost per patient much higher than with electrosurgery and possibly in the long term even with lasers, despite their high capital income at installation.

Although these clinical studies on the animal model are important, it must be understood that an individual surgeon who has acquired skill and experience with a particular instrument is often able to use it to his own advantage. Tulandi et al. (1994) have pointed out quite clearly that results in endoscopic surgery are often more determined by the experience and skill of the operator than the individual energy sources. One of the criticisms of experimental studies with animals is that a power density setting is calculated that might not be the most appropriate in clinical practise and would possibly not be used by an experienced surgeon in a laparoscopic operation, and yet the actual tissue results of standardized power settings might give different results. In practise, most experienced surgeons vary the power sources depending upon the clinical situation and these animal studies must be interpreted with some caution.

Summary

Heat generation for operative and therapeutic destruction or coagulation of biological tissue can be achieved by either electrodiathermy or medical laser systems, or by ultrasonic energy. The effect these methods produce varies according to the amount of energy applied. Electrodiathermy is a very versatile cutting and coagulation method. Tissue effect is, however, dependent on variables such as peak voltage, HF frequency, modulation, cutting and coagulation speed, shape of electrode and type of tissue. The laser systems currently available are well suited to coagulation and/or cutting of tissue in non-contact technique. The Nd:YAG or KTP lasers can also be put to a multitude of uses when applied in contact technique. Ultrasonic energy has recently been redesigned and improved, and is an excellent laparoscopic surgical energy source for myometry and hysterectomy.

References

Amaral JF (1994) The experimental development of an ultrasonically activated scalpel for laparoscopic use. *Surgical Laparoscopic Endoscopy* **4**: 92–99.

Badaway SZA, ElBakry MM, Baggish MS, Choe JK (1986) Pulsed CO_2 laser versus conventional microsurgical anastomosis of the rat uterine horn. *Fertility and Sterility* **46**: 127–131.

Baggish MS, ElBakry MM (1986) Comparison of electronically superpulsed and continuous-wave CO_2 laser on the rat uterine horn. *Fertility and Sterility* **45**: 120–127.

Barbot J, Parent B, Dubuisson JB, Aubriot FX (1987) A clinical study of the CO_2 laser and electrosurgery for adhesiolysis in 172 cases followed by early second-look laparoscopy. *Fertility and Sterility* **48**: 140–142.

Bellina J, Fisher Ross L, Holmquist N, Voros J, Moorehead M (1983) Linear and nonlinear effect of the argon laser on a fallopian tube animal model. *Lasers in Surgery and Medicine* **2**: 343–355.

Bellina JH, Hemmings R, Voros J, Ross LF (1984) Carbon dioxide laser and electrosurgical wound study with an animal model: a comparison of damage and healing patterns in peritoneal tissue. *American Journal of Obstetrics and Gynecology* **148**: 327–334.

Daniell J (1989) Fiberoptic laser laparoscopy. In Sutton C (ed.) *Laparoscopic Surgery.* pp. 545–562. London: Baillière.

Farin G (1990) *Principles of High Frequency Surgery*, 12 pp. Tübingen: Erbe Elektromedizin.

Filmar S, Gomel V, McComb P (1986) The effectiveness of CO_2 laser and electrosurgery in adhesiolysis: a comparative study. *Fertility and Sterility* **45**: 407–411.

Grochmal S (1988) Contact Nd:YAG superior to CO_2 for treatment of ovarian disease. *Laser Practice Report* **3**: 1S–2S.

Hambley R, Hebda PA, Abell E, Cohen BA, Jegasothy BV (1988) Wound healing of skin incisions produced by ultrasonically vibrating knife, scalpel, electrosurgery, and carbon dioxide laser. *Journal of Dermatologic Surgery and Oncology* **14**: 1213–1217.

Keckstein J (1990) *Laser in der operativen Pelviskopie. In-vitro, tierexperimentelle und klinische Studien über Gewebereaktionen und Applikationsarten von CO_2-, Nd:YAG- und Argon-Laser für endoskopische Operationen.* Habilitationsschrift [Postdoctoral thesis], University of Ulm.

Keckstein J, Wolf A, Steiner R (1987) The use of contact laser probe in gynecological endoscopy. *Proceedings of the 7th Congress International Society for Laser Surgery and Medicine*, Munich, pp. 267–272.

Keckstein J, Finger A, Steiner R (1988) Laser application in contact- and non-contact procedures; sapphire tips in comparison to 'bare-fiber' argon laser in comparison to Nd:YAG laser. *Lasers in Surgery and Medicine* **4**: 158–162.

Keye W, Dixon J (1983) Photocoagulation of endometriosis by the argon laser through the laparoscope. *Obstetrics and Gynecology* **62**: 383–386.

Kojiama E, Yanagigori A, Yuda K, Hirakawa S (1988) Nd:YAG laser endoscopy. *Journal of Reproductive Medicine* **33**: 907–911.

Luciano AA, Whitman G, Maier DB, Randolph J, Maenza R (1987) A comparison of thermal injury, healing patterns, and postoperative adhesion formation following CO_2 laser and electromicrosurgery. *Fertility and Sterility* **48**: 1025–1029.

McKenzie AL (1986) A three-zone model of soft tissue damage by a CO_2 laser. *Physics in Medicine and Biology* **31**: 967–983.

Puolakkainen P, Brackett K, Sankar NY, Joffe S, Schröder T (1987) Effects of electrocautery, CO_2 laser, and contact Nd:YAG laser scalpel in the healing of intestinal incision. *Lasers in Surgery and Medicine* **7**: 507–511.

Schemmel M, Haefner HK, Selvaggi SM, *et al.* (1997) Comparison of the ultrasonic scalpel to CO_2 laser and electrosurgery in terms of tissue injury and adhesion formation in a rabbit model. *Fertility and Sterility* **67**: 382–386.

Stringer NH (1994) Laparoscopic myomectomy with the harmonic scalpel: a review of 25 cases. *Journal of Gynecological Surgery* **10**: 241–245.

Tulandi T, Chan KL, Arseneau J (1994) Histopathological and adhesion formation after incision using ultrasonic vibrating scalpel and regular scalpel in the rat. *Fertility and Sterility* **61**: 548–550.

Wallwiener D, Morawski A, Plantener G, Bastert G (1987) Ist die Adhäsiolyse mittels Nd:YAG-Laser eine Alternative zur CO_2-Laser-Adhäsiolyse? *Lasers in Surgery and Medicine* **3**: 142–147.

10

Laparoscopic Use of the Argon Beam Coagulator

JAMES F. DANIELL* AND RICHARD W. DOVER†

*2222 State Street, Nashville, Tennessee, USA
†Department of Gynaecology, Royal Surrey County Hospital, Guildford, UK

Introduction

Over the years, many methods have been used for laparoscopic surgery, including blunt traction, scissors, forceps, and electrosurgical energy by both unipolar and bipolar methods (Murphy, 1987). This last decade, various lasers have been used, including the carbon dioxide (CO_2) (Daniell, 1985), argon (Keye and Dixon, 1983), potassium titanyl phosphate (KTP) (Daniell et al., 1986) and the neodymium:yttrium-aluminum-garnet (Nd:YAG) lasers. Newer mechanical methods for laparoscopic surgery include permanent clips, laparoscopic suturing techniques, and mechanical stapling devices (Daniell et al., 1991a). The advantages and disadvantages of all these types of operative laparoscopic procedures are discussed in this book. This chapter reviews our current experience of the newest form of electrosurgical energy to be used laparoscopically, the argon beam coagulator (ABC).

Method of Action of the ABC

The ABC allows a jet of argon gas to carry electrons from a unipolar electrode through space to impact on tissue that is appropriately grounded, delivering electrosurgical energy as standard unipolar cautery. However, this energy is delivered in a no-touch technique through a plume of argon gas so that no smoke develops with the coagulation. In addition, the plume of argon gas that sprays around the needle electrode and conducts the electrical energy through space has a blast effect on the tissue before impact. Thus, fluids such as blood or irrigation fluids will be momentarily blown away from the tissues to allow the electrosurgical energy to impact on the actual bleeding site instead of coagulating the protein in overlying blood. The flow rates of argon gas can be varied, and although the initial studies used rates of $4 \, l \, min^{-1}$, rates of $2 \, l \, min^{-1}$ can now be used with some devices being capable of delivering gas at a rate of $0.1 \, l \, min^{-1}$ upwards. The spot diameter of the argon gas that delivers the beam can vary, and power settings of 40–150 W are available for clinical use. The electrosurgical principles of this system are the same as unipolar coagulation, the only difference being that electrons carried by argon gas flow from a needle electrode through space to the tissue. The distance that these electrons arc to tissue depends upon the diameter of the plume, the wattage being delivered from the electrosurgical unit, and the conductivity of the tissue. Tissue effects are the same as with unipolar cautery histologically. Animal studies have shown that thermal necrosis at 40 W will extend to 2–3 mm (Rusch et al., 1990).

The diameter of the impact site varies with the diameter of the nozzle that carries the cone of argon gas to the tissue. This diameter expands as the tip of the nozzle is held further away from the tissue impact site. In our preliminary animal studies including both pigs and rabbits, energy passed a distance of 1 cm at laparoscopy with power settings up to 100 W. Early histologic investigations of the effects of laparoscopic use of the argon beam coagulator in both pigs and rabbits demonstrated thermal damage to tissue similar to that seen with unipolar electrosurgery at the same wattage (Bard Electro Medical Systems, 1988).

Investigations of the ABC have begun at open surgery in several specialties, including head and neck surgery (Ward *et al.*, 1989), thoracic surgery (Rusch *et al.*, 1990) and gynecology (Brand and Pearlman, 1990). All investigators have been impressed with the rapidity with which bleeding can be controlled in a non-contact method compared to other methods of hemostasis at surgery.

Early Animal Investigations of the ABC for Laparoscopy

The first laparoscopic investigation of the ABC was begun at Centennial Medical Center in Nashville, Tennessee, in February, 1991 (Daniell *et al.*, 1993a). Using anesthetized pigs undergoing laparoscopic cholecystectomy in training courses in laparoscopic techniques for surgeons, the ABC was used with a prototype 10 mm diameter probe. This probe contained a needle electrode slightly recessed from its tip to provide the electrosurgical spark. The diameter of the probe tip through which the argon gas flowed around the needle electrode was 3 mm. During laparoscopic cholecystectomy in the pigs, the ABC probe was placed through an accessory 10 mm port and used to coagulate the liver bed, both before any bleeding and after intentional or accidental bleeding had occurred from the bed of the liver during manipulations. The pigs underwent general anesthesia with a pulse oximeter being used to monitor oxygen changes. An anesthesiologist and veterinarian were present to carry out careful observations in this initial series of five pigs. All pigs survived the laparoscopic cholecystectomy with use of the ABC with no detectable physiologic changes under anesthesia. Flow rates of argon were regulated at 4 l min^{-1} with simultaneous evacuation of the pneumoperitoneum and argon gas used to deliver the electrosurgical effect to the tissue in the pigs. After successfully using the ABC in the pig model with no evidence of immediate or delayed complications, Investigational Review Board approval was obtained at Centennial Medical Center for early clinical trials of the ABC laparoscopically in humans in both general surgery and gynecology.

Modifications of the ABC for Laparoscopic Use

The initial prototype probe for laparoscopic use of the ABC was made of plastic 10 mm in diameter and attached to the electrosurgical generator by a tube that was approximately 4.5 m. The tip of the disposable probe was coned down to 3 mm in diameter (Figure 10.1). Inside this tip was a standard unipolar needle electrode, which was recessed from the surface of the opening of the cone by approximately 2 mm. Thus, if this probe touched the tissue, there would be no tissue contact with the unipolar electrode. The initial 10 mm probe was disposable and somewhat flimsy, because it was made of plastic. The attachment of the tubing to the probe was particularly weak and would occasionally separate with manipulations at laparoscopy. This resulted in instantaneous cessation of coagulation since the argon gas would leak and not deliver a flow of gas to the needle electrode in the tip of the probe.

Over recent years the range of probes suitable for use with the ABC has increased dramatically. Probes are currently available in either 5 mm or 10 mm diameter and as either reusable or disposable units. Multifunction probes comprising a retractable needle electrode in combination with an ABC port allow rapid cutting, while angled semi-rigid probes have improved access to some areas of the pelvis. The ability to divert the beam of the ABC has led to new clinical applications, with a role being suggested for it in the management of hemorrhage from trocar sites in the anterior abdominal wall (Galen *et al.*, 1994).

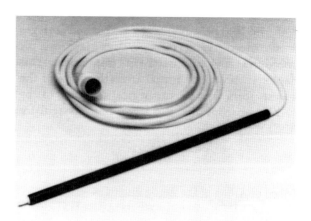

Figure 10.1 The 10 mm prototype disposable probe for laparoscopic use of the argon beam coagulator is shown here. Argon gas from the ABC flows through the instrument at 4 l min^{-1} during coagulation. The white tip of the probe delivers an argon beam 3 mm in diameter for non-touching unipolar coagulation.

Techniques of Laparoscopic Use of the ABC

The ABC is electrosurgical energy and all the standard safety precautions must be followed, such as proper grounding of the patient, correct setting of the desired wattage, and isolation of the unit to minimize electrical problems. At present, for laparoscopy, the ABC must be introduced through an accessory probe. Thus, most laparoscopies require at least three probes, one for the optical channel, one for an accessory probe for manipulation, and a third probe to deliver the argon beam. Before the ABC is fired, it is important to anticipate and prepare for management of the sudden burst of argon gas which will be flowing intraperitoneally through the probe. At present, this flow is 4 litres per minute. It is best to use a high-flow automatic insufflator that shuts off when the intraperitoneal pressure is greater than 20 mm Hg. Just before firing the ABC, we place a 5 mm suction irrigation probe close to the point of impact, and aspirate, using a PumpVac II disposable suction irrigation system for laparoscopy (Marlow Medical, Willoughby, OH, USA). Thus, by actively suctioning as the ABC is fired, we rapidly remove the argon gas from the intraperitoneal cavity and vent it straight into the wall suction system of the operating room. This eliminates accumulation of argon gas in the room, rapidly removes it from the intraperitoneal environment, and helps reduce intraperitoneal pressure. Because of this potential for sudden increased intraperitoneal pressure, the anesthesiologist should always be alerted before the ABC is to be fired laparoscopically.

The concerns relating to the safety of large volumes of argon gas under high pressure are not unfounded. The combination of high intraperitoneal pressures and open blood vessels can lead to the development of gas emboli. These have been described both in animal studies (Palmer et al., 1993) and more recently in human subjects (Anonymous, 1994). It is possible that some of the inherent dangers have now been reduced by further development of the argon delivery systems and the ability to achieve consistent results with flow rates in the region of 2 l min^{-1}.

Electrosurgical energy is invisible, but as electrons flow through the argon gas there is an arcing effect, which is visible. This is similar to the glow seen with neon lights. This gives the operator the ability to see the diameter of the beam when firing laparoscopically. There is a reduction in smoke with coagulation because argon gas completely surrounds the impact site. This allows excellent visibility of tissue effects at laparoscopy compared to other forms of electrosurgery or various lasers. Our method of use is to touch the tip of the probe to the planned impact site, back away 2–3 mm, and then activate the ABC while instantaneously suctioning. We then adjust the distance from the tip of the probe to the tissue, depending upon the tissue effects we see. The 4 l min^{-1} plume of argon gas begins to flow just before the needle electrode is energized. Thus, blood or irrigation fluids are blown away from the impact site, allowing rapid hemostasis by direct coagulation to exposed vessels. Since the spot size is 3 mm, fine cutting is more difficult, but the ability to perform this is also affected by the distance from the tissue, power setting, argon flow rate and the inherent characteristics of the tissue being cut. However, for hemostasis and blunt dissection with coagulation, we have found that the ABC is rapid and effective. After firing the ABC, fresh CO_2 infused via the high-flow insufflator rapidly washes out the residual intraperitoneal argon gas.

Early Clinical Use of the ABC at Laparoscopy in Humans

Our initial clinical trials of the ABC were to evaluate its safety at laparoscopy and its effectiveness for hemostasis. This first series of patients has been reported (Daniell et al., 1993a). In this group of 20 patients, we were able to accomplish hemostasis successfully with the ABC following adhesiolysis, myomectomy, cholecystectomy, and endometriosis ablation. After becoming comfortable with the laparoscopic use of the ABC and its tissue effects, we began to use its coagulation effects as primary therapy for endometriosis, myomectomy, uterosacral ligament transection and presacral neurectomy (Table 10.1). For uterosacral ligament transection with the ABC, a third probe is always needed, so that traction can be placed on the ligament. With such traction, the 3 mm diameter spot of the ABC will successfully coagulate and hemostatically separate the uterosacral ligaments. If there is no tissue traction,

Table 10.1 Laparoscopic use of the argon beam coagulator – early clinical evaluation (20 patients)*

Coagulation of endometriosis	14
Uterosacral nerve abalation	10
Presacral neurectomy	3
Myomectomy	1
Excision of ovarian fibroma	1
Conservative surgery for ectopic pregnancy	1

* Multiple procedures were performed on certain patients

coagulation occurs without adequate separation. For myomectomy we have found that the ABC is an excellent laparoscopic adjuvant to our dissection techniques because of the smoke generated with other forms of dissection in the myometrium and the high potential for bleeding from this operation.

Laparoscopic Presacral Neurectomy with the ABC

Several papers have described the efficacy of laparoscopic presacral neurectomy in treating certain forms of midline pelvic pain (Perez, 1990; Perry and Perez, 1993).

We have performed this procedure in the past, as previously described, but had problems with bleeding retroperitoneally that prolongs the operation and frightens the operator. With the availability of the ABC, we have performed many laparoscopic presacral neurectomies, with a symptomatic relief rate equivalent to that achieved by conventional laparoscopic methods (Daniell et al., 1993b).

We have altered the surgical procedure to accommodate the features of the ABC using a power setting of 80–100 W. The tissue overlying the sacral promontory is coagulated transversely without an incision until the white periosteum is exposed, all tissues between the peritoneum and bone having been coagulated and separated for a distance of at least 1 cm. If a large middle sacral vessel is present, bipolar coagulation is used to occlude it. As the ABC energy is applied to the tissue, gentle traction and countertraction with atraumatic graspers inserted via the lateral ports, results in separation and retraction of the tissue overlying the sacral promontory. With this new neurotomy procedure, a segment of nerves is not excised or removed, but merely coagulated with the ABC and bluntly separated without retroperitoneal dissection. This is important since it has been suggested that failure of pain relief following presacral neurectomy may occur due to reinnervation of the nerve fibers. Although the short-term results achieved with neurotomy are as good as those obtained with neurectomy, it remains to be seen if these benefits are as longlasting.

Although the outcome measures appear to be the same, this new technique has resulted in a major reduction in operating time (64 minutes for ABC neurotomy compared with 92 minutes for conventional laparoscopic techniques). It is pertinent to note that there was one major complication among 15 patients undergoing ABC neurotomy with the left common iliac vein being lacerated during firing of the beam. This necessitated a laparotomy and the prompt assistance of a vascular surgeon. This is thought to have resulted from firing of the beam tangentially across

the sacral promontory, and reflection laterally off the underlying bone onto the medial wall of the exposed vessel. This obviously has major safety implications and has resulted in a change in our current practise – now the beam is only fired directly down onto the sacral promontory.

It should be stressed that the paper described here was a small non-randomized trial, and continued long-term follow-up involving larger numbers of patients is required before meaningful conclusions can be drawn concerning the effectiveness of this new method for performing an old operation.

Laparoscopic Treatment of Endometriosis

There is a long history of effective laparoscopic treatment of endometriosis for both pain relief and enhancement of fertility using electrosurgical energy (Daniell and Christianson, 1981; Murphy et al., 1991). Recently, lasers of various types have become popular for laparoscopic treatment of endometriosis (Daniell and Brown, 1982; Feste, 1985; Martin, 1985; Diamond et al., 1987; Daniell et al., 1991b). After over ten years' experience with lasers for laparoscopic endometriosis treatment, we are now returning to electrosurgical energy for most of our laparoscopic endometriosis treatment. The ease with which the ABC allows us to rapidly coagulate endometriosis without smoke production and with excellent visible observation of the tissue is impressive. Although it is still too soon to conclude that the ABC will replace surgical lasers or conventional electrosurgical techniques for endometriosis ablation via laparoscopy, our early results in 25 patients are promising (Daniell et al., 1993c).

For laparoscopic treatment of endometriosis with the ABC power settings ranged from 40–100 W of current with the flow of argon gas limited to 4 l min^{-1} through a 5 mm or 10 mm disposable second puncture probe held within 10 mm of the tissue to be coagulated. Most implants were coagulated at settings of 80–100 W, but when the endometriotic deposits were involving the bowel or bladder or overlying the ureter, the power was reduced to 40 W. With firing, the tissue coagulation effects can be clearly seen, since there is very little smoke and the probe does not touch the tissues. Each area is ablated with adjacent peritoneal edges coagulated for 2–3 mm. The jet of argon gas blows blood and debris away from the impact site and allows hemostatic coagulation within a 3 mm spot diameter. We have thus been able to treat 90% of all implants with this simple rapid method of coagulation. Actual operating time with the ABC is reduced compared to that with surgical lasers or contact cautery due to less smoke generation, reduced bleeding, and fewer unnecessary delays for reinsufflation. This shortens anesthesia time, reduces operator fatigue, and thus benefits all parties involved.

Laparoscopic Myomectomy

Symptomatic uterine fibroids are common in many women who want to became pregnant or avoid major surgery or hysterectomy. Laparoscopic myomectomy is therefore becoming more commonplace in this era of aggressive endoscopic surgery (Gurley and Daniell, 1991). Present techniques combine preoperative suppression of growth, atraumatic dissection, effective hemostasis, myometrial closure and removal of portions of the myoma by morcellation or colpotomy. Obtaining hemostasis during myomectomy can be tedious and difficult at laparoscopy. Since the availability of the ABC for laparoscopic evaluation in our practise, we have been impressed with its ability to accomplish rapid hemostasis during dissection in the myometrium. Blood loss is reduced and the operation proceeds more easily when the ABC is used to bluntly dissect the fibrous myoma from the vascular myometrium (Daniell *et al.*, 1993d). We now consider the ABC to be our primary method for dissection for both open and laparoscopic myomectomy.

Laparoscopic Enterolysis

Laparoscopic lysis of adhesions to bowel is becoming a common operation (Daniell, 1989; Sutton and MacDonald, 1990). Usually blunt or sharp dissection are satisfactory, but significant bleeding often occurs. This can usually be managed with a variety of techniques including mechanical or electrosurgical or with lasers. Occasionally, laparotomy is the only recourse to successful and safe control of some of these events. The ABC is especially effective for accomplishing hemostasis in oozing areas when vessels are difficult to identify and control. Omental bleeding can be controlled with 60–80 W of power with the ABC with minimal smoke production by merely passing the probe slowly over the bleeding area from a distance of 3–4 mm. The plume of argon gas that blows over the clots allows the electrons to impact on the actual vessels for coagulation. Since this is all done with a non-touching technique, the resulting coagulum is not dislodged, as often occurs with unipolar or even bipolar coagulation. There is only slight smoke, so operator control is excellent. The

depth of tissue coagulation is safely limited to 2–3 mm and irrigation is possible while firing the ABC since the first jet of argon gas blows the fluids off the tissue before actual coagulation. This gives the laparoscopist a valuable new tool for safe effective adhesiolysis.

The Future of the ABC for Laparoscopy

The ABC should become a valuable tool for certain laparoscopic procedures. In our early evaluations, it has proved to be a safe and simple system to deliver laparoscopically. If other laparoscopists find the system as effective for hemostasis and coagulation as we have, it should become commonly used for many laparoscopic operations. All surgeons and operating room personnel are already experienced in the safe use of electrosurgical energy. Thus, introduction of the ABC does not entail extensive new orientation. The ABC can be a very cost-effective addition to the operating room since it provides a combined unipolar, bipolar, and argon beam coagulation system. It can then be used by many surgical disciplines. At present, these multiple use top of the line electrosurgical generators cost less than $15 000 in the USA

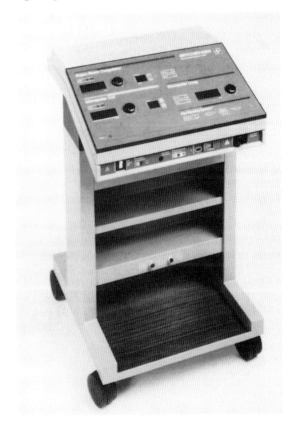

Figure 10.2 The Birtcher model 6400 electrosurgical generator – ABC is seen in this photograph. It can be used for standard unipolar cutting or coagulation or for argon beam coagulation. The power for each mode of use is monitored by a digital readout system.

(Figure 10.2). The combination of reduced capital costs to the hospital and shortened operating time should translate into significant savings to all patients in the health care system. We should all consider cost containment in health care delivery in this era of patient awareness of minimally invasive surgery and spiralling health care costs.

In our opinion, the ABC with an effective delivery system for laparoscopic surgery may possibly have as much impact in the late 1990s as lasers have had over the last decade. In our hands, we have found it to be useful for many laparoscopic procedures without complications. It reduces operating times and eliminates excessive intraperitoneal smoke while increasing our confidence when faced with potential or actual bleeding episodes during laparoscopic manipulations.

Much further evaluation of the ABC is needed in animal models and clinically at both laparotomy and laparoscopy before its true role in surgery is clear. The safety implications of large volumes of intraperitoneal gas at high pressures during the use of the ABC, however, do need to be considered, and the reports of fatal gas embolism do give some cause for concern. This is undoubtedly an area where further research is needed in an attempt to reduce or abolish the incidence of this potentially catastrophic complication. However, all operative laparoscopists should become familiar with the effects of the ABC at laparotomy and consider exploring its potential for assisting at operative laparoscopy. Only time and careful future investigations will be able to determine the true benefits of the ABC for laparoscopic surgery.

References

Anonymous (1994) Fatal gas embolism caused by over-pressurization during laparoscopic use of argon enhanced coagulation. *Health Devices* **23(6)**: 257–259.

Bard Electro Medical Systems (1988) *System 6000 Argon Beam Coagulator Tissue Effects*. Technical document. Englewood, Colorado: Bard Electro Medical Systems, Inc.

Brand E, Pearlman N (1990) Electrosurgical debulking of ovarian cancer: a new technique using the argon beam coagulator. *Gynecologic Oncology* **39**: 115.

Daniell JF (1985) The role of lasers in infertility surgery. *Fertility and Sterility* **45**: 815.

Daniell JF (1989) Laparoscopic enterolysis for chronic abdominal pain. *Journal of Gynecologic Surgery* **5**: 61–66.

Daniell JF, Christianson C (1981) Combined laparoscopic surgery and danazol therapy for pelvic endometriosis. *Fertility and Sterility* **35**: 521.

Daniell JF, Brown DH (1982) Carbon dioxide laser laparoscopy: initial experience in experimental animals and humans. *Obstetrics and Gynecology* **59**: 761.

Daniell JF, Miller SW, Tosh R (1986) Initial evaluation of the use of the potassium-titanyl-phosphate (KTP/532) laser in gynecologic laparoscopy. *Fertility and Sterility* **46**: 373.

Daniell JF, Gurley LD, Chambers JF (1991a) The use of an automatic stapling device for laparoscopic appendectomy. *Obstetrics and Gynecology* **78**: 721.

Daniell JF, Gurley LD, Kurtz B (1991b) Laser laparoscopic management of large endometriomas. *Fertility and Sterility* **55**: 692.

Daniell JF, Fisher B, Alexander W (1993a) Laparoscopic evaluation of the argon beam coagulator – initial report. *Journal of Reproductive Medicine* **38(2)**: 121–125.

Daniell JF, Kurtz BR, Gurley LD, Lalonde CJ (1993b) Laparoscopic presacral neurectomy vs neurotomy: Use of the argon beam coagulator compared to conventional technique. *Journal of Gynecologic Surgery* **9**: 169–173.

Daniell JF, Kurtz BR, Nair S (1993c) Laparoscopic treatment of endometriosis with the argon beam coagulator: initial report. *Gynaecologic Endoscopy* **2**: 13–19.

Daniell JF, Kurtz BR, Taylor SN (1993d) Laparoscopic myomectomy using the argon beam coagulator. *Journal of Gynecologic Surgery* **9**: 207–212.

Diamond MP, Boyers SP, Lavy G et al. (1987) Endoscopic use of the potassium-titanyl-phosphate 532 laser in gynecologic surgery. *Colposcopy and Gynecologic Laser Surgery* **3**: 213.

Feste JR (1985) Laser laparoscopy: a new modality. *Journal of Reproductive Medicine* **30**: 413.

Galen DI, Jacobson A, Weckstein LN (1994) Argon beam coagulation rescue to correct bleeding during pelviscopy. *Journal of the American Association of Gynecologic Laparoscopy* **1(2)**: 146–149.

Gurley L, Daniell JF (1991) Laparoscopic management of clinically significant symptomatic uterine fibroids. *Journal of Gynecologic Surgery* **7**: 37–40.

Keye WR, Dixon J (1983) Photocoagulation of endometriosis by the argon laser through the laparoscope. *Obstetrics and Gynecology* **62**: 383.

Martin DC (1985) CO_2 laser laparoscopy for the treatment of endometriosis associated with infertility. *Journal of Reproductive Medicine* **30**: 409.

Murphy AA (1987) Operative laparoscopy. *Fertility and Sterility* **47**: 6.

Murphy AA, Schlaff WD, Hassiakos D et al. (1991) Laparoscopic cautery in the treatment of endometriosis-related infertility. *Fertility and Sterility* **55**: 246.

Palmer M, Miller CW, van Way CW, Orton EC (1993) Venous gas embolism associated with argon-enhanced coagulation of the liver. *Journal of Investigative Surgery* **6(5)**: 391–399.

Perez JJ (1990) Laparoscopic presacral neurectomy. *Journal of Reproductive Medicine* **35**: 625–630.

Perry CP, Perez J (1993) The role for laparoscopic presacral neurectomy. *Journal of Gynecologic Surgery* **9**: 165–168.

Rusch VW, Schmidt R, Yoshimi S, Fujimura Y (1990) Use of the argon beam electrocoagulator for performing pulmonary wedge resections. *Annals of Thoracic Surgery* **49**: 287.

Sutton C, MacDonald R (1990) Laser laparoscopic adhesiolysis. *Journal of Gynecologic Surgery* **6**: 155–159.

Ward PH, Castro DJ, Ward S (1989) The argon beam coagulator – a significant new contribution to radical head and neck surgery. *Archives of Otolaryngology – Head and Neck Surgery* **115**: 921.

11

Recent Advances in Laparoscopic Tissue Extraction

ANDREW POOLEY* and ROLF STEINER†

*Mayday University Hospital, Surrey, UK
†Kantonales Frauenspital Fontana, Chur, Switzerland

Introduction

The applications of the laparoscope in gynecology have progressed enormously in the last 25 years. In modern practise many of the classical major gynecological procedures are routinely performed without the use of a large abdominal incision, including some procedures for gynecological malignancy. Frequently the need arises to remove quite large volumes of tissue generated by these procedures.

Early methods of laparoscopic tissue removal involving significant enlargement of an abdominal port or a large posterior colpotomy incision seem to negate the rationale for minimal access surgery (i.e. smaller less painful wounds with more rapid recover). However, in the absence of specific extraction techniques, removing large volumes of tissue from the abdomen can be the most time consuming and frustrating part of the operation.

Principles and Pitfalls of Devices and Techniques used for Laparoscopic Tissue Extraction

Before describing the various devices and techniques that have been developed to facilitate laparoscopic extraction of various tissue specimens, it is worth considering certain principles and potential pitfalls.

Significant enlargement of an abdominal port site goes against the principles of minimal access surgery and invites the risk of incisional hernia formation, even if attempts are made to close the fascial defect. The risk of hernia formation rises with the size of the incision (Kadar et al., 1993) and is more common with laterally placed ports (Kurtz et al., 1993; Patterson et al., 1993). The performance of a posterior colpotomy allows large pieces of tissue to be removed, but can be complicated by infection, dyspareunia, adhesion formation and rectal or ureteric injury.

In several of the widely practised gynecologic procedures the tissue for removal has to to be removed completely without spillage if certain complications are to be avoided. The commonest problem encountered after conservative laparoscopic treatment of an ectopic pregnancy has been residual trophoblast within the tube, occurring in 5% of cases (Donnez and Nisolle, 1989) and rising to 16% in cases of laparoscopic tubal milking (Chapron et al., 1991). There is also a potential for trophoblastic tissue to implant in the abdominal wall if the specimen is pulled through a port site without isolation. Similarly, during laparoscopic appendicectomy the transection margin may contaminate the abdomen with fecal material if not isolated carefully and the excised appendix may infect the port site through which it is removed. Simply pulling a specimen through an abdominal port has been reported to lead to implantation in the abdominal wall of both endometriosis (Sutton, 1993) and papillary serous carcinoma of the ovary (Hsiu et al., 1986).

The laparoscopic management of adnexal cystic masses is the subject of considerable debate. Intraoperative spillage of the contents of a mucinous cystadenoma may theoretically initiate pseudomyxoma peritonei, though the risk appears to be small (Mage *et al.*, 1990). Similarly, chemical peritonitis and granuloma formation with intestinal obstruction have been reported after laparoscopic management of benign cystic teratomas (Langebrekke and Urnes, 1994). In this case, however, the entire capsules of bilateral cystic tumors were not removed, and there are several series of laparoscopically managed teratomas without this complication (Mage *et al.*, 1990; Ulrich *et al.*, 1994).

Debate continues as to the dangers of spillage of the contents of borderline and malignant ovarian cysts, with some authors showing no change in prognosis (Sigurdsson *et al.*, 1983; Grogan, 1967), while others suggest that spillage is an important negative prognostic factor (Malkasian *et al.*, 1984). Adequate intra-abdominal isolation and removal of such specimens should avoid this potential problem.

Clearly many of the specimens already mentioned require careful histologic examination, which may be complicated by the mode of removal. Vaginal squames may contaminate an ovary pulled through a posterior colpotomy confusing accurate histology. Although morcellation does not prevent histologic examination of a specimen, it will destroy surgical tissue margins (Clayman *et al.*, 1991) and make orientation more difficult for the pathologist.

If a delay is intended between the excision of a piece of tissue and its subsequent removal from the abdomen, care must be taken not to misplace it. A specimen placed on or allowed to fall onto the loops of bowel in the central abdomen at laparoscopy may sink without trace. It may be possible to recover lost specimens by filling the upper abdomen with fluid with the patient in a Trendelenburg position and then reversing the position with aspiration in the cul-de-sac to flush the tissue into the pelvis. If this is not successful, one would hope to find the specimen in the pouch of Douglas at a later laparoscopy, but the need for a laparotomy to retrieve a transected uterine corpus from beneath the spleen has been described (Semm, 1993).

When it is intended to perform a procedure that will generate tissue needing removal, two aspects must be addressed. Firstly the size or volume of the specimen and secondly, depending upon the likely pathology, the need to isolate the specimen within a retrieval device to avoid contamination during removal. If extraction is to be delayed, parking the specimen in the uterovesical pouch or the pouch of Douglas in a laparoscopic bag or against the abdominal wall with a suture is advisable.

One can debate the point at which an enlarged port site becomes a mini-laparotomy, but it is probably at about 20 mm. This can be done with a knife or with a specific port enlarging device. These port enlargers are designed to enlarge the umbilical incision to facilitate the removal of the gallbladder at laparoscopic cholecystectomy. On no account should they be used to enlarge lateral incisions because of the very real risk of tearing the inferior epigastric vessels which have been so carefully avoided during the initial placement of the lower quadrant ports.

Devices and Techniques for Laparoscopic Tissue Extraction

The simplest method of removal is to grasp the tissue with a strong toothed grasping forceps and pull it up the port cannula and through the valve. Some valves will allow tissue to be pulled through them. If this is not possible the trochar can be used with a screw-locking anchor, which can be left *in situ* with a thumb over the end when the trochar containing the specimen is removed to prevent loss of pneumoperitoneum. If plastic locking devices are used, great care must be taken if monopolar electrosurgical instruments are used. Capacitive coupling can occur if a hybrid port is created in which the plastic locking anchor prevents dispersal of radiofrequency energy through the abdominal wall.

Several devices exist that allow isolation of a specimen. Olympus Keymed (Southend-on-Sea, UK) make simple 5 mm-, 15 mm- and 20 mm-diameter guiding tubes into which a specimen can be drawn, and a 20 mm diameter extractor, which seals the specimen in the shaft. Alternatively a bag or sac can be used, examples of which include the Extraction Bag (Storz, Tuttlingen, Germany), the Lapsac (Cook (UK), Letchworth, UK; Cook Ob-Gyn, Spencer, USA), the Pleatman Sac (Cabot Medical, Langhorne, USA), and the Endocatch (Autosuture, Ascot, UK; US Surgical Corporation, Norwalk, USA). With a range of sizes, all of these devices will allow isolation of a specimen inside the abdomen. If the specimen is sufficiently small and malleable, the bag can be drawn through the port or through the abdominal wall after removing the port. Suitable specimens would be an ectopic pregnancy, a tube, an appendix, an endometrioma or its capsule, or an ovary of normal size of uncertain pathology.

A novel method of removing salpingectomy specimens has been reported using commercially available condoms that have been washed in an antiseptic solution to remove the lubricant and spermicide (Trujillo *et al.*, 1994). Although these are cheap to use, the potential risks include questionable asepsis, latex anaphylaxis (Swartz *et al.*, 1990) and splitting and fragmentation of the condom.

Larger volume specimens require considerable effort if morcellation and removal through a small incision are to be achieved. With patience and ingenuity uterine fibroids up to 15 cm in diameter can be removed laparoscopically (Nezhat *et al.*, 1991). Other authors question the sense of time-consuming extraction of large specimens with prolonged anesthesia and operator fatigue (Daniell and Gurley, 1991). Specimens suitable for simple morcellation include uterine fibroids, subtotal hysterectomies and benign ovaries. It is worth remembering that uterine fibroids can be reduced in volume by up to 40% using gonadotropin-releasing hormone analogues before surgery (Dubuisson *et al.*, 1992).

In its simplest form morcellation can be achieved using graspers and endoscopic scissors, cutting diathermy or laser energy to yield pieces small enough to pull through a port. Alternatively the specimen can be pulled against an abdominal incision or posterior colpotomy through which a small knife is inserted to divide it. This technique can be difficult and potentially dangerous. After any morcellation procedure it is advisable to wash and aspirate the abdomen and pelvis copiously to remove any debris.

Devices exist for both manual and mechanical morcellation. The hand operated Tissue Punch (Storz, Tuttlingen, Germany), first described by Semm in 1978 takes bites of tissue, which are pushed up the 11 mm diameter shaft of the instrument. It is said to be inadequate for large tissue volumes and unable to deal with firm or calcified specimens (Steiner *et al.*, 1993).

Two devices are currently available that will mechanically morcellate large volumes of tissue. The Cook Tissue Morcellator (Cook (UK) Letchworth, UK), was first described for the laparoscopic removal of a 190 g tumor-bearing kidney through an 11 mm port by Clayman *et al.* in 1991. The disposable morcellator is connected to a reusable power unit and a suction supply. The tissue for removal needs to be placed in an isolating bag, the mouth of which is pulled through the abdominal wall. The cutting cannula is then placed into the bag. Using the foot switch the specimen is then morcellated and aspirated from within the bag.

The Steiner Electromechanical Morcellator (Storz, Tuttlingen, Germany) is shown in Figure 11.1. Introduced in 1993 (Steiner *et al.*, 1993), this reusable device allows morcellation inside the abdomen under laparoscopic observation. The instrument has a motor driven cutting tube that is 13 mm in diameter. After inserting the tube, claw forceps are passed down the shaft to grasp the specimen. Using a foot switch the tube is then rotated while pulling the

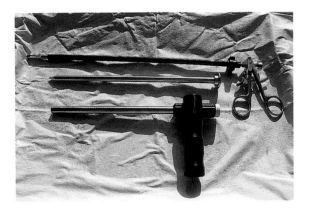

Figure 11.1 The Steiner Electromechanical Morcellator (Storz, Tuttlingen, Germany).

specimen against the mouth of the tube. Cylinders of tissue are cut, which are pulled up the shaft and are suitable for histologic examination. The speed and direction of rotation of the tube can be varied.

With the potential for severe trauma to intra-abdominal organs certain precautions are recommended:

- Only adequately trained surgeons should use the device, which should always be correctly maintained and functioning properly.
- The rotating cylinder should only be in motion when under continuous visual control.
- The sharp tip should be maintained in the same position within the abdomen at all times.

A new version of this device is equipped with a springloaded retractable trocar sleeve, which covers the cutting edge of the cylinder.

Large volumes of tissue that need isolation before removal can be placed within one of the larger laparoscopic bags. Suitable specimens include ovarian teratomas and mucinous cysts, and any ovary that may be neoplastic.

Errors in laparoscopic assessment of ovarian cysts are well documented (Maiman *et al.*, 1991). Others have shown that with strict adherence to guidelines of preoperative ultrasound assessment and intraoperative inspection, laparoscopic management of adnexal cystic masses appears to be safe (Mage *et al.*, 1990). Indeed some now advocate laparoscopic management of Stage 1A and B ovarian carcinoma (Reich *et al.*, 1990).

Once inside a bag cystic masses can be decompressed by incision and aspiration of their contents. This can be done inside the abdomen or after pulling the mouth of the bag outside the abdominal wall. Although malignant tumors can be safely removed using aspiration and morcellation with the mouth of the bag outside the abdomen (Clayman *et al.*, 1991), some authors are against this technique for suspicious masses, advocating intact extraction using a bag and an enlarged abdominal or colpotomy incision (Canis *et al.*, 1994).

Conclusion

With patience and ingenuity the specimens generated by operative laparoscopy can be removed without resorting to enlarged incisions. The use of such techniques for very large specimens and for suspicious and malignant masses clearly needs long-term evaluation of large series before widespread acceptance.

Potential complications of laparoscopic tissue extraction

- Enlargement of a portal
  - vessel trauma
  - hernia

- Posterior colpotomy
  - trauma to adjacent structures
  - adhesions
  - subsequent dyspareunia
  - granulation in the scar

- Spillage or incomplete removal of specimens
  - trophoblastic tissue
  - fecal matter at appendicectomy
  - endometriotic tissue
  - contents of ovarian cysts, mucinous fluid, cystic teratomata

- Morcellation
  - trauma to adjacent structures

References

Canis C, Mage G, Wattiez A *et al.* (1994) The role of laparoscopic surgery in gynaecological oncology. *Current Opinion in Obstetrics and Gynecology* **6**: 210–214.

Chapron C, Querleu D, Crepin G (1991) Laparoscopic treatment of ectopic pregnancies. A one hundred cases study. *European Journal of Obstetrics, Gynecology, and Reproductive Biology* **41**: 4–13.

Clayman R, Kavoussi L, Soper N *et al.* (1991) Laparoscopic nephrectomy: initial case report. *Journal of Urology* **146**: 278–282.

Daniell J, Gurley L (1991) Laparoscopic treatment of clinically significant symptomatic uterine fibroids. *Journal of Gynaecological Surgery* **7**: 37–40.

Donnez J, Nisolle M (1989) Laparoscopic treatment of ampullary tubal pregnancy. *Journal of Gynaecological Surgery* **5**: 157–162.

Dubuisson JB, Lecuru F, Foulot H, Mandelbrot L, Bouquet de la Joliniere J, Aubriot FX (1992) Gonadotrophin-releasing releasing hormone agonist and laparoscopic myomectomy. *Clinical Therapeutics* **14** (Supplement A): 51–56.

Grogan RH (1967) Accidental rupture of malignant ovarian cysts during surgical removal. *Obstetrics and Gynecology* **30**: 716.

Hsiu J, Given FT Jr, Kemp GM (1986) Tumour implantation after diagnostic laparoscopic biopsy of serous ovarian tumours of low malignant potential. *Obstetrics and Gynecology* **3** (Supplement): 90–93.

Kadar N, Reich H, Liu CY, Manko GF, Gimpelson R (1993) Incisional hernia after major laparoscopic gynecological procedures. *American Journal of Obstetrics and Gynecology* **168**: 1493–1495.

Kurtz BR, Daniell JF, Spaw AT (1993) Incarcerated incisional hernia after laparoscopy. A case report. *Journal of Reproductive Medicine* **38**: 643–644.

Langebrekke A and Urnes A (1994) Postoperative complications after laparoscopic removal of benign cystic teratoma. *Gynaecological Endoscopy* **3**: 245–246.

Mage G, Canis M, Manhes H *et al.* (1990) Laparoscopic management of adnexal cystic masses. *Journal of Gynaecological Surgery* **6**: 71–79.

Maiman M, Seltzer V, Boyce J (1991) Laparoscopic excision of ovarian neoplasms subsequently found to be malignant. *Obstetrics and Gynecology* **77**: 563–565.

Malkasian GD, Melton LJ, O'Brien PC, Green MH (1984) Prognostic significance of histologic classification and grading of epithelial malignancies of the ovary. *American Journal of Obstetrics and Gynecology* **149**: 274.

Nezhat C, Nezhat F, Silfen SL, Schaffer N, Evans D (1991) Laparoscopic myomectomy. *International Journal of Fertility* **36(5)**: 275–280.

Patterson M *et al.* (1993) Postoperative bowel obstruction following laparoscopic surgery. *American Surgeon* **59**: 656–657.

Reich H, McGlynn F, Wilkie W (1990) Laparoscopic management of stage I ovarian carcinoma; a case report. *Journal of Reproductive Medicine* **35**: 601–605.

Semm K (1978) Tissue-puncher and loop ligation – new aid for surgical therapeutic pelviscopy (laparoscopy) endoscopic intraabdominal surgery. *Endoscopy* **10**: 119–124.

Semm K (1993) Hysterectomy by pelviscopy: an alternative approach without colpotomy. In Garry R, Reich H (eds). *Laparoscopic Hysterectomy*, pp. 118–132. London: Blackwell Science Ltd.

Sigurdsson K, Alm P, Gullberg B (1983) Prognostic factors in malignant ovarian tumours. *Gynecologic Oncology* **15**: 370.

Steiner A, Wight E, Tadir Y, Haller U (1993) Electrical cutting device for laparoscopic removal of tissue from the abdominal cavity. *Obstetrics and Gynecology* **81(3)**: 471–474.

Sutton CJG (1993) A practical approach to diagnostic laparoscopy. In Sutton CJG, Diamond M (eds).

Endoscopic Surgery For Gynaecologists, pp. 21–27. London: Saunders Company Ltd.

Swartz J *et al.* (1990) Intraoperative anaphylaxis to latex. *Canadian Journal of Anaesthesia* **37**: 589–592.

Trujillo J, Molina A, Parache J (1994) Laparoscopic extraction of a tubal pregnancy using a condom. *Gynaecological Endoscopy* **3**: 241–243.

Ulrich U, Keckstein J, Karageogieva E *et al.* (1994) Ovarian mature teratoma: technical aspects of laparoscopic removal. *Gynaecological Endoscopy* **3**: 169–172.

12

Surgical Modalities and Clinical Results

TOGAS TULANDI

Department of Obstetrics and Gynecology, McGill University, Quebec, Canada

Surgical Modalities

Laparoscopic surgery can be achieved using various modalities such as scissors, electrical energy or surgical lasers. The basic physics of these modalities and their tissue effects are discussed in Chapter 9. In short, coagulating current causes cellular dehydration and its main effect is hemostatic. The current is characterized by intermittent periods of electrical inactivity. The cutting mode is a continuous current that causes actual explosion of the cell membrane due to the intense heat generated within the tissue itself. A blend between cutting and coagulation current is called a blended current.

In the unipolar system, electrons flow from the electrosurgical unit to the active electrode. From the tip of the electrode, the current will flow through the air to the tissue. The current will then be conducted through the body to the ground plate attached to the patient and returns to the electrosurgical unit. In the bipolar system, the current from the electrosurgical unit flows to the active electrode of the bipolar forceps (the shorter paddle of the forceps) through the intervening tissue to the inactive electrode (the longer paddle) and back to the electrosurgical unit. Only tissue in the forceps is affected and no ground plate is required. Thus the effect is focused and damage to adjacent tissues is minimized. A modification of a unipolar system is the argon beam coagulator (ABC). Here, electrons from an electrode flow through space to the tissue via argon gas, therefore the energy is delivered to the tissue in a 'non-touch' technique. This modality does not allow fine cutting. One of the concerns of this surgical modality is an immediate increase in intra-abdominal pressure due to the sudden burst of argon gas during the procedure.

Another surgical modality that has gained in popularity is the laser. The most widely used medical laser today is the carbon dioxide (CO_2) laser. It is the most precise laser and leads to minimal thermal injury. Unlike other lasers such as argon, neodymium:yttrium-aluminum-garnet (Nd:YAG) and potassium titanyl phosphate (KTP) lasers, CO_2 laser has limited coagulation properties. Indeed, lasers with a long wavelength are more effective for tissue vaporization, but poor for coagulation. Lasers with a short wavelength, on the other hand have good coagulation, but poor vaporization properties. The main advantage of using laser via the built-in channel of the laparoscope is that it makes one of the secondary trocars unnecessary. This can be used for an extra ancillary instrument.

A relatively new surgical modality is an ultrasonic scalpel. It is an instrument that potentially causes minimal tissue injury with good hemostasis. Ultrasonically activated, the scalpel blade moves longitudinally at 55 000 vibrations s^{-1} cutting the tissue. Since little heat is produced, thermal injury is minimal. The vibration of the ultrasonic scalpel is said to generate low heat at the incision site and the combination of the vibration and the heat causes the proteins to denature. The denatured proteins form a coagulum that seals the bleeding vessels. The ultrasonic scalpel produces less tissue injury on the porcine skin than electrosurgery or CO_2 laser (Hambley et al., 1988).

Tissue Effects

The use of heat in laser and electrosurgery gives a combination of cutting and coagulation properties, but it is associated with a thermal injury. Some studies suggest that the use of CO_2 laser is associated with minimal tissue damage, minimal scar formation and rapid healing. Subsequent studies have disproved that laser produces less tissue damage than other surgical modalities. In a rabbit model, there were no differences in the depth of thermal damage and in postoperative adhesion following CO_2 laser and electrocautery treatment (Pittaway et al., 1983; Luciano et al., 1987). Filmar et al. (1989a,b) demonstrated that the use of CO_2 laser on the rat's uterine horn produces more tissue necrosis and more extensive foreign body reaction than the use of scissors. However, the use of laser is associated with less particulate carbon than electrosurgery. Other studies suggest that the use of superpulse and ultrapulse CO_2 laser produces a localized thermal necrosis without lateral spread. Lasers such as Nd:YAG and KTP lasers produce more tissue necrosis than the CO_2 laser.

The tissue effects of the ultrasonic scalpel and regular scalpel were compared by Tulandi et al. (1994). Unlike use of a regular scalpel, the use of an ultrasonic scalpel is associated with very minimal bleeding. It causes tissue blanching without charring and with minimal smoke production.

Clinical Results

It was initially believed that the results of laser surgery were superior to those of conventional techniques. However, there are randomized clinical studies comparing reproductive surgery using laser and electrosurgery by laparotomy showing similar results (Tulandi and Vilos, 1985; Tulandi, 1986, 1987). The degree of postsurgical adhesion is also comparable. Thus there is little advantage of using laser by laparotomy. The results of laparoscopic surgery using different modalities are discussed below.

Laparoscopic Salpingo-ovariolysis

It is obvious that women with bilateral tubal occlusion will not spontaneously conceive, but spontaneous pregnancy can occur in women with periadnexal adhesions. However, the chances of conceiving can be increased by salpingo-ovariolysis (Tulandi et al., 1990). Salpingo-ovariolysis is carried out by stretching the adhesions with the help of a laparoscopic forceps and an intrauterine cannula and then dividing them. The adhesions can be lysed with laparoscopic scissors, electrocautery or laser. The results are similar (Table 12.1). The overall pregnancy rate after laparoscopic salpingo-ovariolysis is 60% and the ectopic pregnancy rate is 5%. However, severe and dense adhesions cannot be completely liberated by laparoscopy. In these patients, the pregnancy rate after salpingo-ovariolysis by laparotomy is poor (10–15%). Patients with severe and dense adhesions will gain more from in vitro fertilization than from reproductive surgery.

Laparoscopic Terminal Salpingostomy

Laparoscopic salpingostomy is carried out in a similar manner as that by laparotomy. The tubal opening is created using laser, needle point unipolar

Table 12.1 Results of laparoscopic salpingo-ovariolysis following sharp dissection, laser or electrocautery.

Technique	Authors	Number	Follow-up (years)	Intrauterine pregnancy (%)	Ectopic pregnancy (%)	Total pregnancy (%)
Scissors	Gomel (1983)	92	1	62.0	5.4	67.4
Scissors	Fayez (1983)	50	2	56.0	4.0	60.0
Electrocautery	Mettler et al. (1979)	44	1–6	NA	NA	29.5
Electrocautery	Bruhat et al. (1983)	93	1	51.6	7.5	59.1
CO_2 laser	Donnez et al. (1989)	186	1½	NA	NA	58.0

electrode or laparoscopic scissors. To maintain the eversion of the neoostium, the mucosal flap is everted without tension using a few interrupted sutures of 6/0 polyglactin, laser or electrocoagulation. Laser eversion is done by defocusing the CO_2 laser and directing the beam 0.5 cm from the margin of the flap. Retraction of the mucosal flap creates an eversion. This can also be accomplished using a light electro-coagulation with a bipolar cautery. The same principle may be followed using other types of lasers. Because of the concerns of thermal damage and that a thick hydrosalpinx will not evert with laser or electrical energy, I prefer using sutures. The intussusception technique is also helpful for everting the mucosal flap and minimizing the number of sutures (McComb and Paleologou, 1991).

It is important to evaluate the pregnancy rate after reproductive surgery according to the tube with the least damage. After all, pregnancy tends to occur more often via the better fallopian tube. The outcomes following laparoscopic salpingostomy are shown in Table 12.2. The small number of patients in some of the studies, the different degrees of tubal damage, the variations in length of follow-up and the different operating surgeons make it difficult to compare the results of these various techniques (Gomel, 1977; Daniell and Herbert, 1984; Dubuisson et al., 1990; Canis et al., 1991). Depending upon the degree of tubal damage, the intrauterine pregnancy rate after salpingostomy ranges from 10–80% (Schlaff et al., 1990; Canis et al., 1991). Using salpingoscopy to evaluate tubal mucosa, Marana et al. (1995) reported that the term pregnancy rate in women with normal tubal mucosa was 64%. They found that salpingoscopic assessment of the tubal mucosa is of greater prognostic value than the American Fertility Society classifications for adnexal adhesions and distal tubal occlusion.

In general, better results can be expected for patients with bilateral hydrosalpinx following in vitro fertilization than after salpingostomy by laparotomy. However, laparoscopic salpingostomy is a reasonable alternative for selected patients who do not wish or cannot afford in vitro fertilization or for those who are found to have a hydrosalpinx at the time of diagnostic laparoscopy. The results depend upon the extent of tubal damage and are independent of the surgical modality used.

Recent studies suggest that the presence of hydrosalpinx decreases the success rate of in vitro fertilization (Vandromme et al., 1995; Katz et al., 1996; Voss et al., 1996). Perhaps, this is due to the toxic effect of the hydrosalpinx fluid. Accordingly, a salpingectomy should be considered in women who are undergoing in vitro fertilization or those with severe hydrosalpinx.

Endometriosis

Conservative Laparoscopic Surgical Treatment of Endometriosis

Several studies have shown that the results of conservative surgical treatment for endometriosis by laparoscopy are similar and better than those by laparotomy (Nezhat et al., 1989; Sutton and Hill, 1990; Cook and Rock, 1991; Adamson et al., 1993, 1994; Hughes et al., 1993). Laparoscopic treatment of endometriosis is associated with a high fecundity rate, even in the presence of advanced disease and there is a trend for increased early pregnancy rates. This is achieved by lysis of adhesions, excision of endometriotic implants and excision of endometriomas. The incidence of pregnancy (70%) is independent of the stage of endometriosis (Olive and Martin,

Table 12.2 Outcomes following laparoscopic salpingostomy using sharp dissection, laser or electrocautery.

Technique	Authors	Number	Follow-up (years)	Intrauterine pregnancy (%)	Ectopic pregnancy (%)	Total pregnancy (%)
Scissors	Gomel (1977)	9	1	44.4	0	44.4
Scissors	Mettler et al. (1979)	36	1–6	NA	NA	26.0
Scissors	Fayez (1983)	19	2	0	10.0	10.0
CO_2 laser	Daniell and Herbert (1984)	21	>1	19.0	5.0	24.0
CO_2 laser	Donnez et al. (1989)	25	>1	NA	NA	20.0
Combined	Dubuisson et al. (1990)	34	>1	29.4	2.9	32.4

1987; Nezhat *et al.*, 1989) and of the surgical modality used (Tulandi and Bugnah, 1995), but is directly related to the duration of infertility. Adamson *et al.* (1993) reported that laparoscopic treatment of endometriosis is superior to medical treatment. They also found that the laparoscopic approach is superior to laparotomy. The question whether minimal and mild endometriosis are associated with infertility remains unanswered. Some authors suggest that the pregnancy rate after laparoscopic treatment of minimal and mild endometriosis is higher than after no treatment (Nowroozi *et al.*, 1987). Others could not confirm this association (Hughes *et al.*, 1993; Marana *et al.*, 1995). Well-designed randomized trials of laparoscopic treatment of endometriosis will clarify this uncertainty.

In the treatment of pelvic pain, a randomized double-blind prospective study demonstrated the superiority of laparoscopic uterine nerve transection and laser ablation of endometriotic implants in women with endometriosis Stage I, II and III compared to an untreated control group (Sutton *et al.*, 1994).

Excision of Endometriosis

Endometriotic implants can be coagulated electrosurgically or vaporized with the laser, but excision of the lesions results in a more complete removal (Redwine, 1994). Often a seemingly small endometriotic lesion on the peritoneum represents the tip of a deep endometriotic nodule. This will not be recog-nized without excision of the lesion. Excision is carried out by grasping the peritoneum harboring endometriosis (Figure 12.1). A small incision is made on the peritoneum and the peritoneum is under-mined, separating it from the underlying structures. This is done by blunt dissection and hydrodissection using a solution of Ringer's lactate or physiologic saline under pressure. The abnormal peritoneum, including the endometriotic lesion, is then excised. This technique is applicable for endometriosis over the ureter, the bladder or in the posterior cul-de-sac.

Excision of Ovarian Endometrioma

The technique of removal of an endometrioma is similar to ovarian cystectomy in general. However, rarely, an endometrioma can be enucleated intact. The chocolate-colored content of the cyst often escapes during the dissection. In this situation, the cyst's content should be drained and lavaged. A cleavage plane is created between the cyst wall and the ovarian capsule. Using two grasping forceps for traction and countertraction, the cyst wall is sepa-rated from the ovarian tissue (Figure 12.2). Bleeding from the inner surface of the ovarian defect can be electrocoagulated using a bipolar forceps.

Occasionally, the cyst wall is so intimately adher-ent to the ovarian tissue that a cleavage plane can-not be created. This is not uncommonly found with a small ovarian endometrioma. Here, the content of the cyst is aspirated and repeatedly irrigated. The top of the cyst including the associated 'ovarian

Figure 12.1 The peritoneum adjacent to the endometriosis on the right uterosacral ligament is grasped with a forceps and stretched medially. An incision is made on the peritoneum. The ureter is displaced laterally by the suction irrigator. (Reprinted from Tulandi T (1994) *Atlas of Laparoscopy Technique for Gynecologists.* London: WB Saunders Co. Reproduced with permission.)

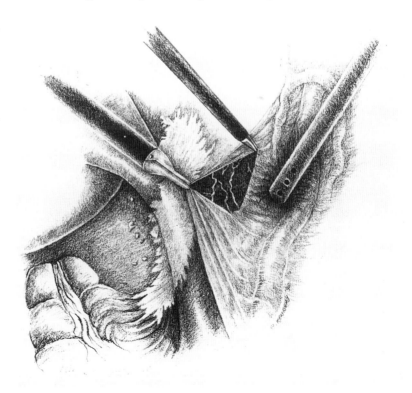

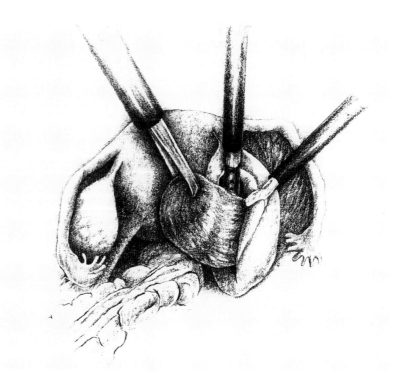

Figure 12.2 Stripping an endometriotic cyst wall using two grasping forceps for traction and countertraction. (Reprinted from Tulandi T (1994) *Atlas of Laparoscopy Technique for Gynecologists.* London: WB Saunders Co. 1994. Reproduced with permission.)

capsule' is decapitated. Care should be taken not to remove excessive ovarian tissue. If a cleavage plane is still not found, and after ascertaining that there is no suspicious lesion, the inner surface of the cyst wall is coagulated either with laser or electrocoagulation. This technique should, however, be rarely used because of the possibility of leaving active endometriotic tissue behind and the destruction of ovarian follicles. Usually, the ovarian defect collapses. If the ovary is gaping, two or three sutures of polydioxanone 4–0 or 5–0 or tissue sealant can be used to approximate the edges of the ovarian tissue. The ovarian capsule can also be inverted by coagulating the inner side of the ovarian opening approximately 1 cm from its margin. Inversion of the ovarian capsule approximates the ovarian opening.

Surgical Laparoscopic Treatment of Ectopic Pregnancy

Surgical treatment of ectopic pregnancy remains the definitive and universal treatment of ectopic pregnancy and it can be safely carried out by laparoscopy. Pouly *et al.* (1991) reported that in a series of 223 women with ectopic pregnancy treated by laparoscopic salpingostomy using electrocautery, the subsequent intrauterine pregnancy rate was 67% and the recurrent ectopic pregnancy was 12%. No complications were encountered. Paulson (1992) used CO_2 laser to perform salpingostomy in 125 patients and found that the intrauterine preg-

nancy rate among 48 women attempting to conceive was 79.2% and the recurrent ectopic pregnancy rate was 31.5%. It appears that the use of laser does not offer any advantage over electrocautery (Figure 12.3).

Laparoscopic Treatment of Polycystic Ovaries

The oldest treatment for polycystic ovarian syndrome (PCOS)-related anovulation is bilateral ovarian wedge resection by laparotomy. A decrease in testosterone secretion occurs after this procedure. This frees the inhibited hypothalamopituitary axis and allows ovulation to occur. It also removes the local intraovarian androgen blockade that prevents normal follicular development. Another possible explanation is reduction in ovarian inhibin or stimulation of growth factor production. Ovarian wedge resection, however, is associated with a high incidence of periadnexal adhesions, which may jeopardize fertility (Donesky and Adashi, 1995).

Gjönnaes (1984) first reported treatment of PCOS by laparoscopic ovarian drilling. Using a unipolar electrode, he created 8–15 craters 2–4 mm deep on the ovarian capsule of each ovary. The ovulatory rate after the procedure was 92% with a pregnancy rate of 84% among women with no other cause of infertility. The ovulatory rate in obese women is lower than in women with lower body weight. Laparoscopic ovarian drilling is a less invasive technique than ovarian wedge resection by laparotomy

Figure 12.3 Reproductive performance after laparoscopic treatment of ectopic pregnancy by electrocautery and by laser.

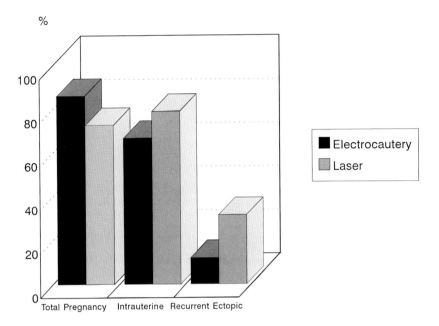

and is associated with less adhesion formation (Naether *et al.*, 1993). Furthermore, the results appear to be superior.

Ovarian drilling can be done using a unipolar needle electrode or laser. The overall ovulation and pregnancy rates after laparoscopic treatment using different modalities are shown in Table 12.3. There are other variables that should be considered including the ovulatory status before surgery, the use of ovulation inducing agents before and after the procedure, and the presence of other infertility factors. However, it appears that electrosurgery provides better results than laser (Figure 12.4). Perhaps, this is due to a better reduction of androgen-producing cells and inhibin by electrocautery.

Among different surgical modalities, the use of a unipolar insulated needle cautery of 40 W for 2 s is preferable. As most of the uninsulated part of the needle is inside the ovary, the risk of sparking is reduced. Furthermore, the thermal damage to the ovarian surface is limited (Figure 12.5). This may decrease adhesion formation. Depending upon the size of the ovary, usually 10–20 'holes' are created in the capsule and stroma of each ovary. Liberal irrigation of the pelvic cavity to remove necrotic debris and carbon materials should be carried out at the completion of an ovarian drilling. In our institution, this technique is limited to anovulatory women with PCOS who have failed gonadotropin treatment or those who have failed to ovulate with high

Table 12.3 Ovulatory and pregnancy rates after laparoscopic treatment of PCOS.

Author		Ovulatory rate	Pregnancy rate
Electrosurgery			
Gjönnaess (1984)		57/62 (92%)	24/35 (69%)
Greenblatt and Casper (1987)		5/6 (83%)	4/6 (67%)
Sumioki *et al.* (1988)		6/7 (86%)	4/7 (57%)
Sakata *et al.* (1990)		8/9 (89%)	3/9 (33%)
Abdel Gadir *et al.* (1990)		25/29 (86%)	14/29 (48%)
Gürgan *et al.* (1991)		7/10 (70%)	4/7 (57%)
Armar and Lachelin (1993)		45/50 (90%)	31/50 (62%)
Naether *et al.* (1993)		90/104 (86%)	73/104 (70%)
Subtotal		**243/277 (88%)**	**157/247 (64%)**
Laser	**Type**		
Daniell and Miller (1989)	CO_2/KTP	60/85 (71%)	48/85 (56%)
Keckstein *et al.* (1990)	CO_2	15/19 (79%)	7/19 (37%)
Rossmanith *et al.* (1991)	Nd:YAG	8/11 (73%)	4/11 (36%)
Gürgan *et al.* (1992)	Nd:YAG	28/40 (70%)	20/40 (50%)
Verhelst *et al.* (1993)	CO_2	14/17 (82%)	11/17 (65%)
Subtotal		**125/172 (73%)**	**90/172 (52%)**

Figure 12.4 Ovulation and pregnancy rates after laparoscopic treatment of polycystic ovaries using electrocautery and laser.

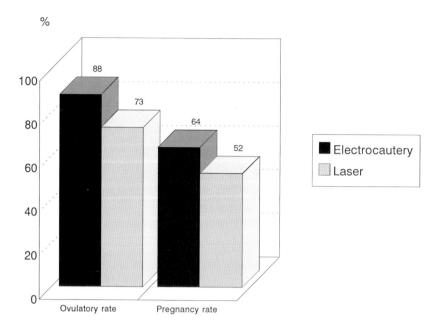

Figure 12.5 A computer-enhanced 3D image of a region of the ovary after ovarian drilling with a unipolar needle electrode at 40 W for 2 s. Burn region, yellow; region of necrotization, orange; normal tissue, dark red to light blue). (Courtesy of Kenneth L. Watkins PhD, Department of Obstetrics and Gynecology, McGill University, Canada.)

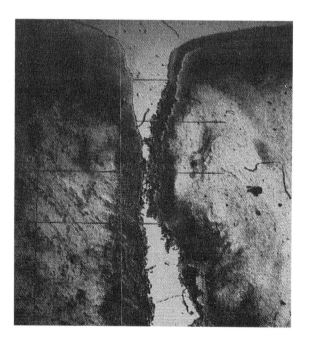

dose clomiphene and cannot afford gonadotropin treatment. The results have been promising and most pregnancies occur within six months of the procedure.

Excessive drilling may cause ovarian atrophy and premature menopause. Creating more than 20 'holes' per ovary and drilling the ovarian hilum should be avoided. This may jeopardize the blood supply to the ovary and may also cause bleeding. Due to concern about adhesion formation, coagulation on the ovarian surface should be minimal.

Miscellaneous Laparoscopic Procedures and Complications

Other procedures, including hysterectomy, myomectomy, presacral neurectomy and urethropexy can be carried out using various surgical modalities. The results appear to be independent of the surgical modality used. Certainly, the risks of post-surgical adhesions in women who are beyond their reproductive age or who have completed their family are of less concern than in younger women. Laparoscopic clips, staples, sutures, laser and electrosurgical energy can be used. For hysterectomy, the use of endoscopic linear staples decreases the operating time. A multiple staple applicator applies six rows of titanium staples. The standard staple compresses on firing to 1.5 mm and the vascular cartridge compresses to 1 mm. However, because blood can seep between the staples, its use during hysterectomy has been associated with hematoma formation. Furthermore, due to its width, ureteral entrapment in the staples can occur (Woodland, 1992). For myomectomy, ultrasonic scalpel may be a promising modality. It cuts with minimal bleeding. Also, because it produces less tissue injury than electrocautery or laser, it may be associated with less adhesion formation.

Among the complications of operative laparoscopy:

- The most common is injury to the blood vessels in the abdominal wall and mesosalpinx (0.7–1.0 per 1000 laparoscopies) (Lehmann-Willenbrock *et al.*, 1992).
- The incidence of mechanical injury to the bowel or ureter is higher than that of electrical injury (0.6 versus 0.1–0.2 per 1000 laparoscopies).
- The incidence of serious bowel or ureteral injury due to bipolar and unipolar coagulation is 0.2–0.4 versus 0.1–0.2 per 1000 laparoscopies, respectively.
- About 50% of the injuries occurring are related to the trocar insertion and another 50% are encountered during the procedure.

Because complications tend to be under-reported, in practise the incidence of complications may be higher. The use of laser is not devoid of complications. Ureteral transection and bladder and bowel injury have occurred. To date there is no comparative study demonstrating that laser injury is less frequent or less severe than electrosurgical injury or injury due to sharp dissection.

Summary

Numerous studies on the success of endoscopic surgery have been published. The majority describe the personal experience of one or several surgeons and the results are often complicated by many variables. Without a randomized trial, it is difficult to evaluate the results of a particular procedure or a surgical modality with certainty. However, a randomized trial is not always easy to conduct or can be impossible. In any event, published reports to date suggest that the results of laparoscopic surgery are independent of the surgical modality used. The surgeon's skill and experience, his or her preference of technique and appropriate patient selection play a more important role.

References

Abdel Gadir A, Mowafi RS, Alnaser HMI, Albrashide AH, Alonezi OM, Shaw RW (1990) Ovarian electrocautery versus human menopausal gonadotrophins and pure follicle stimulating hormone therapy in the treatment of patients with polycystic ovarian disease. *Clinical Endocrinology (Oxford)* **33**: 55–592.

Adamson GD, Hurd SJ, Pasta DJ, Rodriguez BD (1993) Laparoscopic endometriosis treatment: is it better. *Fertility and Sterility* **59**: 35.

Adamson GD, Pasta DJ (1994) Surgical treatment of endometriosis-associated infertility: meta-analysis compared with survival analysis. *American Journal of Obstetrics and Gynecology* **171**: 1488.

Armar NA, Lachelin GC (1993) Laparoscopic ovarian diathermy: an effective treatment for anti-oestrogen resistant anovulatory infertility in women with polycystic ovary syndrome. *British Journal of Obstetrics and Gynaecology* **100**: 161–164.

Bruhat MA, Mage G, Manhes H (1983) Laparoscopic procedures to promote fertility ovariolysis and salpingolysis: results of 93 selected cases. *Acta Europaea Fertilitatis* **14**: 113–117.

Canis M, Mage G, Pouly JL, Manhes H, Wattiez A, Bruhat MA (1991) Laparoscopic distal tuboplasty: report of 87 cases and a 4-year experience. *Fertility and Sterility* **56**: 616.

Cook AS, Rock JA (1991) The role of laparoscopy in the treatment of endometriosis. *Fertility and Sterility* **55**: 663–680.

Daniell JF, Herbert CM (1984) Laparoscopic salpingostomy utilizing the CO_2 laser. *Fertility and Sterility* **41**: 558–563.

Daniell JF, Miller W (1989) Polycystic ovaries treated by laparoscopic laser vaporization. *Fertility and Sterility* **51**: 232–236.

Donesky BW, Adashi EY (1995) Surgically induced ovulation in the polycystic ovary syndrome: wedge resection revisited in the age of laparoscopy. *Fertility and Sterility* **63**: 439.

Donnez J, Nisolle M, Casanas-Roux F (1989) CO_2 laser laparoscopy in infertile women with adnexal adhesions and women with tubal occlusion. *Journal of Gynecologic Surgery* **5**: 47–53.

Dubuisson JB, De Jolinière JB, Aubriot FX, Darai E, Foulot H, Mandelbrot. (1990) Terminal tuboplasties by laparoscope: 65 consecutive cases. *Fertility and Sterility* **54**: 401–403.

Fayez JA (1983) An assessment of the role of operative laparoscopy in tuboplasty. *Fertility and Sterility* **39**: 476–479.

Filmar S, Jetha N, McComb P, Gomel V (1989a) A comparative histologic study on the healing process after tissue transection. I. Carbon dioxide laser and electro-microsurgery. *American Journal of Obstetrics and Gynecology* **160**: 1062–1067.

Filmar S, Jetha N, McComb P, Gomel V (1989b) A comparative histologic study on the healing process after tissue transection. II. Carbon dioxide laser and surgical microscissors. *American Journal of Obstetrics and Gynecology* **160**: 1068–1072.

Gjönnaes H (1984) Polycystic ovarian syndrome treated by ovarian electrocautery through the laparoscope. *Fertility and Sterility* **41**: 20–25.

Gomel V (1977) Salpingostomy by laparoscopy. *Journal of Reproductive Medicine* **18**: 265–268.

Gomel V (1983) Salpingoovariolysis by laparoscopy in infertility. *Fertility and Sterility* **40**: 607–611.

Greenblatt E, Casper RF (1987) Endocrine changes after laparoscopic ovarian cautery in polycystic ovarian syndrome. *American Journal of Obstetrics and Gynecology* **156**: 279–285.

Gürgan T, Kisnisci H, Yarali H, Develioglu O, Zeyneloglu H, Aksu T (1991) Evaluation of adhesion formation after laparoscopic treatment of polycystic ovarian disease. *Fertility and Sterility* **56**: 1176–1178.

Gürgan T, Urman B, Aksu T, Yarali H, Develioglu O, Kisnisci H (1992) The effect of short-interval laparoscopic lysis of adhesions on pregnancy rates following Nd-YAG laser photocoagulation of polycystic ovaries. *Obstetrics and Gynecology* **80**: 45–47.

Hambley R, Hebda PA, Abell E, Cohen BA, Jegasothy BV (1988) Wound healing of skin incisions produced by ultrasonically vibrating knife, scalpel, electrosurgery, and carbon dioxide laser. *Journal of Dermatologic Surgery and Oncology* **14**: 1213–1217.

Hughes EG, Fedorkow DM, Collins JA (1993) A quantitative overview of controlled trials in endometriosis-associated infertility. *Fertility and Sterility* **59**: 963.

Katz E, Akman MA, Damewood MD, Garcia JE (1996) Deleterious effect of the presence of hydrosalpinx on implantation and pregnancy rates with *in vitro* fertilization. *Fertility and Sterility* **66**: 122–125.

Keckstein G, Wolf AS, Börchers K, Lauritzen CH, Steiner R (1990) Pelviskopischer einsatz des CO_2-lasers zur behandlung des polyzystischen ovarsyndroms. *Zentrablatt fur Gynakologie* **112**: 361–368.

Lehmann-Willenbrock E, Riedel HH, Mecke H, Semm K (1992). Pelviscopy/laparoscopy and its complications in Germany, 1949–1988. *Journal of Reproductive Medicine* **8**: 671–677.

Luciano AL, Whitman G, Maier DB, Randolph J, Maenza R (1987) Comparison of thermal injury, healing patterns and postoperative adhesion formation following CO_2 laser and electromicrosurgery. *Fertility and Sterility* **48**: 1025–1029.

Marana R, Rizzi M, Muzii L, Catalano GF, Caruana P, Mancuso S (1995) Correlation between the American Fertility Society Classification of adnexal adhesions and distal tubal occlusion, salpingoscopy and reproductive outcome in tubal surgery. *Fertility and Sterility* **64**: 924–928.

McComb P, Paleologou A (1991) The intussusception salpingostomy technique for the therapy of distal oviductal occlusion at laparoscopy. *Obstetrics and Gynecology* **78**: 443.

Mettler L, Giesel H, Semm K (1979) Treatment of female infertility due to tubal obstruction by operative laparoscopy. *Fertility and Sterility* **32**: 384–388.

Naether OGJ, Fischer R, Weise HC, Delfs T, Rudolf K (1993) Laparoscopic electrocoagulation of the ovarian surface in infertility patients with polycystic ovarian disease. *Fertility and Sterility* **60**: 88–94.

Nezhat C, Crowgey S, Nezhat F (1989) Videolaseroscopy for the treatment of endometriosis associated infertility. *Fertility and Sterility* **51**: 237–240.

Nowroozi K, Chase JS, Check JH, Wu CH (1987) The importance of laparoscopic coagulation of mild endometriosis in infertile women. *International Journal of Fertility* **32**: 442–444.

Olive DL, Martin DC (1987) Treatment of endometriosis-associated infertility with CO_2 laser laparoscopy: the use of one and two-parameter exponential models. *Fertility and Sterility* **48**: 18–23.

Paulson JD (1992) The use of carbon dioxide laser laparoscopy in the treatment of tubal ectopic pregnancies. *American Journal of Obstetrics and Gynecology* **167**: 382–386.

Pittaway DE, Maxson WS, Daniell JF (1983) A comparison of the CO_2 laser and electrocautery on postoperative intraperitoneal adhesion formation in rabbits. *Fertility and Sterility* **40**: 366–368.

Pouly JL, Chapron C, Manhes H, Canis M, Wattiez A, Bruhat MA (1991) Multifactorial analysis of fertility after conservative laparoscopic treatment of ectopic pregnancy in a series of 223 patients. *Fertility and Sterility* **56**: 453–460.

Redwine D (1994) Treatment of endometriosis. In Tulandi T (ed.) *Atlas of Laparoscopy Technique for Gynecologists*, pp. 23–32. London: WB Saunders Company.

Rossmanith WG, Keckstein J, Spatzier K, Lauritzen Ch (1991) Impact of ovarian laser surgery on gonadotropin secretion in women with polycystic ovarian disease. *Clinical Endocrinology (Oxford)* **34**: 223–230.

Sakata M, Tasaka K, Kurachi H, Terakawa N, Miyake A, Tanizawa O (1990) Changes of bioactive luteinizing hormone after laparoscopic ovarian cautery in patients with polycystic ovarian syndrome. *Fertility and Sterility* **53**: 610–613.

Schlaff WD, Hassiakos DK, Damewood MD, Rock J (1990) Neosalpingostomy for distal tubal obstruction. Prognostic factors and impact of surgical technique. *Fertility and Sterility* **54**: 984–990.

Sumioki H, Utsunomyiya T, Matsuoka K, Korenaga M, Kadota T (1988) The effect of laparoscopic multiple punch resection of the ovary on the hypothalamo-pituitary axis in polycystic ovary syndrome. *Fertility and Sterility* **50**: 567–572.

Sutton C, Hill D (1990) Laser laparoscopy in the treatment of endometriosis. A 5 year study. *British Journal of Obstetrics and Gynaecology* **97**: 181–185.

Sutton CJG, Ewen SP, Whitelaw N, Haines P (1994) Prospective, randomized, double-blind, controlled trial of laser laparoscopy in the treatment of pelvic pain associated with minimal, mild and moderate endometriosis. *Fertility and Sterility* **62**: 696–670.

Tulandi T (1986) Salpingo-ovariolysis: A comparison between laser surgery and electrosurgery. *Fertility and Sterility* **45**: 489–491.

Tulandi T (1987) Adhesion reformation after reproductive

surgery with or without the carbon dioxide laser. *Fertility and Sterility* **47**: 704–706.

Tulandi T, Vilos GA (1985) A comparison between laser surgery and electrosurgery for bilateral hydrosalpinx: A 2 year follow-up. *Fertility and Sterility* **44**: 846–848.

Tulandi T, Bugnah M (1995) Operative laparoscopy: surgical modalities. *Fertility and Sterility* **63**: 237.

Tulandi T, Collins JA, Burrows E *et al.* (1990) Treatment-dependent and treatment-independent pregnancy among women with periadnexal adhesions. *American Journal of Obstetrics and Gynecology* **162**: 354.

Tulandi T, Chan KL, Arseneau J (1994) Histopathologic and adhesion formation study after incision using ultrasound vibrating scalpel and regular scalpel. *Fertility and Sterility* **61**: 548–550.

Vandromme J, Chase E, Lejeune B, Van Rysselberge M, Delvigne A, Leroy F (1995) Hydrosalpinges in *in-vitro* fertilization; an unfavourable prognostic feature. *Human Reproduction* **10**: 576–579.

Verhelst J, Joostens M, Van der Meer S, Van Royen E, Mahler C (1993) Clinical and endocrine effects of laser vaporization in patients with polycystic ovarian disease. *Gynecologic Endocrinology* **7**: 49–55.

Voss E, Boldes R, Stark M (1996) Impaired implantation after *in vitro* fertilization treatment associated with hydrosalpinx. *British Journal of Obstetrics and Gynaecology* **103**: 851.

Woodland MB (1992) Ureter injury during laparoscopy-assisted vaginal hysterectomy with the endoscopic linear stapler. *American Journal of Obstetrics and Gynecology* **167**: 756–757.

Laparoscopic Tubal Surgery

13

Salpingostomy and Fimbrioplasty

JEAN-BERNARD DUBUISSON AND CHARLES CHAPRON

Clinique Universitaire Baudelocque, Paris, France

Introduction

The past 30 years have been marked by considerable progress in the management of distal tubal infertility. Under the influence of several teams in the 1970s, involving Swolin, Gomel, Winston, Donnez, Salat-Baroux, Bruhat and Dubuisson, the principles and techniques for microsurgical treatment were laid down, replacing classic surgery methods. Then during a second phase, laparoscopic surgery gradually came to the fore as the treatment of choice for distal tubal infertility. From a medical point of view there has also been very considerable progress. The *in vitro* fertilization (IVF) techniques are now reliable and the results correctly assessed. The goal of this work is to describe the techniques for laparoscopic surgical treatment of distal tubal infertility and to clarify the place of laparoscopic surgery for this indication in relation to the other possible treatments.

Anatomy of the Distal Fallopian Tube

Precise knowledge of the anatomy and physiology of the fallopian tube is essential to understand the mechanisms of each case of tubal infertility and to establish its prognosis. An operative strategy must be decided to avoid inappropriate reconstructive procedures. The ampulla is elastic and sinuous and about 5–8 cm in length. The diameter increases distally, reaching 1–2 cm at the extremity. Its thin walls allow it to be distended readily by fluids. The distal portion or infundibulum measures 2–3 cm in length. It is funnel-shaped and opens into the peritoneal cavity via the abdominal ostium, which is surrounded by 12–15 mobile fimbriae. The internal diameter of the ostium is 2 mm, but is distensible. Microscopic studies have shown that the fimbriae are continuous, with complex longitudinal branching folds. The ampulla includes 3–5 main folds. The columnar epithelium or endosalpinx consists of secretory and ciliated cells.

Pathology of the Distal Fallopian Tube

Lesions to the distal tube are most often secondary to pelvic inflammatory disease. Other causes of distal tubal pathology include tuberculosis, schistosomiasis, endometriosis and congenital anomalies (De Brux, 1982). There are two degrees of obstruction:

- Partial stenosis or phimosis with some degree of tuboperitoneal permeability.
- Total occlusion with hydrosalpinx.

Four main anatomical problems may be observed in stenosis:

- Adhesions encapsulating the fimbrial extremity.
- Adhesions glueing the fimbriae together, which may extend into the ampulla.
- A retracted peritoneal ring strangulating the distal tube.

- Less frequently, adhesions affect the ostium itself, resulting in ampullary dilatation with apparently normal fimbriae. Patency is demonstrated under high-pressure chromotubation.

Histologic evidence of chronic salpingitis is usually observed in the ampulla and infundibulum. In cases with glued fimbriae, more severe lesions of follicular salpingitis are not infrequent.

The anatomical details of hydrosalpinges are related to the degree of damage to the mucosa and tube wall:

- Hydrosalpinx simplex is a moderately dilated ampulla containing clear yellow fluid. The tube wall is thinned and there is atrophy of the mucosa. Mucosal folds may be decreased or absent. The epithelium is usually altered with flattened cells and a marked reduction in the number of cilia.
- In follicular hydrosalpinx, the lumen is divided by adhesions forming septa, which terminate in fimbrial adhesions. This is the most advanced stage of follicular or alveolar salpingitis. The epithelium is often hypertrophic, the cells retaining their morphological characteristics and cilia.
- Hydrosalpinx with pachysalpinx is characterized by a thickened tube wall with local total sclerosis (fibrosis) replacing smooth muscle fibers.
- Inflammatory hydrosalpinges show lymphoplasmocytic infiltration and tube wall edema.

Preoperative Evaluation

A complete clinical examination and psychologic assessment of the couple are essential. The preoperative work-up follows three main lines as follows.

Evaluation of the Couple's Fertility

All possible male and female factors for infertility should always be investigated. Spermocytogram, postcoital testing, temperature charts, hormone assays and testing for infections, including *Neisseria gonorrhoeae* and *Chlamydia trachomatis*, must be systematic. Diagnostic hysteroscopy with carbon dioxide (CO_2) is necessary in order to analyze the uterine cavity and visualize the tubal ostia. A biopsy of the endometrium is required to screen for endometritis and to assess hormonal impregnation. In our institution we carry out this hysteroscopy

on an outpatient basis during a preoperative consultation.

Diagnostic Work-up and Prognosis for the Tube Lesions

Hysterosalpingography is of prime importance. It should be carried out in the absence of infection and under antibiotic cover, and enables the quality of the interstitial and isthmic segments to be assessed, together with the ampullary mucosal folds, the passage to the infundibulum and the peritoneal environment (Maathuis *et al.*, 1972). We will see that the initial diagnostic phase during laparoscopy also contributes to this work-up.

Analysis of How the Lesions are Evolving

Signs for current infection are systematically looked for during the clinical examination and by biologic testing. We check the blood count, sedimentation rate and C-reactive protein. If one of these markers indicates inflammation, corrective surgery is postponed and is preceded by medical treatment. Cervicovaginal bacteriologic samples are always taken to look for gonococcus, *Chlamydia trachomatis*, mycoplasma and common pathogenic microorganisms. Chlamydia serology is essential, as is a check on the partner for infection (e.g. urethral, urine and sperm culture samples). Here again the initial diagnostic phase of the laparoscopy contributes to the work-up by checking for obvious signs of ongoing inflammation and by enabling cytologic and bacteriologic samples to be taken, together with biopsies of the adhesions.

Contraindications for Tubal Repair Surgery

The aim of the work-up is to select those patients who will best benefit from surgical treatment. The main contraindications for tubal repair surgery are:

- Severe pelvic adhesions with a 'frozen pelvis'.
- Past history of extensive ampullo-infundibular tube resections for sterilization.
- Extensive intra-ampullary adhesions suspected at hysterosalpingography and confirmed during the diagnostic phase of laparoscopy after opening the hydrosalpinx.
- Bilateral bifocal tube disease or unilateral on a solitary tube (Dubuisson *et al.*, 1984).
- Ongoing genital tuberculosis or sequelae.

- The existence of associated incurable factors for infertility.
- Medical pathology contraindicating surgery or pregnancy.
- The age of older patients, bearing in mind that each case should be assessed individually.

Operative Techniques

General Equipment for Laparoscopic Surgery

Laparoscopic surgical treatment for distal tubal infertility requires experienced surgeons and theater staff who are well trained in laparoscopic surgery, together with suitable and high-performance equipment. The equipment needed for any laparoscopic surgery (e.g. automatically controlled electronic insufflator, panoramic optics, video system) is well known by now. The basic instrumentation includes atraumatic grasping forceps, a pair of fine scissors with straight or curved blades, a bipolar coagulation forceps (with narrow jaws), a fine monopolar electrode and an irrigation system. All the instruments we use come from Karl Storz (Endoscope, Tuttlingen, Germany).

More Specific Equipment

THE CO_2 LASER

The physical properties of the CO_2 laser mean it can be used both to section and to vaporize. These two effects are useful for adhesiolysis, for incising the tube (sectioning effect) and to enable tubal eversion (vaporization effect). The CO_2 laser can be used either with a bayonet lens via the transumbilical route or with a hand forceps by the suprapubic route.

THE DIATHERMY COAGULATOR

This is recommended by Semm and it enables the tissues to be heated to 100–140 °C for several seconds. This effect is obtained at the point where a probe with a flat end, diameter 5 mm, is applied. We frequently use this possibility to maintain tubal eversion.

Patient Installation

In most cases we use bowel preparation and the following protocol:

- A low residue diet for eight days before hospitalization.
- 1 × 5 g sachet X-Prep (sennosides A and B, Laboratories Plantier, Mérignac, France) each day for two days before hospitalization.
- Normacol enema (1 × 130 ml adult flask (Laboratoire Norgan, Paris, France)) the night before the operation.

This bowel preparation makes it easier to push back the loops of bowel and thus helps to obtain better exposure during the operation.

The laparoscopy is carried out under general anesthesia with endotracheal intubation. The patient is installed flat on her back with buttocks protruding slightly over the edge of the table. A bladder catheter is systematically installed. A cannula introduced through the cervical canal enables a methylene blue test to be carried out. We usually create the pneumoperitoneum by the transumbilical route. If there is a past history of surgery the pneumoperitoneum can be created with no hesitation in the left hypochondrium (Palmer, 1974). The security tests must be carried out systematically to minimize the risk of injury secondary to introduction of the trocars (Chapron *et al.*, 1994c). The three suprapubic trocars must always be inserted under visual control.

The Laparoscopic Surgical Techniques

The first phase in the operation is diagnostic, both for the pelvis and the abdominal cavity. The surgeon looks for inflammatory lesions, ongoing adhesion formation, and lesions suggesting endometriosis. The morphology of the tubes must also be evaluated, and their permeability checked using a methylene blue test. In the abdomen, particular attention is paid to investigating the regions of the appendix and liver (Fitz-Hugh–Curtis syndrome).

Whether fimbrioplasty or salpingostomy is required, the first phase of the operation must always be devoted to freeing adhesions. Adhesiolysis must be atraumatic and should avoid any injury to the peritoneum using microsurgical principles. Whatever the technique used (laparoscopic scissors or CO_2 laser), adhesiolysis must also be carried out according to several rules as follows:

- Place adhesions under tension before sectioning.
- Do the simplest parts first before the more complicated.
- Start by freeing adhesions along the midline of the pelvis before freeing the adnexa.
- Start by freeing superficial adhesions.

This adhesiolysis is essential to restore normal anatomical relationships and perfect mobility of the tube relative to the ovary. Once it has been carried out the tubal lesions can be assessed more accurately.

LAPAROSCOPIC FIMBRIOPLASTY

The principle of fimbrioplasty is to restore the original anatomy of the infundibulum by treating the phimosis.

Section of the adhesions reveals the tubal phimosis. A fine atraumatic forceps inserted via the contralateral trocar to the tube is then cautiously introduced into the phimosis. By gently opening it, the adhesions and bridles in the infundibulum can be observed and exposed. Fimbrioplasty then consists of incising or excising the adhesions using fine scissors, the monopolar electrode or the CO_2 laser. When using the latter, a focused shot will enable section–coagulation to be obtained.

If the infundibular folds are stuck together, in many cases all that is needed is to dilate the stenosis by introducing the fine atraumatic forceps into the existing ostium with the jaws closed and then gently opening the jaws. If this does not work then the bands of sclerotic tissue need to be incised.

After these procedures to restore a normal infundibulum, the next task is to assess the quality of the tubal mucosa and look for any intratubal synechiae, which are evidence from the histologic point of view of alveolar salpingitis, which adversely affects the prognosis. At the end of the operation any slight bleeding should be checked by meticulous peritoneal irrigation with hot (37 °C) normal saline. If there is a small hemorrhage, the infundibulum can be immersed in the hot saline for a few minutes and in most cases the bleeding will stop. If not, the answer is elective coagulation with the fine monopolar electrode.

LAPAROSCOPIC SALPINGOSTOMY

This technique (Figures 13.1–13.5) consists of creating a new ostium in cases where the distal part of the tube is totally occluded (hydrosalpinx). The operation comprises two phases: incision and eversion (Dubuisson *et al.*, 1990).

Opening and Incising the Tube

This exposes the hydrosalpinx. Methylene blue is now injected to make the old ostium show up as a whitish sclerosed area. The ideal is to start opening at this point. The tube is incised using fine laparoscopic scissors or the CO_2 laser with a focused shot.

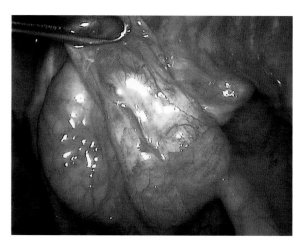

Figure 13.1 Aspect of right hydrosalpinx before salpingostomy.

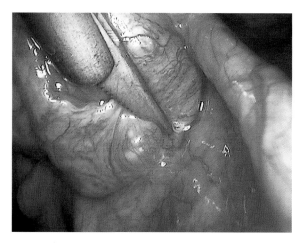

Figure 13.2 Incision of the hydrosalpinx at its apex.

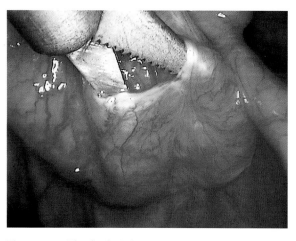

Figure 13.3 The hydrosalpinx is opened atraumatically along the fibrous scars, avoiding the mucosa plicae.

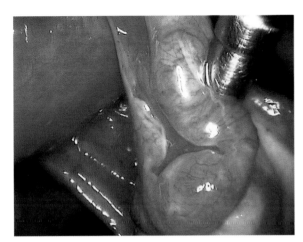

Figure 13.4 Eversion of the hydrosalpinx using the thermocoagulation technique. The probe is placed on the serosa for a few seconds. With retraction of the serosa, the mucosa is everted.

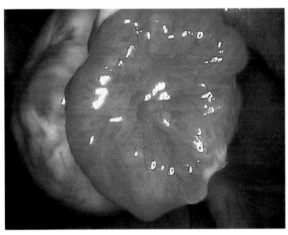

Figure 13.5 Flower aspect after salpingostomy. Mucosa grade 1.

Once the hydrosalpinx has been opened, several incisions (2–4 depending upon what is technically feasible) of about 1–2 cm are made. Care should be taken to locate these incisions between the longitudinal mucosal folds in an avascular area. Theoretically these incisions should not bleed. If there is any bleeding, immersing the infundibulum in hot (37°C) normal saline helps to obtain hemostasis. If this fails then elective coagulation of the vessels with the fine monopolar electrode or the bipolar forceps is needed.

Stabilizing the Eversion

Once the hydrosalpinx has been opened, the neo-ostium is kept in the everted position by creating a retraction of the distal serosa. Several techniques

can be used to perform the distal serosa retraction as follows:

- Vaporization of the tubal serosa with a de-focused shot from the CO_2 laser. Eversion is maintained due to the surface coagulation caused by the laser.
- Bipolar coagulation of the serosa. This enables the same results to be obtained as with the laser. As with the laser method, only the serosa should be coagulated with the lowest power possible to avoid charring the tissues and provoking any lesions in the tubal mucosa.
- Thermocoagulation of the serosa. In this case the 5 mm diathermy probe is applied to the serosa. Once again the serosa whitens and retracts, creating the required eversion very easily. This is the technique we usually use (see Figure 13.4).
- Suture with separate stitches of Vicryl 7/0 (polyglactin 910, Ethicon, Neuilly, France). This technique is the most delicate and is only possible when the tube wall is fine and supple. It is not used very often.

Results

The results of laparoscopic adhesiolysis are difficult to assess because in a number of situations it is associated with distal tuboplasty (fimbrioplasty or salpingostomy). Table 13.1 gives the fertility results after purely laparoscopic adhesiolysis. The intrauterine pregnancy (IUP) rate varies from 12–78% with an average of about 50%. The ectopic pregnancy (EP) rate is 5% on average. Most pregnancies occur within one year of the operation. With respect to infertility, the results of laparoscopic adhesiolysis are comparable to those for microsurgical adhesiolysis (Saravelos *et al.*, 1995).

Very few teams have presented results for laparoscopic fimbrioplasty. The results in Table 13.2 show that the IUP rate is 40% on average, with an 8.5% risk of EP.

The fertility results for laparoscopic salpingostomy are presented in Table 13.3. They are comparable to those obtained with microsurgery by laparotomy (Saravelos *et al.*, 1995). So when salpingostomy needs to be carried out, we suggest that operative laparoscopy is the method of reference (Chapron *et al.*, 1994a) in view of the tremendous advantages of laparoscopy compared with laparotomy (Chapron *et al.*, 1994b).

Table 13.1 Laparoscopic adhesiolysis: fertility results.

Authors	Year	Number	Intrauterine pregnancies		Ectopic pregnancies	
			(N)	(%)	(N)	(%)
Mettler *et al.*	1979	44	13	29	–	–
Palmer	1979	144	34	23.6	11	7.6
Mintz *et al.*	1979	65	34	52.3	–	–
Gomel	1983	92	54	58.7	5	5.4
Audebert	1983	50	15	30	0	0
Fayez	1983	50	30	60	2	4
Bruhat *et al.*	1983	93	48	52	7	7.5
Feste	1985	17	6	35.3	–	–
Diamond *et al.*	1986	9	0	0.0	–	–
Reich	1987	27	21	78	1	4
Serour *et al.*	1989	25	3	12.0	–	–

Table 13.2 Fimbrioplasty by laparoscopy: fertility results.

Authors	Year	Number	Intrauterine pregnancy		Ectopic pregnancy	
			(N)	(%)	(N)	(%)
Gomel	1983	40	20	50	2	5
Dubuisson *et al.*	1990	31	8	25.8	4	12.9
Total		**71**	**28**	**39.4**	**6**	**8.5**

Table 13.3 Salpingostomy by laparoscopy: fertility results.

Authors	Year	Number	Pregnancy (%)	Intrauterine pregnancy (%)	Ectopic pregnancy (%)
Gomel	1977	9		44.4	0
Mettler *et al.*	1979	38	26	–	–
Fayez	1983	19	10	–	10
Daniell and Herbert	1984	21	24	19	5
Audibert *et al.*	1991	55	20	–	15
Canis *et al.*	1991	87		33.3	6.9
McComb and Paleologou	1991	22	22.7	–	?
Nezhat *et al.*	1992	42	35.7	–	15.4
Dubuisson *et al.*	1994	81	37	32.1	4.9

Discussion

The fertility results after distal tubal plasty operations are correlated with the state of the tube. The more the tube has deteriorated, the less chance there is of obtaining an intrauterine pregnancy (Canis *et al.*, 1991; Dubuisson *et al.*, 1994). A Tubal Scoring System has been proposed in France (Mage *et al.*, 1987). Analysis of the fertility results after laparo-scopic salpingostomy according to this score shows that there is a statistically highly significant difference between patients with Stages 1 and 2 and those with Stages 3 and 4 (Table 13.4). Taking these results and the possibilities for IVF into account (FIVNAT, 1995; American Fertility Society, 1994; Benadiva *et al.*, 1995) the following program for treatment can be proposed in cases of distal tubal infertility:

Table 13.4 Salpingostomy by laparoscopy: intrauterine pregnancy rates according to the French Tubal Scoring System (Mage *et al.*, 1987).

Authors	Year	French Tubal Scoring System(%)			
		1	2	3	4
Canis *et al.*	1991	50.0	32.4	8.3	0.0
Dubuisson *et al.*	1994	60.0	51.7	12.5	5.4
Lavergne *et al.*	1996	50.0	60.0	16.6	0.0

• Distal tubal surgery for patients with a score of 1 or 2.

• Immediate referral to IVF for patients with a score of 3 or 4.

We believe that those patients who will benefit from distal tubal plasty should be operated on by laparoscopy because the fertility results are similar to those of microsurgery (Chapron *et al.*, 1994a).

Given that the condition of the tubal mucosa is the main prognostic factor for distal tubal plasty, the problem we are faced with in practise is how to assess this mucosa. Several classifications have been put forward for this purpose. Up until now all of the various classifications (Rock *et al.*, 1978; Mage *et al.*, 1986; American Fertility Society, 1988) have proved complicated to use, including a large number of parameters such as tubal patency (Mage *et al.*, 1986), tubal mucosa (Rock *et al.*, 1978; Mage *et al.*, 1986; American Fertility Society, 1988), the appearance of the fimbriae (Rock *et al.*, 1978), tube wall (Rock *et al.*, 1978; Mage *et al.*, 1986; American Fertility Society, 1988), size of the hydrosalpinx (Rock *et al.*, 1978; American Fertility Society, 1988), type of adhesions and area involved (Rock *et al.*, 1978; American Fertility Society, 1988).

Although the French Tubal Scoring System (Mage *et al.*, 1987) enables two groups of patients to be differentiated who will be offered totally different programs of treatment, the score is complicated to use. It takes several parameters into account with assessment either during the preoperative work-up or during laparoscopy (Table 13.5). With this in mind we have attempted to simplify the assessment of distal tube condition (Dubuisson *et al.*, 1994). To this end we compared our fertility results by analyzing them according to the French Tubal Scoring System (Mage *et al.*, 1987) and according to the Boer-Meisel classification (1986).

This Boer-Meisel classification (Boer–Meisel *et al.*, 1986) relies upon evaluation of the tubal mucosa alone and enables patients to be classed into three groups.

• Patients belonging to Group 1 are those whose mucosa is normal with regular folds.

• Patients in Group 2 have moderate alterations to the ampullary mucosa, with areas of normal mucosa interspersed with areas where the mucosal folds are rare or non-existent (atrophic mucosa).

• The patients in Group 3 are those whose mucosa has deteriorated considerably with

Table 13.5 French Tubal Scoring System (Mage *et al.*, 1987).

Tube permeability	Ampullary mucosa	Wall of ampulla
Phimosis 2	Folds remaining 0	Normal 0
Hydrosalpinx 5	Fold reduced 5	Thin 5
	No folds or alveolar salpingitis 10	Thick or sclerotic 10

Stage 1: 2–5.
Stage 2: 6–10.
Stage 3: 11–15.
Stage 4: > 15.

either complete disappearance of the mucosa or the existence of intratubal synechiae (alveolar mucosa).

The results presented in Table 13.6 demonstrate very clearly that the Boer-Meisel classification (Boer-Meisel *et al.*, 1986) provides a prognosis and orientation tool comparable in value to that of the French Tubal Scoring System. It is far simpler to assess the distal tubal condition by laparoscopic inspection of the ampullary mucosa alone than to take into account all of the parameters in the French Tubal Scoring System. We therefore now use this factor only when deciding which patients should be offered salpingostomy during the same anesthesia or be referred for IVF.

This finding raises the problem of being sure whether our assessment (i.e. simply assessing the tubal condition by laparoscopic evaluation of the infundibular mucosa) is reliable enough. Tuboscopy carried out during laparoscopy (Henry-Suchet *et al.*, 1984; Cornier *et al.*, 1984; Puttemans *et al.*, 1987) has been proposed for exploring the whole of the ampullary mucosa. Whereas there is an excellent correlation between tuboscopic investigation and the anatomopathologic results in cases of severe intratubal lesions, the correlation is not so satisfactory when these lesions are mild or moderate (Herschlag *et al.*, 1991). Nevertheless the prognostic value of tuboscopy is undeniable (De Bruyne *et al.*, 1989; Heylen *et al.*, 1995; Vasquez *et al.*, 1995). So the question we need to answer in the years that come is whether carrying out tuboscopy will provide a better assessment of the tubal condition than simple laparoscopic inspection of the infundibular mucosa when the aim is a more satisfactory selection of patients liable to benefit from salpingostomy.

Referral of patients with considerably deteriorated tubes to medically assisted procreation techniques does not necessarily mean, however, that these patients should not receive any surgery. In this situation adnexal adhesiolysis is necessary to obtain better ovarian stimulation and make oocyte retrieval easier. Furthermore, for patients with hydrosalpinx who are to undergo IVF, salpingectomy would seem to be advisable to prevent the risk of ectopic pregnancy and improve embryo implantation. This salpingectomy can be carried out by laparoscopy (Dubuisson *et al.*, 1987). There is a real risk of ectopic pregnancy after IVF and this occurs more often when the indication for IVF is tube pathology (Dubuisson *et al.*, 1991; Zouves *et al.*, 1991). In addition several teams have demonstrated that the success rates for IVF are lower for patients with hydrosalpinx (Anderson *et al.*, 1994; Strandell *et al.*, 1994; Vandromme *et al.*, 1995; Fleming and Hull, 1996). It would therefore seem to be an advantage to carry out salpingectomy in these situations, particularly as when this procedure is performed

Table 13.6 Salpingostomy by laparoscopy (Dubuisson *et al.*, 1994). Fertility results according to the French Tubal Scoring System (Mage *et al.*, 1987) and the Boer-Meisel classification (Boer-Meisel *et al.*, 1986)

Results according to the French Tubal Scoring System

Tube score	Number	Intrauterine pregnancy (N)	Intrauterine pregnancy (%)	Ectopic pregnancy (N)	Ectopic pregnancy (%)
1	15	9	60.0	0	0.0
2	29	15	51.7	2	6.9
1 + 2	44	24	54.5[a]	2	4.5
3	16	2	12.5	1	6.2
4	21	0	0.0	1	4.7
3 + 4	37	2	5.4[a]	2	5.4

Results according to Boer-Meisel Classification

	Number	Intrauterine pregnancy (N)	Intrauterine pregnancy (%)	Ectopic pregnancy (N)	Ectopic pregnancy (%)
Group 1	32	17	53.1	0	0.0
Group 2	27	9	33.3	4	14.8
Group 1+2	59	26	44.0[b]	4	6.7
Group 3	22	0	0.0[b]	0	0

[a]$p < 0.001$; [b]$p < 0.01$

correctly it has no deterimental effect on ovarian performance during IVF and embryo transfer treatment or on the outcome (Oehninger *et al.*, 1989; Verhulst *et al.*, 1994).

Conclusion

The fundamental changes represented by the development of laparoscopic surgery and medically assisted procreation techniques have modified the way patients with distal tubal infertility can be managed. The fertility prognosis is directly correlated with the condition of the distal tube. Simple laparoscopic evaluation of the tubal mucosa provides an excellent prognostic and strategic tool. Now when surgery is indicated (i.e. normal or atrophic mucosa), we believe that laparoscopic surgery is the technique of reference for periadnexal adhesiolysis and distal tubal plasty (fimbrioplasty or salpingostomy). IVF should be strongly considered from the outset for patients whose tubes are too badly deteriorated (i.e. alveolar mucosa).

Summary

The progress made over the past few years in laparoscopic surgery and *in vitro* fertilization (IVF) has brought about considerable changes in the management of patients presenting with distal tubal infertility. The fertility prognosis is correlated with the severity of the tubal lesions. Simple laparoscopic inspection of the mucosa in the ampulla and infundibulum provides an excellent means of evaluation. Only those patients presenting with moderate deterioration of the tube will draw any benefit from distal tubal surgery, with the others being better referred to IVF. When surgery is indicated, it is our opinion that it should be carried out via laparoscopy because we believe the fertility results are comparable to those for microsurgery via laparotomy.

References

Anderson AN, Yue Z, Meng FJ, Petersen K (1994) Low implantation rate after *in-vitro* fertilization in patients with hydrosalpinges diagnosed by ultrasonography. *Human Reproduction* **9**: 1935–1938.

American Fertility Society (1988) The American Fertility Society classifications of adnexal adhesions, distal tubal occlusion, tubal occlusion secondary to tubal ligation, tubal pregnancies, müllerian anomalies and intrauterine adhesions. *Fertility and Sterility* **49**: 944–955.

American Fertility Society, Society for Assisted Reproductive Technology (1994) Assisted reproductive technology in the United States and Canada: 1992 results generated from the American Fertility Society/Society for Assisted Reproductive Technology Registry. *Fertility and Sterility* **62**: 1121–1128.

Audebert AJ (1983) L'adhésiolyse per-coelioscopique. *Contraception Fertilité Sexualité* **11**: 857–862.

Audibert F, Hedon B, Arnal F *et al.* (1991) Therapeutic strategies in tubal infertility with distal pathology. *Human Reproduction* **6**: 1439–1442.

Benadiva CA, Kligman I, Davis O, Rosenwaks Z (1995) *In vitro* fertilization versus tubal surgery: is pelvic reconstructive surgery obsolete? *Fertility and Sterility* **64**: 1051–1061.

Boer-Meisel ME, Te Velde ER, Habbema JDF, Kardaum JWPF (1986) Predicting the pregnancy outcome in patients treated for hydrosalpinx: prospective study. *Fertility and Sterility* **45**: 23–29.

Bruhat MA, Mage G, Manhes H, Soualhat C, Ropers JF, Pouly JL (1983) Laparoscopic procedures to promote fertility: ovariolysis and salpingolysis; results of 93 cases. *Acta Europaea Fertilitatis* **14**: 113–115.

Canis M, Mage G, Pouly JL, Manhes H, Wattiez A, Bruhat MA (1991) Laparoscopic distal tuboplasty: report of 87 cases and a 4-year experience. *Fertility and Sterility* **56**: 616–621.

Chapron C, Dubuisson JB, Chavet X, Morice P (1994a) Treatment and causes of female infertility. *Lancet* **344**: 333–334.

Chapron C, Dubuisson JB, Morice P, Chavet X, Foulot H, Aubriot FX (1994b) La coeliochirurgie en gynécologie. Indications, bénéfices et risques. *Annales de Chirurgie* **48**: 618–624.

Chapron C, Querleu D, Chevallier L (1994c) Complications chirurgicales de la coeliochirurgie gynécologiques: données statistiques. In Chapron C, Querleu D (eds) *Complications de l'Endoscopie Opératoire en Gynécologie*. pp 101–114. Paris: Editions Arnette.

Cornier E, Feintuch MJ, Bouccara L (1984) La fibrotuboscopie ampullaire. *Journal de Gynécologie Obstétrique et Biologie de la Reproduction* **13**: 49–53.

Daniell JF, Herbert CM (1984) Laparoscopic salpingostomy utilizing the CO_2 laser. *Fertility and Sterility* **41**: 558–563.

De Brux J (1982) Les trompes. In De Brux J (ed.) *Histopathologie Gynécologique*. pp. 257–298. Paris: Editions Masson.

De Bruyne F, Puttemans P, Boeckx W, Brosens Y (1989) The clinical value of salpingoscopy in tubal infertility. *Fertility and Sterility* **51**: 339–340.

Diamond MP, De Cherney AH, Polan ML (1986) Laparoscopic use of the argon laser in non-endometriotic reproductive pelvic surgery. *Journal of Reproductive Medicine* **31**: 1011–1013.

Dubuisson JB, Aubriot FX, Garnier P *et al.* (1984) Faut-il opérer les lésions tubaires distales bifocales en 1984? A propos de 54 cas. *Journal de Gynécologie Obstétrique et Biologie de la Reproduction* **13**: 925–932.

Dubuisson JB, Aubriot FX, Cardone V (1987) Laparoscopic salpingectomy for tubal pregnancy. *Fertility and Sterility* **47**: 225–228.

Dubuisson JB, Bouquet de Joliniere J, Aubriot FX, Darai E, Foulot H, Mandelbrot L (1990) Terminal tuboplasties by laparoscopy: 65 consecutive cases. *Fertility and Sterility* **54**: 401–403.

Dubuisson JB, Aubriot FX, Mathieu L, Foulot H, Mandelbrot L, Bouquet de Joliniere J (1991) Risk factors for ectopic pregnancy in 556 pregnancies after *in vitro* fertilization: implications for preventive management. *Fertility and Sterility* **56**: 686–690.

Dubuisson JB, Chapron C, Morice P, Aubriot FX, Foulot H, Bouquet de Joliniere J (1994) Laparoscopic salpingostomy: Fertility results according to the tubal mucosal appearance. *Human Reproduction* **9**: 334–339.

Fayez JA (1983) An assessment of the role of operative laparoscopy in tuboplasty. *Fertility and Sterility* **39**: 476–479.

Feste JR (1985) Laser laparoscopy. A new modality. *Journal of Reproductive Medicine* **30**: 413–417.

FIVNAT (1995) Bilan FIVNAT 1994. *Contraception Fertilité Sexualité* **23**: 490–493.

Fleming C, Hull MGR (1996) Impaired implantation after *in vitro* fertilisation treatment associated with hydrosalpinx. *British Journal of Obstetrics and Gynaecology* **103**: 268–272.

Gomel V (1977) Salpingostomy by laparoscopy. *Journal of Reproductive Medicine* **18**: 265–267.

Gomel V (1983) Salpingo-ovariolysis by laparoscopy in infertility. *Fertility and Sterility* **40**: 607–611.

Henry-Suchet J, Tesquier L, Pez JP, Loffredo V (1984) Prognostic value of tuboscopy vs hysterosalpingography before tuboplasty. *Journal of Reproductive Medicine* **29**: 602–612.

Hershlag A, Seifer DB, Carcangiu ML, Patton DL, Diamond MP, De Cherney AH (1991) Salpingoscopy: light microscopic and electron microscopic correlations. *Obstetrics and Gynecology* **77**: 399–405.

Heylen SM, Brosens IA, Puttemans PJ (1995) Clinical value and cumulative pregnancy rates following rigid salpingoscopy during laparoscopy for infertility. *Human Reproduction* **10**: 2913–2916.

Lavergne N, Krimly A, Roge P, Erny R (1996) Résultats et indications de la coeliochirurgie tubaire distale. *Contraception Fertilité Sexualité* **24**: 41–48.

Maathuis JB, Horbach JG, Van Hall EV (1972) A comparison of the results of hysterosalpingography and laparoscopy in the diagnosis of fallopian tube dysfunction. *Fertility and Sterility* **23**: 428–431.

Mage G, Pouly JL, Bouquet de Joliniere J, Chabrand S, Riouallon A, Bruhat MA (1986) A preoperative classification to predict the intrauterine and ectopic pregnancy rates after distal tubal microsurgery. *Fertility and Sterility* **46**: 807–810.

Mage G, Bruhat MA, Bennis S *et al.* (1987) Score d'opérabilité tubaire. In Société Francaise de Gynécologie (ed.) *La Part de l'Homme et La Part de La Femme Dans La Stérilité du Couple*. pp. 93–96. Paris: Editions Masson.

McComb PF, Paleologou A (1991) The intussusception salpingostomy technique for the therapy of distal oviductal occlusion at laparoscopy. *Obstetrics and Gynecology* **78**: 443–447.

Mettler LR, Geisel H, Semm K (1979) Treatment of female infertility due to tubal obstruction by operative laparoscopy. *Fertility and Sterility* **32**: 384–388.

Mintz M, Madelenat P, Palmer R (1979) Aspects thérapeutiques de la coelioscopie dans les stérilités tubopéritonéales. In Brosens I, Cognat M, Constantin A, Thibier M (eds) *Oviducte et Fertilité*. p. 279. Paris: Editions Masson.

Nezhat C, Nezhat F, Nezhat C (1992) Operative laparoscopy (minimally invasive surgery): state of the art. *Journal of Gynecologic Surgery* **8**: 111–141.

Oehninger S, Scott R, Muascher SJ, Acosta AA, Jones HW Jr, Rosenwaks Z (1989) Effects of the severity of tubo-ovarian disease and previous tubal surgery on the results of *in vitro* fertilization and embryo transfer. *Fertility and Sterility* **51**: 126–130.

Palmer R (1974) Safety in laparoscopy. *Journal of Reproductive Medicine* **13**: 1–5.

Palmer R (1979) La coelioscopie dans le diagnostic et le traitement des adhérences pelviennes. *Contraception Fertilité Sexualité* **7**: 797–798.

Puttemans P, Brosens IA, Delattin PH, Vasquez G, Boeckx W (1987) Salpingoscopy versus hysterosalpingography in hydrosalpinges. *Human Reproduction* **2**: 535–540.

Reich H (1987) Laparoscopic treatment of extended pelvis adhesions including hydrosalpinx. *Journal of Reproductive Medicine* **32**: 736–742.

Rock JA, Katayama P, Marun EJ, Woodruff JD, Jones HW Jr (1978) Factors influencing the success of salpingostomy techniques for distal fimbrial obstruction. *Obstetrics and Gynecology* **52**: 591–599.

Saravelos HG, Li TC, Cooke ID (1995) An analysis of the outcome of microsurgical and laparoscopic adhesiolysis for infertility. *Human Reproduction* **10**: 2887–2894.

Serour GI, Badraoui MH, EI Agizi HM, Hamed AF, Abdel-Azziz F (1989) Laparoscopic adhesiolysis for infertile patients with pelvic adhesive disease. *International Journal of Gynecology and Obstetrics* **30**: 249–252.

Strandell A, Waldenstrom U, Nilsson L, Hamberger L (1994) Hydrosalpinx reduces *in vitro*-fertilization/embryo transfer pregnancy rates. *Human Reproduction* **9**: 861–863.

Vandromme J, Chasse E, Lejeune B, Van Rysselberge M, Delevigne A, Leroy F (1995) Hydrosalpinges in *in-vitro* fertilization: an unfavourable prognostic feature. *Human Reproduction* **10**: 576–579.

Vasquez G, Boeckx W, Brosens I (1995) Prospective study of tubal mucosal lesions and fertility in hydrosalpinges. *Human Reproduction* **10**: 1075–1078.

Verhulst G, Vandersteen N, Van Sterteghem AC, Devoey P (1994) Bilateral salpingectomy does not compromise ovarian stimulation in an *in-vitro* fertilization/embryo transfer programme. *Human Reproduction* **9**: 624–628.

Zouves C, Erenus M, Gomel V (1991) Tubal ectopic pregnancy after *in-vitro* fertilization and embryo transfer: a role for proximal occlusion or salpingectomy after failed distal tubal surgery? *Fertility and Sterility* **56**: 691–695.

14

Laparoscopic Fertility-promoting Procedures

VICTOR GOMEL* AND MALCOLM MUNRO[†]

*Department of Obstetrics and Gynecology, The Vancouver Hospital, Vancouver, Canada
[†]Department of Obstetrics and Gynecology, University of California, Los Angeles, USA

Introduction

Laparoscopy was introduced into gynecology primarily as a diagnostic tool. Its dissemination among gynecologists of the English-speaking world was largely because of its application to the performance of tubal sterilization. The enthusiasm for laparoscopic sterilization did not initially extend to other operative procedures. However, in recent years, laparoscopy has gained universal acceptance as an operative modality (Gomel, 1989). The universal acceptance of operative laparoscopy was slow in coming and many of the techniques were developed in the 1970s by a handful of workers (Gomel, 1975; Gomel, 1977; Mettler *et al.*, 1979). Laparoscopic procedures to promote fertility in women were among the first to be reported.

This chapter will review periadnexal adhesive disease and distal tubal occlusion, and will discuss in detail the techniques of laparoscopically directed salpingo-ovariolysis, fimbrioplasty, salpingostomy and tubal anastomosis.

Periadnexal Adhesive Disease

Pelvic, and especially periadnexal, adhesions are usually secondary to pelvic inflammatory disease (PID). Another infectious cause is acute ruptured appendicitis. Adhesions resulting from operative procedures can be extensive and are usually more cohesive and dense in nature than adhesions due to PID. Adhesions associated with endometriosis are usually encountered in the more extensive stages of this disease. Detailed discussion of the pathogenesis of such adhesions is not in the purview of this chapter.

Although periadnexal adhesions usually accompany other occlusive tubal conditions, they may be present in the absence of any apparent tubal disease. In such instances, adhesions may prevent the transport of the oocyte into the fallopian tube by enveloping the fimbriated end of the tube, the ovary or both. In other instances, adhesions (even localized) may distort the normal anatomic relationship between the tube and ovary, and thus impair fimbrial ovum pick-up.

Adhesions are composed largely of connective tissue and contain a variable degree of vascularity. Consequently, the appearance of adhesions covers a spectrum ranging from those that are filmy or thick and relatively avascular to those that are richly supplied with blood vessels. Adhesions may also vary in their cohesiveness, that is, the amount of space that exists between the structures abnormally joined and the density of the adhesive process. Highly cohesive adhesions leave virtually no space or 'slack' between the abnormally attached structures; this adhesive process is usually very dense. 'Fatty adhesions' are in fact omentum or appendices epiploicae that have adhered to an organ or the parietal peritoneum.

Salpingitis may cause varying degrees of distal tubal occlusion. Agglutination of the fimbriae may produce phimosis of the distal tubal opening, which may be covered by fibrous scar tissue. In other instances the distal tube may be totally occluded (hydrosalpinx), in which case the ampulla exhibits varying degrees of dilation. Such distal tubal occlusions are usually associated with periadnexal adhesions.

Instruments

Modalities for Cutting

Transection via laparoscopy may be accomplished with scissors, electrosurgery or laser energy.

SCISSORS

Laparoscopic scissors are used principally for mechanical division, even when they possess electrosurgical capability. Since the introduction of laparoscopic techniques, scissors have been our cutting instrument of choice for salpingo-ovariolysis and other fertility-promoting procedures of the oviduct. Although laparoscopic scissors are now available in a number of models, the most important characteristic required is their ability to cut effectively, an attribute that is frequently elusive. Indeed, the maintenance of scissors is difficult. This partially relates to the disproportionate ratio between the length and caliber of the instrument, which largely negates any beneficial effect yielded by sharpening. These characteristics led to the development of disposable scissors. We are, in general, philosophically opposed to the use of disposable instruments, largely because of cost/benefit considerations. However, we believe that because of the difficulties associated with the maintenance of scissors in good working order there is a strong argument in favor of disposable or reusable–disposable scissors.

The hooked or pointed scissors provide certain advantages. They allow the operator to lift an adhesion away from adjacent tissue before cutting it; the pointed tip provides ease of entry into the fallopian tube. It is important, however, to select a type of hooked scissors with points that do not overlap when the jaws are closed. Overlap of the pointed tip(s) may be dangerous when the scissors are employed in retraction or dissection or left unattended within the peritoneal cavity.

Laparoscopic operative instruments, especially those used in fertility-promoting procedures, must be improved. This is largely a matter of engineering, and undoubtedly more functional instruments will be available in the foreseeable future.

ELECTROSURGICAL INSTRUMENTS

A sound knowledge of the principles and bioeffects of electrosurgery is mandatory for the use of this modality. Effective cutting is ideally achieved using low voltage continuous monopolar current (cutting mode) and a fine-pointed electrode. Hemostasis is usually achieved by compression of the vessel while applying the same continuous current, or in limited instances, by fulguration, using the modulated, higher voltage 'coagulation' current. 'Blended' current provides additional thermal coagulating effect along with the cutting action. In adhesiolysis we use electrosurgery principally to coagulate blood vessels encountered along the line of mechanical transection or to stop persistent bleeders at the end of the procedure. Bipolar current may also be used for coagulating blood vessels, although currently available bipolar forceps, even the finer types, are often too wide for tubal microsurgery.

In the late 1970s concerns were raised about the use of monopolar current at laparoscopy because of the risk of inadvertent thermal injury to adjacent organs. However, with the production of improved electrosurgical generators and instruments and a better understanding of the principles of electrosurgery, properly used monopolar surgical techniques should not cause a greater rate of injury than other modalities.

LASERS

Of the four lasers that have been employed in the pelvis for cutting purposes – carbon dioxide (CO_2), potassium titanyl phosphate (KTP), argon and neodymium:yttrium-aluminum-garnet (Nd-YAG) – the CO_2 laser has been the most popular. Because of the properties of CO_2 laser energy, it cannot be effectively propagated along a flexible fiber. Consequently the light beam must at present be guided into the peritoneal cavity through a straight hollow tube (wave guide), which in some instances, limits the direction of effective delivery.

With the other three lasers, the energy may be propagated along a quartz fiber, which can be bent to direct the beam as necessary. Sapphire tips attached to the fiber of the Nd-YAG laser allow the surgeon to operate in contact with tissue. However, this system causes greater thermal damage.

The argon laser system requires water cooling, necessitating the installation of new plumbing into the operating rooms and the fiber tends to burn out as the operation proceeds. The KTP laser can now be air cooled, but the cutting action of both the argon and KTP laser is associated with greater adjacent thermal injury than that of the CO_2 laser.

Other Instruments

The other important instruments used in the performance of fertility-promoting procedures include probes, grasping instruments, uterine manipulators, suction irrigation devices, and needle holders. These are available in different calibers, ranging from 2–5 mm in diameter. Grasping instruments are manufactured in different lengths and with a variety of jaw and handle designs. It is not the purview of this chapter to describe instruments in detail. The suction irrigation device permits effective lavage of the pelvis. In addition, it may be used for dissection by introducing an isotonic solution under pressure (hydrodissection). We use heparinized lactated Ringer's solution for irrigation and pelvic lavage.

Investigation

In addition to appropriate history and physical examination of the couple, preliminary investigation must include semen analysis and determination of the ovulatory status of the woman. Hysterosalpingography (HSG) and laparoscopy are complementary methods of assessing tubal and peritoneal causes of infertility. HSG should be the initial investigation for uterine, tubal and peritoneal factors. It is our opinion that a properly performed HSG can be of inestimable value, while a poorly performed HSG is of little value to the physician and an unnecessary source of discomfort to the patient. The advantages of the initial HSG include:

- Identification of uterine anomalies and intrauterine lesions.
- Identification of cornual occlusion and non-occlusive proximal tubal disease.
- Identification of distal occlusion and assessment of intratubal architecture, which is of prognostic significance.

This information is of great value in deciding whether or not to perform corrective surgery at the time of the initial diagnostic laparoscopy (Gomel *et al.*, 1986). Corrective surgery for distal tubal disease carries a better prognosis in the presence of relatively normal intratubal architecture. A previous HSG demonstrating normal uterine architecture and tubal patency will encourage the surgeon who discovers periadnexal adhesive disease to proceed with immediate salpingo-ovariolysis. An endometrial cavity that appears abnormal generally justifies diagnostic hysteroscopy, which can usually be performed in the office or clinic setting. Collectively, such preoperative information will enable the surgeon to request appropriate operating room time for the procedure.

Surgical Technique

The patient is placed in the low lithotomy position, which allows ready access to the genital tract from below. The uterine manipulator should be one that allows chromotubation as well as adequate manipulation of the uterus during the operative procedure. Manipulation of the uterus enhances pelvic exposure and permits immobilization of the adnexal structure to be operated on and thus facilitates the procedure.

Operative laparoscopy requires the use of multiple puncture technique. We usually use a 6.5 mm or an 8 mm laparoscope inserted intraumbilically. Additional punctures are usually placed suprapubically in the midline and McBurney's point. When circumstances necessitate an additional entry site, it is placed over the left lower quadrant. The separation of the visual and operative axes provided by this technique allows better depth perception, recognizing the loss of binocular vision at laparoscopy. The procedure is performed with the aid of a compatible high-resolution camera and video monitor, allowing appropriate interaction between the surgeon, assistant and operating room personnel. We usually locate the television monitor at the caudal end of the patient. Such placement allows a normal visual orientation to the pelvis and permits all those involved with the case to have a clear view of the screen.

Fertility-Promoting Procedures

The fertility-promoting procedures of proven value include:

- Salpingo-ovariolysis.
- Fimbrioplasty.
- Salpingostomy.

Although there have been a number of reports of laparoscopic tubotubal anastomosis, this approach must still be viewed as experimental.

General Principles

Microsurgery represents the gold standard of reconstructive surgery in gynecology. When such procedures are undertaken laparoscopically it is necessary to emulate microsurgical principles.

Infertility microsurgery is a discipline that uses magnification integrated with the philosophy of tissue care designed to minimize trauma (Gomel, 1983a). Peritoneal trauma, whether mechanical, thermal or chemical, elicits an inflammatory reaction. This inflammatory exudate contains fibrinogen, which is transformed into fibrin. Fibrin deposition and fibroblastic proliferation are the basis for adhesion formation.

With proper positioning of the patient, appropriate instrumentation and adequate distention of the peritoneal cavity, excellent exposure can be obtained at laparoscopy. The ability to bring the laparoscope into the vicinity of the area of interest may render exposure even better than that at laparotomy. In addition, the laparoscope provides a degree of magnification.

Since the procedure is carried out within a closed abdomen, in normal conditions potentially adhesiogenic drying of the peritoneal surfaces is largely prevented. This protective effect of operative laparoscopy may be eliminated by continuous insufflation of the high volumes of CO_2 required to eliminate the smoke (plume) generated by the intraperitoneal use of laser energy.

As in microsurgery, few instruments are used during operative laparoscopy. The design of the end effectors and handles of laparoscopic microsurgical instruments has improved substantially over the last few years. However, the length of these instruments, with the cannula acting as a fulcrum, still increases the force applied to the tissue exponentially, generating unnecessary trauma. Laparoscopic microsurgery is still affected by the limitations of monocular vision, which results in decreased depth perception, and at least for some surgeons, difficulty in instrument and tissue manipulation. The emerging development of stereoscopic endoscopes provides a potential solution to this problem. An additional limitation of laparoscopic imaging relates to the angle of approaching the tissue under reconstruction. This limitation may be partly overcome by mobilization of the uterus and adnexal regions as well as the use of the uterus to immobilize the adnexa in an appropriate position. Access to a specific area may also be improved by the introduction of rectal or vaginal probes and variations in the horizontal and lateral tilt of the operating table.

Laparoscopy permits intraoperative irrigation and thorough pelvic lavage at the end of the procedure. In addition, when appropriate, dissection of tissues can be facilitated by introducing irrigation fluid under pressure (hydrodissection).

Despite the development of relatively fine electrodes (both monopolar and bipolar), laparoscopic hemostasis remains relatively crude in comparison to that of microsurgery. Fortunately, most bleeders encountered during fertility-promoting procedures cease spontaneously; occasionally the use of a very dilute vasopressin solution may be sufficient to overcome the problem.

Another limitation of operative laparoscopy in comparison to microsurgery lies with the precise alignment and approximation of tissue planes. Despite the development of needle holders and suturing techniques, including intra-abdominal suturing techniques (which are our preference), laparoscopic suturing is often awkward and more time-consuming. In view of this limitation and since one invariably uses suture material of at least slightly larger caliber than that used in microsurgery, the tendency is to apply fewer sutures in operative laparoscopy.

Salpingo-ovariolysis

Patients who have had previous abdominal surgery frequently have adhesions between the omentum and anterior abdominal wall. If such adhesions limit pelvic visualization it is necessary to remove them first. Adhesiolysis in this instance should be carried out at the level of the parietal peritoneum. Whereas the omentum is a fatty organ, at its site of adherence to the peritoneum the adhesive process may be relatively velamentous. Successful lysis of these adhesions will be dependent upon optimal exposure of the dissection plane. This is accomplished by retraction of the omentum. If the adhesive process is relatively velamentous it will lend itself to mechanical division with laparoscopic scissors. When the adhesive process is more cohesive it will be necessary to carry out dissection along the appropriate plane. The process does not differ from that carried out at laparotomy.

The first step in salpingo-ovariolysis is to assess the type and extent of the adhesive process and the structures involved. One of the clear prerequisites of surgery is the recognition of structures, especially when the anatomy is distorted. Adherence to this principle reduces unnecessary trauma and avoids complications. Section of adhesions should ideally be performed along the organ that must be freed. Furthermore, adhesiolysis should be carried out one layer at a time, keeping in mind that what superficially appears to be a single layer of adhesion is usually composed of two. Adhesiolysis should be commenced in a well exposed area near the optic. Division must be effected parallel to the affected organ, keeping slightly away from the serosa. This is especially important when adhesiolysis is performed with electrosurgery or laser energy since the thermal energy spreads lateral with both of these modalities.

Effective and safe adhesiolysis requires:

- Recognition of what lies behind the adhesion.
- Retraction of the adhesion with a probe, or traction with grasping forceps applied to the adhesion and not to the target organ.

A small incision is made to elucidate what is behind the adhesion and whether the adhesion is composed of two layers rather than one. Division is accomplished parallel to the organ as indicated earlier (see above). Shallow adhesions are simply divided. Broad adhesions should be removed by dividing them at their outer margin in a similar fashion. Such adhesions are then removed through one of the portals of entry.

We prefer mechanical division of adhesions using laparoscopic scissors, and use electrodesiccation only when significant vessels cross the line of section.

Adhesions encountered secondary to pelvic inflammatory disease are usually relatively avascular and readily amenable to mechanical section or excision. Fatty adhesions are usually those related to the omentum or appendices epiploicae. When such adhesions are stretched it will usually be possible to visualize a relatively avascular or filmy attachment where the omentum or appendices epiploicae meet the serosa of the organ to which they are attached. If the adhesive process is cohesive, one should refrain from using any type of thermal energy. It is necessary to make a small incision at the edge of such adhesions and develop a dissection plane either by spreading the jaws of the scissors and/or using hydrodissection.

The procedure is completed with a thorough pelvic lavage. This process removes blood and debris from the pelvis and enables visualization of persistent bleeders. These are individually electrodesiccated using an appropriate unipolar or monopolar electrode.

With all fertility-promoting procedures, at the close of the operation, we leave 150–200 ml of lactated Ringer's solution containing 500 mg of hydrocortisone succinate in the pelvis.

Fimbrioplasty

Fimbrioplasty refers to the reconstruction of existing fimbriae in a partially or totally occluded distal oviduct. In the majority of such cases periadnexal adhesions are also present, in which case salpingo-ovariolysis is carried out first. Stenosis or obstruction of the distal tube may be the result of agglutination of the fimbriae. As a result, the terminal end of the tube may have a phimotic appearance with a degree of patency. Transcervical chromotubation will distend the ampulla before the escape of the dye solution. In other instances, the agglutinated fimbriated end is also covered by a fibrous layer, which may cause complete occlusion at the site. Less frequently, the stenosis is situated at the level of the abdominal tubal ostium at the apex of the infundibulum (prefimbrial phimosis).

When the fimbriated end is covered by a fibrous layer, it will be necessary to incise or excise this layer to expose the agglutinated fimbriae. This can be accomplished using laparoscopic scissors, laser or electrical energy. To deagglutinate the fimbriae, a closed 2–3 mm alligator forceps is introduced into the fallopian tube through the phimotic opening. The jaws of the forceps are opened within the tube and the forceps withdrawn with the jaws in the open position. This procedure is repeated several times, varying the direction of the jaws until satisfactory fimbrial deagglutination is obtained. With gentle manipulation bleeding is seldom encountered.

Prefimbrial phimosis is best corrected by placing an incision over the antemesosalpingial edge of the fallopian tube from the fimbriated end into the distal ampulla in order to get beyond the stenotic site. The tube is immobilized, and if possible a narrow plastic or Teflon probe is introduced through the fimbriated end into the ampulla. Using an electrosurgical needle electrode the incision is commenced at the fimbriated end of the tube and extended into the distal ampulla beyond the site of stenosis. Bleeders on the incisional edges are individually electrodesiccated. To maintain tubal patency, it may be necessary to evert the flaps by placing 6.0 or 7.0 interrupted sutures at the apex of each of the flaps. A thorough pelvic lavage is then carried out.

Salpingostomy (Neosalpingostomy)

Laparoscopic neosalpingostomy was first reported from Vancouver, British Columbia (Gomel, 1977). Although initially mainly used as an iterative procedure, laparoscopic salpingostomy is gaining wide acceptance for correction of distal tubal occlusion (hydrosalpinx) as a primary approach. This is the result of improvement in techniques, the availability of in vitro fertilization (IVF) and embryo transfer (ET) as a therapeutic alternative, and the better recognition of the factors that affect the surgical outcome. These factors are largely inherent to the status of the fallopian tube at the time of surgery.

Since periadnexal adhesions coexist with most cases of hydrosalpinx, salpingo-ovariolysis constitutes the first phase of the procedure. The next step is a thorough assessment of the distal tube and its relationship with the ovary. It is imperative to determine whether or not the occluded distal tube is free. When the distal tube is free the tubo-ovarian ligament is readily visible. In some instances the terminal end of the tube is adherent to the ovary, in which case the tubo-ovarian ligament is not in view. When the distal tube is adherent to the ovary it is necessary to free the tube from the ovary before performing a neosalpingostomy.

We have generally preferred a salpingostomy technique that attempts to imitate the proven microsurgical approach (Gomel, 1978). The tube is distended by transcervical chromotubation. This confirms patency of the proximal tube up to the distal occlusion site. It also facilitates identification of the scars at the terminal end of the tube, which usually extend from a central dimple in a cartwheel configuration.

The tube is grasped near the occluded distal end with atraumatic forceps and the central dimple is entered with the pointed tips of the scissors (or electrosurgically using a needle electrode). At this point, salpingoscopy may be carried out to assess the ampulla by introducing a hysteroscope through this initial opening. The first incision is carried out towards the ovary to form a new fimbria ovarica. Once entered in this way it becomes possible to view the tube from within and to fashion additional incisions along the circumference of the tube over avascular regions (over the scarred areas). This is achieved by grasping the tube at the edge of the initial incision, retracting the tube and folding it slightly backward. Additional incisions are then placed appropriately using the scissors (or needle electrode). Viewing the tube from within will permit these incisions to be made along the circumference of the tube over avascular regions, avoiding transection of the vascular mucosal folds. Preservation of these folds is essential to maintain the ovum capture potential of the oviduct.

Once a satisfactory neostomy is obtained it is possible to evert the edges by applying two or three 6–0 synthetic absorbable sutures. Eversion of the tubal edges can also be accomplished by focal and superficial shrinkage of the serosa proximal to the ostium using either electrodesiccation or a defocused CO_2 laser beam. It should be noted that there is no evidence to suggest that any eversion technique improves the outcome.

Other successful laparoscopic neosalpingostomy techniques have been described. An 'intussusception' method used by McComb and Paleologou (1991) was similar to that described earlier by Kosasa and Hale (1988) for use at laparotomy. Once the tube is entered at the central dimple, the opening is enlarged and a 'cuff' obtained in the following manner. The cut edges are grasped with forceps and the initial opening enlarged by pulling on the forceps. The distal tube is everted by pulling back on the forceps placed at the cut edge and pushing from the serosal aspect of the ampulla with another instrument. Others have reported the use of the CO_2 laser to effect dissection of the occluded distal tube and eversion of the flaps.

Retrograde Salpingoscopy (Tuboscopy)

Before fimbrioplasty or with salpingostomy, it is possible to inspect at least the ampullary epithelium once the tube is entered in the region of the central dimple, using a narrow rigid or, preferably flexible, endoscope introduced through one of the laparoscopic cannulas. A narrow caliber hysteroscope (including the sheath), a modified ureteroscope with a through lumen, or other similar device is inserted into the distal tube with the aid of an atraumatic forceps. Distending the tube with lactated Ringer's solution, it is possible to inspect most of the ampullary portion of the tube, and depending upon the diameter of the endoscope, at least part of the distal isthmus. In the face of extensive endosalpingial damage there may be an argument in favor of performing a salpingectomy. However, unless there are extensive intratubal adhesions, it may be appropriate to complete the salpingostomy since the mucosa may regenerate and intrauterine pregnancies have occurred in the face of apparently severely damaged oviducts. The information provided by the salpingoscopy may influence the decision to proceed with IVF sooner rather than later.

Some have advocated the use of transcervical salpingoscopy (falloposcopy) before laparoscopic or abdominal surgery, thereby triaging patients either to tubal surgery or IVF and ET depending upon the degree of endosalpingial damage. While promising, the utility of such an approach has yet to be determined.

Results

There is a paucity of data analyzing the relationship of adhesions to pain and the impact of adhesiolysis on such symptoms. Consequently, we will review only the data relating the therapy of adnexal adhesive disease and infertility.

For any type of infertility therapy, the results of clinical investigation may be presented and interpreted in a number of ways. When infertility is presumed or known to be secondary to tubal disease, patency and total pregnancy rates are often suggested or reported as appropriate measures of outcome. However, patency does not equal conception, many gestations are ectopic in location and not all intrauterine pregnancies result in a living baby. Consequently, for the patient and her physician, the only acceptable target is the successful delivery of a healthy baby.

Critical evaluation of the impact of laparoscopic procedures requires distinction between pregnancies that are clearly the result of surgery from those that occur despite such intervention. When surgery is performed on women in whom infertility is secondary to tubal disease that completely occludes both oviducts, subsequent pregnancies may be appropriately attributed to the procedure. However, if there is pre-existing unilateral or bilateral patency, even 'partial' in nature, pregnancy could occur without surgery. Consequently, studies evaluating the effect of laparoscopically directed tubal surgery on women with pre-existing tubal patency that do not have control groups can overestimate the therapeutic effects of the intervention.

Salpingo-ovariolysis

Gomel (1975) provided the initial report on laparoscopic salpingo-ovariolysis and fimbrioplasty. Of the whole group of 39 patients one was lost to follow-up, three avoided pregnancy for various reasons, and 14 achieved one or more intrauterine pregnancies. Among the 24 patients followed for one year or more the intrauterine pregnancy rate was 59%. In 1979, Semm's group from Kiel reported on salpingolysis and ovariolysis (Mettler *et al.*, 1979). The total pregnancy rates were 38% and 21%, respectively. However, the location and outcome of these pregnancies was not stated.

Gomel (1983b) reported a series of 92 patients who underwent laparoscopic salpingo-ovariolysis. Of these 13 had moderate periadnexal adhesions and 79 had severe periadnexal adhesions; all had experienced at least 20 months of infertility. After a follow-up period of at least nine months, 57 (62%) had intrauterine pregnancies and 54 (59%) live births, with half of these 57 women conceiving within six months of surgery. Following this report four additional patients delivered healthy infants. Corroborative outcomes were reported by Fayez (1983) and Bruhat *et al.* (1983). They attained intrauterine pregnancies in 56% of 50 and 52% of 93 patients, respectively. The outcome of these pregnancies was not reported. Similar results were reported by Donnez *et al.* in 1989. We must draw attention to the ectopic gestation rates in the preceding reports which ranged from 4–7.5% for operated patients. These rates suggest that periadnexal disease is not an isolated entity and that in a pro-

portion of cases it is associated with significant damage of the tubal endothelium.

Fimbrioplasty

Relatively few investigators separately classify and report cases where fimbrioplasty is performed. Among 40 patients reported by Gomel (1983c), 19 (47.5%) had successful deliveries and two had ectopic gestations. The Kiel group (Mettler *et al.*, 1979) reported a 31% pregnancy rate among 51 women, although again, the location and outcome of these pregnancies was not revealed. Dubuisson *et al.* (1990) reported intrauterine and ectopic pregnancy rates of 25.8% and 12.9%, respectively, among 31 women followed for 18 months. Surprisingly, these results were inferior to those yielded by their salpingostomy group. No patient conceived between 12 and 18 months. More recently, Canis *et al.* (1991) reported intrauterine pregnancies in 16 of 32 patients (50%) treated by laparoscopic fimbrioplasty, but did not provide further details about the pregnancy outcomes. None of these studies were controlled, but collectively the results are similar to those reported when fimbrioplasty is performed at laparotomy with a microsurgical technique.

Salpingostomy

Demonstration of the efficacy of surgery for bilateral tubal occlusion is not dependent upon controlled studies since virtually all subsequent spontaneous pregnancies may be attributed to the intervention. However, the outcomes when salpingostomy by laparotomy and laparoscopy are compared are of interest. The comparison of results has been facilitated with the introduction of the American Society of Reproductive Medicine's (ASRM) (1988) classification system for prognostic factors (Gomel, 1988). These include the distal ampullary diameter, the thickness of the tubal wall, the status of the oviduct's endothelium and the nature and extent of coexistent adhesions.

Laparoscopic salpingostomy was initially reported by Gomel in 1977; four of nine patients conceived, all with successful pregnancies. Of note is that eight of these women had previous conventional salpingostomy via laparotomy with subsequent reocclusion of the tube(s).

Mettler *et al.* (1979) reported ten pregnancies among 38 patients after laparoscopic salpingostomy with the use of thermal coagulation. The location and outcome of these pregnancies were not specified. Daniell and Herbert (1984) reported on 22 patients in whom salpingostomy was performed using CO_2 laser via laparoscopy. Four patients achieved intrauterine pregnancies, one of which was aborted; one patient had a tubal pregnancy.

Dubuisson *et al.* (1990) reported ten uterine pregnancies (29.4%) and only one tubal pregnancy among 34 patients after laparoscopic salpingostomy. McComb and Paleologou (1991) reported five births and one ectopic pregnancy among 22 patients followed for more than one year.

Canis *et al.* (1991) reported intrauterine pregnancies in 29 (33.3%) of 87 patients, while six experienced ectopic gestation. These authors classified their patients into four groups depending upon the severity of the tubal damage. The fallopian tubes in the most favorable group (32 patients) are described as 'partial occlusion (phimotic tube)'. This group, which yields the best outcome, is in effect a fimbrioplasty group. Of the 55 remaining patients with complete distal occlusion, 13 (23.6%) achieved intrauterine pregnancies, the outcome of which was not reported, while 6 (10.9%) had ectopic gestations.

Dubuisson *et al.* (1994) reported a series of 90 such patients, nine of whom were lost to follow-up and excluded from the analysis. Of the remaining 81, four had ectopic pregnancies and 26 (32.1%) had 'normal delivery'. However, the classification used in these series was the same as in the Canis *et al.* (1991) report. When the 15 ('Stage I') fimbrioplasty cases are excluded from the analysis, only 17 (25.8%), of the remaining 66 salpingostomy patients they were able to follow-up had births.

Oh from Korea recently published a comparative study of 82 women allocated in a non-randomized fashion to one of three techniques (Oh, 1996):

(1) A neosalpingotomy fashioned using scissors and eversion obtained using 4–0 polydioxanone sutures on a ski needle.
(2) A stoma fashioned using electrosurgery with a microelectrode and eversion obtained by electrosurgical desiccation of the serosa.
(3) The intussusception method modified by the routine use of a single 4–0 polydioxanone suture for eversion.

Although the patients were not randomized, they had similar modified ASRM prognostic scores. At HSG two months later, patency rates (at least one tube open) for operations 2 (23/27; 85.1%) and 3 (28/29; 96.2%) were significantly higher than for the type 1 procedure (13/26; 50%). The overall rates of intrauterine conception were 19.2% for type 1, 37.2% and 48.2%, respectively for types 2 and 3, and were even higher in women with favorable prognostic scores (30%, 54.5%, and 64.3%).

Gomel (1990) reported a series 90 women who underwent microsurgical neosalpingotomy through minilaparotomy access. Based upon the ASRM classification cited earlier, only 13 (18%) of 73 patients with poor prognosis, achieved an intrauterine pregnancy, while 12 (71%) of 17 with a good prognosis were successful.

Tubotubal Anastomosis

Anastomosis of the mid-portion of the oviduct is most commonly performed to reverse a previous tubal sterilization and rarely to treat pathologic occlusion. Laparoscopic approaches to tubotubal anastomosis must be held to the high standard set by laparotomy-based microsurgical techniques. Such approaches have been considered to be the ideal application of reconstructive microsurgery in gynecology for they permit meticulous apposition of tissue planes and yield excellent results (with reported live birth rates varying between 60–80%). Furthermore, microsurgical repair may be accomplished through a minilaparotomy incision. This coupled with the use of appropriate pre- and post-operative local anesthesia allows early discharge from hospital (Gomel and Taylor, 1993; Gomel and Taylor, 1995). These patients return to normal activity almost as rapidly as those who have had procedures performed by laparoscopy. The laparoscopic approach to tubotubal anastomosis remains to be proven as an appropriate alternative.

Technique

The principles of tubotubal anastomosis are well known and have been extensively described (Gomel, 1980 and 1983b,c). First, the occluded segment of tube is excised, fashioning the incision so that normal-appearing oviduct can be identified. Although hemostasis must be secured, it is important not to compromise the tubal vasculature or epithelium. The cut edges are then aligned accurately and joined with fine minimally reactive suture.

After the induction of satisfactory anesthesia, the patient is placed in the low lithotomy position using appropriate supportive stirrups. An articulated uterine manipulator that allows chromotubation is inserted into the endometrial cavity and affixed to the uterus. After establishing the pneumoperitoneum and satisfactory positioning of the laparoscope, three ancillary cannulas are positioned in each lower quadrant and suprapubically in the midline. Following detailed examination of the fallopian tubes, any necessary salpingo-ovariolysis is performed.

Tubotubal anastomosis is performed as follows:

- The proximal segment of the tube is distended by chromotubation and the occluded end is grasped with fine laparoscopic forceps.
- Fine scissors are inserted through another laparoscopic cannula. They are used to transect the tube at right angles near the occluded end. The incision starts at the antimesosalpingial border and stops short of the vascular arcade.
- Tubal patency is demonstrated by escape of the dye solution.
- The magnifying capability of the laparoscope is used to inspect the lumen, endothelium and muscularis to confirm that the tissues appear healthy.
- If abnormal tissue is identified or suspected, serial incisions are made until normal healthy-appearing tissue is reached.
- For isthmic–isthmic anastomosis, a similar approach is used to prepare the distal segment of the tube. Patency of this segment is ascertained by the insertion of a fine polyethylene catheter and the injection of dye solution through the fimbriated end.
- The occluded end(s) of tube that remain attached are now freed from the mesosalpinx using scissors or electrosurgically using a needle-tipped microelectrode and blended current. The excised tissue is removed through one of the laparoscopic cannulas.
- Hemostasis of the principal bleeders on the periphery of the muscularis is achieved with electrodesiccation using the microelectrode. Alternatively, 1–1.5 ml of dilute (1 unit in 10 ml) vasopressin solution is injected into the mesosalpinx of the anastomosis site at the onset of the procedure. Endothelial oozing is generally self-limited and is therefore managed expectantly.
- Isthmic–ampullary anastomosis provides a challenge due to the disparity in luminal diameters. In this case, it is necessary to fashion a small opening into the ampullary lumen to permit easy anastomosis. First the ampulla is distended following insertion of the polyethylene catheter through the fimbriated end to identify the tip of the occluded end. Fine scissors are then used to incise the serosa over this tip to expose the underlying muscularis. The muscularis is regrasped and the scissors are used to create an opening with a luminal diameter similar to that of the proximal tubal segment.
- Both isthmic–isthmic and isthmic–ampullary anastomoses are completed in a similar fashion. Fine suture (7–0 or 8–0 synthetic absorbable) swaged to a 3/8 curved needle is inserted through a cannula into the pelvis and grasped with a curved microsurgical needle driver. The initial suture is critical to alignment and is placed at 6 o'clock near the attachment of the mesosalpinx, including both the muscularis and the epithelium. The knot is tied with intracorporeal technique and is kept external to the tubal lumen. Additional sutures are positioned and tied in a similar fashion, their number dependent upon the caliber of the tubal lumen. Upon completion of this step, patency is confirmed with trans-cervical chromotubation.
- The serosa and mesosalpinx are repaired with interrupted and/or continuous sutures of the same material.
- If necessary, the same technique is performed on the other side.
- Pelvic lavage completes the procedure.

In an attempt to reduce operating time related to suturing Sedbon *et al.* (1989) and Auld *et al.* (1993) have reported the insertion of tubal stents, either by laparoscopy or hysteroscopy, followed by joining of the segments with a type of biologic glue (Tissucol Immuno Laboratoire, France). Dubuisson (personal communication 1995) has apposed the two segments of tube using two sutures, the first to approximate the mesosalpinx, and the second the complete thickness of tubal wall at the 12 o'clock position.

Results

Relatively few results of laparoscopic tubotubal anastomosis have been published to date. Reich *et al.* (1993) reported that six of 22 women had at least one pregnancy, while three had at least one tubal ectopic gestation. Their procedure differed from those described above in a number of potentially important ways:

- 4–0 or 6–0 suture material was used.
- Only two such sutures were used and these included the serosa, muscularis and endothelium.
- Only one tube was repaired per patient.

Operating times ranged from 65–240 minutes.

Sedbon *et al.* (1989) did not report any pregnancies with tissue glue apposition. Among the six patients treated by Auld *et al.* (1993), two had intrauterine gestations and one an ectopic pregnancy. For both groups of patients, only one tube was anastomosed.

Conclusions

Pelvic and periadnexal adhesions arise as a result of an inflammatory process secondary to infection, endometriosis or physical or chemical trauma. They are most frequently encountered in association with infertility or pelvic pain. With appropriate planning, case selection, instruments and technique, periadnexal and pelvic adhesions and distal tubal occlusion can be treated laparoscopically safely and effectively. The results obtained by laparoscopically directed salpingo-ovariolysis and fimbrioplasty approach or equal those obtained by microsurgery. The advantages afforded by the described procedures, which can be performed at the time of the initial diagnostic laparoscopy include the avoidance of a second procedure and a laparotomy incision.

The results afforded by laparoscopic salpingostomy may be slightly lower than those yielded by microsurgery, especially when fimbrioplasty cases are excluded from salpingostomy series. However, the principal determinant of the outcome is the status of the tube at the time of surgery. The following factors influence the outcome:

- Distal ampullary diameter.
- Tubal wall thickness.
- Nature of the tubal endothelium.
- Extent of adhesions.
- Type of adhesions.

These factors have been quantified in a scoring system, which permits estimation of the likely surgical outcome (Gomel, 1988). A very important prognostic factor is the status of the tubal epithelium, which can be assessed by salpingoscopy as described earlier (see p. 139). Considering that improvements in the results of salpingostomy with the use of microsurgical techniques by laparotomy have been much less impressive than for other tubal reconstructive procedures and that IVF offers a credible alternative therapeutic option, a strong argument can be made in favor of laparoscopic access to perform salpingostomy in appropriately selected cases, especially since this procedure can be performed during the initial diagnostic laparoscopy.

At the present time the reported results of laparoscopic tubotubal anastomosis do not approach those of traditional microsurgery. Nevertheless with time and the development of adequate surgical techniques and skill the results will improve.

References

Auld BJ, Ahmed E, Wright JT *et al.* (1993) Laparoscopic reversal of sterilization facilitated by hysteroscopic tubal cannulation. Presented at the third biennial meeting of the International Society of Gynecologic Endoscopy. Washington DC.

Bruhat MA, Mage G, Manhes H, Soualhat C *et al.* (1983) Laparoscopy procedures to promote fertility: ovariolysis and salpingolysis results of 93 selected cases. *Acta Europaea Fertilitas* **14**: 113–115.

Canis M, Mage G, Pouly JL *et al.* (1991) Laparoscopic distal tuboplasty: report of 87 cases and a 4-year experience. *Fertility and Sterility* **56**: 616–621.

Daniell JF, Herbert CM (1984) Laparoscopic salpingostomy utilizing the CO_2 laser. *Fertility and Sterility* **41**: 558–563.

Donnez J, Nisolle M, Casanas-Roux F (1989) CO_2 laser laparoscopy in infertile women with adnexal adhesions and women with tubal occlusion. *Journal of Gynecologic Surgery* **5**: 47.

Dubuisson JB, Bouquet de Joliniere J, Aubriot FX *et al.* (1990) Terminal tuboplasties by laparoscopy: 65 consecutive cases. *Fertility and Sterility* **54**: 401–403.

Dubuisson JB, Chapron C, Morice P *et al.* (1994) Laparoscopic salpingostomy: fertility results according to the tubal mucosal appearance. *Human Reproductive* **9**: 334–339.

Fayez JA (1983) An assessment of the role of operative laparoscopy in tuboplasty. *Fertility and Sterility* **39**: 476–479.

Gomel V (1975) Laparoscopic tubal surgery in infertility. *Obstetrics and Gynecology* **46**: 47–48.

Gomel V (1977) Salpingostomy by laparoscopy. *Journal of Reproductive Medicine* **18**: 265–268.

Gomel V (1978) Salpingostomy by microsurgery. *Fertility and Sterility* **29**: 389–387.

Gomel V (1980) Microsurgical reversal of sterilization: a reappraisal. *Fertility and Sterility* **33**: 587–596.

Gomel V (1983a) *Microsurgery in Female Infertility.* pp. 143–149. Boston: Little, Brown and Co.

Gomel V (1983b) Salpingo-ovariolysis by laparoscopy in infertility. *Fertility and Sterility* **340**: 607–610.

Gomel V (1983c) An odyssey through the oviduct. *Fertility and Sterility* **39**: 144–156.

Gomel V (1988) Distal tubal occlusion. *Fertility and Sterility* **49**: 946–948.

Gomel V (1989) Operative laparoscopy: time for acceptance. *Fertility and Sterility* **52**: 1–11.

Gomel V (1995) From microsurgery to laparoscopic surgery: A progress. *Fertility and Sterility* **63**: 464–468.

Gomel V (1997) Reconstructive tubal surgery. In Rock, Thompson (eds) *TeLinde's Operative Gynecology*, 8th edition, Philadelphia, PA: Lippincott–Raven.

Gomel V, Erenus M (1990) The American Fertility Society, 46th Annual Meeting. Program Supplement (Abstracts) P-097, S-106.

Gomel V, Taylor PJ (1993) Reconstructive tubal surgery in the female. In Insler V, Lunenfeld B (eds) *Infertility, Male and Female.* pp. 481–503. Edinburgh: Churchill Livingstone.

Gomel V, Taylor PJ (1995) *Diagnostic and Operative Gynecologic Laparoscopy.* St. Louis: Mosby.

Gomel V, Taylor PJ, Yuzpe AA, Rioux JJ (1986) *Laparoscopy and Hysteroscopy in Gynecologic Practice.* pp. 77–79. Chicago: Year Book Medical Publishers.

Kosasa TS, Hale RW (1988) Treatment of hydrosalpinx using a single incision eversion procedure. *International Journal of Fertility* **33**: 319–323.

McComb P, Paleologou A. (1991) The intussusception salpingostomy technique for the therapy of distal oviductal occlusion at laparoscopy. *Obstetrics and Gynecology* **78**: 443–447.

Mettler L, Giesel H, Semm K. (1979) Treatment of female infertility due to tubal obstruction by operative laparoscopy. *Fertility and Sterility* **32**: 384–388.

Oh ST (1996) Tubal patency and conception rates with three methods of laparoscopic terminal neosalpingostomy. *Journal of the American Association of Gynnecologic Laparoscopists* **3**: 519–523.

Reich H, McGlynn F, Parents C *et al.* (1993) Laparoscopic tubal anastomosis. *Journal of the American Association of Gynnecologic Laparoscopists* **1**: 16–19.

Sedbon E, Bouquet Delajolinieres J, Boudouris O *et al.* (1989) Tubal desterilization through exclusive laparocopy. *Human Reproduction* **4**: 158–159.

15

Strategy for Treatment of Ectopic Pregnancy: Conservative Treatment

JEAN LUC POULY

Département de Gynécologie Obstétrique et Reproduction Humaine, Polyclinique de l'Hôtel Dieu, Centre Hospitalier Universitaire, France

The choice between conservative and radical treatment has long been and is still the subject of debate. The first treatment available was radical. This had the advantage of being quick, easy and efficient at a time when an ectopic pregnancy (EP) could be life-threatening. It was only towards the end of the 1950s that conservative treatment came on the scene. The advent of diagnostic laparoscopy made the diagnosis possible before rupture occurred, and around this time too the world of medicine began to address the problem of infertility. So conservation of the tube was a logical sequence to these two points. The development of operative laparoscopy was a decisive element. The laparoscopic treatment of EP reported for the first time by Manhès and Bruhat in 1977 was conservative (Bruhat *et al.*, 1977; Bruhat *et al.*, 1980). For the first time an operation that was usually carried out by laparotomy was adapted for laparoscopy. Radical treatment returned to the limelight a little later when Dubuisson proposed salpingectomy via laparoscopy (Dubuisson *et al.*, 1987). In parallel to this the development of *in vitro* fertilization (IVF), which enables a pregnancy to be obtained in the absence of tubes, provided some justification for this ablation. Still later the various medical treatments for EP proved that conservative treatment was possible without surgery (Feichtinger and Kemeter, 1987; Stovall and Ling, 1993; Fernandez *et al.*, 1993).

In this chapter we will review conservative surgical treatment for EP via laparoscopy, looking at the technical modalities, the results and indications in turn, before a more general assessment of its place in a wider strategy.

Technical Aspects of Conservative Treatment

The first phase in the laparoscopic procedure is to expose the tube. There are two essential points:

- First that the hemoperitoneum must be evacuated to avoid obscuring laparoscopic vision.
- Second, a suprapubic port must be installed so that a forceps can be used to present and hold the tube.

Different surgeons have different preferences for this port. Manhès recommends placing it on the opposite side to the hematosalpinx. Others prefer to place it next to the EP. A second port with larger diameter is installed on the other side. Ideally this should enable the 'Manhès Triton' to be introduced. This multipurpose device (irrigation, aspiration, electrocoagulation) presents the advantage of providing complete treatment all by itself.

In the description we made in 1983 (Manhès *et al.*, 1983) concerning our modified technique, preventive hemostasis was the second operative phase. Ornithine vasopressin was instilled either in contact with the EP or at each end of the tubal artery. The vasoconstriction thus induced avoided bleeding during the remainder of the surgical procedure without running any risk, however, of postoperative hemorrhage. This technique is still in widespread use outside France, where the product has been banned. To date no other locally acting vasoconstrictor agent has been officially allowed as a replacement, even though other derivatives of vasopressin appear promising.

Once satisfactory vasoconstriction has been obtained, the tube is incised. This salpingotomy is carried out by electrosection. Other means have been proposed. Incision using scissors avoids tissue damage. Incision with the laser is a very expensive process and presents no great advantages. The incision needs to be made at the 1/3 internal, 2/3 external point of the hematosalpinx. It should measure about 10 mm and lie longitudinally along and on the antimesenteric edge of the tube. The trophoblast is aspirated through this salpingotomy incision. The tube diameter must be large enough to permit sufficient traction and to completely evacuate the material. Traction must be progressive to avoid fragmenting the trophoblast.

Hemostasis of the tube is usually satisfactory after extraction and when ornithine vasopressin is used. When vasopressin is not used it is not unusual to see oozing of blood, which originates more from where the EP was implanted than from the edges of the salpingotomy. The simplest way of dealing with this is to wait for spontaneous hemostasis, applying pressure to the tube if necessary. We believe that electrocoagulation should not be used, even if bipolar, because it is so likely to cause irreversible lesions.

The operation is completed by irrigation of the peritoneal cavity to evacuate clots and trophoblast debris. The salpingotomy is not sutured. Although at the beginning of our experience we did not suture for technical reasons, Tulandi and Guralnick (1991) have since demonstrated that suturing is unnecessary and has a slightly negative effect.

This treatment requires no particular laparoscopic equipment apart from a large diameter aspiration device (7 mm minimum), and a means of electrosection. The advantage of the Manhès Triton is that both these functions plus irrigation and aspiration are provided in one instrument.

Criteria for Choosing Conservative Treatment

The choice of conservative treatment depends on four main criteria:

- Operability.
- The risk of failure.
- The desire for pregnancy.
- The fertility prognosis, which includes not only the probability of intrauterine pregnancy (IUP), but also the risk of a recurrence of EP.

Operability

With properly trained and equipped surgeons over 95% of tubal pregnancies can be treated via laparoscopy if ornithine vasopressin is available. If this drug is not available, the percentage drops, but remains well above 80%. Factors that contraindicate or prevent conservative treatment relate to location, hemostasis and the condition of the tube.

For interstitial pregnancy, conservative treatment is very hazardous. The tube incision may result in hemorrhage that cannot be stopped by laparoscopy. Some cases may have been treated successfully, but others have resulted in conversion to laparotomy. Now that the diagnosis is most often made preoperatively, medical treatment by injection *in situ* of methotrexate (MTX) is the simplest and certainly the least dangerous solution.

Tube rupture is not in itself a contraindication. However, there are cases where the tube has been so damaged that it is hopeless to expect satisfactory healing of the tube, in which case salpingectomy is far preferable.

Finally there is the rather more delicate problem of hemostasis, particularly when ornithine vasopressin is not used. At the beginning of our experience we insisted that a small residual hemorrhage should not be a subject for concern. Later the use of vasopressin solved this problem. In the meantime the use of video, which exaggerates the importance of these hemorrhages, prompted surgeons to achieve perfect hemostasis, but there is some question as to whether this is an advantage and totally harmless. Extensive use of electrocoagulation, which generates carbon monoxide, poses a real problem in all types of endoscopic surgery, and where the tube is concerned, coagulation, even if bipolar, causes important tissue damage. In practise after the salpingotomy and aspiration of the trophoblast, the degree of hemorrhage needs to be assessed. If it is slight, we believe it is better to abstain from action and terminate the laparoscopy, leaving a drain as a check in the pouch of Douglas. If there is rather more bleeding, then compressing the tube with a bowel type forceps for ten minutes at least can be enough to solve the problem. However, there are cases where this action is not enough. At this point the tube should be investigated to look for a specific point to coagulate, but usually the bleeding is general and salpingectomy is needed rather than multiple coagulation procedures.

The Risk of Failure

Conservative treatment of EP by laparotomy (Kelly *et al.*, 1979) was known to fail sometimes. However, this did not happen very often and did not seem to affect more than 1% of cases. Right from our first experience we pointed out that there was a greater risk (Bruhat *et al.*, 1980; Pouly *et al.*, 1986b). Incomplete ablation of the trophoblast results in the gradual development of a cystic hematocele, which will not show clinically until 15–30 days later. This persistence of trophoblast material can be detected very early and with this in mind we have published a diagram describing supervision that takes into account the relative drop in hCG concentration (Pouly *et al.*, 1986a, 1992). This incomplete ablation of the trophoblast occurs in about 6% of cases if the main series in the literature are consulted (Table 5.1), but rather than 'cure' these failures, it is better to prevent them.

We also underlined from the outset the increased risk of failure in the following circumstances (Pouly *et al.*, 1986):

- With a tubal pregnancy of more than 4 cm in diameter, with the risk becoming a major risk when it is larger than 6 cm.
- When accessibility of the tube is poor because of obesity or peritubal adhesions.
- When the serum hCG concentration is high (> 20 000 IU ml^{-1}).
- If the tube is 'milked' rather than performing a salpingotomy incision.

However, despite precautions being taken the failure rate has not dropped significantly. A new approach to this problem has recently been proposed by Hagström *et al.* (1994). Failures are mostly explained by the persistence of trophoblast that has invaded the tube wall with a very active EP. So the question is to see which factors indicate how evolutive the EP is. Lindblom uses two factors:

- The change in serum hCG concentrations over 48 hours.
- The progesterone level.

Highly active EP is accompanied by an increase in both the serum hCG concentration and progesterone levels increased over 30 nmol ml^{-1}

(10 ng ml^{-1}). In his series almost all of the failures of conservative treatment of EP presented these characteristics. This new approach has not yet been adopted generally, but it is tempting for two reasons.

- First it evaluates the risk more closely.
- Second it raises the question whether conservative treatment should be managed in a new way.

Indeed they also showed that this type of case also presents an even higher risk when treated by MTX. It is known that over 90% of failures of conservative treatment respond favorably to an intramuscular injection of MTX. So in these cases and if it is desired to keep the tube, it would seem logical to propose a combined medical and laparoscopic surgery treatment. Immediately after the laparoscopy is finished, it is followed by an intramuscular injection of 1.5 mg/kg of MTX. The only objection to this approach is the 48 hour wait required to assess the change in serum hCG concentrations. So once again it is logical to ask whether this kind of treatment could be proposed based on the progesterone level alone as very few cases show a low progesterone level and a falling hCG level.

The Desire for Pregnancy

If there is no desire for pregnancy this is an indication for radical treatment by salpingectomy, which can be associated with contralateral sterilization. However, the sociological evolution of the modern world with its many divorces and remarriages means prudence is required and this attitude should be strictly limited. In addition it is not unusual for an unwanted extrauterine pregnancy to stir a new desire for maternity in particular in patients using an intrauterine contraceptive device (IUD). This criterion is very important in our assessment and when in doubt it is better to be overconservative rather than cause a woman to

Table 15.1 Failure rate after laparoscopic conservative treatment of EP.

Authors	Year	Number of cases	Number of failures	Failure rate (%)
Cartwright *et al.*	1986	20	1	5
Pouly *et al.*	1986b	321	15	4.7
De Cherney and Diamond	1987	79	2	2.5
Reich *et al.*	1988	65	4	6.1
Vermesh	1989	30	1	3.3
Donnez and Nisolle	1989	300	17	5.7
Seifer *et al.*	1990	81	11	13.6
Chapron *et al.*	1991	45	3	6.7
Lundorff *et al.*	1992	52	5	9.6
Total		**993**	**59**	**5.94**

need IVF, especially when we know that there is an excellent fertility prognosis after EP in the presence of an IUD (Pouly *et al.*, 1991a).

The Fertility Prognosis

This has two aspects:

- Offer the maximum chances of IUP.
- Limit the risk of recurrence.

In fact these two factors are linked and evolve in the same direction (see below).

THE RISK OF RECURRENCE

The main argument in favor of radical treatment is to limit the risk of recurrence – but this is not a good idea. There are a number of arguments about evidence with statistics to back them up (Table 15.2). In five important series in the literature the recurrence rate for EP after conservative treatment via laparoscopy is 12% among cases. Compared to this there are two major series in the literature covering salpingectomies only, and here the rate is 11% for 157 cases. The data in the Auvergne records are just as telling, showing a recurrence rate of 7–8% for both treatments (Bouyer *et al.*, 1996). Chapron's analysis of the recurrence of EP is just as interesting. It shows that this recurrence occurs in either tube if there is no major tube pathology, and preferably in the contralateral tube if there is (Chapron *et al.*, 1992).

Finally a simple conclusion becomes evident: unilateral salpingectomy does not prevent recurrence of EP, probably because the first EP most

often occurs in the least pathologically affected tube.

THE PROBABILITY OF IUP

We will deal with this aspect from two angles: that of our own work (Pouly *et al.*, 1991b), and then on a more general study of the literature for which we thank Pansky (1995).

We studied post-EP fertility in a continuous series of 223 patient histories analyzed over a period of 2–15 years during which the possibility of IVF was practically non existent. Of these patients 67% had an IUP subsequent to the EP and the recurrence was 12%. For each case we studied:

- The characteristics of the EP: size of the EP, location, tube wall rupture, quantity of hemoperitoneum.
- The condition of the pelvis apart from the EP: presence of pelvic adhesions, condition of contralateral tube.
- The past history: abdominopelvic surgery, tube surgery, adhesiolysis for infertility, the suspicion of infertility, past history of salpingitis and number of pervious pregnancies.

All of the results of this study have been reported both in English (Pouly *et al.*, 1991b) and in French (Pouly *et al.*, 1991c, 1991d, 1991e, 1991f). The main elements that emerged were as follows:

- With conservative treatment, the characteristics of the EP have no impact on the fertility prognosis. Even tube rupture has no adverse effect on the chances of pregnancy.
- The condition of the contralateral tube is a major factor, together with the presence of

Table 15.2 Fertility after conservative or radical laparoscopic treatment of EP.

Authors	Year	Number of cases	Intrauterine pregnancy (%)	Ectopic pregnancy (%)
Conservative treatment				
De Cherney and Diamond	1987	69	52	16
Donnez and Nisolle	1989	138	51	10
Pouly *et al.*	1991a	223	67	12
Paulson	1992	48	54	31
Lundorff *et al.*	1992	42	52	7
Total		**520**	**58**	**12**
Salpingectomy				
Dubuisson *et al.*	1990	125	24	13
Oelsner *et al.*	1994	32	56	6
Total		**157**	**31**	**11**

adhesions on the tube with the EP. In every case the chances of IUP are reduced, especially if there is no contralateral tube.

- Certain events in the past history have a quite decisive effect on the prognosis, especially a past history of EP, salpingitis, treatment for tubal infertility (tuboplasty or adhesiolysis).
- A past history of other types of abdomino-pelvic surgery has no influence. On the contrary, there is an excellent prognosis for an IUP in a patient using an IUD as 95% of such patients subsequently became pregnant (Pouly *et al.*, 1991a).
- Finally it quite clearly appeared that any element affecting the probability of IUP had a direct corollary: an increased risk of EP.

In order to sort out these various elements, we carried out multivariable analysis, which showed us that the factors that have a real statistical weight for the prognosis are past history of EP, past history of several EPs, past history of laparoscopic adhesiolysis or tube surgery, absence or obstruction of the contralateral tube (single tube), past history of salpingitis, the presence of ipsilateral adhesions and contralateral adhesions. Using this analysis we developed a scoring method which is reported in Table 15.3. We then studied the probability of IUP and the risk of EP in our cases according to this score. The results are given in Figure 15.1. It is clear from this that the probability of IUP and the risk of EP evolve in opposite directions and that from a certain score onwards the risk of recurrence is greater than the probability of IUP. It therefore seemed logical for us to propose not only salpingectomy, but also sterilization of the contralateral tube to prevent the risk of recurrence when faced with a score of over 4.

Pansky (1995) studied the literature for the various factors involved in the prognosis for obtaining an IUP based on 12 articles addressing this subject.

He found 12 factors which have been cited as having an adverse effect on the prognosis for fertility after EP. An overall view of his study is presented in Table 15.4. It is not easy to draw conclusions from this type of analysis. Nevertheless certain points stand out clearly. Certain factors do not affect post-EP fertility, for example age, tube rupture, parity and type of surgery (we will return to this point later). Certain other factors have a definite effect on fertility including the existence of a past suspicion of infertility, the presence of pathologic tubes, a blocked contralateral tube, a past history of EP. Finally opinions differ for certain factors: such as a past history of salpingitis, abdominal surgery or curettage and whether there is a single tube or not.

Finally this study concurs with our own by demonstrating that the decisive factor for the prognosis is the previous condition of the tube, which can be assessed by studying the past history and by the condition of the pelvis at the time of laparoscopy (but without considerations on the status of the pregnant tube, rupture and size).

There is still the question of relative fertility after salpingotomy or salpingectomy. In the absence of random studies, which are difficult to carry out for ethical reasons, we have to refer to comparisons, which are always questionable (Brumsted *et al.*, 1988; Tuomivaara and Kaupilla, 1988; Baumann *et al.*, 1991; Tulandi and Guralnick, 1991). Most conclude that conservative treatment is better without clearly demonstrating this. If we simply compare the series as in Table 15.2, the evidence is in favor of conservative treatment. Indeed in this comparison the rate of IUP is 25% greater after salpingotomy than after salpingectomy. However, this is now increasingly called into question. For Dubuisson the difference is minimal and not significant (Dubuisson *et al.*, 1996). Similarly in the Auvergne records of EP, the treatment does not show up as being a significant factor for the fertility prognosis (Bouyer *et al.*, 1996). In fact only Koninckx

Table 15.3 Therapeutic score for EP.

Factors affecting postoperative infertility	Statistical weight	Score
Previous EP	0.434	2
For each additional EP	0.261	1
Previous laparoscopic adhesiolysis*	0.258	1
Previous tubal plasty*	0.351	2
Solitary tube	0.472	2
Previous salpingitis	0.242	1
Ipsilateral adhesions	0.207	1
Contralateral adhesions**	0.198	1

*Only the worst one of these items.
**If the contralateral tube is absent or blocked, consider as 'solitary tube'

Figure 15.1 IUP probability and EP risk according to therapeutic score.

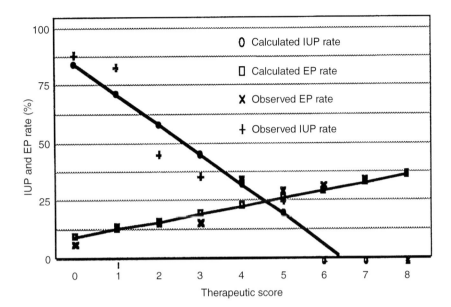

Figure 15.2 Flow chart for therapeutic decision-making between conservative and radical surgical treatment for EP.

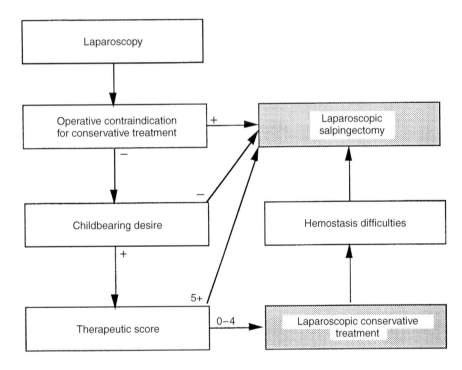

concludes clearly that conservative treatment is better, with figures to support this (Koninckx *et al.*, 1991).

At this point we think it is indispensable to clarify our point of view. It is difficult to see why conservative treatment should have a negative effect. On the contrary it is easier to see that radical treatment should reduce the success rate. So this 'equivalence' of the two treatments should be treated with reserve for at least two reasons. Quite frequently in salpingectomy series, the patients whose contralateral tube is non-existent or blocked are 'removed' from the series, because they have no chance of success, which thus artificially increases the results.

Furthermore the statistics need to be well understood. To say that two treatments are statistically equivalent is not the same as saying there is no statistically significant difference. In the first case the calculation concludes in 'equivalence' while in the second it concludes that it is 'impossible to conclude' because there are not enough cases. So in the Auvergne records the difference is not statistically significant (at 0.05), but it nevertheless shows 15% in favor of salpingotomy (p=0.06).

Finally we believe that it is logical to recommend that treatment should be conservative in as many cases as possible, in agreement with Figure 15.2, which only takes surgical treatment into account

Table 15.4 Infertility factors after EP according to Pansky 1995. Analysed articles: Sherman *et al.*, 1982; Nagamani *et al.*, 1984; Oelsner *et al.*, 1987; Tuomivaara and Kaupilla 1988; Thorburn *et al.*, 1988; Dubuisson *et al.*, 1990; Koninckx *et al.*, 1991; Pouly *et al.*, 1991a; Sultana *et al.*, 1992; Lundorff *et al.*, 1992; Silva *et al.*, 1993; Gruft *et al.*, 1994)

Factor	Numbers of articles[a]	p = significant[b]	Authors[c]
Age	5	1	Sherman
Infertility	5	4	Sherman, Thorburn, Pouly, Sultana
Pathologic tubes	8	4	Sherman, Tuomivaara, Pouly, Silva
Contralateral blocked tube	2	2	Pouly, Lundorff
Previous salpingitis	2	1	Pouly
Tubal rupture	4	1	Sherman
Previous abdominal surgery	2	1	Thorburn
Conservative or radical	7	1	Koninckx
Curettage	1	1	Thorburn
Previous EP	2	2	Pouly, Gruft
Solitary tube	2	1	Pouly
Nulliparity	4	1	Tuomivaara

[a]Number of manuscripts where the factor was analyzed.
[b]Number of manuscripts where the factor was found to be significant.
[c]Authors who have found a difference.

(excludes all medical treatment). Laparotomy remains indicated for a few rare special cases of hemorrhagic shock, but for the rest laparoscopy has proved that it is at least equivalent if not better, particularly with respect to subsequent fertility, as shown by Lundorff *et al.* (1992). Moreover laparoscopy represents major financial savings, as proven by Maruri and Azziz (1993). The only reproach is a slightly higher failure rate due to the persistence of trophoblast material (Seifer *et al.*, 1993), but this can be screened for and treated.

Conclusion

Conservative laparoscopic treatment of EP is the gold standard treatment. It is facing increasing competition from medical treatment using MTX (*in situ* or intramuscularly), but this is only reasonably applicable in 30–40% of cases. The strong movement to bring back salpingectomy does not seem very rational to us. It is often motivated by the simplicity of the procedure and the lower failure rate, whereas conservative treatment is applicable in over 80% of cases and has been proved to safeguard the subsequent fertility of the patients.

Acknowledgement

With grateful thanks to Dr Chapron (Paris) and D Pansky (Tel Aviv) for their help in producing this study.

References

Baumann R, Magos AL, Turnbull A (1991) Prospective comparison of videopelviscopy with laparotomy for ectopic pregnancy. *British Journal of Obstetrics and Gynaecology* **98**: 765–771.

Bouyer J, Job-Spira N, Pouly JL *et al.* (1996) Fertility after ectopic pregnancy. Results of the first three years of the Auvergne Register. *Contraception Fertilité Sexualité* **24**: 475–481.

Bruhat MA, Manhès H, Choukroun J, Suzanne F (1977) Essai de traitement percoelioscopique de la grossesse extra-utérine: a propose de 26 observations. *Revue Française de Gynecologie* **72**: 667–674.

Bruhat MA, Manhès H, Mage G, Pouly JL (1980) Laparoscopic treatment of ectopic pregnancies by means of laparoscopy. *Fertility and Sterility* **33**: 411–414.

Brumsted J, Kessler C, Gibson C, Nakajima D, Riddick DH, Gibson M (1988) A comparison of laparoscopy and laparotomy for the treatment of ectopic pregnancy. *Obstetrics and Gynecology* **71**: 889–892.

Cartwright PS, Herbert CM, Maxson WS (1986) Operative laparoscopy for the management of tubal pregnancy. *Journal of Reproductive Medicine* **31**: 589–591.

Chapron C, Querleu D, Crepin G (1991) Laparoscopic treatment of ectopic pregnancy: a one hundred cases study. *European Journal of Obstetrics and Gynecology* **41**: 187–190.

Chapron C, Pouly JL, Mage G, Canis M, Wattiez A, Bruhat MA (1992) Récidives après traitement coelioscopique d'une première grossesse extra-utérine. *Journal de Gynécologie. Obstétrique et Biologie de Reproduction* **21**: 59–64.

De Cherney A, Diamond MP (1987) Laparoscopic salpingotomy for ectopic pregnancy *Obstetrics and Gynecology* **70**: 948–950

Donnez J, Nisolle M (1989) Laparoscopic treatment of ampullary tubal pregnancy. *Journal of Gynecologic Surgery* **5**: 157–162.

Dubuisson JB, Aubriot FX, Cardone V (1987) Laparoscopic salpingectomy for ectopic pregnancy. *Fertility and Sterility* **47**: 225–228.

Dubuisson JB, Aubriot FX, Foulot H, Bruel D, Bouquet de Jolinière J, Mandelbrot I (1990) Reproductive outcome after laparoscopic salpingectomy for tubal pregnancy. *Fertility and Sterility* **53**: 1004–1007.

Dubuisson JB, Morice P, Chapron C, De Gauffier A, Mouelhi T (1996) Salpingectomy – the laparoscopic surgical choice for ectopic pregnancy. *Human Reproduction* **11**: 1199–1203.

Feichtinger W, Kemeter P (1987) Conservative treatment of ectopic pregnancy by transvaginal aspiration under sonographic control and methotrexate injection. *Lancet* **1**: 381.

Fernandez H, Benifla JL, Lelaidier C, Baton C, Frydman R (1993) Methotrexate treatment of ectopic pregnancy: 100 cases treated by primary transvaginal injection under sonographic control. *Fertility and Sterility* **59**: 773–777.

Gruft L, Bertola E, Luchini L, Azzilonna C, Bigatti G, Parazzini F (1994) Determinants of reproductive prognosis after ectopic pregnancy. *Human Reproduction* **9**: 1333–1336.

Hagström HG, Hahlin M, Bennegarg-Eden B, Sjoblom P, Thorburn J, Lindblom B (1994) Prediction of persistent ectopic pregnancy after laparoscopic salpingostomy. *Obstetrics and Gynecology* **84**: 798–802.

Kelly RW, Martin SA, Strickler RC (1979) Delayed hemorrhage in conservative surgery for ectopic pregnancy. *American Journal of Obstetrics and Gynecology* **133**: 225–228.

Koninckx PR, Witters K, Brosens J, Stemers N, Oosterlynck D, Meuleman C (1991) Conservative laparoscopic treatment of ectopic pregnancies using the CO_2-laser. *British Journal of Obstetrics and Gynaecology* **98**: 1254–1259.

Lundorff P, Thorburn J, Hahlin M, Kallfelt B, Lindblom B (1992) Fertility outcome after conservative surgical treatment of ectopic pregnancy evaluated in a randomized trial. *Fertility and Sterility* **57**: 998–1002.

Manhès H, Mage G, Pouly JL, Ropert JF, Bruhat MA (1983) Améliorations techniques du traitement coelioscopiques de la grossesse extra-utérine. *La Nouvelle Presse Médicale* **12**: 1431–1433.

Maruri F, Azziz R (1993) Laparoscopic surgery for ectopic pregnancy: technology assessment and public health implications. *Fertility and Sterility* **59**: 487–498.

Nagamani M, London S, St-Amand P (1984) Factors influencing fertility after ectopic pregnancy. *American Journal of Obstetrics and Gynecology* **149**: 533–539.

Oelsner G, Morad J, Carp H, Mashiah S, Serr DM (1987) Reproductive performance following conservative microsurgical management of tubal pregnancy. *British Journal of Obstetrics and Gynaecology* **94**: 1078–1083.

Oelsner G, Goldenberg M, Admon D et al. (1994) Salpingectomy by operative laparoscopy and subsequent reproductive performance. *Human Reproduction* **9**: 83–86.

Pansky M (1995) How to Manage Reproductive Problems after E.P. Treatment. References en Gynécologie – Tuboperitoneal Infertility and Ectopic Pregnancy Expert Conference. IFFS 1995 Sattelite Symposium Vichy. *Gynecologic Obstetrics*, Special Issue, **3**: 52–55.

Paulson JD (1992) The use of carbon dioxide laser laparoscopy in the treatment of tubal ectopic pregnancies. *American Journal of Obstetrics and Gynecology* **167**: 382–385 (discussion 385–386).

Pouly JL, Mage G, Gaillard G, Gachon F, Bruhat MA (1986a) La décroissance du taux d'HCG après traitement coelioscopique conservateur de la grossesse extra-utérine. *Journal de Gynécologie, Obstétrique et de Biologie de la Reproduction* **16**: 195–199.

Pouly JL, Manhès H, Mage G, Canis M, Bruhat MA (1986b) Conservative laparoscopic treatment of 321 ectopic pregnancies. *Fertility and Sterility* **46**: 1093–1097.

Pouly JL, Chapron C, Canis M et al. (1991a) Subsequent fertility for patients presenting an ectopic pregnancy with an intrauterine device. *Human Reproduction* **6**: 999–1001.

Pouly JL, Chapron C, Wattiez A, Canis M, Manhès H, Bruhat MA (1991b) Multifactorial analysis of fertility following conservative laparoscopic treatment of ectopic pregnancies. *Fertility and Sterility* **56**: 453–460.

Pouly JL, Chapron C, Wattiez A et al. (1991c) Fertilité après GEU: I – résultats globaux après traitement coelioscopique conservateur. *Contraception Fertilité Sexualité* **19**: 363–367.

Pouly JL, Chapron C, Wattiez A et al. (1991d) Fertilité après GEU: II – valeur pronostique du temps diagnostique de la coelioscopie. *Contraception Fertilité Sexualité* **19**: 367–372

Pouly JL, Chapron C, Wattiez A et al. (1991e) Fertilité après GEU: III – role pronostique des antécédents. *Contraception Fertilité Sexualité* **19**: 373–378.

Pouly JL, Chapron C, Wattiez A, Canis M, Manhès H, Mage G, Bruhat MA (1991f) Fertilité après GEU: IV – Proposition d'un score thérapeutique et d'une stratégie du traitement chirurgical de la GEU. *Contraception Fertilité Sexualité* **19**: 379–386.

Pouly JL, Chapron C, Wattiez A, Canis M, Gaillard G, Bruhat MA (1992) The drop in the level of HCG after conservative laparoscopic treatment of ectopic pregnancy. *Journal of Gynecologic Surgery* **7**: 211–217.

Reich H, Jones DA, De Caprio J, McGlynn F, Reich E (1988) Laparoscopic treatment of 109 consecutive ectopic pregnancies. *Journal of Reproductive Medicine* **33**: 885–890.

Seifer DB, Gutmann JN, Doyle MB, Jones EE, Diamond MP, DeCherney AH (1990) Persistent ectopic pregnancy following laparoscopic linear salpingostomy. *Obstetrics and Gynecology* **76**: 1121–1125.

Seifer DB, Gutmann JN, Grant WD, Kamps CA, DeCherney AH (1993) Comparison of persistent ectopic pregnancy after laparoscopic salpingostomy versus salpingostomy at laparotomy for ectopic pregnancy. *Obstetrics and Gynecology* **81**: 378–382.

Sherman D, Langer R, Sadovsky G (1982) Improved fertility following ectopic pregnancy. *Fertility and Sterility* **37**: 497–502.

Silva P, Schaper A, Rooney B (1993) Reproductive outcome after 143 laparoscopic procedures for ectopic pregnancy. *Obstetrics and Gynecology* **81**: 710–715.

Stovall TG, Ling FW (1993) Single dose methotrexate: an extended clinical trial. *American Journal of Obstetrics and Gynecology* **16**: 1759–1165.

Sultana CJ, Easily K, Collins RL (1992) Outcome of laparo-scopic versus traditional surgery for ectopic pregnancies. *Fertility and Sterility* **57**: 285–289

Thorburn J, Lundorff P, Lindblom B (1988) Fertility after ectopic pregnancy evaluated in relation to background factors and surgical treatment. *Fertility and Sterility* **49**: 595–601

Tulandi T, Guralnick M (1991) Treatment of tubal ectopic pregnancy by salpingotomy with or without tubal suturing and salpingectomy. *Fertility and Sterility* **55**: 53–55.

Tuomivaara L, Kaupilla A (1988) Radical or conservative surgery for ectopic pregnancy? A follow-up study of fertility of 323 patients. *Fertility and Sterility* **50**: 580–588.

Vermesh M (1989) Conservative management of ectopic gestation. *Fertility and Sterility* **51**: 559–567.

16

Techniques of Mass Sterilization

SHIRISH S. SHETH

Sheth Maternity and Gynaecological Nursing Home, Mumbai 400 008, India

Population control is essential in developing countries where a high growth rate of population coupled with poverty has a devastating effect. Thus there is a dire need for a method of permanent contraception or sterilization. Mass voluntary sterilization can be performed on either partner. The demand for female sterilization procedures far surpasses the demand for vasectomies. Globally, more than 120 million couples use sterilization as their contraceptive method of choice.

Choice of Method

Endoscopy has revolutionized the practise of gynecology (Phillips, 1990). Female sterilization on a mass scale can be by tubal occlusion by the laparoscopic method or at mini-laparotomy or by the vaginal route through a posterior colpotomy. Scientific evidence has shown a clear superiority for the laparoscopic method except in the immediate postpartum period.

The laparoscopic method is quick, safe and easy to perform and is therefore the ideal method for mass sterilization and the most acceptable to patients. In the USA, laparoscopic sterilization is the most common laparoscopic procedure as well as the most favored method of sterilization of women (Soderstrom, 1977).

The vaginal method of sterilization was popular briefly before the advent of the laparoscope (Sheth et al., 1973). It now only has a limited role in tubal sterilization (e.g. when a laparoscope or expertise in its use are not available).

According to Bhiwandiwala et al. (1982), the surgeon should continue to use the method with which he is most familiar and comfortable; differences in techniques can usually be overridden by experience.

Methods of Tubal Occlusion

The tubes may be occluded by:

- Cautery, unipolar or bipolar.
- Clip, Filshie (Filshie, 1983) or Hulka (Hulka, 1990).
- Ring (Yoon, 1990).

The choice will depend upon the operator's experience, the relative advantages and disadvantages, and the cost.

Electrocoagulation without transection or resection of the fallopian tube has the largest record of practise of all the methods of sterilization in the USA (Levy and Soderstrom, 1990). Using endocoagulation Semm (1987) destroys only 1 cm of the tubes, which can later be re-anastomosed should the need arise.

The disadvantages of cautery are burns of the abdominal wall and bowel, and problems caused by accidental stepping on the footswitch and erratic power supply in developing countries.

The clip technique is preferred in the young, particularly if the option of reversal is to be considered.

However, in poorer nations where cost plays a major role, the ring is used.

The Sterilization Camp

A 'camp' provides expert medical or surgical assistance to many people in a short time in an orderly organized manner. The patients do not usually have access to even basic facilities. In developing countries this mass scale approach is used for the diagnosis and treatment of cataract, plastic and orthopedic procedures for the handicapped, and for male and female sterilization. A successful outcome enhances the reputation of such a program and generates more volunteers. These camps can be held under the auspices of the government, local authorities or service organizations such as Rotary or Lions organizations or Women's Community groups.

Prerequisites

The prerequisites for a sterilization camp are:

- A large number of willing women – less than 25 operations per day may not be an incentive for the visiting team who come from afar.
- Surgeons with experience of laparoscopic sterilization.
- Trained an anesthesiologist and Boyle's apparatus.
- Availability of running water to clean the instruments.
- A continuous supply of electricity.
- Facilities for laparotomy should the need arise.
- A doctor to assess the patients preoperatively and a social worker to ascertain the number of living children. In some parts of the world with high pediatric mortality, two children are preferred, of which at least one should be a son aged more than four years. This is for cultural and religious reasons.
- Local support from the government and/or municipality is essential.

The Team

The team consists of:

- Experienced surgeons – one or more depending upon the size of the camp.
- Theater nursing staff – one or more.
- Theater assistants – one or more.

The reputation and experience of the team are the pillars upon which the success of the camp is built. Local nursing and other staff can be an asset if included in the program.

Preparations for Holding a Camp

It is necessary to have adequate propaganda by means of pamphlets, posters, banners and visits by social workers. Details of the method of sterilization help to motivate the women. They are told that:

- The abdomen is not cut open.
- There is only one stitch.
- The vagina is left intact.
- The stay is only for a few hours and does not usually involve an overnight absence from home.

Buses, jeeps, ambulances, vans, cars and even bullock carts have been used to fetch the patients from the surrounding countryside and take them back. They need to be reassured about return transport and medical help, should it be required. Well-maintained public relations ensure the success of the camp and any future camps in the area. In some countries, incentive money is paid to the patient, the surgeon and the motivator.

Many of the women are uneducated and illiterate. A patient and understanding chat about their apprehensions, queries and doubts is needed as are satisfactory answers. The failure rate and available alternatives if the need should arise should be explained.

Women with severe anemia (hemoglobin < 7 g dl^{-1}), cardiac disease or severe malnutrition are not accepted. A routine urine examination should be done. Tetanus toxoid is given and sensitivity to lignocaine tested. Pregnancy must be excluded as sterilization with termination of pregnancy performed in an unfamiliar set-up can predispose to sepsis and can prove risky. It is advisable not to hold a mass diagnostic camp for other diseases along with a mass sterilization camp as a mix up can be disastrous (e.g. tubal occlusion mistakenly performed on an infertile patient).

Naturally an operating theater is the ideal place to perform this procedure. However, in the camp scenario, school halls, classrooms, guest houses or parts of an auditorium are temporarily converted into operating rooms. The space allotted should be at least 15×12 feet. The tables are sometimes regular operation tables, but often ordinary tables are used with blocks or bricks at the foot end to achieve the Trendelenburg position. The number of tables varies from two to six, depending upon the number of operations to be performed. A patient is operated on one table and while that patient is being moved, the surgeon starts the pneumoperitoneum for the next patient on the second table. In the meantime, another patient is positioned on the third table, so that an assistant can carry out intravenous premedication, painting, draping and infiltration of local anaesthesia (Table 16.1, Figure 16.1).

Table 16.1 Mass laparoscopic sterilization camps.

Feature	Number or time
Operation tables	2–6
Operations per table per hour	6–15
Working hours per day	8–14
Surgical time for each operation	2–10 min
Operations per day	100–500
Postoperative stay	6–18 hours

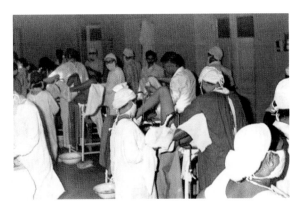

Figure 16.1 Operating room scenario.

Equipment

This consists of:

- Single-puncture operating laparoscopes and/or double-puncture laparoscopes.
- Falope ring applicators, Veress needles, trocar and cannula.
- Fiberoptic light source or a variant.
- A pneumoperitoneum apparatus or a variant (e.g. an air pump).

In operative laparoscopy, the single puncture technique is not recommended (Sutton, 1990), However, for mass sterilization by the laparoscopic method, single-puncture equipment is preferred because:

- Tubal occlusion is the only operation to be performed.
- One stitch is preferred by patients.
- The time for operation is less.
- Less manipulation is required.
- A second set of trocar and cannula is not needed.

The equipment needed is dependent upon the number of tables. One pneumoperitoneum apparatus and a light source between two tables can suffice. These can be operated by a single paramedic or a non-medical person.

The equipment used needs to be cleaned under running water and kept for at least ten minutes in sterilizing solution (Cidex or formalin). If this is not possible, a compromise can be made by cleaning the trocar thoroughly in soapy water, preferably containing 1000 ppm of chlorine and then rinsing and boiling in clean water for five minutes (Woodford, 1989). The laparoscope should be rinsed in 80% ethanol and dried. It helps to have a greater number of those instruments that come into direct contact with body tissue (such as the peritoneum and the fallopian tubes) available as possible.

Light

A fiberoptic light source is ideal for laparoscopic tubal sterilization, but is cumbersome for a visiting team to carry and can easily be damaged while travelling on bumpy roads. Mini-light sources (Figure 16.2) which are handy and easy to transport, may be used (Bhatt *et al.*, 1983). They can also work on a battery, which is an advantage in case of power failure.

Anesthesia

In the vast majority of patients, laparoscopic sterilization can be performed under local anesthesia and premedication. General anesthesia is not necessary unless:

- Premedication and local anesthesia prove inadequate.
- The patient is highly strung and apprehensive.

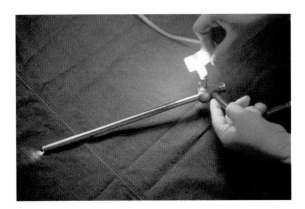

Figure 16.2 Mini-light with laparoscope.

- There is extreme obesity.
- Extra manipulation is needed.

It is mandatory to have a competent anesthesiologist and Boyle's apparatus in the operating theater. The choice of premedication is best left to the anesthesiologist. Usually, atropine 0.6 mg subcutaneously, 50 mg meperidine and either 10–20 mg trifluopromazine hydrochloride or 10 mg diazepam are given. Local infiltration with 3–5 ml of 1% lignocaine hydrochloride around the site for surgery supplements the premedication.

Pneumoperitoneum

The ideal gas, carbon dioxide (CO_2), may not be available in some parts of the world and alternatives such as nitrous oxide or oxygen are expensive. In such circumstances, atmospheric air is an acceptable compromise. Room air can be freely instilled using an air pump similar to the one used in a fish tank to release air bubbles (Figure 16.3). An inexperienced operator should not use air. Even experienced operators must exercise caution as there is a greater chance of embolism and death. The use of cautery is contraindicated when a combustible gas is used.

The amount of gas used can be measured by an air indicator or by clinical judgement. If one fails to create a pneumoperitoneum, the Veress needle is inserted through the pouch of Douglas by colpopuncture. If there is no contraindication, this should pave the way for a successful pneumoperitoneum. Sheth (1976) created pneumoperitoneum by this method in the obese and those with a history of multiple abdominal operations so that such women are not deprived of tubal sterilization.

Procedure

The tables are placed parallel to each other with one light and gas source in between to service the two tables. Each operator manages one table, but the more experienced staff, particularly the speedier ones, usually manage two. The painting, draping and local infiltration of 3–5 ml of 1% lignocaine hydrochloride is done by an assistant. The patient either walks to the table or is carried on a stretcher if premedication has been given earlier. Pneumoperitoneum is created in the usual manner. Single-puncture laparoscopes are preferred through which the chosen occluding device is applied at a distance of 3 cm from the cornual ends. An assistant, usually a highly experienced nurse, inserts the uterine manipulator and almost feeds the fallopian tube to the applicator. Where a population is particulary prudish about external genitalia some operators have performed all tubal sterilization without using uterine manipulators, but with the help of a steep Trendelenburg position.

When the tubes have been occluded, the abdomen is deflated as much as possible and one mattress stitch inserted. The patient is usually lifted bodily by one person (Figure 16.4) and carried to the recovery area.

When a mass laparoscopic sterilization is performed, one may come across unexpected abnormalities, for example a congenital malformation, a mass, pelvic inflammatory disease, and particularly abdominal or pelvic tuberculosis. Women with these conditions should be referred for appropriate therapy and follow-up.

Postoperatively, the patient is observed for 6–12 hours, and may stay overnight if operated on in the evening as travel can be difficult in rural areas. At times, due to the paucity of facilities, patients lie on the floor or share a bed (Figures 16.5, 16.6).

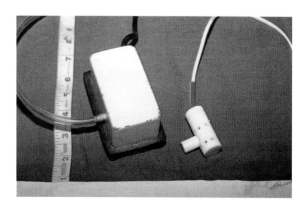

Figure 16.3 Mini-light and air pump device.

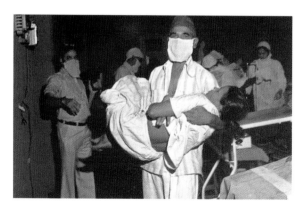

Figure 16.4 Postoperatively the patient is lifted by one person due to the constraints of space and time.

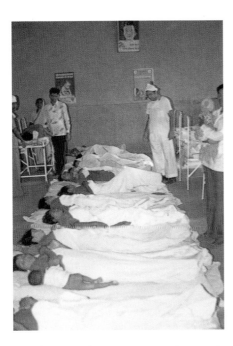

Figure 16.5 Postoperative recovery area in a rural camp.

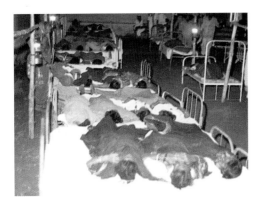

Figure 16.6 Many postoperative patients sharing a bed at a rural camp.

Complications

Brooks and Marlow (1977) have rightly said that 'While laparoscopy is a relatively safe procedure, there are times when its use can be extremely hazardous. Hence the procedure must be treated with respect and done with the utmost care'. Chamberlain and Brown (1978) found a complication rate of 4.1% among 29 661 laparoscopic sterilizations. A World Health Organization multicenter multinational randomized study (1982) found that the incidence of complications at the time of operation is greater with the laparoscopic approach, with 7% of women experiencing major or minor complications. Quilligan and Zuspan (1986) found minor

complications occur less frequently with laparoscopic sterilization than with sterilization via colpotomy or at laparotomy.

The complication rate is higher in the postpartum and postabortal periods (Hughes, 1977). However, the patients at a mass voluntary sterilization camp are the so-called interval, non-obstetric or gynecological cases. In a mass sterilization program for 9066 illiterate women, Bhathena *et al.* (1985) had an overall complication rate of 5.3%. Mehta (1989) had a major complication rate of 3.2 per 100 000. In a series of 30 000 laparoscopic sterilizations (Table 16.2), Sheth (1988) reported complications in 4.7% of cases.

There is a risk of transmission of bloodborne viral infections, particularly hepatitis B and C and also the human immunodeficiency virus (HIV). This necessitates extra care to avoid contamination with blood or needle stick injury.

Mortality

A sterilization death is one that can be directly attributed to sterilization or one that occurs within 30 days of the procedure and cannot be explained satisfactorily by any other cause. Cardiorespiratory complications during general anesthesia are the leading cause of such deaths (Peterson *et al.*, 1982). Bhatt *et al.* (1983) found a mortality rate of 7.15 per 10 000 sterilizations performed by different methods, although there were none when the laparoscopic method was used.

At mass voluntary sterilization rural camps where the laparoscopic method was used, Mehta (1989) reports a death rate of 4.8 per 100 000, while

Table 16.2 Complications in 30 000 laparoscopic sterilizations in rural camps. Wound infections were mild, and there were no deaths. (Courtesy of the *Lancet* **ii**: 1415–1416 (1988).)

Complications	Number
Perforation of uterus	268
Transection of tube	56
Mesosalpingeal hematoma	74
Slight bleeding from tube mesosalpinx	194
Extraperitoneal pneumoperitoneum	118
Failed pneumoperitoneum	60
Failure to apply the silicone rubber band	96
Trocar injury	
Intestinal injury (laparotomy required)	3
Abdominal wall hematoma (evacuation required)	1
Wound infection	560
Total	**1430**

Table 16.3 Laparoscopic sterilizations and mortality.

Report	Number of laparoscopic sterilizations	Failed attempts per 1000	Complication rate (%)	Laparotomy rate per 1000	Death rate per 100 00
AAGL, 1976 (Phillips et al., 1977)	77 103	–	–	2.7	4
RCOG, 1976–1977 (Chamberlain and Brown, 1978)	29 577	7.50	4.1	12.10	10.2
Bhathena et al.* (1985)	9 066	5.0	5.3	2.0	0
Mehta* (1989)	250 136	0.2	1.5	0.003	4.8
Sheth* (1988)	30 000	2.1	4.7	0.10	0

*Mass sterilizations report.

Bhathena *et al.* (1985) had no deaths among 9066 cases and neither did Sheth (1988) among 30 000 cases, though three women had to have a laparotomy (Table 16.3).

In the developing world, maternal mortality is very high, ranging from 100–700 per 100 000 in contrast to 4–6 per 100 000 in developed countries. A significant number of deaths can thus be prevented by mass sterilization (Figure 16.7).

Follow-up

In the developing world, follow-up of women who have taken part in a mass sterilization program is poor, and in the rural areas it is worse. The local health officers are usually in charge, and any major complication would be magnified and compensation may be demanded. Women in the rural areas have remarkable resistance and wound infections are usually mild.

Failure

Phillips *et al.* (1977) report that in a substantial proportion of failures, the pregnancy is ectopic. However, the incidence of ectopic pregnancy is much less (2–8 per 1000) when the occluding device is a clip, as shown by an international multicenter study (Hulka, 1990).

Mehta (1989) had a failure rate of 0.1% with the falope ring, while Rock mentions a pregnancy rate of 0.2–0.5% (Rock *et al.*, 1987). In a mass sterilization program, the incidence of luteal phase pregnancy will be higher.

Reversal

Besides remarriage, in the developing world, the high incidence of infant mortality may also be the reason for reversal. However, the laparoscopic method of tubal sterilization must be considered as permanent and therefore irreversible, despite its well-known high reversibility rate.

Factors that Adversely Affect the Camp

The patient and relatives can be easily displeased if positioning of the patient, internal examination, or lifting the patient after the operation are carried out in an undignified manner. Shouting or screaming by the patient during the operation or complications can upset the large apprehensive crowd waiting for the outcome of the operation. If a death occurs, the news will spread rapidly and the entire crowd will promptly decide against the procedure and vanish from the

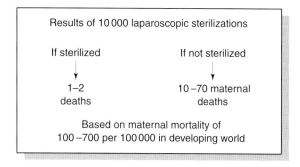

Figure 16.7 Laparoscopic sterilizations and mortality.

scene. A mishap at a camp can become unduly magnified and bring the procedure into disrepute. Any indifference or non-cooperation on the part of the local authorities towards the holding of a camp in the area can also adversely affect the outcome.

Economic Considerations

The equipment required for laparoscopic sterilization is expensive. However, with mini-laparotomy, the cost of the hospital stay is considerable. Laparoscopic mass sterilization, for which patients need to stay for only a few hours, is thus far more economical.

Summary

In the overpopulated countries of the developing world, a large proportion of the population living in rural areas is deprived of the facility of gynecologic specialists and good hospital care. Despite social, cultural and religious taboos, many women in these areas are now aware of the advantages of sterilization. Without the facilities provided by mass sterilization camps, these women would in most cases continue procreating and adding to the population. Laparoscopic sterilization on a mass scale is the ideal method for interval cases, provided there are skilled surgeons and staff and appropriate equipment. Although some compromises have to be made in the developing world, the technique achieves the purpose with very good results, not the least of which is the gratitude of the patients. It is to be hoped that countries with such problems will use the skills of experienced laparoscopists to control their population.

Acknowledgement

My sincere thanks go to Dr V Karani, MD for her painstaking help in compiling this manuscript.

References

Bhathena RK, Jassawalla MJ, Patel DN (1985) Laparoscopic sterilization in camps in rural India. *British Journal of Family Planning* **10**: 121–126.

Bhatt RV, Dawn CS, Gogoi MP *et al.* (1983) Immediate sequelae following tubal sterilisation: A multicentre study of the ICMR Task Force on Female Sterilisation. *Contraception* **28**: 369–384.

Bhiwandiwala PP, Mumford SD, Feldblum PJ (1982) A comparison of different laparoscopic sterilisation occlusion techniques in 24,439 procedures. *American Journal of Obstetrics and Gynecology* **144**: 329–331.

Brooks PG, Marlow J (1977) *Indications and Contraindications in Laparoscopy*. pp. 52–59. Baltimore, USA: Williams & Wilkins.

Chamberlain GVP, Brown JC (eds) (1978) *The Report of the Working Party of the Confidential Enquiry into Gynaecological Laparoscopy*. pp. 3, 8, 27, 109, 116, 152. London: Royal College of Obstetricians and Gynaecologists.

Editorial (1980) Female sterilisation – no more tubal coagulation. *British Medical Journal* **280**: 1037.

Filshie GM (1983) The Filshie clip. In Van Lith DAF, Keith LG, Van Kall EV (eds) *New Trends in Female Sterilisation*. Chicago: Year Book Medical Publishers.

Hughes GJ (1977) Sterilisation failure. *British Medical Journal* **ii**: 1337–1339.

Hulka JV (1990) Technique of Sterilisation: Manual of Endoscopy, pp 63–71, California, USA: American Association of Gynecologic Laparoscopists.

Levy BS & Soderstrom RM (1990) Electrical Techniques of Sterilisation: Manual of Endoscopy, pp 57–61, California, USA: American Association of Gynecologic Laparoscopists.

Mehta PV (1989) A total of 250,136 laparoscopic sterilisations by a single operator. *British Journal of Obstetrics and Gynaecology* **96**: 1024–1034.

Peterson HB, Greenspan JR & DeStefano F (1982) Death associated with laparoscopic sterilisation in the United States. *Reproductive Medicine* **27**: 345–347.

Phillips J, Hulke B, Hulke J *et al.* (1977) Laparoscopic procedures: the American Association of Gynecologic Laparoscopists: membership survey for 1975. *Journal of Reproductive Medicine* **18**: 227–232.

Phillips JM (1990) Preface. In *Manual of Endoscopy*. California, USA: American Association of Gynecologic Laparoscopists.

Quilligan EJ & Zuspan F (1986). *Operative Obstetrics*. pp. 795–803. New York: Appleton Crofts.

Rock JA, Guzick DS, Katz E *et al.* (1987) Tubal anastomosis: Pregnancy success following reversal of falope ring or monopolar cautery sterilisation. *Fertility and Sterility* **48**: 13–17.

Semm K (1987) Surgical pelviscopy: Review of 12 060 pelviscopies. In *Progress in Obstetrics and Gynecology*, Vol. 6. pp. 333–345. London: Churchill Livingstone.

Sheth SS (1976) Transvaginal induction of pneumoperitoneum prior to laparoscopy. *Asian Journal of Obstetrics and Gynaecology* **5**: 50–54.

Sheth SS (1988) Round the world: Laparoscopic female sterilisation camps. *Lancet* **ii**: 1415–1416.

Sheth SS, Kothari ML & Munshi V (1973): Postabortal colpotomy and sterilisation. *Journal of Obstetrics and Gynaecology of the British Commonwealth* **80(3)**: 274–275.

Soderstrom RM (1977) *Operative Sterilisation: An Overview*, Vol. 15. pp. 159–166. Baltimore, Maryland: Williams & Wilkins.

Sutton C (1990) The treatment of endometriosis. In

Progress in Obstetrics and Gynaecology. pp. 251–272. London: Churchill Livingstone.

World Health Organization Task Force on Female Sterilisation (1982) Mini-laparotomy or laparoscopy for sterilisation – a multi-centre, multi-national randomised study. *American Journal of Obstetrics and Gynecology* **143**: 645.

Woodford FP (1989) Decontamination of instruments and appliances used in the vagina. *British Journal of Obstetrics and Gynaecology* **96**: 1024–1034.

Yoon I (1990) Yoon falope ring technique of sterilisation. In *Manual of Endoscopy.* pp. 73–75. California, USA: American Association of Gynecologic Laparoscopists.

17

Laparoscopic Female Sterilization

G. M. FILSHIE

Queen's Medical Centre, Nottingham, UK

Introduction

Laparoscopy is one of the most widely used surgical procedures in gynecology and is now used extensively by general surgeons. Female sterilization is the most common operative procedure and is generally well accepted by both patients and gynecologists. More women throughout the world are protected from pregnancy by tubal ligation than by any other contraceptive method. Over 140 million women throughout the world have been sterilized (Population Report, 1990). Nevertheless, laparoscopy is a sophisticated technique, the success of which depends upon both the skill of the surgeon and the adequacy of the equipment.

Historical Background

Although Kelling from Hamburg first reported the use of a Nitze cystoscope to inspect the abdominal cavity of a dog in 1923, in 1911 Jacobeus from Sweden was the first to inspect the abdominal cavity of a human when he conceived the phrase 'laparoscopy'. The first surgeon to report a laparoscopic female sterilization was Ruddock in 1934. Anderson, in 1937, developed a purpose-built electrode for tubal fulguration. Power and Barnes in 1941 described the technique of tubal fulguration in detail. Little advance was made over the next 20 years. However, as a result of the introduction of the cold light source by Forestier, Galdu and

Vulmier in 1952, and later the Hopkins rod lens laparoscopic system in 1976, laparoscopy became predictably easier and safer. Raoul Palmer is known as the founder of modern day laparoscopy and published extensively on the use of laparoscopy, both as a diagnostic procedure and as a simple method of tubal cautery. Using the biopsy forceps for tubal cautery, he popularized female sterilization, particularly in France (Palmer, 1962). Frankenheim (1964) popularized the procedure in Germany and similarly Steptoe popularized laparoscopy in the UK in 1965 (Steptoe, 1965). Later Wheeless (1972), was responsible for popularizing laparoscopic tubal cautery in the USA. There was an immense surge of interest in the use of unipolar coagulation as patients could be treated on an outpatient basis. Inevitably, problems emerged, particularly those involving inadvertent burns to bowel (Thompson and Wheeless, 1973; Rioux, 1977). This prompted the development of bipolar cautery by Rioux and Cloutier (1974) and subsequently by Kleppinger (1977) and by Hirsch and Roose in 1974. Semm described a 'thermal coagulator' in 1973 that limited the temperature to approximately 140°C and further improved the safety of electrocoagulation. However, anxiety about thermal injuries promoted the development of a number of mechanical methods to occlude the tubes. The Hulka Clemens clip was introduced in 1973 (Hulka *et al.*, 1973) and the falope (Yoon) ring was introduced in 1975 (Yoon and King, 1975). The Bleier clip (Bleier, 1973) and the Tupla clip (Babenerd and Flehr, 1978) were introduced about the same time and more recently, in 1981, the Filshie clip was introduced (Filshie *et al.*, 1981; Filshie, 1983). As a result of these technologies gynecologists have been able to offer women a variety of methods of female sterilization that are relatively simple and safe and can be performed predictably as a day case procedure.

Laparoscopic Instrumentation

A vast number of instruments are now available for female sterilization. Their use depends upon personal preference and availability. Essentially there is a need for a laparoscope to visualize the pelvis, an insufflator and a uterine manipulator. A Veress needle is optional for those who do not like to insert the laparoscopic trocar and cannula in the absence of a pneumoperitoneum. Insufflation is not required when a gasless laparoscopic technique is used (Maher, 1995); however, this technique requires special instrumentation. Some laparoscopes have an operating channel and those without need a second puncture trocar and cannula for the appropriate sterilization instrument to pass through. Where a double-puncture technique is employed there is a trend to use smaller laparoscopes ranging from 7 mm, 5 mm, 2.7 mm and 1.9 mm (micro-laparoscopy) (Bauer et al., 1995). The smaller the laparoscope the less robust it is for general use. A 12 mm operating laparoscope has an operating channel of 8 mm (Wolf) and 7.4 mm (Storz), while a 10 mm operating laparoscope has an operating channel of 5–6 mm. There are many applicators for the different methods of sterilization. For Filshie clip application the three different single puncture applicators are 8 mm, 7.4 mm and 6 mm for the appropriate operating channel. There are also two double-puncture applicators of 7 and 8 mm, respectively. The Hulka clip applicators go down an 8 mm operating channel or cannula and the falope ring may be applied down an 8, 7 or 6 mm operating channel or trocar and cannula. Cautery, either bipolar or unipolar, can usually go down a 5–6 mm operating channel or cannula. The Veress needle for insufflation is available in two sizes, the larger one being suitable for overweight patients. If the abdominal route is unsuccessful for producing a pneumoperitoneum the Veress needle may be introduced through the pouch of Douglas (Seth, 1976) or through the fundus of the uterus (Sanders and Filshie, 1974). There are now a number of excellent insufflators and carbon dioxide (CO_2) is commonly used when a general anesthetic is employed and is particularly necessary when coagulation techniques are used. When a local anesthetic is used, nitrous oxide is the gas of choice as it offers less discomfort to the abdomen and

shoulders, but its use is limited to mechanical methods. Uterine manipulators are also useful for elevating the uterus so that the operator can clearly see the posterior aspect of the uterus, tubes and broad ligament. The tubes can therefore be easily visualized and occluded correctly. However, with an anteverted uterus and the use of a steep Trendelenburg position the tubes can be visualized easily and occluded safely without manipulation. This is particularly satisfactory when the operator is using a local anesthetic technique as the patient can lie supine and not in an uncomfortable lithotomy position.

Open laparoscopy involves a small incision below the umbilicus and dissecting down directly through to the peritoneal layer. Once through the peritoneum a special blunt cannula (Hasson, 1974) is inserted and sutured in place. Insufflation can then take place and the laparoscopy proceeds as normal. In a recent survey 8% of laparoscopies are performed this way (Hulka et al., 1995). The technique might be expected to minimize the risk of damaging bowel, but studies have so far not demonstrated this.

Review of Current Methods of Female Sterilization

Electrocautery

UNIPOLAR COAGULATION

This was originally used laparoscopically to cauterize the fallopian tubes. However, it is now rarely used because of its potential for causing bowel or other intra-abdominal burns (Rioux, 1977). The temperature between the jaws of the forceps may reach 3–400°C and 3 cm of the isthmic portion of the tube are desiccated with multiple burns. Concomitant transection of a tube appears to increase the failure rate. The failure rate in the first 12 months is approximately 0.37% per 100 woman years (Vessey et al., 1983), going down to 0.1% thereafter.

BIPOLAR COAGULATION

This was developed to reduce the problems related to unipolar coagulation. The electrical current only passes between the two jaws of the grasping forceps, eliminating the more extensive track of current from the forceps through the body to the earthing plate on the leg or buttock. The technique is essentially the same as for unipolar coagulation as 3 cm of tube should be coagulated and desiccated. The isthmic portion of the tube is coagulated a number of times adjacent to the isthmic portion. Tubal transection is again not recommended. Large series have shown that the early failure rate is approximately 1.1 per 1000 patients with a complication rate of 2.6 per 1000 cases (Hirsch and Nesser, 1983). This figure has been shown to be much higher with long-term follow-up of ten years (US Collaborative Review of Sterilization, 1996).

Thermal or Cold Coagulation

A low voltage and low temperature technique has been developed to further decrease thermal complications. The temperature between the jaws is elevated to approximately 120–140°C. When the forceps have become heated they are kept in place for 20 seconds. The short-term failure rate is approximately 0.2–0.4 per 1000 women months (Semm, 1977).

Mechanical Techniques

To avoid electrical burns a number of mechanical methods have been developed. There has been an assortment of clips and rings, although at present there are only two clips and the ring currently available: the Hulka clip, the Filshie clip and the falope (Yoon) ring. The Weck clip, Tupla clip and Bleier clip are no longer used for female sterilization (Figure 17.1).

THE FALOPE RING TECHNIQUE

This is the most commonly used mechanical device throughout the developing world. It is an ingenious technique and can be made relatively cheaply for developing countries. A small ring made of silicone rubber 1 × 2.2 × 36 mm is expanded onto the end of a cannula (Figure 17.2). Forceps grasp the isthmic portion of the fallopian tube and pull the tube into the lumen of the cannula. The expanded ring is then pushed off the cannula to contract around a knuckle of approximately 3 cm of the fallopian tube, resulting in a Madlener type of technique. The failure rate varies from 1.7 (Rubin *et al.*, 1982) to 9.3 (Bhiwandiwala *et al.*, 1982) per 1000, although this can be much higher when performed by trainees (Stovall *et al.*, 1991). Surgical difficulties affect 0.7 (Chi *et al.*, 1980) to 1.2% (McCann and Cole, 1980)

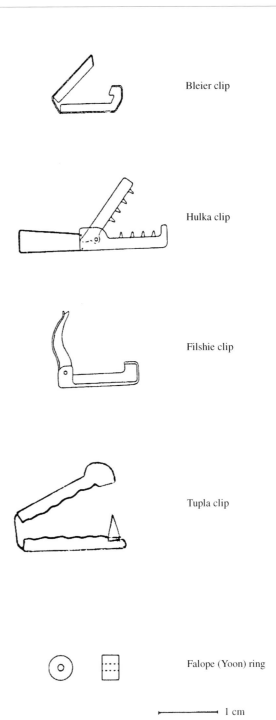

Figure 17.1 Mechanical methods of female sterilization.

of cases and include tubal transection or incomplete occlusion of a fallopian tube.

HULKA CLEMENS CLIP

This is a springloaded clip first described by Hulka and Umran in 1972. The clip is made of lexan plastic and has interdigitating teeth on the jaws to prevent expulsion of the tube during closure of the clip. The clip is kept closed by a spring, which is gold-plated stainless steel. This clip maintains pressure between

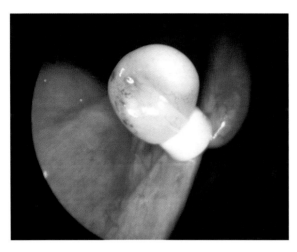

Figure 17.2 Laparoscopic view of a falope ring in place.

the jaws of the clip holding the enclosed tube resulting in pressure necrosis. The clip is 3 mm wide and 15 mm long. It has a short-term failure rate of up to five per 1000 cases (Newton, 1984), long-term follow-up figures are higher. Only 3 mm of tube are destroyed, making reversal more feasible than with other methods (Hulka and Noble, 1982).

FILSHIE CLIP

This is made of titanium with an inner cushion lining of silicone rubber. It has a front locking mechanism to reduce the chances of the tube slipping out of the jaws when correctly applied (Figure 17.3) and is the most widely used method in the UK, Canada and Australia. It has been available in the USA since the end of September 1996. The clip is 4 mm wide and 13 mm long. The failure rate when applied laparoscopically is between 1.7 (Green-Thompson *et al.*, 1993) and 2 (FDA Advisory Panel Meeting, 1996) per 1000 and, like the Hulka clip, failures are mostly due to operator error. Since 1982 nearly 2¼ million clips have been applied, and to date there

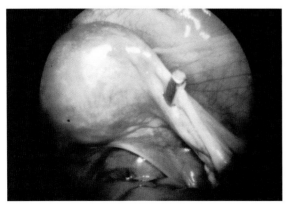

Figure 17.3 Laparoscopic view of the insertion of a Filshie clip.

are no published reports showing that a correctly applied clip has failed by recanalization within the jaws of the clip when the specimen has been histologically scrutinized rather than just being observed. In a recent survey from Scotland it has been regarded as the method of choice (Pennev *et al.*, 1997).

Anesthesia for Laparoscopic Sterilization

Both general and local anesthetics may be employed. Although local anesthetic is probably much safer, in a recent survey only 8% of cases were performed under local anesthesia (Hulka *et al.*, 1995).

General Anesthesia

Short-acting agents are generally employed, together with intubation and administration of a muscle relaxant. There is, however, no statistical evidence that there is any increased morbidity when intubation is not used (Chamberlain and Brown, 1978).

Local Anesthesia

For safety reasons this could and possibly should be used more often, and ideally patients should be given the choice. Its use for both the application of clips and rings and cautery are well documented (MacKenzie *et al.*, 1987; Lipscomb *et al.*, 1992; Green-Thompson *et al.*, 1993). Essentially 10 ml of 1% lignocaine with 1 in 200 000 epinephrine is injected into the skin and underlying fascia to the peritoneum where the puncture sites are to be. A pneumoperitoneum with nitrous oxide is produced using a standard technique. Nitrous oxide produces less shoulder discomfort than with carbon dioxide. 1 ml of 2–4% lignocaine or 0.5% bupivacaine is slowly dropped onto each fallopian tube – the Veress needle is extremely useful for this step. In a recent study patients were given 800 mg ibuprofen 30 minutes preoperatively and midazolam 3 mg, alfentanil 1 mg and atrophine 0.6 mg intravenously immediately preoperatively to allay anxiety and for further analgesia (Lipscomb *et al.*, 1992) and gave very satisfactory results. Postoperatively ibuprofen 800 mg may be given eight-hourly for postoperative discomfort. If tubal cautery is used, CO_2 should be used as the insufflation gas.

Mortality

The Royal College of Gynaecology Laparoscopy Survey reported a mortality of 10.2 per 100 000 cases (Chamberlain and Brown, 1978). Peterson *et al.*, 1983 reviewed 29 cases and found 11 related to a complication of anesthesia and seven cases were due to sepsis, of which three were associated with bowel injury with unipolar coagulation. Two further bowel injuries occurred: one following a postpartum laparotomy and one following an open laparoscopy. Hemorrhage occurred in four patients: three followed major vessel laceration with the trocar and Veress needle, while one vessel was injured during incision of the skin with a scalpel blade. Incidental causes include myocardial infarction, pulmonary embolus and cardiac complications, and a possible CO_2 embolus. Peterson estimates that the overall mortality is probably in the region of 3.6 per 100 000 cases.

Long-Term Failures (8–14 years)

Long-term follow-up for female sterilization has only recently been made available by the Crest Study conducted by the Center for Disease Control (US Collaborative Review of Sterilization, 1996). As this is an American study, Filshie clip data were not included. However, a long-term study is presently being conducted. The long-term follow-up results of unipolar coagulation, bipolar coagulation, falope

rings and Hulka clips are now available. In the US Crest collaborative study 10 863 people were enrolled and 10 685 patients were followed up. Data were collected at 1, 3, 5 and 8–14 years following the operation. Cumulative ten-year morbidities of pregnancy were highest for the Hulka clip method (36.5 per 1 000 cases) and lowest for unipolar coagulation (7.5 per 100 000). Young women had the highest rate of failure and this included 53.3 per 1000 for bipolar coagulation and 52.1 per 1000 for Hulka clip application. With the mechanical methods, failures were in the first three to four years following the operation, whereas pregnancies occurred fairly evenly throughout the ten years following bipolar cautery.

Ectopic Pregnancy Following Sterilization

Ectopic pregnancies are potentially life-threatening complications, particularly in developing countries where access to surgery may be limited. Stock (1984) has described three types of fistula leading to ectopic pregnancy:

- A direct tuboperitoneal fistula deriving from the stump of the tube following any method of tubal ligation.
- As fistula due to endosalpingiosis following tubal ligation.
- A tubotubal fistula causing an ectopic pregnancy to lodge along the line of a tubotubal fistula.

Table 17.1 Ectopic pregnancies by method per 1000 procedures and per 100 pregnancies overall safety population.*

Method	Ectopic pregnancies		Total pregnancies	Ectopic pregnancies per 100 pregnancies
	n	Per 1000 procedures	*n*	
Filshie[†] *n* = 5454	1	0.2	24	4
Falope ring *n* = 1480	1	0.7	5	20
Hulka clip *n* = 1062	0	–	9	–
Pomeroy *n* = 722	0	–	2	–
Bipolar *n* = 471	2	4.3	3	67
Secuclip *n* = 85	0	–	3	–

*Presented by Professor Theodore King at the FDA Advisory Panel Meeting, 26 February, 1996
[†]Pooled interval and post partum data

Electrocoagulation appears to be associated with the highest rate of ectopic pregnancies in relationship to failures (FDA Advisory Panel Meeting, 1988) (Table 17.1) whereas mechanical failures are associated with the lowest rates in this recent study. Filshie clip failures are associated with a 4% ectopic pregnancy rate, compared to 20% for the tubal ring and 67% for electrocautery. In this study the Hulka clip was not associated with any ectopic pregnancy (FDA Advisory Panel Meeting, 1988).

Other Long-Term Problems

Long-term effects on menstrual function have been conflicting. Increased loss and spotting has been reported (Fowkes and Chamberlain, 1985; Rulin et al., 1985; Shain et al., 1989) as has an increased reporting of pelvic pain (Fowkes and Chamberlain, 1985; Rulin et al., 1989; Shain et al., 1989); whereas absence of pain and no menstrual dysfunction have also been reported (Lieberman et al., 1978; Bhiwandiwala et al., 1982; Fortney et al., 1983). Some studies have involved over 10 000 subjects. A prospective study of 5000 patients followed up for five years revealed an increased number of menstrual disturbances, including pain, bleeding and spotting compared with controls (Wilcox et al., 1992). These problems were not related to the degree of tissue destruction at the time of the original operation. The disturbances became increasingly common with time following the procedure. Hysterectomy has been reported in an increased number of women who have been sterilized compared with controls. It has also been concluded that women who have been sterilized accept a future hysterectomy more easily than those who have not been sterilized.

Torsion of the lateral aspect of the fallopian tube may occur after the sterilization, and migration of clips has been commonly observed. Tubal abscesses involving the inguinal canal have been recorded with the Filshie clip in one patient (Robson and Kerin, 1993) and expulsions of the Hulka clip have been reported (Gooden et al., 1993). In a study of 6000 patients, three patients have passed a clip per urethrum, rectum and vaginum. All three patients were subsequently examined and no cause or morbidity was found (FDA Advisory Panel Meeting, 1996). Migration is therefore a common problem and is only very rarely associated with morbidity.

Medico-legal Aspects of Laparoscopic Sterilization

A failure of a sterilization procedure is the most common cause of medico-legal complaints. The Medical Protection Society in the UK reports that this accounts for 29% of claims in obstetrics and gynecology. The three areas of litigation involve:

- Failure to warn patients that there is a failure or complication rate.
- Negligence in performing the sterilization.
- Inadvertent injury during the course of the procedure.

Litigation could be considerably reduced if the following three areas are addressed.

Adequate Counselling

Patients should be informed about the approximate realistic failure rate. They should accept that the operation is permanent and that it should be considered irreversible, even though methods involving minimal tissue destruction have a high reversal potential. Ideally patients should have discussed all alternative methods of family planning, including vasectomy. The type of procedure should be explained and should include type of access and possible complications, including the possibility of having to convert a laparoscopy to a laparotomy. The extent as to how many complications should be discussed is controversial as too much detail can cause unnecessary harm and fear. A complication rate greater than 1% could be regarded as reasonable to discuss with the patient (Brown, 1985), although this is only a view and there are exceptions to this as a failure rate of 2–3 per 1000 is often quoted. Obesity, previous abdominal surgery and current medical problems increase morbidity. Following counselling a dedicated consent form that summarizes the counselling points should be used. Patients should read the consent form thoroughly before signing it. A general leaflet incorporating the counselling points is helpful and if available should be given to each couple.

Negligence in Employing the Technique Used

All surgeons should be appropriately trained and the procedure should be performed using all due care and attention. Whatever method is employed it is important to check that the tubal structure being occluded is the fallopian tube. Fimbrial ends should therefore be clearly identified and the tube should be confluent with the tubal occlusion site. Clips and rings should be applied to the mid-isthmic portion of the tube and meticulous attention should be exercised to ensure that the whole tube has been encompassed within the jaws of the clip and that a small knuckle of tube is completely gathered by the falope ring. Should there be any doubt about correct application (e.g. due to the presence of adhesions obscuring a proper check) then a further clip or ring should be placed appropriately close to the original clip or ring. The patient should then be told to continue to use contraception until a hysterosalpingogram has been performed to establish the success of the operation.

Inadvertent Injury at the Time of Operation

This could involve damage to the gut, bladder or large vessels in the abdomen or pelvis. Ureteric damage has been recorded, but is rare. Damage may occur during the insertion of the Veress needle or trocar and cannula. Thermal injuries due to electrocoagulation are always a danger. Intra-abdominal adhesions, obesity and faulty equipment can all contribute to intraoperative injury. Regular maintenance of equipment should be mandatory, and strict attention should always be paid to the correct laparoscopic technique.

Pregnancy Relating to a Sterilization Operation

Being pregnant at the time of operation has been estimated to account for as much as 9% of the total sterilization litigation cases. It is the author's belief that patients should be told to take the responsibility of not becoming pregnant before the procedure. Ideally the operation should be performed in the first ten days of the menstrual cycle, but this causes a logistical problem. If a woman is overdue at the time of the sterilization procedure a sensitive pregnancy test should be performed. If a patient does become pregnant following a tubal ligation and she has a repeat sterilization procedure, then ideally a colleague should take the responsibility of the repeat operation, and if not there should always be a second gynecologist to observe independently exactly what had happened. If a specimen is obtained (e.g. at salpingectomy), then the tube occluded in the sterilization area should be reviewed by a histopathologist competent in examining the tube appropriately. It is not sufficient to state that the adjacent tube is normal. Multiple sections should be taken to identify the exact cause of failure and a fistula should be looked for.

Histopathologists should be aware that the report will subsequently be thoroughly scrutinized by lawyers.

References

Anderson ET (1937) Peritoneoscopy. *American Journal of Surgery* **35**: 136–139.

Babenerd J, Flehr I (1978) Erfahrungen mit dem tuplaclip zur tubensterilisation per laparascopiam. *Geburtsitilfe und Frauenheilkunde* **38**: 299

Bauer O, Devroey P, Wisanto A, Gerting W, Kaisl M, Diedrich K (1995) Small diameter laparoscopy using a microlaparoscope. *Human Reproduction* **10**: 1461–1464.

Bhiwandiwala PP, Mumford SD, Feldblum PJ (1982) A comparison of different laparoscopic sterilization techniques in 24,439 procedures. *American Journal of Obstetrics and Gynecology* **144**: 319–331.

Bleier W (1973) *Tubensterilisation mit einem Polyacetalclip.* London: Planned Parenthood Foundation.

Brown ADG (1985) Discussion: Female sterilization. In Chamberlain GVP, Urr CJB, Sharp F (eds) *Litigation and Obstetrics and Gynaecology.* p. 187. London: Royal College of Obstetrics and Gynaecology.

Chamberlain G, Brown JC (eds) (1978) Gynaecological Laparoscopy – The Report of the Working Party of the Confidential Enquiry into Gynaecological Laparoscopy. London: Royal College of Obstetricians and Gynaecologists.

Chi IC, Laufe LE, Gardner SD *et al.* (1980) An epidemiological study of risk factors associated with pregnancy following female sterilization. *American Journal of Obstetrics and Gynecology* **136**: 768–773.

FDA Advisory Panel Meeting (presentation made by Professor Theodore King), 26 February, 1996.

Filshie GM (1983) The Filshie clip. In Van Lith DAF, Keith LG, Van Hall EV (eds). *New Trends in Female Sterilisation.* pp. 83–90. Chicago/London: Year Book Medical.

Filshie GM, Casey D, Pogmore JR *et al.* (1981) The titanium/silicone rubber clip for female sterilisation. *British Journal of Obstetrics and Gynaecology* **88**: 655–662.

Fortney JA, Cole IP, Kennedy KI (1983) A new approach to measuring menstrual pattern change after tubal sterilization. *American Journal of Obstetrics and Gynecology* **147**: 830–836.

Fowkes J, Chamberlain G (1985) Effects of sterilization on menstruation. *South African Medical Journal* **78**: 544–547.

Frankenheim H (1964) Die tuben sterilisation unter sicgh mit dem lapauscope. *Geburtsitilfe und Frauenheilkunde* **24**: 470–473.

Gooden MD, Hulka JF, Cristman GM (1993) Spontaneous vaginal expulsion of Hulka clips. *Obstetrics and Gynecology* **81(5 Part 2)**: 884–886.

Green-Thompson RW, Popis M, Cairncross NWA (1993) Outpatient laparoscopic tubal sterilization under local anaesthesia. *Obstetrics and Gynaecological Forum* 4–14.

Hasson HM (1974) Open laparoscopy: a report of 150 cases. *Journal of Reproductive Medicine* **12**: 234

Hirsch HA, Nesser E (1983) Bipolar high frequency. In Van Lith DAF, Keith LG, Van Hall EV (eds) *New Trends* in Female Sterilization. pp. 83–90. Chicago/London: Year Book Medical.

Hirsch HA, Roose E (1974) Laparoskopische tuben-sterilisation mit einer neuen bikoagulationsange. *Geburtsitilfe und Frauenheilkunde* **34**: 340

Hopkins HH (1976) *Optical principles of the endoscope.* In Berci G (ed.) *Endoscopy.* pp. 3–27. New York: Appleton-Century-Crofts.

Hulka JF, Umran KF (1972) Comparative tubal occlusion: rigid and springloaded clips. *Fertility and Sterility* **23**: 633–638.

Hulka JF, Noble AD (1982) Reversibility of clip steriliza-tion. *Lancet* **11**: 927.

Hulka JF, Fishbourne J, Mercer JP et al. (1973) Laparoscopic sterilisation with a spring clip. A report of the first fifty cases. *American Journal of Obstetrics and Gynecology* **116**: 715

Hulka JF, Herbert B et al. (1995) Operative laparoscopy: American Association of Gynecologic Laparoscopists' 1993 membership survey. *Journal of the American Association of Gynecologic Laparoscopists* **2**: 137–138.

Jacobeus HC (1911) Kurze ubersicht uber meine erfahrun-gen mit der laparoskopie. *Munchener Medizinische Wuchenschrift* **58**: 2017–2019.

Kelling G (1923) Zue Colioskopie. *Archives Klinische Chirurgie* **126**: 226–229.

Kleppinger RK (1977) Ancillary uses of bipolar forceps. *Journal of Reproductive Medicine* **18**: 254

Lieberman BA, Belsey F, Gordon AG et al. (1978) Menstrual patterns after laparoscopic sterilization using a spring-loaded clip. *British Journal of Obstetrics and Gynaecology* **85**: 376–380.

Lipscomb GH, Stovall TG, Ramanathan JA, Ling FW (1992) Comparison of silastic rings and electro-coagulation for laparoscopic tubal ligation under local anaesthesia. *Obstetrics and Gynaecology* **80(4)**: 645–649.

MacKenzie IZ, Turner E, O'Sullivan GM, Guillebaud J (1987) Two hundred outpatient laparoscopic clip sterilizations using local anaesthesia. *British Journal of Obstetrics and Gynaecology* **94**: 449–453.

Maher PJ (1995) The place of gasless laparoscopy? *Gynaecological Endoscopy* **4**: 155–158.

McCann MF, Cole LP (1980) Laparoscopy and mini-laparotomy: two major advances in female steriliza-tion. *Studies in Family Planning* **11**: 119.

Newton JR (1984) Contraception update. In Newton JR (ed.) *Clinics in Obstetrics and Gynaecology* **11(3)**: 603–640.

Palmer R (1962) Essai de sterilisation tubaire coelio-scopique par electrocoagulation isthmique. *R.C. Soc Franc Gynaecol* **5**: 3.

Pennev GC, Souter V, Glasier A, Templeton AA (1997) Laparoscopic sterilisation: opinion and practice among gynaecologists in Scotland. *British Journal of Obstetrics and Gynaecology* **104**: 71–77.

Peterson HB, DeStefano F, Rubin GL et al. (1983) Deaths attributable to tubal sterilization in the United States: 1977–1981. *American Journal of Obstetrics and Gynecology* **164**: 131–136.

Peterson HB, Xia Z, Hughes JM et al. (1996) The risk of pregnancy after tubal sterilization: Findings from the US Collaborative Review of Sterilization. *American Journal of Obstetrics and Gynecology* **174(4)**: 1161–1179.

Population Report (1990) *Voluntary Female Sterilization,* Series C, No. 10. **1**: 2–23.

Power FH, Barnes AC (1941) Sterilization by means of peritoneoscopic tubal fulguration. *American Journal of Obstetrics and Gynecology* **41**: 1038.

Rioux JE (1977) Late complications of female sterilisation. A review of the literature and a proposal for further research. *Journal of Reproductive Medicine* **19(6)**: 329–340.

Rioux JE, Cloutier D (1974) Bipolar cautery for sterilisa-tion by laparoscopy. *Journal of Reproductive Medicine* **13**: 6

Robson S, Kerin J (1993) Recurrence of pelvic abscess asso-ciated with a detached Filshie clip. *Australia and New Zealand Journal of Obstetrics and Gynaecology* **33(4)**: 446.

Rubin G, Lian A, DeStefano F et al. (1982) Failure Rate of Electrocoagulation and Silastic Band Sterilization. Presented at the Annual Meeting of the American Association of Gynecologic Laparoscopists. San Diego: Downey.

Ruddock JC (1934) Peritoneoscopy. *Western Journal of Surgery* **35**: 136–139.

Rulin MC, Turner JH, Dunworth R et al. (1985) Post tubal ligation syndrome – a misnoma. *American Journal of Obstetrics and Gynecology* **151**: 13–19.

Rulin MC, Davidson AR, Philliben SG et al. (1989) Menstrual symptoms amongst sterilized and compari-son women. *Obstetrics and Gynaecology* **24**: 149–154.

Sanders RR, Filshie GM (1974) Transfundal induction of pneumoperitoneum prior to laparoscopy. *Journal of Obstetrics and Gynaecology of the British Commonwealth* **8(10)**: 829–830.

Semm K (1973) Thermal coagulation for sterilisation. *Endoscopy* **5**: 218

Semm K (1977) *Atlas of Gynecologic Laparoscopy and Hysteroscopy.* Philadelphia: Saunders.

Shain RN, Miller WB, Mitchell GW (1989) Menstrual pat-tern change one year after sterilization – results of a controlled prospective study. *Fertility and Sterility* **52**: 192–203.

Sheth SS (1976) Transvaginal induction of pneumoperi-toneum prior to laparoscopy. *Asian Journal of Obstetrics and Gynaecology* **5**: 50–54.

Steptoe PC (1965) Gynaecological endoscopy, laparoscopy and culdoscopy. *General Obstetrics and Gynaecology for the British Commonwealth,* vol. **72**: 535–543.

Steptoe PC (1967) *Laparoscopy in Gynaecology.* Edinburgh: E & S Livingstone.

Stock RJ (1984) Ectopic pregnancy subsequent to sterilisa-tion: histologic evaluation and clinical implications. *Fertility and Sterility* **42**: 211–215.

Stovall JG, Ling FW, Henry GM, Ryan GM (1991) Method factor of laparoscopic tubal sterilization in a residency training program – a comparison of the tubal ring and springloaded clip. *Journal of Reproductive Medicine* **36(4)**: 283–286.

Thompson BH, Wheeless CRJ (1973) Gastrointestinal complications of laparoscopic sterilization. *Obstetrics and Gynaecology* **41**: 669.

Vessey M, Huggins G, Lawless M, McPherson K, Yeates D (1983) Tubal sterilization: findings in a large prospec-tive study. *British Journal of Obstetrics and Gynaecology* **90**: 203–209.

Wheeless CRJ (1972) The status of out-patient sterilization

by laparoscopy: improved techniques and review of 1,000 cases. *Obstetrics and Gynaecology* **39**: 635.

Wilcox L, Martinez-Schnell B, Peterson HB *et al.* (1992) Menstrual function after sterilisation. *American Journal of Epidemiology* **135**: 1368–1381.

Yoon I, King TM (1975) A preliminary and immediate report on a new laparoscopic tubal ring procedure. *Journal of Reproductive Medicine* **15**: 54.

18

Laparoscopic Microsurgical Tubal Anastomosis

CHARLES H. KOH

Reproductive Specialty Center, Milwaukee, Wisconsin, USA

Introduction

The advent of microsurgical techniques for infertility surgery began with Swolin (1967), who proposed the use of magnification and delicate instrumentation for adhesiolysis and neosalpingostomy. Gomel (1977) and Winston (1977) separately published their first series of microsurgical reversal of sterilization with better results compared to those of macrosurgical techniques. Microsurgical techniques have become the gold standard for reproductive surgery in the last two decades.

We began exploring the feasibility of performing true microsurgery through the laparoscope in 1990. Our first laparoscopic microsurgical tubal anastomosis was performed in February 1992 using 7–0 and 8–0 nylon with microlaryngoscopic graspers and a modified needle holder. The adaptations and early instrumentation have been described (Koh and Janik, 1996a).

Principles of Microsurgery

Microsurgery employs two strategies, namely:

- Microsurgical technique.
- Microsuturing.

Microsurgical technique is a delicate surgical style that uses fine atraumatic instrumentation, magnification for accurate dissection and reconstruction, intermittent irrigation to avoid desiccation and achieve pinpoint hemostasis, and a precise energy source. The aim is to remove abnormal pathology with as little damage as possible to adjacent normal tissue to encourage better healing and less adhesion formation. Microsuturing involves the use of 6–0 to 10–0 microsutures to effect repair or anastomosis. Small needles (less than 200 μm chord diameter) minimize entry trauma and are an appropriate size for lumen being anastomosed, which can be as small as 500 μm. Microsutures of nonabsorbable material (e.g. nylon) have been shown to reduce foreign body reaction (Winston, 1975), which may compromise repair. Gomel et al. (1980) found that while there was more multinucleated giant cell formation at 24 days to 10–0 polyglactin than to 10–0 nylon and polyethylene, by 80 days this was absent. However, the presence of an early histologic reaction to absorbable material may have significance with intramucosal sutures for anastomosis in that many cases with laparoscopic anastomosis achieve pregnancy within 1–2 months following surgery. For this reason we only use 8–0 nylon or polypropylene for intramucosal suturing and caution patients to avoid pregnancy in the first month.

Laparotomy Versus Laparoscopy

Traditional microsurgery was performed via laparotomy and as long as there was no alternative access route the inherent disadvantages of the technique could not be improved. These included the laparotomy exposure itself, which predisposed to desiccation and foreign body introduction, and the need for retraction and pelvic and bowel packing with its adhesiogenic potential. Furthermore, the operating microscope could only be directed vertically downward at the pelvic organs and could not access structures that were deep and beneath organs such as ovaries, tubes or uterus. Therefore, often mobilization had to be performed macroscopically until it was possible to elevate the adnexa for actual microsurgery. Another disadvantage of the operating microscope was the limited depth of field and the small field of view.

In contrast, with laparoscopy, the varied angle of approach of the telescope allowed multiple angles of view as well as the ability to look underneath organs to effect continuous microsurgery. The absence of stereoscopic vision is initially troublesome, but adaptation occurs rapidly. The closed environment and use of patient positioning and pneumoperitoneum to obtain exposure without retractors or packing are probably responsible for the reduction in *de novo* adhesion formation as shown in animal (Luciano *et al.*, 1989; Maier *et al.*, 1992) and clinical studies (Operative Laparoscopy Study Group, 1991). The superiority of laparoscopy in decreasing adhesion reformation has not been established. With reversal of sterilization one usually starts with few adhesions so the problem of reformation is less of an issue.

The advantages of laparoscopic or minimal access surgery in terms of patient comfort and recovery are well documented and are additive to the above therapeutic advantages.

Laparoscopic Microsurgery – A New Tool for Continuous Microsurgery

We believe that laparoscopic microsurgery is a technique that synergizes the potential of classical microsurgery and laparoscopy. It can overcome the deficits inherent in both. The concerns that crude macrosurgical laparoscopic surgery could cause irreparable tissue damage that would be avoided by conventional open microsurgery (Gomel, 1995; Brosens, 1995) are legitimate and are addressed by this new tool. In fact as our experience and technique of laparoscopic microsurgery has evolved and improved, it is becoming evident that we are progressing from Brosens' characterization of laparoscopic surgery as 'new access, old technique' (Brosens, 1995) into the era of what we would now call 'new access, new technique'. Reproductive surgery can now be performed in ways that were not possible with either operative laparoscopy or classical microsurgery. In the performance of tubal anastomosis, one can be truly minimally interventionist by omitting the use of

retractors and packing, while the treatment of severe adhesions, endometriosis of the cul-de-sac and microsurgical repair of the ureters, for example, were not previously achievable under conditions of continuous microsurgery and minimal collateral trauma. With the further evolution of technology, this tool is poised for as yet undiscovered applications.

Preoperative Work-Up

Semen Analysis

Severe oligospermia or teratospermia may point to the need for assisted reproduction and may contraindicate anastomosis.

Day 3 Serum FSH Concentration and Basal Body Temperature Chart

The ovarian reserve, irrespective of age, is usefully predicted by the day 3 serum follicle stimulating hormone (FSH) concentration and will assist in counseling women with impending ovarian failure. The basal body temperature is an inexpensive way of monitoring and confirming ovulatory and anovulatory cycles.

Hysterosalpingogram

This is useful for differentiating cases that will need a tubocornual anastomosis by indicating the length of the proximal tube. However, it does not indicate the length of the distal tube. If one is equipped to perform tubocornual anastomosis at the same sitting, it is not necessary to perform a preoperative hysterosalpingogram routinely.

Preliminary Micro- or Mini-laparoscopy

We advise this in all cases of electrosurgical sterilization, whether by unipolar or bipolar current. The length of available tube is unpredictable and may be too short for meaningful anastomosis. With all other methods of sterilization it is not necessary to perform a preliminary laparoscopy.

The Operative Report

This is the most important prognostic indicator for the feasibility of performing surgery and the feasibility of good results. It gives an indication of how much tube is available for anastomosis and how easy or difficult the proposed anastomosis will be. Mechanical sterilization by clip or loop and Pomeroy-type sterilizations are the most favorable to reverse, both from a technical and pregnancy rate standpoint. With electrosurgical sterilization, there is often a need to perform tubocornual anastomosis. We do not perform postcoital tests or endometrial biopsies as part of the work-up as deficiencies in these tests can be remedied.

Indications for Laparoscopic Tubal Anastomosis

These are:

- Reversal of sterilization.
- Mid-tubal block secondary to pathology.
- Tubal occlusion secondary to treatment of ectopic pregnancy.
- Salpingitis isthmica nodosa.
- Failed tubal cannulation for proximal block.

Equipment and Instruments Needed for Laparoscopic Microsurgery

Magnification, Resolution, Digital Enhancement

Magnification of 25–40-times is essential to identify healthy mucosa and muscularis before anastomosis can be performed. For microsuturing, magnification at 10–15-times is adequate. The telescope has a magnification factor of 3–5-times and this is increased to 7-times when the telescope is brought very close to tissue. The use of an endoscopic camera with a television monitor provides a 'multiplier' effect, which further magnifies the image. Recent cameras with a zoom factor further enlarge the image. We therefore find it more practical to measure magnification by using a 20-inch monitor and determining the ratio of the size of the image on the monitor to actual life size. We call this the 'magnification factor of video laparoscopy'.

Magnification requires a corresponding high resolution to be usable, and this is provided by the three-chip cameras available today, which are capable of 800 lines of horizontal resolution, and this is complemented by monitors capable of 800 lines of resolution. The three-chip camera is also indispensable for accurate color resolution. An 8–0 suture, which is 45 μm in diameter, is easily seen using such a video system.

To further enhance contrast, some companies have built in digital enhancement in their cameras or as an add-on unit. This enhances small vessels and edge detail, thus improving discrimination. An extremely sensitive auto-iris built into the camera provides rapid control of illumination, avoiding the dreaded 'white-out' when the telescope is brought close to tissue. This is particularly important in microsuturing as the telescope has to be frequently panned in and out during the case.

Microinstrumentation

We have designed microinstrumentation that will allow laparoscopic microsuturing with precision and ease. They are collectively known as the 'Koh Ultramicro Series' with the following design elements featured in the graspers:

- Sand-blasted tips reduce glare when the telescope is brought close to it, thus allowing the suture and magnified tissue to be visible without distraction.
- The terminal serration of the jaw is specially designed to be able to pick tissue atraumatically, leaving no petechia or abrasion. Jaw apposition occurs precisely over its whole length so that 8–0 suture may be grasped anywhere without slippage. This greatly aids intracorporeal suturing as there is no need to grasp the suture at a designated portion of the jaw.
- The serrations and edges of the jaw have been treated so that 8–0 nylon or Prolene is not crushed or cut during normal use for suturing.
- The handle design has been chosen as having least friction and maximal transmission of finger movement to the instrument tip, another prerequisite for precision microsurgery. The handle angle to the shaft of 130° complements the set-up described above and allows the elbows to be at rest and adducted to the body during microsurgery.

The Ultramicro Series is depicted in Figures 18.1–18.12, together with a description of their function.

Sutures and Needles

From extensive trials and not infrequent tribulations we have found that a slightly more rigid needle is necessary for laparoscopic microsuturing than for classical microsurgery. Furthermore, it is often easier to insert the needle directly into tissue without the use of a counterpressing grasper. To achieve this the needle needs low force penetration

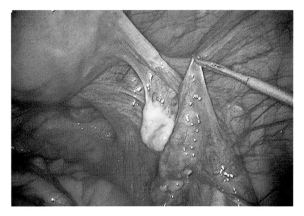

Figure 18.1 The right fallopian tube before anastomosis.

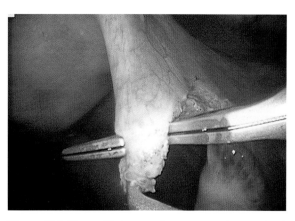

Figure 18.2 The guillotine used to transect the proximal tube.

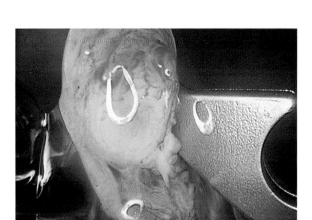

Figure 18.3 The transected proximal tube at laparoscopic magnification. Normal mucosa and muscularis is evident.

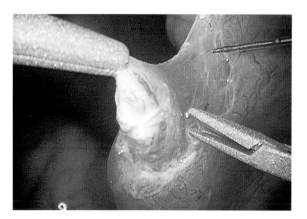

Figure 18.4 Proximal stump of distal tube. The serosa has been dissected off using the microelectrode. Ultramicro-graspers I and II are demonstrated.

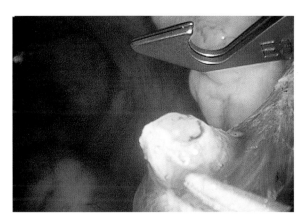

Figure 18.5 The distal tube after transection, revealing an appropriate ostium.

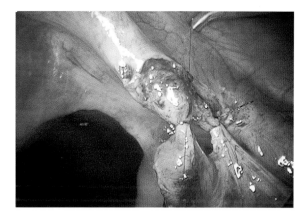

Figure 18.6 Polypropylene has been placed and tied at 6 o-clock.

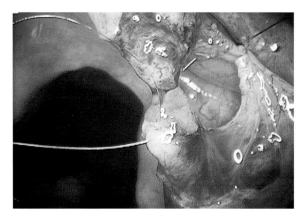

Figure 18.7 Polypropylene placed at 12 o'clock.

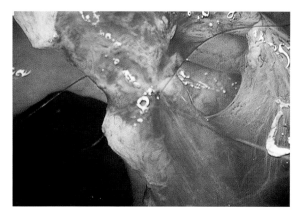

Figure 18.8 3 o'clock 8–0 Polypropylene tied. 12 o'clock Polypropylene shown untied.

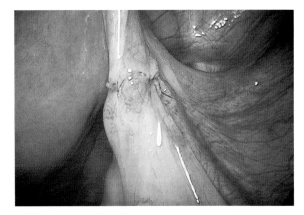

Figure 18.9 Serosal closure with 7–0 Polypropylene interrupted.

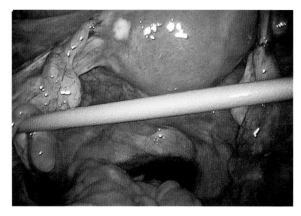

Figure 18.10 Completion of bilateral microsurgical anastomosis.

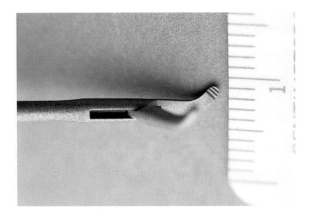

Figure 18.11 Ultramicro I (curved) showing atraumatic serration design.

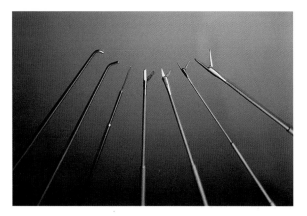

Figure 18.12 KOH Ultramicro Instrument Series.

characteristics and superior rigidity. Suitable examples include the BV 175–6 needle swaged to 7–0 and 8–0 polypropylene or a BV 130–5 needle swaged to 8–0 polypropylene (Ethalloy TruTaper needle, Ethicon Endo-surgery, Cincinnati, OH). Another excellent needle we have used recently is the Surgipro 135–5 needle swaged to 8–0 polypropylene (US Surgical Corporation, Norwalk, CT). Although black nylon would give better discrimination laparoscopically, the needle is not ideal. Plain polyglactin is the most difficult to see laparoscopically and becomes limp when wet. Monofilament sutures tend not to fray and allow easier intracorporeal suturing.

Other Equipment

Other equipment includes:

- Trocars – reusable 3 mm trocars are available with the Ultramicro Series or 5 mm trocars with 3 mm reducers may be used.
- Suction irrigation – 3 mm suction irrigators are available and provide a more suitable jet for microsurgery than the 5 mm counterparts.

Stents are not used as it can be traumatic to can-

nulate the distal fallopian tube, and hysteroscopic cannulation creates a distraction to the rhythm of surgery and the possibility of contamination. If necessary, we use a vessel occluder (Florestor vessel occluder: Biovascular Inc., St Paul, MN) as a guide to the lumen. We find it more expedient and accurate to place sutures accurately under high magnification without the use of stents.

- Uterine manipulator – the Rumi uterine manipulator with its superior anteversion mechanism is indispensable for tubal anastomosis as multiple permutations of uterine position can be obtained, thereby presenting the proximal tube at a favorable angle for microsuturing. While at laparotomy the needle holder can approach the fallopian tube from an unlimited number of positions and angles, the needle holder for laparoscopic microsurgery can only be delivered through one of the three portals, mostly the right lower quadrant. Therefore, the uterine manipulator needs to display the uterine cornua and tube at various angles to compensate. Less sturdy uterine manipulators tend to bend during prolonged usage or slip around within the uterine cavity. The lateral openings of the Rumi intrauterine tip facilitate retrograde chromopertubation. Uterine manipulators having a terminal opening tend to be lodged in the endometrium and cause intravasation of dye and a false diagnosis of a proximal block.

- Energy – a $150\,\mu m$ microneedle tip unipolar electrode is used for incision and dissection, powered from a low voltage generator. Power settings of 15–20 W for cutting and 15 W for fulguration are adequate. When the mesenteric vasculature is inadvertently cut causing more vigorous bleeding, a microbipolar electrode of 1 mm diameter is used.

Prerequisites of Surgeon

Classical Microsurgery

The aspiring laparoscopic microsurgeon has to be highly experienced in classical microsurgery. It is often necessary for the operator to compensate for unanticipated difficulties encountered during the laparoscopic approach by falling back on previous microsurgical experience to employ alternative strategies and devices to complete the operation laparoscopically.

Laparoscopic Skills

The surgeon should have highly developed two-handed laparoscopic skills and should routinely be using both hands for laparoscopic dissection and macrosuturing before attempting laparoscopic microsurgery. Advanced suturing skills with 4–0 to 6–0 sutures are also necessary before embarking on 7–0 and 8–0 microsuturing. Intracorporeal knotting is indispensable as extracorporeal techniques for 7–0 and 8–0 sutures are impractical and crude and cause 'cutting through' or disruption of tissue.

The art of laparoscopic microsuturing is highly skills based. The Ultramicro instrumentation prevent frustration from broken sutures and facilitate the correct technique of intracorporeal microsuturing. However, they do not 'do the job' for the surgeon like semiautomatic devices and force the laparoscopic microsurgeon to upgrade his skills. The end result of this, however, is a much more versatile suturing approach than can be obtained by automatic devices, and once the steep learning curve has been overcome all manner of suturing is possible.

Types of Anastomosis

Isthmic–Isthmic Anastomosis

Although the lumen may be as small as $500\,\mu m$ to 1 mm, equal luminal size and a thick muscularis allows a technically easier anastomosis, particularly if 8–0 suture is used.

Isthmic–Ampullary Anastomosis

Luminal disparity is a potential problem. Using the technique as described above for fashioning the proximal opening of the distal tube, it is possible to create a lumen only slightly larger than the proximal ostium.

Ampullary–ampullary Anastomosis

The awkwardness in these cases is due to the thin muscularis and the tendency for prolapse or extrusion of the mucosal folds. The angled probe can be used to delineate the muscularis as well as push the redundant mucosa back into the lumen after tying the muscularis sutures.

Tubal–Cornual Anastomosis

A linear slit at 12 o'clock is made in the cornual muscularis using the microneedle electrode after synthetic vasopressin injection. This allows some mobility of the interstitial tube so that it can be aligned to the needle and needle holder to effect suturing.

Selection of Cases for the Inexperienced Operator

The easiest cases for performing laparoscopic microsurgical anastomosis are the mechanical sterilizations. The tissue damage is predictable and there is enough proximal and distal tube available. In particular, the availability of proximal tube allows its mobilization to conform with the needle position, whereas with cornual anastomosis, extra steps are needed to mobilize the intramural tube and the suture placement may be inaccurate without considerable experience. Therefore, cases of electrosurgical sterilization, salpingitis isthmica nodosa and failed tubal cannulation are not suitable for anastomosis by an operator until the operator has carried out more than 40 cases of mid-tubal anastomosis with a good outcome. A preoperative

Ipsilateral Intracoporeal Suturing

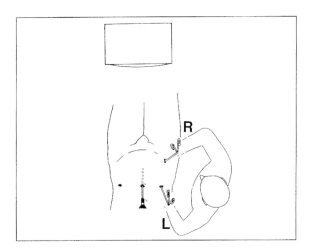

Figure 18.13 In this method, both arms remain on the ipsilateral side of the patient. The left arm of the surgeon does not have to cross over to the contralateral side and, therefore, fatigue is decreased. This is the most advanced form of intracorporeal suturing and requires considerably more dexterity and experience than the contralateral method. When properly mastered, it is rapid and allows the assistant to assist with the contralateral grasper. (Reproduced from Koh, C, whitepaper on *Laparoscopic Microsuturing*, with permission from Karl Storz Endoscopy America, Inc.)

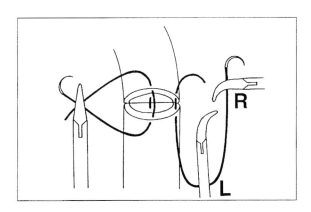

Figure 18.15 The contralateral grasper rotates the tube counterclockwise to expose the 3 o'clock area to aid in suture placement. The suture has passed from proximal to distal tube, and pulled through. The 'U' address is now prepared by the right grasper (R) holding up the needle end. (Reproduced from Koh, C, whitepaper on *Laparoscopic Microsuturing*, with permission from Karl Storz Endoscopy America, Inc.)

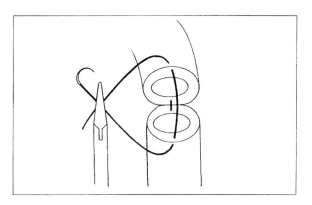

Figure 18.14 The 6 o'clock suture has been tied. The 12 o'clock suture has been placed and is held by the contralateral grasper by the assistant. (Reproduced from Koh, C, whitepaper on *Laparoscopic Microsuturing*, with permission from Karl Storz Endoscopy America, Inc.)

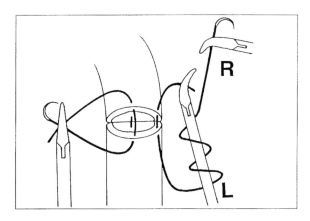

Figure 18.16 A double clockwise loop has been thrown over the left (L) Ultramicro grasper, which then picks the short end of the suture. (Reproduced from Koh, C, whitepaper on *Laparoscopic Microsuturing*, with permission from Karl Storz Endoscopy America, Inc.)

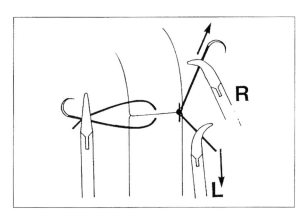

Figure 18.17 The knot is cinched by pulling in the direction of the arrows. (Reproduced from Koh, C, whitepaper on *Laparoscopic Microsuturing*, with permission from Karl Storz Endoscopy America, Inc.)

hysterosalpingogram may therefore be a screening procedure.

Setup

The position of the ports is critical in enabling fluent two-handed operating as well as suturing. The so-called 'fulcrum effect' is virtually eliminated by adopting these port positions (Figure 18.13). The lower pelvic ports are 5 mm with a 3 mm reducer and are placed 2 cm medial to the anterior superior iliac spine after the pneumoperitoneum has been created. The right upper port is paraumbilical at the same level as the umbilicus and laterally at the same displacement as the right lower port. Very rarely, a fourth paraumbilical port may be necessary on the left.

If right-handed the primary surgeon stands on the right side of the patient and operates the instruments from the right ports using his or her left and right hand. The assistant stands on the patient's left and holds the camera and operates the left lower instrument portal. In rare cases, a third person has to hold the camera while the assistant uses both hands for the extra portal at the left paraumbilical area. The table height should be adjusted after a Trendelenburg position has been attained. This should be such that the operator has his or her elbows comfortably adducted and the lower arms are almost parallel to the floor. This position is possible only by having the lateral ports as lateral as possible as described above. This ensures a relaxed stance and efficiency in two-handed surgery that approaches the ease of open laparotomy. The fulcrum effect becomes nonexistent and movement is by the use of the wrists and fingers as in classical microsurgery.

Surgical Technique

After insertion of a Foley catheter, the Rumi uterine manipulator with the appropriate tip is inserted into the uterus for mobilization. The intrauterine balloon is inflated with 3 ml normal saline. Dilute methylene blue is attached via a syringe to the chromopertubation port. After sterile preparation and draping, the trocars are inserted. We employ the direct puncture technique using a 10 mm disposable trocar through the umbilical incision. The secondary ports are then placed after the pneumoperitoneum has been created under direct visu-

alization. The secondary ports can be reusable or disposable, but should be able to accommodate 3 mm instruments without leakage. Following this, the uterus is mobilized and anteverted and retroverted to inspect the pelvis. The lengths of the proximal and distal tube are examined as well as the condition of the fimbriae. Any paratubal and periovarian adhesions are treated at this point, using the microelectrode. If all conditions are satisfactory for anastomosis, the operation proceeds.

The synthetic vasopressin injector is inserted through the right lower port and 1:30 dilute synthetic vasopressin is injected into the terminal serosa of the proximal tube – just enough to bulge the serosa. Next, using the Ultramicro I grasper with the left hand to stabilize the tip of the tube, the operator introduces the microneedle electrode through the right lower port to circumscribe the serosa of the proximal tube about 5 mm away from the tip. If the tubal length is generous and there is obvious bulbous dilatation of the tip, more tube can be sacrificed and the serosal cut would be 1 cm away from the tip. Following this, the microneedle is used to divide the tubal mesentery up to the chosen point for transection. By keeping this incision close to the tube, the mesosalpingial vessels are not damaged and do not therefore require cautery, which may compromise the blood supply to the fallopian tube.

At this point, the microelectrode is removed from the right lower port and the guillotine is inserted into the right lower port. Again, the primary operator uses the Ultramicro I grasper to hold the tip of the tube, and by moving it, one is able to position the guillotine so that a right-angled cut is made of the proximal tube. After this is achieved, chromopertubation is performed retrogradely by means of the syringe attached to the Rumi uterine manipulator. When dye emerges freely from the proximal tube, the laparoscope is brought to within 1 cm of the tissue and using the zoom magnification, one is able to obtain a 40-times magnification on the video monitor. This allows examination of the muscularis and the mucosa. Normal isthmic tissue is depicted by the mucosa taking up the blue stain and having the normal 3–4 folds. The muscularis is found to be circular and nonfibrotic. Methylene blue should emerge without undue pressure on injection. Pinpoint hemostasis can be achieved using irrigation and the modulated current of the unipolar microelectrode sparingly. Preparation of the proximal tube is now complete.

The proximal end of the distal tube is now held up and the synthetic vasopressin injector is reintroduced via the right lower port and subserosal injection is performed using dilute synthetic vasopressin. Following this, the microelectrode is introduced and careful incision is performed around the tube. The serosa is incised and care is taken not to incise the muscularis. The serosa can then be dissected to expose the proximal stump of the distal tube, which is regrasped using the Ultramicro II grasper at the very tip. At this point, the tubal lumen is compared to that of the proximal tube by using the straight chromopertubator, which has 1 mm markings along its tip. The aim is to obtain a distal lumen that is no more than 1 mm larger than the proximal stump. The guillotine is then reintroduced to cut the distal stump, the curved chromopertubator is introduced through the proximal lumen gently and methylene blue dye is injected carefully, paying attention to see that it emerges through the fimbriae. When this has been achieved it confirms patency of the distal tube without the need for cannulation, which is more difficult to achieve laparoscopically and traumatic. The lumen is inspected to ensure that the size is adequate and if not, further cuts are made with the guillotine. Pinpoint hemostasis is performed as necessary. Any redundant segment of fallopian tube with attached loop or clip may now be removed using the unipolar electrode.

An 8 cm-length of 6–0 nylon or polypropylene is now introduced by holding the suture 2 cm from the needle. This is introduced using the Ultramicro I through the right upper quadrant with the operator's left hand. The needle holder in the operator's right hand is introduced into the right lower quadrant. The needle is grasped by the needle holder and positioned with the help of the grasper as shown. The mesosalpinx is sutured together using an intracorporeal knot tying about 5 mm away from the fallopian tube. Care should be taken not to approximate the mesosalpinx too near the tube as it will hinder subsequent anastomosis.

A 6 cm-length of 7–0 or 8–0 suture is now introduced in the same way as previously and the needle is positioned on the needle holder similarly. Using clockwise rotation of the wrist, the muscularis is pierced at 6 o'clock on the distal tube avoiding the mucosa. The needle is then inserted at 6 o'clock of the proximal tube from submucosa through muscularis, again maintaining the clockwise motion of the wrist. Intracorporeal knot tying is performed with three knots thrown. This is then cut using the suture scissors. Another 7–0 or 8–0 suture is placed at 12 o'clock of the proximal tube from muscularis to submucosa and then to the 12 o'clock position of the distal tube with the needle entering from submucosa through muscularis. This suture is now held by the assistant (Figure 18.14) and together with the use of the uterine manipulator, one is able to rotate the tube so that both the 3 and 9 o'clock positions become available for accurate suture placement (Figures 18.15–18.17). These are placed next and tied, and finally, the 12 o'clock suture is tied. Chromopertubation is performed via the uterine manipulator and patency of the tube can now be demonstrated. Slight leakage at the anastomotic site is no cause for concern as long as dye emerges from the distal fimbriae. 6–0 polypropylene or nylon is then used to place two or three interrupted serosal sutures. These sutures should also incorporate the outer muscularis to maintain the strength of the anastomosis. Any evident gaps in the mesosalpinx are similarly closed using 6–0 nylon.

The other tube is then treated in the same way.

Discussion

The pool of patients suitable for reproductive surgery is continually being reduced with better selection processes using microendoscopy (falloposcopy, salpingoscopy), which predict the functional status of the fallopian tube. Furthermore, the increasingly low threshold for *in vitro* fertilization further reduces this pool. Therefore the remaining candidates for surgery require the best efforts of the expert reproductive surgeon employing the best techniques and technology on their behalf.

Validation of laparoscopic microsurgery as a discipline requires that the results of reversals of sterilization performed with this technique are equal or better than those with the open microsurgical technique. Our cumulative pregnancy rates are 35.5% at three months, 54.8% at six months, 67.7% at nine months, and 71% at 12 months with an ectopic pregnancy rate of 5% (Koh and Janik, 1996). The surgical duration in the first ten cases fell from a mean of 5.9 hours in the first five to 3.1 hours in the later five cases. Current operating times range from 60–120 minutes for midtubal anastomosis, and up to 240 minutes for difficult cornual cases. The patients are discharged the same day (75%) or the next morning within 23 hours (25%). Currently the total cost (US $8000–9000) is 20–30% below a comparable laparotomy. Cumulative pregnancy rates at six and 12 months are shown in Table 18.1. In this era of assisted reproduction, it is important to be able to counsel patients on their pregnancy chances within a specific time frame.

In contrast, exigent techniques for laparoscopic reversal of sterilization by the use of a single stitch with or without glue (Sedbon *et al.*, 1989; Dubuisson and Swolin, 1995) or the use of macrosuturing (Reich, 1989; Reich *et al.*, 1993) have not yielded pregnancy rates comparable to those of open microsurgery, which is not surprising as techniques that

Table 18.1 Cumulative pregnancy rates at 6 and 12 months following laparoscopic microsurgery.

Cumulative pregnancy rate (%)		Study
6 months	12 months	
63	80	Jansen, 1986
39	55	Prado and Venegas, 1993
40	53	Putman et al., 1990
55	71	Koh and Janik, 1996

have not been successful at laparotomy will not work any better when introduced through the laparoscope.

The indications of operative laparoscopy will continue to expand as technical feasibility continues to increase, driven both by hardware advances and increased surgical dexterity. It is essential to ensure that clear operative goals are always maintained. The attainment of high laparoscopic skills through laparoscopic microsurgery will allow the advanced laparoscopist to transfer this technique to other applications, both within and beyond gynecology. Diseases like salpingitis isthmica nodosa and other cornual blocks may now be attempted. It has been possible to perform ureteric microdissection and anastomosis, vascular repair, intramural myomectomy repair, and bowel repair using the techniques described above. Intrauterine fetal surgery and pediatric surgery will also find applications, as will vascular and coronary surgery in time.

Laparoscopic microsurgery will introduce a new dimension to reproductive surgery and over time will replace laparotomy for microsurgery. It is important to realize, however, that the learning curve is considerable and the technique may not be attainable by all despite their best efforts. The reproductive surgeon of tomorrow will be an expert in microendoscopy and laparoscopic microsurgery with sufficient numbers of cases to maintain and develop his expertise.

References

Brosens IA (1995) Risks and benefits of endoscopic surgery in reproductive medicine. *Proceedings of the 15th World Congress on Fertility and Sterility* **47**: 339–343.

Dubuisson JB, Swolin K (1995) Laparoscopic tubal anastomosis (the one stitch technique): preliminary results. *Human Reproduction* **10(8)**: 2044–2046.

Gomel V (1977) Tubal reconstruction by microsurgery. *Fertility and Sterility* **28**: 59.

Gomel V (1995) From microsurgery to laparoscopic surgery: A progress. *Fertility and Sterility* **63**: 464–468.

Gomel V, McComb P, Boer-Meisel MD (1980) Histologic reactions to polyglactin-910, polyethylene and nylon microsuture. *Journal of Reproductive Medicine* **25**: 56.

Jansen RP (1986) Tubal resection and anastomosis 1. Sterilization reversal. *Australian and New Zealand Journal of Obstetrics and Gynaecology* **26(4)**: 294–299.

Koh CH, Janik GM (1996a) Laparoscopic microsurgical tubal anastamosis. In Adamson GD, Martin DC (eds) *Endoscopic Management of Gynecologic Disease*. pp. 119–145. Philadelphia: Lippincott, Raven.

Koh CH, Janik GM (1996b) Laparoscopic microsurgical tubal anastomosis. Results of 40 consecutive cases. (Abstract). American Society of Reproductive Medicine 52nd Annual Meeting. Boston, USA.

Luciano AA, Maier DB, Koch EL, Nulsen JC, Whitman GF (1989) A comparative study of postoperative adhesions following laser surgery by laparoscopy versus laparotomy in the rabbit model. *Obstetrics and Gynecology* **74**: 220.

Maier DB, Nulsen JC, Klock A, Luciano AA (1992) Laser laparoscopy versus laparotomy in lysis of pelvic adhesions. *Journal of Reproductive Medicine* **37(12)**: 965–968.

Operative Laparoscopy Study Group (1991) Postoperative adhesion development following operative laparoscopy: evaluation of early second look procedures. *Fertility and Sterility* **55**: 700–704.

Prado J, Venegas J (1993) Application of microsurgical principles of the reversal of tubal sterilization. *Revista Chilena de Obstetricia y Ginecologia* **58(4)**: 298–303.

Putnam J, Holden A, Olive D (1990) Pregnancy rates following tubal anastomosis: Pomeroy partial salpingectomy versus electrocautery. *Journal of Gynecologic Surgery* **6(3)**.

Reich H (1989) Laparoscopic reversal of sterilization (Abstract). Presented at *Second World Congress of Gynecological Endoscopy, Clermont–Ferrand, France, June 5–8*.

Reich H, McGlynn F, Parente C, Sekel L, Levie M (1993) Laparoscopic tubal anastomosis. *Journal of the American Association of Gynecologic Laparoscopists* **1(1)**: 16–19.

Sedbon E, Delajoulinieres JB, Boudouris O, Madelenat P (1989) Tubal desterilisation through exclusive laparoscopy. *Human Reproduction* **4**: 158.

Swolin K (1967) *Fifty Fertilatiasoperationen. Vols 1, 2.* Microsurgical Concepts for Infertility Surgery.

Winston RML (1975) Microsurgical anastomosis of the rabbit Fallopian tube and its functional and pathological sequelae. *British Journal of Obstetrics and Gynaecology* **82**: 513–522.

Winston RML (1977) Microsurgical tubocornual anastomosis for reversal of sterilization. *Lancet* **1**: 284.

19

Falloposcopy and Other Tubal Cannulation Techniques

I.W. SCUDAMORE* AND I.D. COOKE[†]

*Leicester General Hospital, Leicester, UK
[†]Jessop Hospital for Women, Sheffield, UK

Introduction

The fallopian tube is a dynamic organ with an important role in the transport of sperm and ova. It is the site of fertilization and early embryonic growth, indicating that the tubal environment is important for early nurture of the pre-implantation pregnancy (Murray and DeSouza, 1995). Until the advent of *in vitro* fertilization (IVF) techniques the tube was essential for successful reproduction. Much of the physiology of normal tubal function is poorly understood as access to the tubal lumen *in vivo* has not been available. There is reported to be a tubal factor in 14–50% of couples with infertility (Lederer, 1993; Jaffe and Jewelewicz, 1991) with the damaged tube having been known to have a role in causing infertility since the early nineteenth century (Burns, 1809). In recent years many methods of transcervical cannulation of the proximal fallopian tube have been developed and reported in the literature. The purpose of this chapter is to review these techniques and their potential uses in modern practise. The reader is also referred to four previous review publications of interest (Lederer, 1993; Flood and Grow, 1993; Risquez and Confino, 1993; Valle, 1995).

Reasons for Tubal Cannulation

Assessment of Tubal Patency and Potential Treatment of Proximal Occlusion

The wide range of reported incidence of tubal factor contributing to infertility probably reflects the lack of specificity of the tests available to detect tubal abnormality. In modern practise the most commonly used investigations are contrast hysterosalpingography (HSG) and laparoscopy with hydrotubation, although a wide range of tests of tubal patency and function have been used. An excellent review of tests to assess the fallopian tube was recently published by Maguiness *et al.* (1992). Stallworthy (1948) argued that rates of proximal tubal occlusion of 26–50% diagnosed by HSG were grossly inflated and could be reduced to 12.8% by repeat testing and the use of spasmolytics. Muscular spasm as a cause of false positive assessment of proximal tubal patency is still somewhat controversial. At best, spasmolytic drugs seem to assist in demonstrating proximal tubal patency in 30–50% of tubes thought to be occluded proximally (Winfield and Wentz, 1987; Lang, 1991) and at worst have little effect (World Health Organization, 1983; Thurmond *et al.*, 1988).

Histologic examination of excised proximal segments thought to have been proximally occluded have repeatedly found a low incidence of fibrotic tubal occlusion (Grant, 1971; Fortier and Haney, 1985; Sulak *et al.*, 1987). These reports have identified other 'non-occlusive' pathology such as the presence of a 'plug' of amorphous material in association with tubal fibrosis or inflammation. Such isthmic plugs have subsequently been identified as reversible causes of proximal obstruction and characterized histologically (Kerin *et al.*, 1991; Kindermann *et al.*, 1993). It is well documented that the likelihood of pregnancy after HSG is improved for at least several months (DeCherney *et al.*, 1980), presumably due to the ability of HSG to 'flush' through some of the displaceable tubal debris. Selective salpingography in tubes with a suggestion of proximal tubal blockage is claimed to be effective in 39–80% of cases in demonstrating tubal patency (Lang *et al.*, 1990; Capitanio *et al.*, 1991; Thurmond., 1991). This is presumed to be due to the higher pressure overcoming relative tubal occlusion or displacing an occlusive plug.

As long ago as 1849 attempts were made to 'unblock' the proximal end of the fallopian tube using a device designed to allow transcervical transuterine access to the tubal ostium (Tyler-Smith, 1849). Tubal cannulation as treatment for proximal occlusion has been proposed by many authors in recent years using techniques guided by hysteroscopy and radiology, which will be discussed in more depth in this chapter. Ultrasound (Stern *et al.*, 1991; Breckenridge and Schinfeld, 1991; Lisse and Sydow, 1991; Maroulis and Yeko, 1992), 'digital road mapping' (Eckstein *et al.*, 1992) and other bespoke devices (Confino *et al.*, 1990; Ataya and Thomas, 1991) have also been reported. More recently still, falloposcopy has provided the facility for visually assessing the proximal tubal lumen, enabling cannulation of the proximal tube or classification of the cause of the tubal occlusion on the basis of the tubal appearances.

Traditional treatment for proximal tubal occlusion has been tubal microsurgery. Marana and Quagliarello (1988) concluded that term pregnancy rates of 'about 50%' could be achieved after microsurgical tubocornual anastomosis (TCA) making this the treatment of choice for cornual occlusion. The efficacy of tubal surgery is influenced by the presence of proximal and distal disease. McComb *et al.* (1991) reported that surgery for proximal and distal disease in the same tube has a uniformly poor outcome, a sentiment reiterated with respect to multisite disease in the tube by Novy (1994). Selective salpingography and tubal recanalization have been reported as so successful in achieving tubal patency that the American Fertility Society has recommended that such a noninvasive technique should be tried before major tubal surgery in patients with a diagnosis of proximal tubal occlusion (Thurmond, 1994). Not all authors have been happy with such 'blind' techniques of tubal recanalization, with much less consistent cannulation rates reported (Hercz *et al.*, 1994). Although successful in achieving patency of the proximal tube, poor post-recanalization pregnancy rates have been reported (Gleicher *et al.*, 1994; Hayashi *et al.*, 1994). This suggests that the tubes that are not patent by selective salpingography and require guidewire recanalization are a different group with a poorer prognosis than those that are patent after selective salpingography alone. Indeed, the success of recanalization

(measured by pregnancy rates) seems to relate to the likelihood of distal disease (Gleicher *et al.*, 1993; Sowa *et al.*, 1993) suggesting advantages to techniques that can visualize the tubal lumen in the proximal and distal segments directly as well as cannulate the tube. Furthermore, from histologic assessment of resected proximal segments it is known that there is a considerable incidence of nonocclusive pathology that may compromise tubal function subsequent to successful guidewire cannulation (Fortier and Haney, 1985; Sulak *et al.*, 1987).

Falloposcopy has provided the facility for visually assessing the proximal tubal lumen, enabling cannulation of the proximal tube or classification of the cause of tubal occlusion on the basis of the tubal appearances (Kerin *et al.*, 1991; Kovacs *et al.*, 1992; Grow *et al.*, 1993; Dunphy, 1994; Scudamore *et al.*, 1994a). The direct visualization of the proximal tubal lumen by falloposcopy enables confirmation of the positioning of the device. Added to this, visual assessment of the state of the luminal epithelium in the proximal segment can be supplemented by assessment of the distal tubal lumen if the proximal segment is patent.

Assessment of Condition of Intratubal Epithelium in Patients with Distal Tubal Disease

Surgery for distal tubal disease is a potential 'cure' for tubal disease, enabling several pregnancies if successful (Evans, 1995). However, the results of indiscriminant distal tubal surgery have been criticized as undoubtedly they are poor and assisted reproductive techniques may be more appropriate in many patients (Afnan *et al.*, 1991). Appropriate selection of patients for distal surgery should enable postoperative pregnancy rates of 50% or greater (Gomel and Yarali, 1992). Salpingoscopic assessment of the condition of the tubal epithelium has been demonstrated to be of significant prognostic value in the surgical treatment of patients with distal tubal disease (Cornier, 1985; Henry-Suchet *et al.*, 1985; Boer-Meisel *et al.*, 1986; De Bruyne *et al.*, 1989; Henry-Suchet *et al.*, 1989; Dubuisson *et al.*, 1994) and has been found to provide more precise and accurate assessment of the condition of the tubal mucosa than HSG (Puttemans *et al.*, 1987). Falloposcopic assessment of the intratubal epithelium has been demonstrated to correlate well with tubal assessment by salpingoscopy (Scudamore *et al.*, 1994b), which requires laparoscopy and is limited to the assessment of the distal two-thirds of the tube. In their original series of falloposcopic assessment of patients with tubal disease, Kerin *et al.*

Table 19.1 Relationship of tubal score and subsequent pregnancy rates. (Adapted from Kerin *et al.*, 1992)

Falloposcopy	12-month pregnancy rates
No tubal disease (score = 20)	6/28 (21%)
Mild/moderate disease (score = 21–30)	2/22 (9%)
Severe disease (score > 30)	0/16 (0%)

(1992) demonstrated that subsequent pregnancy was more likely if falloposcopy indicated tubal health and less likely if the epithelium appeared damaged (Table 19.1). Within 12 months of falloposcopy 6/28 (21%) of the women with at least one apparently normal tube had conceived, 2/22 (9%) of those with mild to moderate disease had conceived and none of the 16 patients with severe disease had achieved a pregnancy. Transcervical evaluation of the intratubal epithelium by falloposcopy may therefore be a valuable tool in the selection of patients appropriate for distal tubal surgery.

Use of the Tubal Environment for Fertilization or Early Embryo Growth

There is evidence that co-culture of embryos with tubal epithelium results in improved early embryo development in treatment with assisted reproduction techniques (Bongso *et al.*, 1992; Yeung *et al.*, 1992), indicating a facilitating role of the tubal epithelium. Techniques of assisted reproduction using gamete transfer to the tube (Asch *et al.*, 1985; Braeckmans *et al.*, 1987; Palermo *et al.*, 1989; Murdoch *et al.*, 1991) achieve good pregnancy rates and the results of transfer of postfertilization zygotes to the tube appeared to be promising (Jansen *et al.*, 1988; Devroey *et al.*, 1989; Palermo *et al.*, 1989; Rotsztejn *et al.*, 1990; Scholtes *et al.*, 1990). At the present time, there does not appear to be a significant advantage in using tubal embryo transfer (Scholtes *et al.*, 1990) and so it has not replaced more conventional methods of intrauterine transfer of embryos in assisted reproduction treatments.

Contraception

Early approaches to causing sufficient damage to the fallopian tube to achieve sterility in women wanting long-term contraception used a transcervi-cal approach. These were not very successful and the development of laparoscopy led to laparoscopic occlusion of the isthmic portion of the tube becoming the standard method of female sterilization. As this carries a risk of bowel and vessel damage associated with the transabdominal approach and in most hands is performed under general anesthesia, a transcervical approach is an attractive alternative and interest in such a method has been rekindled. Various agents of tissue destruction (cauterization, application of chemicals such as formaldehyde) and tubal occlusion (methyl cyanoacrylate, plastic plugs) have been used with limited success (Valle, 1989; Risquez and Confino, 1993). Most recently persistent bilateral tubal occlusion four months after the procedure has been demonstrated in 88% of cases when the proximal tubes were injected with methyl-2-cyanoacrylate using a special balloon cannula designed to prevent reflux during injection of the occlusive material (Shuber, 1989). Successful long-term tubal occlusion will, however, have to be very much better before laparoscopic sterilization is replaced.

Diagnosis and Treatment of Ectopic Pregnancy

The diagnosis of ectopic pregnancy at early gestation (less than six weeks) is often difficult despite the availability of vaginal ultrasound scan and quantitative human chorionic gonadotropin (hCG) assays. In theory, diagnosis of ectopic pregnancy as early as possible ought to maximize the efficacy of conservative surgical or medical treatment and enable maximum preservation of tubal anatomy and function with minimal morbidity for the patient. The potential of tubal cannulation techniques in the diagnosis and treatment of ectopic pregnancy is discussed by Risquez and Confino (1993). Essentially, these authors suggest that selective tubal cannulation may aid localization of an early ectopic pregnancy and enable accurate local application of a small dose of medication with an expected increased cytoreductive effect as a result of direct administration. If patient selection is restricted to those with very early ectopic gestations characterized by a low static or falling serum hCG level and the absence of fetal heart motion, these authors argue that treatment failures will be minimal. In an uncontrolled study of tubal catheterization and local instillation of methotrexate 27/31 (87%) resolved with only 4/31 (13%) requiring surgery (Risquez et al., 1992a). Falloposcopy is an attractive option in the diagnosis and treatment of ectopic pregnancy. It could enhance the assessment of the site and nature of the intratubal lesion by direct visualization and has reportedly been performed successfully (Risquez et al., 1992b). In our experience, cannulation and falloposcopy of the tube have proved difficult in pregnancy, perhaps because of decidual overgrowth. Distention of the uterine cavity in order to identify the tubal ostium is not appropriate in many cases as an alternative diagnosis may be an intrauterine pregnancy.

Anatomy

The ability to cannulate the fallopian tube successfully from its proximal end is significantly influenced by the anatomy of the tube itself. The intrauterine (intramural) section of the tube has been measured at 1.5–2.5 cm in length by fresh dissection (Sweeney, 1962) with a maximum diameter of less than 1 mm. Measuring from the histologically evident change in the epithelium from endometrium to the single columnar layer of the intramural segment, the distance to the outer margin of the uterus is somewhat less than 1 cm (Lisa et al., 1954). It is often at the junction of the intramural section and the isthmus of the tube that an acute angulation of the tube occurs.

There has been much speculation regarding the presence or otherwise of a discrete sphincter mechanism, either muscular or epithelial, at the uterotubal junction. Kennedy (1925) believed there was an anatomic sphincter, which contributed to dysmenorrhea, infertility and ectopic pregnancy, and Lee (1928) described well-developed muscular folds around the tubal opening, which he believed were consistent with such a mechanism. This was refuted by the study of Lisa et al. (1954) who described inner longitudinal and outer circular layers of muscle, but denied the presence of an anatomic sphincter.

Subsequently the tubal muscle layers were described as being three, merging continuously into the uterine wall without interruption and without any clearly defined muscular sphincter (Vasen, 1959). The arrangement of these layers was reported to be such that contraction of the different muscle bundles would cause an effect varying from occlusion of the intramural lumen to peristalsis with intramural flow toward the uterine cavity. This observation is given some support in that kymographic recording of pressure changes during transcervical carbon dioxide (CO_2) tubal insufflation demonstrates a resistance consistent with rhythmic contractions of up to 7–9 min^{-1} (Rubin, 1939).

Early studies of the uterotubal junction were conducted on non-human species and the observation that mucosal folds at the uterotubal ostium were capable of closing the ostium (Kelly, 1927; Lee, 1928) was not made in the human model. There may, however, be endometrial epithelial folds at the human uterotubal junction (Lisa et al., 1954; Hafez, 1973; Rocca et al., 1989), which may well play a role in the control of sperm and egg transport and storage (Hafez, 1973). These are liable to extend into the intramural portion of the tube where there is a change in epithelial histology to a flat single columnar layer (Lisa et al., 1954; Rocca et al., 1989).

The intramural passage of the fallopian tube was originally described as having a gently curving course in 40–50% of cases and a tortuous path through the uterine wall in the remainder (Geist and Goldberger, 1925). This was confirmed by a dissection study of fresh hysterectomy specimens, which found the tubal course to be gently curved or straight in 31/100 cases and tortuously curved in the remaining 69 (Sweeney, 1962). These findings led the latter author to comment 'Probing or catheterising the interstitial portion of the tubes at the time of tuboplasties is practically impossible, damages the tubes, and is probably of little value.' Certainly the reported diameter of the intramural and isthmic sections of the tube of less than 1 mm would lend support to this contention.

The anatomic factors that must therefore be taken into account when attempting transcervical tubal cannulation are multiple. The uterine cavity has to be accessed via the cervix, which must be patent and readily cannulated. A catheter must be used to gain access to the uterotubal ostium if a non-hysteroscopic technique of tubal cannulation is to be attempted. Such a catheter benefits from being shaped so that its distal end curves toward the tubal ostium when directed into either the left or right cornu of the uterus. If the intention of proximal cannulation is to perform selective salpingography using higher pressure contrast injection to try and demonstrate tubal patency (Gleicher et al., 1992) then such a catheter can be 3–4 mm in diameter, often with a 'ball-tip' on the end. Cannulation of the proximal tube achieves occlusion of the tube behind the 'ball-tip' of the catheter, preventing backflow of contrast material. Alternatively, advancement of a catheter, wire or endoscope into and along the tube as far as the ampulla may be desirable for gamete or embryo transfer, recanalization of an 'occluded' tube or endoscopy of the lumen. In such cases, if a guidewire or catheter is used it must be rigid enough to achieve forward movement when advanced, but flexible enough to follow curves in the proximal segment and to minimize the risk of tubal perforation. It must also have a diameter considerably less than 1 mm as otherwise it will be wider than the proximal segment of the majority of normal fallopian tubes, and must have a smooth blunt tip so that the risk of 'catching' in the tubal wall is minimal. Many tubal cannulation techniques use a coaxial method to overcome some of these difficulties. Usually a flexible guidewire is threaded through a fine diameter catheter and then the guidewire advanced into the proximal tube, either under hysteroscopic visualization or imaging (e.g. fluoroscopy, ultrasound) control. If the guidewire curls on itself, then advancing the outer catheter to shorten the length of guidewire protruding from it stiffens the guidewire and can aid its advancement. In this situation care must be taken as the resistance to guidewire advancement may indicate tubal occlusion or tortuosity, and forcing the guidewire may cause tubal damage.

A novel alternative to such direct 'probing' is provided by the linear eversion catheter (LEC) (Pearlstone *et al.*, 1992). This is a plastic polymer catheter of 2.8 mm outer diameter with a sliding stainless steel inner body 0.8 mm in diameter. The outer and inner bodies are connected at their tips by a polyethylene membrane or balloon some 20 cm long and 50 μm thick. There is a closed space confined by the outer and inner bodies and the membrane ('the balloon space'), to which access is gained via a Luer Lock tap near the rear of the outer body. All these features are illustrated in Figure 19.1. A fluid-filled syringe fitted with a pressure gauge is attached to this Luer lock tap and allows the pressure within this space to be controlled. Instillation of fluid will increase the pressure resulting in outward pressure on the balloon wall exerted in a radial fashion at right angles to the polyethylene membrane. Advancing the inner body tip into the outer body results in membrane eversion beyond the end of the catheter as a balloon-like tube with a pressurized two-layered wall (Figure 19.2). This everting tube unrolls as the inner body is advanced further until the inner body tip reaches the tip of the outer body. At this point the balloon will be everted a full 10 cm.

An advantage of this technique is that the balloon unrolls, laying the polymer membrane down against the tubal wall without exerting shear forces. Hence, the risk of direct tubal damage is minimized, and is aided in negotiating tubal curves and strictures as the balloon 'lifts' the tube open in front of it. Furthermore, because the balloon unrolls as a tubular structure with a pressurized double-layer polymer wall it has a lumen down which a 0.48 mm diameter fiberoptic falloposcope can be carried. The balloon wall supports the fragile endoscope and protects it from snapping and also prevents the sharp tip from impacting directly on the tubal wall, thus minimizing the risk of tubal damage and the examination being compromised. The LEC system of cannulation offers an atraumatic method of tubal cannulation with features that enable it to overcome difficulties inherent in guidewire techniques or related to anatomic irregularities.

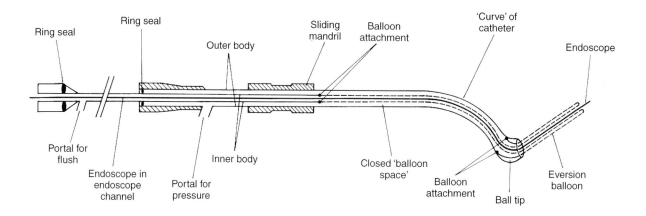

Figure 19.1 Linear eversion catheter (Imagyn Medical, USA), partially everted and containing the 0.5 mm endoscope (not to scale). (Reproduced with kind permission from *British Journal of Obstetrics and Gynaecology*, 1992.)

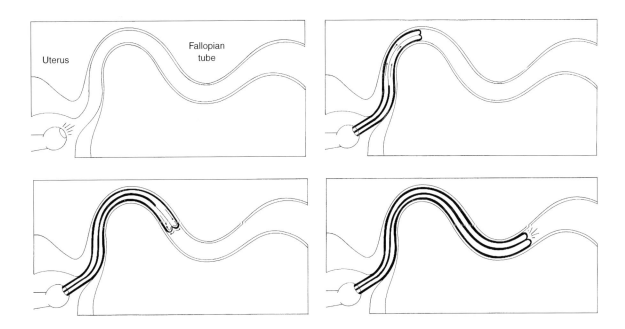

Figure 19.2 Eversion of the balloon cannulates the fallopian tube and carries the endoscope along with minimal risk of trauma, even in a tortuous segment. The sequence shown is read from left to right, demonstrating progressive eversion of the balloon into the tube carrying the endoscope with it. (Reproduced with kind permission from the *British Journal of Obstetrics and Gynaecology*, 1992.)

Methods of Tubal Cannulation

Many different methods of tubal cannulation have been attempted and reported since the mid-1960s, most in the interests of attempting to relieve proximal tubal occlusion. Unfortunately few have been submitted to rigorous randomized scientific assessment and the vast majority of reports simply detail the success rates of cannulation with or without subsequent pregnancy rates. It is only recently that the value of such reporting in establishing practise has been questioned with some authors raising questions about the efficacy and place of relatively 'blind' tubal cannulation procedures (Gleicher *et al.*, 1994; Hayashi *et al.*, 1994; Hercz *et al.*, 1994). However, it is probable that some patients will benefit from cannulation procedures by improved tubal patency rates.

Hysteroscopy

Hysteroscopically-guided tubal cannulation for the treatment of proximal tubal occlusion was reviewed by Valle (1995). In his review of series reported to 1994, 183/244 (75%) tubes were cannulated successfully. Of 191/215 (89%) patients at least one tube was successfully treated, the perforation rate was 6.5% and there were 105 pregnancies (50%). Similar

outcomes were reported by Das *et al.* (1995) when comparing hysteroscopic tubal cannulation with proximal resection and tubocornual anastamosis as treatment for proximal occlusion, leading these authors to propose cannulation as a preferable first choice treatment. Assuming adequate diagnosis of proximal tubal occlusion before the procedure these would be very good results. Unfortunately we have no data about the treatment independent pregnancy rates, a recurring problem in examining the published work on tubal cannulation techniques.

Hysteroscopic techniques require a rigid or flexible hysteroscope with an operating channel sufficiently wide to allow passage of a 5-French (1 mm) diameter catheter. The coaxial method of tubal cannulation employs a flexible guidewire of less than 0.5 mm loaded into a 3-French catheter all passed through the 5-French catheter. Once the guidewire has been used to cannulate the tube under hysteroscopic vision the 3-French inner catheter is advanced over the guidewire, which is then removed, allowing injection of dye to confirm tubal patency. Such a procedure usually needs concurrent laparoscopy and needs to be performed under general anesthesia.

More recent reports of hysteroscopic cannulation have used the technique to facilitate tubal transfer of embryos or gametes (Patton *et al.*, 1991; Seracchioli *et al.*, 1995). In this case laparoscopy is not necessary and so despite a probable lower pregnancy rate with hysteroscopic versus laparoscopic gamete intrafallopian transfer (29.8% versus 43.3%) Seracchioli *et al.* (1995) argue that the hysteroscopic approach is easier, quicker, more cost-effective and less distressing for the patients.

Fluoroscopy

Fluoroscopy is generally used as an adjunct to 'standard' contrast HSG and can be used for selective salpingography and then also for control of guidewire tubal cannulation. Selective salpingography is a relatively straightforward procedure to perform and carries very little risk. It is convenient to perform standard HSG assessment of tubal patency and to follow this with selective fluoroscopic ostial cannulation and injection of contrast to assess tubal patency where there is no tubal fill with contrast by the standard method. Such sequential assessment of the proximal tube is illustrated in Figures 19.3–19.5. If selective salpingography fails to achieve patency then fluoroscopic guidewire cannulation can be attempted, followed again by contrast injection. Such an approach to diagnosis (with a component of treatment) is discussed by Thurmond (1994). In this paper she argues the case for fluoroscopic procedures as part of the diagnostic armamentarium in the investigation of tubal disease. She reviews the reported data of fluoroscopic catheterization in the literature, indicating that tubal patency rates of over 80% at the time of the procedure are consistently achieved with 40–72% remaining patent at 6–12 months. Reported postprocedure intrauterine pregnancy rates vary from 9–37%. Thurmond attempts to explain these differences by highlighting problems in the definition of the denominator used to make such calculations, emphasizing the importance of adequate precatheterization HSG in patient selection. She also stresses the role of non-tubal factors contributing to infertility, their influence on post-recanalization pregnancy rates and the negative effect of distal tubal disease on pregnancy rates despite proximal patency. Once again the data presented are limited in their value because of a paucity of controlled studies. Despite this she indicates that the American Fertility Society has recommended that tubal catheterization should be attempted in the presence of suspected proximal tubal occlusion before using proximal tubal resection and tubocornual anastomosis or assisted reproduction techniques.

Since this report several more papers about selective salpingography and fluoroscopic guidewire cannulation have been published, although as before these are reports of treatment results rather than properly controlled studies. The largest of these reports is that of Lang and Dunaway (1996). This report is difficult to interpret as the patient group studied was heterogeneous with varied pathologic reasons for proximal tubal occlusion. The aim of the study appears to have been to achieve at least one patent tube by sequential use of repeat HSG, selective salpingography and guidewire cannulation. Of 187 patients with bilateral occlusion after selective salpingography, at least one tube was successfully recanalized by guidewire in 145 (78%). Of these 145, 24 (17%) subsequently became pregnant. Selective salpingography had been successful in achieving patency of at least one tube in 131/318 (41%) patients (Lang and Dunaway, 1996). Woolcott *et al.* (1995) reported on attempted treatment of 113 tubes. Selective catheterization and salpingography resulted in 91 (81%) patent tubes in 52 patients of whom 23 (44%) became pregnant. Guidewire cannulation was attempted in the remaining 22 tubes, with 10 (45%) successfully canalized in seven patients and only one subsequent pregnancy, which was ectopic. Sowa *et al.* (1993) reported successful recanalization of 56/92 (61%) fallopian tubes in 58 patients with at least one tube rendered patent in 41/58 (71%). They reported a pregnancy rate after treatment of 22%. Motta *et al.* (1995) reported similar results with 28/40 (70%) tubes in 23 patients successfully recanalized using a coaxial guidewire technique, with at least one tube patent after the procedure in 18 (78%) and overall six subsequent live births – 26% of the group studied. Thurmond *et al.* (1995) reported on a group of patients with salpingitis isthmica nodosa diagnosed by HSG, achieving patency in 52/65 (80%) tubes with six live births in 19 patients (32%), who only had recanalized tubes for achieving pregnancy. Success rates reported by Thompson *et al.* (1994) were rather less impressive. Of 35 tubes still apparently occluded after repeat HSG, only 6 (17%) were recanalized by selective salpingography and 9/29 (31%) remaining tubes were patent after guidewire cannulation.

These variable results are potentially explained by the heterogeneous nature of the reported patient groups, the techniques used and the varied experience of the operators. In the multicenter trial of balloon tuboplasty, patency was achieved in 167/205 (82%) tubes in 95/106 (90%) patients with 37 (35%) pregnancies (Gleicher *et al.*, 1993). However, the authors also describe a group of 28 patients who did not have balloon tuboplasty as their tubes were patent on repeat HSG or selective salpingography. Of these patients eight (29%) subsequently became pregnant. Unfortunately, even this study does not have a control group for balloon tuboplasty. This would have required randomizing those patients

Figure 19.3 Selective salpingography demonstrating patency of the right fallopian tube in a patient who had demonstrated bilateral proximal occlusion by conventional HSG assessment immediately before the selective salpingography. Selective salpingography of the left tube was initially not successful in demonstrating patency.

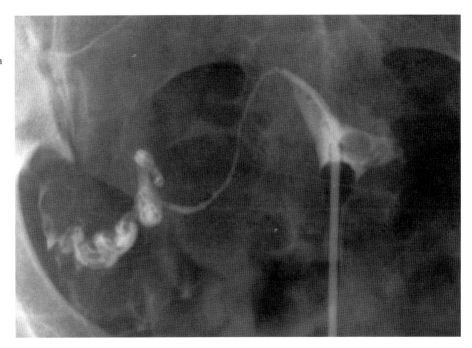

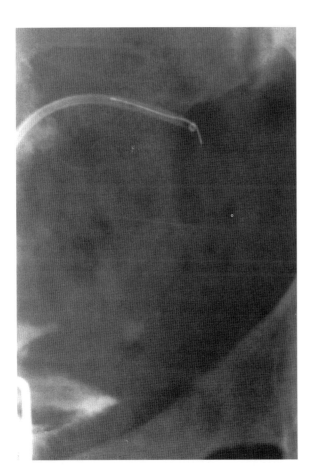

Figure 19.4 Cannulation of the left proximal tube in the same patient using a flexible guidewire coaxial system (Conceptus, San Carlo, USA) under fluoroscopic control.

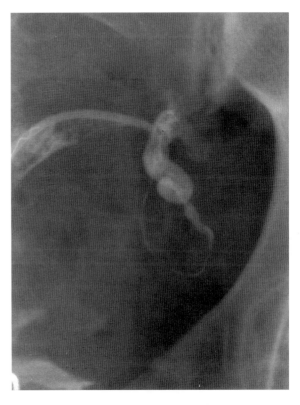

Figure 19.5 Demonstration of patency of the left tube in the same patient by selective salpingography after guidewire recanalization is complete.

with apparent tubal occlusion after repeat HSG to a treatment or a no-treatment group. However, this study does illustrate that tubal appearances after recanalization that suggest distal disease as well as proximal disease are likely to result in compromised subsequent pregnancy rates. Overall, it suggests that such an approach to proximal occlusion is likely to improve tubal patency and pregnancy rates while carrying minimal risk and being relatively inexpensive.

Two other reports are worthy of note. Gleicher *et al.* (1994) performed guidewire cannulation in 35 occluded tubes of 25 women without passing a catheter or balloon over the guidewire following tubal cannulation. The intention was to test whether it was the guidewire or the coaxial passage of the catheter/balloon over the guidewire that was effective in improving subsequent pregnancy rates. Unfortunately there was no untreated control group and no randomization to a group in which the catheter/balloon was passed to enable direct comparison of the two methods of treatment. The authors argue that the patency rate of 27/35 (77%) tubes in 20/25 (80%) patients is consistent with previous reports of coaxial procedures. They believe that the subsequent occurrence of only one pregnancy indicates that the guidewire is not sufficient to improve proximal tubal function and passage of a catheter/balloon over the guidewire is of clinical importance. Of course other non-tubal factors could influence the outcomes in this small group when compared to the outcomes in other reports.

Ferraiolo *et al.* (1995) reported on 117 patients treated by the coaxial technique. In 77 (66%) the procedure was deemed to be successful as it achieved patency in at least one tube with no evidence of distal disease. Of these patients 56 were followed up and 21 (38%) became pregnant. In 23 patients the procedure failed to demonstrate proximal tubal patency and left the patient with no apparently useful tubes. Of these patients 19 were followed up and three (16%) had become pregnant. There were 17 patients with evidence of distal disease and of the 12 of these who were followed up, three had ectopic pregnancies and there were no intrauterine pregnancies. This report illustrates that pregnancy rates are poor if there is evidence of proximal and distal disease. It places a premium on assessing the distal tube as carefully as possible. Also, although not a controlled study, the failed cannulation group still achieved pregnancy, questioning the benefit of recanalization after what is at best an indirect assessment of proximal tubal pathology.

These variable reports indicate that high rates of tubal patency rates can be achieved by selective salpingography and coaxial guidewire balloon/ catheter tubal cannulation. The absence of properly conducted, controlled, randomized studies precludes the conclusion that they cure proximal disease that would otherwise have prevented pregnancy. They emphasize the importance of non-tubal factors (ovulation, maternal age, male factor) as well as the poor prognosis when additional distal disease is present. As relatively simple cheap procedures it is not unreasonable to consider them as an early option in the presence of apparent proximal occlusion on the premise that they are likely to cause more good than harm.

Falloposcopy

Falloposcopy is the transcervical cannulation and imaging of the lumen of the fallopian tube. It provides the opportunity for direct visualization of cannulation and also of the tubal lumen. In the presence of proximal disease the technique enables direct assessment of the likely tubal condition, rather than the indirect assessment provided by HSG. Furthermore, assessment of the lumen of the distal segments is likely to be of prognostic value in predicting tubal epithelial function. This is supported by the evidence that salpingoscopic assessment of the distal tubal lumen is of value in predicting prognosis after tubal surgery for distal tubal disease (Henry-Suchet *et al.*, 1985; Henry-Suchet *et al.*, 1989; Vasquez *et al.*, 1995) and that falloposcopic classification of distal tubal condition correlates well with that provided by salpingoscopy (Scudamore *et al.*, 1994b). This is in contrast to HSG, which has been found to correlate poorly with the findings of salpingoscopy (Puttemans *et al.*, 1987). Therefore falloposcopy has the potential to make a direct and complete assessment of the tubal lumen in both the proximal and distal segments. It can be used without general anesthesia (Scudamore *et al.*, 1992) and with good patient acceptance (Scudamore and Cooke, 1995). Its diagnostic role can include the assessment of tubal condition to identify those patients best treated by surgery, IVF or gamete/ embryo tubal transfer, while a therapeutic role is inherent in proximal cannulation and tuboplasty, which is part of the procedure itself.

First attempts at falloposcopy in 1970 resulted in failure due to the limited technology available for imaging (Mohri *et al.*, 1970). Subsequent advances in technology have led to the development of the coaxial and LEC techniques described earlier. Concurrent laparoscopy is helpful with the coaxial technique as there can be no visualization during advancement of the endoscope and laparoscopy will confirm placement of the endoscope. Manipulation to straighten the tube is useful as even the most flexible guidewire can have difficulty

Table 19.2 Comparison of falloposcopic assessment with HSG and laparoscopy. (H, healthy appearances; D, appearances of disease)

		HSG						Laparoscopy				
		Proximal		Distal		Overall		Proximal		Distal		Overall	
		H	D	H	D	H	D	H	D	H	D	H	D
Falloposcopy	H	106 (75%)	27 (52%)	37 (67%)	25 (42%)	45 (64%)	50 (41%)	102 (84%)	33 (45%)	33 (75%)	49 (49%)	25 (76%)	75 (45%)
	D	35 (25%)	25 (48%)	18 (33%)	34 (58%)	25 (36%)	73 (59%)	19 (16%)	41 (55%)	11 (25%)	51 (51%)	8 (24%)	90 (55%)
Total		**141**	**52**	**55**	**59**	**70**	**123**	**121**	**74**	**44**	**100**	**33**	**165**

negotiating acute bends and flexures of the tube and will exert shear forces against the tubal wall. The LEC technique enables intermittent visualization of the tubal lumen during forward advancement of the endoscope. Also, the advancing balloon tends to follow curves in the tube and prevents the endoscope from exerting such shear forces on the tubal wall (see Figure 19.2). This enables falloposcopy to be performed without laparoscopy as positioning of the endoscope is confirmed directly and the tube does not need straightening.

Using a coaxial technique similar to hysteroscopic guidewire tubal recanalization, Kerin *et al.* (1992) reported a technical failure rate of 7% in 112 tubes of 75 women with a history of infertility thought likely to be related to tubal disease after HSG and laparoscopic assessment. The paper also provides a useful attempt to 'score' the appearances seen objectively. Using this system the subsequent 12-month pregnancy rates correlated inversely with the severity of tubal disease (see Table 19.1).

This scoring system provided for a score of 1 (normal), 2 (mild to moderate disease) or 3 (severe damage) to be ascribed to each of five variables in each of the four segments of the fallopian tube examined: intramural, isthmic, ampullary or fimbrial. These variables included the degree of patency, the epithelial appearances, the endotubal vascularity, the presence and type of adhesions and the presence and degree of dilatation. This method of scoring of the tubal status was presumably based on the methods reported as being of prognostic significance in the treatment of distal tubal disease by various authors (Henry-Suchet *et al.*, 1985; Boer-Meisel *et al.*, 1986; Mage *et al.*, 1986).

Early comparison of LEC falloposcopy with HSG suggested that there were differences in assessment in up to 60% of tubes examined (Venezia *et al.*, 1993). In most, the falloposcopy suggested tubal damage while the HSG had appeared normal. In our own series of 193 tubes of patients thought to have tubal disease there were significant differences in the assessment made by falloposcopy in compar-

ison to that made by HSG and laparoscopy (Scudamore *et al.* (1997) thesis – unpublished data). These data are represented in Table 19.2. Both HSG and laparoscopy concurred best with falloposcopic assessment when they assessed the tube as healthy. Nevertheless falloposcopy identified luminal abnormalities in up to 36% of normal HSGs and 24% of laparoscopies. If tubal disease was diagnosed by HSG or laparoscopy, falloposcopy demonstrated normal appearances of the tubal epithelium in 41–52% of tubes or tubal segments.

These data confirm the potential value of falloposcopy previously reported by Kerin *et al.* (1992) in the assessment of the tubal lumen. Indirect assessment of the tubal lumen by laparoscopy or HSG is likely to be less specific in identifying the presence of intratubal damage than direct visualization. Hence, falloposcopy is potentially useful for achieving patency of tubes diagnosed as proximally occluded (Kovacs *et al.*, 1992; Grow *et al.*, 1993) perhaps caused by displaceable endotubal 'plugs' of the type previously reported by Kerin *et al.* (1991) and Kindermann *et al.* (1993). Direct visual assessment of the proximal and distal segments provides diagnostic information that may be important in subsequent treatment choices (Winston, 1982). The real clinical value of falloposcopy awaits assessment by well-conducted randomized trials as most publications to date are only reports of findings in groups of patients and as such do not prove the value of the technique beyond doubt.

Conclusion

Tubal cannulation techniques have developed greatly in the past 25–30 years. They now have potential use in a number of areas of assessment and treatment of infertile couples. In the presence of apparent proximal tubal occlusion, tubal cannulation techniques enable more specific assessment of tubal damage and often result in tubal patency. Although no well-controlled data are available, proximal recanalization is relatively cheap, may result in subsequent tubal patency and probably improves the chances of 'spontaneous' pregnancy. Tuboplasty with balloon or coaxial techniques may be more effective than guidewire cannulation alone. Falloposcopy is more technically demanding and more expensive, but may provide more complete tubal assessment by visualization of the tubal lumen in both the proximal and distal segments. The proper place of such techniques in modern practise is not clear and will depend upon the results of well-designed and controlled studies.

References

Afnan M, Mastrominas M, Margara RA, Winston RML (1991) The place of *in vitro* fertilisation in the treatment of tubal disease (letter). *Fertility and Sterility* **56**: 582.

Asch RH, Balmaceda JP, Ellsworth LR, Wong PC (1985) Gamete intra-fallopian transfer (GIFT): A new treatment for infertility. *International Journal of Fertility* **30**: 41–45.

Ataya K, Thomas M (1991) New technique for selective transcervical ostial salpingography and catheterization in the diagnosis and treatment of proximal tubal obstruction. *Fertility and Sterility* **56**: 980–983.

Boer-Meisel ME, te Velde ER, Habbema JDF, Kardaun JWPF (1986) Predicting the pregnancy outcome in patients treated for hydrosalpinges: A prospective study. *Fertility and Sterility* **45**: 23–29.

Bongso A, Ng SC, Fong CY *et al.* (1992) Improved pregnancy rate after transfer of embryos grown in human fallopian tubal cell coculture. *Fertility and Sterility* **58**: 569–574.

Braeckmans P, Devroey P, Camus M *et al.* (1987) Gamete intra-fallopian transfer: evaluation of 100 consecutive attempts. *Human Reproduction* **2**: 201–205.

Breckenridge JW, Schinfeld JS (1991) Technique for US-guided fallopian tube catheterization. *Radiology* **180**: 569–570.

Burns J (1809) *Principles of Midwifery.* London: Longman, Hurst, Rees & Orme.

Capitanio GL, Ferraiolo A, Croce S, Gazzo R, Anserini P, de Cecco L (1991) Transcervical selective salpingography: a diagnostic and therapeutic approach to cases of proximal tubal injection failure. *Fertility and Sterility* **55**: 1045–1050.

Confino E, Tur-Kaspa I, DeCherney A *et al.* (1990) Transcervical balloon tuboplasty. A multicenter study. *Journal of the American Medical Association* **264**, 2079–2082.

Cornier E (1985) L'Ampulloscopic per-coelioscopique. *Journal de Gynécologie, Obstétrique et Biologie de la Reproduction* **14**: 459–466.

Das K, Nagel TC, Malo JW (1995) Hysteroscopic cannulation for proximal tubal obstruction: a change for the better? *Fertility and Sterility* **63**: 1009–1015.

De Bruyne F, Puttemans P, Boeckx W, Brosens I (1989) The clinical value of salpingoscopy in tubal infertility. *Fertility and Sterility* **51**: 339–340.

DeCherney AH, Kort H, Barney JB, DeVore GR (1980) Increased pregnancy rate with oil-soluble hysterosalpingography dye. *Fertility and Sterility* **33**: 407–410.

Devroey P, Staessen C, Camus M, De Grauwe E, Wisanto A, Van Steirteghem AC (1989) Zygote intrafallopian transfer as a successful treatment for unexplained infertility. *Fertility and Sterility* **52**: 246–249.

Dubuisson JB, Chapron C, Morice P, Aubriot FX, Foulot H, de Joliniere JB (1994) Laparoscopic salpingostomy: fertility results according to the tubal mucosal appearance. *Human Reproduction* **9**: 334–339.

Dunphy BC (1994) Office falloposcopic assessment in proximal tubal occlusive disease. *Fertility and Sterility* **61(1)**: 168–170.

Eckstein N, Orron DE, Vagman I *et al.* (1992) Digital road mapping image – a novel fluoroscopic real-time guide for selective transcervical catheterization in the treatment of proximal tubal obstruction. *Fertility and Sterility* **58**: 850–853.

Evans D (1995) Infertility and the NHS. *British Medical Journal* **311**: 1586–1587.

Ferraiolo A, Ferraro F, Remorgida V, Gorlero F, Capitanio GL, de Cecco L (1995) Unexpected pregnancies after tubal recanalization failure with selective catheterization. *Fertility and Sterility* **63**: 299–302.

Flood JT, Grow DR (1993) Transcervical tubal cannulation: a review. *Obstetrical and Gynecological Survey* **48**: 768–776.

Fortier KJ and Haney AF (1985) The pathological spectrum of uterotubal junction obstruction. *Obstetrics and Gynecology* **65(1)**: 93–98.

Geist SH, Goldberger MA (1925) A study of the intramural position of normal and diseased tubes with special reference to the question of sterility. *Surgery, Gynecology and Obstetrics* **41**: 646–654.

Gleicher N, Parrilli M, Redding L, Pratt D, Karande V (1992) Standardization of hysterosalpingography and selective salpingography: a valuable adjunct to simple opacification studies. *Fertility and Sterility* **58**: 1136–1141.

Gleicher N, Confino E, Corfman R *et al.* (1993) The multicentre transcervical balloon tuboplasty study: conclusions and comparison to alternative technologies. *Human Reproduction* **8**: 1264–1271.

Gleicher N, Redding L, Parrilli M, Karande V, Pratt D (1994) Wire guide cannulation alone is no treatment of proximal tubal occlusion. *Human Reproduction* **9**: 1109–1111.

Gomel V, Yarali H (1992) Infertility surgery: microsurgery. *Current Opinion in Obstetrics and Gynecology* **4**: 390–399.

Grant A (1971) Infertility surgery of the oviduct. *Fertility and Sterility* **22**: 496–503.

Grow DR, Coddington CC, Flood JT (1993) Proximal tubal occlusion by hysterosalpingogram: a role for falloposcopy. *Fertility and Sterility* **60**: 170–174.

Hafez ESE (1973) Anatomy and physiology of the mammalian uterotubal junction. In Greep RO, Astwood EB (eds) *Handbook of Physiology. Endocrinology II, Part II.* pp. 87–95. Washington DC: American Physiological Society.

Hayashi N, Kimoto T, Sakai T *et al.* (1994) Fallopian tube disease: limited value of treatment with Fallopian tube catheterization. *Radiology* **190**: 141–143.

Henry-Suchet J, Loffredo V, Tesquier L, Pez J (1985) Endoscopy of the tube (=tuboscopy): its prognostic value for tuboplasties. *Acta Europaea Fertilitatis* **16**: 139–145.

Henry-Suchet J, Veluyre M, Pia P (1989) Statistical study of the factors influencing the prognosis in tuboplasty operations. Importance of the status of the ampullary mucosa and of chlamydial infection. *Journal de Gynécologie, Obstétrique et Biologie de la Reproduction* **18**: 571–580.

Hercz P, Vine SJ, Walker SM (1994) Experience with transcervical fallopian tube catheterization. *Fertility and Sterility* **61**: 551–553.

Jaffe SB, Jewelewicz R (1991) The basic infertility investigation. *Fertility and Sterility* **56**: 599–611.

Jansen RPS, Anderson JC, Sutherland PD (1988) Nonoperative embryo transfer to the fallopian tube. *New England Journal of Medicine* **319**: 288–291.

Kelly GL (1927) The uterotubal junction in the guinea-pig. *American Journal of Anatomy* **40**: 373–385.

Kennedy WT (1925) Isthmospasm of the fallopian tube. *Journal of the American Medical Association* **85**: 13–17.

Kerin JF, Surrey ES, Williams DB, Daykhovsky L, Grundfest WS (1991) Falloposcopic observations of endotubal isthmic plugs as a cause of reversible obstruction and their histological characterization. *Journal of Laparoendoscopic Surgery* **1**: 103–110.

Kerin JF, Williams DB, San Roman GA, Pearlstone AC, Grundfest WS, Surrey ES (1992) Falloposcopic classification and treatment of fallopian tube lumen disease. *Fertility and Sterility* **57**: 731–741.

Kindermann D, Bauer O, Fischer HP, Dietrich K (1993) Histological findings in a falloposcopically retrieved isthmic plug causing reversible proximal tubal obstruction. *Human Reproduction* **8**: 1429–1434.

Kovacs G, Kerin J, Scudamore I, Wood C (1992) Falloposcopy – a non-invasive method of salpingostomy. *Gynaecological Endoscopy* **1**: 159–160.

Lang EK (1991) Organic vs functional obstruction of the fallopian tubes: differentiation with prostaglandin antagonist- and beta 2-agonist-mediated hysterosalpingography and selective ostial salpingography. *American Journal of Roentgenology* **157**: 77–80.

Lang EK, Dunaway HH (1996) Recanalization of obstructed fallopian tube by selective salpingography and transvaginal bougie dilatation: outcome and cost analysis. *Fertility and Sterility* **66**: 210–215.

Lang EK, Dunaway HE Jr, Roniger WE (1990) Selective ostial salpingography and transvaginal catheter dilatation in the diagnosis and treatment of fallopian tube obstruction. *American Journal of Roentgenology* **154**: 735–740.

Lederer KJ (1993) Transcervical tubal cannulation and salpingoscopy in the treatment of tubal infertility. *Current Opinion in Obstetrics and Gynecology* **5**: 240–244.

Lee FC (1928) The tubo-uterine junction in various animals. *Bulletin of the Johns Hopkins Hospital* **42**: 335–357.

Lisa JR, Gioia JD, Rubin IC (1954) Observations on the interstitial portion of the Fallopian tube. *Surgery, Gynecology and Obstetrics* **99**: 159–169.

Lisse K, Sydow P (1991) Fallopian tube catheterization and recanalization under ultrasonic observation: a simplified technique to evaluate tubal patency and open proximally obstructed tubes. *Fertility and Sterility* **56**: 198–201.

Mage G, Pouly J, Bouquet de Joliniere J, Chabrand S, Riouallon A, Bruhat M (1986) A preoperative classification to predict the intrauterine and ectopic pregnancy rates after distal tubal microsurgery. *Fertility and Sterility* **46**: 807–810.

Maguiness SD, Djahanbakhch O, Grudzinskas JG (1992) Assessment of the fallopian tube. *Obstetrical and Gynecological Survey* **47**: 587–603.

Marana R, Quagliarello J (1988) Proximal tubal occlusion: microsurgery versus IVF – A review. *International Journal of Fertility* **33**: 338–340.

Maroulis GB, Yeko TR (1992) Treatment of cornual obstruction by transvaginal cannulation without hysteroscopy or fluoroscopy. *Fertility and Sterility* **57**: 1136–1138.

McComb PF, Lee NH, Stephenson MD (1991) Reproductive outcome after microsurgery for proximal and distal occlusions in the same fallopian tube. *Fertility and Sterility* **56**: 134–135.

Mohri T, Mohri C, Yamadori F (1970) Flexible glass fibre endoscope for intratubal observation. *Endoscopy* **2**: 226–230.

Motta EL, Nelson J, Batzofin J, Serafini P (1995) Selective salpingography with an insemination catheter in the treatment of women with cornual fallopian tube obstruction. *Human Reproduction* **10**: 1156–1159.

Murdoch AP, Harris M, Mahroo M, Williams M, Dunlop W (1991) Is GIFT (gamete intrafallopian transfer) the best treatment for unexplained infertility? *British Journal of Obstetrics and Gynaecology* **98**: 643–647.

Murray MK, DeSouza MM (1995) Messenger RNA encoding an estrogen-dependent oviduct secretory protein in the sheep is localized in the apical tips and basal compartments of fimbria and ampulla epithelial cells implying translation at unique cytoplasmic foci. *Molecular Reproduction and Development* **42**: 268–283.

Novy M (1994) Concurrent tuboplasty and assisted reproduction. *Fertility and Sterility* **62(2)**: 242–245.

Palermo G, Devroey P, Camus M *et al.* (1989) Zygote intrafallopian transfer as an alternative treatment for male infertility. *Human Reproduction* **4**: 412–415.

Patton PE, Hickok LR, Wolf DP (1991) Successful hysteroscopic cannulation and tubal transfer of cryopreserved embryos. *Fertility and Sterility* **55**: 640–641.

Pearlstone AC, Surrey ES, Kerin JF (1992) The linear everting catheter: a nonhysteroscopic, transvaginal technique for access and microendoscopy of the fallopian tube. *Fertility and Sterility* **58**: 854–857.

Puttemans P, Brosens I, Delattin P, Vasquez G, Boeckx W (1987) Salpingoscopy versus hysterosalpingography in hydrosalpinges. *Human Reproduction* **2**: 535–540.

Risquez F, Forman R, Maleika F *et al.* (1992a) Transcervical cannulation of the fallopian tube for the management of ectopic pregnancy: prospective multicenter study. *Fertility and Sterility* **58**: 1131–1135.

Risquez F, Pennehouat G, Foulot H *et al.* (1992b) Transcervical tubal cannulation and falloposcopy for the management of tubal pregnancy. *Human Reproduction* **7**: 274–275.

Risquez F, Confino E (1993) Transcervical tubal cannulation, past, present, and future. *Fertility and Sterility* **60**: 211–226.

Rocca M, el Habashy M, Nayel S, Madwar A (1989) The intramural segment and the uterotubal junction: an anatomic and histologic study. *International Journal of Gynaecology and Obstetrics* **28**: 343–349.

Rotsztejn DA, Remohi J, Weckstein LN *et al.* (1990) Results of tubal embryo transfer in premature ovarian failure. *Fertility and Sterility* **54**: 348–350.

Rubin IC (1939) The influence of the hormonal activity of the ovaries upon the character of tubal contractions as determined by uterine insufflation. A clinical study. *American Journal of Obstetrics and Gynecology* **37**: 394–404.

Scholtes MC, Roozenburg BJ, Alberda AT, Zeilmaker GH (1990) Transcervical intrafallopian transfer of zygotes. *Fertility and Sterility* **54**: 283–286.

Scudamore IW, Cooke ID (1995) Can falloposcopy be performed as an outpatient procedure? *Tubo-Peritoneal Infertility and Ectopic Pregnancy, Experts Conference and I.F.F.S. Satellite Symposium, Clermont-Ferrand, France, Sept. 14–16 1995.* London: Mosby-Wolfe.

Scudamore IW, Dunphy BC, Cooke ID (1992) Outpatient falloposcopy: intra-luminal imaging of the fallopian tube by trans-uterine fibre-optic endoscopy as an outpatient procedure. *British Journal of Obstetrics and Gynaecology* **99**: 829–835.

Scudamore IW, Dunphy BC, Cooke ID (1994a) Falloposcopic comparison of unilateral and bilateral proximal tubal occlusive disease. *Human Reproduction* **9**: 340–342.

Scudamore IW, Dunphy BC, Bowman M, Jenkins J, Cooke ID (1994b) Comparison of ampullary assessment by falloposcopy and salpingoscopy. *Human Reproduction* **9**: 1516–1518.

Seracchioli R, Porcu E, Ciotti P, Fabbri R, Colombi C, Flamigni C (1995) Gamete intrafallopian transfer: prospective randomized comparison between hysteroscopic and laparoscopic transfer techniques. *Fertility and Sterility* **64**: 355–359.

Shuber J (1989) Transcervical sterilization with use of methyl 2-cyanoacrylate and newer delivery system (the FEMCEPT device). *American Journal of Obstetrics and Gynecology* **160**: 887.

Sowa M, Shimamoto T, Nakano R, Sato M, Yamada R (1993) Diagnosis and treatment of proximal tubal obstruction by fluoroscopic transcervical fallopian tube catheterization. *Human Reproduction* **8**: 1711–1714.

Stallworthy J (1948) Fact and fantasy in the study of female infertility. *Journal of Obstetrics and Gynaecology of the British Empire* **55**: 171–180.

Stern JJ, Peters AJ, Coulam CB (1991) Transcervical tuboplasty under ultrasonographic guidance: a pilot study. *Fertility and Sterility* **56**: 359–360.

Sulak PJ, Letterie GS, Coddington CC, Hayslip CC, Woodward JE, Klein TA (1987) Histology of proximal tubal occlusion. *Fertility and Sterility* **48**: 437–440.

Sweeney WJ (1962) The interstitial portion of the uterine tube – its gross anatomy, course, and length. *Obstetrics and Gynecology* **19**: 3–8.

Thompson KA, Kiltz RJ, Koci T, Cabus ET, Kletzky OA (1994) Transcervical fallopian tube catheterization and recanalization for proximal tubal obstruction. *Fertility and Sterility* **61**: 243–247.

Thurmond AS (1991) Selective salpingography and fallopian tube recanalization. *American Journal of Roentogenology* **156**: 33–38.

Thurmond AS (1994) Pregnancies after selective salpingography and tubal recanalization. *Radiology* **190**: 11–13.

Thurmond AS, Novy M, Rosch J (1988) Terbutaline in diagnosis of interstitial fallopian tube obstruction. *Investigative Radiology* **23**: 209–210.

Thurmond AS, Burry KA, Novy MJ (1995) Salpingitis isthmica nodosa: results of transcervical fluoroscopic catheter recanalization. *Fertility and Sterility* **63**: 715–722.

Tyler-Smith W (1849) New method of treating sterility by the removal of obstructions of the fallopian tubes. *Lancet* **1**: 116–118.

Valle RF (1995) Tubal cannulation. *Obstetrics and Gynecology Clinics of North America* **22**: 519–540.

Valle RR (1989) Hysteroscopic sterilization. In Baggish HS (ed.) *Diagnostic and Operative Hysteroscopy.* pp. 145–203. Chicago: Yearbook Medical Publishers.

Vasen LCLM (1959) The intramural part of the fallopian tube. *International Journal of Fertility* **4**: 309–314.

Vasquez G, Boeckx W, Brosens I (1995) Prospective study of tubal mucosal lesions and fertility in hydrosalpinges. *Human Reproduction* **10**: 1075–1078.

Venezia R, Zangara C, Knight C, Cittadini E (1993) Initial experience of a new linear everting falloposcopy system in comparison with hysterosalpingography. *Fertility and Sterility* **60**: 771–775.

Winfield AC, Wentz AC (1987) *Diagnostic Imaging in Infertility.* Baltimore: Williams & Wilkins.

Winston R (1982) Reconstructive microsurgery at the lateral end of the fallopian tube. In Chamberlain G, Winston R (eds) *Tubal Infertility. Diagnosis and Treatment.* pp. 79–104. Oxford: Blackwell Scientific Publications.

Woolcott R, Petchpud A, O'Donnell P, Stanger J (1995) Differential impact on pregnancy rate of selective salpingography, tubal catheterization and wire-guide recanalization in the treatment of proximal fallopian tube obstruction. *Human Reproduction* **10**: 1423–1426.

World Health Organization (1983) A new hysterographic approach to the evaluation of tubal spasm and spasmolytic agents. *Fertility and Sterility* **39**: 105–107.

Yeung WS, Ho PC, Lau EY, Chan ST (1992) Improved development of human embryos *in vitro* by a human oviductal cell co-culture system. *Human Reproduction* **7**: 1144–1149.

Laparoscopic Ovarian Surgery

20

Laparoscopic Ovarian Surgery: Preoperative Diagnosis and Imaging

LACHLAN DE CRESPIGNY

Royal Women's Hospital, Melbourne, Australia

Introduction

The appropriate selection of a patient for laparoscopic ovarian surgery depends upon the availability of reliable information on the etiology of the pelvic mass. A high-quality ultrasound service is therefore essential as it is the imaging modality of choice for the assessment of pelvic pathology. Continuing refinements in technology with resultant improvements in the resolution of ultrasonic equipment has made it an accurate method for assessing a pelvic mass, having the flexibility to allow any suspicious area to be scrutinized from different angles. In relative terms it is a low cost investigation.

A most important advance in the diagnosis of pelvic pathology using ultrasound is the development of the endovaginal transducer. Not only does this avoid the necessity of an uncomfortably distended bladder as a prerequisite to imaging the ovaries, but it also provides improved resolution since the transducer is closer to the area under investigation. More recently color and power Doppler have been introduced with their capacity to demonstrate the presence or absence of neovascularization in the wall of a cyst. This feature is proving to be of value in determining whether a cyst is benign or malignant.

Equipment and Technique

Although detailed technique is not relevant to this chapter, several points are worth making.

- The best results using ultrasound are obtained with 'state of the art' high-resolution equipment, including a Doppler facility. The necessary expertise in interpreting the images is not always widely available.
- A transducer with a small 'footprint' is usually preferred for transabdominal gynecological scanning – the bones of the pelvis limit access if a large transducer is used.
- An endovaginal scanner is essential. A transvaginal ultrasound examination is used for most gynecological scans and is of particular value when transabdominal images are suboptimal (e.g. due to obesity) and in the evaluation of a pelvic mass (Liebman et al., 1988). These workers showed that transvaginal images are better than improved images of adnexal masses in 78% of cases and of uterine fibroids in 74%.
- The results obtained by viewing hard copy images will not be as good as when the sonologist who is preparing the report does the scanning personally (Benacerraf et al., 1990). Indeed, the reports of ultrasound images from hard copy may not be as accurate as the results of clinical examination (O'Brien et al., 1984). When the sonologist does the scanning then even transabdominal scanning alone (without transvaginal scanning) is superior to clinical examination (Andolf and Jorgensen, 1988).

Transvaginal images are superior to transabdominal images in early pregnancy and gynecological scanning of the pelvis. This has been translated into

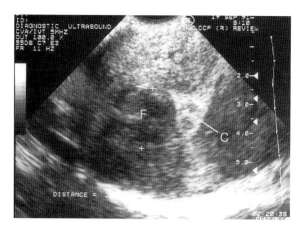

Figure 20.1 A transvaginal section of the uterus which virtually fills the image. The cavity line (C) is demonstrated with a fibroid (F marked with calipers) abutting the cavity line.

who have had a hysterectomy (Coleman *et al.*, 1988). Ovaries situated in the pouch of Douglas are more readily visualized with transvaginal ultrasound, while those high above the uterine fundus may be better seen transabdominally.

Logic dictates that transvaginal scanning should provide improved clinical information (Figure 20.3). Unfortunately the two methods of scanning have not commonly been compared in a study setting. Lande *et al.* (1988) performed transvaginal ultrasound when transabdominal views were suboptimal or the diagnosis uncertain and found that transvaginal ultrasound added diagnostically useful information for 25 of 28 patients with adnexal cysts. Liebman *et al.* (1988) compared transabdominal and transvaginal ultrasound in patients with a

earlier diagnosis of pregnancy (de Crespigny *et al.*, 1988), and more accurate assessment of patients with a suspected ectopic pregnancy (de Crespigny, 1988; Kivikoski *et al.*, 1990). The improved resolution of transvaginal scanning provides the ability to diagnose uterine fibroids more accurately, especially if small, and to define their position. In particular, the proximity of a fibroid to the uterine cavity line can be precisely defined (Figure 20.1). Difficulty in distinguishing a solid ovarian tumor from a fibroid is not uncommon using transabdominal scanning but unusual with transvaginal scanning. The ability to move a pelvic mass with the end of the transducer is a further aid to diagnosis.

The exclusion of an ovarian cyst using ultrasound necessitates clear visualization of each ovary (Figure 20.2). Transvaginal scanning allows the ovaries to be identified more often than transabdominal scanning when the uterus is enlarged, such as when there are uterine fibroids (especially in peri- and postmenopausal women) and in women

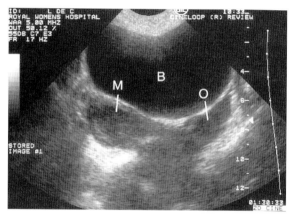

(a)

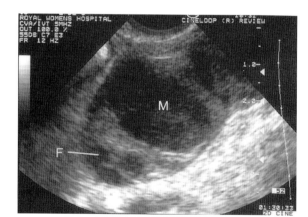

(b)

Figure 20.3 (a) A transverse transabdominal section of the pelvis. Behind the bladder (B) is a normal right ovary (O) and a left mass (M), which is poorly defined and centrally echo poor. (b) On transvaginal ultrasound this same mass (M) is a clearly defined relatively echo free cyst. The adjacent follicles (F) in the cyst wall indicate that the cyst is ovarian, the features being those of a benign blood-filled cyst.

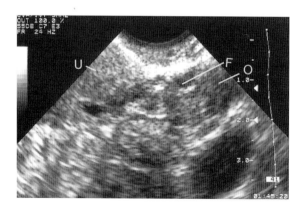

Figure 20.2 A transvaginal image of a normal ovary (O) containing small atretic follicles (F), adjacent to the uterus (U).

palpable mass and found that transvaginal ultrasound delineated the internal architecture of the lesion or its relationship to other pelvic structures better in 81%. Transvaginal ultrasound should therefore be part of the ultrasound examination of a pelvic mass unless declined by the patient.

Indications for Ultrasound

The major indications for gynecological ultrasound include the following.

Pelvic Pain

Although an ovarian cyst is not often found in the absence of a clinically detected mass, ultrasound is particularly valuable when the clinical examination is difficult or impossible such as when the patient is obese or refuses a vaginal examination. In other situations, diagnostic ultrasound may enable the clinician and patient to continue with conservative treatment with confidence when no mass is detected, rather than resort to diagnostic laparoscopy. In this regard it is worth emphasizing that while ultrasound is expected to detect even a small pelvic mass, the examination may be normal if the cause of the pain is not associated with a mass (e.g. pelvic adhesions or small areas of endometriosis). In addition, while a dilated fallopian tube may be seen, especially using a vaginal transducer, a normal tube is not usually visualized with ultrasound. Valuable information is obtained by using the vaginal transducer to move pelvic organs to assess mobility and tenderness and so localize the site of pain.

Pelvic Mass

The major areas in which ultrasound can influence management in patients with a clinical suspicion of a pelvic mass may be summarized as:

- Confirmation of a mass: is a pelvic mass present? Appropriate use of diagnostic ultrasound in such patients avoids the necessity for surgery if there is clinical uncertainty (e.g. in an obese patient).
- Site of a mass: is a palpable mass ovarian in origin or does it arise from the uterus or other pelvic organs?
- Insignificant masses: when a mass is palpable is it significant? Small transient fluid-filled

ovarian cysts are common in both pre-menopausal and postmenopausal women.
- Assessment of possible malignancy: ultrasound cannot provide a pathologic diagnosis, but is valuable in helping to determine the likelihood of malignancy. Some benign ovarian cysts have characteristic features (e.g. benign cystic teratoma).
- Treatment: what is the appropriate management? Treatment may be more rationally planned in the light of the findings above. Is treatment necessary and if so, is ultrasound guided cyst aspiration, laparoscopy or laparotomy appropriate? If laparotomy is indicated, the ultrasound findings assist in determining the degree of urgency and whether a gynecological oncologist should be present, and depending upon the likelihood of malignancy, may help in the decision about which incision to use.

Ultrasound Screening for Ovarian Cancer

Less than 30% of primary ovarian cancers are confined to the ovary at the time of diagnosis and the overall five-year survival rate is less than 25%. Ovarian cancer screening aims to detect lesions at an early stage when the five-year survival is around 80% (Sigurdsson et al., 1983). The detection rate is low with population screening: Campbell et al. (1989, 1990) identified five patients with primary ovarian cancer in 15 977 screening examinations of women aged 45 and above. To detect these primary tumors, the chance of detecting an ovarian cancer at a single examination was 0.03%, while the incidence of false positives was 3.6% at the first ultrasound examination, but lower with subsequent examinations. Such a program therefore generates a large workload of benign pathology requiring management, much of which with careful patient selection could be managed using laparoscopy or even cyst aspiration.

On close examination of the cost/benefit of ultrasound screening for ovarian cancer Creasman and Di Saia (1991) conclude that it is premature to recommend population screening. It is worth nothing that the American College of Obstetricians and Gynecologists Committee consider that 'no available techniques are currently suitable for routine screening', a view supported by Westhoff and Randall (1991). Creasman and Di Saia (1991) suggest that only a minority (<5%) of patients with ovarian cancer have a positive family history, but in this group ultrasound screening may be justified. It should probably be commenced at a young age because the onset of hereditary forms of cancer is usually between the ages of 35 and 45 (Lynch et al., 1982). Women with a first degree relative with ovarian cancer have a 5% risk of developing it themselves. There is a 30% lifetime risk for women with two affected close relatives (Webb, 1993). Ultrasound studies and clinical practise increasingly focus on women with a positive family history of ovarian or related cancer. An ultrasound ovarian cancer screening program showed that the odds of finding an ovarian cancer in self-referred symptomless women who came to surgery were increased from one in 50 in an unselected population to one in 12 among those with a family history of the disease. These odds may be increased further by careful ultrasonic classification of ovarian cysts (Bourne *et al.*, 1993). However, familial cancers form a small percentage of all ovarian cancers, so screening such women has little impact on the disease prevalence (Webb, 1993).

A Normal Ovary

The normal ovary is ovoid in outline (see Figure 20.2) and measures an average of 6.5 ml (5.4–7.6 ml) in premenopausal women (Munn *et al.*, 1986), but is smaller following the menopause (3.6 ± 1.4 ml, Goswamy *et al.*, 1988) and before the menarche. Before ovulation in spontaneous cycles the ovarian follicle may reach up to 2.5 cm (O'Herlihy *et al.*, 1980), but may be larger in stimulated cycles. In addition, the ovary usually contains several small, mostly peripheral 'cysts' of up to 10 mm diameter. These are seldom seen following the menopause.

The number of small 'cysts' is increased in polycystic ovarian disease. The ovaries in this condition have been described as having multiple cysts (ten or more) 2–18 mm in diameter distributed around the ovarian periphery with an increased amount of stroma (Figure 20.4). Less commonly there are multiple small cysts 2–4 mm in diameter distributed throughout abundant stroma (Adams *et al.*, 1985).

Both ovaries should be visualized using ultrasound in nearly all women. In a series of 321 consecutive patients the author was able to locate both ovaries (when present) in all but one patient who had had a hysterectomy for whom there was uncertainty as to whether a single ovary had or had not been removed. Of these patients 240 who had the ultrasound examination for follicular assessment in either stimulated or non-stimulated cycles, 15 patients were postmenopausal, 13 had a transabdominal scan only, eight had transabdominal plus transvaginal scans, and the remainder had transvaginal scans only.

The ovary may be readily differentiated from bowel by watching for peristalsis. Localized collections of tortuous adnexal vessels may occasionally be confused with the ovary, but are differentiated easily by examination using color Doppler. The ovaries may be more difficult to visualize following hysterectomy and after the menopause.

Differential Diagnosis of an Ovarian Mass

The major method of differentiating an ovarian from a non-ovarian pelvic mass is to visualize a normal ovary separate from the mass. If the ovary is moved with the vaginal transducer, an extra-ovarian mass will usually not move with it. A further diagnostic feature is the shape of the ovary – if the ovary is visible adjacent to the mass and is the normal ovoid shape, then the mass is likely to be extra-ovarian; if the ovary is flattened around the mass then it is usually ovarian (Figure 20.5).

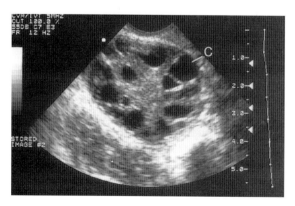

Figure 20.4 A transvaginal section of a polycystic ovary with multiple small, mostly peripheral, cysts (C).

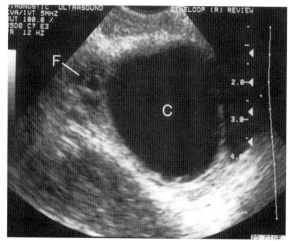

Figure 20.5 A 'simple' ovarian cyst (C) with the ovary containing small atretic follicles (F) in the cyst wall.

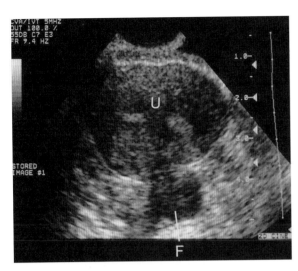

Figure 20.6 A transvaginal image of the uterus (U) with a subserous fibroid (F) posteriorly. The ovaries were visible separately.

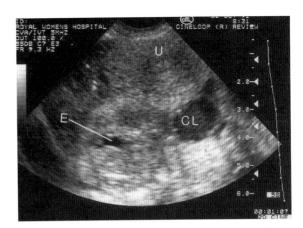

Figure 20.8 Behind the uterus (U) is a 5 mm cystic lesion surrounded by an echo-dense rim of tissue, which is the typical appearance of an ectopic pregnancy (E). A small blood-filled cyst, presumably the corpus luteum (CL), is visible adjacent to the ectopic pregnancy.

The most frequent differential diagnosis of an ovarian mass on clinical examination is a uterine fibroid, especially if the fibroid is pedunculated. On transvaginal ultrasound the fibroid can be seen as part of the uterus and if pedunculated, the pedicle visualized (Figure 20.6). The fibroid moves with the uterus and the normal ovary is visualized separately. Other fibroids may also be seen.

A hydrosalpinx can be difficult to distinguish from an ovarian cyst. On ultrasound section both appear to be spherical, thin-walled, fluid-filled structures, but by examining sections at different angles the tortuous shape of the dilated tube is usually identifiable and its epithelial infolding noted (Figure 20.7). The ovary should be visible separately. This also applies to other non-ovarian masses such as a fimbrial cyst or an ectopic pregnancy (Figure 20.8). It is often difficult to identify the site of origin of an extra-ovarian cyst.

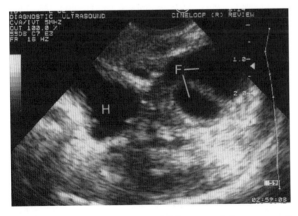

Figure 20.7 The ovary is visible containing several follicles (F). A separate fluid-filled lesion with epithelial folds is visible (H), which was subsequently confirmed to be a hydrosalpinx.

Ovarian Cysts

It is worth noting that diagnostic ultrasound frequently offers more information about the nature of a cyst than inspection of its surface at laparoscopy or laparotomy. Using ultrasound, the cyst contents can be carefully scrutinized and magnified – so-called 'sonomicroscopy' (Goldstein, 1990) – and the presence and characteristics of any solid areas and vascularity studied.

UNILOCULAR SIMPLE CYSTS

In a spontaneously cycling woman, any cyst greater than 2.5 cm diameter should be considered as being too large to be a follicle (see Figure 20.5). The significance of such a 'simple' cyst depends upon its size and the patient's age.

The histologic diagnoses include follicular cysts, simple serous cysts, endometriosis, benign mucinous and serous cystadenomas. Few are malignant – of 57 patients with advanced ovarian cancer, in no case was the primary tumor entirely cystic (Paling and Shawker, 1981).

Only some 5% of ovarian cancers are less than 5 cm at the time of diagnosis (Scully, 1982) – larger ovarian cysts are more likely to be malignant, even when the cyst is unilocular with no solid element. Herrmann *et al.* (1987) found no malignancies among 48 'simple' cysts of less than 10 cm diameter, but one malignancy among nine patients with a cyst greater than 10 cm diameter. Similarly, Meire *et al.* (1978) found no malignancies among 23 unilocular cysts of less than 5 cm in diameter, but two malignancies among the 19 patients in whom the cyst was greater than 5 cm in diameter.

Even in older women, small 'simple' cysts are rarely malignant. In 1989 two series were published, which together totalled 100 patients with anechoic, unilocular thin-walled, fluid-filled cysts of less than 5 cm in diameter. The patients in one study were all over 50 years of age (Andolf and Jorgensen, 1989) and in the other were all postmenopausal (Goldstein et al., 1989). On follow-up none was found to be malignant. In an earlier study (1983–85) of 13 postmenopausal patients who had a cyst of less than 10 cm in diameter, one borderline malignancy was found using transabdominal ultrasound (Hall and McCarthy, 1986). It is reasonable to expect that even this tumor would have been more likely to be suspected using the improved equipment now available, especially transvaginal ultrasound and color Doppler.

The management of a small 'simple' ovarian cyst therefore depends more on its malignant potential than the very small risk of actual malignancy. It has been suggested that serous and mucinous cystadenomas only occasionally undergo malignant change – surface epithelial inclusion glands are thought to be the source of most of the common epithelial carcinomas of the ovary (Scully, 1982). There can therefore be little justification in treating all small 'simple' ovarian cysts as potential cancers.

SIMPLE CYSTS WITH ECHOES IN THE FLUID

The presence of fine echoes throughout the cyst fluid frequently indicates that blood is present, either as a result of hemorrhage into the cyst (Reynolds et al., 1986) or endometriosis. Endometriotic or other blood-filled cysts may contain dense echoes (Figure 20.9) or fine echoes – there is

some relationship between the viscosity of the blood-filled cyst and its echodensity on ultrasound. However, not all blood-filled cysts contain such echoes and not all cysts with uniform echoes contain blood (de Crespigny et al., 1989).

FEATURES OF MALIGNANCY

Multilocular cysts, particularly when the septa are thick and those with solid areas within the cyst are more likely to be malignant. Even small solid areas are of concern (Moyle et al., 1983). These features have been combined into a scoring system by Sassone et al. (1991), which confirms the empirical results of others – namely that using ultrasound one can effectively select out a group at extremely low risk of malignancy (their classification showed a negative predictive value of 100%). However, many benign cysts have some of the adverse features, for example they may be large, multilocular (Figure 20.10) or have solid areas (Figure 20.11) – Sassone et al. (1991) found a positive predictive value of 37%. There is, however, undoubtedly a group with many of the adverse features that clearly has a very high chance of malignancy (e.g. complex-looking solid and cystic multilocular ovarian tumors, Figure 20.12).

Refinements to the scoring system of Sassone et al. (1991) include a weighted system (Lerner et al., 1994) and adding Doppler information (Timor-Tritsch et al., 1993). While such systems may be valuable as a guide, it would be foolhardy to treat an ovarian cyst with papillary excrescences as benign even if there were no other adverse factors and no neovascularization.

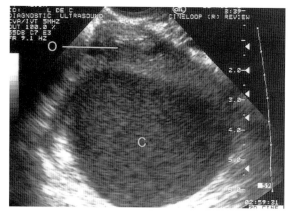

Figure 20.9 An adnexal cyst (C) contains dense echoes. The ovary (O) is in the cyst wall and contains several small cystic lesions of <5 mm diameter. The cyst was removed surgically and proved to be an endometrioma.

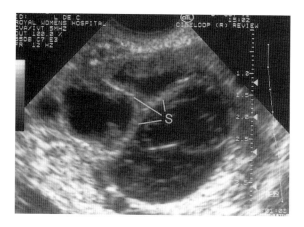

Figure 20.10 This trilocular cyst has thick septa (S). The patient had a past history of endometriosis and this was subsequently confirmed at surgery.

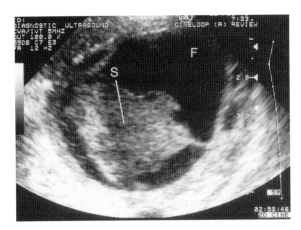

Figure 20.11 This cyst contains a large solid area (S) as well as fluid (F). The solid area wobbled within the cyst when the ovarian cyst was shaken with the vaginal transducer. This represents clot and the cyst subsequently resolved.

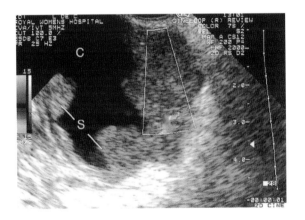

Figure 20.12 A solid (S) and cystic (C) ovarian tumor. The colored area indicates neovascularization within the solid areas. The resistance index (RI) was low and the pathology later indicated a mucinous cystadenocarcinoma.

SPECIAL TUMORS WITH CHARACTERISTIC FEATURES

On first appearances a benign cystic teratoma may appear suspiciously malignant since it is a complex solid and cystic lesion. Dermoid cysts, even when large, may be missed, as their echodense contents may reflect ultrasound and they are mistaken for normal bowel. On closer inspection the bizarre echo pattern is characteristic. Bronshtein *et al.* (1991) have shown that individual hair fibers seen with transvaginal ultrasound are hyperechoic sparkling dots or delicate white lines. An awareness of this characteristic allowed the group to diagnose 25 dermoid cysts with 100% accuracy (Figure 20.13).

Other cysts with characteristic appearances include thecomas – a hypoechoic mass with

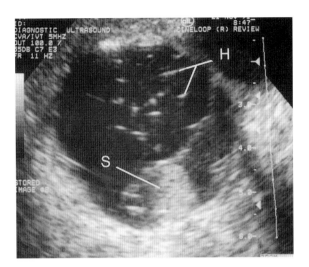

Figure 20.13 A benign cystic teratoma. The dense solid area (S) and the cyst containing fine dense echogenic lines – hair (H) – are characteristic.

acoustic shadowing (Athey and Malone, 1987) – and Krukenberg tumors whose pattern includes irregular hyperechoic areas and moth-eaten cyst formation (Shimizu *et al.*, 1990).

Colorflow and Duplex Doppler

High-quality vaginal ultrasound transducers now have a colorflow imaging capability. This allows the imaging of small blood vessels, which would not be visible without color and are often too small to be seen, even with transabdominal colorflow imaging. Colored areas within a tumor show the presence of neovascularization (see Figure 20.12) – benign tumors and normal ovarian tissue do not usually show areas of color. The presence of blood flow within even small ovarian tumors correlates well with laboratory work showing that angiogenesis occurs in hyperplastic tissue and is important for the conversion of normal epithelium into cancer (Folkman *et al.*, 1989). There is, however, increased vascularity within the ovarian parenchyma in the luteal phase of the cycle, around the time of ovulation and during pregnancy; hence it is suggested that examinations are performed between day 1 and day 8 of the cycle (Bourne *et al.*, 1989).

Duplex Doppler is combined ultrasound imaging with pulsed Doppler. This allows an area of interest to be identified on the B-mode image then examined with pulsed Doppler. Using transvaginal color Doppler to identify small vessels within a lesion, the blood flow characteristics within that vessel may be examined with duplex Doppler. A number of formulas have been used to relate the systolic and diastolic blood flow within a vessel. The pulsatility index (PI) and resistance index (RI) are two such measures and reflect the blood flow impedance distal to the point of sampling. A low PI or RI indicates a low impedance to blood flow in the distal vasculature, as seen in neoplasia; a high PI or RI associated with absent intratumoral neovascularization with color or power Doppler indicates a low risk of ovarian cancer.

It has become clear that transvaginal color Doppler (Figure 20.14) is a valuable method of differentiating benign and malignant ovarian tumors (Bourne et al., 1989; Fleischer et al., 1991; Kurjak et al., 1991). Kurjak and his colleagues found colorflow to be present and the RI to be less than or equal to 0.4 in 54 of 56 malignant adnexal tumors, and no colorflow and an RI higher than 0.4 in 623 of 624 benign adnexal tumors, although others have been unable to reproduce these results. It has been suggested that use of this technology should provide an improved method of selection of those patients suitable for conservative treatment for an ovarian cyst such as cyst aspiration (Editorial, 1990). Perhaps the most important contribution by color

Doppler will prove to be its capacity to demonstrate that a cyst with an adverse feature such as large size, multilocularity or possession of solid areas is likely to be benign.

The normal corpus luteum can closely mimic a solid ovarian tumor. Using color Doppler, however, the typical pericystic luteal blood flow can be seen with great reliability, and if present, may allow one to ignore an otherwise worrying-looking lesion.

Despite all the exaggerated claims and controversy of Doppler for ovarian cysts, it has nevertheless been noted that 'colour Doppler provides interesting insights into tumour pathology and part of the diagnostic picture, but it is still not clear whether it should be used to change the clinical management of patients' (Bourne, 1994).

Power (or amplitude) Doppler uses the Doppler information differently to produce a Doppler image that is direction-independent. It is particularly good at assessing low flow and will therefore be increasingly used in the assessment of ovarian lesions. It is available on many current generation ultrasound machines.

Other Imaging Modalities

Ultrasound remains the imaging method of choice for the assessment of ovarian lesions and in clinical practise other modalities are rarely used. The advantages of ultrasound include its relatively low cost and its high resolution (particularly with transvaginal ultrasound). In addition Doppler provides the ability to assess blood flow, and real-time technology provides great versatility. However, both computerized tomography (CT) and magnetic resonance imaging (MRI) also have a role.

CT provides high-quality images of the ovaries, but does not provide more information than ultrasound (Walsh et al., 1978). Both CT and ultrasound are similarly accurate in evaluating pelvic masses, but CT is better at detecting abdominal metastatic disease since bowel gas interferes with ultrasound images (Sommer et al., 1982).

There are few studies comparing transvaginal ultrasound with MRI, but prospective studies suggest that ultrasound is better than pre-contrast MRI since the latter does not depict the fine internal details as clearly. Contrast-enhanced MRI, however, depicts the internal detail of some lesions and is especially useful for differentiating malignant and benign lesions (Yamashita et al., 1995).

Fat saturation techniques allow the zonal anatomy of normal ovaries to be visualized with the lower signal of the cortex and the high signal

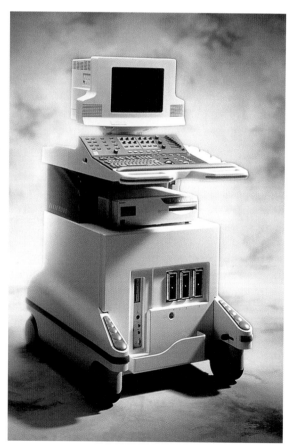

Figure 20.14 Advanced Technology Laboratories color Doppler machine.

intensity of the medulla. Postmenopausal ovaries tend to appear more homogeneous, making them more difficult to see unless they contain small cysts. Small ovarian cysts are visible in most post-menopausal ovaries.

It has been suggested that diagnostic accuracy with contrast-enhanced MRI is better than either pre-contrast MRI or transvaginal ultrasound because of the improved internal details and soft tissue contrast, although ultrasound Doppler techniques may further enhance the accuracy of ultrasound.

Management of the Pelvic Mass

An ultrasound examination by an experienced sonologist using 'state of the art' equipment should be part of the preoperative assessment of patients undergoing laparoscopic surgery for an ovarian cyst. When septations are present it is recommended that a technique is used that avoids rupturing the mass (Levene, 1990). In a report of a survey of ovarian neoplasms that had been treated laparo-scopically Maiman *et al.* (1991) suggested that 'strict uniform sonographic criteria must be adhered to in patient selection for the laparoscopic approach to ovarian masses'.

The 'Simple' Cyst

The management of a patient with a unilocular thin-walled ovarian cyst without any solid areas (and preferably no neovascularization detectable using color Doppler and a high RI depends upon both the size of the cyst and the age of the patient. Spontaneous resolution of a small simple ovarian cyst is common, even in postmenopausal women (Andolf and Jorgensen, 1989). Expectant manage-ment is therefore often appropriate if the cyst is asymptomatic. However, if associated with pain, treatment may become necessary.

Ultrasound-guided cyst aspiration in carefully selected patients has been shown to relieve pain with a low incidence of cyst recurrence (de Crespigny *et al.*, 1989). Aspiration is applicable in a premenopausal woman if the cyst is less than 10 cm, as malignancy is then rare. Surgery is commonly the treatment of choice for an ovarian cyst in a post-menopausal woman, since functional cysts are not expected, but cyst aspiration may sometimes be a reasonable alternative if the cyst is no greater than 5 cm diameter and appears 'simple' using a high-quality transvaginal scanner. Aspirated cyst fluid

should be submitted for cytologic examination and estradiol estimation (i.e. increased serum estradiol concentration), the latter giving support to a diag-nosis of a functional cyst. A follow-up ultrasound examination is advocated to exclude cyst recur-rence. More invasive treatment such as laparo-scopic surgery is indicated in the presence of severe pain since this is uncommon in an uncomplicated cyst or for a recurrent or large cyst. Such an approach allows complete removal, or at least a biopsy of the cyst wall. The ongoing controversy in relation to the role of ultrasound-guided ovarian cyst aspiration must be acknowledged. Although there are many advocates (de Crespigny, 1995), there are others who see no role for this procedure (Nicklin *et al.*, 1994). Careful patient selection is undoubtedly the key to safe aspiration.

Blood-filled Cysts

When fine echoes are visible throughout the cyst, usually indicating a blood-filled cyst, ultrasound-guided aspiration may still be performed; however, not infrequently some or all of the contents may be too viscous to allow aspiration. Cyst aspiration provides pain relief, but recurrence is common, although acceptable results have been obtained with this technique (Giorlandino *et al.*, 1994). Surgery is usually considered to be the treatment of choice.

Other Apparently Benign Cysts

Benign cystic teratomas and cysts with several thin-walled locules are best treated surgically.

Possibly Malignant Cysts

Cysts that show adverse features such as large or multilocular cysts (especially if thick-walled), those with solid areas, those with neovascularization seen with color Doppler and a low RI on duplex Doppler require surgery.

Summary

High-resolution ultrasound equipment has allowed gynecologists to develop a more rational approach to the management of an adnexal mass. This is pos-sible in centers in which 'state of the art' ultrasound equipment is available, including a vaginal transducer and color Doppler, together with an experienced sonologist. No longer can there be any justification in recommending surgery for all pre-menopausal women with a palpable ovarian mass that persists for one month, as advocated in the classic textbook of *Bonney's Gynaecological Surgery* (Howkins and Stallworthy, 1974). Similarly, laparo-tomy and total abdominal hysterectomy and bilateral salpingo-oophorectomy is not necessarily essential for all postmenopausal women with a palpable ovary on clinical examination (Barber and Graber, 1971).

An ultrasound examination should now be part of the diagnostic work-up of an ovarian cyst. A decision can then be made between conservative management, cyst aspiration, laparoscopic surgery or laparotomy depending upon the patient's symp-toms and age, the clinical findings and the ultra-sound features.

References

Adams J, Polson DW, Abdulwahid N *et al.* (1985) Multifollicular ovaries: clinical and endocrine features and response to pulsatile gonatropin releasing hor-mone. *Lancet* **2**: 1375–1378.

Andolf E, Jorgensen C (1988) The prospective comparison of clinical ultrasound and operative examination of the female pelvis. *Journal of Ultrasound in Medicine* **7**: 617–620.

Andolf E, Jorgensen C (1989) Cystic lesions in elderly women diagnosed by ultrasound. *British Journal of Obstetrics and Gynaecology* **96**: 1076–1079.

Athey PA, Malone RS (1987) Sonography of ovarian fibromas/thecomas. *Journal of Ultrasound in Medicine* **6**: 431–436.

Barber HRK, Graber FA (1971) PMBO syndrome (post-menopausal palpable ovary syndrome). *Obstetrics and Gynecology* **38**: 921–923.

Benacerraf BR, Finkler NJ, Wojciechowski C, Knapp RC (1990) Sonographic accuracy in the diagnosis of ovar-ian masses. *Journal of Reproductive Medicine* **35**: 491–495.

Bourne TH (1994) Should clinical decisions be made about ovarian masses using transvaginal colour Doppler? *Ultrasound in Obstetrics and Gynecology* **4**: 357–360.

Bourne T, Campbell S, Steer C, Whitehead MI, Collins WP (1989) Transvaginal colour flow imaging: a possible new screening technique for ovarian cancer. *British Medical Journal* **299**: 1367–1370.

Bourne TH, Campbell S, Reynolds KM *et al.* (1993) Screening for early familial ovarian cancer with trans-vaginal ultrasonography and colour blood flow imag-ing. *British Medical Journal* **306**: 1025–1029.

Bronshtein M, Yoffe N, Brandes JM, Blumenfeld Z (1991) Hair as a sonographic marker of ovarian teratomas: improved identification using transvaginal sonogra-phy and simulation model. *Journal of Clinical Ultrasound* **19**: 351–355.

Campbell S, Bhan V, Royston P, Whitehead MI, Collins WP (1989) Transabdominal ultrasound screening for early ovarian cancer. *British Medical Journal* **299**: 1363–1367.

Campbell S, Royston P, Bran V, Whitehead MI, Collins WP (1990) Novel screening strategies for early ovarian cancer by transabdominal ultrasonography. *British Journal of Obstetrics and Gynaecology* **97**: 304–311.

Coleman BG, Arger PH, Grumbach K *et al.* (1988) Transvaginal and transabdominal sonography: prospective comparison. *Radiology* **168**: 639–643.

Creasman WT, Di Saia PJ (1991) Screening in ovarian cancer. *American Journal of Obstetrics and Gynecology* **165**: 7 10.

de Crespigny L (1988) Demonstration of ectopic preg-nancy with transvaginal ultrasound. *British Journal of Obstetrics and Gynaecology* **95**: 1253–1256.

de Crespigny L (1995) Letter to editor. *Australian and New Zealand Journal of Obstetrics and Gynaecology* **35**: 233–234.

de Crespigny L, Cooper D, McKenna M (1988) Early detection of uterine pregnancy with ultrasound. *Journal of Ultrasound in Medicine* **7**: 7–10.

de Crespigny L, Robinson HP, Davoren RAM, Fortune D (1989) The 'simple' ovarian cyst: aspirate or operate? *British Journal of Obstetrics and Gynaecology* **96**: 1035–1039.

Editorial (1990) First catch your deer. *Lancet* **336**: 147–149.

Fleischer AC, Rogers WH, Rao BK, Kepple DM, Jones HW (1991) Transvaginal color Doppler sonography of ovarian masses with pathological correlation. *Ultrasound in Obstetrics and Gynaecology* **1**: 275–278.

Folkman J, Watson K, Ingber D, Hanahan D (1989) Induction of angiogenesis during the transition from hyperplasia to neoplasia. *Nature* **339**: 58–61.

Giorlandino C, Taramanni C, Muzii L *et al.* (1994) Ultrasound-guided aspiration of ovarian endometri-otic cysts. *Obstetrical and Gynecological Survey* **49**: 249–250.

Goldstein SR (1990) Early pregnancy failure – appropriate terminology. *American Journal of Obstetrics and Gynecology* **163**: 1093.

Goldstein SR, Subramanyam B, Snyder JR *et al.* (1989) The postmenopausal cystic adnexal mass: the potential role of ultrasound in conservative management. *Obstetrics and Gynecology* **73**: 8–10.

Goswamy RK, Campbell S, Royston JP *et al.* (1988) Ovarian size in postmenopausal women. *British Journal of Obstetrics and Gynaecology* **95**: 795–801.

Hall DA, McCarthy KA (1986) The significance of the postmenopausal simple adnexal cyst. *Journal of Ultrasound in Medicine* **5**: 503–505.

Herrmann UJ, Locher GW, Goldhirsch AA (1987) Sonographic patterns of ovarian tumours: prediction of malignancy. *Obstetrics and Gynecology* **69**: 777–781.

Howkins J, Stallworthy J (1974) *Bonney's Gynaecological Surgery*, p. 586. London: Baillière Tindall.

Kivikoski AI, Martin CM, Smeltzer JS (1990) Transabdominal and transvaginal ultrasonography in the diagnosis of ectopic pregnancy: a comparative study. *American Journal of Obstetrics and Gynecology* **163**: 123–128.

Kurjak A, Zulad I, Alfirevic Z (1991) Evaluation of adnexal masses with transvaginal colour ultrasound. *Journal of Ultrasound in Medicine* **10**: 295–297.

Lande IM, Hill MC, Cosco FE, Kator NN (1988) Adnexal and cul-de-sac abnormalities: transvaginal sonography. *Radiology* **166**: 325–332.

Liebman AJ, Kruse B, McSweeney MB (1988) Transvaginal sonography: comparison with transabdominal sonography in the diagnosis of pelvic masses. *American Journal of Roentgenology* **151**: 89–92.

Lerner JP, Timor-Tritsch IE, Federman A, Abramovich G (1994) Transvaginal ultrasonographic characterisation of ovarian masses with an improved weighted scoring system. *American Journal of Obstetrics and Gynecology* **170**: 81–85.

Levene RL (1990) Pelviscopic surgery in women over forty. *Journal of Reproductive Medicine* **35**: 597–600.

Lynch HT, Albano WA, Lynch JF, Lynch PM, Campbell A (1982) Surveillance and management of patients at high genetic risk for ovarian carcinoma. *Obstetrics and Gynecology* **59**: 589–596.

Maiman M, Seltzer V, Boyce J (1991) Laparoscopic excision of ovarian neoplasms subsequently found to be malignant. *Obstetrics and Gynecology* **77**: 563–565.

Meire HB, Farrant P, Guha T (1978) Distinction of benign from malignant ovarian cysts by ultrasound. *British Journal of Obstetrics and Gynaecology* **85**: 893–899.

Moyle JW, Rochester D, Sider L, Shrock K, Krause P (1983) Sonography of ovarian tumours: predictability of tumour type. *American Journal of Roentgenology* **141**: 985–991.

Munn CS, Kiser LC, Wetzner SM, Baer JE (1986) Ovary volume in young and premenopausal adults: US determination. *Radiology* **159**: 731–732.

Nicklin JL, Van Eijkeren M, Athanasatos P *et al.* (1994) A comparison of ovarian cyst aspirate cytology and histology. The case against aspiration of cystic pelvic masses. *Australian and New Zealand Journal of Obstetrics and Gynaecology* **34**: 546–549.

O'Brien WF, Buck DR, Nash JD (1984) Evaluation of sonography in the initial assessment of the gynaecologic patient. *American Journal of Obstetrics and Gynecology* **149**: 598–601.

O'Herlihy C, de Crespigny L, Lopata A *et al.* (1980) Preovulatory follicular size: a comparison of ultrasound and laparoscopic measurements. *Fertility and Sterility* **34**: 24–26.

Outwater EK, Mitchell DG (1996) Normal ovaries and functional cysts: MR appearance. *Radiology* **198**: 397–402.

Paling MR, Shawker JH (1981) Abdominal ultrasound in advanced ovarian carcinoma. *Journal of Clinical Ultrasound* **9**: 435–441.

Reynolds T, Hill MC, Glassman LM (1986) Sonography of haemorrhagic ovarian cysts. *Journal of Clinical Ultrasound* **14**: 449–453.

Sassone AM, Timor–Tritsch IE, Artner A, Westhoff C, Warren WB (1991) Transvaginal sonographic characterization of ovarian disease: evaluation of a new scoring system to predict ovarian malignancy. *Obstetrics and Gynecology* **78**: 70–76.

Scully RE (1982) Minimal cancer of the ovary. *Clinics in Oncology* **1(2)**: 379–387.

Shimizu H, Yamasaki M, Ohama K, Nozaki T, Tanaka Y (1990) Characteristic ultrasonographic appearance of the Krukenberg tumour. *Journal of Clinical Ultrasound* **18**: 697–703.

Sigurdsson K, Alm P, Gullberg B (1983) Prognostic factors in malignant epithelial ovarian tumours. *Gynecologic Oncology* **15**: 370–380.

Sommer FG, Walsh JW, Schwartz PE *et al.* (1982) Evaluation of gynecologic pelvic masses by ultrasound and computed tomography. *Journal of Reproductive Medicine* **27**: 45–50.

Timor-Tritsch IE, Lerner JP, Monteagudo A, Santos R (1993) Transvaginal ultrasonographic characterization of ovarian masses by means of color flow-directed Doppler measurements and morphologic scoring system. *American Journal of Obstetrics and Gynecology* **168**: 909–913.

Walsh JW, Taylor KJW, Wasson JFM (1978) Prospective comparison of ultrasound and computed tomography in the evaluation of gynecologic pelvic masses. *American Journal of Roentgenology* **131**: 955–959.

Webb MJ (1993) Screening for ovarian cancer. Still a long way to go. *British Medical Journal* **306**: 1015–1016.

Westhoff C, Randall MC (1991) Ovarian cancer screening: potential effect on mortality. *American Journal of Obstetrics and Gynecology* **165**: 502–505.

Yamashita Y, Torashima M, Hatanaka Y *et al.* (1995) Adnexal masses: accuracy of characterization with transvaginal ultrasound and pre contrast and post contrast MR imaging. *Radiology* **194**: 557–565.

21

Laparoscopic Ovarian Surgery and Ovarian Torsion

ALAIN J.M. AUDEBERT

Institut Robert B. Greenblatt, Bordeaux, France

Ovarian surgery is one of the most frequently performed laparoscopic procedures (Peterson *et al.*, 1990); in routine practise the increased use of pelvic imaging (sonography) for cases with any gynecologic symptom or as a screening exploration in women at risk explains why more and more ovarian masses are encountered. The diagnostic and therapeutic challenge for the clinician has to be solved in order to provide the best immediate and long-term benefits for the patient.

In trying to simplify the situation, the major objective is to identify:

- The functional ovarian cyst, requiring in most cases no treatment if a rigorous clinical and sonographic observation can be achieved.
- The borderline cases and malignant ovarian neoplasms requiring a conventional and adequate surgical approach by laparotomy.
- The benign ovarian neoplasm for which, under rigorous conditions, there is a major role for a therapeutic approach by laparoscopy.

In fact, at any step in the presently available diagnostic strategy one cannot be sure of the true nature of an ovarian lesion in the absence of a complete pathological report; this means that at any moment one has to be prepared to change the planned therapeutic approach in order to give the patient the best treatment according to the new situation.

Ovarian torsion requires an early diagnosis for conservative treatment and this is easily achieved by laparoscopy.

Oncologic Considerations

Careful selection of appropriate cases for laparoscopic surgery is mandatory because there is a risk of treating an unsuspected ovarian malignancy by laparoscopy. In a recent survey, 42 such cases were reported (Maiman *et al.*, 1991). The main difficulty is the identification of early ovarian cancer, especially in young women. With an advanced lesion the diagnosis is usually suspected before laparoscopy or when the ovarian neoplasm is ultrasonically visualized before any additional procedure is undertaken. The risk of spreading the cancer in the event of rupturing an ovarian malignancy may compromise the patient's survival unless additional cytotoxic therapy is administered (Schwartz, 1991a). However, the literature is controversial; puncture of an ovarian malignancy immediately followed by laparotomy probably bears less risk of dissemination than a spontaneous rupture.

The incidence of malignant epithelial ovarian neoplasms is variable. In northern America and northern Europe the reported rates are close to ten per 100 000 women. The incidence is correlated with the age of the patient. For women aged under 35 years with a 'simple' ovarian cyst the incidence of malignancy is 4.5 per 100 000 women. In cases of unilocular cyst less than 10 cm in diameter the risk of malignancy appears to be very low (Meire *et al.*, 1978).

Borderline ovarian tumors represent 9.2–16.3% of epithelial ovarian neoplasms (Chambers *et al.*, 1988). After ovarian cystectomy the risk of recurrence for stages Ia and Ib is around 10% (Lim-Tan *et*

Table 21.1 Risk factors for ovarian malignancy.

Absence of child, low parity, infertility
Middle or upper socioeconomic class
Caucasian
Age > 50 years
Family history of ovarian, breast or endometrial
cancer
No oral contraceptive use
Regular coffee drinking
Perineal exposure to talcum powder

Table 21.2 Incidence of malignancy in two large series of laparoscopic surgical removal of ovarian neoplasms.

Author	Numbers of cases	Cancer	Borderline	Operated by laparoscopy
Canis *et al.* (1992)	652	6	6	0
Audebert (1994)	700	17	8	2 borderline (intentional)

al., 1988). The reported frequency of microscopic tumors with a grossly normal-appearing contralateral ovary varies from 5–10% (McGowan *et al.*, 1985). Immediate formal surgery in the event of puncturing such a lesion does not seem to hamper the prognosis (Tasker and Langley, 1985).

The known risk factors for ovarian malignancy are listed in Table 21.1.

One large published series of ovarian cysts managed by laparoscopy included 652 cysts (Canis *et al.*, 1992); six ovarian cancers and six borderline malignant neoplasms were identified at the time of the diagnostic laparoscopy and treated immediately by laparotomy (Table 21.2).

Our own data evaluated in November 1994 included 700 adnexal masses, some bilateral lesions; 25 malignant or borderline neoplasms were demonstrated by the pathologic report. Only two patients with borderline tumors were managed by laparoscopy. These patients are carefully and regularly checked and the second ovary was removed in one patient three years later; no evidence of malignancy was detected.

These two important series demonstrate that with a careful approach the risk of operating on an undetected malignancy is very low.

Pre-Laparoscopic Assessment of an Ovarian Mass

The pre-laparoscopic assessment of an ovarian mass is more efficient with the newer developments in pelvic imaging. Abdominal ultrasound and more recently transvaginal ultrasound are the best diagnostic tools presently available. Significant progress has been made in establishing satisfactory guidelines for detecting a suspected malignant ovarian neoplasm in addition to other information (risk factors, age, clinical examination, tumor markers).

The main ultrasound findings suggesting malignancy are size (> 5 cm in diameter), the presence of thick septa, solid parts or papillary projections, bilaterality, indefinite margins and the presence of ascites (Herrmann *et al.*, 1987; Grandberg *et al.*, 1990). Trained operators, using strict ultrasonic criteria are able to predict benign masses accurately in 96% of patients studied (Herrmann *et al.*, 1987). When a clear unilocular cyst is diagnosed by ultrasound, the predictability for benign neoplasms is in the range of 90–95% (Meire *et al.*, 1978; Herrmann *et al.*, 1987). In 152 women aged 50 years or more, no malignancy was detected in pure cystic lesions less than 5 cm in diameter (Andolf and Jorgensen, 1989). In another series of 102 postmenopausal women who had abdominal ultrasonic evaluation of adnexal masses before surgery, a negative predictive value of 94% was established (Luxman *et al.*, 1991), meaning that six of 100 postmenopausal women with a 'simple' cyst may have a malignant tumor; two of 33 patients with a 'simple' cyst smaller than 5 cm in diameter had a malignant ovarian tumor. These controversial results illustrate the limits of the ultrasonic assessment. The diagnostic role of color Doppler sonography has yet to be evaluated in this situation. The subject is covered in more detail in Chapter 20 by Lachlan de Crespigny.

The present serologic markers have a variable specificity according to the nature of the ovarian neoplasm; they are relatively specific for ovarian germ cell malignancies, but these malignancies are rare (Schwartz, 1991b). CA 125 (cancellation of

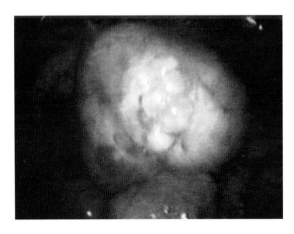

Figure 21.1 External excrescences on the surface of a borderline malignant ovarian neoplasm.

antigen) is the most commonly used marker for epithelial ovarian neoplasms. Its poor sensitivity and specificity limit its use except in post-menopausal women. In this group of patients an elevated CA 125 in association with any other positive diagnostic test has a positive predictive value approaching 100%. When used alone, CA 125 has a positive predictive value of 36% for pre-menopausal women and 87% for postmenopausal women with pelvic masses (Finkler *et al.*, 1988). In serous subtypes of epithelial ovarian neoplasms CA 125 is the most appropriate marker and is found to be elevated in approximately 85% of ovarian cancers of this type (Morgensen *et al.*, 1989).

If the role of ultrasonography in diagnosing suspected malignancy is important, a common practical question to be answered in the case of a unilocular cyst identified in a young woman by ultrasonography is 'Is it a functional ovarian cyst?' When uncomplicated, these cysts frequently undergo spontaneous resolution and do not need any form of treatment. In women with a persisting ovarian cyst submitted to laparoscopy the incidence of functional cysts varies from 16–43.5%. Every effort should be made to reduce this incidence. On some occasions the cyst may be aspirated under ultrasound control in order to obtain cytologic confirmation; this procedure has to be performed with caution because cytologic examination of cystic fluid is frequently unreliable. In a series of 59 ovarian cysts the sensitivity and specificity of cytology alone was 67% and 91%, respectively (Diernaes *et al.*, 1987). Cytologic examination of fluid of 35 functional cysts was found to be concordant with the pathologic examination in only 22 cases (Abeille *et al.*, 1988); the risks of failing to identify an ovarian malignancy and implantation of malignant cells along the needle track have to be further evaluated. Cyst fluid can be used to determine the concentration of steroids and tumor markers: in functional cysts steroid concentrations are elevated and CA 125 concentrations are usually low (Abeille *et al.*, 1988). A combination of these various tests with the gross appearance of the fluid allows a correct diagnosis to be established in most cases. Ultrasound-guided cystoscopy with a 0.5 mm scope is presently being evaluated. At present transvaginal ultrasonography appears to be the most accurate tool for predicting which masses are benign and which are malignant (Maiman, 1994). It must be remembered that palpatation of an asymptomatic adnexal mass during routine pelvic examination is still the most common method of detecting early-stage ovarian cancer.

Laparoscopic Assessment of an Ovarian Neoplasm

Before any procedure, any ovarian neoplasm to be treated by operative laparoscopy has to be carefully assessed according to a predefined protocol (Table 21.3):

1. The first procedure is inspection and aspiration of fluid in the pouch of Douglas for cytology before any contamination.
2. The surface of the pelvic and abdominal peritoneum is then carefully exposed for a thorough and complete visual examination with a probe; the same procedure is performed for the digestive tract, the omentum and the liver. Some lesions may provide the diagnosis (endometriotic implants) or directly lead to a laparotomy.
3. The ovarian surface of both ovaries is scrutinized and other masses originating from the tube (hydrosalpinx) or the paraovarian region (vestigial cyst) are identified. External papillary projections are easily detected. Ovarian connections with surrounding structures are determined; if there are adhesions partially or totally obscuring the ovary a gentle adhesiolysis may first be necessary. Lengthening of the utero-ovarian ligament is usually an indirect sign of a non-functional ovarian cyst. At this stage one has to be able to identify a malignant or borderline malignant ovarian neoplasm indicating immediate laparotomy. If this is not necessary, additional diagnostic procedures are then performed.
4. The ovary is gently grasped with a forceps and mobilized in order to select the most appropriate site for puncture (Figure 21.2), preferentially at the apex of the cyst and at a distance from the ovarian blood supply. If internal papillary projections have been eliminated by the ultrasonic examination, a fine needle can be used to aspirate the fluid content, avoiding any spillage, and identification according to its characteristics frequently orienting the diagnosis when typical. In a series of 144 cases the macroscopic appearance of

Table 21.3 Laparoscopic assessment of ovarian neoplasms: procedures performed systematically (benign neoplasm)

Aspiration of peritoneal fluid for cytology
Inspection of the abdominal cavity, omentum, liver
Inspection of ovarian surface and ovarian ligaments
Puncture of the ovarian cyst
Cystoscopy
Frozen sections

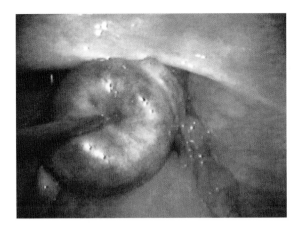

Figure 21.2 Puncture of a benign ovarian cyst.

the cystic fluid correlated with the pathological report in 82% of the cases (Abeille *et al.*, 1988).

5. If a 'cystoscopy' is planned it is better to introduce an appropriate trocar directly into the cyst for aspiration and lavage with a cannula, then replace by the small endoscope to visualize all the internal surface of the cystic wall (Figure 21.3) and look for any excrescence. Another possibility is to enlarge the site of puncture with scissors and expose the interior of the cyst with two grasping forceps. Any suspicious lesion may halt the laparoscopic procedure, except lavage of the pouch of Douglas (which theoretically contains 60 ml), and a laparotomy is immediately performed. In some cases, if it is preferable to remove an intact cyst or the whole ovary, no puncture is performed before the excision procedure. In other cases absolute identification of the nature of the ovarian neoplasm is impossible.

6. It is then recommended that frozen sections are taken for accurate diagnosis.

At the end of this diagnostic stage any evident or suspected malignancy of the ovarian neoplasm must have been excluded in order to proceed with a laparoscopic treatment. In our series of 700 adnexal masses, the 25 malignant or borderline malignant ovarian neoplasms were correctly identified; three other patients who were operated on by laparotomy because of a high suspicion of malignancy were found to have a benign lesion on pathologic examination.

In another report of 652 ovarian cysts, 6 malignant lesions were recorded and immediately treated by laparotomy; in 6 other cases a laparotomy was performed for benign neoplasm thought to be malignant at the time of the laparoscopic assessment (Canis *et al.*, 1992). In a previous series by the same authors the positive predictive diagnosis of being benign was accurate in all cases (100% specificity); the sensitivity for diagnosing a malignant lesion was also 100% (Mage *et al.*, 1987). The correlation between laparoscopic presumptive diagnosis and pathologic examination is not as good, with a correct identification in only 80% of the cases.

Only macroscopic benign-appearing neoplasm will be treated by laparoscopy (unilocular lesions, cysts with a smooth wall). Severe dense adhesions may oblige the surgeon to perform a laparotomy on some occasions, but this is not specific for ovarian surgery. This indicates that all patients have initially to give their consent to a laparotomy in case it is required. All benign ovarian neoplasms can be treated by laparoscopy, including ovarian endometriomas and teratomas (Nezhat *et al.*, 1989), depending upon the experience of the operator and the use of appropriate technique. During the past three years we, like others, have been able to remove all ovarian endometriomas (> 100) and teratomas (25 cases) by laparoscopy.

Laparoscopic Ovarian Surgery

We include only major procedures with complete intraperitoneal removal or destruction of the ovarian neoplasm as laparoscopic ovarian surgery and exclude simple ovarian puncture and biopsy or excision of part of a cyst wall (fenestration), which we consider to be diagnostic.

General Principles

All of the general principles described for laparoscopic surgery are applied for ovarian surgery including:

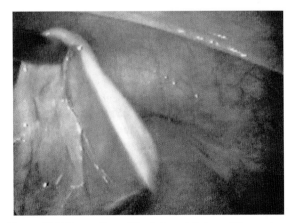

Figure 21.3 Inspection of the internal lining of the cyst

- Proper selection and preoperative counselling of patients.
- General endotracheal anesthesia.
- Urinary drainage with a Foley catheter.
- Capability to perform immediate laparotomy if necessary.
- Uterine manipulator placed inside the uterus.
- Experience in operative laparoscopy.

Equipment

Mandatory equipment for laparoscopic ovarian surgery includes:

- A video camera and monitor system.
- A high-flow controlled insufflator.
- Bipolar cautery forceps and generator.
- A suction and irrigating system.
- A needle for suction, laparoscopic scissors and grasping forceps.
- An 11-mm grasping forceps for extraction of excised tissues.
- Endoscopic sutures and endoscopic stapling device.
- A monopolar instrument for cutting or laser.
- A small endoscope for 'ovarian cytoscopy'.
- Biologic tissue glue.

The last two in this list are still undergoing development and evaluation.

Technique of Ovarian Cystectomy

The technique of ovarian cystectomy has been previously described in detail (Bruhat *et al.*, 1989; Johns, 1991), so we will only focus on certain aspects. With possible malignancy having been certainly ruled out, the ovary is gently mobilized with grasping forceps, on some occasions after preliminary adhesiolysis. The size and the intraovarian location of the cyst are determined in order to select the proper site for the incision of the ovarian albuginea. The ideal site is the antimesenteric portion of the ovary, away from the blood vessels of the hilus.

Two different approaches can be used depending upon whether a previous puncture and cystoscopy have been performed: in the case of puncture, the opening is enlarged with scissors, unipolar electrode or laser and the cyst wall grasped (Figure 21.4), the ovary being stabilized by another pair of grasping forceps. The length of the incision is adapted to the size of the cyst. The cystic wall is then progressively and gently stripped from the ovary (Figure 21.5). The ease with which this procedure can be performed depends upon the strength of the wall (functional cysts are usually very

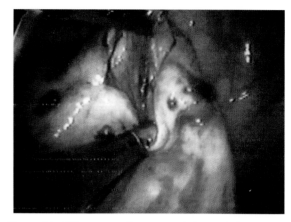

Figure 21.4 The cyst wall is grasped through the ovarian incision.

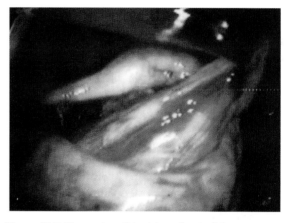

Figure 21.5 The cyst wall is stripped out of the ovary.

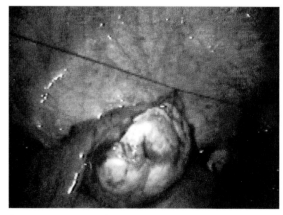

Figure 21.6 Suture of the ovary after cystectomy.

smooth) and its adherence to the adjacent ovarian cortex. On some occasions, excision of the adjacent ovarian cortex is necessary. Hemostasis is attained when necessary with fine bipolar forceps.

The dissection can also be achieved with a laser or facilitated by aquadissection with an irrigating probe. The ovarian wound is irrigated and hemostasis completed when necessary. The ovarian

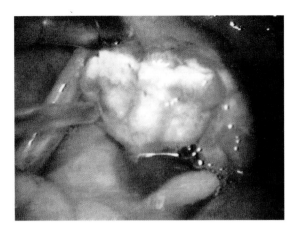

Figure 21.7 End result after suture of the ovary.

incision can be left open or approximated by three techniques: fine monofilament suture of the edges (Figures 21.6, 21.7), tissue glue or coagulation of the ovarian cortex adjacent to the surface, which will in some instances evert the opening. The excised tissue is removed from the abdominal cavity through an adapted trocar (11 mm sleeve in most cases) with strong grasping forceps. Fragmentation with scissors or a tissue morcellator is performed if the amount of tissue is excessive. Lavage of the pelvis and aspiration of all debris with warmed Ringer's lactate completes the procedure as hemostasis is re-checked by underwater inspection. A large volume of warmed Ringer's lactate is left *in situ* to reduce the risk of postoperative adhesion formation. The solution should stay clear, otherwise the pelvis should be irrigated again.

When the ovarian cyst has not been punctured, the same procedures can be applied with great care to avoid rupture of the cyst wall. The ovarian incision is larger in this case. This technique is preferred if leakage of cystic fluid is not advisable, as with a teratoma or mucinous cyst. The cyst can be removed from the abdominal cavity, although not always easily, through an enlarged abdominal incision used to introduce one of the trocars or through a colpotomy incision. Another possibility is to aspirate the cyst contents and to fragment the cyst which is first placed in a plastic bag held by two grasping forceps. Properly done this procedure avoids any spillage and may be safer than the other techniques when unexpected rupture of the cyst can occur at the time of removal if the incision is not large enough.

In all the cases the removed tissues are submitted for pathologic evaluation.

Both techniques have advantages and disadvantages (Table 21.4). The removal of an intact ('closed' technique) cyst with 'in bag' extraction is the recommended technique, especially in older women and for all cysts containing peritoneal-irritating fluid.

Destruction of the Ovarian Cyst Lining *in situ*

This method is usually used when stripping out the wall cyst is difficult and when there is definitely no suspected malignancy (endometrioma, functional cyst). Contrary to some authors (Donnez, 1989; Fayez and Vogel, 1991), however, we avoid this procedure if possible because only a part of the cyst wall can be evaluated by the pathologist.

The top of the cyst is removed, the content of the cyst is aspirated and irrigated, and the whole surface of the lining is carefully inspected. Ablation is then attained with any type of laser or by bipolar coagulation; for large cysts it is not always easy to expose the whole surface properly and this is mandatory to reduce the risk of recurrence, especially in the case of endometrioma. One has to be very careful when the cyst is adherent to the pelvic wall to avoid damaging underlying structures. The depth of destruction must be accurately determined beforehand for the selected method. It is then important to check that hemostasis has been achieved and that ablation of the wall cyst is fully attained.

Table 21.4 Advantages and disadvantages of the two techniques of cystectomy.

	Advantages	Disadvantages
Punctured cyst	Smaller ovarian incision No size limit Faster to perform Easy extraction	Spillage of fluid content
Intact cyst	No fluid spillage	Larger ovarian incision Size limit Longer to perform Accidental rupture Extraction more difficult

Laparoscopic Oophorectomy

Laparoscopic oophorectomy or salpingo-oophor-ectomy are preferred when the cyst fills the ovary and in postmenopausal women. The first report was published in 1979 (Semm, 1979). The availability of endoscopic sutures and stapling devices has facilitated this type of laparoscopic surgery.

It is important to mobilize the ovary or the adnexa to evaluate whether the vessels are easily exposed and skeletonized at a sufficient distance from the pelvic wall and to facilitate identification of important structures such as the ureter through the peritoneum. If the ovary cannot be mobilized sufficiently, an irrigating probe is passed into the retroperitoneal space through a small incision in an avascular area of the anterior leaf of the broad ligament; the peritoneum is dissected away from the sidewall by Ringer's lactate.

The skeletonized infundibulopelvic vessels and utero-ovarian ligaments are ligated with Endoknot suture or application of clips and transected. The pedicles have to be checked; it is safer in addition to apply an Endoloop suture. An alternative method is the use of bipolar coagulation (Figure 21.8) or thermocoagulation. The forceps are carefully applied on the pedicles at a safe distance from the sidewall. When proper desiccation has been obtained the pedicles are transected; we preferentially use this technique.

If the fallopian tube is to be removed the same approach is applied. Hemostasis is inspected and completed. The removal is performed as previously described. Irrigation and lavage of the pelvic cavity complete the procedure.

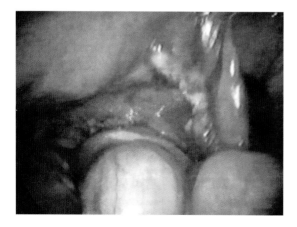

Figure 21.8 Laparoscopic oophorectomy with bipolar coagulation technique.

Complications

As in other surgical laparoscopic procedures various complications may occur, but are rarely reported in the literature.

During the operation uncontrolled bleeding, injury to other structures, or unsuccessful removal will require adequate treatment by laparotomy. In our experience and in another series (Mage *et al.*, 1987), with a combined number of cases close to 1000, no such complication was encountered. In a prospective study comparing different methods for treating 124 ovarian endometriomas, no intraoperative complication was recorded (Fayez and Vogel, 1991). Laparotomy was performed only for unsuspected malignant neoplasm identified at the time of the laparoscopy.

Rupture of the cyst with spillage of its fluid content may be deleterious with mucinous lesions, teratomas or endometriomas.

In order to avoid postoperative adhesion formation or peritonitis a long and meticulous lavage is required until the irrigation solution is completely clear. Subsequent abdominal pain and ovarian abscess have been reported (Mage *et al.*, 1987). The occlusive syndrome and postoperative hemorrhage may also occur.

The incidence of postoperative adhesion has been properly evaluated only for endometriomas. Adhesions are statistically more frequent with excision techniques (100%) than with stripping of the lining (37%), laser ablation (30%) or drainage (27%) (Fayez and Vogel, 1991). For other types of ovarian neoplasms it is difficult to gather a sufficient number of second-look laparoscopies. Excluding endometriomas, the fertility after laparoscopic management of ovarian cysts is satisfactory: 34 (89.5%) of 38 patients wishing conception had a subsequent pregnancy (Canis *et al.*, 1992). Recurrence of the cyst is also more frequent with endometriomas; it has not been proved that complementary medical treatment following the laparoscopy reduces the risk.

In a prospective study of 700 adnexal masses we have evaluated the feasibility of ovarian laparoscopic surgery (Audebert, 1994). After exclusion of laparotomies for oncologic reasons, the global rate of conversion into laparotomies was 2.9% for patients and 3.1% for cysts. The rate of conversion was higher for endometriomas (6.2%) and dermoid cysts (14.7%). The main reasons for conversion into laparotomy were adhesions and the need for a microsurgical approach to better preserve fertility potential in cases with large bilateral lesions. Size of the cyst, pregnancy and adnexal torsion accounted for only a few cases. No laparotomy was required for a peroperative complication. Thus the laparoscopic approach can properly treat more than 90% of ovarian cysts depending upon the type of patient selected by any one center to undergo laparoscopy.

Laparoscopic Treatment of Ovarian Torsion

Acute abdominal pain originating from the ovary is due in most cases to an ovarian abscess, intracystic hemorrhage, with or without rupture, or ovarian torsion, which is rare and may also be associated with subacute or chronic pain. Ultrasonography may help the diagnosis with a predictive value of 88% (Graif and Itzchak, 1988); laparoscopy is promptly indicated for early diagnosis and treatment and possibly salvage of the ovary (Manhès *et al.*, 1984).

Usually ovarian torsion is due to an abnormality of the adnexa (ovarian cyst, ectopic pregnancy, paraovarian cyst or long utero-ovarian ligament).

Untwisting the ovary or the adnexa is simply attained with a blunt probe or grasping forceps. Conservative treatment is preferred when the condition of the tissues appears favorable, but tissue necrosis indicates a need for complete removal.

Causal factors must be adequately treated as previously described. It is not always easy to identify the causal abnormality when ischemia is present. The utero-ovarian ligament can be shortened if indicated by laparoscopy using the same techniques used by laparotomy; ovarian fixation can be achieved by adequate suturing with two endoscopic needle holders and fine monofilament suture.

Second-look laparoscopy a few weeks later is mandatory when conservative treatment has been provided for severe lesions (Bruhat *et al.*, 1989).

After conservative treatment normal follicular development has been observed in 94.2% of cases (Shalev *et al.*, 1995).

The risk of recurrence was 10% in a series of 40 treated patients followed during a period varying from ten months to 12 years (Manhès *et al.*, 1984).

Conclusion

The great majority of benign ovarian neoplasms can be properly treated laparoscopically. The advantages of laparoscopic surgery are now well established, but such surgery requires adequate instrumentation and training.

Laparoscopic operative techniques for ovarian neoplasms are now standardized and the results compare favorably with surgery by laparotomy.

Careful selection of patients is necessary to exclude malignant neoplasms requiring conventional treatment by laparotomy. A fear of missing a diagnosis of malignancy dictates a policy of meticulous evaluation until laparoscopic treatment is indicated. However, guidelines have still to be established and validated.

References

Abeille JP, Mintz M, Pez JP (1988) Intérêt de certains dosages dans les liquides des kystes annexiels: à propos de 144 cas. *Contraception Fertilité Sexualité* **16**: 3315–3320.

Andolf E, Jorgensen C (1989) Cystic lesions in elderly women, diagnosed by ultrasound. *British Journal of Obstetrics and Gynaecology* **96**: 1076–1079.

Audebert AJM (1994) Les limites techniques du traitement coeliochirurgical des kystes annexiels – à propos d'une série de 700 kystes. *JOBGYN* **2**: 409–414.

Bruhat MA, Mage G, Pouly JL *et al.* (1989) *Coélioscopie Opératoire*, Vol. 1. Paris: Medsci/McGraw-Hill.

Canis M, Mage G, Wattiez A *et al.* (1992) Résultats à court terme et long terme après traitement coélioscopique des kystes de l'ovaire. *Contraception Fertilité Sexualité* (In press).

Chambers JT, Merino MJ, Kohorn EI, Schwartz PE (1988) Borderline ovarian tumors. *American Journal of Obstetrics and Gynecology* **159**: 1088–1094.

Diernaes E, Rasmussen J, Soerensen T, Hasch E (1987) Ovarian cyst management by puncture. *Lancet* **1**: 1084.

Donnez J (1989) *Laser Operative Laparoscopy and Hysteroscopy*, Vol. 1. Leuven, Belgium: Nauwelaerts Printing.

Fayez JA, Vogel MF (1991) Comparison of different treatment methods of endometriomas by laparoscopy. *Obstetrics and Gynecology* **78**: 661–665.

Finkler NJ, Benacerreraf B, Lavin PT, Wojciechowski C, Knapp RC (1988) Comparison of serum CA 125, clinical impression and ultrasound in the preoperative evaluation of ovarian masses. *Obstetrics and Gynecology* **72**: 659–664.

Gabriel R, Quereux C, Wahl P (1989) Kystes fonctionnels de l'ovaire. *Encyclopédie Médico-Chirugicale (Paris-France), Gynécologie* **158**: A10,7-1989, 4 p.

Graif M, Itzchak Y (1988) Sonographic evaluation of ovarian torsion in childhood and adolescence. *American Journal of Roentgenology* **150**: 647–649.

Grandberg S, Norstrom A, Wikland A (1990) Tumors in the pelvis as imaged by vaginal sonography. *Gynecologic Oncology* **37**: 224.

Herrmann UJ, Locher GW, Goldhirsch A (1987) Sonographic patterns of malignancy: prediction of malignancy. *Obstetrics and Gynecology* **69**: 777–781.

Johns A (1991) Laparoscopic oophorectomy/oophorocystectomy. *Clinical Obstetrics and Gynecology* **34**: 460–466.

Lim-Tan SK, Cajigas HE, Scully RE (1988) Ovarian cyst-ectomy for serous borderline tumors: a follow-up study of 35 cases. *Obstetrics and Gynecology* **72**: 775–780.

Luxman D, Bergman A, Sagi J, David MP (1991) The post-menopausal adnexal mass: correlation between ultrasonic and pathologic findings. *Obstetrics and Gynecology* **77**: 726–728.

Mage G, Canis M, Manhès H, Pouly JL, Bruhat MA (1987) Kystes ovariens et coélioscopie – A propos de 226 observations. *Journal de Gynécologie, Obstétrique et Biologie de la Reproduction* **16**: 1053–1061.

Maiman M (1994) Laparoscopic removal of the adnexal mass: the case for caution. *Clinical Obstetrics and Gynecology* **38**: 370–379.

Maiman M, Seltzer V, Boyce J (1991) Laparoscopic excision of ovarian neoplasms subsequently found to be malignant. *Obstetrics and Gynecology* **77**: 563–565.

Manhès H, Canis M, Mage G, Pouly JL, Bruhat MA (1984) Place de la coélioscopie dans le diagnostic et le traite-ment des torsions d'annexes. *Journal de Gynécologie, Obstétrique et Biologie de la Reproduction* **13**: 825–829.

McGowan L, Lesher LP, Norris HJ *et al.* (1985) Misstaging of ovarian cancer. *Obstetrics and Gynecology* **65**: 568–572.

Meire HB, Farrant P, Gutha T (1978) Distinction of benign from malignant ovarian cysts by ultrasound. *British Journal of Obstetrics and Gynaecology* **85**: 893.

Morgensen O, Morgensen B, Jakobsen A, Sell A (1989) Perioperative measurement of cancer antigen (CA-125) in the differential diagnosis of ovarian tumors. *Acta Oncologica* **28**: 471–473.

Nezhat C, Winer WK, Nezhat F (1989) Laparoscopic removal of dermoid cysts. *Obstetrics and Gynecology* **73**: 278–280.

Peterson H, Hulka J, Phillips J (1990) American Association of Gynecologic Laparoscopists 1988 mem-bership survey on operative laparoscopy. *Journal of Reproductive Medicine* **35**: 587–589.

Schwartz PE (1991a) An oncologic view of when to do endoscopic surgery. *Clinical Obstetrics and Gynecology* **34**: 467–472.

Schwartz PE (1991b) Ovarian masses: serologic markers. *Clinical Obstetrics and Gynecology* **34**: 423–432.

Semm K (1979) Changes in the classic gynecologic surgery: review of 3,300 pelviscopies in 1971–1976. *International Journal of Fertility* **24**: 13–18.

Shalev E, Bustan M, Yarom I, Peleg D (1995) Recovery of ovarian function after laparoscopic detorsion. *Human Reproduction* **10**: 2965–2966.

Tasker M, Langley FA (1985) The outlook for women with borderline epithelial tumours of the ovary. *British Journal of Obstetrics and Gynaecology* **92**: 969–976.

22

Laparoscopic Treatment of Ovarian Endometriomas

IVO BROSENS* AND CHRIS SUTTON†

*Leuven Institute for Fertility and Embryology, Belgium
†Royal Surrey County Hospital, Guildford, The Chelsea and Westminster Hospital, London and
Imperial College School of Medicine, University of London, UK

How the Endometrial Cyst of the Ovary was Discovered

It took more than 20 years before a specific type of hematoma of the ovary was recognized as an endometrial cyst (Benagiano and Brosens, 1991). The first case of such an ovarian endometrial cyst was described by Russel in 1899 in a premenopausal woman who underwent surgery for a cystic adeno-carcinoma of the left ovary in whom the right ovary was 'enveloped in adhesions of the posterior face of the broad ligament'. On microscopic examination Russel was 'astonished to find areas which were an exact prototype of uterine glands and interglandu-lar connective tissue'. Another case, which can be rec-ognized as ovarian endometriosis is that of Casler (1919), who described the presence of 'uterine mucosa in remaining ovary' after hysterectomy. In the discussion that followed Casler's presentation to the American Gynecological Society, Norris (1921) reported a case of a 29-year-old woman who under-went surgery for severe pelvic pain. On gross exam-ination the 'ovary showed a number of adhesions' and on histologic examination an area of endo-metrium about 6–7 mm in diameter was found. The endometrium of the ovary was similar to that removed from the uterus by curettage and was of the same cyclic change. However, despite these accurate descriptions it took more than two decades before the pathogenesis of the cysts, which were described as 'hemorrhagic cysts or hematomas of the ovary' was elucidated (Sampson, 1921).

The evidence that the perforating hemorrhagic cyst was of endometrial origin was based on the observations that the lining of the cyst was similar to endometrial tissue and that in two patients who underwent surgery at the time of the menstrual period, the histologic changes in the ovarian 'endometrial' tissue corresponded to the phase of the menstrual cycle. Both structural and functional features therefore indicated the endometrial origin of these cysts. It is therefore not surprising that the endometrioma has been described as a pseudo-uterine cavity. As in the uterus, the vessels of free superficial implants with a surface epithelium show cyclic changes that fully correspond with the vascular changes in the upper functional layer of eutopic endometrium, including menstrual flow (Nieminen, 1962).

The escape of chocolate-colored fluid while free-ing the ovary from adhesions and the identification of endometrial implants with the full characteristics of superficial endometrium at the site of perforation led Sampson (1921) to belief that perforation of these cysts was a frequent phenomenon, leading to spilling, adhesions and spread of peritoneal endometriosis.

From serial sections of endometriotic ovaries Hughesdon (1957) demonstrated that in 90% of the cases the endometriotic cyst wall consisted of ovarian cortex, as demonstrated by the presence of primordial follicles (Figure 22.1). This observation supported a surface origin of the lesions by implan-tation or metaplasia and subsequent invagination of the ovarian cortex. The so-called site of perforation, as described by Sampson, represents the stigma of invagination. These findings contradict Sampson's

Figure 22.1 Diagram of a typical ovarian endometrioma. The wall is the inverted or inner cortex, which is lined by endometrial tissue, and the pseudocyst is sealed off at the site of inversion by retraction and adhesions (Hughesdon, 1957). (By courtesy of Brosens and Gordon, *Tubal Infertility*, Gower Medical Publishing.)

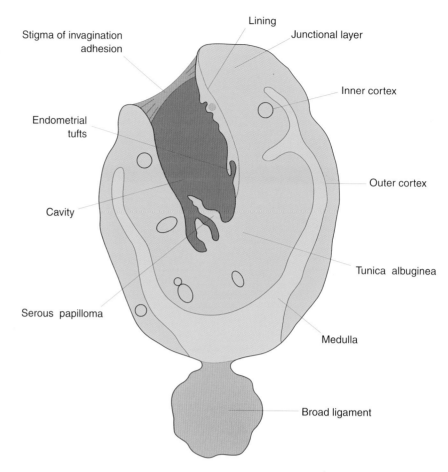

original hypothesis and suggest that adhesions are not the consequence, but the cause of endometrioma formation by sealing off active implants on the surface of the ovary. In fact when Sampson in 1927 formulated the hypothesis that peritoneal endometriosis was due to the menstrual dissemination of endometrial tissue into the peritoneal cavity, he came to suggest that the endometrial cyst of the ovary 'can be explained . . . by endometrial tissue developing on the surface of the ovary caused adhesions . . . which fused the ovary to the uterus and an endometrial cavity developed in this situation'. The potential role of the adhesions in the formation of the endometrioma was well recognized by Sampson when he formulated his classic theory on the pathogenesis of endometriosis.

Surgical Pathology

Macroscopic Features

The endometrioma has typical features, which make the visual diagnosis very reliable with a sensitivity, specificity and accuracy of 97%, 95% and 96%, respectively (Vercellini *et al.*, 1990). These features include:

- Size not more than 12 cm in diameter.
- Adhesions to the pelvic sidewall and/or the posterior broad ligament.
- 'Powder burns' and minute red or blue spots with adjacent puckering on the surface of the ovary.
- Tarry, thick chocolate-colored fluid content.

In contrast with other ovarian cysts the walls of the small endometrioma do not usually collapse after opening the cyst, and in the absence of fibrosis have the pearl-white appearance of ovarian cortex (Figure 22.2). Removal of the walls can be difficult, but with persistence they can be removed completely by segments. Large ovarian endometriomas are characteristically adherent to the posterior side of the uterus or broad ligament or the lateral pelvic wall. Adhesiolysis often results in opening of the cyst and spilling of the chocolate content. Removal of a large cyst from the underlying ovarian stroma is relatively easy except at the site where the capsule is adherent (Nezhat *et al.*, 1992). At this site the adhesions are often very dense and in the absence of a plane of cleavage, removal can be difficult.

Microscopic Features

In small endometriomas the endometrial lining is easily identified by the presence of a surface epithelium with

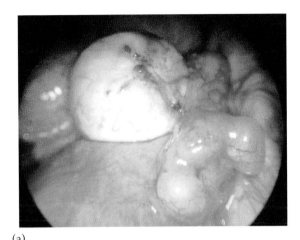

(a)

(b)

Figure 22.2 (a) A typical small endometrioma with the puckered scar closing the invagination of the ovarian cortex. The ovary is rotated and manipulated to rest on the anterior side of the uterus exposing the anterior face. (b) The inside wall is ovarian cortex, which has a slightly pigmented appearance.

stroma. Large endometriomas, however, are rarely completely lined by endometrial tissue and the endometrial layer is rarely typical glandular endometrium. Biopsies from the wall can therefore show different linings, which are all compatible with endometriosis, such as ovarian cortex, fibroreactive tissue with hemosiderin-laden macrophages and endometrial surface epithelium with or without stroma. Foci with glandular endometrium occur at or about the stigma of inversion (Sampson 1921; Brosens *et al.*, 1994).

These microscopic features explain the late discovery of the endometrial cyst:

- First, the endometrial layer rarely completely lines a large hemorrhagic cyst.
- Second, the endometrial layer in most areas represents not more than an epithelium with or without stroma and glandular endometrium is found in a few sites only.

- Third, the foci with glandular endometrium occur at the site of adhesions in small niches, which are frequently destroyed during adhesiolysis of the ovary.

Association with Luteal Cysts

It is well known that large endometriomas are frequently multilocular and that luteal cysts pose a diagnostic and surgical problem. Excisional specimens of presumed large endometriomas are frequently revealed to be luteal (unilocular) or combined with an endometrial (multilocular) cyst at microscopic examination (Table 22.1). In the multilocular endometrioma the luteal cyst can be found separate or communicating with the endometrial cyst (Sampson, 1921). The combination of luteal and endometrial cysts therefore poses a specific diagnostic and surgical problem for large (> 3 cm) unilocular and multilocular hemorrhagic cysts.

Table 22.1 Excisional specimens of presumed endometriomas showing luteal lining.

Authors	Number	Percentage
Martin and Berry (1990)	41	27%
Nezhat *et al.* (1992)	216	33%*

*8% combined with endometrial lining

Classification

The terminology of deep endometriosis used in the American Fertility Society's revised classification of endometriosis (1985) is inappropriate for the majority of endometriomas in which endometrial tissue is not invading the ovary, but only colonizing the wall of a pseudocystic structure such as the inverted cortex. The presence of adhesions is also an essential feature of endometriosis and an important factor in determining the function of the ovary. In addition, the size of the cyst has less bearing on the operability in reconstructive surgery than the extent of adhesions (Canis *et al.*, 1992).

Pre-operative Imaging of Ovarian Tumors

Ultrasound

It is vital to have reliable information on the pelvic mass before proceeding to laparoscopic ovarian surgery and one must be as certain as possible that the mass does not have any of the ultrasonic features of malignancy (see below). Ovarian ultrasound requires special expertise and the best results are obtained by using high-resolution equipment, but also requires considerable expertise in interpreting the images, which is not widely available except at referral centers.

The most important advance in the diagnosis of pelvic pathology using ultrasound has been the development of the endovaginal transducer. Not only does this avoid the necessity of requiring the patient to have a full bladder to provide optimum imaging of the ovaries, but it provides improved resolution since the transducer is closer to the area under investigation. A more recent development has been the introduction of color Doppler, which will demonstrate the presence or absence of neovascularization in the wall of the cyst, which helps to determine whether a cyst is benign or malignant.

The main way of differentiating an ovarian from a non-ovarian pelvic mass is to visualize a normal ovary separate from the mass. Thus, if an ovary is moved by a vaginal ultrasound transducer an extra-ovarian mass will usually not move with it. The shape of the ovary is also important, and if the ovary is visible adjacent to the mass, but has its normal ovoid shape, then the mass is likely to be extra-ovarian, but if the ovary is flattened around the mass, then it is usually ovarian. In practise it can sometimes be difficult to differentiate a hydrosalpinx from an ovarian cyst, but if the tube is examined at different angles, then the tortuous shape of the dilated tube can usually be identified and its epithelial infolding noted.

The presence of fine echoes throughout the cyst fluid usually indicates that blood is present, either as a result of hemorrhage into the cyst or endometriosis. The viscosity of the hemosiderin-laden material will give rise to dense or fine echoes in an endometrioma, depending on the echo density of the fluid. It is important to note, however, that not all blood-filled cysts contain such echoes and not all cysts with uniform echoes contain blood (de Crespigny et al., 1989). Equally it is important to realize that the ultrasonic appearance of an echogenic cystic structure is not pathognomonic of an endometrioma (Schwarz and Seifer, 1992). The reader is referred to Chapter 20 on laparoscopic ovarian surgery: preoperative diagnosis and imaging by Lachlan de Crespigny.

Magnetic Resonance Imaging (MRI)

Initial studies of MRI with endometriosis proved disappointing, but if its use is limited to women with adnexal masses, the sensitivity, specificity and predictive accuracy of this technique for the identification of endometriomas are 90%, 98% and 96%, respectively (Togashi et al., 1991). As with ultrasonography, the appearance of endometriosis on MRI is not pathognomonic, but this technique may be valuable for identifying endometriosis obscured by pelvic adhesions, particularly those involving the bowel. It may also be a valuable method for monitoring the response to medical therapy once the diagnosis has been more securely established (Sawin et al., 1989, 1990).

In the future MRI promises to offer improved diagnosis of some forms of ovarian endometriosis. Ovarian endometriomas show up with a high signal on T1 and T2 sequences because of the blood and the diagnosis can be further refined by additional sequences such as STIR (fat saturation) sequences, which suppress signals from fat in the pelvis, since fat can also give high signals on T1 sequences. Visualization can also be improved by oral and rectal magnetic contrast to eliminate high signals from the bowel (see Chapter 20).

Exclusion of Malignancy

The most important reason for performing preoperative ultrasound is to exclude any features of malignancy, particularly with multilocular endometriomas, and those with thick septa or solid areas within the cyst are more likely to be malignant. An effort should be made to make a tissue diagnosis by fine-needle aspiration or ultrasonically-guided biopsy before embarking on any surgery. If there is any suspicion of malignancy, then laparotomy is the procedure of choice rather than laparoscopic surgery. The ultrasonic features suggesting malignancy of ovarian cysts are discussed in detail by Lachlan de Crespigny in Chapter 20, but it must be understood that there is a wide overlap, and benign lesions such as a leiomyoma or endometrioma can sometimes appear similar to certain carcinomas. Malignant disease is overdiagnosed by ultrasound and it is important to realize that aspiration cytology may miss malignant cells.

Ovarian Cystoscopy

Ovarian cystoscopy has recently been proposed as a useful diagnostic technique for preoperative identification of endometriotic implants and for the selection of site for biopsy of large ovarian endometriomas (Brosens et al., 1994). The technique described by Brosens and Puttemans (1989) uses a small optical instrument such as the 4 mm 30° rigid Hamou II hysteroscope with an operating channel (Karl Storz Endoscopy, Tüttlingen, Germany). After careful inspection of the pelvis and in the absence of signs suggesting malignancy, the cyst is first punctured and an aspiration sample is obtained. The cyst is subsequently flushed abundantly with sterile saline at body temperature until the fluid becomes clear using a suction irrigator. The small endoscope is introduced through a suprapubic port into the cyst and a saline infusion is allowed to run freely to distend the cyst. The 30° angle of the endoscope allows nearly complete visualization of the inside wall of the cyst.

This technique allows *in situ* identification of the characteristics of the wall of the cyst. The typical features of the large endometriotic cyst are:

- Retraction of the wall with the formation of crypts or pockets at the caudal and posterior side of the cyst.
- The presence of old and recent hemorrhage.
- Irregular distribution of a network of red implants and superficial vessels, which tend to be more concentrated in the caudal and posterior side of the cyst (Figure 22.3).

The color of the wall varies from pearl white to yellow–pigmented or brown–black depending upon the degree of fibrosis and hemopigmentation. In the non-fibrotic endometrioma the thin endometrial mucosa can be easily dislodged from the wall by manipulation. These endoscopic features make it easy to distinguish the endometrioma from other hemorrhagic cysts (Figure 22.4). However, biopsies should be obtained in all cases to confirm the diagnosis.

At histology the red hemorrhagic foci represent vascularized endometriotic stroma with a surface epithelium (Martin and Berry, 1990). However, in large (> 3 cm) endometriomas much of the wall can be devoid of red implants or vascularization. It is therefore not surprising that microbiopsies of 2 mm size obtained under ovarioscopic guidance from the red foci produce endometriotic tissue more frequently than large random biopsies or even resected specimens. Glandular endometrial tissue is occasionally found at or around the site of the inversion stigma, and absence of the classical type of endometriosis may explain the failure of some authors to detect endometriosis in resected specimens (Fayez and Vogel, 1991).

Laparoscopic Surgical Technique

The technique for extraovarian reconstruction of the ovary with a typical endometrioma has recently

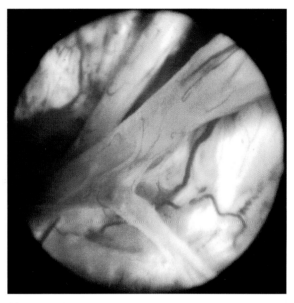

(a)

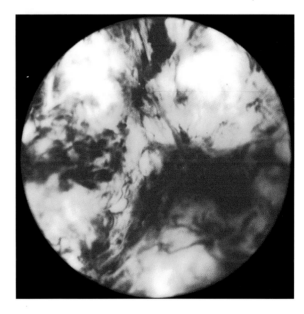

(b)

Figure 22.3 Ovarian cystoscopy of an endometrioma. (a) Detail of the retraction at the site of invagination. Note the red hemorrhagic implant and the vascularization at the site of invagination. (b) Superficial red implants and their vascularization.

been described by Brosens *et al.* (1996). The technique includes the following steps:

- Full adhesiolysis of the ovary and identification of the invagination site.
- Wide opening of the invagination site and resection of the fibrotic ring (Figure 22.5).
- Destruction of the superficial endometriotic

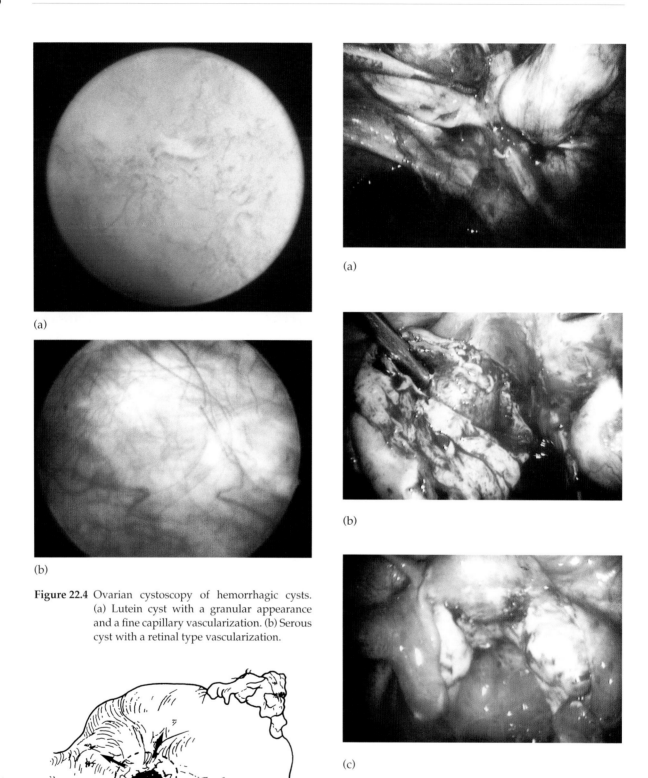

(a)

(b)

Figure 22.4 Ovarian cystoscopy of hemorrhagic cysts. (a) Lutein cyst with a granular appearance and a fine capillary vascularization. (b) Serous cyst with a retinal type vascularization.

Figure 22.5 Diagram of the site of invagination of the endometrioma. The cyst is widely opened at this site by resection of the fibrotic ring.

(a)

(b)

(c)

Figure 22.6 Extraovarian technique for reconstruction of the ovary with a large endometrioma. (a) Dense adhesions at the site of invagination are dissected following the plane between the ovary and the pelvic wall. (b) After wide opening of the pseudocyst the superficial red implants are coagulated using bipolar coagulation. (c) A second-look laparoscopy is performed after 2–3 months when the ovary has regressed to its normal size, and remaining implants and adhesions are removed.

implants by bipolar coagulation or laser photocoagulation or vaporization.

The technique can be applied laparoscopically, for both small and large endometriomas (Figure 22.6). However, a large endometrioma is preferably treated by a two-step laparoscopic technique (Table 22.2) for two reasons.

- First, large chocolate cysts are frequently a combination of an endometrioma and one or more hemorrhagic functional cysts. The second step is performed 2–3 months after the first procedure and during this period the cystic structures regress and the ovary resumes an almost normal size. This avoids the excision or coagulation of functional cysts.
- Second, after regression the cystic wall can be fully inspected and any remaining superficial neovascularization and implants are easily coagulated and adhesions are removed.

In contrast with other reconstructive techniques, the extraovarian technique makes use of the stigma of inversion to enter and open the cavity while avoiding additional trauma to the ovary. Closing by apposition of the walls and suturing of the cortex is not indicated because the ovarian stroma is not exposed and the ovarian cortex is preserved. Theoretically, closure of the walls could carry the risk of burying cortex with follicles deep into the ovary and create a risk of functional cyst formation.

The use of ovarian suppressive therapy before or after endometriosis surgery is still controversial. Some authors have recommended the use of GnRH agonist therapy between the cystectomy procedure and the second-look laparoscopy (Donnez *et al.*, 1990;

Table 22.2. Two-step endoscopic technique for reconstruction of the ovary with a large or multilocular endometrioma.

Step	Components of Step
First step:	Combined explorative and operative procedure
	Inspection for typical features of endometrioma
	Adhesiolysis and full mobilization of ovary
	Wide opening of inversion site and resection of fibrosis
	Representative biopsies
	Bipolar coagulation of neovascularization and implants
	2–3 month interval to allow spontaneous involution of pseudocyst
	The use of a gonadotropin releasing hormone (GnRH) agonist can be beneficial.
Second step:	Adhesiolysis
	Coagulation of remnant neovascularization and implants

Vercellini *et al.*, 1992). This may have the advantage of avoiding the presence of follicles or a corpus luteum at the time of second-look laparoscopy and theoretically of reducing the inflammatory condition of the peritoneum and therefore decreasing the risk of postoperative adhesion formation. However, the primary prevention of postoperative adhesion formation is achieved by avoiding any unnecessary surgical procedure such as incision of normal cortex or excision of functional structures. Simplification of the surgical technique by the extraovarian approach results in minimal surgical trauma and the long-term follow-up has shown a low incidence of recurrent cyst formation (Brosens *et al.*, 1996).

The basic principle of the surgical treatment of small and large ovarian endometriomas therefore includes adhesiolysis first to achieve full mobilization of the ovary and relief of the invagination and, second, the selective destruction of superficial endometriotic implants. In young women the wall is usually not fibrotic and the superficial implants can be eliminated by superficial bipolar coagulation or laser photocoagulation or vaporization causing minimal damage to the ovarian cortex.

Laparoscopic Laser Surgery for Large Endometriomas

Recent advances in minimal access surgery together with the increased magnification afforded by the laparoscope have made it possible to treat large endometriomas and severe endometriosis by endoscopic surgery, which is associated with less adhesion formation (Luciano *et al.*, 1989; Lundorff *et al.*, 1991), faster recovery and impressive results in terms of pain relief and fecundity.

A recent prospective study has shown an increase in postoperative adhesion formation following excisional techniques (Fayez and Vogel, 1991) and mere drainage of endometriomas under ultrasonic control is associated with an unacceptable recurrence rate, as is the case with ultrasound-guided aspiration of benign-appearing ovarian cysts generally (Lipitz *et al.*, 1992). A more logical approach is to use the photovaporization ability of the laser, either the carbon dioxide (CO_2) laser, the potassium titanyl phosphate (KTP/532) laser (Figure 22.7) or argon laser, but not the deeply penetrating Nd:YAG laser (Sutton and Hodgson, 1992).

Laparoscopic Surgical Technique using Lasers

All patients undergoing advanced laparoscopic surgery should be consented for laparotomy in the

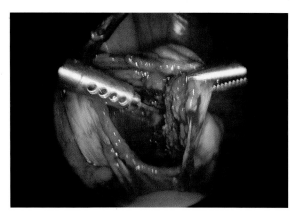

Figure 22.7 KTP/532 emerald green laser is an excellent laser for the photovaporization of an endometrioma capsule. It works well in the presence of blood and hemosiderin and yet due not penetrate as deeply as the neodymium:yttrium-aluminum-garnet (Nd:YAG) laser and causes less thermal injury than electrosurgery.

unlikely event of uncontrollable bleeding or bowel perforation while performing adhesiolysis. With recent developments in bipolar electrosurgical technology (Odell, 1993) bleeding can virtually always be controlled by these means. With increasing experience most of the hazards can be avoided and the procedure described below is essentially very safe; however, even in the best hands, accidents can occasionally occur and patients should be made aware of this possibility mainly for medicolegal reasons.

Large endometriomas are usually associated with endometriosis in other sites and often with associated adhesions, and attention should be directed to adhesiolysis and removal of the ectopic implants before tackling the endometrioma. Some patients who have had a previous rupture of an endometrioma will have brown specks of tissue on the peritoneal surface from the released hemosiderin, but this is not endometriosis *per se* and biopsy will not reveal any glands or stroma as these deposits are essentially inactive and can be left alone.

Peritoneal surface endometriosis can be excised surgically to provide pathologic proof of the extent of the disease, but this is time-consuming and laborious and we therefore prefer to use the laser to photocoagulate or photovaporize tissue. We use the CO_2 laser with its established accuracy for localized deposits, especially if they are over the bladder, ureter or bowel, since with skill and a knowledge of the laser tissue effects it is possible to vaporize these lesions with only 50 μm of irreversible tissue damage from the edge of the impact crater (Sutton and Hodgson, 1992). For more diffuse disease and the endometrioma itself we prefer to use the KTP/532 laser (Laserscope, San Jose, California, USA;

Cwmbran, UK; HGM Lasers, Salt Lake City, Utah, USA; Litechnica, Manchester, UK) since it works well in the presence of blood and hemosiderin and the operating wavelength of 532 nm coincides with the absorption peak of hemoglobin and red-colored lesions. If lasers are not available then electrosurgical techniques can be used. However, these have the disadvantage that the depth of penetration is difficult to assess and high-frequency current follows the path of least resistance and is particularly drawn by tissues rich in fluids and electrolytes, which includes the blood vessels, ureter, bladder and bowel. In addition care must be taken to avoid indirect damage by capacitative coupling (Odell, 1993) causing electrical burns, which are often outside the operator's field of vision and are therefore unrecognized at the time.

Endometriomas that form in accordance with the Hughesdon theory (Hughesdon, 1957) are invariably densely adherent to the pelvic sidewall over the ovarian fossa. Using a strong stainless steel round-ended atraumatic probe placed in a 5 mm suprapubic midline port and an aquadissector introduced through another 5 mm port in one or other of the iliac fossae lateral to the inferior epigastric vessels, the ovary can usually be teased away from the dense adhesions binding to the ovarian fossa. Sometimes the adhesions are particularly dense and require laser dissection or scissor dissection, but great care should be taken during this step because the ureter is extremely close: its course should have been previously identified and in certain cases it is worth using an illuminated ureteric stent introduced through an operating cystoscope before the procedure is commenced (Phipps and Tyrell, 1991). However, in severe endometriosis the tissues are thickened by infiltrating disease and the illumination cannot be seen. An alternative technique therefore is to open the peritoneum medial to the ureter nearer the pelvic brim with a CO_2 laser or microsurgical electrode and using hydrodissection carry the incision caudad to display the course of the ureter (Nezhat *et al.*, 1996)

During the course of this manipulation to free the ovary, the endometrioma almost invariably ruptures and the thick viscous hemosiderin-laden fluid escapes. It is vital to have a good-quality wide-bore suction irrigator such as the Nezhat–Dorsey device (Sigmacon Heriots Wood, UK) to remove all the chocolate fluid at this stage and to prevent its escape into the upper abdomen. This material can induce a painful chemical peritonitis and it is essential that it is removed by copious irrigation with warm heparinized Ringer's lactate solution until the effluent runs clear. The edges of the cyst are then grasped by two pairs of traumatic grasping forceps introduced into the 5 mm ports that had previously been used for the probes and irrigator, and a further 5 mm trocar is inserted in the contralateral iliac fossa to introduce the suction irrigator with the laser fiber passing through the central channel. At this stage the laparoscope is introduced into the interior of the ovarian endometrioma and the internal architecture is carefully inspected and biopsies taken. If there are any suspicious areas, the result of a frozen section should be awaited.

The KTP/532 laser fiber (600 µm) is used at 18 W to photovaporize the entire surface of the endometrioma lining (Figure 22.8). This laser will penetrate to about 3 mm and is frequently flushed with the irrigator to avoid any unnecessary thermal damage. This laser is particularly effective at preventing hemorrhage during the procedure and can be used through a flexible fiber introducer to get at awkward areas of the cyst. However, in practise it is usually employed with the straight irrigation sucker and the assistants manipulate the grasping forceps to bring each area of the cyst lining at right angles to it.

At the end of the procedure, copious irrigation is employed and an underwater inspection performed to make sure there is no bleeding. Any ongoing hemorrhage that has failed to be contained by the laser can be stopped with bipolar electrosurgery and at the end of the procedure about one liter of warm heparinized Ringer's lactate is left *in situ* to prevent subsequent adhesion formation, which usually occurs during the initial stages of the healing process. The idea of this aquaflotation is to prevent surfaces adhering during this phase (Reich, 1989).

Adhesion formation has always been one of the most regrettable aftermaths of surgery and is particularly unfortunate if the aim of the surgery has been to promote fertility. Research has suggested that a reduction in mesothelial plasminogen activator activity in the presence of trauma, infection or tissue ischemia is the likely pathway in post-surgical adhesion formation (Buckman *et al.*, 1976; Raftery, 1981; Menzies and Ellis, 1989). Trauma is inevitably associated with any surgical insult, but the biologic inter-action between lasers and living tissue minimizes this. Infection is less likely with laparoscopy than laparotomy and the ischemia produced by surgical knots can be largely avoided by the use of lasers. It is therefore not surprising that laparoscopic surgery is associated with less adhesion formation, both in experimental animals (Luciano *et al.*, 1989) and in clinical practise (Lundorff *et al.*, 1991).

It seems illogical to us to deliberately induce tissue ischemia with surgical knots and to bury the invaginated ovarian cortex so we leave the ovarian defect open and always finish our procedures by leaving about one liter of heparinized Hartmann's solution in the peritoneal cavity in the hope of preventing the initial phase of fibrinous adhesion formation, which usually occurs in the first 4–20 hours following surgery (Sutton and MacDonald, 1990). When we have had an opportunity to have a second-look procedure we have been gratified to find that in the vast majority there has been little or no adhesion formation to the previous scar. This is in marked contrast to second-look procedures we have witnessed when patients have been referred to us to clear up the adhesions resulting from formal laparotomy, even when performed with microsurgical techniques.

Risks and Complications of Reconstructive Surgery of the Ovary with an Endometrioma

Such surgery poses specific surgical problems.

Incomplete Surgery

Incomplete surgery occurs when the superficial endometrial implants are not completely removed or destroyed. Implants of glandular endometrium are often found at the site where the cystic ovary is densely adherent to other pelvic structures. The site is very often caudal and lateral and its accessibility can be difficult. Incomplete surgery results from incomplete adhesiolysis and incomplete exposure of the ovary. Small or minute endometriomas can be located at the hilus of the ovary, and full mobilization and inspection of the hilus of the ovary are necessary to detect these lesions.

Excessive Surgery

Excessive surgery can result from two causes.

- First, not all chocolate cysts are of endometrial origin. Although peroperative inspection is

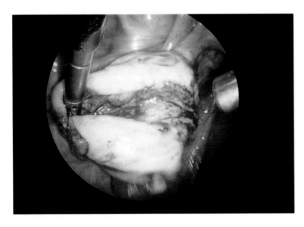

Figure 22.8 Internal view of endometrioma after photocoagulation with KTP/532 laser.

supposedly reliable, excisional specimens reveal luteal lining in approximately one-third of cases.

- Second, excision specimens frequently reveal ovarian cortex with follicles at microscopic examination. Therefore the excisional technique carries the risk of removing ovarian follicles and functional cysts.

Specific Complications

Specific complications of ovarian surgery for endometriomas include:

- Severe bleeding from the hilus of the ovary; excessive coagulation of the ovarian hilus can lead to ovarian atrophy.
- Trauma to the ureter during dissection.
- Postoperative adhesions with partial or complete encapsulation of the ovary resulting in pain and recurrent functional cyst formation.
- Immobilization of the ampullary segment of the fallopian tube by adhesions.
- Distal occlusion of the fallopian tube by external compression resulting in a mechanical hydrosalpinx.
- Ovarian resistance during stimulation for *in vitro* fertilization and premature menopause due reportedly to repeat excision of ovarian endometriomas (Maruyama *et al.* 1996).
- Ovarian remnant syndrome due to a failure of radical surgery of the encapsulated ovary.

The first surgical procedure in a young woman with an ovarian endometrioma therefore frequently determines the ultimate outcome of her reproductive life.

Results of Lapaparoscopic Laser Surgery

We have reported our experience over ten years between 1982 and 1992 with the CO_2 and the KTP laser (Sutton, 1993). During that time we treated 102 patients with proven endometriomas with pain, infertility or both. The endometriomas were usually large, varying between 3–18 cm and the mean American Fertility Society score was 45. The mean duration of infertility was 53 months and most of the patients were tertiary referrals and had been treated with numerous previous treatments, including attempts at assisted conception. Of the 84 presenting with pain 66 (78%) reported a marked improvement or even complete resolution, and many patients remarked on the gratifying absence

of the very unpleasant pain as soon as the effects of anesthesia had worn off. We were even more surprised to find that even though most of these patients were in the severe endometriosis category on the revised American Fertility Society classification, 24 of 42 (57%) achieved a pregnancy. The majority of those who conceived did so within eight months of the surgical procedure and most were natural conceptions, although a few patients had been referred from assisted conception clinics, specifically for treatment of the endometrioma before a planned treatment cycle. The overall recurrence rate during the course of the study and the subsequent two-year follow-up was 19%, and not all endometriomas recurred in the same situation or indeed in the same ovary. We have recently updated this series and calculated the cumulative conception rates, which have remained excellent, particularly when one considers that this group represents women with severe (stage IV) endometriosis with gross anatomical distortion and usually a long duration of infertility and relatively advanced age (Sutton *et al.*, 1997).

Photocoagulation of the endometrioma capsule with the KTP/532 laser has been reported by other authors and Marrs (1991) reported a low recurrence rate, while Daniell *et al.* (1991) reported a significant relief of pain and a pregnancy rate of 37.5% in 32 patients trying for conception.

The KTP laser works particularly well on an unprepared endometrioma since it will function in the presence of blood and fluids, which can seriously impede the action of the CO_2 laser due to the high absorption of laser energy at this wavelength by the water molecule. For this reason Donnez has advocated a three-stage approach to the treatment of large endometriomas involving drainage at the initial laparoscopy followed by a three-month course of GnRH analogs to decrease the vascularity and shrink the endometrioma down to a sufficiently small size so that it can be efficiently vaporized with the CO_2 laser (Donnez *et al.*, 1989).

Results of Conventional Laparoscopic Surgery

When reviewing their data, Bruhat's team from Clermont Ferrand, found that adhesions were the main factor limiting complete treatment. They achieved complete treatment for 89% of cysts larger than 3 cm, but only 73.3% of cysts diagnosed in patients with an overall adhesion score of more than 50. They found that using their intraperitoneal cystectomy technique resulted in adhesion formation in 21% of the adnexa treated and complete or partial recurrence of adhesions treated at laparoscopy occurred in 82.3% of the cases. They concluded that postoperative adhesion formation was largely a result of poor surgical technique and strict guidelines should be adhered to to minimize postoperative adhesion formation. In a retrospective study of 163 patients followed for more than one year the recurrence rate was 15.9%, all of whom were confirmed pathologically. Most recurrences occurred within the first postoperative year or after the end of the second postoperative year. Early recurrences were attributed to incomplete treatment whereas late recurrences were thought to be due to *de novo* endometrioma formation as part of the natural history of this disease (Canis *et al.*, 1992).

Comparison of Laparoscopic Surgery versus Laparotomy

Recently Bateman has reported a retrospective case–control study comparing the surgical management of patients with endometriomas managed by endoscopic surgery versus laparotomy. The outcome parameters in terms of operating time, estimated blood loss and recovery time were all in favor of endoscopic surgery. The recurrence rate was 11% for those treated endoscopically and 19% for those treated by laparotomy, and the pregnancy rates were as expected very similar, with 42.8% for endoscopy and 46.6% for laparotomy, which is not statistically different (Bateman *et al.*, 1994). Their findings support the findings of a larger study by Adamson *et al.* (1992) that most endometriomas can be treated safely and appropriately by laparoscopic surgery.

Conclusion

Both ovarian endometriomas and deeply infiltrating endometriosis are best treated by surgery, preferably laparoscopically. We have recently (Sutton *et al.*, 1994) reported our results of a randomized double-blind controlled study comparing the efficacy of laparoscopic laser surgery for peritoneal endometriosis stages I–III compared with a control arm who received no treatment and undoubtedly laser vaporization results in convincingly superior results as far as pelvic pain is concerned. Since ovarian endometriomas and deeply infiltrating disease are less responsive in the long term to medical therapy the argument in favor of

surgery is even more convincing for these conditions. There is an urgent need to perform randomized prospective studies to evaluate the place of postoperative suppression with GnRH analogs, but it is likely, certainly in the foreseeable future, that laparoscopic surgery will remain the mainstay of treatment.

References

Adamson GD, Subak LL, Pasta DJ, Hurd SJ, von Fraque O, Rodriguez BD (1992) Comparison of CO_2 laser laparoscopy with laparotomy for treatment of endometriomata. *Fertility and Sterility* **57**: 965–973.

American Fertility Society (1985) Revised American Fertility Society classification of endometriosis. *Fertility and Sterility* **43**: 351–352.

Bateman BG, Kolp LA, Mills S (1994) Endoscopic versus laparotomy management of endometriomas. *Fertility and Sterility* **62(4)**: 690–695.

Benagiano G, Brosens I (1991). The history of endometriosis: identifying the disease. *Human Reproduction* **7**: 963–968.

Brosens IA, Puttemans PJ (1989) Double-optic laparoscopy. Salpingoscopy, ovarian cystoscopy and endo-ovarian surgery with the argon laser. *Baillière's Clinical Obstetrics and Gynaecology* **3**: 595–608.

Brosens IA, Puttemans PJ, Deprest J (1994) The endoscopic localisation of endometrial implants in the ovarian chocolate cyst. *Fertility and Sterility* **61**: 1034–1038.

Brosens IA, Van Ballaer P, Pettemans P, Deprest J (1996) Reconstruction of the ovary containing large endometriomas by an extraovarian endosurgical technique. *Fertility and Sterility* **66**: 517–521.

Buckman RF, Woods M, Sargent L, Gervin AS (1976) A unifying pathogenic mechanism in the aetiology of intraperitoneal adhesions. *Journal of Surgical Research* **20**: 1–5.

Canis M, Mage G, Watiez A, Chapron C, Pouly JL, Bassil S (1992) Second-look laparoscopy after laparoscopic cystectomy of large ovarian endometriomas (see comments). *Fertility and Sterility* **58**: 617–619.

Casler DB (1919) A unique, diffuse uterine tumor, really an adenomyoma, with stroma, but no glands: menstruation after complete hysterectomy due to uterine mucosa remaining in the ovary. *Transactions of American Gynecologic Society* **44**: 69–84.

Daniell JF, Kurtz BR, Gurley LD (1991) Laser laparoscopic management of large endometriomas. *Fertility and Sterility* **55**: 692–695.

de Crespigny L, Robinson HP, Davoren RAM, Fortune D (1989) The 'simple' ovarian cyst: aspirate or operate? *British Journal of Obstetrics and Gynaecology* **96**: 1035–1039.

Donnez J, Nisolle M, Clerckx F et al. (1990) The ovarian endometrial cyst: The combined (hormonal and surgical) therapy. In Brosens I, Jacobs HS, Runnebaum B (eds) *LNRH-analogues in Gynaecology*. pp. 165–175. Carnforth: Parthenon Publishing.

Donnez J, Nisolle M, Wayembergh M, Clerckx F,

Casanas-Roux F (1989) CO_2 laser laparoscopy in peritoneal endometriosis and in ovarian endometrial cysts. In Donnez J (ed.) *Laser Operative Laparoscopy and Hysteroscopy.* pp. 53–78. Belgium: Nauwelaerts Printing.

Fayez JA, Vogel MF (1991) Comparison of different treatment methods of endometriomas by laparoscopy. *Obstetrics and Gynecology* **78**: 660–665.

Hughesdon PE (1957) The structure of endometrial cysts of the ovary. *Journal of Obstetrics and Gynaecology of the British Empire* **44**: 481–487.

Lipitz S, Seidman PS, Menczer J *et al.* (1992) Recurrence rate after fluid aspiration from sonographically benign ovarian cysts. *Journal of Reproductive Medicine* **37**: 845–848.

Luciano AA, Mayer D, Koch E, Nillsen J, Whitman F (1989) A comparative study of post-operative adhesions following laser surgery by laparoscopy and laparotomy in the rabbit model. *Obstetrics and Gynecology* **74**: 220–224.

Lundorff SP, Harlin M, Kiallfelt B, Thorburn J, Lindblom B (1991) Adhesion formation after laparoscopic surgery in tubal pregnancy: a randomised trial versus laparotomy. *Fertility and Sterility* **55**: 911–915.

Marrs RP (1991) The use of the KTP laser for laparoscopic removal of ovarian endometrioma. *Journal of Obstetrics and Gynaecology* **164**: 1622–1626.

Martin DC, Berry JD (1990) Histology of chocolate cysts. *Journal of Gynecological Surgery* **6**: 43–46.

Maruyama M, Yano T, Morita Y *et al.* (1996) Effect of ovarian cystectomy on outcome of IVF-ET treatment in endometriosis patients. Proceedings of Vth World Congress on Endometriosis, 21–24 October, Yokohama, Japan, Abstract, p. 118.

Menzies D, Ellis H (1989) Intra-abdominal adhesions and their prevention by topical tissue plasminogen activator. *Journal of the Royal Society of Medicine* **82**: 534–535.

Nezhat F, Nezhat C, Allan CJ, Metzger DA, Sears DL (1992) A clinical and histologic classification of endometriomas: implications for a mechanism of pathogenesis. *Journal of Reproductive Medicine* **37**: 771–776.

Nezhat C, Nezhat F, Nezhat CH, Nasserbakh TF, Rosat M, Seidman DS (1996) Urinary tract endometriosis treated by laparoscopy. *Fertility and Sterility* **66(6)**: 920–924.

Nieminen J (1962) Studies on the vascular pattern of ectopic endometrium with special reference to cyclic changes. *Acta Obstetricia et Gynecologica Scandinavica* **41 (Suppl 3)**: 1–81.

Norris CC (1921) Ovary containing endometrium. *American Journal of Obstetrics and Gynecology* **1**: 831–834.

Odell RC (1993) Electrosurgery. In Sutton C, Diamond M (eds) *Endoscopic Surgery for Gynaecologists.* pp 51–59. London: W.B. Saunders.

Phipps J, Tyrell N (1991) Transilluminating ureteric stents for preventing operative ureteric injury. *British Journal of Obstetrics and Gynaecology* **9**: 81–83.

Raftery AT (1981) Effect of peritoneal trauma on peritoneal fibrinolytic activity and intraperitoneal adhesion formation. An experimental study in the rat. *European Surgical Research* **13**: 397–401.

Reich H (1989) New techniques in advanced laparoscopic surgery. *Baillière's Clinical Obstetrics and Gynaecology. Laparoscopic Surgery* **13**: 655–681.

Russell WW (1899) Aberrant portions of the Mullerian duct found in the ovary. *Johns Hopkins Hospital Bulletin* **10**: 8–10.

Sampson JA (1921) Perforating haemorrhagic (chocolate) cysts of the ovary. *Archives of Surgery* **3**: 245–323.

Sampson JA (1927) Peritoneal endometriosis due to the menstrual dissemination of endometrial tissue into the peritoneal cavity. *American Journal of Obstetrics and Gynecology* **14**: 422–469.

Sawin M, McCarthy S, Acoutt L, Comite F (1989) Endometriosis: Appearance and detection at MR imaging. *Radiology* **171**: 693–696.

Sawin M, McCarthy S, Acoutt L *et al.* (1990) Monitoring therapy with a gonadatrophin releasing hormone analogue: utility of MR imaging. *Radiology* **175**: 503–506.

Schwarz LB, Seifer DB (1992) Diagnostic imaging of adnexal masses; a review. *Journal of Reproductive Medicine* **37**: 63–71.

Sutton CJG (1993) Lasers in infertility. *Human Reproduction* **8(8)**: 133–146.

Sutton CJG, MacDonald R (1990) Laser laparoscopic adhesiolysis. *Journal of Gynaecological Surgery* **6**: 155–160.

Sutton CJG, Hodgson R (1992) Endoscopic cutting with lasers. *Minimally Invasive Therapy* **1**: 117–205.

Sutton CJG, Ewen SP, Whitelaw N, Haines P (1994) Prospective, randomized double-blind, controlled trial of laser laparoscopy in the treatment of pelvic pain associated with minimal, mild, and moderate endometriosis. *Fertility and Sterility* **62(4)**: 696–700.

Sutton CJG, Even SP, Jacobs SA, Whitelaw NL (1997) 10 years' experience of laser laparoscopic surgery in the treatment of ovarian endometriomas. *Journal of the American Association of Gynecologic Laparoscopists* **4(3)**: 319–323.

Togashi K, Niscimura K, Kimura I *et al.* (1991) Endometrial cysts; diagnosis with MR imaging. *Radiology* **180**: 73–78.

Vercellini P, Vendola N, Bocciolone L, Rognoni M, Carinelli S, Candiani G (1990) Reliability of the visual diagnosis of ovarian endometriosis. *Fertility and Sterility* **53**: 1198–1200.

Vercellini P, Vendola N, Bocciolone L, Colombo A, Rognoni MT, Bolis G (1992) Laparoscopic aspiration of ovarian endometriomas. Effect with postoperative gonadotropin releasing hormone agonist treatment. *Journal of Reproductive Medicine* **37**: 577–580.

23

Polycystic Ovaries, Surgical Management

GABOR T. KOVACS

Box Hill Hospital, Monash University, Victoria, Australia

The surgical treatment of polycystic ovary syndrome (PCOS) to restore regular menstruation and lead to subsequent pregnancy was first reported by Stein and Leventhal in 1935. This was the only treatment available for anovulatory women with PCOS and therefore became widely used. By 1964 Stein reported on a series of 108 women with a 95% cyclic menstruation rate and 86% pregnancy rate (Stein, 1964). This treatment became widely accepted and the first suggestion of a problem was in 1981 when Adashi *et al.* reported on finding significant pelvic adhesions subsequent to wedge resection. With the availability of clomiphene citrate to induce ovulation, there was an alternative to the operative treatment of polycystic ovaries (Kistner, 1968) and with the availability of human gonadotropins to induce ovulation (Gemzell *et al.*, 1960), surgical treatment became truly obsolete.

Renewed interest in the surgical approach for the treatment of PCOS commenced with a report by Gjönnaess in 1984. In this initial report involving 62 women, 92% ovulated within three months and there was a conception rate of 80%. Not only was this cheaper and easier than the hormonal approach, but the risk of multiple pregnancy was also eliminated (Box 23.1). Furthermore, initial reports suggested that the risk of adhesion formation was far less after laparoscopic surgery than after laparotomy and wedge resection. In 1989 Dabirashrafi reported adhesions in only one out of nine women who had undergone electrocautery followed by second-look laparoscopy. Some workers preferred the use of laser, and carbon dioxide (CO_2), argon, neodymium:yttrium-aluminum-garnet (Nd:YAG) and potassium titanyl phosphate (KTP)

> **Box 23.1 Benefits of ovarian drilling**
>
> - Once only procedure
> - No ongoing monitoring (biochemistry and ultrasound)
> - No increase in multiple pregnancy

have all been used (Feste, 1990). It was believed that laser would cause less tissue damage with better hemostasis and therefore lower the risk of adhesion formation. Daniell and Miller reported on 85 women who were treated with the KTP or CO_2 lasers, resulting in an ovulation rate of 71% and conception rate of 56%. They advocated that this treatment was effective, safe and without the risk of postoperative adhesions. To determine the efficacy of ovarian cautery compared to gonadotropin treatment Abdel Gadir *et al.* (1990a) carried out a controlled trial of ovarian electrocautery against human menopausal gonadotropins (hMG) and follicle stimulating hormone (FSH) and found that ovarian electrocautery was as effective as the two hormonal therapies. As ovarian electrocautery needs only gynecological surgical expertise and not the availability of ultrasound or hormonal monitoring equipment, they recommended it as the primary method of treatment for clomiphene non-responding PCOS patients.

The early 1990s therefore saw the reintroduction of surgical management for the treatment of PCOS associated with anovulation and subfertility

(Gurgan *et al.*, 1994). The techniques of laparoscopic surgery included electrocautery (Gjönnaess, 1984), laser vaporization (Daniell and Miller, 1989), capsule resection (Campo *et al.*, 1993) and multiple ovarian punch biopsies (Sumioki *et al.*, 1988).

The reported ovulation and pregnancy rates from several series are summarized in Table 23.1. This shows ovulation rates of 41–92% and pregnancy rates of 20–75%. These papers were reviewed and the 'worst case scenario' ovulation and pregnancy rates have been recalculated. This means that if patients were lost to follow-up they were considered as 'unsuccessful', and comments such as 'women who only had ovulatory problems' were ignored and all treated women were considered to make up the denominator. The ovulation and pregnancy rates were clinically acceptable, and there appeared to be no significant difference between the various techniques. Unipolar electrocautery was the method that was most widely used, as it was available in every operating theater.

Table 23.1 Reported ovulation and pregnancy rates following laparoscopic treatment of PCOS.

Reference	Women treated	Method	Ovulation	Pregnancy	Comments
Farhi *et al.* (1995)	22	Cautery	(41%)		
Gjöannaess (1994)	252	Cautery	201 (92%)	145 (58%)	
Gjöannaess (1984)*	65	Cautery	57 (88%)	24 (37%)	
Heylen *et al.* (1994)	44	Argon laser	35 (80%)	24 (55%)	1 out of 3 women had adhesions
Verhelst *et al.* (1993)	17	CO_2 laser	14 (82%)	11 (65%)	
Naether *et al.* (1993)*	133	Cautery		73 (55%)	Adhesions in 26% of second-look patients
Naether and Fischer (1993)	199	Cautery			62 second-look patients, 19.3% adhesions
Tiitinen *et al.* (1993)	10	Cautery	3 (30%)	2 (20%)	Four clomiphene responsive subsequently
Armar and Lachelin (1993)	50		43 (86%)	33 (66%)	0 adhesions in nine women investigated
Ostrzenski (1992)	12	CO_2 laser wedge		(75%)	8% of women studied had adhesions
Gurgan *et al.* (1992)	40	Nd:YAG laser		20 (50%)	Adhesions in 13 (68%) of second-look patients
Kovacs *et al.* (1991)	10	Cautery	7 (70%)	3 (30%)	
Keckstein *et al.* (1990)	19 11	CO_2 or YAG laser		8 (42%) 3 (27%)	11 examined, 3 adhesions after CO_2 laser 0 adhesions after YAG laser
Abdel Gadir *et al.* (1990a)	29	Cautery	71%	10 (34%)	
Daniell and Miller (1989)	85	Argon, CO_2 or KTP laser	60 (70%)	48 (56%)	

*Presumably included in later data.

Complications

The only reservations about the use of laparoscopic surgery for PCOS were the reported complications of subsequent adhesion formation and the concern about the theoretic risk of premature ovarian failure and the risk of intraoperative complications (Box 23.2).

Box 23.2 Intraoperative and postoperative complications of ovarian drilling

Intraoperative complications
    Anesthetic
    Trauma to viscus
    Bleeding

Postoperative complications
    Pelvic adhesions
    Ovarian atrophy (??)
    Premature menopause (???)
    Failure to respond

Intraoperative Complications

With the advent of operative laparoscopy, surgeons have become disciplined about minimizing visceral damage, and intraoperative complications are rare. None of the papers report any episodes of thermal damage to adjoining tissues. Bleeding from the ovary does not seem to be reported, although it must occur and is probably the reason for subsequent ovarian adhesions.

Adhesion Formation

As many patients conceived after treatment, the rate of 'second-look' laparoscopy or laparotomy was low and therefore information on the rate of adhesion formation is only available for a small proportion of patients with the incidence varying from 0% (none of eight patients from 85 treated by CO_2, KTP or argon laser) (Daniell and Miller, 1989); up to 100% after electrocautery in all eight patients treated (Greenblatt and Casper, 1993), and 80% (eight of ten patients treated by laser therapy) (Gurgan et al., 1991). I personally have identified a woman who was successfully treated by ovarian electrocautery after PCOS was diagnosed who conceived ten weeks after the procedure, and was again oligomenorrheic and infertile after the birth of her child, delivered by cesarean section. After failure

to respond to clomiphene citrate a repeat laparoscopy was again performed, and ovarian adhesions were identified (Figure 23.1) and divided. Electrocautery was again carried out and ovulation resumed, with pregnancy occurring seven weeks later. It would appear that adequate hemostasis and peritoneal post-drilling lavage are important factors in minimizing adhesion formation.

Naether and Fischer (1993) found a decrease in the incidence of postoperative adhesions from 19.3% to 16.6% when abdominal lavage was introduced. Their expanded series (Naether, 1995) showed a decrease in the incidence of postoperative adhesions from 35% pre-lavage to 10.8% when lavage was undertaken. In a group of five patients who underwent a third-look 259–1204 days (mean 623 days) after cautery with lavage, no adhesions were identified.

Another approach to minimize postoperative adhesion formation is short-interval second-look laparoscopy to lyse any adhesions that may have occurred. Gurgan et al. (1992) reported that 68% of 19 patients who underwent second-look laparoscopy four weeks after Nd:YAG laser photocoagulation of the ovaries had mild adhesions that were easily lysed. However, when this group was compared to a control group without second-look laparoscopy, the pregnancy rates were the same.

Despite frequent reporting of adhesions it does not seem to affect conception rates. In Greenblatt and Casper's series (1993) where 100% of women developed some adhesions, seven of eight managed to conceive.

Despite the wide variation in the incidence of postoperative adhesions it would appear that they are common. Their significance is debatable as conception rates are not affected by their presence. Nevertheless patients undergoing any method of

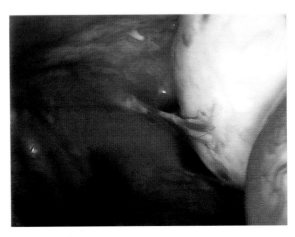

Figure 23.1 Post operative adhesions after ovarian electrocautery for polycystic ovaries.

ovarian surgery for PCOS should be warned that adhesions may occur. Although there is no consensus, a second-look laparoscopy four weeks postoperatively should be considered.

Premature Menopause or Ovarian Atrophy

Although it has been postulated that the destruction of follicles may result in an earlier exhaustion of ovarian function, there is no clinical study reporting on the occurrence of premature menopause, although ovarian atrophy as an incidental finding after ovarian drilling has been reported. There have also been concerns that laser energy could have a deleterious effect on ovarian follicles, and some rabbit work showed that laser wedge resection of rabbit ovaries resulted in fewer follicles than electrocoagulation. The long-term consequences of ovarian drilling on reproductive function are yet to be evaluated. Gjönnaess (1994) did, however, report on a woman who had five pregnancies subsequent to ovarian cautery.

Mechanism of Action

The mechanism of action of the classical wedge resection has never been understood, but there are a number of theories (Box 23.3):

- Stein and Leventhal (1935) initially postulated that wedge resection decreased the mechanical crowding of the cortex by cysts, which then allowed the progression of normal follicles to the surface, with the resumption of normal ovulation.
- Gjönnaess postulated that cautery destroyed an inhibitory substance within the ovarian

---

Box 23.3 Mechanism of Action of Surgical Treatment of PCOS

Poorly understood, but multiple theories including

- Decreased crowding of cortex
- Inhibitory substance from capsule destroyed
- Reduced negative/increased positive feedback
- Transient reduction in inhibin
- Restoration of putative gonadotropin surge attenuating factor
- Removal of androgenic fluid

---

capsule, thus allowing ovulation to occur (Gjönnaess, 1984).

- Another theory is that ovarian damage results in reduced negative or increased positive feedback (Farhi et al., 1995).
- The theory that the resultant ovarian androgen production results in declined luteinizing hormone (LH) secretion has been countered by the observation that the reduction of androgens in non-PCOS patients does not alter LH secretion (Gjönnaess and Norman, 1987).
- Yet another theory is that the transient reduction of inhibin (Kovacs et al., 1991) results in increased secretion of follicle stimulating hormone (FSH) with the recruitment of a new cohort of follicles (Keckstein, 1989).
- A recent theory is that normal production of the putative gonadotropin surge attenuating factor from the ovary may be restored after electrocautery (Balen and Jacobs, 1991), with a subsequent postoperative surge of LH and FSH followed by normal patterns of secretion of gonadotropins and gonadotropin surge attenuating factor during the follicular phase.
- The removal of androgenic fluid from the ovarian environment, thus removing the block for ovulation (Daniell and Miller, 1989) has also been suggested as a possible mechanism.

Thus although there are many theories, the mechanism of action of ovarian drilling as a treatment for anovulation is still not understood.

Hormonal Changes

The hormonal changes associated with ovarian wedge resection or with ovarian drilling are no better understood than the mechanism of action. There does appear to be consensus that there is a decrease in circulating androgenic hormones after surgery (Greenblatt and Casper, 1987; Abdel Gadir et al., 1990b; Keckstein et al., 1990; Ruutiainen and Seppala, 1991; Naether et al., 1993; Tiitinen, 1993; Verhelst et al., 1993), with most studies reporting decreased levels of LH (Abdel Gadir et al., 1990a; 1990b; Sakata et al., 1990; Farhi et al., 1995).

An increase in serum insulin levels after ovarian cautery has been noted (Ruutiainen and Seppala, 1991). Szilagyi et al. (1993) studied the effect of ovarian laser vaporization on opioidergic and dopaminergic activity in women with PCOS and found no alteration, although dopaminergic inhibition of prolactin was enhanced after ovarian surgery. A study of inhibin levels (Kovacs et al., 1991) found a transient fall followed by a rise and then a return to normal after six weeks.

Methodology of Ovarian Drilling

Whatever mode of ovarian drilling is used it is carried out under conditions of operative laparoscopy, usually under general anesthesia. Equipment for operative laparoscopy includes a high-flow gas source. A triple-puncture system at least should be used, with the laparoscope being introduced subumbilically, a grasping forceps suprapubically, and the third port for the diathermy instruments or the laser delivery channel. In order to minimize adhesion formation, it is probably advisable to use a four-puncture technique with a suction irrigator being inserted through a fourth cannula. Another option is to withdraw the diathermy forceps or the laser delivery channel to enable the suction irrigator to be inserted intermittently, but this is not as satisfactory.

The principles of endoscopic gynecological surgery should be followed. Bowels should be scooped out of the way to minimize the risk of accidental damage and the ovary should then be grasped so that it can be easily manipulated. Grasping the ovary at its hilus may cause vascular damage and it is, if at all possible, better to grasp it at a less vascular site. The use of videolaparoscopy is highly desirable, as this enables the assistant to see the operative field. The ovarian surface can then be drilled using either electrocautery or laser energy.

The Use of Ovarian Electrocautery with Unipolar Diathermy

This method will be discussed in detail as all of the equipment and the skill required are part of the everyday armory of the operating gynecologist; in addition most of the cases that have been reported in literature have been carried out by electrocautery.

Once the ovary has been visualized and grasped it should be isolated from other tissues. The instrument of choice to carry out the ovarian drilling is a Corson needle (Figure 23.2). This has the advantage that it is insulated except for its distal 1 cm and has a sharp point. The electrocautery unit should be set between 25–30 W. The Corson needle enables the cyst to be punctured and at the same time an electric current is passed down it to burn some of the stroma. It is the author's policy to diathermy each

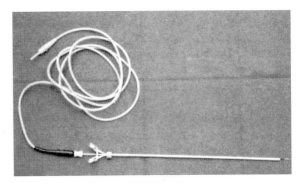

Figure 23.2 The unipolar Corson needle – the instrument of choice for ovarian cautery.

ovary 10–20 times, although a more conservative approach has been advocated (see below). The ovaries should be regularly irrigated and the smoke produced aspirated to enable a clear field of view. Great care should be taken that other tissue, especially bowel, in close proximity to the ovary is not damaged. Another possible complication is that the needle can actually perforate the ovary, being pushed through its distal side and inadvertently burning tissue behind the ovary. This should be avoided by adequate visualization. The ovarian tissue also heats up and it should not be released until it has cooled to prevent it from coming into contact with other tissues while hot. This cooling can be accelerated by irrigating with the suction irrigator. It is also recommended that the diathermy source is turned off at all times, except when burning is actually being carried out. The routine safety procedures for laparoscopic surgery should always be followed.

It is debatable how many times the ovary should be burnt. Gjönnaess (1984) increased the number of burns to each ovary from three initially, to four or five, and finally to eight, using 200–300 W for three seconds. Armar and Lachelin (1993) recommend four burns to each ovary, whereas I usually burn each ovary at least ten times (Kovacs *et al.*, 1991). Naether and Fischer (1995) with an experience of 250 cases recommend adjusting the number of coagulation sites according to ovarian size, the number of cysts, and the preoperative responsiveness to stimulation. They burn the ovary in 5–10 sites, depending upon the above criteria. An interesting observation was reported by Balen and Jacobs (1994) when they found that unilateral cautery of one ovary only (at four sites at 40 W for four seconds) resulted in ovulation in three of four patients treated, but from both ovaries. They therefore concluded that damage to one ovary has effects on the contralateral ovary, presumably by correcting abnormalities in ovarian–pituitary feedback.

Ovarian Cautery with Bipolar Diathermy

In principle bipolar electrocoagulation is safer than unipolar as the current does not pass through the patient, but only between the two electrodes of the bipolar instrument. Possible damage is therefore restricted to heat to surrounding tissues, with electrical burns being virtually eliminated. The disadvantage of bipolar diathermy is that there is no suitable instrument available with which to grasp the ovarian capsule. Unless a special instrument is developed, bipolar coagulation is not a suitable method for ovarian drilling.

The Use of CO_2 Laser for Ovarian Drilling

The technique of CO_2 laser drilling is described in detail by Daniell and Miller (1989). They recommend introducing the laser through an operating laparoscope with a two-puncture technique and grasping the ovary with forceps inserted suprapubically. I personally prefer to introduce the laser through an Infraguide (Laserscope, Santa Clara, CA) coupled to the laser through a third puncture. This enables easy manipulation through the pelvic cavity. Daniell and Miller recommend a 25 W continuous mode laser to vaporize and drain all visible subcapsular follicles, and drill randomly placed craters in each ovary. Each crater takes 5–10 seconds of firing to develop. About 25–40 vaporization sites are formed in each ovary. They recommend irrigating the ovary with heparinized Ringer's lactate, and any excessive bleeding is stopped by unipolar electrocautery. The laser plume is vented off regularly. It was postulated that CO_2 laser drilling would be less likely to cause adhesions than conventional electrocautery. This theory was supported by an experimental study on sheep that showed a total absence of postoperative adhesions (Petrucco, 1988). However, as early as 1989 Keckstein et al. reported adhesions in three of seven women who underwent CO_2 laser treatment for PCOS. It therefore has to be recognized that all forms of ovarian drilling may result in adhesion formation postoperatively.

A different technique was reported by Ostrzenski (1992) who used translaparoscopic CO_2 laser ovarian wedge resection on 12 women with a 75% conception rate and 8% postsurgical adhesion rate.

The Use of Other Lasers

KTP, Nd:YAG, and argon lasers have all been used laparoscopically for the surgical treatment of PCOS (Gurgan et al., 1994). When using a KTP or argon laser, a flexible fiber is used to deliver the energy to the ovary.

Heylen et al. (1994) reported their experience with the argon laser in 44 women with PCOS resulting in an overall conception rate of 73%, and compared classical vaporization of the ovarian capsule with simple perforation and subcapsular destruction of the ovarian stroma. There was no difference with respect to ovulation or pregnancy rates postoperatively between the two groups. When using the KTP or argon laser the flexible fiber is introduced 5 cm below the telescope through a third 5.5 mm trocar, which has a dual channel enabling smoke to be evacuated close to its source. When the Nd:YAG laser is used, 25 W of power, a sapphire tip and a minimum of 15 holes penetrating the stroma into each ovary have been recommended (Feste, 1990).

Other Benefits of Surgical Treatment of PCOS

The place of ovarian drilling as a reasonable alternative to the use of gonadotropins was proven by the controlled study of Abdel Gadir et al. in 1990 (1990a). This is in the best tradition of 'evidence based medicine', a routine which has not been followed in many other areas of infertility therapy. A further possible benefit shown in their study is the decreased early pregnancy wastage, with spontaneous abortion rates of 21% after cautery and 53% after hMG, with 40% after Metrodin therapy (Serono, Geneva, Switzerland; Abdel Gadir et al., 1990a). The mechanism for this explained by Balen and Jacobs (1995) is the decrease in circulating LH levels removing the main endocrine disturbance that is related to the risk of miscarriage (Balen et al., 1993).

Although the aim of ovarian drilling is to restore regular ovulation with the chance of pregnancy, this will only occur in 40–90% of women treated. However, there is also a potential benefit in those women who do not resume regular spontaneous ovulation. Some will become clomiphene responsive, and even those women who need to change to or return to gonadotropin therapy will need less hormone (Farhi et al., 1995).

Another possible application of ovarian drilling is before controlled hyperstimulation associated with in vitro fertilization (IVF) techniques. It has been recognized that women with PCOS have an increased risk of ovarian hyperstimulation syndrome (OHSS) when undergoing stimulation, and Fukaya et al. (1995) have reported that laser vaporization before IVF resulted in lower rates of OHSS and higher pregnancy rates in a series of 17 patients (Fukaya et al., 1995).

Conclusions

The treatment of PCOS has gone around full circle, and has started going around again! Initially surgical treatment with wedge resection was the only option. This was superseded by the availability of clomiphene citrate and gonadotropins (Box 23.4). However, the gonadotropins are expensive and require intensive monitoring, and even in the most careful hands is associated with a multiple pregnancy rate of about 20%. The controlled trial of Abdel Gadir *et al.* (1990) showed that ovarian cautery was as good if not better because of a lower early pregnancy loss rate than gonadotropin treatment. The cloud on the horizon appeared with the reports that postoperative adhesions were common, even after ovarian drilling, though these do not seem to affect pregnancy rates. There has therefore evolved a new resistance to this form of therapy.

What is the place of ovarian drilling for the treatment of PCOS associated with anovulatory infertility in the late 1990s? I believe that the first line of therapy should be clomiphene citrate. Women with PCOS who do not respond to clomiphene citrate (at 150 mg per day for five days) should then be offered ovarian drilling. This can be combined with checking tubal normality, and excluding other pelvic pathology. As electrocautery appears as effective as laser treatment, and is readily and cheaply available, this should be the method of choice. The number and depth of drill sites should be between four and ten. Unilateral cautery, I believe, cannot yet be dogmatically recommended as the series of Balen and Jacobs is too small, but may become the routine once their results are confirmed by larger studies.

Because the occurrence of adhesions after ovarian cautery seems to be significantly frequent, patients should have this explained to them before they decide on the procedure. They can be reassured that these adhesions are usually minor and do not seem to affect pregnancy rates. The risk of adhesions should be minimized by careful hemostasis, and irrigation lavage, as well as postoperative artificial ascites with normal saline. The possibility of a 'second-look' laparoscopy 2–6 weeks after electrocautery should be considered.

Finally the advantages of a prolonged effect for several potential pregnancies and normalization of LH levels with a lower early pregnancy loss rate should also be considered when the method of treatment is considered for clomiphene-resistant PCOS.

Acknowledgment

Thanks to Mrs Lee McLaren for typing the manuscript.

References

Abdel Gadir A, Mowafi RS, Alnaser HM *et al.* (1990a) Ovarian electrocautery, human menopausal gonadotrophins and pure follicle stimulating hormone therapy in the treatment of patients with polycystic ovarian disease. *Clinical Endocrinology (Oxford)* **33**: 585–592.

Abdel Gadir A, Khatim MS, Mowafi RS, Alnaser HMI, Alzaid HGN, Shaw RW (1990b) Hormonal changes in patients with polycystic ovarian disease after ovarian electrocautery or pituitary desensitization. *Clinical Endocrinology (Oxford)* **32**: 749–754.

Adashi EY, Rock JA, Guzick D *et al.* (1981) Fertility following bilateral ovarian wedge resection: a critical analysis of 90 consecutive cases of the polycystic ovary syndrome. *Fertility and Sterility* **36**: 320–325.

Armar NA, Lachelin GC (1993) Laparoscopic ovarian diathermy: an effective treatment for anti-oestrogen resistant anovulatory infertility in women with polycystic ovary syndrome. *British Journal of Obstetrics and Gynaecology* **100**: 161–164.

Balen AH, Jacobs HS (1991) Gonadotrophin surge attenuating factor: a missing link in the control of LH secretion? *Clinical Endocrinology (Oxford)* **35**: 399–402.

Balen AH, Jacobs HS (1994) Prospective study comparing unilateral and bilateral laparoscopic ovarian diathermy in women with polycystic ovary syndrome. *Fertility and Sterility* **62**: 921–925.

Balen AH, Jacobs HS (1995). Conception rates after laparoscopic electrocautery of the ovarian surface. *Fertility and Sterility* **63**: 1358–1359.

Balen AH, Tan SL, Jacobs HS (1993). Hypersecretion of luteinising hormone – a significant cause of subfertility and miscarriage. *British Journal of Obstetrics and Gynaecology* **100**: 1082–1089.

Campo S, Felli A, Lamanna MA, Barini A, Garcea N (1993). Endocrine changes and clinical outcome after laparoscopic ovarian resection in women with polycystic ovaries. *Human Reproduction* **8**: 359–363.

Dabirashrafi H (1989). Complications of laparoscopic ovarian cauterization. *Fertility and Sterility* **52**: 878.

Daniell JF, Miller W (1989). Polycystic ovaries treated by laparoscopic laser vaporization. *Fertility and Sterility* **51**: 232–236.

Box 23.4 Management of PCOS

- Wedge resection
- Clomiphene citrate induction
- Ovarian drilling
- Gonadotropin therapy

Farhi J, Soule S, Jacobs HS (1995). Effect of laparoscopic ovarian electrocautery on ovarian response and outcome of treatment with gonadotropins in clomiphene citrate-resistant patients with polycystic ovary syndrome. *Fertility and Sterility* **64**: 930–935.

Feste JR (1990) General aspects of CO_2 laser laparoscopy. In Baggish MS (ed.) *Endoscopic Laser Surgery.* pp. 67–68. New York: Elsevier.

Fukaya T, Murakami T, Tamura M, Watanabe T, Terada Y, Yajima A (1995). Laser vaporization of the ovarian surface in polycystic ovary disease results in reduced ovarian hyperstimulation and improved pregnancy rates. *American Journal of Obstetrics and Gynecology* **173**: 119–125.

Gemzell CA, Diczfalusy E, Tilliger KG (1960). Human pituitary follicle stimulating hormone. Clinical effect of a partially purified preparation. Ciba Foundation colloquia. *Endocrinology* **13**: 191–208.

Gjönnaess H (1984). Polycystic ovarian syndrome treated by ovarian electrocautery through the laparoscope. *Fertility and Sterility* **41**: 20–25.

Gjönnaess H (1994). Ovarian electrocautery in the treatment of women with polycystic ovary syndrome (PCOS). Factors affecting the results. *Acta Obstetricia et Gynecologica Scandinavica* **73**: 407–412.

Gjönnaess H, Norman N (1987). Endocrine effects of ovarian electrocautery in patients with polycystic ovarian disease. *British Journal of Obstetrics and Gynaecology* **94**: 779–782.

Greenblatt EM, Casper RF (1987). Endocrine changes after laparoscopic ovarian cautery in polycystic ovarian syndrome. *American Journal of Obstetrics and Gynecology* **156**: 279–285.

Greenblatt EM, Casper RF (1993). Adhesion formation after laparoscopic ovarian cautery for polycystic ovarian syndrome: lack of correlation with pregnancy rate. *Fertility and Sterility* **60**: 766–770.

Gurgan T, Kisnisci H, Yarali H, Devegliou O, Zeyneloglu H, Aksu T (1991). Evaluation of adhesion formation after a laparoscopic treatment of polycystic ovarian disease. *Fertility and Sterility* **56**: 1176–1178.

Gurgan T, Urman B, Aksu T, Yarali H, Develioglu O, Kisnisci H (1992). The effect of short-interval laparoscopic lysis of adhesions on pregnancy rates following Nd-Yag laser photocoagulation of polycystic ovaries. *Obstetrics and Gynecology* **80**: 45–47.

Gurgan T, Yarali H, Urman B (1994). Laparoscopic treatment of polycystic ovarian disease. *Human Reproduction* **9**: 573–577.

Heylen SM, Puttemans PJ, Brosens IA (1994). Polycystic ovarian disease treated by laparoscopic argon laser capsule drilling: comparison of vaporization versus perforation technique. *Human Reproduction* **9**: 1038–1042.

Keckstein J (1989) Laparoscopic treatment of polycystic ovarian syndrome. In Sutton CJG (ed.) *Baillière's Clinical Obstetrics and Gynaecology. Laparoscopic Surgery* **3(3)**: 563–581.

Keckstein J, Rossmanith W, Spatzier K, Schneider V, Borchers K, Steiner R (1990). The effect of laparoscopic treatment of polycystic ovarian disease by CO_2 laser or Nd:YAG laser. *Surgical Endoscopy* **4**: 103–107.

Kistner RW (1968). Induction of ovulation with clomiphene citrate. In Behrman SH, Kistner RW (eds) *Progress in Infertility.* p. 407. Boston: Little, Brown & Co.

Kovacs G, Buckler H, Bangah M *et al.* (1991). Treatment of anovulation due to polycystic ovarian syndrome by laparoscopic ovarian electrocautery. *British Journal of Obstetrics and Gynaecology* **98**: 30–35.

Naether OGJ (1995). Significant reduction of adnexal adhesion following laparoscopic electrocautery of the ovarian surface (LEOS) by lavage and artificial ascites. *Gynaecological Endoscopy* **4**: 17–19.

Naether OGJ, Fischer R (1993). Adhesion formation after laparoscopic electrocoagulation of the ovarian surface in polycystic ovary patients. *Fertility and Sterility* **60**: 95–98.

Naether OGJ, Fischer R (1995). Conception rates after laparoscopic electrocautery of the ovarian surface. *Fertility and Sterility* **63**: 1357–1358.

Naether OGJ, Fischer R, Weise HC, Geiger-Kotzler L, Delfs T, Rudolf K (1993). Laparoscopic electrocoagulation of the ovarian surface in infertile patients with polycystic ovarian disease. *Fertility and Sterility* **60**: 88–94.

Ostrzenski A (1992). Endoscopic carbon dioxide laser ovarian wedge resection in resistant polycystic ovarian disease. *International Journal of Fertility* **37**: 295–299.

Petrucco OM (1988) Laparoscopic CO_2 laser drilling of sheep ovaries – interval assessment of histological changes and adhesion formation. *Abstracts of the Seventh Scientific Meeting of The Fertility Society of Australia, Newcastle.* p. 21.

Ruutiainen K, Seppala M (1991). Polycystic ovary syndrome: evolution of a concept. *Current Opinion in Obstetrics and Gynecology* **3**: 326–335.

Sakata M, Tasaka K, Kurachi H, Terakawa N, Miyake A, Tanizawa O (1990). Changes of bioactive luteinizing hormone after laparoscopic ovarian cautery in patients with polycystic ovarian syndrome. *Fertility and Sterility* **53**: 610–613.

Stein FI (1964). Duration of fertility following ovarian wedge resection – Stein–Leventhal syndrome. *Western Journal of Surgery, Obstetrics and Gynecology* **78**: 237.

Stein FI, Leventhal ML (1935). Amenorrhea associated with bilateral polycystic ovaries. *American Journal of Obstetrics and Gynecology* **29**: 181–191.

Sumioki H, Utsumomyiya K, Korenaga M, Kadota T (1988). The effect of laparoscopic multiple punch resection of the ovary on hypothalamo-pituitary axis in polycystic ovary syndrome. *Fertility and Sterility* **50**: 567–572.

Szilagyi A, Hole R, Keckstein J, Rossmanith WG (1993). Effects of ovarian surgery on the dopaminergic and opioidergic control of gonadotropin and prolactin secretion in women with polycystic ovarian disease. *Gynaecological Endocrinology* **7**: 159–166.

Tiitinen A, Tenhunen A, Seppala M (1993). Ovarian electrocauterization causes LH-regulated but not insulin-regulated endocrine changes. *Clinical Endocrinology (Oxford)* **39**: 181–184.

Verhelst J, Gerris J, Joostens M, Van der Meer S, Van Royen E, Mahler C (1993). Clinical and endocrine effects of laser vaporization in patients with polycystic ovarian disease. *Gynaecological Endocrinology* **7**: 49–55.

24

Laparoscopic Treatment of Tubo-ovarian Abscess

D. ALAN JOHNS

Richland Medical Center, Fort Worth, Texas, USA

The accepted treatment for pelvic inflammatory disease and tubo-ovarian abscess has changed very little in the last 15 years. Newer, more potent antibiotic regimens have been used, but the mainstay of treatment remains laparotomy with drainage of the abscess and excision of the affected organs in those patients unresponsive to antibiotic therapy. Most recently, the trend has been toward treating suspected unruptured tubo-ovarian abscesses solely with aggressive antibiotic therapy (Kaplan *et al.*, 1967; Landers and Sweet, 1985). The common result of this approach is extensive dense pelvic adhesive disease with resultant pain and infertility. The alternative course of therapy (intervention by laparotomy) often results in sterility from hysterectomy or adhesive disease from both the infectious process and the laparotomy. Complications of laparotomy in these patients include wound infection and dehiscence, bowel injury, embolism, sepsis, and recurrence of the pelvic abscess (Pedowitz and Bloomfield, 1964). Thus, the treatment of pelvic abscess remains a challenge.

Pelvic abscesses most commonly occur as a result of infection within the fallopian tube with resultant drainage of pus and bacteria into the abdominal cavity. The most common organisms involved are *Neisseria gonorrhoeae*, *Chlamydia trachomatis*, and the facultative and obligate anaerobes (Faro, 1991). Most often, an intense inflammatory response involving the surrounding tissues (usually bowel, peritoneal surfaces, and omentum) occurs. These adhesions are initially very friable and avascular, but become more dense and vascular with time.

Other causes of pelvic abscesses include ruptured appendix, diverticulitis, postoperative pelvic infection related to pelvic surgery, traumatic injury to the bowel or pelvis, and iatrogenic surgical injuries.

Diagnosis

The diagnosis of tubo-ovarian abscess should be considered in any female presenting with significant pelvic pain (with or without a palpable mass), fever and/or leukocytosis. Ultrasound, radiography, computerized tomography (CT), and nuclear magnetic resonance imaging (NMRI) may be helpful in making the diagnosis. Laboratory evaluations including complete blood count (CBC) and erythrocyte sedimentation rate may also be useful.

Using the most advanced and sophisticated assays and scans coupled with a thorough physical examination, 35% of patients diagnosed with acute pelvic inflammatory disease are found to have other conditions when laparoscopy is used to confirm the diagnosis (Binstock *et al.*, 1986). Because of this, many authors advocate routine use of laparoscopy to confirm the diagnosis when pelvic inflammatory disease is suspected (Jacobson and Westrom, 1969; Chaparro *et al.*, 1978). The most common diagnoses confused with pelvic inflammatory disease and tubo-ovarian abscess include endometriomas (both ruptured and intact), bleeding corpus luteum cysts, mesenteric adenitis and ectopic pregnancy.

Treatment: Traditional Approach

When a tubo-ovarian abscess is suspected, the patient should be admitted to hospital immediately and appropriate laboratory evaluation initiated and specimens taken. After hospital admission but before laparoscopy, baseline laboratory evaluation includes a CBC, including white cell count and differential, liver function studies and clotting studies. Cervical cultures for *N. gonorrhoeae* and *C. trachomatis* are obtained.

At the time of laparoscopy, fluid from the abscess cavity is sent for both aerobic and anaerobic culture and sensitivity assays. Intravenous antibiotic therapy should be started at the time of admission. After laboratory evaluation has been obtained and antibiotics started, laparoscopy should be performed to confirm the diagnosis and document the extent of the infectious process. At this point, 35–40% of these patients will be found to have conditions other than pelvic infection producing their symptoms (Binstock *et al.*, 1986; Levine and Sanfilippo, 1989).

It was traditionally believed that surgical treatment of an acute pelvic infection often resulted in greater risk of injury to the bowel and reproductive tract than conservative therapy (antibiotics and observation). This was based on literature dating back 20–25 years (Pedowitz and Bloomfield, 1964; Kaplan *et al.*, 1967). Although in the past 10–20 years antibiotic therapy has progressed and surgical risks have decreased dramatically, this concept remains firmly entrenched.

Initial therapy includes high-dose intravenous antibiotics, which are continued until the patient remains afebrile for 48–72 hours. Some authors have recommended continued antibiotic therapy (after the patient has become afebrile) until the pelvic mass has diminished significantly in size by ultrasound examination or CT scan.

If the abscess is visible with ultrasound or palpable in the cul-de-sac, drainage through the cul-de-sac has been advocated (Franklin *et al.*, 1973). Abscesses higher in the pelvis may be drained transabdominally with ultrasound guidance (Gerzoff *et al.*, 1981). The abscess cavity should be thoroughly irrigated until the effluent is clear, and a drain is placed within the abscess cavity. Treatment by these methods is occasionally associated with recurrence of the abscess or significant morbidity.

Surgical intervention is recommended for those patients with multiloculated abscesses since multiple abscess cavities are difficult to drain vaginally. Those patients unresponsive to intravenous antibiotic therapy and those with multiloculated abscesses are also subjected to laparotomy with excision of the affected organs, often including hysterectomy and salpingo-oophorectomy. This regimen results in excellent cure rates, but significant morbidity, infertility from pelvic adhesive disease or extirpative pelvic surgery, and long-term hypo-estrogenic problems. In addition, the cost of long-term, in-hospital intravenous therapy with or without laparotomy is significant.

Laparoscopic Treatment: Modern Approach

In an effort to avoid the cost, morbidity and subsequent infertility problems associated with traditional treatment of tubo-ovarian abscesses, a regimen of laparoscopic treatment of pelvic abscesses (regardless of cause) and the associated acute fibrinous adhesions has evolved (Henry-Suchet *et al.*, 1984). When the laparoscopic approach is used it can be extremely cost-effective and benefit the patient.

Preoperative Evaluation and Treatment

The patient with a presumptive diagnosis of pelvic abscess is admitted to hospital immediately, appropriate laboratory evaluations are obtained, and intravenous antibiotics initiated. The choice of antibiotics should take into consideration the most common organisms producing pelvic abscesses. In the first instance, I recommend the use of simple broad-spectrum intravenous antibiotics (cefoxitin 2 g I.V. every four hours until the patient becomes afebrile). Oral doxycycline is used as soon as the patient is taking fluids orally (doxycycline 100 mg every 12 hours) for a total of ten days. Other single agents which could be used include ticarcillin/clavulanate (Timentin), ampicillin/sulbactam (Unasyn), or imipenem/cilastatin (Primaxin). In the rare patient who fails to respond to the combination of laparoscopic surgery and single dose agents, combination therapy (clindamycin and metronidazole) may be used. Once an adequate level of intravenous antibiotics has been attained, laparoscopy is performed for confirmation of the diagnosis and therapy.

Equipment

The laparoscopic treatment of pelvic inflammatory disease and tubo-ovarian abscess requires a minimum of laparoscopic equipment, but extraordinary patience.

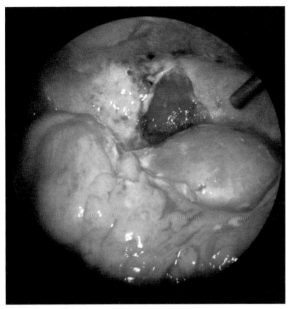

(a)

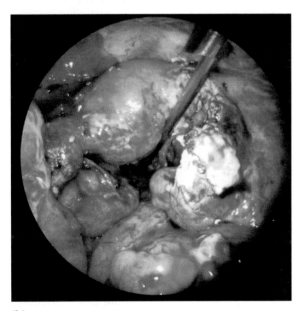

(b)

Figure 24.1 (a) The laparoscopic appearance of tubo-ovarian abscesses prior to conservative laparoscopic therapy. (b) The same patient after laparoscopic aspiration of abscess material and adhesiolysis.

A high-flow insufflator is mandatory to maintain an adequate pneumoperitoneum. A uterine manipulator is placed. Occasionally, electrocautery will be necessary for hemostasis, but bleeding is rarely a problem.

The single most important instrument used in the procedure is a hollow blunt dissecting probe through which irrigation fluid can be forced. This probe is invaluable for careful blunt dissection of

adhesions involving bowel and pelvic structures. Coupled with aquadissection (dissection of tissue planes with fluid under minimal pressure), the manipulation/dissection probe eliminates the need for scissors, lasers, or other more traumatic (and expensive) instruments.

Any intravenous fluid may be used for aquadissection, but the surgeon should know if this irrigating fluid encourages, supports or retards bacterial growth. Ringer's lactate is the most common fluid used for this dissection. It does not facilitate the growth of most bacteria in pelvic abscesses.

Technique

Under general anesthesia, the 10 mm diagnostic laparoscope is inserted through an intraumbilical incision. Two suprapubic incisions (5 mm) are made on either side of the midline, medial to the inferior epigastric vessels.

The patient is placed in the Trendelenburg position and the pelvis and upper abdomen are visually examined. If the diagnosis of pelvic abscess is confirmed, cultures are obtained (Figure 24.1a). The entire abdominal cavity is then thoroughly rinsed with irrigating fluid to remove blood, pus and debris. The pelvis is carefully inspected and evaluated. The most appropriate course of dissection is then planned.

Using the blunt dissection probe, omentum, small bowel and large bowel are carefully dissected away from pelvic structures. Irrigating fluid forced through the irrigation/dissection probe will often allow dissection planes between bowel and pelvic structures to be identified more easily. These planes may then be opened and extended bluntly or with aquadissection. Most often the abscess cavity will be entered during this initial dissection.

Once the abscess cavity has been entered, the patient should immediately be placed in the reverse Trendelenburg position and cultures obtained. The abscess cavity is then thoroughly irrigated and aspirated until all pus is totally removed. Copious amounts of irrigating fluid are used to cleanse the entire abdominal cavity of pus and debris. In the reverse Trendelenburg position there is minimal contamination of the upper abdomen.

The adnexal structures are then carefully dissected free. Since these adhesions are filmy and avascular, scissors dissection, laser dissection, and electrosurgery are rarely necessary. Very minimal bleeding will be encountered when careful blunt aquadissection is used. Once all structures have been identified and dissected, as much inflammatory exudate lining the abscess cavity should be removed as possible. This is accomplished with aquadissection and tissue grasping forceps. Aquadissection is most helpful in separating the necrotic abscess cavity from pelvic structures and bowel wall.

After dissection of all pelvic structures and removal of inflammatory exudate, the entire abdominal cavity is irrigated with copious amounts of warmed irrigation fluid. After each irrigation, the patient is placed in the reverse Trendelenburg position and the irrigating fluid is aspirated. The process of irrigation and aspiration is continued until the aspirated fluid is clear (Figure 24.1b).

When careful aquadissection is used (and scissors are avoided), very little bleeding will be encountered at the end of the dissection/irrigation process. Any residual bleeding can be controlled easily with microbipolar cautery. At the completion of the procedure, 1–2 litres of irrigation fluid is left in the abdomen in an attempt to 'float' pelvic structures and minimize subsequent adhesive disease. The intra-abdominal fluid also dilutes any remaining bacteria.

The umbilical incision is closed with absorbable sutures. The lower incisions are approximated with collodion. This allows fluid to escape from the lower incisions should abdominal distention occur. Abdominal and vaginal drains are not used.

Postoperative Care

Intravenous antibiotics are continued for 24 hours or until the patient is afebrile. Oral antibiotics are then continued for five days. No postoperative dietary restrictions are used and the patient's activity is not limited. Those patients desiring pregnancy are encouraged to undergo a second-look laparoscopy within two months of their initial procedure for treatment of any residual adhesive disease.

Aspiration of Pelvic Abscesses by Invasive Radiology

While laparoscopy represents a minimal invasive approach to the treatment of pelvic abscesses in contrast to laparotomy, radiological guided aspiration of these abscesses is another alternative, which is even less invasive. Several small series now exist of patients with abdominopelvic abscesses drained under CT or ultrasonographic guidance. Anecdotally, these reports suggest that drainage very often represents adequate therapy to treat the infectious process; however, the extent of adhesion development after these aspiration procedures

remains to be defined. Additionally, several brief reports have described transvaginal ultrasound guided drainage of abscesses. The cases described in the literature to date are primarily women with pelvic inflammatory disease; the applicability of these observations to infections of other etiologies remains to be established. Future studies will be needed to define the appropriate role of abscess aspiration, especially when considering long-term clinical outcome.

Conclusions

Compared to traditional treatment, laparoscopic treatment of pelvic abscess offers many potential advantages including the following:

- More precise dissection of pelvic structures using the magnification capability of the laparoscope.
- More through removal of pus and necrotic material from the pelvic cavity than would be possible at laparotomy.
- More thorough and precise irrigation of the upper abdomen by direction of fluid through the dissection/irrigation probe.
- Minimal intraoperative bleeding due to the use of magnification and aquadissection (as opposed to gross scissors and blunt dissection used at laparotomy).
- Decreased risk of bowel perforation due to more precise dissection of tissue planes using the magnification capabilities of the laparoscope.
- Elimination of the risk of wound infection and possible evisceration.
- A shortened patient recovery period – the patient recovers from the abscess, infectious process, and adhesiolysis, not from laparotomy.
- Decreased pelvic pain and infertility due to decreased pelvic adhesions as a result of laparoscopic treatment.

Our goal in treating pelvic abscess should include prevention of infertility and pelvic pain from resultant adhesive disease. The combination of laparoscopic treatment of pelvic abscesses and intravenous antibiotics offers an effective alternative to traditional long-term antibiotics or laparotomy with radical extirpative pelvic surgery.

Both anecdotal and published data imply significant advantages of the laparoscopic approach to pelvic abscess with few of the hazards of laparotomy in the acutely infected patient (Henry-Suchet et al., 1984; Reich and McGlynn, 1987; Reich, 1989). Large controlled randomized studies comparing laparotomy and laparoscopy for the treatment of pelvic abscesses with second-look data are needed to confirm this perceived advantage.

Major Complications Associated with Laparoscopic Treatment of Tubo-Ovarian Abscess

Complications include:

- Bowel perforation from the primary intra-umbilical trocar intraabdominal inflammatory processes may adhere the small or large bowel to the anterior abdominal wall.
- Sepsis and multisystem abscess formation as a result of 'seeding' the venous system with bacteria during dissection of the abscess cavity.
- Bowel perforation during dissection and drainage of the abscess.
- Excessive damage to adnexal structures from dissection.
- Intraoperative hemorrhage which can be extremely difficult to control due to edematous, friable, vascular tissue.

This procedure requires careful, meticulous, and gentle dissection techniques to minimize the risk of worsening an already compromised patient.

References

Binstock M, Muzsnai D, Apodaca L, Goldman L, Keith L (1986) Laparoscopy in the diagnosis and treatment of pelvic inflammatory disease. A review and discussion. *International Journal on Fertility* **31**: 341.

Chaparro MV, Ghosh S, Nashed A *et al.* (1978) Laparoscopy for the confirmation and prognostic evaluation of pelvic inflammatory disease. *International Journal of Gynecology and Obstetrics* **15**: 307.

Faro S (1991) Why pelvic abscesses form. *Contemporary Obstetrics and Gynecology* **36**: 69–71.

Franklin EW, Hevron JE, Thompson JD (1973) Management of the pelvic abscess. *Clinical Obstetrics and Gynecology* **16**: 66.

Gerzoff SG, Robbins AG, Johnson WC *et al.* (1981) Percutaneous catheter drainage of abdominal abscesses. *New England Journal of Medicine* **305**: 653.

Henry-Suchet J, Soler A, Loffredo V (1984) Laparoscopic treatment of tuboovarian abscesses. *Journal of Reproductive Medicine* **29**: 579.

Jacobson L, Westrom L (1969) Objectivized diagnosis of acute pelvic inflammatory disease: Diagnostic and prognostic value of routine laparoscopy. *American Journal of Obstetrics and Gynecology* **105**: 1088.

Kaplan AL, Jacobs WM, Ehresman JB (1967) Aggressive management of pelvic abscess. *American Journal of Obstetrics and Gynecology* **98**: 482.

Landers DV, Sweet RL (1985) Current trends in the diagnosis and treatment of tuboovarian abscess. *American Journal of Obstetrics and Gynecology* **151**: 1098.

Levine R, Sanfilippo J (1989) Endoscopic management of tubo-ovarian abscess and pelvic inflammatory disease. In Sanfilippo J, Levine R (eds) *Operative Gynecologic Endoscopy*. pp. 118–132. Berlin: Springer-Verlag.

Pedowitz P, Bloomfield RD (1964) Ruptured adnexal abscess (tuboovarian) with generalized peritonitis. *American Journal of Obstetrics and Gynecology* **88**: 721.

Reich H (1989) Role of laparoscopy in treating TOA and pelvic abscess. *Contemporary Obstetrics and Gynecology* **34**: 91.

Reich H, McGlynn F (1987) Laparoscopic treatment of tuboovarian and pelvic abscess. *Journal of Reproductive Medicine* **32**: 747.

Laparoscopic Uterine Surgery

25

Laparoscopic Uterine Nerve Ablation for Intractable Dysmenorrhea

CHRIS SUTTON

Royal Surrey County Hospital, Guildford, The Chelsea and Westminster Hospital, London and Imperial College School of Medicine, University of London, UK

Dysmenorrhea continues to be a problem in modern society and some 14% of all visits to the general practitioner of women between the ages of 15 and 50 years is related to this as the primary complaint (Richards, 1979). It is a major cause of periodic absenteeism from the workplace (Sundell *et al.*, 1990) and in the USA it has been estimated that 600 million hours are lost annually because of dysmenorrhea (Ylikorkala and Dawood, 1978). Those women who continue to work despite significant menstrual pain have a reduced productivity, increased accident rate and produce work of diminished quality (Lumsden, 1985; Dawood, 1990). In the UK around 6.8 million women are thought to have this problem and of these 2.6 million have such unpleasant symptoms that they have to discontinue their normal activities and retire to bed with strong analgesics (Anderson, 1981).

The actual incidence of dysmenorrhea in different populations is difficult to assess and depends upon many complex and variable factors, including prevailing social and sexual attitudes in different societies. Prevalence rates vary in different studies from 3–90%, but probably the best population study comes from Sweden where all 19-year-old girls from the town of Gothenburg were questioned with a 90% response rate (Andersch and Milsom, 1982). Of the girls 73% had primary dysmenorrhea and 15% had severe dysmenorrhea, which affected their working ability and could not be controlled adequately by analgesics or ovulation suppression. It is for this group of patients that surgery is recommended either by presacral neurectomy, the uterosacral ligament division technique of Doyle (Doyle, 1955) or more simply by laparoscopic uter-ine nerve ablation (LUNA). Before describing this technique it is worth considering the relevant anatomy and to describe in some detail Doyle's procedure, which we are trying to imitate with the laser or electrodiathermy at laparoscopy rather than using a scalpel at laparotomy.

Anatomy of the Uterine Nerve Supply

The sensory parasympathetic fibers to the cervix and the sensory sympathetic fibers to the corpus traverse the cervical division of the Lee-Frankenhauser plexus (Frankenhauser, 1864), which lies in, under and around the attachments of the uterosacral ligament to the posterior aspect of the cervix. Sympathetic fibers can also be found in this area and reach the cervix by accompanying the uterine and other arteries.

The parasympathetic components originate from the first to the fourth sacral nerves, reaching the plexus by the pelvic nerves (nervi erigentes). In a study of 33 cadavers Campbell (1950) confirmed the finding of earlier workers (Latarjet and Roget, 1922; Davis, 1936) by identifying parasympathetic fibers in the anterior two-thirds of the uterosacral ligaments and demonstrated the presence of small ganglia around the area where the ligaments attach to the cervix.

Theoretically, therefore, division of the uterosacral ligaments at the point of their attachment to the cervix should interrupt most of the cervical sensory fibers and some of the corporal sensory fibers and lead to reduced uterine pain at the time of menstruation. It is important at the outset for the surgeon and the patient to realize that division of the uterosacral ligaments will not obliterate all the afferent sensory nerve supply and cannot therefore be expected to provide completely painless periods or, indeed, painless childbirth.

Doyle's Procedure

In 1963 Joseph Doyle described the procedure of paracervical uterine denervation, which bears his name (Doyle and Des Rosiers, 1963). The procedure could be performed vaginally or abdominally and Doyle suggested that gynecologists may be more comfortable with the former approach while general surgeons would prefer the latter. Employing the vaginal approach a suture was placed through the posterior lip of the cervix at the apex of the vagina and traction on this suture increased the distance of the cervix from the ureter, which is clearly demonstrated in his article by a very convincing radiograph of a cervi-coureteterogram. The attachments of the uterosacral ligaments to the cervix were then divided between two Heaney clamps and to prevent regrowth of the bisected nerve trunks the posterior leaf of the peritoneal incision was interposed between them. The abdominal approach was recommended if endometriosis was suspected or any gross pathology, such as fibroids, were felt. The pathologic tissue was then excised (which may, of course, have had a significant effect on the results) and then traction was applied to the uterosacral ligaments by means of a suture placed in the cervix just above the point of their insertion. He carefully scrutinized the course of the ureters and found that they lie close to the ligaments, usually running 1–2 cm laterally. As before, the ligaments were divided between two clamps, and in a further refinement of the technique he sutured the ligaments together with stainless steel sutures to the isthmus of the cervix in the midline about 1 cm higher than their original attachment.

Doyle's results were extremely impressive with complete pain relief in 63 of 73 cases (86%): 35 had primary dysmenorrhea (85.7% success) and 38 had secondary dysmenorrhea (86.8% success). Relief was partial in six cases and there were four failures (Doyle, 1954, 1955). With such a satisfactory outcome it is difficult to see why the operation sank into obscurity. Possibly the advent of powerful prostaglandin synthetase inhibitors reduced the demand for relatively drastic forms of intervention. Interest in Doyle's work has revived with the development of surgical lasers and electrosurgical instruments, which can be used endoscopically to perform much the same tissue effect without the need for major surgery.

Counselling and Consenting the Patient

It is important to inform women of the likely success of the procedure and to make it clear that pain relief cannot be guaranteed and that it is intended to ameliorate the discomfort of dysmenorrhea rather than alleviate it completely. It certainly cannot be guaranteed to work in all cases and although we have no instances of patients being made worse by the procedure in our own series, Daniell (1989) has reported this and patients should probably be advised accordingly.

As with all laparoscopic procedures there is a definite, albeit small, risk of unexpected complications and patients should be consented for a laparotomy should the need arise.

Initial Pelvic Inspection

Before embarking on operative laparoscopy the surgeon should perform an anatomical tour of the pelvis to identify any structures that could be harmed if inadvertently hit with the laser or radiofrequency energy. This first step is vital to ensure the safety of operative laparoscopy and should never be omitted since no two pelvises are identical and anatomical variations, particularly concerning the course of the ureter, are not unusual.

The posterior leaves of the broad ligaments are carefully inspected to try to identify the course of the ureters, which can rarely lie close to the uterosacral ligaments, but commonly run 1–2 cm laterally. They can usually be 'palpated' via a probe and often the characteristic peristaltic movements can be recognized beneath the peritoneal surface. The operator should also take note of some thin-walled veins, which often lie just lateral to the uterosacral ligaments; if these veins are accidentally punctured they can cause troublesome bleeding, which can be very difficult to stop with the carbon dioxide (CO_2) laser. Hemostatic clips, bipolar diathermy or an endocoagulator should be immediately available if required.

Operative Procedure

Since laparoscopic surgery developed independently in several different centers it is not surprising that there are many different approaches to essentially the same operation. The description given here (Sutton, 1989a) is the method that I have developed and adapted over the past ten years using the double-puncture technique employing lasers for precise surgical destruction of tissue. The reasons for this preference are given, but alternative methods are described for those who do not have access to laser technology.

Laser Uterine Nerve Ablation (LUNA)

The uterosacral ligaments are encouraged to 'standout' by the assistant manipulating the uterus to one or other side with an 8 mm Hegar dilator or preferably with a Valtchev uterine mobilizer (Conkin Surgical Instruments, Toronto, Canada). If this fails to delineate them clearly a rigid metal probe is inserted through the suprapubic trocar and pressed on the posterior aspect of the cervix. The position of the ureters should be checked again and any large vessels in the vicinity of the ligaments noted.

The most precise way to ablate the uterosacral ligaments is to vaporize them with a CO_2 laser transmitted down the central channel of the laparoscope (Donnez and Nisolle, 1989) or via the iliac fossa trocar (Sutton, 1986; Figure 25.1). The disadvantage of the single-puncture approach is that a considerable amount of the cross-sectional diameter has to be sacrificed to the laser channel, inevitably resulting in reduced visibility. Furthermore, the actual view is not exactly the same as the path of the laser beam and there have been reports of accidental injury due to unrecognized interposition of a loop of bowel (Borten and Friedman, 1986).

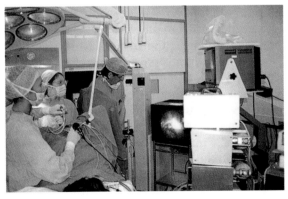

Figure 25.1 CO_2 laser laparoscopy being used for LUNA with double-puncture technique.

The laser is set at a relatively high power density setting of 10 000–15 000 W/cm^2 and the uterosacral ligaments are vaporized near the point of their attachment to the posterior aspect of the cervix. The idea of the procedure is to destroy the sensory nerve fibers and their secondary ganglia as they leave the uterus, and because of the divergence of these fibers in the uterosacral ligament they should be vaporized as close to the cervix as possible (Figure 25.2). A crater about 1 cm in diameter and 5 mm deep is formed and great care must be taken to vaporize medially rather than laterally to avoid damage to the vessels already identified coursing alongside the uterosacral ligaments (Figure 25.3). A further refinement is to laser the posterior aspect of the cervix superficially between the insertion of the ligaments to interrupt fibers crossing to the contralateral side (Daniell, 1989).

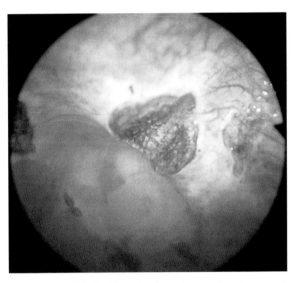

Figure 25.2 LUNA. Vaporization of the right uterosacral ligament showing depth of vaporization until nerve fibers stop splitting.

Vaporization continues until the nerve fibers stop splitting, but care should be taken not to go too deep since a relatively large artery often lurks in the depth of the ligament and if transected it can bleed copiously. It is relatively easy to vaporize to the correct depth when the uterosacral ligaments are well formed, but sometimes their limits are poorly defined and the procedure is less than satisfactory simply because it is difficult to be sure that the area vaporized is in the same place as the uterine nerve fibers.

FLEXIBLE FIBER LASERS

We are increasingly using the potassium titanyl phosphate (KTP)/532 laser (Laserscope, San Jose, California, USA) for uterosacral ligament transection

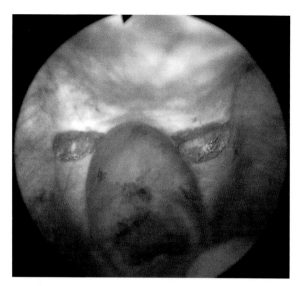

Figure 25.3 LUNA on well-developed uterosacral ligaments. Note that a large artery is just visible at the base of the crater on the left.

because it is very quick and effective and is associated with less bleeding. This laser is a frequency doubled neodymium:yttrium-aluminum-garnet (Nd:YAG) laser and is transmitted down flexible reusable silicone quartz optical fibers as a visible emerald green light. When dragged across stretched tissue the end of the fiber will vaporize tissue – probably a thermal effect (Keckstein, 1989) – and provides effective cutting, but if bleeding occurs the fiber can be held a few millimetres away from the bleeding point and fired to photocoagulate the vessel and seal it. Sometimes it is necessary to flush away the blood with irrigant solution, which passes down the same introducer as the laser fiber, to achieve hemostasis. If large vessel hemorrhage is encountered it is possible to interpose a mirror at a flick of a switch and seal the artery with the deeper penetrating Nd:YAG laser energy, which is produced in the same laser generator.

The argon laser can also be employed, but in my experience, although of similar wavelength to the KTP, is not so effective at cutting and produces a blanched zone of coagulation, which makes it difficult to assess the depth of penetration. The Nd:YAG laser on its own should be used with considerable caution because of its deep penetration, but in skilled hands has been associated with good results (Corson, 1992). Nevertheless I have seen video recordings from other institutions showing catastrophic bleeding with the use of the Nd:YAG laser over the internal iliac artery – a sobering example of the effect this laser has deep below the surface. In order to get around these problems manufacturers have devised artificial sapphire tips and sculpted quartz fibers to focus the energy, but such devices only work when contaminated with blood and

tissue debris and then heat to 600°C, so the effect is purely a thermal one and could be achieved much more cheaply with an electrodiathermy needle or probe (Keckstein *et al.*, 1988). Indeed, laser manufacturers seem to have realized that they have produced a sophisticated 'hot wire' with the introduction of the fibretom (Medilas, MBB, Germany), which incorporates an optoelectronic control system to regulate the heat applied to the tissue. A sensor in the laser measures the temperature of the fiber tip during cutting and a servomechanism automatically controls the laser power to keep the temperature of the tip below the meltdown threshold (Sutton and Hodgson, 1992).

ELECTRODIATHERMY AND ENDOCOAGULATION

If laser technology is not available electrodiathermy and endocoagulation can be employed, but the depth of tissue destruction is difficult to assess and studies in experimental animals and humans show that healing is less efficient than after laser surgery (Bellina *et al.*, 1984).

If electrosurgery is employed it is more efficacious to use a microdiathermy needle on pure cutting current to excise a segment of the uterosacral ligament just before it enters the posterior aspect of the cervix. This is particularly important if the uterosacral ligament is involved in deeply infiltrating implants, which can result in disabling dysmenorrhea. Martin *et al.* (1989) showed that 61% of their patients had clinically recognized lesions penetrating deeper than 2 mm, 43% had lesions penetrating deeper than 3 mm, and 25% had lesions penetrating deeper than 5 mm; some even went as deep as 15 mm. Thus, laser vaporization to 5 mm would have missed the full depth of endometriotic lesions in 25% of the patients if a mere depth was aimed at, but in practise we continue to vaporize until we are down to normal tissue. A more satisfactory technique, however, is to use the CO_2 laser in a superpulse or ultrapulse mode in order to excise tissue effectively, or to use an electrosurgical needle or scissors to excise all the tissue involved in the endometriotic disease process and submit the specimen for histologic examination to check that excision is complete. Konninckx *et al.* (1991) have shown that this deeply infiltrating disease is associated with the most pelvic pain and the deeper the implant the more severe the pain. Many specialized centers treating advanced endometriosis are using excisional techniques, either with the laser or with electrosurgery to remove these deposits since they are invariably unresponsive to drug therapy. Redwine (1991) has shown excellent long-term results, which indicate a maximum occurrence of new disease of 19% over a five-year period of meticulous follow-up.

Endocoagulation (Semm, 1966; Semm and O'Neill-Freys, 1989) is undoubtedly safer (Semm and Mettler, 1980), but much slower than electrodiathermy. Tissue is heated to about 100°C and when this temperature is reached the acoustic signal changes frequency and is present until the tissue cools to 60°C. This can be rather tedious although the process can be accelerated by flushing the tip with cool saline solution. If the crocodile forceps are removed before this temperature is reached the instrument sticks to the tissue with resultant bleeding when the jaws are opened.

Although electrosurgical equipment is getting safer, there have been many reports of accidents occurring when:

- The hot tip of the electrode at about 600°C inadvertently touches bowel.
- Radiofrequency current follows the path of least resistance and damages bowel distant to the site of application (Di Novo, 1983) due to its high electrolyte content.

Ureteric injuries have also occurred when electrocautery has been used for laparoscopic sterilization (Irvin et al., 1975), during electrosurgical resection of endometriosis (Gomel and James, 1991) and, more pertinently, during electrofulguration of an endometriotic implant on the uterosacral ligament (Cheng, 1976).

Lichten and Bombard (1987) used electrosurgery to perform LUNA and 81% of a small group of 11 patients reported relief from dysmenorrhea.

COMPLICATIONS

Apart from the risks of electrosurgery alluded to above, the main problem is hemorrhage either from the thin-walled veins just lateral to the uterosacral ligaments or from arterial bleeding from large vessels lying deep in the uterosacral ligaments. If bleeding does occur attempts should be made to stem the flow by the usual techniques of pressure with a blunt probe and then firing the laser in a rosette fashion around the bleeding point using a defocused beam and a lower power density. If this is unsuccessful other endoscopic techniques of hemostasis should be instantly available, either endocoagulation (Semm, 1966), bipolar desiccation (Reich, 1989) or laparoscopic endoclips (Semm and O'Neill-Freys, 1989). If there is any uncertainty about the effectiveness of hemostasis a redivac drain should be inserted through the suprapubic cannula before withdrawing it to lessen the chance of hematoma formation

and to monitor any ongoing blood loss. If hemorrhage continues it is safer to resort to laparotomy to stop the bleeding. Two patients have died as a result of postoperative hemorrhage following this procedure in the USA (Daniell, 1989) and patients should never be discharged from a day-care facility if there is a possibility of ongoing intraperitoneal bleeding.

RESULTS

The first laser laparoscopy in the UK was performed in Guildford, Surrey, in October 1982 using a Sharplan CO_2 laser (Litechnica, Manchester, UK). Since then we have treated more than 4500 women with CO_2 laser laparoscopy and during the past eight years we have also used a combined KTP and Nd:YAG laser (Laserscope, San Jose, California, USA). Most of the patients treated have had endometriosis and about 20% of the women have had laparoscopic LUNA performed for secondary dysmenorrhea associated with endometriosis or for primary dysmenorrhea unresponsive to medical treatment. During the first five years we conducted a careful longitudinal study of the patients with endometriosis (Sutton and Hill, 1990) and as an offshoot of this enquiry we also followed a group of patients who had severe dysmenorrhea without pelvic pathology. These patients with primary dysmenorrhea were asked to record the intensity of their pain on a linear analogue scale, marked from 0–10, before the operation and at the follow-up visit four months later. All patients were warned that the first period might be slightly more uncomfortable, possibly due to edema around the nerve fibers during the healing process after laser surgery. The follow-up interview was conducted by one of the vocational trainees from general practise in order to minimize subjective bias that might have been introduced had the surgeon himself seen the patient at the follow-up visit. Patients with secondary (congestive) dysmenorrhea were informed that if endometriosis was discovered at diagnostic laparoscopy all visible implants would be vaporized and the uterosacral ligaments would also be vaporized if this was technically feasible. Sometimes only one of the ligaments was anatomically obvious and in that case the procedure was recorded as a partial LUNA.

In the course of this longitudinal study we followed 100 consecutive patients with dysmenorrhea associated with endometriosis and 26 patients with no obvious pelvic pathology. We deliberately did not include patients with secondary dysmenorrhea due to other causes such as fibroids or pelvic congestion.

For patients with primary dysmenorrhea we used a linear analogue scale to judge the response to treatment. The initial score on average was 9.2. The symptoms improved in 16 patients (73%) with an average score among the successful patients of 3.4. Of these, 15 had a complete neurectomy and one had a partial neurectomy due to poor formation of the uterosacral ligament on one side.

No patients were made worse by the procedure, but six patients failed to show any improvement, though for three of these a partial neurectomy was performed, suggesting an element of technical failure. Of the three patients who failed to show any improvement one subsequently had a hysterectomy and the pathologist noted marked adenomyosis in the myometrium (endometriosis interna), explaining her lack of response to nerve severance. Four patients were lost to follow-up.

Of the 100 women with dysmenorrhea associated with endometriosis six were lost to follow-up. Of those who were followed up 81 (86%) reported an improvement in symptoms even though 26 (32%) of them had a partial (unilateral) neurectomy. In three patients the symptoms returned at 6–12 months following the procedure. No patients were made worse, but 13 reported no improvement, and interestingly, nine of these had incomplete or partial neurectomies (Sutton, 1989b).

There were no serious complications in this group of patients and all were treated on a day case or overnight stay basis. Troublesome bleeding was encountered in two patients, requiring endocoagulation or hemostatic clips and the insertion of a redivac drain in the pelvis for 12 hours.

Division of the autonomic nerves and ganglia in the Lee-Frankenhauser plexus does not appear to have any adverse effect on bowel or bladder function and no patients have reported any reduction in the ability to enjoy sexual intercourse or achieve orgasm (Daniell, 1992).

Discussion

Although many women are able to cope with the symptoms of dysmenorrhea, a sizeable proportion of the female population have to take to their bed for a few days each month and use potent analgesics to obtain pain relief (Anderson, 1981).

Before 1960 many patients were treated surgically with interruption of the inferior hypogastric nerve plexus as it ramifies over the sacral promontory (Black, 1964; Counseller, 1934) or simple division of the uterosacral ligaments, performed either abdominally or vaginally (Doyle, 1955). Early reports of presacral neurectomy yielded disappointing results with failure rates of around 11–15% for primary dysmenorrhea and 25–40% for secondary dysmenorrhea (Tucker, 1947; Ingersoll and Meigs, 1948). In 1952 White pointed out that the nerve supply to the cervix is not usually interrupted by the presacral neurectomy procedure (White, 1952). For this reason and because of the development of powerful prostaglandin synthetase inhibitors and new steroids to inhibit ovulation, the procedure was all but abandoned by most gynecologists.

A significant reduction in the prevalence of dysmenorrhea was noted with the advent of the combined oral contraceptive pill (Royal College of General Practitioners, 1974), a greater influence being exhibited by those preparations with dominant progestogen activity (Dygdeman et al., 1979).

The discovery that many prostaglandins are raised in women with dysmenorrhea (Chan et al., 1981; Lumsden et al., 1983; Milsom and Andersch, 1984) led to the widespread use of non-steroidal anti-inflammatory drugs (NSAIDs) to treat this condition and surgical procedures virtually shrank into obscurity.

Nevertheless there remains a significant proportion of sufferers, as many as 20%, who fail to respond to such pharmacologic manipulation (Anderson, 1981; Dawood, 1985; Henzl, 1985), and for these women some form of surgical intervention remains an option. Several recent reports of presacral neurectomy from specialist centers have given excellent results, but have involved a large midline incision and all the disadvantages of major surgery (Lee et al., 1986; Tjaden et al., 1990; Fliegner and Umstead, 1991); although with ancillary instruments like the argon beam coagulator it is possible to perform this procedure laparoscopically (Daniell, 1992). This is the subject of Chapter 26.

With the increasing popularity of operative laparoscopy in recent years there has been a revival of interest in Doyle's procedure because it is possible to transect or destroy the uterosacral ligaments with either diathermy coagulation and laparoscopic scissors (Lichten and Bombard, 1987), the CO_2 laser (Daniell and Feste, 1985; Feste, 1985; Donnez and Nisolle, 1989; Sutton, 1989a) or the KTP/532 laser (Daniell, 1989).

The study of Lichten and Bombard (1987) is particularly interesting because it is the only randomized prospective double-blind study performed in this rapidly developing branch of operative gynecology. A relatively homogeneous group of women were selected who had severe or incapacitating dysmenorrhea and no demonstrable pelvic pathology at laparoscopy and who were unresponsive to NSAIDs and oral contraceptives prescribed concurrently. Coexisting psychiatric illness was evaluated with the Minnesota Multiphasic Personality Inventory and those with an abnormal psychologic profile were excluded from the study. The remaining 21 patients were randomized to uterine nerve ablation or control group at the time of diagnostic laparoscopy. Neither the patient nor the clinical psychologist who conducted the interview and the follow-up was aware of the group to which the patient had been randomized. No patient in the control group reported relief from dysmenorrhea whereas nine of the 11 patients (81%) who had LUNA reported almost complete relief at three months and five of them had continued relief from dysmenorrhea one year after surgery. Interestingly, those that reported surgical success also reported relief from the associated symptoms of nausea, vomiting, diarrhea and headaches. Although there were no reported complications in this study the numbers involved were small and the use of thermocautery in this area is potentially hazardous because of the proximity of the ureter.

We originally chose the CO_2 laser because of its ability to vaporize tissue precisely causing a zone of thermal necrosis only 100 µm beyond the impact site (Wilson, 1988), and employing the new ultra-pulse lasers (Coherent Lasers, Cambridge, UK) the zone of irreversible tissue damage is less than 50 µm. The laser craters in the uterosacral ligaments produce very little postoperative pain – no more than that associated with a diagnostic laparoscopy because all tissue debris is removed in the laser smoke plume and residual carbon is flushed away by a jet of irrigant solution. There is very little inflammatory reaction, no edema and

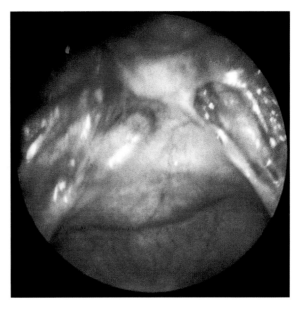

Figure 25.5 LUNA crater at second-look laparoscopy – three months after KTP/532 laser treatment. (Photograph courtesy of Jim Daniell.)

healing occurs with virtually no fibrosis, contracture or adhesion formation (Figures 25.4, 25.5). The main disadvantage of the CO_2 laser is the almost total absorption by water, rendering it ineffective in the presence of anything more than capillary bleeding. Any gynecologist attempting LUNA should be able to use endoscopic operative skills to deal with hemorrhage by suture, endo-coagulation, clips or diathermy or be prepared to perform a laparotomy to stop the bleeding, and the patient should be forewarned of this possible complication.

Because of its ease of use, limited penetration and ability to deal with bleeding we have recently favored the KTP/532 laser (Figure 25.6), which was initially pioneered in gynecology by James Daniell in Nashville, Tennessee (Daniell, 1986, 1989). His

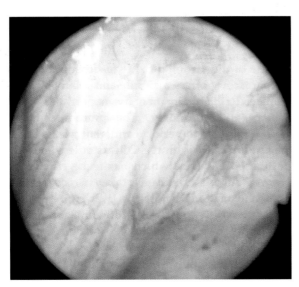

Figure 25.4 LUNA crater at second-look laparoscopy – three months after CO_2 laser vaporization.

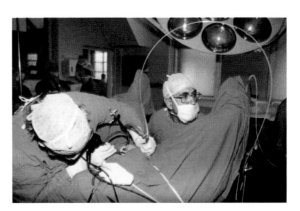

Figure 25.6 KTP/532 emerald green flexible fiber laser.

Table 25.1 LUNA results with KTP laser. (Data from Daniell, 1989.)

	Improved	Same	Worse
Endometriosis 80 patients	60 (75%)	17 (21%)	3 (4%)
Primary dysmenorrhea 20 patients	12 (60%)	6 (30%)	2 (10%)
Total 100 patients	72 (72%)	23 (23%)	5 (5%)

initial results for LUNA employing the KTP laser are shown in Table 25.1. To anyone who has visited his surgical facility in Nashville it is abundantly clear that his patients are very well informed: he carefully counsels his patients and tells them that the first period might still be painful; he also tells them that some of them may be made worse by the procedure, and this does appear to be the case for 4% of patients with endometriosis and 10% with primary dysmenorrhea. The relatively high number in this latter group without pelvic pathology suggests that there may be considerable psychological overlay. We do not tell patients that the procedure may make their periods worse and so far no patients have complained of a deterioration in dysmenorrhea.

Although LUNA technique is frequently used by laser laparoscopists during the investigation of dysmenorrhea and dyspareunia there are only a few reported series in the literature. Feste (1985) reported his results with 12 patients in a review of 202 patients treated by laser laparoscopy. In a review article Daniell and Feste (1985) reported on their combined results with CO_2 laser

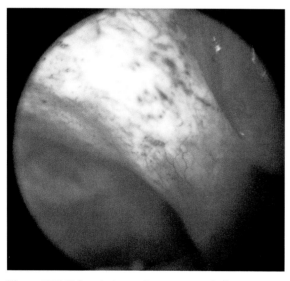

Figure 25.7 Telangiectases in uterosacral ligaments – atypical appearance of endometriosis.

laparoscopy in a series of 50 patients: 64% with endometriosis and 50% with primary dysmenorrhea were cured. Feste (1989) presented an update of his work at the World Endometriosis Congress in Houston. He performed laser neurectomy on 196 patients with intractable dysmenorrhea associated with endometriosis (Figure 25.7), and in the 124 patients that he managed to follow up the success rate was 87% – almost exactly the same as our result even though at the time neither surgeon was aware of the technique or laser power used by the other (Table 25.2). It is also interesting that the result is almost exactly the same as that obtained by Doyle in 1963 by laparotomy (Doyle and Des Rosiers, 1963).

Table 25.2 LUNA results with CO_2 laser. (Sutton, 1989b.)

	Lost to follow up	Improved	Same	Worse
Endometriosis 100 patients	6	81 (86%)	13	—
Primary dysmenorrhea 26 patients	4	16 (73%)	6	—
Total 126 patients	10	97 (84%)	19	—

Donnez has reported a series of 100 patients who have been followed for more than one year (Donnez and Nisolle, 1989). There was complete relief of symptoms in 50% of the patients while 41% reported mild to moderate relief. There was no change in the symptoms of 9%, but no patient said that their dysmenorrhea was worse following the procedure. In this study they also found that many patients complaining of dyspareunia experienced relief from this symptom and we have also noticed this in the absence of endometriosis especially in patients with very taut and well-demarcated uterosacral ligaments. Donnez's group may, however, have another explanation for this finding since they have found histologic evidence of endometriosis in biopsies of the uterosacral ligaments in 52% of patients with pelvic pain when there was no laparoscopic evidence of the disease (Nisolle *et al.*, 1990). There is considerable controversy in the literature about the significance of random peritoneal biopsies, but if it is eventually shown that endometriosis exists without its usual outward appearances it calls into question the whole philosophy of vaporizing the deposits with lasers or electrocautery and certainly explains some of our treatment failures.

GUILDFORD PROSPECTIVE RANDOMIZED
DOUBLE-BLIND CONTROLLED TRIAL OF LASER
LAPAROSCOPY FOR STAGES I–III ENDOMETRIOSIS

In order to investigate the role of laser laparoscopy in the treatment of endometriosis, it was necessary to perform a double-blind prospective randomized controlled study comparing laparoscopic ablation of endometrial implants and LUNA with diagnostic laparoscopy and no other treatment. The placebo effect of any new treatment, especially that associated with new high-technology inventions such as lasers, can be significant. It was therefore essential that a prospective study was performed comparing laser treatment with a sham (no treatment) arm to determine whether or not this therapy really worked. The study was approved by the Hospital Ethics Committee, but they reasonably felt that it was unethical to withhold treatment from patients in severe pain due to Stage IV disease, particularly because our previous experience had shown 80% pain relief in this group, most of whom had failed to respond to medical therapy (Sutton *et al.*, 1993).

There were 63 patients with pain (dysmenorrhea, pelvic pain or dyspareunia) and minimal to moderate endometriosis enrolled in the study and randomized at the time of laparoscopy by a computer generated randomization sequence to either laser ablation of endometriotic deposits and LUNA or expectant management alone. Pain symptoms were recorded subjectively and by visual analogue scale. The women were unaware of the treatment allocated as was the nurse who assessed them at three and six months after surgery. The main outcome measure was improvement or resolution of pain symptoms assessed both subjectively by a pain score and by a visual analogue score on a scale of 0–10, 10 representing the most severe pain in their life. The code was broken at six months and we discovered somewhat to our dismay that at three months there was little difference between either arm of the study; 18 of 32 (56%) in the laser-treated group reported that their pain was better or improved compared with 15 of 31 (48%) in the expectant group (z = 0.37, P = 0.35, Fisher's exact test). However at the six month follow-up, 20 of 32 (62.5%) in the laser group were better, which was significantly different from seven of 31 (22.6%) in the expectant group (z = 2.92, P < 0.01, Fisher's exact test) (Figures 25.8, 25.9).

The median value of visual analogue scores related to time are illustrated in Figure 25.9. At three months the median decrease in pain score was 2.6 for the laser group and 1.2 for the expectant group; this was not significant (P = 0.9,

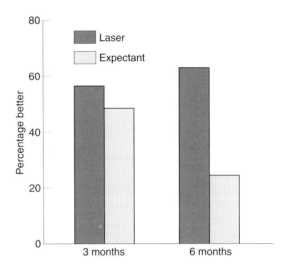

Figure 25.8 Proportion of patients with pain symptom alleviation at all stages. From Sutton CJG *et al.* 1994. Reproduced with permission of the publisher, the American Society for Reproductive Medicine.

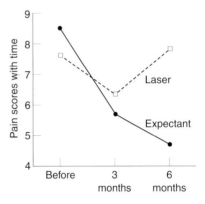

Figure 25.9 Median visual analogue pain scores (with time). From Sutton CJG *et al.* 1994. Reproduced with permission of the publisher, the American Society for Reproductive Medicine.

Mann–Whitney U test). When the decrease in pain score from baseline to six months is analyzed, the median decrease was 2.9 for the laser group and 0.1 for the expectant group. This difference was significant (P = 0.01, Mann–Whitney U test). When successful outcome after laser laparoscopy was analyzed stage by stage it was apparent that the poorest results were for Stage I; it may well be that some of these minimal appearances do not in fact represent endometriosis at all. Biopsy was not permitted because in itself it would have acted as cytoreductive surgery. If patients with Stage I disease were excluded from analysis, 14 of 19 (73.7%) patients experienced pain relief at six months after laser laparoscopy compared with only three of 15 (20%) in the group managed expectantly.

In this study all patients who still had pain at the end of six months were offered an immediate laser laparoscopy and the one-year follow-up of this group shows a 75% relief of pain symptoms.

The study is interesting because it is the first time that laser laparoscopy has been subjected to the true scientific test of efficacy, namely a randomized prospective double-blind controlled study comparing the treatment with a sham arm where no treatment was given apart from the removal of the serosanguineous fluid in the pelvis in order to complete the diagnostic examination. It is interesting to speculate whether or not the removal of this fluid was responsible for the relatively good results at three months and possibly it took some considerable time for the noxious substances and pain-mediating hormones found in that fluid to reaccumulate; or possibly it is a phenomenon well-known to psychologists called 'pain memory', which appears to be beneficial at least for three months after feeling some therapeutic intervention has been performed.

A further subjective interest is whether or not the uterine nerve ablation contributed to the good results at six months and at the time of writing we are near to completing a further randomized prospective study, but on this occasion there is no sham arm and it merely compares patients treated by laser vaporization of peritoneal implants on the one hand and those who additionally had uterine nerve ablation. Hopefully this will elucidate the role of laparoscopic uterine nerve ablation in the management of these patients.

Summary

The use of the CO_2 or fiberoptic lasers at laparoscopy offers a simple and relatively safe approach to the treatment of dysmenorrhea, both primary and secondary. The procedure takes about five minutes to perform and generates a large amount of smoke with the CO_2 laser (less so with the fiberoptic lasers), which has to be efficiently removed. However, as long as care is taken in recognizing the pelvic anatomy before the laser is fired there should be little possibility of damage to the ureters or the thin-walled veins coursing just medial to the uterosacral ligaments.

Prospective double-blind randomized controlled studies have shown that laparoscopic transection of the uterosacral ligaments close to their insertion in the posterior aspect of the cervix is an effective treatment for dysmenorrhea that has been unresponsive to drug therapy. Further trials are needed on larger numbers of patients to establish the long-term results,

but available evidence suggests that this relatively simple procedure is a useful technique in laparoscopic surgery and confers considerable benefit on patients with recalcitrant dysmenorrhea.

Complications of laparoscopic uterine nerve ablation for intractable dysmenorrhoea

- Injury to the ureter.
- Injury to the internal iliac artery.
- Venous bleeding from plexus of vessels just lateral to the uterosacral ligament.
- Arterial bleeding from deep down in the uterosacral ligament.
- Injury to the rectum if the rectum is tethered by endometriosis with partial or complete obliteration of the cul-de-sac.

Before performing LUNA, the laparoscopic surgeon must undertake a careful anatomical check on the structures of the pelvic sidewall. There are several structures running in parallel with the uterosacral ligament, including the ureter and the internal iliac artery. It is important to trace the course of the ureter from the pelvic brim, making sure that the characteristic peristaltic movements can be seen, which will always identify it unless the patient is very obese or there is considerable distortion of the anatomy due to endometriosis. It is particularly the medial part of the uterosacral ligaments that must be removed in order to perform uterine neurectomy and it is important that the irrigation and suction equipment (as well as bipolar diathermy) are available and are working, before performing the procedure in the event of encountering troublesome bleeding.

Finally, remember that 5% of patients have duplication of the ureter, which can place it perilously close to the uterosacral ligament.

References

Andersch B, Milsom I (1982) An epidemiologic study of young women with dysmenorrhoea. *American Journal of Obstetrics and Gynecology* **144**: 655.

Anderson A (1981) The role of prostaglandin synthetase inhibitors in gynaecology. *The Practitioner* **225**: 1460–1470.

Bellina JH, Hemmings R, Voros IJ, Ross LF (1984) Carbon dioxide laser and electrosurgical wound study with an animal model. A comparison of tissue damage and healing patterns in peritoneal tissue. *American Journal of Obstetrics and Gynecology* **148**: 327.

Black WT Jr (1964) Use of pre-sacral sympathectomy in the treatment of dysmenorrhoea: a second look after 25 years. *American Journal of Obstetrics and Gynecology* **89**: 17.

Borten M, Friedman EA (1986) Visual field obstruction in single puncture operative laparoscopy. *Journal of Reproductive Medicine* **31(12)**: 1102–1105.

Campbell RM (1950) Anatomy and physiology of sacrouterine ligaments. *American Journal of Obstetrics and Gynecology* **59**: 1.

Chan WY, Dawood MY, Fuchs F (1981) Prostaglandins in primary dysmenorrhoea. *American Journal of Medicine* **70**: 535–540.

Cheng YS (1976) Ureteral injury resulting from laparoscopic fulguration of endometriotic implant. *American Journal of Obstetrics and Gynecology* **126**: 1045–1046.

Corson SL (1992) Neodymium-YAG laser laparoscopy. In Sutton CJG (ed.) *Lasers in Gynaecology*. pp. 141–154. London: Chapman and Hall.

Counsellor V (1934) Resection of the pre-sacral nerves: evaluation of end results. *American Journal of Obstetrics and Gynecology* **28**: 161.

Daniell JF (1986) Laparoscopic evaluation of the KTP/532 laser for treating endometriosis – initial report. *Fertility and Sterility* **46**: 373.

Daniell JF (1989) Fibreoptic laser laparoscopy. In Sutton C (ed.) *Baillière's Clinical Obstetrics and Gynaecology. Laparoscopic Surgery* **3(3)**: 545–562.

Daniell JF (1992) Advanced operative laser laparoscopy. In Sutton CJG (ed.) *Lasers in Gynaecology*. pp. 119–139. London: Chapman and Hall.

Daniell JF, Feste J (1985) Laser laparoscopy. In Keye WR (ed.) *Laser Surgery in Gynecology and Obstetrics*. Chapter 11, pp. 147–165. Boston MA: GK Hall.

Davis A (1936) Intrinsic dysmenorrhoea. *Proceedings of the Royal Society of Medicine* **29**: 931.

Dawood YM (1985) Dysmenorrhoea. *Pain and Analgesia* **1**: 20.

Dawood YM (1990) Dysmenorrhoea. In Reiter RC (ed.) *Chronic Pelvic Pain. Clinical Obstetrics and Gynaecology* **33(1)**: 168–178.

Di Novo JA (1983) Radiofrequency leakage current from unipolar laparoscopic electrocoagulators. *Journal of Reproductive Medicine* **28(9)**: 565–575.

Donnez J, Nisolle M (1989) Carbon-dioxide laser laparoscopy in pelvic pain and infertility. In Sutton CJG (ed.) *Baillière's Clinical Obstetrics and Gynaecology. Laparoscopic Surgery* **3(3)**: 525–544.

Doyle JB (1954) Paracervical uterine denervation for dysmenorrhoea. *Transactions of the New England Obstetrical and Gynecological Society* **8**: 143.

Doyle JB (1955) Paracervical uterine denervation by transection of the cervical plexus for the relief of dysmenorrhoea. *American Journal of Obstetrics and Gynecology* **70**: 1.

Doyle JB, Des Rosiers JJ (1963) Paracervical uterine denervation for relief of pelvic pain. *Clinical Obstetrics and Gynecology* **6**: 742–753.

Dygdeman M, Bremme K, Gillespie A, Lundstrom V (1979) Effects of prostaglandins on the uterus. *Acta Obstetricia et Gynecologica Scandinavica Supplement* **87**: 33–38.

Feste JR (1985) Laser laparoscopy. *Journal of Reproductive Medicine* **30**: 414.

Feste JR (1989) *Proceedings of the 2nd World Congress of Gynaecological Endoscopy*. p. 35. Basel: Karger.

Fliegner JRH, Umstead MP (1991) Presacral neurectomy – a reappraisal. *Australian and New Zealand Journal of Obstetrics and Gynaecology* **31**: 76–79.

Frankenhauser G (1864) Die Bewegungenerven der Gerbarmutter. *Zeitschrift fur Medizinische Nat. Wissemburg* **1**: 35.

Gomel V, James C (1991) Intraoperative management of ureteral injury during laparoscopic surgery. *Fertility and Sterility* **55**: 416–419.

Henzl MR (1985) Dysmenorrhoea: achievements and challenges. *Sex Medicine Today* **9**: 8.

Ingersoll F, Meigs JV (1948) Presacral neurectomy for dysmenorrhoea. *New England Journal of Medicine* **238**: 357.

Irvin TT, Goligher JC, Scott JS (1975) Injury to the ureter during laparoscopic tubal sterilization. *Archives of Surgery* **110**: 1501.

Keckstein J (1989) Laparoscopic treatment of polycystic ovarian syndrome. In Sutton CJG (ed.) *Baillière's Clinical Obstetrics and Gynaecology. Laparoscopic Surgery.* **3(3)**: 563–582.

Keckstein J, Finger A, Steiner R (1988) Laser application in contact and non-contact procedures: sapphire tips in comparison to 'bare-fibre', argon laser in comparison to Nd:YAG laser. *Lasers in Medicine and Surgery* **4**: 158–162.

Konninckx PR, Meuleman C, Demeyere S, Lesaffre E, Cornillie FJ (1991) Suggestive evidence that pelvic endometriosis is a progressive disease, whereas deeply infiltrating endometriosis is associated with pelvic pain. *Fertility and Sterility* **55**: 759–765.

Latarjet A, Roget P (1922) Le plexus hypogastrique chez la femme. *Gynécologie et Obstétrique* **6**: 225.

Lee RB, Stone K, Magelssen D, Belts RP, Benson WL (1986) Presacral neurectomy for chronic pelvic pain. *Obstetrics and Gynecology* **69**: 517–521.

Lichten EM, Bombard J (1987) Surgical treatment of dysmenorrhoea with laparoscopic uterine nerve ablation. *Journal of Reproductive Medicine* **32(1)**: 37–42.

Lumsden MA (1985) Dysmenorrhoea. In Studd JWW (ed.) *Progress in Obstetrics and Gynaecology*, Vol. 5. pp. 276–292. Edinburgh: Churchill Livingstone.

Lumsden MA, Kelly RW, Baird DT (1983) Primary dysmenorrhoea: the importance of both prostaglandins C2 and F2 alpha. *British Journal of Obstetrics and Gynaecology* **90**: 1135–1140.

Martin DC, Hubert GD, Levy BS (1989) Depth of infiltration of endometriosis. *Journal of Gynecological Surgery* **5**: 55–60.

Milsom I, Andersch B (1984) Effect of various oral contraceptive combinations on dysmenorrhoea. *Gynecologic and Obstetric Investigation* **17**: 284–292.

Nisolle M, Paindeveine B, Bourdon A *et al.* (1990) Histological study of peritoneal endometriosis in infertile women. *Fertility and Sterility* **53**: 984–988.

Redwine DB (1991) Conservative laparoscopic excision of endometriosis by sharp dissection: life table analysis of re-operation and persistent or recurrent disease. *Fertility and Sterility* **56**: 628–634.

Reich H (1989) Advanced operative laparoscopy. In Sutton CJG (ed.) *Baillière's Clinical Obstetrics and Gynaecology. Laparoscopic Surgery* **3(3)**: 655–682.

Richards DH (1979) A general practice view of functional disorders associated with menstruation. *Research Clinical Forums* **1**: 39–45.

Royal College of General Practitioners (1974) *Oral Contraceptives and Health.* London: Pitman Medical.

Semm K (1966) New apparatus for 'cold-coagulation' of benign cervical lesions. *American Journal of Obstetrics and Gynecology* **95**: 963–967.

Semm K, Mettler L (1980) Technical progress in pelvic surgery via operative laparoscopy. *American Journal of Obstetrics and Gynecology* **138**: 121–127.

Semm K, O'Neill-Freys I (1989) Conventional operative laparoscopy. In Sutton CJG (ed.) *Baillière's Clinical Obstetrics and Gynaecology. Laparoscopic Surgery* **3(3)**: 451–486.

Sundell G, Milsom I, Andersch B (1990) Factors influencing the prevalence and severity of dysmenorrhoea in young women. *British Journal of Obstetrics and Gynaecology* **97**: 588–594.

Sutton CJG (1986) Initial experience with CO_2 laser laparoscopy. *Lasers in Medical Science* **1**: 25–31.

Sutton CJG (1989a) Carbon dioxide laser laparoscopy in the treatment of endometriosis. In Sutton CJG (ed) *Baillière's Clinical Obstetrics and Gynaecology. Laparoscopic Surgery* **3.3**: 499–523.

Sutton CJG (1989b) Laser laparoscopic uterine nerve ablation. In Donnez J (ed) *Operative Laser Laparoscopy and Hysteroscopy*, pp 43–52. Louvain, Belgium: Nauwelaerts Publishers.

Sutton CJG & Hill D (1990) Laser laparoscopy in endometriosis: a 5-year study. *British Journal of Obstetrics and Gynaecology* **97**: 901–905.

Sutton CJG & Hodgson R (1992) Endoscopic cutting with lasers: a review article. *Journal of Minimally Invasive Therapy* **1**: 197–205.

Sutton CJG, Nair S, Ewen SP, Haines P (1993) A comparison between the CO_2 and KTP lasers in the treatment of large ovarian endometriomas. *Gynaecological Endoscopy* **2**: 113–116.

Sutton CJG, Ewen SP, Whitelaw N, Haines P (1994) Prospective randomized, double-blind, controlled trial of laser laparoscopy in the treatment of pelvic pain associated with minimal, mild and moderate endometriosis. *Fertility and Sterility* **62**: 696–700.

Tjaden B, Schlaff WD, Kimball A, Rock JA (1990) The efficacy of pre-sacral neurectomy for the relief of mid-line dysmenorrhoea. *Obstetrics and Gynecology* **76**: 89–91.

Tucker AW (1947) Evaluation of pre-sacral neurectomy in the treatment of dysmenorrhoea. *American Journal of Obstetrics and Gynecology* **53**: 226.

White JC (1952) Conduction of visceral pain. *New England Journal of Medicine* **246**: 686–688.

Wilson EA (1988) Surgical therapy for endometriosis. *Clinical Obstetrics and Gynecology* **31(4)**: 857–865.

Ylikorkala O, Dawood YM (1978) New concepts in dysmenorrhoea. *American Journal of Obstetrics and Gynecology* **130**: 833.

26

Laparoscopic Surgery for Pelvic Pain

E. DANIEL BIGGERSTAFF

The Advanced Surgery Center at Candler Hospital, Savannah, Georgia, USA

Introduction

Pelvic pain is one of the more common conditions addressed in gynecological practise. The etiology of pain may be simple and the location specific, or the pain may be multifactorial in origin and diffuse in location. The pain may be affected by a variety of physiological events including ovulation, menstruation, urination, digestion, defecation and coitus. A detailed discussion on pelvic pain can be found in Bonica's (1990) text, *The Management of Pain*.

History

Presacral neurectomy (PSN) has been used successfully to treat women experiencing midline pelvic pain and dysmenorrhea for almost 100 years (Fontaine and Herrmann, 1932; Cotte, 1937; Black, 1964). Black (1964) summarized case reports from the literature and calculated an overall success rate of 79% for previously reported studies. He surveyed 800 physicians (472 responded) and 43 of his former patients who had been treated with PSN at least 10 years before his study. The physician responses showed a 75% success rate for patients' pain relief following treatment with PSN, while 80% of Black's former patients were pain free ten or more years after treatment for dysmenorrhea with PSN.

Doyle (1955) described a procedure for paracervical uterine denervation by transection of the cervical plexus. He reported an 86% success rate for complete relief, and a 95% success rate for complete or partial relief of pelvic pain in 73 patients followed from four months to four years postoperatively. Lichten and Bombard (1987) described a laparoscopic approach to Doyle's procedure. However, they reported that over 50% of the subjects treated with laparoscopic uterosacral nerve ablation (LUNA) in a double-blind study perceived the same or a greater level of pain 12 months postoperatively. Gürgan *et al.* (1992) used LUNA to treat 20 patients with primary dysmenorrhea. Of these women, 14 were seen for follow-up after one year: 8 (57%) required medication for pain during menstrual periods, and only five were free of significant pain (one additional patient was pregnant).

Introduction of the oral contraceptive pill (OCP) in the early 1960s had a major impact on the treatment of dysmenorrhea as has the subsequent widespread use of non-steroidal anti-inflammatory drugs (NSAIDs). NSAIDs taken on a regular basis, especially before the onset of symptoms, are effective for many women in relieving dysmenorrhea. Danazol was a mainstay in the medical therapy of pain and dysmenorrhea associated with endometriosis (Greenblatt *et al.*, 1971); however, Fedele *et al.* (1989) reported that over 90% of subjects treated with danazol experienced a recurrence of endometriosis symptoms one year after stopping treatment. Gonadotropin releasing hormone (GnRH) analogs were described as treatment by medical oophorectomy for endometriosis by Meldrum *et al.* (1982), but Fedele *et al.* (1990) found a 42% recurrence rate of pain symptoms within one year of cessation of treatment of pelvic pain with buserelin acetate. Both danazol and GnRH analogs are expensive, require six months of therapy and can have significant side effects. Danazol may cause weight gain, acne, hirsutism, voice change, vaginal dryness, emotional lability and menstrual irregularities. GnRH analogs may cause side effects related to hypoestrogenism including hot flushes, headaches, emotional lability, acne, vaginal dryness and a decrease in bone density (these side effects may be decreased with low dose estrogen replacement, but some of the bone loss may not be preventable or reversible). Medical suppression will decrease the size of the lesions of endometriosis and diminish or eliminate pain, but the lesions remain and respond to cyclic hormonal stimulation when therapy is discontinued (Steingold *et al.*, 1987).

Recent developments in laparoscopic surgery have enabled physicians to perform PSN laparoscopically in conjunction with other conservative surgical procedures for the treatment of endometriosis or pelvic pain. Perez (1990) reported the results of the first 25 cases treated with laparoscopic presacral neurectomy (LPSN). The patients reported a significant decrease in their pain symptoms postoperatively, and there were no serious complications or side effects from the procedure. Nezhat and Nezhat (1992) performed a retrospective investigation of 52 patients from 1990 to 1992 who underwent LPSN for the treatment of midline pain. They concurred with previous reports (Cotte, 1937; Doyle, 1955; Polan and DeCherney, 1980; Rock and Jones, 1983; Perez, 1990; Candiani *et al.*, 1992) that PSN significantly reduces midline pelvic pain and pain associated with intractable primary dysmenorrhea or secondary dysmenorrhea and has little effect on adnexal pain. All authors recommend that physicians select candidates for PSN or LPSN carefully and that only those patients who have previously attempted medical therapy without relief of midline pain should undergo the procedure (Fontaine and Herrmann, 1932; Counsellor and Craig, 1934; Black, 1964; Mahfoud and Hewitt, 1981; Fliegner and Umstad, 1991; Hill and Maher, 1991; Daniell *et al.*, 1993; Perry and Perez, 1993; Biggerstaff and Foster, 1994). The authors also agree that the most common reason for failure of PSN or LPSN is incomplete resection of the nerve plexus.

Indications for PSN

In recent years, medical therapy (especially with OCPs and NSAIDs) has significantly reduced the need for surgical intervention for primary dysmenorrhea. Many cases of pelvic pain have specific etiologies amenable to medical therapy such as infection or irritable bowel syndrome, and should be treated appropriately. LPSN is indicated for the treatment of severe midline pelvic pain including dysmenorrhea that does not respond to medical or other appropriate therapy.

The treatment of endometriosis is covered in great detail elsewhere in this book. Therefore, this information will not be duplicated, but special attention will be placed on discussing adenomyosis. Adenomyosis was first described by Cullen (1908) as a deep proliferation of normal endometrium. It is well known that adenomyosis:

- May cause menorrhagia and dysmenorrhea.
- May be totally asymptomatic.
- Is often found in association with uterine myomas as an incidental finding at pathologic examination (Bird *et al.*, 1956; Bird and Molitor, 1971).

Dysmenorrhea in association with the so-called boggy uterus is often characteristic of adenomyosis (Bird *et al.*, 1972). In a more recent study, Nishida (1991) presented data suggesting that dysmenorrhea is directly related to the amount and size of the areas of adenomyosis in addition to the extent of muscle invasion. He also noted a low incidence of dysmenorrhea in patients with adenomyotic lesions only on the serosal surface of the uterus compared to those who had lesions extending from within the uterus.

Most authors concur that PSN significantly reduces midline pelvic pain and pain associated with intractable primary dysmenorrhea or secondary dysmenorrhea, but has little effect on lateral pain. In most cases it is recommended that surgical intervention should be considered only after failure of medical therapy. One exception to this rule may be pain associated with infertility when known or suspected endometriosis is the culprit. In this case primary surgical intervention (not necessarily with PSN) is appropriate since medical suppression simply delays the ability to conceive and does not significantly improve the fecundity rate (Olive and Martin, 1987). In addition to unsuccessful medical therapy, many physicians reserve PSN for those patients who have also had failed previous conservative surgical treatment including ablation of endometriosis and lysis of adhesions. In the author's recent study of 28 patients (Biggerstaff and Foster, 1994), the potential benefits of using LPSN as an initial surgical procedure to alleviate significant midline pain are presented. If a procedure such as PSN requires laparotomy along with its accompanying recovery time and expense, all other avenues for therapy should be exhausted before proceeding. On the other hand, if PSN can be performed laparoscopically, why should the patient who has significant midline pain come back for another procedure requiring an additional anesthetic and expense when the procedure could be performed at the time of the initial ablation of the endometriosis?

Surgical Skills

The learning curve for laparoscopic procedures is significantly longer than for the same procedures performed at laparotomy. A surgeon should demonstrate proficiency in performing a procedure at laparotomy before performing it laparoscopically, and must be able to manage associated complications should they arise.

Because of the anatomical area in which PSN is performed there is a greater likelihood of significant complication with PSN than with most other gynecological procedures unless a meticulous dissection technique is used. Without appropriate training and skills, it is best that a surgeon either refers a patient for PSN to a surgeon with the ability to perform the procedure safely or considers another appropriate treatment if that alternative exists.

Anatomy

A thorough understanding of the relevant anatomy is imperative to perform a procedure that is both safe and complete. It is also important to note the relative locations of vital structures may vary considerably. For example, the left ureter was found within the area of dissection (not outside, as expected) in the third laparoscopic presacral neurectomy the author performed.

The so-called presacral nerve (Figure 26.1) is found in a triangular area known as the interiliac trigone (Elaut, 1933). The lower limit of the trigone is the sacral promontory, and the lateral

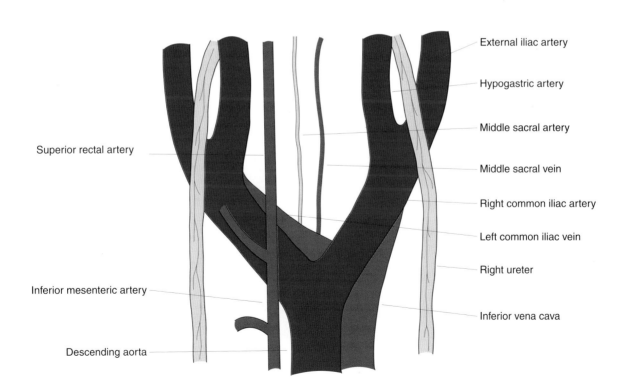

External iliac artery

Hypogastric artery

Middle sacral artery

Middle sacral vein

Right common iliac artery

Left common iliac vein

Right ureter

Inferior vena cava

Superior rectal artery

Inferior mesenteric artery

Descending aorta

Figure 26.1 Deep anatomy in the area of the interiliac trigone.

boundaries are formed by the common iliac arteries meeting at the bifurcation of the aorta above. The right ureter is usually seen at the lateral limit of the dissection as it crosses the common iliac artery just before or at its bifurcation into the external iliac and hypogastric vessels. The corresponding veins course under the arteries. On the left side there is most often a similar positional relationship between the ureter and the common iliac artery on that side. During presacral neurectomy, caution must be exercised to avoid damage to the left common iliac vein since it runs much more medially than the artery and forms a portion of the trigone floor on this side.

The dissection on the left side is not usually carried far enough laterally to visualize the ureter. Since the ureter on the left side may occasionally be seen more medially than described, care must be taken during dissection to avoid damaging it.

The normal limits of dissection on the left side are the inferior mesenteric artery and the base of the sigmoid mesocolon. The inferior mesenteric artery arises approximately 4 cm above the bifurcation, then descends in front of and finally alongside the left side of the aorta. At the level of the left common iliac artery, the inferior mesenteric artery splits into several branches. It continues into the pelvis as the superior rectal (hemorrhoidal) artery and branches laterally into the left colic and 2–4 sigmoid arteries.

The middle sacral artery is a very thin vessel that arises from the posterior aspect of the aorta (before it bifurcates) and continues over the fourth and fifth lumbar vertebrae, the sacrum and the coccyx. The middle sacral vein, which can be a significant source of blood loss if damaged, arises from the left common iliac vein and parallels the path of the middle sacral artery.

Figure 26.2 Nerve supply to the pelvis.

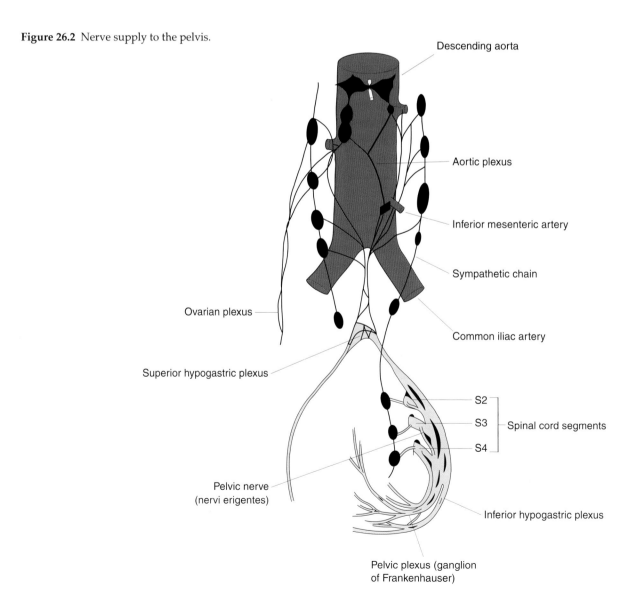

The lower colon, bladder and pelvic organs have an abundant nerve supply arising from the thoracic, lumbar and sacral levels of the spinal cord. There are both afferent (or sensory) and efferent (or sympathetic and parasympathetic) components. Bonica (1990) demonstrates the afferent supply of the entire uterus and proximal fallopian tubes accompanies other sympathetic nerves (Figure 26.2). The uterine and cervical plexuses combine to form the pelvic plexus (ganglion of Frankenhauser) and on each side course posteriorly over the lateral surface of the rectal ampulla. They then join the inferior hypogastric nerve plexuses near the sacral end of the uterosacral ligaments. Travelling cephalad these plexuses form the middle hypogastric plexus or hypogastric nerve on either side just below the level of the sacral promontory.

The hypogastric nerve may be a single nerve or several fibers connected by anastomosing elements. This plexus becomes the superior hypogastric plexus or so-called 'presacral nerve'. A network of veins lies under the middle hypogastric plexus and can cause troublesome bleeding if they are damaged during surgery. The superior hypogastric plexus is in loose areolar tissue overlying the sacral promontory and middle sacral vessels, and under the peritoneum. The breadth of the plexus may vary considerably, as can the degree of condensation of fibers. The plexus can also be in multiple layers. Most often there are 2–4 incompletely fused nerve trunks in a broad flat plexus (Figure 26.3). The

plexus tends to be off center, more frequently to the left. The superior hypogastric plexus leads to the aortic plexus. The afferent fibers course through the lumbar sympathetic chain and cephalad through the lower thoracic sympathetic chain. The fibers leave the chain via the rami communicans of the T10, T11, T12, and L1 spinal nerves and go through the posterior roots to synapse with interneurons in the dorsal horn.

When considering treatment of pelvic pain, it is important to realize that the sensory nerve supply of the ovaries, distal fallopian tubes and posterior broad ligaments is separate from that of the uterus (see Figure 26.2). The nerve fibers from these structures follow the same course as the ovarian vessels and terminate in the ovarian plexus on each side. The ovarian plexuses arise from the aortic and renal plexus. The close proximity of the nerves and vascular supply prevents ovarian denervation from being a practical procedure.

Awareness of the innervation of the remaining pelvic viscera (see Figure 26.2) is important when considering interrupting the nerves to treat pelvic pain and when considering other possible effects of this nerve interruption (Renaer and Guzinski, 1978; Bonica, 1990). The sympathetic nerve supply for the lower colon and rectum in addition to the majority of that for the bladder is derived from the sacral splanchnic nerves, which in turn arise from the sacral portion of the sympathetic chain. A portion of the sympathetic nerve supply of the bladder also travels through the inferior, middle and superior hypogastric plexus. The parasympathetic supply for the lower colon, rectum and bladder comes mainly from direct branches of the pelvic splanchnic nerves originating in spinal cord segments S2, S3, and S4. Afferent fibers from the lower colon accompany the parasympathetic nerves and enter the spinal cord in the same segments. The sensory supply to the rectum is through the pudendal nerve as is that to the external and internal vesicle sphincters and adjacent parts of the bladder. The peritoneum of the dome of the bladder is supplied by afferent fibers of the T11–L1 spinal nerves.

Alternative Therapies and Considerations

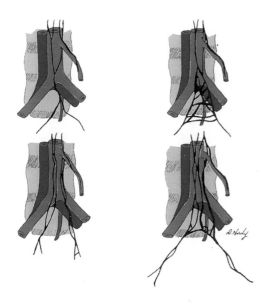

Figure 26.3 Different configurations of the superior hypogastric plexus.

Medical therapy for pelvic pain and dysmenorrhea and paracervical uterine denervation and the LUNA procedure have been presented previously (see page 261). Any obstruction to the flow of menstrual discharge may cause or worsen dysmenorrhea. The completely intact hymen and associated hematocolpometra is an unusual cause of cyclic midline pain, but one that lends itself to easy surgical correction in most cases. Dilation and curettage is rarely indicated as a treatment of dysmenorrhea, but dilation of a significantly stenotic cervix may improve or eliminate dysmenorrhea. Depending upon the cause of the stenosis, the patient should be advised that the dilation may be only temporary and that the pain may return with recurrence of the stenosis. Hysteroscopy should be performed at the time of cervical dilation to look for evidence of adenomyosis. Diagnosing adenomyosis is not easy at hysteroscopy and requires careful scanning of the endometrial surface. If the lesions extend from the surface of the endometrium, one can visualize the ostia of the diverticula as dark depressions that vary in size. The openings may be obscured by the endometrium or may be seen just under the surface of the endometrium when they lie not too far from it (Barbot, 1989). Laparoscopy to ablate endometriosis, if present, along with PSN, should be considered at the same time as cervical dilation for severe cervical stenosis, especially when there is known or suspected adenomyosis.

'Definitive' surgical treatment for midline pelvic pain and dysmenorrhea has traditionally required hysterectomy with or without the removal of the fallopian tubes and ovaries. Certain cases may lend themselves to a vaginal approach, including removal of the adnexa if desired. The author recommends that this approach is not taken when the indication (or one of the indications) is significant pelvic pain because endometriosis may be left *in situ* and be a persistent source of pain. This is of special concern when endometriosis may be left and buried in the cuff at closure, making subsequent removal of the endometriosis more difficult. For these reasons, laparoscopically assisted vaginal hysterectomy is preferred over the vaginal approach to increase the likelihood of complete removal of any endometriosis if present.

Removal of the ovaries should be considered when hysterectomy is chosen as the treatment for endometriosis. In a recent study, Namnoum *et al.* (1993) presented data suggesting ovarian conservation at the time of hysterectomy increases the risk of persistence of symptoms if the surgery is performed to treat pain secondary to endometriosis. In a series of 147 women, 117 had all ovarian tissue removed while 30 had some preservation of ovarian tissue at the time of hysterectomy. Of those patients with no ovarian conservation, 7%

had recurrent symptoms and 1.7% required reoperation for persistent symptomatology. With conservation of some ovarian function, 63% had recurrent symptoms and 30% required reoperation. In addition to recurrent pain, other factors, such as the risk of developing ovarian cancer and other pelvic pathology (e.g. adhesions) must be considered and discussed with the patient. Additionally, the psychological impact of oophorectomy should be addressed. If the ovaries are not removed and there is subsequent need for oophorectomy, current techniques will usually allow laparoscopic removal as an outpatient rather than requiring laparotomy unless there is malignancy.

Preoperative Evaluation and Therapy

A thorough preoperative evaluation is necessary before any surgery is undertaken. The patient's age, health status, weight and fertility desires all have a major bearing on whether a definitive procedure is appropriate (e.g. hysterectomy with removal of fallopian tubes and ovaries) or whether a more conservative approach is desirable. The psychological and cultural impact of removal of the uterus, tubes and ovaries must be considered. A complete history should also include questions regarding the possibility of childhood physical and sexual abuse, which have been shown to have a direct correlation with pelvic pain in women during adulthood (Walker *et al.*, 1988).

Preoperatively, the patient should have a bowel preparation unless it is known from recent surgical evaluation that there is no bowel involvement with endometriosis or adhesions. Preoperative bowel preparation is becoming almost standard with all gynecological surgery whether it is done by laparotomy or laparoscopy since it seems to reduce the incidence of postoperative ileus and provides a margin of safety should the bowel be accidentally or intentionally entered.

Procedure

LPSN is performed under general anesthesia. The patient is placed in the low lithotomy position and a uterine manipulator is used to facilitate adequate endoscopic examination and treatment. A four-puncture technique is preferred:

- An umbilical incision for inserting a 10 mm operating or diagnostic laparoscope.
- Three incisions made just below the pubic hair line for sleeves accommodating 5 mm instruments – one in the midline, and the other two just lateral to the rectus muscles, taking care to avoid both the superficial and deep vessels of the abdominal wall.

A video camera with adequate resolution and color separation is attached to the laparoscope. If monopolar electrocautery is to be used, conductive metal sleeves should be used through all incisions to minimize the chance of accidental injury to vital adjacent structures.

The LPSN is begun after any other procedures necessary to treat pelvic disease have been completed. The goal of surgical therapy for pelvic pain should be complete removal of all typical and atypical endometriosis and adhesions (Martin *et al.*, 1989) in addition to other procedures deemed appropriate, such as PSN. Various instruments can be used for the peritoneal incision and subsequent dissection. Due to the vascularity of the presacral area in addition to personal preference, the author most commonly employs scissors with and without cutting current, in addition to bipolar cautery to control large vessels. Blunt dissection may be carried out with various forceps, irrigation/aspirators and scissors.

A transverse incision is made in the peritoneum overlying the sacral promontory, extending from the ureter on the right side to the inferior mesenteric and superior hemorrhoidal arteries and sigmoid colon on the left side. The landmarks on the right side are usually easily identifiable through the peritoneum, but not on the left side. The inferior mesenteric and superior hemorrhoidal arteries are found in fatty connective tissue and may be difficult to locate. Additionally, care must be taken to avoid damage to the sigmoid colon itself. In a series of 28 cases (Biggerstaff and Foster, 1994), the left ureter was found within the limits of dissection only once; caution is needed to avoid ureteric injury. The sigmoid colon must be retracted to a left lateral position to obtain adequate exposure for the PSN. This is most easily accomplished with an atraumatic grasping forceps introduced through the left suprapubic sleeve, which simultaneously elevates the left end of the incision and retracts the sigmoid colon.

When the limits of the dissection are difficult to identify (almost always on the left side), a T incision should be used, beginning at the middle of the transverse incision in the peritoneum and carrying the incision cephalad to the bifurcation of the descending aorta and inferior vena cava. There is no advantage in exposing the operative field below the

prominence of the sacrum since dissection in this area will very likely result in venous bleeding that is difficult to control. The dissection is usually begun on the right side and carried to the left. Connective and fatty tissue containing the nerve plexus is dissected both sharply and bluntly and isolated in small longitudinal bunches, cauterized in two places 1–2 cm apart, removed, and sent to pathology to confirm removal of nerve elements. When the dissection is complete, the sacral promontory has the appearance of a 'baby's bottom', with the intact middle sacral vein running down the middle. The peritoneum is usually left open as spontaneous reperitonealization will occur in a short period of time.

Unless there are other reasons for hospitalization, most patients can be discharged home the same day once they are voiding and ambulatory after LPSN. Oral pain medication and an antiemetic are prescribed, and the patient is seen within one week of the surgery. Most patients are able to return to all but the most strenuous activities within one week, and may resume sexual activity within several weeks.

Complications

Potential complications of LPSN include those common to all laparoscopic procedures and those unique to LPSN. Complications specific to LPSN are related to the possible effects of cutting the 'presacral nerve' or superior hypogastric plexus and to the anatomical site where the procedure is performed. Careful dissection technique along with knowledge of the relative anatomy and its possible variances will help in avoiding most complications, including injury to the bowel, vessels and ureters. Along with dissection technique, the surgeon must have a full knowledge of the limitations and potential hazards of the energy modalities used.

The most significant intraoperative complication reported is hemorrhage, usually from the middle sacral vein or its branches, or from a larger vessel, most often the left common iliac vein. Interruption of the middle sacral vein or its companion artery can cause significant blood loss. Careful dissection will usually avoid damage to these relatively small vessels, which can often be visualized through the peritoneum before the initial incision is made. If occlusion of either of these vessels is necessary, it can usually be accomplished with bipolar cautery or with a laparoscopically placed suture. Appropriate suture would be a 3–0 braided polyglycolic acid or silk suture on a small curved taper needle transfixed to the periosteum. Placing the suture through the periosteum decreases the likelihood of tearing the vessel and its branches, which will result in further bleeding. Pastner and Orr (1990) reported the use of stainless steel thumbtacks to control intractable venous hemorrhage at the time of conventional PSN. Several small branches of the presacral venous plexus were lacerated and could not be controlled with bovie cautery, suture ligation, packing with bone wax or attempted occlusion with hemaclips. LPSN offers the distinct advantage over conventional PSN of close visual proximity with magnification, which should decrease the chance of accidentally lacerating these vessels. If the dissection is either begun or carried just below the sacral promontory, bleeding from the venous plexus in this location is significantly increased.

The left common iliac vein is the large vessel most often reported to be damaged at LPSN. The vessel frequently runs more medially than anticipated and actually forms a lateral portion of the floor of the interiliac trigone. If there is uncertainty regarding the location of this vessel or of any structure, the initial transverse incision in the peritoneum overlying the sacral promontory should be converted to a T incision as previously described. Previous authors have noted that laceration of the left common iliac vein has required laparotomy for repair, usually with significant blood loss requiring blood transfusion. The author recently reported laparoscopic repair of this vessel using a series of hemaclips

(Biggerstaff and Foster, 1994). An unplanned 1 cm incision was made with scissors in the left common iliac vein and venous blood immediately obscured the operative field. In order to repair the vessel, the vessel was quickly grasped where the laceration occurred with a smooth forceps and gently lifted to stop the bleeding. Adequate exposure and a dry field are mandatory for successful laparoscopic repair in this situation. Once the bleeding was temporarily stopped, the laparotomy set was opened, type and cross-match of blood was begun, and a vascular surgeon was consulted. A row of parallel hemaclips (Figure 26.4) was used to close the laceration using the method agreed upon by the author and the vascular surgeon. An alternate method for closure is the use of precise intracorporeal suturing and knot tying techniques performed in a manner similar to that at laparotomy. The resultant blood loss was less than 50 ml. If it is possible to immediately grasp and occlude the vessel, the patient will be likely to lose less blood than if one proceeds to immediate laparotomy. If the bleeding cannot be controlled laparoscopically, laparotomy should be performed without hesitation. The temptation to grasp a large vessel with a bipolar cautery instrument and apply electrical current should always be avoided. This will inevitably result in a larger hole in the vessel than the initial injury. Prevention of accidental laceration of vessels at laparoscopy is the most important step in treating the complication. Additionally, careful dissection will, in most cases, prevent damage to the ureters or colon.

Figure 26.4 Repair of large vessel laceration with hemaclips.

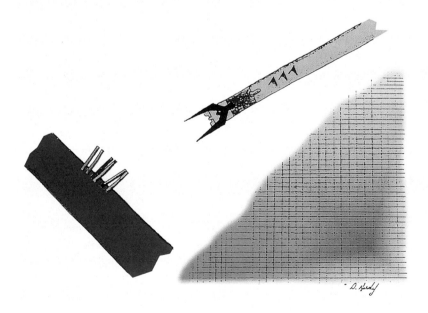

A number of authors have reported side effects of LPSN related to the possible effects of interrupting the presacral nerve, with most lasting two weeks to six months. They include voiding dysfunction, constipation, sexual dysfunction, and backache (Rock and Jones, 1983; Lee et al., 1986; Olive and Martin, 1987; Tjaden et al., 1990; Candiani et al., 1992; Perry and Perez, 1993). Urinary complaints have included urge incontinence, urinary incontinence without urgency, difficulty initiating urination, continual leakage of a small amount of urine requiring a sanitary pad, and loss of the feeling of a full bladder. Constipation is one of the more common postoperative complaints, and is usually easily managed with stool softeners and laxatives. The only form of sexual dysfunction reported is that of occasional vaginal dryness; again this is temporary. Low back pain, if present, most often disappears after 1–3 weeks.

Discussion

LPSN performed by a skilled trained surgeon is an effective procedure for providing long-term relief for women with midline pelvic pain and dysmenorrhea. Compared to other treatment interventions such as medical treatment with GnRH analogs or LUNA, LPSN provides more consistent and complete pain relief over longterm follow-up. When performed in conjunction with appropriate adjunct procedures such as ablation of endometriosis and lysis of adhesions, LPSN is an effective method for an initial surgical treatment of midline dysmenorrhea and pelvic pain.

Only two prospective studies have examined the efficacy of PSN in a controlled setting. Tjaden et al. (1990) randomly assigned four patients to a PSN group, and four patients to a non-PSN group. In addition 13 other women selected PSN to treat moderate to severe midline dysmenorrhea, and five more women selected non-PSN treatment alternatives. All 26 subjects completed an 80-item questionnaire before surgery and a second questionnaire six months following surgery. The eight patients who were randomly assigned to treatment were not informed of the protocol that they had received until after they had completed the six-month follow-up questionnaire. All four of the patients who were randomly assigned to the PSN group reported relief of midline pain at six months, while none of the patients assigned to the non-PSN group reported

pain relief. Overall results indicated that 15 of the 17 women (88%) who underwent PSN experienced pain relief at six months, while none of the nine women who did not have PSN experienced pain relief. The study was stopped by the experimental monitoring committee after the first 26 patients were treated because of concerns about the ethics of depriving future patients of the option of PSN for pain relief for midline dysmenorrhea.

Candiani et al. (1992) examined the efficacy of PSN with adjunct concurrent procedures to provide relief from pain secondary to moderate to severe endometriosis: 78 women were randomly assigned to an experimental group (PSN plus conservative surgery) or a control group (conservative surgery only). A multidimensional instrument for measuring the severity of dysmenorrhea and pelvic pain by functional impact on working ability and the need for analgesics, and a tenpoint linear rating scale to classify pain symptoms (none to severe) were administered to each woman before surgery and at six months and one year following surgery. One year following surgery, 80% of the patients who were treated with PSN and adjunct conservative procedures experienced successful pain relief, while 75% of the women who only had conservative surgical procedures had successful pain relief. Candiani and his colleagues concluded that because women with endometriosis often experience lateral pain in addition to midline pain, this study was inconclusive on the increase in effectiveness of PSN and adjunct conservative over conservative surgery alone. However, they reinforced the assertion that PSN is effective for relieving midline pain associated with dysmenorrhea, and that although their findings were inconclusive PSN would be indicated for patients with endometriosis and significant midline pain. Because of the small number of prospective studies and the absence of systematic long-term follow-up in existing retrospective and prospective studies, additional research is needed to show the efficacy of LPSN for long-term pain relief.

It cannot be overemphasized that LPSN should only be performed by an advanced endoscopic surgeon who has previously demonstrated proficiency in performing PSN at laparotomy and who has demonstrated sufficient skills at laparotomy and laparoscopy to manage potential complications such as accidental laceration of major vessels. The most common side effects of LPSN are transient; however, the potential for significant complications from damage to vessels or other structures means that the surgeon needs to proceed with caution when performing dissection during LPSN. The best method for treating a complication is prevention.

References

Barbot J (1989) Hysteroscopy for abnormal bleeding. In Baggish MS, Barbot J, Valle RF (eds) *Diagnostic and Operative Hysteroscopy: A Text and Atlas*. pp. 147–155. Chicago: Year Book Medical Publishers, Inc.

Biggerstaff ED, Foster SN (1994) Laporoscopic presacral neurectomy for treatment of midline pelvic pain. *Journal of the American Association of Gynecologic Laparoscopists* 2: 31–35.

Bird CC, Molitor JJ (1971) Adenomyosis: A clinical and pathologic appraisal. *American Journal of Obstetrics and Gynecology* 110: 275–284.

Bird CC, McElin TW, Manalo-Estrella P (1956) Problems in the diagnosis of adenomyosis uteri, with special reference to dysfunctional bleeding. *Western Journal of Surgery, Obstetrics and Gynecology* 64: 291–305.

Bird CC, McElin TW, Manalo-Estrella P (1972) The elusive adenomyosis of the uterus – revisited. *American Journal of Obstetrics and Gynecology* 112: 583–593.

Black WT (1964) Use of presacral sympathectomy in the treatment of dysmenorrhea. *American Journal of Obstetrics and Gynecology* 89: 16–22.

Bonica JJ (ed.) (1990) *The Management of Pain*, 2nd edition. Philadelphia: Lea and Febinger.

Candiani GB, Fedele L, Vercellini P, Bianchi S, Di Nola G (1992) Presacral neurectomy for the treatment of pelvic pain associated with endometriosis: A controlled study. *American Journal of Obstetrics and Gynecology* 167: 100–103.

Cotte G (1937) Resection of the presacral nerve in the treatment of obstinate dysmenorrhea. *American Journal of Obstetrics and Gynecology* 33: 1034–1040.

Counsellor VS and Craig McK W (1934) The treatment of dysmenorrhea by resection of the presacral sympathetic nerves: Evaluation of end-results. *American Journal of Obstetrics and Gynecology* 28: 161–172.

Cullen TS (1908) *Adenomyoma of Uterus*. Philadelphia: WB Saunders.

Daniell JF, Kurtz BR, Gurley LD, Lalonde CJ (1993) Laparoscopic presacral neurectomy vs neurotomy: Use of the argon beam coagulator compared to conventional technique. *Journal of Gynecologic Surgery* 9: 169–173.

Doyle JB (1955) Paracervical uterine denervation by transection of the cervical plexus for the relief of dysmenorrhea. *American Journal of Obstetrics and Gynecology* 70: 1–16.

Elaut L (1933) The surgical anatomy of the so-called presacral nerve. *Surgery, Gynecology and Obstetrics* 57: 581–589.

Fedele L, Arcaini L, Bianchi S, Baglioni A, Vercellini P (1989) Comparison of cyproterone acetate and danazol in the treatment of pelvic pain associated with endometriosis. *Obstetrics and Gynecology* 73: 1000–1005.

Fedele L, Bianchi S, Bocciolone L, Di Nola G, Franchi D (1990) Buserelin acetate in the treatment of pelvic pain associated with minimal endometriosis: a controlled study. *Fertility and Sterility* 59: 516–521.

Fliegner JRH, Umstad MP (1991) Presacral neurectomy –

A reappraisal. *Australian and New Zealand Journal of Obstetrics and Gynaecology* 31: 76–79.

Fontaine R, Herrmann LG (1932) Clinical and experimental basis for surgery of the pelvic sympathetic nerves in gynecology. *Surgery, Gynecology and Obstetrics* 54: 133–163.

Greenblatt RB, Dmowski WP, Mahesh VB, Scholer HFL (1971) Clinical studies with an anti-gonadotropin – danazol. *Fertility and Sterility* 22: 102–112.

Gürgan T, Urman B, Aksu T, Develioglu O, Zeyneloglu H, Kisnisci HA (1992) Laparoscopic CO_2 laser uterine nerve ablation for treatment of drug resistant primary dysmenorrhea. *Fertility and Sterility* 58: 422–424.

Hill DJ, Maher PJ (1991) Letter to the editor. *Australian and New Zealand Journal of Obstetrics and Gynaecology* 31: 290.

Lee RB, Stone K, Mageissen D, Betts RP, Benson WL (1986) Presacral neurectomy for chronic pelvic pain. *Obstetrics and Gynecology* 68: 517–521.

Lichten EM, Bombard J (1987) Surgical treatment of dysmenorrhea with laparoscopic uterine nerve ablation. *Journal of Reproductive Medicine* 32: 37–41.

Mahfoud HK, Hewitt SR (1981) A place for presacral neurectomy. *Irish Medical Journal* 74: 198–199.

Martin DC, Hubert GD, Vander Zwaag R, El-Zeky FA (1989) Laparoscopic appearance of peritoneal endometriosis. *Fertility and Sterility* 51: 63–67.

Meldrum DR, Chang RJ, Lu J, Vale W, Rivier J, Judd HL (1982) Medical oophorectomy using a long-acting GnRH agonist: A possible new approach to the treatment of endometriosis. *Journal of Clinical Endocrinology and Metabolism* 54, 1081–1083.

Namnoum AB, Hickman TN, Goodman SB, Gelback DL, Rock JA (1993) Incidence of symptom recurrence following hysterectomy for endometriosis. Scientific paper presented at the Conjoint Meeting of the American Fertility Society and the Canadian Fertility and Andrology Society, October 11–14, 1993, Montreal, Quebec, Canada. The American Society: Birmingham, Alabama (1993)

Nishida M (1991) Relationship between the onset of dysmenorrhea and histological findings in adenomyosis. *American Journal of Obstetrics and Gynecology* 165, 229–231.

Nezhat C, Nezhat F (1992) A simplified method of laparoscopic presacral neurectomy for the treatment of central pelvic pain due to endometriosis. *British Journal of Obstetrics and Gynaecology* 99, 659–663.

Olive DL, Martin DC (1987) Treatment of endometriosis-associated infertility with CO_2 laparoscopy: The use of one and two parameter exponential models. *Fertility and Sterility* 48, 18–23.

Pastner B, Orr JW (1990) Intractable venous sacral hemorrhage: Use of stainless steel thumbtacks to obtain hemostasis. *American Journal of Obstetrics and Gynecology* 162, 452.

Perez JJ (1990) Laparoscopic presacral neurectomy: Results of the first 25 cases. *Journal of Reproductive Medicine* 35, 625–630.

Perry CP, Perez J (1993) The role for laparoscopic presacral neurectomy. *Journal of Gynecological Surgery* 9, 165–168.

Polan ML, DeCherney A (1980) Presacral neurectomy for pelvic pain in infertility. *Fertility and Sterility* 34, 557–560.

Renaer M, Guzinski GM (1978) Pain in gynecologic practice. *Pain* **5**, 305–331.

Rock J, Jones H (1983) Endometriosis externa. In Jones HW (ed.) *Reparative and Constructive Surgery of the Female Generative Tract.* pp. 136–138. Baltimore: Wilkins & Wilkins.

Steingold KA, Cedars L, Lu JKH, Randle D, Judd HL, Meldrum DR (1987) Treatment of endometriosis with a long-acting gonadotropin-releasing hormone agonist. *Obstetrics and Gynecology* **69**, 403–411.

Tjaden B, Schlaff WD, Kinball A, Rock JA (1990) The efficacy of presacral neurectomy for the relief of midline dysmenorrhea. *Obstetrics and Gynecology* **76**, 89–91.

Walker E, Katon W, Harrop-Griffiths J (1988) Relationship of chronic pelvic pain to psychiatric diagnoses and childhood sexual abuse. *American Journal of Psychiatry* **145**, 75–80.

27

Laparoscopic Myomectomy

JEAN-BERNARD DUBUISSON, CHARLES CHAPRON
AND ARNAUD FAUCONNIER

Clinique Universitaire Baudelocque, Port-Royal, Paris, France

Summary

The indications for operative laparoscopy have greatly increased in recent decades as its many advantages over laparotomy have been recognized. Laparoscopic myomectomy (LM) as a technique is now clearly defined. A monopolar hook is used to make the uterine incision. After atraumatic enucleation of the myoma, the myometrium and serosa are usually sutured, especially if the incision is deep or more than 2 cm long. Myomas can be removed by posterior colpotomy. However, the development of an electrical cutting device allows quicker and easier removal of the myoma through the suprapubic puncture site. Only complicated myomas and those that give rise to persistent symptoms in spite of appropriate medical treatment, together with those that grow rapidly, require surgery. The satisfactory preliminary results obtained must not mask the fact that LM is a lengthy and difficult procedure, reserved for experienced surgeons who are thoroughly familiar with endoscopic sutures. LM is possible under these conditions, even for large myomas (measuring 5 cm or more) and even if they are located exclusively intramurally. There are limits, however, and it is preferable to schedule myomas measuring over 8 cm and multiple myomectomy (more than two myomas) for laparotomy. If the preliminary results are encouraging, the risk of adhesiogenesis on the uterine scar, the quality of the uterine suture and the fertility results need to be assessed in the near future.

Introduction

Uterine myomas are extremely frequent, occurring in 20–25% of sexually active women (Novak et al., 1970). The diagnosis of uterine myoma should in no case be taken as synonymous with the need for surgery. Asymptomatic myomas and those discovered by chance should be left alone, requiring simple supervision. Only myomas causing symptoms (e.g. menorrhagia, pain or dragging feeling in the pelvis, urinary dysfunction) are an indication for surgery. In the field of gynecological surgery, the past few years have been marked by the considerable development of endoscopic surgery. The possibilities offered by the new surgical approaches (hysteroscopy, laparoscopy) have brought the management of uterine myomas back into the spotlight (Dubuisson and Chapron, 1995). This technological progress now means that myomectomies can be carried out by laparoscopy. This technique is still very new and has only been reported by a few teams (Daniell and Gurley, 1991; Dubuisson et al., 1991; Nezhat et al., 1991; Hasson et al., 1992). The main objective of these preliminary series was to evaluate the feasibility of this operation. As this has now been proved, the indications, results and risks of the operation now need to be identified. This is what we intend to do in this chapter, after presenting the operating technique that we use to perform laparoscopic myomectomies.

Operative Procedure

Anesthesia and Positioning of the Patient

LM is performed under general anesthesia. The patient is placed in lithomy stirrups at the beginning of the procedure. This enables a uterine cannula to be introduced and a dilute dye solution to be injected (Dubuisson *et al.*, 1993). The injection of methylene blue colors the endometrium and facilitates both cleavage of myomas close to the uterine cavity and closure of the myometrium after accidental or voluntary opening of the cavity. After injection, we replace the cannula by a curet for mobilization of the uterus. For the LM, we use the same cannula as that we recommend for performing a laparoscopic hysterectomy (Chapron *et al.*, 1994). This cannula is vital for correct positioning of the uterus. The uterus is positioned to provide optimum access to the myomas: anteverted position for a posterior myoma and retroverted position for an anterior myoma. To facilitate the handling of the ancillary instruments, low lithotomy stirrups are used.

Positioning of the Suprapubic Trocars

Correct location of the three suprapubic trocars is essential for safety with this operative technique, and is dependent upon the size of the uterus, and the number, location and size of the myomas. The trocars must be introduced 3 cm above the uterine fundus. The lateral trocars are introduced outside the epigastric pedicles.

Instrumentation

A 5 mm monopolar hook is used for coagulation and sectioning of the uterus. An electrosurgical unit may be set up to deliver 50 W of power. Two atraumatic forceps, a pair of 10 mm grip forceps, curved scissors and a pelvicleaner (Storz–France, Paris, France) are used for enucleation of the myoma. A pair of 5 mm bipolar forceps permits hemostasis to be completed during the hysterotomy and the enucleation. A 5 mm needle holder is used to close the uterus, with 2–0, 3–0 or 4–0 polyglactin 910 20 mm straight or curved needle (Ethicon, Neuilly, France) intraperitoneal sutures. Extra-abdominal sutures may also be used. Instrumentation used for mini-laparotomy and vaginal surgery may be necessary to remove the myoma. An electrical cutting device is now used to remove the myoma (Steiner *et al.*, 1993).

Principles of the Technique

The myomas must be located accurately (in relation to ligaments, tubes, bladder) as must the ureter in cases of lateral myomas. As myomectomy is a conservative and minimally invasive procedure performed in relatively young women, it is important to bear in mind the principles of atraumatic infertility surgery at every stage of the technique. Magnification, meticulous hemostasis and impeccable closure of the myometrium are necessary. A 'microsurgical' technique prevents bleeding, adhesions and postoperative complications. The technique differs depending upon the location of the myomas:

- With pedunculated myomas, the technique is easy and consists of coagulation and sectioning of the implantation surface. When the implantation surface is small, no sutures are needed. A loop suture may also be used.
- With sessile subserous or interstitial myomas, a hysterotomy is performed at the site of the myoma. The direct incision limits the bleeding. A vertical incision is usually used, although in some cases, a horizontal incision may be performed. We use the monopolar hook for the incision.

Complementary coagulation of the vessels of the myometrium is often performed using bipolar forceps. Vasoconstrictor agents are not used in our practise. Atraumatic enucleation is performed using large forceps, a monopolar hook, curved scissors and a pelvicleaner. The uterine cavity is not opened, except by accident. The hysterotomy is closed if the incision is deep, long (> 2 cm) or bleeding. We use sutures to prevent rupture of the myometrium in a subsequent pregnancy and to reduce the risk of adhesion formation on a large raw surface. We usually close the uterus in one layer with interrupted (or running) polyglactin 910, sometimes in two layers (Dubuisson *et al.*, 1995a). Extraperitoneal sutures may also be used. Sutures are usually placed every 5 mm along the hysterotomy.

Removal of the Myoma

The myomas must always be extracted to avoid peritoneal reimplantation, which causes postoperative pain, and also to carry out histology. The myoma may be removed through the suprapubic puncture site after enlargement of the incision (20 mm) with a one- or two-tooth tenaculum. The myoma is brought to the suprapubic incision and pressed against the peritoneum to prevent loss of

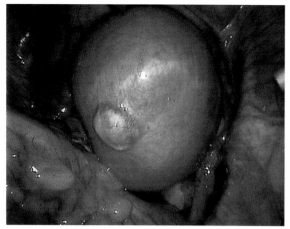

Figure 27.1 Two intramural myomas (7 cm, 4 cm in size) and one subserous myoma (2 cm).

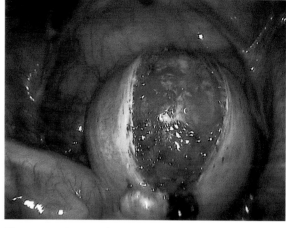

Figure 27.2 Longitudinal incision.

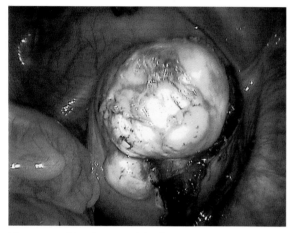

Figure 27.3 Enucleation of the first myoma.

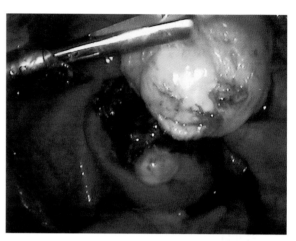

Figure 27.4 The myoma is isolated.

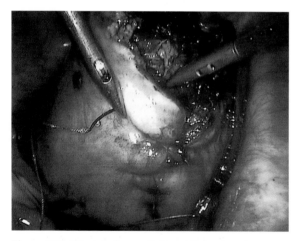

Figure 27.5 Uterine closure (interrupted sutures).

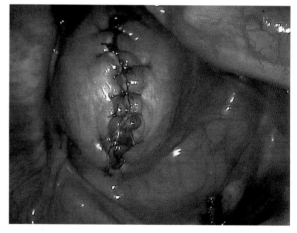

Figure 27.6 Final result.

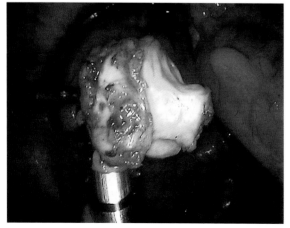

Figure 27.7 Morcellation of the myoma using the electrical morecellator.

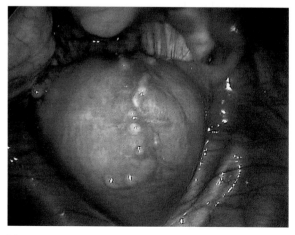

Figure 27.8 Second-look laparoscopy after LM for a large subserous interstitial myoma of the fundus.

carbon dioxide (CO_2). The myoma is then fragmented under laparoscopic control using a small blade passed through the incision. The myoma may also be removed through a posterior colpotomy. More recently, an electrical cutting device has been used to fragment the myoma (Steiner et al., 1993). After removal of the myoma, the peritoneal cavity is irrigated with saline solution and a further check is made for complete hemostasis. No drainage is used.

Results of Our Experience

From January 1990 to June 1995, we carried out 213 LMs using the technique described above. The average age of the patients was 37.5 years ± 6.7 years (range 20–64).

The indications for the LM, which were sometimes combined in the same patient, were as follows:

- Menometrorrhagia (40 cases, 18.8%).
- Pain or dragging feeling in the pelvis (45 cases, 21.1%).
- Large polymyomatous uterus (68 cases, 31.9%).
- Infertility (69 cases, 32.4%).

Laparoscopic procedures were associated with the LM in 89 patients (41.8%). These procedures were as follows:

- Ovarian cystectomy (23 cases).
- Unilateral adnexectomy (ten cases).
- Tubal ligation (15 cases).
- Salpingo-ovariolysis (24 cases).
- Bowel lysis (four cases).
- Distal tuboplasty (nine cases).
- Salpingectomy (five cases).
- Bipolar coagulation of peritoneal endometriosis (24 cases).

The average duration of the operation was 130 ± 56.1 minutes (range 30–300). The mean drop in hemoglobin levels was 1.4 ± 1.1 g 100 ml^{-1} (range 0–6 g 100 ml^{-1}). In these 213 operations, 437 myomectomies were carried out. The average number of myomas removed per patient was 2.05 ± 1.5 (range 1–10). A polymyomectomy was performed in 108 (50.7%) of the cases: in 46 cases (21.6%), two myomas were removed; in 29 cases (13.6%), three myomas were removed; and in 33 cases (15.5%), four or more myomas were removed during the operation. The average size of the largest myoma removed was 5.3 ± 2.2 cm (range 1–12 cm). The average size of the largest myoma removed was less than 4 cm in 22.6% of cases (48 patients), 4–9 cm in 70.4% of cases (150 patients) and larger than 9 cm in

7% of cases (15 patients). The location of the largest myoma removed was interstitial in 47.4% of cases (101 patients), unpedunculated subserous in 40.8% of cases (87 patients) and pedunculated subserous in only 11.8% of cases (25 patients). The site of the largest myoma removed was posterior in 46.5% of cases (99 patients), anterior in 28.6% of cases (61 patients), fundal in 21.6% of cases (46 patients) and on the broad ligament in 3.3% of cases (7 patients).

The failure rate (i.e. rate of conversion to laparotomy) was 7.5% (16 patients) (Table 27.1). Of the cases converted to laparotomy, nine (56.25%) were indicated when difficulties were encountered in obtaining an acceptable quality uterine suture, while five (31.25%) were indicated due to peroperative hemorrhage. However, none of the patients in this series required transfusion. One case of hypercapnia obliged us to interrupt the laparoscopic operation although no surgical complications had been encountered. The remaining conversion to laparotomy was because the cleavage plane for the myoma could not be found. The final histologic results showed that it was a voluminous adenomyoma measuring 8 cm. There is significant statistical correlation between the risk of conversion to laparotomy and the average size and location of the largest myoma removed. When myomas are larger and located anteriorly, the operation becomes more difficult. The risk of conversion to laparotomy is three times greater when the myoma measures 8 cm or more (17.1%, six cases versus 5.6%, ten cases). When the myoma is located anteriorly, the risk of conversion to laparotomy is three times greater than if the myoma is located in the posterior or fundal positions (14.7%, nine cases versus 4.8%, seven cases) (Dubuisson et al., 1996a).

The complication rate for LM is 11.3% (24 cases) (see Table 27.1). Apart from the 16 patients for whom a conversion to laparotomy was necessary and who we consider as having complications, eight other patients had complications. These complications are presented in Table 27.1. Among the 34 patients in this series who had an intrauterine pregnancy (IUP) following the LM, there was one case of uterine rupture (Dubuisson et al., 1995b). This is the only major postoperative complication that we observed. During the same operation, this same patient also underwent a bilateral salpingostomy and LM for an intramural posterior wall myoma measuring 3 cm. The uterine suture was performed by separate 3–0 stitches polyglactin 910 (Ethicon, Neuilly, France). The patient was seen as an emergency due to pelvic pain after 34 weeks of amenorrhea. The diagnosis of uterine rupture was immediately made and an emergency operation was carried out. A large uterine rupture at the uterine scar was observed. It was apparent that the

Table 27.1 Complications of laparoscopic myomectomy. (From Dubuisson *et al.*, 1996a.)

Complication	Number	%
Peroperative complications responsible for conversion to laparotomy	16	7.5
Difficulties with uterine suture	9	4.2
Hemorrhage	5	2.3
Non cleavable adenomyoma	1	0.5
Hypercapnia	1	0.5
Peroperative complications without conversion to laparotomy	1	0.5
Hypercapnia	1	0.5
Immediate postoperative complications	6	2.8
Transient high fever	4	1.8
Phlebitis	1	0.5
Hepatitis	1	0.5
Long-term postoperative complications	1	0.5
Uterine rupture during pregnancy	1	0.5
Total	24	11.3

placenta and the body of the fetus had delivered into the abdominal cavity through a large postero-fundal uterine rupture. The rupture was enlarged with a scalpel and the baby was delivered. The post operative course was uneventful for the mother and the baby. For the 33 other patients, the course of IUP was as follows:

- Premature miscarriage (three cases).
- Second trimester miscarriage (one case).
- Death *in utero* after 28 weeks amenorrhea (one case).
- Full-term pregnancy (27 cases).

In 20 cases (71.4%), the birth was vaginal and in eight cases (29.6%) by cesarean. The indications for cesarean were:

- Uterine scar (five cases).
- Pathological pelvis (one case).
- Dynamic dystocia (one case).
- Maternal counterindications to vaginal delivery (one case).

The rate of postoperative adhesions following LM in our experience was 20%. The uterine scar was checked in 31 patients following LM. This check was made using laparoscopy for 23 cases and during laparotomy for eight cases, six of which were indicated for a cesarean section (Table 27.2).

Discussion

Diagnosing a uterine myoma does not necessarily imply surgery. Only complicated or voluminous myomas, those that increase rapidly in volume and

Table 27.2 Adhesions on uterine scar after laparoscopic myomectomy (Dubuisson *et al.* 1996a).

Operative procedure	Number	No adhesions on uterine scar Number	%
Second-look laparoscopy	23	18	78.3
Laparotomy	8	7	87.5
Cesarean section	6	6	100.0
Other laparotomies	2	1	50.0
Total	31	25	80.6

those causing persistent symptoms in spite of correct medical treatment should be treated surgically. When surgery is indicated, which technique should be used? The development of endoscopic surgery techniques allow the operation to be carried out by either hysteroscopic or laparoscopic methods in certain cases. The indications for these two surgical techniques are completely different:

- Hysteroscopic surgery is indicated to treat submucous myomas, but only if the intra cavity portion of the fibroma represents at least 50% of the volume of the myoma and the fibroma is not larger than 5 cm. It may consist of resection with a diathermy loop (Neuwirth, 1978; Siegler and Valle, 1988; Corson and Brooks, 1991; Parent *et al.*, 1994) or neodymium:yttrium-aluminum-garnet (Nd:YAG) laser myolysis (Baggish *et al.*, 1989; Parent *et al.*, 1994).
- Myomectomy of intramural myomas (subserous or interstitial) as well as pedunculated myomas, previously carried out by laparo-

tomy may in certain situations be performed by laparoscopic surgery.

LM is a difficult technique. In our experience, the rate of conversion to laparotomy is 7.5% and the complication rate is 11.3% (Dubuisson *et al.*, 1996a). LM as an operation involves four specific difficulties:

- The location of the hysterotomy.
- The type of hysterotomy.
- The uterine suture.
- The removal of the myoma.

The choice of site for the hysterotomy is fundamental because it affects the rest of the procedure. The larger the subserous portion of an intramural myoma, the easier it is to identify the site of the hysterotomy. For myomas deeply embedded in the myometrium or for purely interstitial myomas, it is essential to refer to the preoperative ultrasonography. As this locates the myoma very accurately, the hysterotomy may then be made exactly opposite the myoma. In order for the abdominal and transvaginal ultrasound examination to provide as much information as possible, it is carried out during the luteal phase. It is during this period of the menstrual cycle that the endometrium, which is the essential landmark for locating the myomas, can best be seen as a fine echogenic line. Ultrasound also enables the distances between the myoma and the serosa membranes to be measured, together with those between the myoma and the endometrium.

The second difficulty lies in the choice of direction for the uterine incision. The standard option is a vertical hysterotomy (Verkauf, 1992). However, given that the arteries and arterioles of the myometrium run almost transversely and not vertically (Farrer-Brown *et al.*, 1970; Igarashi, 1993), it seems more logical to make a transverse incision. This type of incision would reduce blood loss especially when the intramural myoma is deep and richly vascularized.

The third difficulty with this operation is the uterine suture. In our experience, 56.2% of the conversions to laparotomy were indicated because of difficulties encountered with suturing the hysterotomy (Dubuisson *et al.*, 1996a). The uterine suture may be made in different ways, with either continuous suturing or individual stitches, while the knots may be tied either intra- or extracorporeally, in which case they are taken down the pelvis with a knot pusher. The choice of technique depends mainly upon the surgeon's experience and the surgeon should use the technique that he or she has mastered. There is no gold standard for this, and we ourselves use separate stitches, as we do for laparo-

tomy. If the myomas are deeply embedded in the myometrium, the suture can be made along two planes (Dubuisson *et al.*, 1995a). The quality of the scar after LM has yet to be assessed. Whereas the risk of uterine rupture after myomectomy via laparotomy is low (Brown *et al.*, 1956; Davids, 1952), to our knowledge two cases of uterine rupture have occurred after LM (Harris, 1992; Dubuisson *et al.*, 1995b). In both cases the observations were comparable, with uterine rupture occurring during pregnancy (34 weeks of amenorrhea) after laparoscopic ablation of a small (3 cm) intramural myoma, which had been sutured.

Extraction of the myoma is the fourth difficulty of this operation. Different possibilities are available:

- Extraction via mini laparotomy following laparoscopic morcellation.
- Extraction via one of the suprapubic trocar ports following intraperitoneal fragmentation.
- Extraction via posterior colpotomy.

We carried out extraction using the first two techniques initially, but abandoned them in favor of the posterior colpotomy, which is much more elegant and more rapid. However, extraction via posterior colpotomy is not always easy because:

- The presentation of the fibroma in the pouch of Douglas with respect to the colpotomy site is not always straightforward.
- Then, once the colpotomy has been carried out, the significant CO_2 leak makes the presentation and therefore identification of the fibroma via the vagina difficult.
- Finally, the extraction of the myoma is not always very easy to perform. In the case of limited vaginal access or a voluminous myoma, the myoma may need to be morcellated via the vagina in order to remove it.

At present, this operation is greatly assisted by the electric morcellator (Steiner *et al.*, 1993), which we use in many cases. It permits voluminous myomas to be removed rapidly. The system is made up of a rotating cutting cylinder, which is protected by a sheath and linked to an electric machine. A 10 mm forceps inserted inside the cylinder allows the myoma to be gripped and pulled towards the cylinder so that it can be cut up. The excised tissue is thus extracted in the form of a number of cylindrical carrots (from 1–30 cm long). This instrument takes 3–20 minutes to morcellate myomas of 4–8 cm in size (Dubuisson and Chapron, 1996).

Although our results show that LM is a difficult technique, the feasibility of this operation has nevertheless been definitively proven. Moreover, it is a reproducible technique as other teams have also reported very encouraging results (Daniell and Guerly, 1991; Nezhat *et al.*, 1991; Hasson *et al.*, 1992). Factors that appear to limit the use of this technique seem to be the size and number of the myomas. We consider that the fibromas should not exceed 8 cm in size and that there should be less than three so that LM can be performed satisfactorily (Dubuisson and Chapron, 1996).

The operative technique for LM is now well defined and the indications for this operation are increasingly specific. In the coming years, the risk of adhesions, the quality of the uterine suture and the results of this technique for infertile patients must be analyzed.

As far as the risk of adhesions is concerned, our preliminary results are encouraging, with only 20% of the patients having adhesions on the uterine scar. These results need to be confirmed with a larger series of patients and evaluated in terms of the size and location of the myomas, and whether or not there is a uterine suture. This work is currently in progress and will be published in the near future.

As far as the quality of the uterine suture is concerned, this appears to be satisfactory. Among the 34 patients in our series who had an IUP following LM (Dubuisson *et al.*, 1996a), only one serious complication due to rupture of the uterine scar was observed (Dubuisson *et al.*, 1996a). These encouraging results are comparable to those reported by two other teams (Nezhat *et al.*, 1991; Hasson *et al.*, 1992).

As far as fertility following LM is concerned, to our knowledge only one study deals with this question specifically (Dubuisson *et al.*, 1996b). The preliminary results show that for patients without any other factors for infertility other than myomas, the percentage of IUPs following LM is comparable to that following myomectomy by laparotomy (Table 27.3).

Table 27.3 Reproductive outcome in infertile patients after myomectomy.

Authors	Number of infertile patients*	Intrauterine pregnancy	
		Number	%
Myomectomy by laparotomy			
Brown *et al.* (1956)	21	11	52.4
Babaknia *et al.* (1978)	46	22	47.8
Ranney and Frederick (1979)	9	8	88.9
Berkeley *et al.* (1983)	6	1	16.7
Rosenfeld (1986)	23	15	65.2
Gatti *et al.* (1989)	20	10	50.0
Verkauf (1992)	3	2	66.7
Total	128	69	53.9
Laparoscopic myomectomy			
Dubuisson *et al.* (1996b)	9	4	44.4

* Patients without associated infertility factors.

Conclusion

It is now established that LM is feasible. This technique requires experienced laparoscopic surgeons with total mastery of endoscopic sutures. Providing all contraindications (i.e. myomas of 8 cm or less and less than 3 fibromas) are observed, LM is an effective operation. Preliminary results with respect to the risk of adhesiogenesis, the quality of the laparoscopic uterine suture and fertility are encouraging. However, larger series are needed to confirm these initial results.

Major potential complications of laparoscopic myomectomy.

1. Burn of the bowel during hysterotomy performed with the monopolar hook or scissors.
2. Severe uterine bleeding after incision.
3. Uterine fistula (inadequate uterine suture or abnormal healing).
4. Uterine rupture during pregnancy.
5. Postoperative bowel occlusion (due to uterine adhesions).

References

Babaknia A, Rock JA, Jones HW (1978) Pregnancy success following abdominal myomectomy for infertility. *Fertility and Sterility* **30**: 644–647.

Baggish MS, Sze EHM, Morgan G (1989) Hysteroscopic treatment of symptomatic submucous myomata uteri with the Nd:YAG laser. *Journal of Gynecologic Surgery* **5**: 27–31.

Berkeley AS, De Cherney AH, Polan ML (1983) Abdominal myomectomy and subsequent fertility. *Surgery, Gynecology and Obstetrics* **156**: 319–322.

Brown AB, Chamberlain R, Te Linde RW (1956) Myomectomy. *American Journal of Obstetrics and Gynecology* **71**: 759–763.

Chapron C, Dubuisson JB, Aubert V *et al.* (1994) Total laparoscopic hysterectomy: preliminary results. *Human Reproduction* **9**: 2084–2089.

Corson SL, Brooks PG (1991) Resectoscopic myomectomy. *Fertility and Sterility* **55**: 1041–1044.

Daniell JF, Gurley LD (1991) Laparoscopic treatment of clinically significant symptomatic uterine fibroids. *Journal of Gynecologic Surgery* **7**: 37–40.

Davids A (1952) Myomectomy: Surgical technique and results in a series of 1150 cases. *American Journal of Obstetrics and Gynecology* **63**: 592–604.

Dubuisson JB, Chapron C (1995) Laparoscopic myomectomy and myolysis. *Baillière's Clinical Obstetrics and Gynaecology* **9**: 717–728.

Dubuisson JB, Chapron C (1996) Laparoscopic myomectomy: a good technique when correctly indicated. *Human Reproduction* **11**: 934–935.

Dubuisson JB, Lecuru F, Foulot H, Mandelbrot L, Aubriot FX, Mouly M (1991) Myomectomy by laparoscopy: a preliminary report of 43 cases. *Fertility and Sterility* **56**: 827–830.

Dubuisson JB, Chapron C, Mouly M, Foulot H, Aubriot FX (1993) Laparoscopic myomectomy. *Gynaecological Endoscopy* **2**: 171–173.

Dubuisson JB, Chapron C, Chavet X, Morice P, Aubriot FX (1995a) Laparoscopic myomectomy: Where do we stand? *Gynaecological Endoscopy* **4**: 83–86.

Dubuisson JB, Chavet X, Chapron C, Morice P (1995b) Uterine rupture during pregnancy after laparoscopic myomectomy. *Human Reproduction* **10**: 1475–1477.

Dubuisson JB, Chapron C, Levy L (1996a) Difficulties and complications of laparoscopic myomectomy. *Journal of Gynecologic Surgery* **12**: 159–165.

Dubuisson JB, Chapron C, Chavet X, Gregorakis SS (1996b) Fertility after laparoscopic myomectomy of large intramural myomas: preliminary results. *Human Reproduction* **11**: 518–522.

Farrer-Brown G, Beilby JOW, Tarbit MH (1970) The vascular patterns in myomatous uteri. *Journal of Obstetrics and Gynaecology of the British Commonwealth* **77**: 967–970.

Gatti D, Falsetti L, Viani A, Gastaldi A (1989) Uterine fibromyoma and sterility: Role of myomectomy. *Acta Europaea Fertilitatis* **20**: 11–13.

Harris WJ (1992) Uterine dehiscence following laparoscopic myomectomy. *Obstetrics and Gynecology* **80**: 545–546.

Hasson HM, Rotman C, Rana N, Sistos F, Dmowski WP (1992) Laparoscopic myomectomy. *Obstetrics and Gynecology* **80**: 884–888.

Igarashi M (1993) Value of myomectomy in the treatment of infertility. *Fertility and Sterility* **59**: 1331–1332.

Neuwirth RS (1978) A new technique for an additional experience with hysteroscopic resection of submucous fibroids. *American Journal of Obstetrics and Gynecology* **131**: 91–95.

Nezhat C, Nezhat F, Silfen SL, Schaffer N, Evans D (1991) Laparoscopic myomectomy. *International Journal of Fertility* **36**: 275–280.

Novak ER, Jones GS, Jones HW (1970) Myomes utérins. In Novak ER, Jones GS, Jones HW (eds) *Gynécologie Pratiquue*. pp. 309–322. Paris: Editions Maloine.

Parent B, Barbot J, Guedj H, Nodarian P (eds) (1994) *Hystéroscopie Chirurgicale. Lasers et Techniques Classiques*. pp. 48–60. Paris: Editions Masson.

Ranney B, Frederick I (1979) The occasional need for myomectomy. *Obstetrics and Gynecology* **53**: 437–441.

Rosenfeld DL (1986) Abdominal myomectomy for otherwise unexplained infertility. *Fertility and Sterility* **46**: 328–330.

Siegler AM, Valle RF (1988) Therapeutic hysteroscopic procedures. *Fertility and Sterility* **50**: 685–701.

Steiner RA, Wight E, Tadir Y, Haller U (1993) Electrical device for laparoscopic removal of tissue from the abdominal cavity. *Obstetrics and Gynecology* **81**: 471–474.

Verkauf BS (1992) Myomectomy for fertility enhancement and preservation. *Fertility and Sterility* **58**: 1–15.

28

Laparoscopic Leiomyoma Coagulation – Myolysis

DOUGLAS R. PHILLIPS

Department of Obstetrics and Gynecology, School of Medicine, State University of New York at Stony Brook, New York, USA

Leiomyomas, the most common solid pelvic tumors, occur in 25–30% of women during their reproductive years. Approximately 20–50% of these women experience symptoms that require treatment, with the most common complaints being menorrhagia, metrorrhagia, pelvic pressure and the appreciation of a pelvic mass (Buttram and Reiter, 1981).

Determining the appropriate treatment of uterine leiomyomas involves assessing not only the size, location and growth rate of the tumors, but also the symptoms and coexisting pelvic pathology as well as the age, reproductive status and desires of the patient. No treatment is required for peri-menopausal patients with asymptomatic leiomy-omas unless there is a concern about future complications. Therapy is warranted, however, if a woman experiences symptoms that interfere with her health or the quality of her life. Treatment may be medical, surgical or a combination of both. Before the development of hysteroscopic and laparoscopic procedures, symptomatic leiomyomas in perimenopausal women were successfully man-aged by hysterectomy and occasionally by abdominal myomectomy. Of the more than 600 000 hysterectomies performed annually in the USA, leiomyoma is an indication in about 25% of cases, while 18 000 abdominal myomectomies are per-formed annually as conservative treatment of symptomatic uterine leiomyomas (Pokras and Hufnagel, 1987). For women who do not contem-plate childbearing, the treatment of choice has been hysterectomy. Patients of reproductive age who were infertile, unable to carry a pregnancy to term, and/or suffering from symptomatic leiomyomas were also treated with abdominal or laparoscopic myomectomy. Even though these procedures are invasive and morbid, they were the only surgical remedies available.

Laparoscopic leiomyoma (myoma) coagulation (myolysis) was developed in Germany in 1986 (Gallinat and Leuken, 1993) and was first reported in the literature and first performed in the USA in 1990 (Goldfarb, 1992). It involves using either a neodymium:yttrium-aluminum-garnet (Nd:YAG) laser bare fiber (Goldfarb, 1992, 1994, 1995a, b, 1996; Nisolle et al., 1993; Phillips, 1995a; Phillips et al., 1997b), monopolar needle (Wood et al., 1994) or bipolar coagulation needles (Goldfarb 1992, 1994, 1995a, b, 1996; Phillips, 1995a; Phillips et al., 1997b), hyperthermia elec-trode (diathermy) (Chapman, 1993), or recently, hypothermia probe (cryomyolysis) (Zreik et al., 1998) to destroy the stroma and vascular supply of the targeted leiomyoma. This results in significant shrinkage or even disappearance of the leiomyoma and resolution of its former associated symptoms.

Selection of Patients

Usually, the candidate for myolysis is the peri-menopausal woman presenting with pelvic pres-sure or pain, which is often associated with one or more of the following symptoms: heavy or prolonged menses documented by history, anemia or both; intermenstrual bleeding; or the appreciation of a pelvic mass. She has the required inclusion criteria for hysterectomy, but wants to avoid it or abdominal myomectomy. In most cases, a laparoscopic myomectomy would be time-consuming, technically difficult or unnecessary for pathologic evaluation. Occasionally, a woman with similar symptom(s) who is infertile or who wishes to retain her capacity to bear a child may also be a candidate.

The diagnosis of uterine leiomyoma is usually made by abdominopelvic examination. Location and size of the leiomyoma are determined by ultrasonography, hysteroscopy, sonohysterography, and/or occasionally by magnetic resonance imaging (MRI). Endometrial sampling is required to determine whether endometrial cancer or a precursor lesion is present as these are contraindications to conservative pelvic surgery.

Before myolysis, leuprolide acetate depot 3.75 mg or goserelin depot 3.6 mg, is usually administered in three monthly treatments. Two groups of women should not be considered candidates for myolysis: those who remain symptomatic after three months of this GnRH agonist pretreatment, even if there is significant shrinkage in the uterine and leiomyoma volumes, and those whose total uterine volume (TUV) is not reduced by at least 25% after GnRH agonist therapy because there is a possibility of leiomyosarcoma.

Sarcomatous degeneration is present in 0.04–0.29% of uterine leiomyomas removed surgically (Corscaden and Singh, 1958; Montague et al., 1965). Myolysis may delay the diagnosis and treatment of a leiomyosarcoma, since leiomyomatous tissue would not be routinely obtained via laparoscopy for pathologic examination. Furthermore, for women who have been infertile or who desire the capacity to have a child, it should also be emphasized that the long-term results of conception, success of carrying to term and appropriate mode of delivery have not been sufficiently studied and that the subsequent pregnancy risk is not yet known. Therefore, appropriate written informed consent explaining the aforementioned information should be obtained.

Pelvic and vaginal ultrasonography should be performed preoperatively before and after GnRH agonist pretreatment and between three and six months postoperatively. Measurements of the volume of the uterus and of each leiomyoma are calculated using the prolate ellipse equation: Volume = $(0.523)(D_1)(D_2)(D_3)$, where D_1, D_2 and D_3 represent the three largest diameters (length, transverse, and anteroposterior) (Goldstein et al., 1988).

Technique

Patients are placed in the low dorsolithotomy position in the Trendelenburg position at $10-20°$ under general endotracheal anesthesia. Prophylactic antibiotics are administered routinely. Immediately before myolysis, women with chronic menorrhagia have concomitant transcervical resection of endometrium (TCRE) if childbearing is not a consideration, and transcervical resection of leiomyoma (TCRL) for any existing submucous leiomyoma(s). Some 20 ml of vasopressin (0.05 U ml^{-1}) is used intracervically to reduce blood loss and distension fluid absorption and to facilitate dilation of the cervix (Phillips et al., 1996, 1997a).

During TCRL, the submucous leiomyoma(s) is resected to the level of the endometrium with a 7 mm wireloop electrode at 110–140 W of blended cutting current. If concomitant TCRE is performed, strips of endometrium and underlying myometrium are systematically resected to a thickness of approximately 5 mm, except at the tubal ostia, where either the resection is 2 mm or less or spot coagulation is done using a rollerball electrode at 40–60 W of pure coagulation current. The TCRE is completed by coagulating the entire denuded surface of the cavity with the rollerball electrode at the same wattage (Phillips, 1994, 1995b; Phillips et al., 1995; Wortman and Daggett, 1994).

Following the hysteroscopic portion of the surgery, either a Valtchev uterine mobilizer (Conklin Surgical Instruments, Toronto, Canada) or a Pelosi uterine mobilizer (Nova Endoscopy, Palm, PA, USA) is placed onto the cervix to manipulate the uterus into an optimum position for the laparoscopic surgery. At this time, if there is any pedunculated subserosal leiomyoma present, it is removed by first desiccating its base with bipolar coagulation and then excising it using scissors, knife or unipolar electrode. At the completion of myolysis, the intact or morcellated leiomyoma may be delivered either from one of the laparoscopic ports or through a culdotomy incision.

Laparoscopic leiomyoma coagulation is performed using either the Nd:YAG laser bare fiber or bipolar coagulation needles. Because of the fragility of the bare fiber and its inferior hemostatic effect, a bipolar coagulation technique is now exclusively used. This method uses a 32 cm long (or a 45 cm long, if it is used through the 5 mm operative channel of an operative laparoscope) bipolar coagulation instrument (J.E.M.D. Medical, Hicksville, NY, USA; Figure 28.1) connected to an electrosurgical generator. The active electrodes are two parallel 5 cm long needles.

The proper placement of the ancillary ports and stabilization of the uterus are of paramount

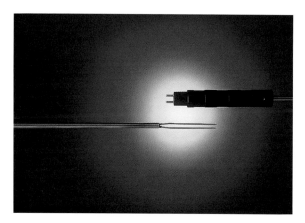

Figure 28.1 Bipolar coagulation needles (32 cm long with two parallel 5 cm long needles).

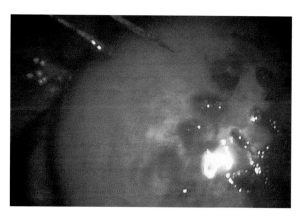

Figure 28.2 Perforation of leiomyoma with bipolar needles.

importance. At least two ports should be developed in the lower right and lower left abdominal regions, lateral to the deep epigastric blood vessels and sufficiently cephalad so that the leiomyoma(s) can be approached perpendicularly. The coagulation instrument is passed through one of these ports; 70 W of power is used. The uterus is usually stabilized by directly anchoring the leiomyoma or uterus with a 5 or 10 mm myoma drill (WISAP, Sauerlach, Germany), a corkscrew-grasping device delivered through either a 5 or 10 mm lower abdominal port. Occasionally, if applying high-flow suction and irrigation is warranted to facilitate the procedure, a third 5 mm trocar is placed suprapubically. Alternatively, a 10 mm bipolar coagulation needle instrument with irrigation and suction can be used, usually obviating the need for a third 5 mm puncture site.

Some 5–20 ml of a dilute vasopressin solution (0.05 U ml⁻¹) are administered transabdominally with an 18-guage needle to just beneath the serosal surface of the uterus overlying the leiomyoma; this provides a chemical tourniquet to reduce blood loss (Goldfarb, 1992, 1994, 1995b; Phillips, 1995a, Phillips *et al.* 1997b; Wood, 1994). Either the laser fiber or bipolar needles are used to systematically perforate subserous or intramural leiomyomas in 5–10 mm increments, which extend across the serosal surface to the base, forming parallel cylinders of desiccated denatured tissue. To maximize the coagulation effect to the leiomyoma, all passes are done slowly (10–15 mm s⁻¹) and are directed perpendicularly to the serosal surface to minimize the force necessary for entry (Figure 28.2). An effort is made to reduce coagulation of the uterine serosal surfaces by applying energy after the electrodes have pierced approximately 3–5 mm below the surface and by discontinuing the energy

just before removing the needles when the pass has been completed. When technically feasible, the leiomyoma is perforated in perpendicular planes to destroy the stroma and vasculature more completely. At the endpoint of the procedure almost the entire leiomyoma surface is paled and blanched.

A modification of this laparoscopic technique may be used on patients who wish to bear a child. Instead of perforating the entire leiomyoma with the bipolar coagulation needles, only the circumference of the base of the leiomyoma is perforated every 5 mm in an attempt to destroy the blood supply to the lesion while minimizing the damage to the overlying serosal surface (Goldfarb, 1996).

Results

From February 1992 to March 1995 our studies with myolysis involved 167 women with a mean age of 44.7 years, gravidity of 2.2 and a weight of 60.2 kg. The TUV decreased from 620 cm³ before leuprolide medication to 297 cm³ one month after the third dose and immediately before surgery (Table 28.1).

Of the 52 women with chronic menorrhagia, 50 had TCRE and 22 women who had submucous myomas had these lesions resected concomitantly. Two other patients who wanted to preserve their fertility underwent TCRL without TCRE.

Amenorrhea, hypomenorrhea and eumenorrhea were considered satisfactory menstrual results after TCRE and eumenorrhea a satisfactory menstrual result after TCRL. Six months after surgery, satisfactory results had been achieved in 50 of the 52 women (96.2%). Hysteroscopic procedures added a mean of 29.4 minutes to the total operating time,

Table 28.1 Uterine leiomyoma measurements.* (TUV, total uterine volume; LLD, longest leiomyoma diameter; LLC, laparoscopic leiomyoma coagulation (myolysis); TLV, total leiomyoma volume.)

Measurement	Surgery	Premedication	Postleuprolide	3–6 months postoperative	7–12 months postoperative
TUV	LLC	637 ± 35.7; 105–2002	291 ± 11.9; 87–1133	121 ± 7.8; 6–601	139 ± 8.0; 6–605
	LLC with TCRE and/or TCRL	582 ± 25.1; 126–2116	311 ±13.6; 84–989	99 ± 6.4; 9–588	113 ± 6.9; 6–590
	Both groups	620 ± 28.4; 110–2312	297 ± 13.0; 78–1011	114 ± 6.5; 6–601	131 ± 7.2; 6–605
LLD	LLC	6.7 ± 0.2; 2.6–12.4	5.4 ± 0.2; 2.3–11.9	2.6 ± 0.1; 0–5.6	2.9 ± 0.2; 0–5.9
	LLC with TCRE and/or TCRL	6.5 ± 0.2; 2.7–11.3	5.3 ± 0.2; 2.4–10.8	2.6 ± 0.1; 0–5.8	2.8 ± 0.2; 0–6.0
	Both groups	6.6 ± 0.2; 2.6–13.4	5.4 ± 0.2; 2.3–11.7	2.6 ± 0.1; 0–5.8	2.9 ± 0.2; 0–6.1
TLV	LLC	198 ± 13.9; 9–602	83 ± 4.5; 7–367	26 ± 2.4; 0–168	31 ± 2.5; 0–177
	LLC with TCRE and/or TCRL	181 ± 10.9; 7–577	84 ± 4.5; 5–361	23 ± 2.2; 0–167	27 ± 2.3; 0–179
	Both groups	193 ± 11.5; 6–602	83 ± 4.6; 4–367	25 ± 2.3; 0–171	30 ± 2.4; 0–183

* Based on 115 women having LLC and 52 women having LLC with TCRE and/or TCRL. All volumes are expressed in terms of mean ± SEM; range, cm³; all diameters in cm. The two surgery groups, LLC and LLC with TCRE and/or TCRL, showed no statistically significant differences ($P >0.05$).

which was determined from when the resectoscope was inserted to when the resection was completed. There were no intraoperative or postoperative complications arising from this portion of the surgery.

TUV decreased significantly ($P<0.0001$) from 620 cm³ before leuprolide medication to 131 cm³, 7–12 months postoperatively (see Table 28.1). Similarly, the mean longest leiomyoma diameter (LLD) decreased from 6.6 cm to 2.9 cm ($P<0.0001$), and the mean total leiomyoma volume (TLV) decreased from 193 cm³ to 30 cm³ ($P<0.0001$). There were no statistically significant changes in mean TUV, LLD or TLV determined by ultrasonography 7–12 months after surgery when compared with the results 3–6 months postoperatively.

Of the 19 women who had second-look laparoscopy six months after surgery, 14 showed no adhesions at the myolysis sites. However, all sites of previous surgery showed areas of increased superficial serosal vascularization in a radial pattern (Figure 28.3). The other five women had thick and thin avascular adhesions extending from the bowel to some of the uterine serosal surgical sites; the adhesion score was a mean of 1.15 ± 0.6 (range 0–10; Surgical Membrane Study Group, 1992). Although these patients were asymptomatic, these adhesions were electrosurgically lysed to evaluate the under-

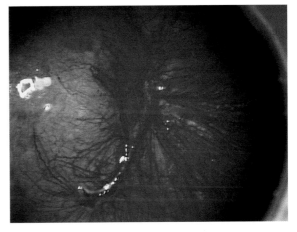

Figure 28.3 Elective second-look laparoscopy six months postoperatively after myolysis showing the radial pattern of superficial blood vessels.

lying uterine tissue. After adhesiolysis, the serosal surfaces overlying the treated leiomyomas appeared white and avascular; the uterine walls appeared smooth with no obvious structural defects.

The two women who wanted to retain their childbearing options underwent myolysis and TCRL; one woman conceived seven months

Table 28.2 Subsequent gynecologic surgery performed after six months.*

Initial surgery	TCRE n (%)	Repeat LLC n (%)	Hysterectomy n (%)	Total number (%)
LLC		1 (0.6)	1 (0.6)‡	2 (1.2)
LLC/TCRL	2 (1.2)†	1 (0.6)	4 (2.4)‡	7 (4.2)
TCRE				
Both groups	2 (1.2)	2 (1.2)	5 (3.0)	9 (5.4)

* Based on a follow-up of 36.0 ± 1.2 months (mean ± SEM; range 18–54 months) of 115 women initially having myolysis and 52 having myolysis and TCRE and/or TCRL.
† One patient had repeat TEMR and then a subsequent hysterectomy.
‡ This difference was significant ($P = 0.01$).

postoperatively and the other eight months postoperatively. They both had uneventful pregnancies and vaginal deliveries of healthy male infants weighting 2796 g and 3211 g, respectively.

Reoperation

More than 6 months postoperatively, eight women (4.8%) complained that one or more of the following symptoms had recurred: pain, pressure or menorrhagia. Although a repeat conservative endoscopic procedure or medical therapy was offered, only the two patients complaining of menorrhagia chose a repeat TCRE at seven and nine months postoperatively, respectively (Table 28.2). One of the patients who had a repeat procedure, subsequently became hypoamenorrheic; the other continued to have symptoms and ultimately chose to have a laparoscopically assisted vaginal hysterectomy (LAVH) five months after the repeat hysteroscopic procedure. During the laparoscopic procedure, no pelvic adhesions were noted. However, there was an elliptical ovoid superficial depression approximately 4 cm wide at its largest diameter on the serosal surface of the uterus at the site of the previous myolysis. Pathologic review of the myometrium revealed severe diffuse adenomyosis with multifocal areas of microcysts containing chocolate-brown fluid, predominantly at the area of serosal defects.

A 37-year-old woman had laser myolysis of a 4.5 cm posterior fundal intramural leiomyoma that was undetectable clinically or by ultrasound three months postoperatively, but 15 months after surgery she suddenly developed lower abdominal pressure and an appreciation of a rapidly growing abdominal mass. MRI revealed a 14 cm predominantly low-density pelvic mass with multiple foci of hyperintensity. She underwent a total abdominal hysterectomy since there was a possibility of leiomyosarcoma. A 5 mm wide filmy adhesion was noted that extended from the site of the previous myolysis to the anterior abdominal wall. Pathology revealed a benign leiomyoma.

Three of five women chose hysterectomy, and the other two chose a repeat myolysis for recurrent symptoms of pelvic pressure and pain from 7–27 months postoperatively (see Table 28.2). One hysterectomy was performed laparoscopically and two vaginally. During the LAVH, thick adhesions were noted on the posterior wall of the uterus between the site of the previous myolysis, the large bowel and the anterior abdominal wall. Pathologic evaluation of the three uteri revealed diffuse adenomyosis and leiomyomas in all specimens. None of the extirpated uteri from the five women who had hysterectomy or the two uteri examined during the repeat myolysis showed evidence of regrowth of leiomyomas at the site of previous myolysis surgery; however, all sites of previous surgery showed areas of increased superficial serosal vascularization in a radial pattern. The patients who underwent repeat myolysis have since remained asymptomatic 12 and 22 months postoperatively.

Complications

None of the women had any intraoperative complications; they all were discharged from the ambulatory surgery unit within a mean of 5.1 hours after surgery was completed. Eight patients (4.8%) complained of a transient pyrexia up to a maximum of 102.8°F for a mean of 7.5 days postoperatively with minimal elevations of erythrocyte sedimentation rates (ESRs) and white blood cell counts (WBCs) and without pelvic or abdominal discomfort (Table 28.3). They were placed on antibiotics and analgesics and responded well to this conservative therapy.

One of the three women who refused GnRH agonist pretreatment had laparoscopic laser myolysis without hysteroscopic surgery. She developed symptoms of acute leiomyoma degeneration one day postoperatively: these included moderate to

Table 28.3 Complications.*

Complication	LLC n (%)	LLC with TCRE and/or TCRL n (%)	Total number (%)	Statistical significance, P†
Transient pyrexia	4 (3.5)	4 (7.7)	8 (4.8)	0.21
Myoma degeneration	1 (0.9)	0	1 (0.6)	0.69
Abdominal wall hematoma	0	2 (3.8)	2 (1.2)	0.10
Urinary tract infection	2 (1.7)	1 (1.9)	3 (1.8)	0.68
Total	7 (6.1)	7 (13.5)	14 (8.4)	0.10

* Based on 115 women initially having myolysis and 52 having myolysis with TCRE and/or TCRL.
† Data did not reach the level of significance.

severe abdominal cramps, a WBC count as high as 23 543 mm^{-3}, as ESR as high as 37 mm h^{-1}, and a fever that rose to 102.2°F. She responded well to oral antibiotics, analgesics, and bed rest and became asymptomatic five days postoperatively. Two women developed a suprapubic abdominal wall hematoma, which limited ambulation for 2–3 weeks. They responded well to conservative therapy and resumed normal activities within three weeks.

Discussion

Perimenopausal patients with asymptomatic leiomyomas require no treatment unless there is a concern about future complications. Therapy is warranted, however, if a woman experiences symptoms that interfere with her health or quality of life. Medical options have included iron supplementation and GnRH agonist therapy.

GnRH agonist therapy reversibly inhibits the pituitary–gonadal axis to produce a hypogonadal state consistent with menopausal estrogen levels. Since leiomyomas are estrogen-dependent tumors, in most cases GnRH agonist therapy reduces TUV by 35–50%, usually within three months (Coddington *et al.*, 1986; Friedman, 1989; Friedman *et al.*, 1991; Phillips, 1994; 1995a; Phillips *et al.*, 1995, 1997b). In addition to reducing uterine volume, GnRH agonist therapy results in cessation or reduction of menorrhagia, allowing spontaneous recovery from anemia, especially when it is associated with oral iron supplementation, and permits autologous blood collection. GnRH agonist therapy may also facilitate subsequent surgery and expand surgical alternatives. The therapy reduces or eliminates leiomyoma symptoms, perhaps allowing patients to wait for spontaneous menopause.

However, within 3–6 months after GnRH agonist therapy is discontinued, 80% of women experience a regrowth of leiomyomas to pretreatment size (Coddington *et al.*, 1986; Friedman, 1989; Friedman *et al.*, 1991). After three months of GnRH agonist therapy (during which time the maximum reduction in TUV usually occurs), researchers have shown that the addition of estrogen either alone or with progestin prevents osteoporosis and vasomotor symptoms without increasing the size of the leiomyoma (Friedman and Hornstein, 1993). However, cost-effectiveness analysis and further long-term studies of the safety of GnRH agonist therapy are needed before its routine use can be advocated.

Depending upon the symptoms, surgical treatment options of symptomatic leiomyomas include hysterectomy, abdominal or laparoscopic myomectomy, endometrial ablation or TCRE, and TCRL. Although hysterectomy has been considered the treatment of choice for perimenopausal patients with symptomatic leiomyomas who do not contemplate childbearing, less morbid, more cost-effective and more patient-acceptable procedures could be offered. Myomectomy, when carried out through the laparoscope or through an abdominal incision may be considered if there is a desire to retain fecundity or the uterus. However, there are drawbacks associated with a myomectomy:

- It can be a difficult operation if there are large multiple leiomyomas.
- There is a 5–30% recurrence rate.
- 20–25% of patients require subsequent surgical therapy, usually a hysterectomy (Candiani *et al.*, 1991).

In 45–68% of cases, marked adhesions form after myomectomy (Nezhat *et al.*, 1991; Gehlbach *et al.*, 1993), but there is little information to suggest that they affect fertility. A 3% adhesion rate has been reported (Nezhat *et al.*, 1991) when sutures were not used to close the uterine defects compared to a 45% adhesion rate when sutures were used. Although they were asymptomatic, 19 of our myolysis patients agreed to an elective second-look laparoscopy procedure six months postoperatively to evaluate adhesion formation after myolysis. Two of the women who had undergone laser myolysis had adhesions and three of them who had bipolar myolysis had adhesions. A substantially higher incidence of adhesion formation has been reported (Nisolle et al., 1993) with very dense adhesions observed in seven (100%) patients during second-look laparoscopy six months after Nd:YAG laser myolysis. When myomectomy is performed for primary infertility in the absence of other causal factors, the subsequent pregnancy rate is approximately 40% (Buttram and Reiter, 1981). Whether or not the rates of adhesion formation and of pregnancy following laparoscopic myolysis are comparable to the rates following a myomectomy remains to be determined. Randomized double-blind, prospective studies using 'adhesion prevention' substances such as Interceed (Ethicon, Cincinnati, OH, USA) or fibrin sealant (Tissucol, Immuno, Austria) are needed to address this issue.

Laparoscopic myomectomy has the advantages of an outpatient surgical procedure. Pedunculated subserous leiomyomas can be readily removed, but if large multiple sessile subserous and intramural leiomyomas are present, this procedure is often technically difficult, time-consuming and requires the expertise of an advanced laparoscopic surgeon. It may lead to an undesired laparotomy, hysterectomy or blood transfusion. A vaginal hysterectomy or a laparoscopic hysterectomy may be an option, if it is technically feasible. The addition of a course of GnRH analogues may permit this surgical choice.

The success of myolysis to resolve symptomatic leiomyomas has been confirmed by many investigators (Goldfarb, 1992, 1994, 1995a,b, 1996; Chapman 1993; Gallinat and Leuken, 1993; Nisolle et al., 1993; Wood et al., 1994; Phillips, 1995a, 1997b). The first report to discuss the use of a Nd:YAG laser bare fiber to perforate leiomyomas as large as 10 cm in diameter described the perforation of the leiomyoma every 5 mm to produce contiguous cylinders of denatured and devascularized stroma (Goldfarb, 1992). Women were pretreated for 3–6 months with leuprolide acetate depot, which reduced leiomyoma volumes 40–60%. Within 6–9 months postoperatively, the diameters of the leiomyomas continued to decrease approximately 50–70%. There was no regrowth of leiomyomas during a 12-month follow-up period, and no subsequent hysterectomies or abdominal surgeries were performed on the 75 patients studied. The same investigator later reported an expansion to a series of 300 myolysis cases, 150 performed using a Nd:YAG laser and an equal number performed using bipolar coagulation six months postoperatively. There was

leiomyoma shrinkage of 30–50% beyond the effect of the leuprolide depot (Goldfarb, 1995a,b, 1996). There were no cases of myoma regeneration; therefore, no patient required a repeat procedure or hysterectomy for this reason. One patient, however, developed a pelvic abscess and subsequently underwent hysterectomy. Another patient developed bacteremia and responded well to intensive antibiotic therapy. Six patients developed myoma degeneration, but responded well to conservative therapy.

The cost-effectiveness of myolysis compared to the more traditional surgical methods of hysterectomy and abdominal myomectomy has to be ascertained. Myolysis has the obvious economic benefits of outpatient surgery and rapid recovery with consequent return to a normal life style. Unfortunately, long-term reoperation rates for previously treated or new leiomyoma regrowth or for recurrent or persistent symptoms are unknown. However, since most of the women undergoing myolysis are perimenopausal, the anticipated need for additional surgery for symptoms due to an increase in the volume of leiomyoma is probably minimal. Although myolysis follow-up studies have been limited in duration (Goldfarb, 1992, 1994, 1995a,b, 1996; Chapman, 1993; Gallinat and Leuken, 1993; Nisolle et al., 1993; Wood et al., 1994; Phillips, 1995, 1997b; Zreik et al., 1998), the subsequent reoperation rates for recurrence or persistence of symptoms are acceptably low. A prospective randomized multicenter trial comparing myolysis with hysterectomy for women who no longer desire fertility is underway to ascertain cost-effectiveness, efficacy and long-term sequelae.

The issue of whether to offer myolysis to women who wish to bear children is controversial. Although studies have been limited in the number of women undergoing various procedures to destroy their leiomyomas, the data have clearly demonstrated that conception and viable pregnancies are possible after laparoscopic myolysis (Chapman, 1993; Wood et al., 1994; Phillips et al., 1997b) or hysteroscopic laser myolysis (Donnez et al., 1990). However, it is not known whether the integrity and the tensile strength of the uterine walls are maintained after myolysis. Recently, of two women who conceived within two months of myolysis, one experienced spontaneous uterine rupture at 32–33 weeks' gestation and the other, at term during labor (Joseph Daly, personal communication, 1995). The first case resulted in a fetal demise delivered by a hysterotomy; in the second case, a healthy infant was delivered during an emergency cesarean section and the uterus was repaired uneventfully. Both women had uneventful postoperative courses. Furthermore, it was reported that a spontaneous rupture of a gravid uterus occurred at 26 weeks gestation (Arcangeli, 1997). The woman, who had complained of primary infertility and pelvic pain, underwent bipolar myolysis of a 3-cm intramural fundal leiomyoma; she conceived on her third cycle of clomiphene citrate. Emergent laparotomy for severe abdominal pain suggestive of intra-abdominal hemorrhage revealed a rupture in the fundal area. Although the uterine repair and the mother's postoperative course were uneventful, the infant died after 27 weeks of intensive care from multiple disorders related to prematurity and anemia.

It is also not known whether the integrity and tensile strength of the uterine walls are retained after laparoscopic myomectomy. Uterine rupture during subsequent pregnancies is a complication of myomectomy (Dubuisson *et al.*, 1995), but it is relatively rare when myomectomy is carried out via laparotomy (Davids, 1952; Brown *et al.*, 1956; Garnet, 1964; Palerme and Friedman, 1966; Georgakopoulos and Bersis, 1981; Golan *et al.*, 1990). Laparoscopic myomectomy, however, is a relatively new technique with limited numbers of patients and inconclusive follow-up. There have been two cases of uterine rupture after laparoscopic myomectomy reported (Harris, 1992; Dubuisson *et al.*, 1995) in which pregnancies at 34 weeks resulted in spontaneous rupture of the uterus. In both cases, the monopolar hook was used to incise the uterus, bipolar coagulation was used for hemostasis of the uterine edge, and suturing was accomplished with interrupted polyglactin 3–0 or 4–0. Arguably, conception after myolysis or laparoscopic myomectomy should be delayed for an adequate postoperative time period, and an elective cesarean section should be contemplated, especially when conception occurs in the immediate postoperative period or the uterine surgery was extensive or both. In order to ascertain cost-effectiveness, efficacy and long-term sequelae, a prospective randomized multicenter trial to compare myolysis with myomectomy in women desiring either to retain their fertility or childbearing is in progress. Until the data become available from these studies, myolysis and even laparoscopic myomectomy should be offered to women desiring childbearing only after careful consideration of the advantages and disadvantages.

For the perimenopausal woman who wishes to retain her uterus, myolysis, a technically easy procedure to perform with a minimal complication rate, provides symptomatic relief by markedly reducing the sizes of the subserosal and intramural leiomyomas as well as the size of the uterus. Patients with chronic menorrhagia can undergo concomitant TCRE, TCRL or both.

References

Arcangeli S, Pasquarette MM (1997) Gravid uterine rupture after myolysis. *Obstetrics and Gynecology* **89**: 857.

Brown AB, Chamberlain R, Telinde RW (1956) Myomectomy. *American Journal of Obstetrics and Gynecology* **71**: 759–763.

Buttram VC, Reiter RC (1981) Uterine leiomyomata: etiology, symptomatology and management. *Fertility and Sterility* **36**: 433–435.

Candiani GB, Fedele L, Parazzini F *et al.* (1991) Risk of reoccurrence after myomectomy. *British Journal of Obstetrics and Gynaecology* **98**: 385–389.

Chapman R (1993) Treatment of uterine myomas by interstitial hyperthermia. *Gynaecological Endoscopy* **2**: 227–234.

Coddington CC, Collins RI, Shawker TH *et al.* (1986). Long acting gonadotropin hormone-releasing hormone analog use to treat uteri. *Fertility and Sterility* **45**: 624–629.

Corscaden JF, Singh BP (1958) Leiomyosarcoma of the uterus. *American Journal of Obstetrics and Gynecology* **75**: 149–155.

Davids A (1952) Myomectomy: surgical technique and results in a series of 1150 cases. *American Journal of Obstetrics and Gynecology* **63**: 592–604.

Donnez J, Gillerot S, Bourgonjon D *et al.* (1990) Neodymium:YAG laser hysteroscopy in large submucous fibroids. *Fertility and Sterility* **54**: 999–1003.

Dubuisson JB, Chavet X, Chapron C *et al.* (1995) Uterine rupture during pregnancy after laparoscopic myomectomy. *Human Reproduction* **10**: 1475–1477.

Friedman AJ (1989) Treatment of leiomyomata uteri with short-term leuprolide followed by leuprolide plus estrogen-progestin hormone replacement for 2 years: a pilot study. *Fertility and Sterility* **51**: 526–528.

Friedman AJ, Hornstein MD (1993) Gonadotropin-releasing hormone agonist plus estrogen progestin 'add-back' therapy for endometriosis-related pelvic pain. *Fertility and Sterility* **60**: 236–241.

Friedman AJ, Hoffman DI, Comire F *et al.* (1991) Treatment of leiomyomata uteri with leuprolide acetate depot: A double-blind, placebo-controlled, multicenter study. *Obstetrics and Gynecology* **77**: 720–725.

Gallinat A, Leuken RP (1993). Addendum – Current trends in the therapy of myomata. In Leuken RP, Gallinat A (eds) *Endoscopic Surgery in Gynecology*. pp. 69–71. Berlin: Demeter Verlag.

Garnet JD (1964) Uterine rupture during pregnancy. *Obstetrics and Gynecology* **23**: 898–904.

Gehlbach DL, Sousa RC, Carpenter SE *et al.* (1993) Abdominal myomectomy in the treatment of infertility. International Journal of Gynecology and Obstetrics **40**: 45–50.

Georgakopoulos PA, Bersis G (1981) Sigmoido-uterine rupture in pregnancy after multiple myomectomy. *International Journal of Surgery* **66**: 367–368.

Golan D, Aharoni A, Gonon R *et al.* (1990) Early spontaneous rupture of the post myomectomy gravid uterus. *International Journal of Gynecology and Obstetrics* **31**: 167–170.

Goldfarb, HA (1992) Nd: YAG laser laparoscopic coagulation of symptomatic myomas. *Journal of Reproductive Medicine* **36**: 636–638.

Goldfarb HA (1994) Removing uterine fibroids laparo-scopically. *Contemporary Obstetrics and Gynecology* **39**: 50–72.

Goldfarb HA (1995a) Bipolar laparoscopic needles for myoma coagulation. *Journal of the American Association of Gynecologic Laparoscopists* **2**: 175–179.

Goldfarb HA (1995b) Laparoscopic coagulation of myoma (myolysis). In Hutchins FL, Greenberg MD (eds) *Obstetrics and Gynecology Clinics of North America. Uterine Fibroids.* pp. 807–819. Philadelphia: W.B. Saunders.

Goldfarb HA (1996) Laparoscopic coagulation of myoma (myolysis). In Tolandi T (ed.) *Infertility and Reproductive Medicine Clinics of North America. Uterine Myomas.* pp. 129–141. Philadelphia: W.B. Saunders.

Goldstein SR, Horii SC, Snyder JR *et al.* (1988) Estimation of nongravid uterine volume based on a nomogram of gravid uterine volume: Its value in gynecological abnormalities. *Obstetrics and Gynecology* **72**: 86–90.

Harris WJ (1992) Uterine dehiscence following laparo-scopic myomectomy. *Obstetrics and Gynecology* **80**: 545–546.

Montague A, Schwartz A, Woodruff J (1965) Sarcoma arising in a leiomyoma of the uterus. *American Journal of Obstetrics and Gynecology* **92**: 421–427.

Nezhat C, Nezhat F, Silfen S *et al.* (1991) Laparoscopic myomectomy. *International Journal of Fertility* **36**: 275–280.

Nisolle M, Smets M, Malvaux V *et al.* (1993) Laparoscopic myolysis with the Nd:YAG laser. *Journal of Gynecologic Surgery* **9**: 95–99.

Palerme GR, Friedman EA (1966) Rupture of the gravid uterus in the third trimester. *American Journal of Obstetrics and Gynecology* **94**: 571–576.

Phillips DR (1994) A comparison of endometrial ablation using the Nd:YAG laser or electrosurgical techniques. *Journal of the American Association of Gynecology Laparoscopists.* **1**: 235–239.

Phillips DR (1995a) Laparoscopic leiomyoma coagulation (myolysis). *Gynaecologic Endoscopy* **4**: 5–12.

Phillips DR (1995b) Endometrial ablation for post-menopausal uterine bleeding induced by hormone replacement therapy. *Journal of the American Association of Gynecologic Laparoscopists* **2**: 389–393.

Philips DR, Nathanson HG, Meltzer SM *et al.* (1995) Transcervical electrosurgical resection of submucous leiomyomas for chronic menorrhagia. *Journal of the American Association of Gynecologic Laparoscopists* **2**: 147–153.

Phillips DR, Nathanson HG, Milim SJ *et al.* (1996) The effect of dilute vasopressin solution on blood loss during operative hysteroscopy: A randomized, controlled trial. *Obstetrics and Gynecology* **88**: 761–766.

Phillips DR, Nathanson HG, Milim SJ *et al.* (1997a) The effect of dilute vasopressin solution on cervical dilatation: A randomized controlled trial. *Journal of Obstetrics and Gynecology* **89**: 507–511.

Phillips DR, Nathanson HG, Milim SJ *et al.* (1997b) Experience with laparoscopic leiomyoma coagulation and concomitant operative hysteroscopy. *Journal of the American Association of Gynecologic Laparoscopists* **4**: 425–433.

Pokras R, Hufnagel VG (1987) Hysterectomies in the United States, 1965–1984. Vital and health statistics. In *National Center for Health Statistics.* Series 13. No. 92. Washington, D.C.: Government Printing Office. (DHOWS publication no. (PAS) 88–1753).

Surgical Membrane Study Group (1992) Prophylaxis of pelvic sidewall adhesions with Gore-Tex surgical membrane: A Multicenter clinical investigation. *Fertility and Sterility* **57**: 921–923.

Wood C, Maher P, Hill D (1994) Myoma reduction by electrocautery. *Gynaecological Endoscopy* **3**: 163–165.

Wortman M, Daggett A (1994) Hysteroscopic endomyo-metrial resection: A new technique for the treatment of menorrhagia. *Obstetrics and Gynecology* **83**: 295–298.

Zreik TG, Rutherford T *et al.* (1998) Cryomyolysis: A new procedure for the conservative treatment of uterine fibroids. *Journal of the American Association of Gynecologic Laparoscopists* (In press).

29

Avoidance of Complications of Laparoscopic Hysterectomy

Jeffrey H. Phipps

George Eliot Hospital, Nuneaton, Warwickshire, UK

Introduction

Some skepticism still surrounds the laparoscopic approach to hysterectomy, but it seems that acceptance of this form of operation as a valuable and viable alternative to laparotomy for certain carefully selected cases is becoming more widespread. It therefore follows that an increasing number of gynecologists, both at consultant and training grades will attempt one form or another of laparoscopic hysterectomy. Although there is little doubt that a large proportion of hysterectomies can be carried out by the unassisted vaginal route, there will always be cases where the use of the laparoscope will enable the surgeon to avoid a laparotomy for hysterectomy (Phipps *et al.*, 1993). The presence of severe adhesive disease, a co-indication for oophorectomy with hysterectomy in the absence of prolapse or difficult vaginal access are factors that prompt most surgeons to list the patient for an abdominal operation rather than a vaginal procedure. However, it must be recognized that the current enthusiasm for laparoscopic hysterectomy has led many to reconsider their indications and contraindications for vaginal surgery, with a substantial increase in the number of vaginal operations carried out as a result of an increase in the skill and experience of the surgeons.

The most vital prerequisite to safe endoscopic surgery is patient selection. Patients must be offered operations that are both appropriate for the disease and for the ability of the surgeon at that particular stage of his or her training.

Given the rising popularity of laparoscopic surgery, it is of paramount importance that every possible step should be taken to minimize complications. There can be little doubt that the best way to achieve this is by properly conducted and adequate training of gynecologists in the skills necessary for safe practise in endoscopic surgery.

We are concerned here with those maneuvers that have been shown to reduce the incidence of complications during laparoscopic hysterectomy by trained and experienced endoscopic surgeons. Some of the issues will be controversial to some degree, but this is bound to happen with any discussion of relatively new techniques. I can only say that the recommendations included here have proved of great value in the author's experience, and have been formulated both from extensive personal work in the field and from observation and discussion with experts in endoscopic gynecological surgery.

Imaging Systems

The single most important factor in the success of any endoscopic procedure is that the surgeon must be able to see, not just well, but with total and utter clarity. The image must be of the highest quality, and this can only be achieved with the best laparoscopes and imaging equipment. The laparoscope must be in perfect condition, without chipped or cracked lenses, and without any water vapor trapped within its structure, which may lead to intermittent haziness of the image. The camera, control system, light source and light guide cable must be in good working order, and therefore must be handled only by those who understand that such instruments are delicate, and who require at least a basic knowledge of how they work. There are many high-quality systems now on the market, and the surgeon is to some extent spoilt for choice. Specifications vary, and in many cases the only deciding factors are price and quality of back-up and repair services should anything go wrong.

It cannot be overstressed that if the image is not adequate, if the equipment is faulty or a picture quality problem arises that cannot be dealt with immediately, the laparoscopic approach must be abandoned. It is very tempting to struggle on in the presence of substandard imaging because one feels obliged to please the patient. The careful surgeon will never succumb to this and will stop the moment the appearance of the screen does not make perfect anatomical sense in perfect clarity.

Sterility

It goes without saying that all instruments used in surgery must be sterile. However, in the case of laparoscopic surgery, the concern for sterility must be tempered with concern for care of the delicate intrumentation used. For example, it is only the distal end of the laparoscope that is actually introduced into the abdomen, not the eyepiece. In times past the eyepiece was actually in contact with the surgeon's face! It is important that personnel in the endoscopic operating theater understand this. The repeated heat sterilization of laparoscopes and even camera heads will without doubt eventually compromise their function and lead to a deterioration of the image presented to the surgeon. This places patients far more at risk than for example failing to cover the camera head with a sterile plastic hood. The author has never seen a case of intra-abdominal infection following any laparoscopic procedure where the vaginal vault remains unbreached and bowel perforation has not occurred. With this in mind, theater personnel must be encouraged to weigh the continued function of instruments against an unfounded obsession with 'sterility'.

Gaining Access to the Peritoneal Cavity

First Entry

It may be safely said that there is probably more dispute and argument about the safest way into the abdominal cavity than any other single aspect of laparoscopic surgery. Methods of entering the cavity for introducing the laparoscope ('first entry') have been described ranging from the so-called 'open laparoscopy' technique (where the entry site is formally dissected openly until the cavity is reached, which involves at least some degree of larger incision), to the use of self-guarding trocar/cannulae, which purport to shield their points on introduction of the tip into the potential space of the intraperitoneal compartment (but see below). Whether or not pre-insufflation of the cavity with carbon dioxide (CO_2) using a Veress needle before introducing the (usually) 10 mm first entry trocar/cannula reduces the risk of damage to intra-abdominal structures, especially in the presence of adhesions, remains contentious.

The following method, which has been employed without undetected visceral injury in over 3000 laparoscopies in this unit, is as follows:

- The abdomen is not pre-insufflated with a Veress needle, but instead a 'direct entry' approach is used. The abdominal wall is elevated by the surgeon's grasping hand (in order to create a negative pressure within the potential space of the peritoneal cavity), and the 10 mm trocar/cannula is thrust through all layers of the abdominal wall in the midline subumbilically.
- The laparoscope is then immediately introduced and the tissue lying at the end of the cannula inspected. Intraperitoneal fat or bowel serosa is easily recognized, and the surgeon already knows that he is in the correct location, eliminating the risk of inappropriate introduction of gas into the abdominal wall or into any viscus or blood vessel inadvertently breached. If intraperitoneal contents are not evident, then the cannula must be re-sited.
- The abdomen is then insufflated in the usual way. It is important to have the gas tap in the 'open' position when introducing the trocar/cannula so that as soon as the peritoneum is entered, the negative pressure is released, and the bowel falls safely away from the anterior abdominal wall.

With the advent of the 'microlaparoscope' (i.e. 3 mm overall diameter or less, with sheath), in difficult cases (e.g. due to previous surgery or adhesions) it is now possible to enter the peritoneal cavity and then insufflate. Once this is achieved, a second entry point may be selected under direct vision that is known to be definitely free of adherent bowel. The microlaparoscope may then be re-sited, and the first entry site inspected to make certain that adherent bowel has not been damaged in an 'in and out' fashion (i.e. that the first entry has not passed in through one side of the bowel and out through the opposite side, thus going undetected). Any trauma that was caused by the first entry will be of only 3 mm (or less) diameter.

Once the operation is finished using the standard 10 mm laparoscope (i.e. when exiting the abdomen), the cannula is slid up the shaft of the laparoscope, leaving the laparoscope itself 'naked' inside the abdomen. The laparoscope itself is then slowly withdrawn under direct vision at all times. The peritoneum should eventually close over the end of the laparoscope like a pair of curtains, followed by clear views of the layers of the abdominal wall. This maneuver is another safeguard against undetected perforation of bowel adherent to the anterior abdominal wall where the lumen of the bowel has been entered and then exited as the trocar passes completely through one side and out of the other. Gas is allowed to escape via the drain, which we invariably leave in the abdominal cavity (vaginally) after hysterectomy. The alternative method for releasing the gas is to slide the laparoscope and then the cannula back into the cavity (under direct vision), allow the gas to escape, and then exit in the usual way. We have detected two cases of small bowel injury in this fashion out of several thousand laparoscopies and these might well have otherwise gone undetected at the time of operation.

Many traditionalists draw back in horror at the suggestion that a Veress needle is of little value, but let us consider the following. First of all, when the Veress needle is placed through the abdominal wall where the end of the needle lies is a completely unknown factor. Relying on pressure measurements or the 'sucking in' of drops of saline is of no value at all. If the end of the needle lies in the lumen of bowel or even within the lumen of great veins, the pressure at the tip of the needle may well be zero or below. Hence the bowel, or worse, large veins, may be filled with gas if this method is relied upon. The argument that the needle is of sufficiently small diameter that bowel perforation is of no significance may well be true per se, but the question 'what follows?' must be asked. The most dangerous situation and that which most often leads to serious complication is when the bowel is adherent to the anterior abdominal wall or nearby. Even if the abdominal cavity has been filled with gas first the passage and withdrawal of the needle is immediately followed by the passage of the first entry trocar/cannula (usually 10 mm in diameter), which will obviously penetrate the same pathway (or very close to it, which may include the adherent

bowel) as the pathway of the needle itself. Nothing is therefore gained by passing the needle first. Although it is often quoted that the (so-called) 'guarded tip' of the Veress needle self-shields on entering the abdominal cavity and thus perforation of intra-abdominal structures is less likely, this is not true. If the tissues of the abdominal wall present sufficient shear resistance to cause the guard to retract and the point to be exposed, then so will any adherent structures deep to the peritoneum. The tip of the needle will just as easily pass through 'captured' (by adhesions) bowel wall as it will pass through the abdominal wall layers.

Each surgeon must decide which method suits both him or herself and the individual patient. As an aside, it is most certainly not true that the direct entry approach leaves the surgeon open to medicolegal difficulty should complications arise. This technique has now been used by many authorities on very large series of patients.

A number of blunt-ended cannulae are now available on the market, but the reduced risk of accidental perforation of deep tissues must be weighed against the inevitable increased tissue trauma as the blunt instrument is negotiated through the abdominal wall. A number of 'laparoscope-monitored' transparent-ended cannulae are now also available (e.g. 'Visiport', Auto Suture Company, CT, USA), which allow the operator to continuously monitor the progress of the tip as it passes through the layers of the abdominal wall. Entry is effected by a centrally mounted, remotely controlled blade at the distal end of the device. However, although this may sound ideal, the transparent section always becomes contaminated by fat and blood, and visibility is often poor at best. This device requires a considerable amount of experience to master, and it is easy for the unwary to 'lose their way'. This may end in disaster if a major blood vessel is encountered.

Second Entry

Placing other ports in the abdomen is much safer than the first entry because they may be introduced under direct vision. However, there are a number of rules to observe if complications are to be avoided. It is vitally important that the abdomen is fully insufflated (especially in small or thin patients) before any second entry ports are placed. Full distention provides the greatest clearance between the anterior abdominal wall peritoneal surface and both intra-abdominal contents and most especially the posterior wall peritoneum (and the great retroperitoneal blood vessels). It is often surprising just how close the iliac vessels are to the point of entry, particularly when ports are placed very laterally. The use of 'self-guarding' or shielded, trocar/cannulae is no guarantee that accidental laceration of great vessels or bowel will not occur. As the tip of the self-guarding trocar/cannula is introduced, it is essential to follow the progress of the sharp end laparoscopically first as it inwardly distends the peritoneum, then as it perforates the latter, and finally after full entry is gained and the shield engages and covers the sharp section. There is a finite length of time before the guard has a 'chance' to lock forward, when the unguarded tip is exposed inside the abdomen due to 'holding back' of the shield by the peritoneum.

When placing lateral ports, especially, the presence of the inferior epigastric vessels must be borne in mind. The major vessels of the anterior abdominal wall may not be detected solely by transillumination, especially in a patient who is even modestly obese. They are, however, often easily visible by direct inspection of the peritoneum with the laparoscope, and always lie lateral to the landmarks of the obliterated umbilical arteries. Transillumination should also be used to avoid the (sometimes of significant diameter) superficial vessels. Accidental trauma to the inferior epigastric artery in particular may result in a surprisingly brisk loss of blood, which almost always leaks into the abdomen and infiltrates the layers of the abdominal wall, reducing laparoscopic vision effectively to zero. If this occurs, the situation is not irremediable in the hands of an experienced laparoscopist. If the surgeon is still learning the best option may well be to explore the wound immediately using traditional open techniques to avoid significant blood loss. The situation may be rescued after first restoring laparoscopic vision with copious irrigation/suction by using a 'J' shaped peritoneal closure needle (Phipps and Taranissi, 1994a, b) by passing the device through the wound and taking bites of tissue from either side of the primary incision, thereby controlling the bleeding and allowing placement of a hemostatic suture.

The Safe Use of Methods of Tissue Dissection and Hemostasis

Diathermy

The safe use of diathermy in endoscopic surgery is a separate subject in itself and cannot be dealt with in detail here. The advantages and disadvantages of mono- and bipolar diathermy relative to each other and to other methods of dissecting tissues without bleeding are well known. The potential complications and a guide to understanding diathermy electrosurgery appear elsewhere (Phipps, 1994). It is vital that the surgeon has some understanding of the nature of diathermy and the elementary physics that determine how radiofrequency electricity behaves in a biologic environment. Essentially, monopolar diathermy is a highly flexible modality that may be used to great effect during laparoscopic surgery both to cut and effect hemostasis. By manipulating any given laparoscopic instrument so that the area of contact between the instrument and the target tissue varies, a highly efficient cutting or coagulation effect may be obtained, without repeatedly changing instruments or from 'cutting current' to 'coagulation current'. Laparoscopic scissors and hook-type instruments are good examples of this phenomenon.

The disadvantages are that because monopolar diathermy relies on the passage of current through the whole patient, the opportunity for unwanted current flow and undesired tissue heating arises and may lead to serious complications. However, monopolar diathermy is remarkably safe if:

- Good-quality instruments with sound electrical insulation are always used to deliver monopolar diathermy.
- Metal cannulae are never inserted through plastic grip collars into the abdomen (which may cause bizarre and dangerous currents to flow and burns due to capacitative coupling).
- The laparoscope itself is always passed through metal cannulae (to prevent possible energization of the laparoscope with diathermy and consequent burns).

Bipolar diathermy is electrically safer than monopolar diathermy in general terms, and especially with regard to current flow since current is only passing through the target tissue rather than the whole patient. However, the deposition of several hundred joules of energy into a small volume of tissue (which is 95% water) inevitably causes a rise in temperature of several hundred degrees, and the degree of thermal spread and subsequent tissue necrosis may be considerable (Phipps, 1993b). Damage to the ureter when coagulating the uterine artery is a particular theoretical problem, and the surgeon must be aware of the potential dangers. Bipolar instruments to cut tissue, despite the recent design of several ingenious devices, by their very nature must always be inferior to those armed with monopolar diathermy.

In conclusion, diathermy (whichever modality is used) is very safe provided that the surgeon understands its nature and bears in mind that the interface between the instrument and the patient is only one part of an electrical circuit. He or she must make certain that that interface (i.e. where desired heating occurs) is accurately placed and that the rest of the circuit is functioning correctly.

Lasers

The subject of lasers in laparoscopic surgery is now vast. Lasers in general terms, with the exception of dealing with endometriosis, have little advantage over diathermy, in the author's opinion. Safety in laparoscopic surgery concerns those factors pertaining to surgical laser use in general.

Staples

There are now a number of devices on the market capable of delivering multiple rows of titanium staples while simultaneously dividing tissue that has been stapled. There is a considerable debate at the present time as to whether their use is justified in view of their high cost. However, it is the opinion of the author that when used correctly they consistently provide perfect and safe hemostasis without the potential risks and long operation time of 'all diathermy' methods of tissue dissection. Their use in safe laparoscopic hysterectomy provides the surgeon with precise and clean dissection of tissues, including large diameter arteries – the uterine artery – when the surgeon may be assured that hemostasis is reliably secure. Reports of 'imperfect hemostasis' are always due to improper application, as the author has witnessed on many occasions. The off-stated maxim 'you cannot use diathermy in the presence of staples' is wrong. If a minor degree of bleeding does occur along a staple line (though with proper application this should be rare), there is no reason at all why the tissue edge should not be 'touched up' with diathermy. The secret is that when grasping the staple line, it is vital that the tissue as well as the staples themselves are grasped when the diathermy is activated. Delicate gripping of small volumes of tissue is likely to lead to only the staples themselves being grasped. This of course creates a voltage between the staples and the tissue in which they are embedded causing current to flow between the two and instant vaporization of the staple(s).

There are a number of golden rules about the safe use of staples in laparoscopic hysterectomy:

- Do not overload the jaws of the device. There is a temptation to get as much tissue as possible in 'one bite,' but this may well lead to loss of hemostasis.

- Use the correct closure height of staple cartridge. There are two closure heights available for the EndoGIA (Auto Suture Company, CT, USA), blue coded (1.5 mm closure height) and white coded (1.0 mm closure height). It is the opinion of the author that the white cartridge should be applied at every first application for any tissue. If the tissue turns out to be too thick for satisfactory application, then a blue cartridge may be substituted. The tissue gauge devices available (e.g. Endo Gauge, Auto Suture) are not sufficiently accurate to guarantee proper staple application and should not be used. More than 95% of cartridges used in the author's series of more than 1000 laparoscopic hysterectomies have been white coded – the smaller (i.e. tighter and more hemostatic) 1.0 mm closure height.

- Be certain that the gun is correctly placed before 'firing' the device. This goes without saying, but the position of the ureter during laparoscopic hysterectomy is especially vital to determine, since staples form a very watertight seal.

- Always open and close the device under direct vision. Pieces of bowel and omentum will not then be inadvertently torn as the gun is exited through one of the ports because the jaws have trapped a vital structure when being closed after moving from the target area.

Sutures

There is little specific to discuss about sutures in laparoscopic hysterectomy regarding safety other than ensuring their accurate and secure placement. One point is worth mentioning – once the suture is placed, the subsequent (medial) incision should be made as far from the suture as is practicably possible. A common mistake is to place a suture only to divide it inadertently, because tissue 'bunching' means that the thread 'sinks' into the tissue and becomes hidden.

Injury to Bowel

Bowel injury is the worst and potentially the most lethal of all complications encountered with laparoscopic hysterectomy. The surgeon must assiduously ensure that all possible precautions are taken, and especially that any trauma that does occur is diagnosed at the time of operation, since later leakage of bowel content is disastrous. Although in the author's experience it is not necessary to prepare the patient facing laparoscopic hysterectomy with a fluid-only diet in an effort to reduce bowel gas distention to a minimum (some authorities claim that this is essential), taking precautions to keep the bowel 'out of the way' is wise. To this end the patient should be operated upon in a steep Trendelenburg position. The anesthesiologist should avoid any introduction of anesthetic gases into the gastrointestinal tract due to injudicious placement (however transitory) of an endotracheal tube or laryngeal mask. It should be mentioned that just occasionally one gains entrance to the peritoneal cavity only to encounter loop upon loop of gas-filled bowel. The mechanism of this is not clear, but the wise laparoscopic surgeon retreats. The majority of bowel injuries occur at the time of trocar placement, and a strategy to make gaining entry to the abdomen and subsequent operative port placement as safe as possible has already been described. However, in the presence of adhesions the integrity of the bowel wall may become compromised as a result of difficult dissection from other structures, and the surgeon must be vigilant. Should problems with the bowel arise it is recommended that the surgeon should have a very low threshold for reverting to 'open' surgery in order to resolve the difficulty unless the laparoscopist is highly experienced. In the presence of endometriosis particularly, tissue planes can be very difficult to define laparoscopically, and may be absent in the presence of infiltrating disease. With very few exceptions, injury or suspected injury to bowel should be dealt with by open surgery.

In the hands of an expert senior laparoscopic surgeon, repair by laparoscopically placed sutures to inadvertently incised bowel is permissible provided the extent and margins of the incision are clearly defined. Like any other tissue, bowel is highly sensitive to thermal injury, and diathermy (mono- or bipolar) must be applied with great care. It is vital to remember that tissue necrosis after exposure to heat may be delayed by up to 48 hours. The zone of 'whitening' that one sees after application of diathermy does not delimit the zone of necrosis. In other words 'what you see is not what you get'. The limit of tissue destruction is considerably beyond that seen as the blanching of protein denaturation due to mechanisms discussed elsewhere (Phipps, 1994). A sensible maneuver to minimize thermal spread is to copiously irrigate the area immediately after diathermy application, which has the added advantage of maintaining clear vision. The author routinely uses a 1% glycine solution for this purpose. The advantage of this over using conductive solutions such as saline or Hartmann's solution is that diathermy may be delivered 'underwater'. This

is especially useful when dealing with bleeding points on a flat surface where a continuous flow of washing solution is necessary to identify the bleeding area. Very little glycine is left behind after surgery (it is aspirated out), and since (unlike during endometrial resection) the glycine solution is not pressurized, systemic absorption is not problematic.

The tips of diathermy instruments may well remain histotoxically hot for several seconds after use (especially if arcing has occurred). Capacitative coupling and insulation failure have often been quoted as potentially serious problems that may lead to thermal injury of non-target tissue, especially bowel. Although it is important not to overemphasize the potential dangers of these phenomena, it is only good sense to avoid their occurrence. A detailed description of them is available elsewhere (Phipps, 1994), but essentially both mechanisms of unwanted current flow may lead to injury to bowel outside the view of the surgeon. While the active tip of any diathermy instrument is used only under direct vision, leakage of current from other parts of the instrument may occur due to:

- Faulty insulation – this may be eliminated by using either disposable instruments or only those of excellent quality for their defined life span.
- Capacitative current flow from the conductive core of the instrument to the isolated metal tube section of the surrounding cannula – this may be totally avoided by never using plastic abdominal wall grips/collars with metal cannulae.

Devices that constantly monitor current leakage (Electroshield, Boulder, Colorado, USA) are available, and this innovation may go some way to reducing problems related to aberrant current flow.

Injury to the Urinary Tract

The bladder and ureters are easily damaged during laparoscopic hysterectomy unless certain precautions are taken. The ureters are most often compromised as they lie just below the uterine artery, but may also fall victim to an injudiciously placed staple, diathermy forceps or suture much more proximally. The variability of the path of the ureter is quite extraordinary, as anyone who routinely uses transilluminating ureteric stents will attest. It is not uncommon for the ureter to stray into the folds of the peritoneum of the infundibulopelvic ligament so that even simple oophorectomy may cause trouble if the ureter is not constantly monitored. It is the practise of the author to pass transilluminating ureteric stents ('Uriglow', Rocket of London, Watford, UK) (Phipps and Tyrrell, 1991) at the start of every case of laparoscopic hysterectomy. We have had no ureteric injuries in over 1000 cases of laparoscopic hysterectomy and ovarian cystectomy where the uterus has been previously removed. It is important that nonheating atraumatic stents are used. There are a number of copies on the market that are not ideal for this purpose. Indeed, reports are beginning to be seen of ureteric edema and even obstruction after such stenting. Attempting use of such devices without the infra-red filtering coupling device is dangerous, as heating of the ureters may result. Passing the stents too far (i.e. as far as the renal pelvis) is likewise bound to cause trouble, since the delicate renal pelvis may bleed profusely with the gentlest of provocation from the end of a stent.

With stents in, the ureter becomes visible as a row of points of light running parallel to the uterosacral ligaments. Naturally, it is not possible to visualize the ureter as it lies in the ureteric tunnel (where it is most likely to be injured), but this is not important. The correct use of the device is to monitor the movement of the points of light as they lie under the peritoneum proximal to the point at which the uterine artery is being secured (most safely by staples or suture). As the staple gun is slowly closed, the stents are gently agitated back and forth as they leave the external urethral meatus. Loss of movement of the points of light means that the ureter is trapped. Continued movement guarantees that the ureter is safe. The increasing popularity of supracervical hysterectomy may mean that ureteric injuries become less common, but this may not be the case, since the ureter lies very close to the point at which the uterus is separated from the cervix. This point is contentious.

Damage to the bladder is less common. Careful dissection of the bladder from the anterior aspect of the uterus during hysterectomy and clear identification of tissue planes, especially in a patient with a history of previous gynecological surgery is mandatory, and the mucosa should rarely be breached. Diathermy or other thermal energy sources must be used sparingly and with caution. It must be remembered that tissue destruction due to the effects of hyperthermia may only be manifest after 48 hours following the original tissue insult. If a defect is accidentally created, it is not a difficult matter to rectify by means of a laparoscopically delivered suture. If the surgeon is unsure of where the bladder margin lies during dissection, a useful maneuver is to place a cystoscope (preferably a simple small gauge diagnostic one without a stent manipulating bridge, which tends to be more traumatic) connected to a cold light source into the bladder transurethrally and to gently probe the superior margin of the bladder. The light from the cystoscope easily transilluminates the tissues, and the boundaries of the bladder are thereby elucidated. It is essential to check the bladder for integrity at the end of the operation (i.e. at the time of 'second-look' after completion of the vaginal part of the procedure).

It is standard practise to leave a catheter in the bladder for 7–10 days after closure of a defect in the mucosa, but with a small hole that is clearly defined and closed immediately this is probably unnecessary. Provided the defect is small, the margins are clearly defined and closure is assured, our practise is not to leave a catheter longer than 48 hours. The risks of urinary tract infection associated with prolonged catheterization must be weighed in the risk: benefit equation.

Vascular Injuries

(with Mr B.R. Bullen, Consultant Vascular Surgeon)

Two main types of vascular structure are at risk during laparoscopic surgery:

- Those lying in the abdominal wall.
- Those lying retroperitoneally in the pelvic sidewall and posterior abdominal wall.

Injuries are almost always caused by injudicious placement of trocar/cannulae, but occasionally vascular trauma may arise because an instrument is overenthusiastically thrust into the abdomen or someone accidentally pushes an instrument deep into the abdomen because it has been left lying through a cannula. For this reason, instruments must never be left 'dangling' inside the abdomen, and should always be removed from the cannula when not in active use by the surgeon. Diathermy injuries may also be avoided by following this golden rule.

The important difference between the two sites of vessel is that those lying in the retroperitoneum are (or in the event of injury, should be assumed to be) mainly 'anatomically critical'. In other words, if they are traumatized, meticulous repair is required to maintain essential blood supply to other structures rather than simple staunching of hemorrhage by ligation. This must always be in the forefront of the laparoscopist's mind if a vascular complication does occur, since inappropriate action can lead to further and unnecessary problems.

A strategy for avoiding damage to the inferior epigastric vessels and other vessels of the abdominal wall has already been outlined, as has 'first aid' management – control of hemorrhage with a 'J' needle – if it does occur. Injury to the vessels of the great vascular tree demand a completely different approach. Having a workable protocol to deal with major vascular injury is essential. Failure to do so can cost the patient her life, and all surgeons passing trocar/cannulae into the peritoneal cavity must be quite certain of what they are going to do should problems arise. Evidence of severe bleeding may occur at any stage of the laparoscopic operation, and there are certain maneuvers peculiar to each circumstance, which may save life and at the very least severe morbidity. It is vital that all operating theaters undertaking laparoscopic surgery have a set of sterile vascular instruments and that all personnel know their location.

Obvious Hemorrhage Detected at the Time of First Entry into the Abdomen

This occurs because either:

- The trocar/cannula (or Veress needle) has been introduced into the abdomen at an angle too perpendicular to avoid the aorta and vena cava.
- The tip of the trocar has been allowed to 'wander' off the mid-line during penetration of the abdominal wall and the iliac vessels are traumatized (more common).

If removal of the trocar from the cannula (now resting in the abdominal wall) is accompanied by a gush of blood, the cannula must never be removed. There is a great temptation to pull the offending instrument out when severe bleeding occurs, but this can lead to disaster, especially if the end of the cannula has breached the aorta. The cannula should be pushed in slightly and the surgeon must place his thumb over the cannula's open end. This means that hemorrhage is at least to some degree controlled, and equally importantly, the defect in the great vessel is easily identified by the immediately-called vascular surgeon. Removal of the cannula from the defect in a vessel lying retroperitoneally may lead to massive blood loss both intraperitoneally and, worse still, retroperitoneally. Retroperitoneal bleeding rapidly leads to hematoma formation, obscuring the site of the injury, and such hematoma is often difficult to evacuate as it quickly tracks up the retroperitoneal space.

Once the cannula is held in position, a mid-line incision is made as quickly as possible, and the bleeding point identified. Simple compression of the defect should be applied either with a thumb or finger or with a large tightly wrapped pack. Under no circumstances should a non-vascular surgical clamp be applied to vital blood vessels. Again, it is tempting for the gynecologist to stop bleeding in the manner with which he is most familiar (i.e. call for a Spencer–Wells hemostatic clamp). Crushing of great vessels damages the intima and later leads to thrombosis. Crushed vessels often need grafting rather than simple closure of the traumatized section, so it is essential that no further damage is done. A single application of a gynecological instrument to a great vessel may turn a simple repair job for the vascular surgeon into a highly complex procedure.

Severe Hemorrhage Occurring Under All Other Circumstances

With few exceptions, the only other uncommon problem encountered with vascular injury is the placement of the second entry ports. Meticulous care in avoiding the vessels of the abdominal wall and scrutiny of every step of the penetration process with the laparoscope should minimize this type of problem. However, accidents do happen, but when a vascular injury occurs with a laparoscope already in the abdomen the surgeon knows where the injury is. For example, if there is profuse bleeding from the iliac artery because of a port injury, a transverse suprapubic incision is quite sufficient for access to effect a vascular repair.

Anesthetic Problems

A good account of the anesthetic perspective on laparoscopic hysterectomy is given by Miller (1993). In essence, the prolonged CO_2 pneumoperitoneum and the extreme degree of Trendelenburg position are the factors giving rise to most anesthetic anxiety. These may lead to splinting of the diaphragm, difficulty maintaining ventilation and hypercapnia. These points are discussed in full elsewhere and in fact rarely present a significant problem.

The important point is that the anesthesiologist must be aware of the potential problems associated with laparoscopic surgery and their management. When surgeon training is discussed, education of the anesthesiologist who will be dealing with such cases must not be neglected.

Prevention of Problems Associated with Exiting the Peritoneal Cavity

It has become apparent that the laparoscopist cannot rest from his or her efforts in preventing complications of laparoscopic surgery even when the operation is almost over. The simple removal of the cannulae from the abdominal cavity itself must be addressed as a separate and important part of the operation to maintain an operative record as close to free from complication as possible. If port sites of 10 mm or over are not closed throughout the thickness of the abdominal wall, there is a small, but significant risk of hernia of intra-abdominal contents, notably bowel (Kadar *et al.*, 1993). The consequences of trapped and obstructed bowel may be catastrophic for the patient, and it is essential that all ports of 10 mm diameter or over are closed, with the possible exception of the laparoscope port. Hernias through the subumbilical port site are very rare and the mechanism(s) are obscure. It may be that the anatomy of the abdominal wall in the midline is less liable to allow egress of gut or omentum than breaches of the wall away from the mid-line, but this is not known. Closing the umbilical port site without the benefit of direct vision to monitor the process is fraught with risk to bowel, since a suture may inadvertently trap it. Lengthening the umbilical skin incision and formally closing the sheath using conventional techniques seems self-defeating, although this technique is recommended by several authorities. In the opinion of the author, closure of the umbilical site is unnecessary, or at the very least not worth the attendant risks. In thin patients, the inner layers of the abdominal wall may be identified simply by reaching through the skin incision of the port site with dissecting forceps, although this is rarely easy. Routine use of one of the two designs of 'J'-shaped peritoneal closure needle (Phipps and Taranissi, 1994a, 1994b) or some other similar device to close the breaches in the lateral sheath and peritoneum is safe, quick and easy, and is therefore strongly recommended. Once the surgeon is practised, operation time is only increased by a few minutes.

Postoperative Care

Close observation of patients who have undergone major surgery is obviously mandatory in all cases, whether laparoscopic or otherwise. However, it is a wise precaution to emphasize to all paramedical and nursing staff involved that small incisions do not mean small operations, although in a unit specializing in endoscopic surgery they will already be well aware of this.

The early detection of complications in the case of major laparoscopic surgery, like any other operation is essential if severe morbidity and mortality are to be avoided. The laparoscopist should have a very low threshold for re-laparoscoping the patient where hemorrhage is suspected. Preoperative cross-match of at least two units of blood is routine in our unit for all major laparoscopic procedures. It is our practice to leave a 10 mm semi-rigid tube drain through the vault of the vagina in all cases of laparoscopic hysterectomy, and this provides an excellent detection mechanism in case of bleeding after surgery involving transection of large blood vessels. Provided the surgeon is experienced, there is almost never any need to resort directly to laparotomy if primary hemorrhage is suspected, although this may subsequently become necessary if the surgeon is unable to deal satisfactorily with the bleeding laparoscopically.

A point of practise worth mentioning concerns the reintroduction of laterally sited ports, which under these circumstances will be attempted only a few hours after they have previously been removed. The previously placed deep sutures (hernia prevention sutures) are often very difficult to divide, and it is easier not to attempt this in most cases. The same skin incisions may be used to re-enter the abdomen, but the point of the trocar should be guided slightly lateral to the previously closed peritoneum to eliminate the risk of injuring to the inferior epigastric vessels.

In the case of significant bleeding, early diagnosis and investigation means that blood clot inside the abdomen will not have had time to organize and become tenaciously adherent to the pelvis as it does after more than 12 hours, and thus washing out the operative site is much easier. For this purpose a combined high-pressure jet of water (5 mm washer–sucker device) combined with a large-bore aspirator (10 or 12 mm) is essential. Once the clot has been broken up and aspirated, meticulous peritoneal toilet will usually elucidate the cause of bleeding, which may then be dealt with. Final inspection of the whole abdomen before closing again is vital to ensure that no large blood clots are left inside as these may predispose to abscess formation. In cases where significant venous 'ooze' is encountered, we use a technique where the operative site is inspected under zero-pressure pneumoperitoneum (Phipps, 1993a) using a 'C' bar retractor. Positive pressure pneumoperitoneum may mask venous bleeding.

Detection of Injury to the Urinary Tract

Damage to the ureter cannot usually be detected immediately postoperatively unless there is bilateral obstruction. Urine output is normal in the presence of unilateral obstruction. Ureteric obstruction due to an injudiciously placed staple or suture will manifest at 7–10 days, usually as pain and low-grade fever, although fistulation and incontinence are also possible. Light hematuria following laparoscopic surgery is a regular feature if the ureters have been stented, and should not alarm the surgeon or nursing staff. It is transitory, and usually lasts less than a few hours. Gross hematuria may signal bladder injury and is an indication for immediate cystoscopy.

If urinary symptoms arise, the surgeon should have a low threshold for requesting an intravenous urogram (IVU) to make certain that the ureters and bladder are intact. Insensible incontinence is an absolute indication for an IVU as soon as possible in order to differentiate between bladder and ureteric damage. Symptoms suggestive of ureteric obstruction are similarly a signal to perform an IVU. It seems that ureteric obstruction may be the most common urinary tract-related problem after laparoscopic hysterectomy, although comprehensive figures are as yet unavailable. We have recently described a technique for early management and correction of low uncomplicated (i.e. in the absence of urinary leakage) ureteric obstruction following hysterectomy, which may be used to rescue the situation. This maneuver is recommended only for those experienced in urologic procedures (Phipps and Desai, 1994):

- Once a diagnosis is made on the basis of an IVU and cystoscopy, the patient is returned to theater and the help of a urologic surgeon obtained.
- The vault of the vagina is opened, and hemostasis is meticulously achieved.
- Transilluminating ureteric stents are passed first into the normal ureter, then into the obstructed ureter as far as possible (i.e. until the obstruction is reached).
- Inspection of the bladder base using a low powered ENT-type headlight allows the point of the lighted tip of the catheter to meet the obstruction. The offending object causing the obstruction may then be located. If it is a suture, it is not difficult to remove, but if staples are involved, removal can be very tedious.
- Once the obstruction is cleared, a 'pig-tail' ureteric catheter is then left *in situ* for four weeks and subsequently removed under local anesthetic.

Normal anatomy is thus restored without ureteric re-implantation, which may leave the patient with long-term problems such as urinary reflux and stone formation. It must be borne in mind, however, that the constricted part of the ureter after transvaginal 'freeing' may develop a stricture in the long term.

Detection of Injury to Bowel

This has already been dealt with. Bowel injury is not recognizable in the immediate postoperative period. Any suspicion that arises must be dealt with immediately, usually by laparotomy, with the help of a general surgeon.

Conclusions

The laparoscopic approach to hysterectomy offers the patient very considerable advantages over the open surgical approach, although the majority of hysterectomies may be achieved by the unassisted vaginal route. For safe practise, the surgeon must be properly trained and experienced before attempting advanced laparoscopic surgery and patients must be carefully selected for their suitability to undergo such operations. There are a number of specific precautions and maneuvers detailed here that may greatly enhance the safety of laparoscopic hysterectomy and reduce complications to an absolute minimum in the hands of the trained laparoscopic surgeon.

Summary of major complications

1. Poor quality imaging and/or equipment failure.
2. Intra-abdominal injury due to first entry trochar.
3. Intra-abdominal injury during second entry trochar.
4. Bowel injury.
5. Injury to great blood vessels, particularly at trochar entry.
6. Injury to urinary tract, especially the ureters.
7. Inappropriate application of energy sources (diathermy, lasers, high intensity ultrasound).
8. 'Electrical leakage' of diathermy energy leading to burns. It is essential for the surgeon to understand electrosurgery in order to prevent this problem.
9. Inappropriate placement of CO_2 gas.
10. Herniae of bowel/omentum into port sites.

References

Kadar N, Reich H, Lui CY, Manko G, Gimpelson R (1993) Incisional hernias after major laparoscopic gynecologic procedures. *American Journal of Obstetrics and Gynecology* **168**: 1493–1495.

Miller RM (1993) Anaesthetic problems in laparoscopic hysterectomy. In Phipps JH (ed.) *Laparoscopic Hysterectomy and Oophorectomy: A Colour Atlas and Practical Manual.* p. 65. Edinburgh: Churchill–Livingstone.

Phipps JH (1993a) C-bar abdominal wall retractor for laparoscopic surgery without positive pressure pneumoperitoneum. *Gynecological Endoscopy* **2**: 183–184.

Phipps JH (1993b) *Laparoscopic Hysterectomy and Oophorctomy: A Colour Atlas and Practical Manual* Edinburgh: Churchill–Livingstone.

Phipps JH (1994) Diathermy electrosurgery – a working model for gynaecologists and endoscopic surgeons. *Gynecologic Endoscopy* **4**: 159–168.

Phipps JH (1996) Synchronous combined transvaginal/ laparoscopic repair of iatrogenic vesicovaginal fistulae. *Gynaecologic Endoscopy* **5(2)**: 123–124.

Phipps JH, Tyrrell NJ (1991) Transilluminating ureteric stents for preventing operative ureteric injury. *British Journal of Obstetrics and Gynaecology* **99**: 81.

Phipps JH, Desai K (1994) Synchronous combined cystoscopic/vaginal correction of iatrogenic ureteric obstruction following hysterectomy. *British Journal of Obstetrics and Gynaecology* **102(2)**: 168–169.

Phipps JH, Taranissi M (1994a) Laparoscopic peritoneal closure needle for prevention of port herniae and management of abdominal wall vessel injury. *Gynaecologic Endoscopy* **3**: 189–191.

Phipps JH, Taranissi M (1994b) A modified device for full-thickness closure of laparoscopic port incisions. *New Techniques in Gynaecology.*

Phipps JH, John M, Nayak S (1993) Laparoscopically assisted vaginal hysterectomy and bilateral salpingo-oophorectomy versus abdominal hysterectomy and bilateral salpingo-oophorectomy. *British Journal of Obstetrics and Gynaecology* **100**: 698–670.

30

Laparoscopic Assisted Vaginal Hysterectomy

D. ALAN JOHNS

Richland Medical Center, Fort Worth, Texas, USA

Hysterectomy remains one of the most common inpatient surgical procedures performed in the USA. Of these procedures, approximately 70% are performed using the abdominal approach and 30% vaginally (Kovac *et al.*, 1990). Since most hysterectomies are performed for benign disease, the choice of surgical route depends almost entirely upon the surgeon's experience and skill (Dorsey *et al.*, 1995).

Traditional contraindications to vaginal hysterectomy are numerous and varied, most determined more by operator experience than true technical considerations (Isaacs, 1990; Smith and Thompson, 1986; Kovac *et al.*, 1988). Factors often cited as relative or absolute contraindications to the vaginal approach include:

- Previous pelvic surgery.
- Endometriosis.
- Previous cesarean section.
- Significant uterine enlargement.
- Limited uterine mobility.
- Pelvic pain.
- Suspected pathology of the adnexa.
- Ectopic pregnancy.
- Acute or chronic pelvic inflammatory disease.
- Suspected bowel or appendiceal disease.
- Previous uterine suspension.
- Invasive cervical or endometrial carcinoma.

Many of these preoperative diagnoses are based on history, pelvic examination, and ultrasound or computerized tomographic (CT) scans of the pelvis. However, these parameters may be inaccurate when predicting the extent of pelvic pathology (Kovac *et al.*, 1990) and may surreptitiously dictate an abdominal approach.

In their study published in 1990, Kovac *et al.* performed diagnostic laparoscopy in patients scheduled for abdominal hysterectomy. Based on preoperative evaluation, these patients were thought to have contraindications to the vaginal approach. At laparoscopy, however, the majority of these patients did not have pathology precluding vaginal hysterectomy. In this circumstance, the laparoscope provided an accurate assessment of pelvic pathology, and many laparotomies were avoided.

Over the past decade, techniques permitting laparoscopic treatment of extensive pelvic endometriosis, uterine myoma, pelvic adhesive disease, ectopic pregnancy, pelvic abscess, and adnexal disease have been developed. By combining operative laparoscopy with skillful vaginal surgery, most patients with these benign pelvic conditions can avoid laparotomy. The surgeon must, however, attain sufficient skills in both advanced operative endoscopy and vaginal surgery before attempting these potentially difficult cases.

Laparoscopic Approach for Patients with Traditional Contraindications to Vaginal Hysterectomy

Specific techniques for laparoscopic assisted vaginal hysterectomy (LAVH) will be discussed later in this chapter.

Previous Pelvic Surgery

Adhesions are common sequelae to pelvic and abdominal surgery. Iatrogenic adhesions involving the uterus, adnexal structures, or bowel can make vaginal hysterectomy difficult and risky. Although adhesive disease of any clinical significance may or may not exist in any particular patient, the possibility often prevents consideration of a vaginal approach. As shown by Kovac *et al.*, pelvic adhesive disease (when present) is often not as severe as anticipated by the surgeon and is not usually an impediment to simple vaginal hysterectomy. Laparoscopy performed immediately before hysterectomy therefore allows the surgeon to accurately assess pelvic adhesions and plan the appropriate surgical approach.

When significant adhesions are present, the surgeon may either choose an abdominal approach or treat adhesions laparoscopically to the point that vaginal hysterectomy is possible. When tissue is 1–2 cm from the laparoscope, the surgical field is magnified as much as six times, an advantage not enjoyed during laparotomy. This magnification combined with precise microsurgical and dissection techniques gives the surgeon significant advantages in dissecting adhesions involving vital structures. Once adnexal or bowel adhesions are treated, vaginal hysterectomy is more feasible.

Endometriosis

During vaginal hysterectomy, endometriotic nodules may be out of view or technically impossible to remove. Even during abdominal hysterectomy, subtle implants of endometriosis are often missed. As a result, the patient's pain may persist despite hysterectomy and salpingo-oophorectomy.

As mentioned above, laparoscopic inspection of the pelvis, including peritoneal surfaces, ovaries and bowel, is an examination under magnification and endometrial implants are therefore less likely to be missed. When implants are identified, they are destroyed (by electrosurgery or laser) or excised (depending upon depth of penetration) before removal of the uterus or ovaries. Remember, the pain from endometriosis is probably from the implants themselves, not necessarily the uterus or ovaries.

Complete laparoscopic removal of pelvic endometriosis before vaginal hysterectomy is more likely to alleviate the patient's symptoms than simple hysterectomy alone. In addition, adhesive disease, which often accompanies endometriosis can also be treated endoscopically.

Previous Cesarean Section

Patients who have undergone previous cesarean section often have adhesions involving the anterior cul-de-sac, lower uterine segment, and bladder. Some gynecologists believe these adhesions are best approached at laparotomy. The laparoscopic technique for dissection of the bladder from the lower uterine segment is virtually identical to that used at laparotomy. Scissors, blunt dissection and aquadissection all work equally well in freeing the uterus from the bladder in preparation for vaginal hysterectomy. The only difference is the size of the abdominal incision.

Pelvic Pain

Patients with pelvic pain unexplained by preoperative investigation have traditionally been treated by abdominal hysterectomy since the vaginal approach does not allow a thorough evaluation of the pelvic cavity and may leave significant pathology untreated. Additionally, some findings (e.g. endometriosis) might preclude a vaginal approach. Although these points are well taken, they were promulgated before the widespread use of laparoscopy as a diagnostic tool.

When the surgeon performs diagnostic laparoscopy immediately prior to hysterectomy, an accurate etiology for the pain can be identified and treated. The appropriate surgical procedure can then be tailored to those findings.

Suspected Adnexal Pathology (Including Adnexal Mass)

Adenexal masses – most of which are benign and do not require removal – can easily be evaluated laparoscopically. Hysterectomy for an adnexal mass should therefore be well suited to a laparoscopic approach.

Thorough preoperative evaluation and transvaginal ultrasound should help identify those masses most likely to be malignant. These patients are evaluated by laparotomy. The remaining masses, most of which are benign, can be diagnosed laparoscopically, freed, and removed vaginally with the uterus. This can be accomplished without spillage of the ovarian contents into the abdominal cavity. When there is no obvious evidence of malignancy on initial laparoscopic examination, the ovary is freed, decompressed transvaginally and removed for definitive pathologic diagnosis. If malignancy is found, the patient should undergo immediate laparotomy and appropriate surgical therapy. If the mass proves to be benign, laparotomy has been avoided.

Often adnexal pathology (e.g. adhesions, endometriosis) is suspected when none exists

(Kovac *et al.*, 1990). Laparotomy is not indicated simply because the surgeon suspects adnexal pathology. If none exists, the patient is a candidate for simple vaginal hysterectomy. Adnexal adhesions or endometriosis (when encountered) are treated with laparoscopic techniques, followed by vaginal hysterectomy.

Uterine Myoma

Uterine enlargement – most commonly caused by myoma – has been a traditional contraindication to vaginal hysterectomy. The American College of Obstetricians and Gynecologists (1994) suggests that a 12-week-size (or larger) uterus may require an abdominal approach for removal. Several authors, however, dispute this size limit (Kovac and Stovall, 1986). Using morcellation and coring techniques, Kovac and Stovall commonly remove 20-week-size uteri vaginally.

Patients with large – over 14-week-size – uteri present the laparoscopist with unique problems. The uterine size may prevent laparoscopic access to the uterine vessels or cul-de-sac. In these circumstances, the only advantage offered by laparoscopy lies in controlling the infundibulopelvic vessels before transvaginal morcellation of the uterus. This may decrease blood loss while the uterus and myoma are being fragmented. If the uterine arteries are accessible, laparoscopic control of these vessels will definitely decrease blood loss during the remainder of the procedure.

In order to remove these large uteri vaginally, the surgeon must possess considerable skill and experience in vaginal surgery. Laparoscopy may offer some advantages, but the majority of this procedure is performed vaginally.

Ectopic Pregnancy

Occasionally, a patient presents with an ectopic pregnancy and other gynecologic pathology best treated by hysterectomy. As long as she is hematologically stable, the ectopic pregnancy can be treated by laparoscopic salpingectomy and the hysterectomy completed vaginally. This combination of techniques avoids laparotomy while treating all pelvic pathology in a single operation.

Acute or Chronic Pelvic Inflammatory Disease

Pelvic inflammatory disease with associated adhesions or abscess may be treated laparoscopically. These techniques are discussed elsewhere in Chapter 24. If hysterectomy, salpingo-oophorectomy, or both are clinically indicated in the presence of pelvic inflammatory disease or abscess, these conditions are treated laparoscopically to the point where vaginal hysterectomy is possible. Neither adhesive disease from chronic pelvic inflammatory disease nor abscess from acute pelvic inflammatory disease are absolute contraindications to the combination of laparoscopic and vaginal procedures.

Minimal Uterine Mobility and Limited Vaginal Access

One of the most common indications for abdominal hysterectomy is 'minimal uterine mobility', the definition of which is extremely vague. Since there is no reproducible method for measuring uterine mobility, this is strictly a subjective assessment by the operating physician. The same applies when considering 'limited vaginal access'. In these patients, laparoscopic techniques are employed until there is sufficient 'descensus' or 'access' to allow vaginal completion of the operation.

In rare patients, there is not sufficient descensus of the cervix to even begin a vaginal hysterectomy. Similarly, there may not be sufficient room in the vagina to place a tenaculum on the cervix, regardless of descensus. In these patients, the only alternative to abdominal hysterectomy is total laparoscopic hysterectomy (complete removal of the uterus by laparoscopic techniques). The freed uterus is morcellated and removed through an abdominal port. The vaginal cuff is closed laparoscopically.

Most often, laparoscopic techniques are used to free adnexal and uterine support structures to the point that the operation can be completed vaginally. This rarely requires freeing the uterus below the uterine artery.

Technique of LAVH

After introduction of the 10 mm diagnostic laparoscope through an intraumbilical incision, two 5 mm suprapubic incisions are made approximately 4–5 cm on either side of the midline. These secondary ports are placed medial or lateral to the inferior epigastric artery, depending upon uterine size and other pelvic pathology. Placement lateral to the epigastric vessels allows better access to the pelvic sidewalls, but makes the cul-de-sac less accessible. Placement medial to the epigastric vessels provides the best angle to access the cul-de-sac, but makes dissection of pelvic sidewall structures and vessels more difficult, particularly when a large uterus is present.

The entire abdominal cavity is thoroughly inspected and all pathology documented and evaluated. The anterior and posterior cul-de-sac and pelvic sidewall surfaces must be examined very carefully. Subtle implants of endometriosis can be easily overlooked during a cursory inspection.

While placing the uterine manipulator, the surgeon assesses both the 'mobility' of the uterus and the intravaginal 'area' through which the uterus must be removed. This information, coupled with knowledge of pelvic pathology identified at laparoscopy determines how much of the hysterectomy must be completed laparoscopically (Figure 30.1). Remember, the object of LAVH is to perform a vaginal hysterectomy with as little laparoscopic work as is necessary. As more of the procedure is performed laparoscopically, both cost and operative time increase.

If the adnexa are to be removed, the retroperitoneal approach offers the best protection for the ureter and the least risk of leaving an ovarian remnant. This begins by entering the retroperitoneal space between the round ligament and the infundibulopelvic ligament. Apply medial traction to the ovary and tube, stretching the peritoneum lateral to the broad ligament. The retroperitoneal space can then be easily entered with scissors or electrosurgery. The peritoneum is opened cephalad to the infundibulopelvic ligament and caudad to the round ligament. Using a blunt dissection probe and aquadissection, the peritoneum is dissected medially between these structures. This should allow the ureter to be easily identified. If the ovary is adherent to the pelvic sidewall, it is taken along with the peritoneum, lessening the chances of leaving an ovarian remnant. Endometrial implants on the pelvic sidewall are also removed with the peritoneum.

The key to safe and thorough desiccation (coaptation) of the ovarian artery and vein lies in opening the peritoneum overlying these structures, dissecting the vessels, and removing as much surrounding retroperitoneal fat and connective tissue as possible. Electrosurgical desiccation and coaptation of these vessels then becomes very safe and effective. If possible, a non-electrolyte solution should be passed through the bipolar forceps during the desiccation process. This will cool the tissue, limit lateral thermal injury and minimize tissue adherence to the metal bipolar electrodes. Endoscopic sutures can also be used to ligate the skeletonized vessels. Metal clips and staples are also available for this purpose, but are rarely (if ever) necessary and add significant cost to the procedure.

The posterior leaf of the broad ligament is opened (parallel to the ureter) to the level of the uterine artery (Figure 30.2). The round ligament is electrosurgically desiccated then transected. Careful blunt aquadissection is used to dissect and identify the uterine artery as it crosses over the ureter.

If the pelvic examination under anesthesia or pelvic pathology indicates that the uterine artery cannot be controlled transvaginally it should be ligated just lateral to the point where it crosses the ureter. Attempts to control this vessel further medially (after it crosses the ureter) can be more difficult because it divides into several branches as it nears

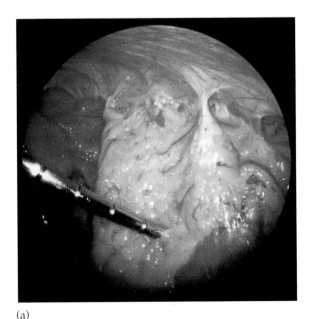

(a)

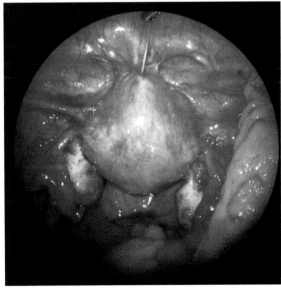

(b)

Figure 30.1 (a) Preoperative view of the pelvis. (b) The same patient after adhesiolysis (LAVH Stage 1).

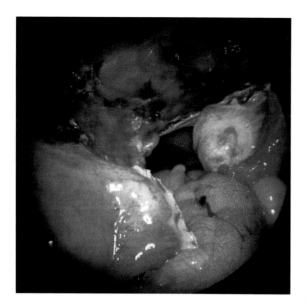

Figure 30.2 Uterine artery dissected and identified.

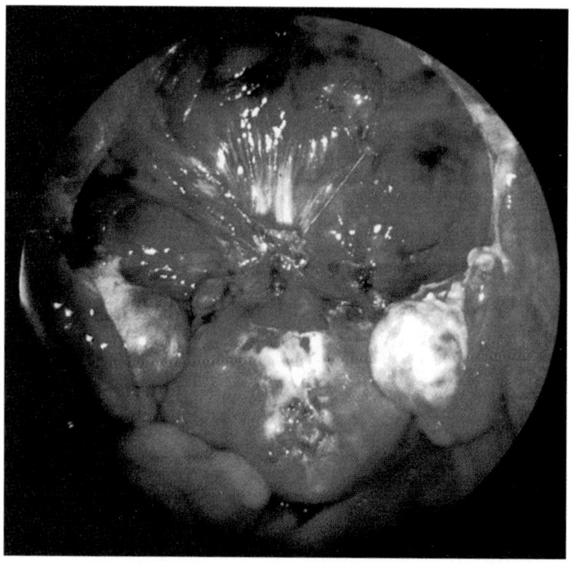

Figure 30.3 Bladder peritoneum entered and the bladder has been dissected from the lower uterine segment (LAVH Stage 3).

the uterus. If the uterine artery is difficult to identify, follow the umbilical ligament from the abdominal wall through the retroperitoneal space to the level of the ureter. The uterine artery lies in this anatomic area. Dissect the vessel from the surrounding tissue and ligate it with suture and a knot pusher. Because of the close proximity of the ureter, it is safer to dissect and ligate the uterine artery than use electrosurgery or staples.

Next, the bladder is dissected from the lower uterine segment. This can be accomplished vaginally, but may be associated with less risk of bladder injury when done laparoscopically under direct vision. Using the uterine manipulator, the uterus is pushed cephalad, thereby stretching the peritoneum overlying the bladder and lower uterine segment. The peritoneum overlying this area is elevated upward with grasping forceps and the junction of the bladder and lower uterine segment identified. The peritoneum is opened with scissors or monopolar electrosurgery. While maintaining cephalad pressure on the uterus, the bladder is dissected from the lower uterine segment with blunt aquadissection. Completion of this step simplifies entry into the anterior cul-de-sac during the vaginal portion of the operation (Figure 30.3).

If the posterior cul-de-sac is obliterated, the rectum should be carefully dissected from the posterior uterus, uterosacral ligaments and rectovaginal septum. Since endometriosis is the most common etiology for this problem, endometriotic nodules should be identified and removed. Since this dissection always involves the rectum, it should never be undertaken unless the patient has had a preopera-

tive bowel preparation. Although some surgeons perform this dissection with electrosurgery, most prefer the carbon dioxide (CO_2) laser. Because this procedure is technically difficult and fraught with potential complications, it should be undertaken only by the most experienced laparoscopic surgeons.

At this point, the vast majority of cases can be completed vaginally. The patient should be repositioned as she would be for vaginal hysterectomy. With experience, the operating room personnel should be able to accomplish this in less than ten minutes. Repositioning is critical to facilitate the remaining vaginal portion of the procedure.

In rare circumstances, none of the operation can be performed vaginally, requiring the uterus to be completely freed and removed laparoscopically (total laparoscopic hysterectomy) as first reported by Reich *et al.* in 1989. It should be kept in mind, however, that total laparoscopic hysterectomy requires the highest level of technical skill and is associated with prolonged operative times. It should only be undertaken in those patients in whom no part of the hysterectomy can be completed vaginally.

The anterior cul-de-sac is entered first. The vaginal wall is identified after the bladder has been dissected from the lower uterine segment and cervix. It is entered with unipolar electrosurgery or laser. Scissors can also be used, but may result in more arterial bleeding from vessels in the vagina. After the rectal wall has been positively identified, the posterior cul-de-sac is entered, again with electrosurgery or laser. During this portion of the procedure, pneumoperitoneum is maintained by placement of a moistened sponge or inflated Foley catheter bulb in the vagina.

The uterosacral ligaments are carefully identified, desiccated and transected above the rectum and medial to the ureters. The remaining attachments of the cervix to the apex of the vagina are cut with unipolar electrosurgery.

Now completely freed, the uterus is removed through the vaginal cuff or morcellated and removed through a larger suprapubic port. The vaginal cuff is then closed laparoscopically.

Once the procedure is completed, the abdomen is reinflated and the operative field closely inspected. This usually requires repositioning of the patient's legs. The entire abdominal cavity is thoroughly cleansed, removing all blood, clots and debris (Figure 30.4). Bleeding sites are identified and controlled. Approximately 1000 ml of isotonic irrigating fluid is left in the abdomen. Trocar wounds are then closed, including fascial closure in all sites greater than 5 mm in diameter.

LAVH without Salpingo-oophorectomy

A slightly different approach is necessary if the adnexa are to be preserved. As large veins are often found within the broad ligament, great care is required while freeing the ovary and tube from the uterus.

The round ligament is grasped at the point it attaches to the uterus and pulled medially. It is desiccated and transected 2–3 cm lateral to this location. The fallopian tube is desiccated and transected at a similar point. This leaves the remaining broad ligament and utero-ovarian ligament still intact.

Through the incision in the anterior leaf of the broad ligament – at the transected end of the round ligament – the posterior leaf of the broad ligament is identified by careful blunt dissection. During this dissection, care must be taken to avoid injury to the large veins in this area. If the walls of these vessels are inadvertently breached, very brisk bleeding ensues and can be very difficult to control.

Once identified, the posterior leaf of the broad ligament is opened medial to the ureter, near the utero-ovarian ligament. The remaining broad and utero-ovarian ligaments can then be controlled by passing a suture through the window in the medial leaf of the broad ligament and around the 'pedicle', securing it with a laparoscopic knot pusher. The attachments to the uterus are then cut and a second suture secured around the pedicle. Similarly, these attachments can be controlled by electrosurgical desiccation. If this energy source is used on the broad ligament, however, the surgeon must be prepared to handle bleeding from these veins if the coaptation process fails. Stapling devices can also be used for this procedure, but they are very expensive and require 12 mm ports.

Once the adnexa are freed from the uterus (Figure 30.5), the remainder of the procedure proceeds as previously described.

Postoperative Care

The majority of patients will be able to void spontaneously within 6–8 hours, therefore an indwelling

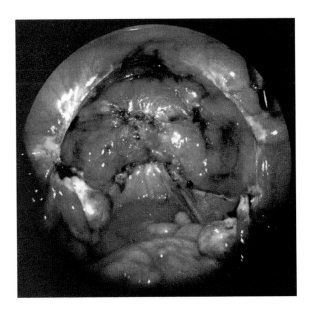

Figure 30.4 Postoperative view of the pelvis.

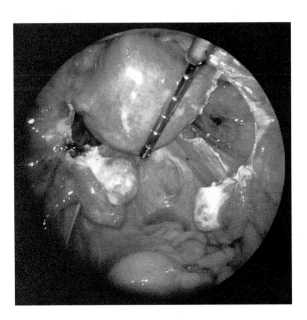

Figure 30.5 Both adnexa have been freed (LAVH Stage 2).

catheter is unnecessary. Intermittent 'in-and-out' catheterization is used until spontaneous voiding occurs.

Isotonic fluid left in the abdomen will prevent dehydration, so intravenous fluids are unnecessary beyond the first few postoperative hours. Pain is controlled with intramuscular or intravenous analgesics until postoperative nausea resolves (usually within 8–10 hours). The patient is then begun on oral fluids and oral analgesics.

Since there is little intraoperative bowel manipulation, postoperative ileus is extremely uncommon. Patients are begun on an unrestricted diet as soon as they desire. By 24 hours postoperatively, patients are voiding spontaneously, have no intravenous line, are on a general diet and taking oral analgesics. Most are dismissed 24–36 hours after their procedure.

In an attempt to standardize terminology with reference to LAVH, a staging system for LAVH has been devised and published (Table 30.1). Using this system, surgeons can easily categorize the extent of laparoscopic surgery performed in any particular patient. Operative parameters (e.g. operative time, costs, complication rates, blood loss) can then be more accurately compared between surgeons and patients.

Conclusions

For the appropriately selected patient, combining the techniques of operative laparoscopy with those

Table 30.1 Laparoscopically assisted vaginal hysterectomy (LAVH) staging (Johns and Diamond, 1992).

Stage 0	Laparoscopy done – no laparoscopic procedure performed before vaginal hysterectomy
Stage 1	Procedure included laparoscopic adhesiolysis and/or excision of endometriosis (see Figure 30.1)
Stage 2	Either or both adnexa freed laparoscopically (see Figure 30.5)
Stage 3	Bladder dissected from uterus (see Figure 30.3)
Stage 4	Uterine artery transected laparoscopically
Stage 5	Anterior and/or posterior colpotomy or entire uterus freed
Subscript 0	Neither ovary excised
Subscript 1	One ovary excised
Subscript 2	Both ovaries excised

Note: If the extent of the procedure performed laparoscopically varies on the right and left pelvic sidewalls, stage the procedure by the most advanced side.

of vaginal surgery benefits the patient, hospital and health care system. The potential benefits include the following:

- Those patients who would otherwise be committed to abdominal procedures enjoy less postoperative pain and a shorter recovery.
- The decision for laparotomy or vaginal surgery can be made based on accurate knowledge of the pathology to be addressed, not guesswork.
- When the patients are properly selected (those in whom simple vaginal hysterectomy is not reasonable) and reusable laparoscopic equipment and electrosurgery are used, LAVH can be performed at a cost equal to or less than that of abdominal hysterectomy (Johns et al., 1995). These savings benefit everyone.
- Those patients with pain from endometriosis benefit from a more complete excision and destruction of the implants than would be possible during vaginal hysterectomy.
- Since the bladder is dissected from the lower uterine segment with the laparoscope under direct vision, the incidence of bladder perforation may be lower.
- Since the cul-de-sac has been inspected laparoscopically, the risk of rectal injury during vaginal colpotomy should be decreased. Cul-de-sac adhesions or obliteration are identified and treated before the colpotomy is performed.
- Laparoscopic inspection of the operative field at the conclusion of the procedure permits identification and control of any bleeding areas before the patient reaches the recovery room. This bleeding may go undiscovered during vaginal hysterectomy. Thorough irrigation of the operative field may also decrease the risk of postoperative infection.
- In some studies, when compared to abdominal hysterectomy, vaginal hysterectomy and LAVH are both associated with a 48-hour shorter hospital stay and significant savings in hospital costs (Johns et al., 1995).
- From morbidity and mortality studies, both LAVH and vaginal hysterectomy are associated with fewer complications than abdominal hysterectomy (Bolsen, 1982; Johns et al., 1995).

It must be remembered, however, that LAVH is associated with one unique group of complications, which never occur during either abdominal or vaginal hysterectomy – trocar injuries. A trocar injury to an iliac vessel or large bowel quickly negates any potential benefit of LAVH. This single complication, unique to laparoscopy, mandates that we select only those patients with unquestioned contraindications to vaginal hysterectomy for LAVH. Placement of a trocar into a patient who could undergo simple vaginal hysterectomy simply adds risk and cost, and provides no proven offsetting benefit.

As we move into the next century, our goal should be to perform the vast majority of hysterectomies for benign disease via the vaginal route, using laparoscopic assistance when necessary. The abdominal approach should be used for only a very small proportion of patients requiring hysterectomy. As our skills and experience in operative laparoscopy and vaginal surgery increase, this should be achievable.

References

American College of Obstetricians and Gynecologists (1994) *Uterine Leiomyomata*. Technical bulletin no. 192.

Bolsen B (1982) Study suggests vaginal hysterectomy is safer. *Journal of the American Medical Association* **247**: 13.

Dorsey JH, Steinberg EP, Holfz PM (1995) Clinical indications for hysterectomy route: Patient characteristics or physician preference? *American Journal of Obstetrics and Gynecology* **173(5)**: 1452–1460.

Isaacs JH (1990) *Gynecology and Obstetrics. Clinical Gynecology*, vol. 1. Ch. 50, pp. 1–11. Philadelphia: JB Lippincott Company.

Johns DA, Diamond M (1992) Laparoscopically assisted vaginal hysterectomy (LAVH) staging. *Journal of Reproductive Medicine* **39(6)**: 424–428.

Johns DA, Carrera B, Jones J (1995). The medical and economic impact of laparoscopically assisted vaginal hysterectomy in a large, metropolitan, not-for-profit hospital. *American Journal of Obstetrics and Gynecology* **172(6)**: 1709–1715.

Kovac SR and Stovall (1986). Intramyometrial coring as an adjunct to vaginal hysterectomy. *Obstetrics and Gynecology* **67(1)**: 131 136.

Kovac SR, Cruikshank SH, Retto HF (1990) Laparoscopy-assisted vaginal hysterectomy. *Journal of Gynecologic Surgery* **6**: 185.

Kovac SR, Pignotti BJ, Binduetel GA (1988). Hysterectomy: a comparative statistical study of abdominal v. vaginal approaches. *Missouri Medicine* **85**: 312–316.

Reich H and Decapno J (1989). Laparoscopic hysterectomy. *Journal of Gynecologic Surgery* **5**: 213–216.

Smith HO, Thompson JD (1986) Indications and technique for vaginal hysterectomy. *Contemporary Obstetrics and Gynecology* **10**: 125.

31

Laparoscopic Supracervical Hysterectomy

THOMAS L. LYONS

Center for Women's Care and Reproductive Surgery, Atlanta, Georgia, USA

Currently hysterectomy is the third most frequently performed procedure in the USA with approximately 650 000 performed in 1993. Adequate data have been accumulated to demonstrate the efficacy of a minimally invasive approach to this procedure (Maher *et al.*, 1992; Levy *et al.*, 1994; Ou *et al.*, 1994). However, the acknowledged penetration of laparoscopic hysterectomy is only 10+% and the apparent lack of conversion – total abdominal hysterectomy (TAH) to laparoscopic assisted vaginal hysterectomy (LAVH) – leaves some proponents of this minimally invasive procedure to consider what is necessary to accomplish the desired goal (Ou *et al.*, 1994). The goal of this conversion is to reduce the acknowledged higher morbidity of abdominal hysterectomy (TAH) to at least that of vaginal hysterectomy (VH) or perhaps lower if the procedure will allow.

Various minimally invasive technique alternatives have been offered to accomplish this goal including the laparoscopic assisted Doderlein hysterectomy (LADH) (Garry, 1994), the classic intrafascial Semm hysterectomy (CISH) of Kurt Semm (Semm, 1991), and the laparoscopic supracervical hysterectomy (LSH) offered first by Thomas Lyons in 1990 (Lyons, 1993). Each of these procedures has some strengths and weaknesses, but all seem to provide the practitioner with viable alternatives and the opportunity to convert more hysterectomies to less invasive, lower morbidity procedures.

It is this author's contention with the data presented that LSH is the most versatile and simple of these alternatives, can accommodate large myomas or the significant scarring of pelvic inflammatory disease or endometriosis and still leaves the patient with the lowest overall morbidity (Lyons, 1993). The following discussion presents a more detailed rationale and technique for performing this procedure and a series of 236 patients who underwent LSH during the initial experience in this author's clinic.

Indications

Although not every hysterectomy patient is a candidate for laparoscopic supracervical hysterectomy, the clinical presentations which are accommodated by this procedure encompass a wide range of patients. Indications for hysterectomy via this laparoscopic approach are as follows:

- Dysfunctional bleeding – but, patients who are candidates for endometrial ablation should be excluded.
- Pelvic or abdominal pain.
- Adnexal masses with indications for hysterectomy.
- Uterine leiomyomas with indications for hysterectomy – patients may not need preoperative suppressive therapy despite large uterine size, although potentiation of red cell count may be indicated for severe anemia.
- Endometriosis requiring definitive surgery – these patients may have extensive cervical disease necessitating removal of the cervix during the procedure.

- Known or suspected adhesive disease or pelvic inflammatory disease.
- Indicated appendectomy with indications for hysterectomy.
- The difficult vaginal hysterectomy requiring removal of the adnexa (i.e. in a nulligravida or if there are vaginal or anatomic abnormalities).
- Tubo-ovarian abscess.

Patients who have endometrial cancer or invasive cervical cancer or other absolute indications for removal of the cervix should be excluded from this procedure. Cervical intraepithelial neoplasia (CIN) I or II does not exclude the patient from consideration and the transformation zone can be excised at the time of surgery.

Description of Procedure

Patient Preparation

Consent is given for total hysterectomy and laparotomy in addition to LAVH and LSH. The attendant risks and benefits of leaving the cervix *in situ* are discussed with the patient during the consent interview. All attendant laparoscopic technologies are prepared for this procedure including Contact neodymium:yttrium-aluminum-garnet (Nd:YAG) laser system (Surgical Laser Technologies, PA, USA), ultrasonically activated scalpel (very useful for large myomas), bipolar forceps, endoloops, ligatures and ligaclips. The procedure can be performed using any method of large vessel occlusion and any cutting device, but sound surgical principles of traction and counter-traction facilitated by appropriate trocar placement and continuous monitoring of anatomic landmarks is essential. The patient is positioned in the modified dorsal lithotomy position in Allen stirrups (Allen Medical, Inc., Boston, MA, USA) as shown in Figure 31.1. A uterine manipulator is placed. The Pelosi or Valchev (Apple Medical Corp., Trenton, NJ, USA) uterine manipulator has been found to be most suited to this procedure by this author.

The open laparoscopy technique is used as it aids in speedy removal of the specimen at the end of the case. The Hassan cannula or a disposable open trocar (Ethicon Endo Surgery, Inc., Cincinnati, OH, USA) may be used. Secondary trocars of 5 mm are placed bilaterally, well lateral to the rectus muscles and avoiding the epigastric vasculature, and a third secondary trocar at 3–4 fingerbreadths above the symphysis pubis is placed in the midline of 10–11 mm in diameter (Figure 31.2). Curved needle suturing may be performed using this lower midline trocar as well as passage of endoclips or endoscopic stapling devices. Also, the laparoscope may be placed through this trocar to address upper abdominal adhesive disease or other epigastric or mild abdominal pathology problems. If a large uterus is encountered, trocars must be placed at higher levels in the abdomen in order to create exposure of the vascular pedicles and the ureters. Placement of the open 'Hasson' trocar at the umbilicus first, even in the presence of large masses, facilitates final trocar placement, even if upper abdominal trocars are necessary.

Figure 31.1 Operating theater set-up for laparoscopic hysterectomy.

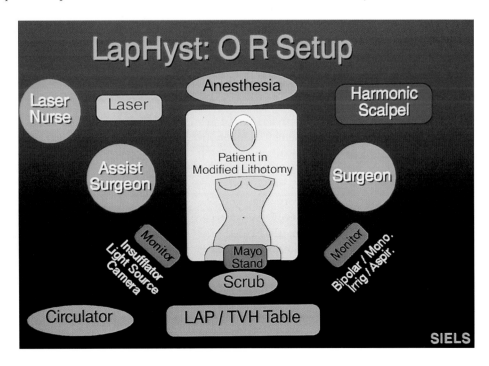

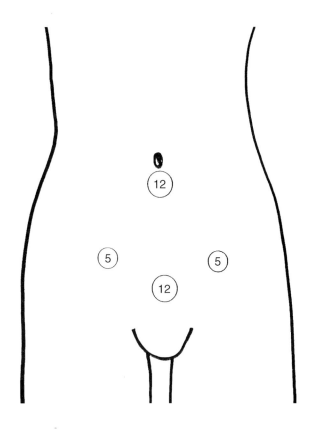

Figure 31.2 Trocar placement for LSH.

Exploratory laparoscopy is performed, pathology is identified and adhesiolysis is accomplished as necessary at the onset of the case. After careful identification of the ureters at the pelvic brim, the infundibulopelvic ligaments are desiccated with bipolar cautery, divided with the Nd:YAG laser scalpel or scissors and can be ligated using Endoloop (Ethicon Endo Surgery Inc.) of 0 polydioxanone. Back-bleeding from the specimen side is carefully controlled with bipolar cautery. This important step is performed before division of any pedicles by desiccating the specimen side of the round ligament, tube, and utero-ovarian pedicles. If any pedicles can not be freed, careful lateral sidewall dissection and ureterolysis is first performed, then ligatures are passed and extracorporeal knotting techniques may be used to ligate these vascular pedicles. The round ligament is desiccated and divided in similar fashion. The uterovesical fold is dissected using the Nd:YAG laser scalpel, harmonic scalpel or scissors, and blunt and sharp dissection of the bladder flap are carefully accomplished. An endoscopic kittner/ pledget (Ethicon Endo Surgery) may be employed in this blunt dissection as this is atraumatic and may decrease the tendency for

bladder injury. It is imperative that this portion of the procedure is carefully carried out because this opens the uterine vessel fossa for dissection of the uterine vasculature. It is of further importance to note that aquadissection in this area may be a difficult or impossible technique to use due to dense adherence of the bladder flap in cases of previous cesarean section. Also, the distortion of the anatomy, which is incumbent with aquadissection, can make identification of vital structures (i.e. the uterine arteries and the ureter) very difficult. Division and dissection/ligation of these structures may therefore be more difficult if aquadissection is used extensively. The laparoscopic coagulating shears (LCS) (Ultracision Inc., Providence, RI, USA) device can be used to coagulate and divide the larger vascular pedicles of the infundibulopelvic (IP) and utero-ovarian ligament if the operator desires. The posterior leaf of the broad ligament is dissected carefully allowing the ureter to splay laterally. This posterior leaf dissection allows the surgeon, along with good countertraction on the uterine fundus from the contralateral port to maximize the distance from the ureter to the uterine vessels at their insertion into the uterus (Figure 31.3).

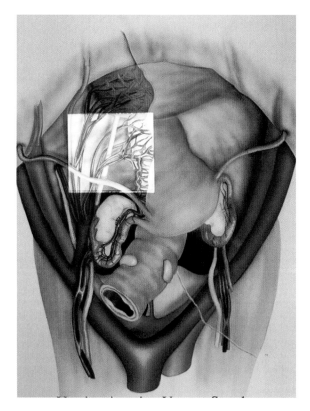

Figure 31.3 Anatomic diagram representing the relationship of the uterine vasculature and the ureter, and the effects of countertraction on these structures.

After the uterine arteries have been dissected carefully and the ureter is identified well away from these structures, the uterine arteries are desiccated with the bipolar forceps and divided. Occasionally, suture ligatures or ligaclips may be placed if a pedicle can be developed in this area. However, high ligation of the uterine artery is usually unnecessary unless this area of anatomy has become obscured due to endometriosis or previous surgery. Once these vascular structures have been occluded, the uterus will become cyanotic, denoting that the vascular supply has been eliminated. At this time, the Nd:YAG laser scalpel is used to divide the uterine artery and veins, and to cut down on the uterine manipulator, which was placed preoperatively into the cervix. This procedure can also be performed with a monopolar spoon or needle electrode using high power density cutting current or the harmonic scalpel. The surgeon should note that this division of the cervix is at or below the endocervical os. The remainder of the dissection is then performed in a coring manner with removal of the upper end of the cervical canal. The uterine manipulator can facilitate this amputation.

After removal of the uterus, the cuff is inspected and any areas of bleeding are coagulated using the bipolar cautery. The anterior and posterior folds of the peritoneum and the anterior pubocervical fascia and posterior cervix are plicated together using an interrupted mattress suture of polyglactin 910 or using the EMS endoscopic stapler (Ethicon Endo Surgery Inc.).

Before peritoneal closure the endocervical canal should be ablated using the Nd:YAG laser, bipolar cautery or a monopolar ball electrode to decrease postoperative leukorrhea and reduce the risk of dysplasia. At this point, the abdomen is lavaged and inspected for signs of bleeding while decreasing intra-abdominal pressure to less than 8 mm Hg. Any areas of bleeding are carefully attended to using the bipolar forceps or the Nd:YAG hemostasis tip. The uterus is then bifurcated or morcellated using sharp dissection with the ultrasonically activated scalpel or large scissors. Removal is accomplished through the subumbilical open laparoscopy port (Figure 31.4). This port is chosen as it can be easily extended to accommodate a larger uterine corpus. During this process, the scope is moved to the lower 10 to 11 trocar for direct visualization of removal of the uterus and/or other pathologic specimens. Appendectomy or other procedures may be performed as necessary at this time. A modified McCall's posterior culdoplasty may be accomplished by plicating the uterosacral ligaments that remain intact and the posterior fascia using an O-Ethibond (Ethicon Inc., Somerville, NS, USA) purse

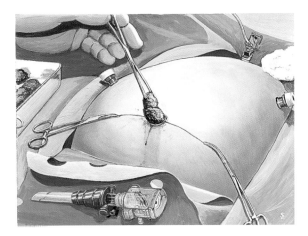

Figure 31.4 Removal of the specimen through the subumbilical site. The open trocar has been removed and the tissue is extracted via a small extension of this site.

string suture and an extracorpeal knotting technique. The patient is then allowed to recover with the catheter in place and is observed for approximately 18 hours postoperatively before discharge.

Patients are allowed to return to normal activity at home within 2–3 days and are able to return to work within 7–10 days with normal activity. There is no evidence of significant vaginal discharge postoperatively and intercourse may be resumed at two weeks.

Results

In our clinic a total of 236 LSH procedures have been performed over a four year period from February 1990 to February 1994. Results of these patients are shown in Table 31.1. A learning curve was demonstrated for cases 1–50, which resulted in steadily decreasing operative times; however, this is the only variable that changed during this time period. Complications were no more frequent in year one versus year four. Also, the learning curve may not have been as dramatic because LAVH or technically laparoscopic hysterectomy (LH) had been performed in 25 cases before initiating LSH. It should be noted that at no time did procedures extend beyond four hours (average time now 85 minutes) and no injury occurred to bowel, bladder, ureter or major vasculature. Febrile morbidity was less than 1%, no transfusions were required (average blood loss 55 ml) and only three patients needed hospital re-admission. One patient underwent trachelectomy

Table 31.1 Clinical outcome results of the initial series of LSH procedures (n=236). (DUB, dysfunctional uterine bleeding; PID, pelvic inflammatory disease).

(n=236)		
Age	43.4 years (27–86)	
Parity	2.1 (0–9)	
Weight	68.7 kg (41–77)	

	Preoperative	*Postoperative*
Diagnosis (Average uterine weight 178 g)	DUB 69%	Leiomyomata uteri 69%
	Myomas 53%	Adenomyosis 68%
	Pain 53%	Endometriosis 36%
	Pelvic relaxation 45%	Pelvic inflammation 21%
	Endometriosis 23%	Ovarian adenocarcinoma <1%
	PID 11%	Normal pathology 31%
	Ovarian cancer <1%	
Associated procedures	Unilateral or bilateral salpingoophorectomy	117
	McCalls/modified Moschowitz	216
	Burch colposuspension	54
	Appendectomy	65
	Adhesiolysis	205
	Sacral culpopexy	2
	High rectocele repair	12
Estimated blood loss	55 ml (25–125)	
Operating time	85 min (59–235)	
Hospital stay	17 h (3–38)	
Readmission	2 (both with signs of bowel obstruction at 7–10 days postoperatively – spontaneous resolution with hydration)	
Conversion to open	0	
Recurrent bleeding	1 (ceased with treatment of canal with HgNO$_3$)	
Acute complications of surgery	Infection	4 trocar site infections requiring drainage 2 urinary tract infections
	Bleeding	0 (no transfusions were required)
	Bowel injury	0
	Urinary tract injury	0
	Subcutaneous emphysema	1 (mild)
Reoperations to remove cervix	3 (1 because endometrial cancer was diagnosed on pathologic examination at the time of surgery; 2 for subsequent reconstruction)	

and node dissection two weeks postoperatively due to the presence of a microscopic focus of endometrial carcinoma found on pathology examination following a hysterectomy for painful menses. There were no cases of conversion to open surgery despite a group of 30 patients with uteri weighing over 500 g (eight patients had uteri weighing more than 1000 g). Hospital stay averaged 16 hours and resumption of normal activity was within 2–3 days. Return to work was at two weeks for the entire series. Increasingly, later in the series other procedures for pelvic support (Burch, rectocele, and enterocele repair) were performed, which combined with LSH gave this patient population a significant improvement in overall morbidity when compared with similar vaginal or abdominal approaches.

Discussion

Today, laparoscopic hysterectomy is an appropriate therapeutic alternative in an era when the gynecologist is able to evaluate and treat cervical disease with local therapies including Papanicolaou smear, colposcopy with directed biopsy, cold knife conizations, laser therapy, and/or large loop excision of transformation zone (LLETZ) therapy. The advent of TAH in 1888 as first described by Jones (Rock and Thompson, 1997) was an attempt to control and prevent deaths from carcinoma of the cervix. Of course, at that time Papanicolaou smears were not available as a diagnostic tool for cervical disease as the use of this screening procedure did not become

Figure 31.5 Graph showing relationship between deaths from cervical cancer and increased use of total hysterectomy in the USA. The onset of routine Papanicolaou smears is shown in 1958 and the human papillomavirus epidemic is superimposed.

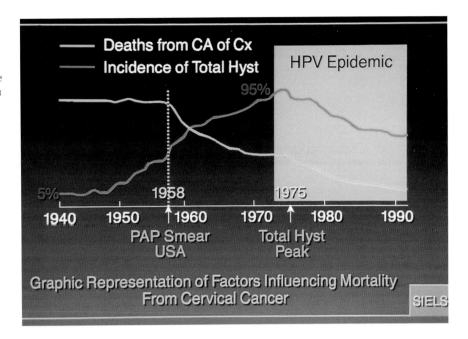

routine in the USA until 1958. As can be seen in Figure 31.5 this procedure (total hysterectomy) did not significantly change the mortality from cancer of the cervix, but routine Papanicolaou smears did. A report by Cutler in 1949 (Cutler and Zollinger, 1949) suggested that the incidence of cancer in the cervical stump after supracervical hysterectomy is 0.4% (n=6600). Kilkku et al. (1985) confirmed these data in Finland showing a cervical cancer risk after supracervical hysterectomy of 0.11% when the endocervical canal is treated with monopolar diathermy. This is comparable to the incidence of vaginal cuff carcinoma and other dysplastic conditions, which would be considered a follow-up risk after TAH (Gallup and Morley, 1975; Jimerson and Merrill, 1976; Stuart et al., 1981).

It is thought that since the attendant morbidity of LSH is less than LAVH (Lyons, 1993) and certainly less than TAH, that LSH should be an appropriate alternative for patients requiring removal of the uterine corpus. It has been shown in several reports that injuries to the ureter occur most frequently during attempts to remove the cervix. Therefore sparing this structure should reduce this morbidity further.

Laparoscopic procedures have in most cases, where tested, proved to be efficient and effective methods of dealing with pelvic pathology – ectopic pregnancy (Brumsted et al., 1986), endometriosis (Martin, 1990), and pelvic inflammatory disease. With a skilled operator these procedures not only reduce medical morbidity, but also financial requirements. LSH provides a versatile simple approach to the removal of the uterine corpus with

the known reduced morbidity of the subtotal approach. The series presented in this chapter clearly demonstrates these facts. The present data feature procedures accomplished by a single surgeon working in a standard operating suite using equipment available to virtually all surgeons and is inexpensive when compared with some other emerging technologies. These results can be compared favorably with any existing data or retrospective review. In order to accomplish the desired goal (i.e. to present the patient with the appropriate, most efficient and least invasive procedure with the least morbidity) it would seem that this alternative should be considered. Laparoscopic hysterectomy or LAVH have not so far resulted in conversion of the desired percentage of abdominal hysterectomies to the less morbid vaginal approach. Possibly, therefore, other minimally invasive procedures should be considered to accomplish this goal.

It was somewhat fortuitous that the present author proposed the subtotal procedure in an attempt to provide a more readily accessible alternative to patients and surgeons. If this had not been the case these data might not have been re-examined. Careful inspection of the data shows clearly that total hysterectomy does not prevent deaths from cervical cancer as expected (Figure 31.5) and, as importantly, that the subtotal method may provide a number of positive effects (Table 31.1). Current studies show a decreased morbidity (LSH and LAVH) and both current and previous data show a decreased risk of cervical cancer, decreased urinary tract and bowel symptomology, improved vault support and improved sexual performance (when subtotal hysterectomy is compared with total hysterectomy) (Kilkku *et al.*, 1981, 1983, 1987; Kilkku, 1985).

Advanced operative laparoscopy procedures require some retraining and practice to develop the skills necessary to produce a quality product in the operating theater. However, these requirements have never been a barrier to the ongoing educational process that is crucial to the practice of medicine. The directive to the practitioner remains the same as proposed by William Mayo decades ago that 'Concern for the benefit of the patient is the primary concern of the physician'. If our goal as operative gynecologists is to meet the needs of our patients in the 1990s and into the twenty-first century, we must re-examine our practice and, where possible, offer our patients all possible choices regarding their ongoing reproductive health care.

References

Brumsted J, Kessler C, Gibson C *et al.* (1986) A comparison of laparoscopy and laparotomy for the treatment of ectopic pregnancy. *Obstetrics and Gynecology* **71**: 889–892.

Cutler EC, Zollinger RM (1949) *Atlas of Surgical Operations.* New York: Macmillan.

Gallup DG, Morley GW (1975) Carcinoma *in situ* of the vagina: A study and review. *Obstetrics and Gynecology* **46**: 334–340.

Garry R (1994) Laparoscopic hysterectomy. Definitions and indications. *Gynaecological Endoscopy* **3**: 1–3.

Jimerson GK, Merrill JA (1976) Cancer and dysplasia of the post hysterectomy vaginal cuff. *Gynecologic Oncology* **4**: 328–332.

Kilkku P (1985) Supravaginal amputation versus hysterectomy with reference to bladder symptoms and incontinence. *Acta Obstetrica Gynecologica Scandinavica* **64**: 375–379.

Kilkku P, Hirvonen T, Gronoos M (1981) Supracervical uterine amputation vs. abdominal hysterectomy: The effects in urinary symptoms with special reference to pollakiuria, nocturia, and dysuria. *Maturitas* **3**: 197.

Kilkku P, Gronoos M, Hirvonen T *et al.* (1983) Supravaginal uterine amputation vs. hysterectomy: Effects on libido and orgasm. *Acta Obstetrica Gynecologica Scandinavica* **62**: 141–146.

Kilkku P, Gronoos M, Taina E *et al.* (1985) Culposcopic, cytological, and histological evaluation of the cervical stump 3 yrs after supravaginal uterine amputation. *Acta Obstetrica Gynecologica Scandinavica* **64**: 235–240.

Kilkku P, Lehtinen V, Hirvonen T *et al.* (1987) Abdominal hysterectomy vs. supravaginal amputation: psychic factors. *Annales Chirurgiae et Gynaecologiae* **202**: 62–66.

Levy BS, Hulka JF, Peterson HB, Phillips JM (1994) Operative laparoscopy. AAGL 1993 membership survey. *Journal of the American Association of Gynecologic Laparoscopists* **1(4)**: 301–305.

Liu CY (1992) Laparoscopic hysterectomy. Report of 215 cases. *Gynecological Endoscopy* **1**: 73–77.

Lyons TL (1991) Laparoscopic supracervical hysterectomy. *Proceedings of the 20th Annual Meeting AAGL*, Las Vegas, Nevada, November 1991. AAG

Lyons TL (1993) Laparoscopic supracervical hysterectomy – A comparison of morbidity and mortality results with laparoscopically assisted vaginal hysterectomy. *Journal of Reproductive Medicine* **38**: 763–767.

Maher PJ, Wood EC, Hill DJ *et al.* (1992) Laparoscopically assisted hysterectomy. *Medical Journal of Australia* **156**: 316–318.

Martin DC (1990) *Laparoscopic Appearance of Endometriosis.* Memphis: Resurge Press.

Ou CS, Beadle E, Presthus J, Smith M (1994) A multicenter review of 839 laparoscopically assisted vaginal hysterectomies. *Journal of the American Association of Gynecologic Laparoscopists* **1(4)**: 417–422.

Rock A, Thompson JD (eds) (1997) *Telinde's Operative Gynecology*, 8th edn., p. 773. Philadelphia, PA: Lippincott–Raven.

Semm K (1991) Hysterectomy via laparotomy or pelviscopy. A new CASH method without culpotomy. *Geburtshilfe Frauenheilkd* **51**: 996–1003.

Stuart GCE, Allen HH, Anderson RJ (1981) Squamous cell carcinoma of the vagina after hysterectomy. *American Journal of Obstetrics and Gynecology* **139**: 311–315.

Thompson JT (1992) In Thompson JT, Rock J (eds) *Telinde's Operative Gynecology.* pp. 758–759. Philadelphia: J. Lippincott.

32

Laparoscopic Assisted Doderlein Hysterectomy

MARK D. WHITTAKER AND RAY GARRY

St James's University Hospital, Leeds, UK

Background

Doderlein described a technique of vaginal hysterectomy (Doderlein and Kronig, 1906) that involved delivering the uterine fundus through a colpotomy incision before performing the hysterectomy. Saye reported a form of this operation in which the upper uterine pedicles were mobilized with laparoscopic techniques before delivering the uterus through the anterior colpotomy (Saye *et al.*, 1993). The operation Saye described used expensive stapling devices to secure the laparoscopic pedicles. These are rapid in action and easy to apply, but are expensive and so we suggested a modification of the technique using bipolar diathermy for the pedicles (Garry, 1994). This approach was found to be more cost-effective because it used simpler, more readily available and less expensive equipment. We subsequently reported our early encouraging experience with this technique (Garry and Hercz, 1995).

Before the introduction of the laparoscopic assisted Doderlein hysterectomy (LADH), we performed most of our laparoscopic hysterectomies with a standard laparoscopic assisted vaginal hysterectomy (LAVH) technique in which the uterine vessels, lower uterine supports and vaginal cuff were all secured from below with vaginal techniques. A formal audit of our early experience with this approach confirmed our clinical impression that we were encountering a higher than expected complication rate. The main difficulties were of vault hematoma, the need for blood transfusion and bladder and ureteric damage. The principle anatomic problem is that the vaginal vault has a very rich vascular supply, the main vessels of which are very close to the ureter. As in every other method of hysterectomy the principle technical problem is to ensure complete hemostasis, not only of the major uterine vessels, but also of the small vessel plexus around the uterus without damaging the adjacent urinary tract. The complication rate we encountered with the LAVH approach was unacceptable to us and so we reviewed the literature to find a simpler and safer approach.

The LADH described by Saye appealed to us because of a number of practical advantages:

- The laparoscopic portion of the procedure is discontinued cephalad to the uterine artery as it crosses the ureter. If the laparoscopic dissection stops above the uterine artery, it must also stop above the ureter. The ureter cannot therefore be injured at this stage when it is traditionally most vulnerable.
- When the uterus is inverted, the uterine arteries are clearly visualized outside the peritoneal cavity. The action of tipping the uterus also removes the arteries far from the ureter, so that when the arteries are clamped with standard vaginal instruments, the ureter cannot be damaged at this time.
- The third advantage of the approach is that the vascular posterior wall of the vagina, which in most methods of hysterectomy must be incised before it can be secured, can with this approach, be secured with clamps before section reducing the risk of operative bleeding and postoperative hematoma formation.
- An unexpected difficulty of the standard

LAVH is that it is sometimes difficult to ensure that the top of the vaginal incision precisely meets the bottom of the laparoscopic incision. With a traditional LAVH the pedicle containing the uterine artery is the last one to be secured and is often contained in a very thin pedicle, which can easily be avulsed during manipulation. The Doderlein adaptation of the LAVH technique allows clamping and securing of the uterine arteries before division of the uterosacral/cardinal complex, thus protecting these vessels from accidental injury.

Classification of LADH Hysterectomy

With the LADH technique the upper uterine pedicles are secured laparoscopically, but the uterine arteries are secured by the vaginal route. As defined by the classification of Garry, Reich and Liu (Figure 32.1), the LADH is therefore a variant of the LAVH (Garry *et al.*, 1994).

Patient Suitability

The LADH is suitable for almost any woman requiring a hysterectomy. The main use for this technique is to replace the total abdominal hysterectomy. The main reasons for not adopting a LADH approach are because the patient is suitable for vaginal hysterectomy or has very large fibroid uterus. Morbid

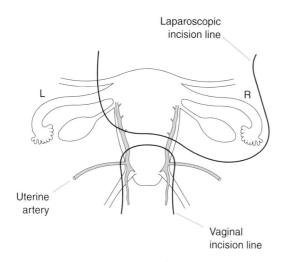

Figure 32.1 Classification of laparoscopic hysterectomy. (Reproduced with permission from Garry *et al.*, 1994.)

obesity can be a problem with any method of hysterectomy, but all laparoscopic approaches may be impaired by an inability to ventilate the patient due to a diaphragmatic splinting effect and also possible difficulties with entry because of the thickness of the abdominal wall.

Operative Technique: LADH

Patient Preparation

Following administration of general anesthesia, the patient is placed in a modified lithotomy position with only minimal flexion of the legs at the hip (Figure 32.2). Hyperflexion of the hip will reduce

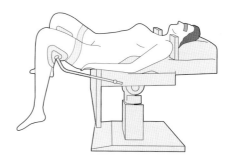

Figure 32.2 Patient position at beginning of the hysterectomy.

access to the abdomen and the legs will restrict movement of the laparoscopic instruments. The patient is cleaned with aqueous iodine solution, catheterized and a Valtchev uterine manipulator (Valtcher, Conkin Surgical Instruments, Toronto, Canada) is inserted (Figure 32.3). The ability to adjust the uterine position effectively during the procedure is essential to achieve good exposure of the operative site and adequate tissue tensions for dissection and cutting. It is essential that the main surgeon performs a vaginal examination immediately before surgery to obtain an accurate assessment of uterine size. Such estimation of size is very difficult at the subsequent laparoscopy.

Laparoscopic Component of LADH

The laparoscopic component of the procedure is commenced by gaining laparoscopic access to the abdominal cavity. The technique of insertion of the

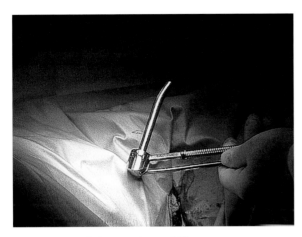

Figure 32.3 Valtchev uterine mobilizer.

primary trocar is that described by Reich using an incision at the base of the umbilicus. The Veress needle is inserted with care, gripping low down on the shaft of the instrument to increase the feel of the point penetrating the various layers of the abdomen. The initial insufflation pressure is raised to 25 mm Hg with the patient flat. A short, sharp 10 mm trocar is held guarded in the palm of the hand with only the tip exposed and is inserted vertically through the intraumbilical incision until the sharp tip enters the cavity (Figure 32.4). The sharp trocar is then withdrawn from the cannula and the cannula screwed more firmly into position (Hulka and Reich, 1994). Three secondary 5 mm ports are used in the lower abdominal wall and are inserted under direct vision after identifying the inferior epigastric vessels.

The pelvis is inspected to determine the extent and nature of any pathology present. If endometriosis is found this is excised during the course of the laparoscopic dissection, usually by wide excision of the peritoneal disease. Deep infiltrative disease in

the pouch of Douglas involving the uterosacral ligaments or pararectal spaces is dissected out early in the procedure with the aim of excising these lesions together with the uterus. Some smaller lesions may be excised separately and removed before the hysterectomy. The presence of large leiomyomas (> 18 weeks) may alter the planned approach to the uterine vessels. Large fibroids low in the uterus with poor laparoscopic and vaginal access may be an indication for securing the uterine vessels out on the pelvic sidewall close to their origin and lateral to the ureter in the manner suggested by Kadar (Kadar, 1995). Alternatively the uterine vessels may be secured from below as with a standard LAVH to occlude the uterine blood supply before commencing morcellation via the vaginal route. A third approach has been suggested by Donnez (Donnez, personal communication) in which a subtotal hysterectomy is performed, again occluding the relevant blood supply before morcellation by a laparoscopic approach. The LAVH method may also be preferred when large fibroids are present because it can be difficult to deliver a grossly enlarged uterus through the colpotomy incision. The largest we have dealt with by LADH weighed 730 g. A total abdominal hysterectomy may be offered to the patient for a very large fibroid uterus rather than a laparoscopic approach.

The hysterectomy is commenced by dividing the right round ligament. Bipolar Kleppinger forceps (Kleppinger, Wolf, Germany) at 25 W (unmodulated waveform) are used to desiccate the ligament before dividing it with scissors (Figure 32.5). The bladder flap is developed by extending the incision down into the uterovesical pouch (Figure 32.6). The left round ligament is divided in an identical manner and the bladder is reflected by continuing the peritoneal incision down to meet with the contralateral incision. The peritoneum is desiccated with bipolar electrosurgery during this dissection. The

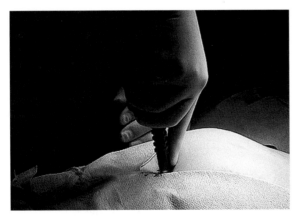

Figure 32.4 Controlled insertion technique for the umbilical trocar.

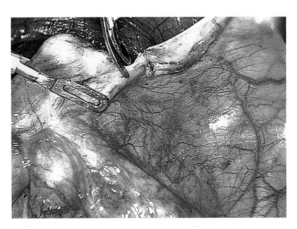

Figure 32.5 Cutting the right round ligament with scissors.

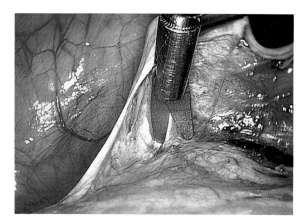

Figure 32.6 Dividing the peritoneum in the uterovesicular pouch.

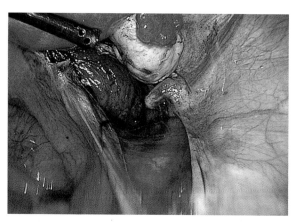

Figure 32.8 Laparoscopic view at the end of the laparoscopic component of the hysterectomy.

bladder is usually easily separated from the cervix and upper vagina, but may require sharp dissection after previous cesarean section.

The course of the pelvic ureter is identified by inspection – the ureter is most easily located as it enters the pelvis at the pelvic brim. The infundibulopelvic ligament/utero-ovarian pedicle is then desiccated and transected with scissors (Figure 32.7). It may be necessary to mobilize an ovary adherent to the pelvic sidewall and it is especially important to identify that the ureter is clear before desiccating the pedicle.

The laparoscopic dissection is continued down to the level of the uterine artery, but this structure is not divided laparoscopically. Once the vessel is identified entering the uterus, the contralateral infundibulopelvic ligament is divided in an identical manner using bipolar desiccation and scissors. The dissection is continued down to the level of the uterine vessels. The laparoscopic component is complete once hemostasis of all the pedicles has been confirmed (Figure 32.8).

The gas is evacuated from the peritoneal cavity and the gas line detached to prevent contamination of the gas line or insufflator. The instruments and camera are stored safely so as not to injure the patient or risk damage to the equipment by falling to the ground during the vaginal surgery. The legs are adjusted by loosening the leg supports and elevating the legs to achieve increased flexion at the hip to permit better vaginal access. The uterine manipulator is removed.

Vaginal Component of LADH

The vaginal component of the procedure is commenced by infiltrating the upper anterior vaginal wall with dilute adrenaline or vasopressin solution. An anterior colpotomy is performed with an incision from the nine o'clock to the three o'clock positions only (Figure 32.9). No attempt is made to open up the posterior cul-de-sac. When the incision is opened care is taken to ensure that the bladder is pushed up particularly laterally. The pubocervical fascia is divided and the peritoneal cavity entered – this is particularly easy if the bladder has been reflected during the laparoscopic part of the operation. A Vienna type retractor is then inserted to ensure that the bladder remains out of the operative field.

The uterus is then inverted through the anterior colpotomy: this is achieved by grasping the low anterior uterine wall with toothed forceps. We have found Braun forceps (Endosafe Technologies, Leeds, UK), which are modified thyroid forceps, to be particularly useful for this as they grasp tissue firmly without tearing it. The technique is to march two of these over each other up the anterior uterine wall by applying a second Braun a little higher and then removing the first and grasping even higher. This is continued until the uterine fundus is

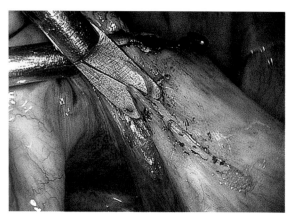

Figure 32.7 Cutting the right infundibulopelvic ligament.

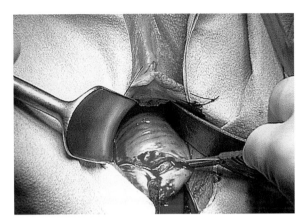

Figure 32.9 Anterior colpotomy performed with an incision from the nine o'clock to the three o'clock positions only.

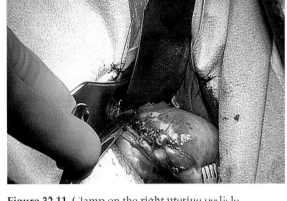

Figure 32.11 Clamp on the right uterine pedicle.

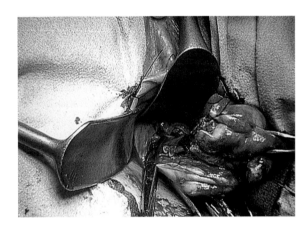

Figure 32.12 Clamp on the right uterosacral/cardinal pedicle.

reached. While maintaining firm downward traction with the Braun, a vulsellum applied to the posterior leaf of the cervix should be pushed posteriorly into the pouch of Douglas. This combined action has the effect of rotating the uterus forwards. The uterine fundus is then pulled out through the colpotomy (Figure 32.10). This is possible even with fairly large fibroid uteri (see previous section).

The uterine arteries can then be clamped, divided and suture ligated under direct vision in the vagina (Figure 32.11). This is the most important and satisfying step in this approach to hysterectomy. The major vessels can be secured in full view and in the certain knowledge that the ureter is well clear and is in fact completely outside the operating field. The uterosacral/cardinal complex is then clamped incorporating the vaginal angle and it is divided and suture ligated (Figure 32.12). This suture is left long so that it can be used to approximate the ligaments and support the vaginal vault later. The remaining vagina is divided after first applying clamps. This allows the uterus to be freed without the risk of ooz-

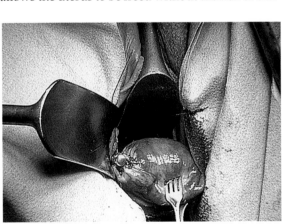

Figure 32.10 Uterus delivered out through the anterior colpotomy.

ing from this very vascular area. The ligaments are approximated with a continuous suture, which also brings together the vaginal skin edges. No attempt is made to close the peritoneum, which is left open to facilitate subsequent laparoscopic inspection. The vaginal vault is further supported by tying together the long sutures attached to the uterosacral/cardinal ligaments. They may be reattached to the rectovaginal septum by suturing them into the posterior vaginal vault. The vagina is closed with absorbable sutures. Vaginal packs are not used.

The abdomen is then re-insufflated and the pedicles and vaginal vault are inspected for any bleeding points, which are coagulated using bipolar electrosurgery. Copious warm heparinized normal saline irrigation is used to remove any blood clots and confirm hemostasis. A drain is passed down the suprapubic port to remove irrigant, blood and any residual carbon dioxide gas. The skin incisions are closed with interrupted sutures. A Foley catheter is used to drain the bladder and confirm clear urine.

In the more difficult cases (e.g. extensive excision of endometriosis from the pelvic sidewalls), a cystoscopy is performed at the completion of the procedure to ensure passage of urine from each ureteric orifice. This can be assisted by injecting indigo carmine intravenously and observing its excretion in the urine within about five minutes. This reassures the surgeon that the ureter has not been transected or completely occluded, but cannot fully exclude kinking of the ureter low in the pelvis. When pararectal endometriosis has been excised a rectal integrity test is performed by instilling 50–150 ml of methylene blue into the rectum via a Foley catheter and observing the rectum laparoscopically to ensure no leaks.

Postoperative Care

The Foley catheter and pelvic drain are removed the following morning. The intravenous cannula is left *in situ* until the patient is tolerating oral fluids, which is usually the same morning. The patient is encouraged to mobilize early and told that she may go home when she feels fit to do so, the majority of our patients currently choosing to return home 48–72 hours postoperatively. The patient is advised to avoid heavy lifting for six weeks, but can resume lighter duties much sooner and return to work as soon as she feels ready. The patient is offered an outpatient appointment for six weeks.

Results

The results of the first 100 patients undergoing LADH are given here. The hysterectomies were performed at South Cleveland Hospital, Middlesbrough and St James's University Hospital, Leeds between January 1994 and March 1995. The mean age was 41.8 years (range 26–73 years). Some 27% of the patients had undergone a previous laparotomy mainly for either cesarean section, appendicectomy or adnexal surgery. During the hysterectomy only 14% of the patients required no other surgery in addition to the hysterectomy, with the other 86% undergoing either bilateral/unilateral salpingo-oophorectomy, adhesiolysis or excision/ablation of endometriosis.

The mean operative time was 97.1 minutes (range 54–183 minutes). The mean uterine weight was 160.9 g (range 30–710 g). The pathology was fibroids 36%, endometriosis 31%, adenomyosis 11%, atypical hyperplasia 3%, carcinoma of the endometrium 2%, tuberculosis 1%, cervical intraepithelial neoplasia II

1% and endometrial polyp 1%. No pelvic pathology was identified in 28% of the group. Blood transfusion was required for six patients, with two of these patients being anemic preoperatively.

There were no complications in 92% of the patients. None of the patients required conversion to total abdominal hysterectomy and none required a laparotomy to manage any complication. Of the complications there were:

- Three vault hematomas
- Two patients complained of vaginal discharge, which was treated with antibiotics.
- Two patients had inadvertent cystotomy, which occurred during the vaginal dissection and these were both repaired vaginally without further problem in either patient.

Information on one patient was missing. The mean hospital stay was 74.4 hours (range 48–168 hours).

Summary

The LADH is a variant of the LAVH. Audit of the introduction of the LADH into our practise has assured us that this approach to hysterectomy is widely applicable to our patients and can be used with low complication rates, even in patients with complex pelvic pathology. Currently this approach is used for most of our hysterectomies, and we have found that it can be readily learnt by trainees in our unit. The Doderlein approach offers an optimal approach to securing the uterine arteries and allows direct clamping of the posterior vaginal wall. The laparoscopy at the completion of the procedure allows confirmation of complete hemostasis. The procedure may take longer than performing a total abdominal hysterectomy and this has associated theater cost implications, but we believe that the postoperative advantages for the patient, including short hospital stay, outweigh the operative time disadvantages.

References

Doderlein A, Kronig S (1906) *Die Technik der Vaginalen Bauchholen-Operationen*. Leipzig: Verlag von S. Hirzel.
Garry R, Reich H, Liu CY (1994) Laparoscopic hysterectomy: definitions and indications. *Gynaecological Endoscopy* 3: 1–3.

Garry R (1994) The evolution of a technique for laparoscopic hysterectomy: laparoscopic assisted Doderlein's hysterectomy. *Gynaecological Endoscopy* **3**: 123–128.

Garry R, Hercz P (1995) Initial experience with laparoscopic-assisted Doderlein hysterectomy. *British Journal of Obstetrics and Gynaecology* **102**: 307–310.

Hulka JF, Reich H (1994) *Textbook* of *Laparoscopy*, 2nd edition. pp. 85–102. Philadelphia: W.B. Saunders Company.

Kadar N (1995) *Atlas of Laparoscopic Pelvic Surgery.* pp. 101–114 Oxford: Blackwell Science.

Saye WB, Epsy GB, Bishop MR *et al.* (1993) Laparoscopic Doderlein hysterectomy: a rational alternative to traditional abdominal hysterectomy. *Surgical Laparoscopy and Endoscopy* **3**: 88–94.

Laparoscopic Pelvic Floor Repair and Incontinence Procedures

33

Laparoscopic Colposuspension

ANTHONY R.B. SMITH* AND THIERRY G. VANCAILLIE[†]

*Saint Mary's Hospital, Manchester, UK
[†]Royal Hospital for Women, Sydney, Australia

Introduction

Urinary incontinence is common and in over 50% of women is caused by failure of the urethral sphincter mechanism producing genuine stress incontinence. Stress incontinence may be managed by conservative therapy employing pelvic floor physiotherapy or by surgical treatment. Over the last two decades it has been recognized that colposuspension gives the best chance of surgical cure of stress incontinence, though the immediate surgical morbidity may be greater with an abdominal incision than with the vaginal incision used for the anterior vaginal repair. Use of the laparoscope at colposuspension enables the suprapubic approach to the bladder neck to be used without the need for laparotomy and may confer advantages in postoperative recovery. Randomized trials with long-term follow-up are required to establish the value of this approach to colposuspension.

Literature Review

Experience with retropubic bladder neck suspension procedures has led to the recognition that the higher cure rate may be accompanied by an increased risk of postoperative voiding difficulty, detrusor instability and vaginal prolapse. Study has shown that use of minimally invasive techniques for colposuspension such as those described by Pereyra (1959) and Stamey (1973) have not proved as effective or

longlasting (Elia and Bergman, 1994) as the colposuspension first described by Burch in 1961. To date there are insufficient data to determine whether laparoscopic colposuspension represents an advance in the surgical management of stress incontinence in terms of cure and postoperative recovery or merely a further procedure in a long list of procedures that have promised but failed to produce a high cure rate with low morbidity.

Burch (1961) experienced technical difficulty reproducing the colposuspension described by Marshall et al. (1949) whereby the peri-urethral fascia was sutured to the periosteum of the pubis. Cooper's ligament proved to be an easier fixed point than either the periosteum of the pubis or the arcus tendineus fascia. Burch (1961) reported 'satisfactory results' in 93% of 143 patients, only 12 of whom had undergone previous surgery. No cystometric studies were performed. Burch noted at an early stage that postoperative enterocele was common and incorporated obliteration of the cul-de-sac into the procedure, but still reported postoperative enteroceles in 7.6% of cases. Burch employed chromic catgut #2 suture for colposuspension and reported failure of bladder neck suspension in only two of 143 cases at follow-up. Currently, most surgeons prefer a stronger more durable suture material and many use a non-absorbable suture. No trial has established the optimal suture material. A non-absorbable suture material carries a risk of stone formation if placed or if it migrates into the bladder.

Numerous reports on Burch colposuspension have been published over the past 35 years, but most do not include a large number of patients with pre- and postoperative urodynamic assessment with long-term follow-up including documentation of complications. In 1993 Kiilholma *et al.* reported on a two-year follow-up of 186 women after colposuspension. Of the women undergoing colposuspension as a primary procedure 95% were cured or markedly improved compared with 82% who had undergone previous bladder neck surgery. Postoperatively 9% of patients experienced voiding difficulty, 12% developed a rectocele or enterocele and 19% described urinary urgency *de novo*, which is the same incidence of detrusor instability as found by Cardozo *et al.* (1979) in a study of 92 patients following colposuspension. Thus, there are good data to indicate that open colposuspension provides a good chance of curing stress incontinence, particularly as a primary procedure, but problems with abnormal bladder function, voiding and vaginal prolapse may follow surgery.

In a five-year follow-up of 127 women undergoing primary bladder neck surgery, Elia and Bergman (1994) reported a higher success rate for colposuspension than vaginal repair or Stamey procedure. Twice as many women were continent at five years following colposuspension than following the vaginal repair or Stamey procedure (82% vs 37% and 43%, respectively). Alcalay *et al.* (1994) investigated a group of 109 women with a mean follow-up time of 14 years following colposuspension. They reported a time-dependent fall in cure over ten years after which a plateau was reached.

In summary it would appear that open colposuspension produces the highest success rate with greatest longevity of cure. The less invasive needle colposuspension undoubtedly results in less surgical trauma to the patient, but appears to result in a lower short-term cure rate and a higher risk of recurrence. Since all studies indicate that primary surgery is more likely to be successful than subsequent surgery there is a good argument for opting for open Burch colposuspension as a primary procedure. Balanced against this, however, must be the incidence of postoperative detrusor instability, voiding dysfunction and vaginal prolapse. Unfortunately, there are no good comparative data on the incidence of these problems, but it would seem logical that voiding dysfunction will become increasingly prevalent with increasing bladder neck elevation. It is possible that the paravaginal defect repair is the compromise approach. Shull and Baden (1989) reported a cure rate of 97% for stress incontinence in a series of 149 women undergoing predominantly primary bladder neck surgery. Voiding problems were not encountered, presumably because it does not produce anatomic distortion, but vaginal vault prolapse was noted in 6% of patients postoperatively.

There is no doubt that the view of the retropubic space through the laparoscope introduced through or without the peritoneal cavity can be excellent. The value of gaining access to the retropubic space in this way, with the apparent shorter convalescence, has to be matched against the capital cost of the equipment, the additional technical expertise required by the surgeon and the risk inherent in laparoscopic surgery. Even if a technically excellent result is achieved by the laparoscopic approach, the early return to normal activity commonly seen in such patients may be placing more stress on the surgical site, actually resulting in more frequent recurrence of symptoms, as seen with needle suspension.

The first report on laparoscopic colposuspension by Vancaillie and Schuessler in 1991 included nine patients. Two of the first four patients required laparotomy to complete the procedure, indicating the technical difficulty of the operation. Since then there have been more than 25 reports on various laparoscopic techniques. Most of the publications are case report studies. In 1993 Liu reported on a series of 58 patients who all had demonstrable primary stress incontinence and normal bladder function on simple office cystometry. The intraperitoneal approach was employed and the cul-de-sac obliterated with prolene sutures, termed a 'Moschowitz' procedure (Moschowitz, 1912). The retropubic space was then opened through an incision 2.5–3.5 cm above the symphysis pubis on the anterior abdominal wall peritoneum between the obliterated umbilical artery folds in the peritoneum. After bladder mobilization two Gortex (Gore, USA) sutures, including a full-thickness double-bite in the anterior vaginal wall, were fixed to Cooper's ligament on each side. The peritoneal defect was closed and cystoscopy performed. Of the 58 cases reported, one sustained a bladder injury during surgery, which was repaired laparoscopically and another bled from a suprapubic catheter insertion. The suprapubic catheter was removed in all cases one week after surgery and no cases of voiding difficulty were reported. No patient leaked with a standing stress test three months after surgery, but three patients had increased incontinence due to detrusor instability, although it is not made clear how this was defined. The paper states that all patients were allowed to drive and return to work one week after surgery provided that their job did not require much physical exertion. It is not made clear what tasks the patients were actually able to perform and indeed did perform following surgery.

In order to overcome the difficulty of laparoscopic suturing, Ou *et al.* (1993) developed a technique of laparoscopic colposuspension using prolene mesh fixed to the paraurethral fascia and Cooper's ligaments with titanium staples. The staples are applied through a disposable hernia stapling gun, the cost of which may be regained through reduced operating time. No case of failure was reported in a series of 40 patients with a mean of six months' follow-up. No complications of staples in the anterior wall were reported.

Another modification of laparoscopic colposuspension has been described by Harewood (1993). In a series of seven patients, a Stamey type procedure was performed under laparoscopic vision. The author suggests that the advantage of the laparoscopic approach is that it allows direct examination of the bladder and observation of the bladder neck during tying of the sutures. Despite this, bladder perforation occurred in one case.

Burton (1994) performed the first published randomized control trial of laparoscopic and open colposuspension. In a series of 60 patients undergoing primary treatment for stress incontinence full postoperative subjective and objective assessment was performed at six and 12 months. The procedure was performed through the peritoneal cavity and four polyglycolic acid sutures were placed with a 12-mm curved needle in all cases. One bladder perforation occurred in each group. Cure of stress incontinence was only 60% at 36 months, compared with 93% for the open approach. Although Burton performed ten laparoscopic colposuspensions before the study to familiarize himself with the technique, many surgeons would suggest more experience is advisable before conducting such a study. Having performed several hundred laparoscopic colposuspensions, the authors would suggest that the learning curve is longer than for open surgery, predominantly due to the difficulty with suturing. This is well illustrated by a 50% reduction in mean operating time noted over the first 50 cases.

Two further prospective studies are currently available. One published by McDougall et al. (1995) compares laparoscopic bladder neck suspension to vaginal needle suspension. The author notices no difference in outcome on a short-term basis, but points out the significantly longer operating room time for the laparoscopic procedure. A study performed at Johns Hopkins Hospital (Polascik et al., 1995) shows that patients do better after laparoscopic colposuspension than after open Burch.

The data are therefore conflicting with the exception that all studies highlight the increased technical difficulty and the lower short-term morbidity of the laparoscopic approach.

Technique of Laparoscopic Bladder Neck Suspension

There are many variations of the laparoscopic retropubic bladder neck suspension. An effort will be made to present an eclectic array of technical variations.

Anesthesia

General endotracheal anesthesia is as a rule preferred, although the preperitoneal approach could be performed under regional block. The usual concerns of anesthesia for laparoscopy obviously apply here.

Positioning of the Patient on the Operating Table

The most important impact positioning has for the surgery is allowing or limiting access to the operating field. A classic lithotomy position is the optimal position for easy access to both the suprapubic and vaginal areas. It is also recommended to tuck the patient's arms alongside her body. This needs to be discussed with the anesthesiologist as access to the intravenous lines to the arm or hand are often made more difficult when the arms are tucked alongside the body. If a concomitant vaginal procedure is needed, such as colporrhaphy or large enterocele repair, the lithotomy position may be slightly modified into what is termed the 'frog' position. In this position, the legs are bent a little more and the knees are abducted to increase access to the vagina.

Access to the Retropubic Space

There are three variations of abdominal endosurgical access to the space of Retzius:

- The classical transperitoneal laparoscopy.
- The preperitoneal laparoscopy with insertion of the main trocar at the umbilicus.
- The so-called 'Retziusscopy', in which the main trocar is inserted suprapubically at the approximate site of the suprapubic catheter, directly into the space of Retzius.

TRANSPERITONEAL ('CLASSIC') APPROACH

The most important advantage of the transperitoneal approach is that a general inspection of the abdominal and pelvic cavity is possible. Ensuing from this is the surgical access to the cul-de-sac and rectovaginal fossa in cases where such access is needed. Other procedures involving the pelvis can be performed at the same time. There are some disadvantages too – mainly those related to blind entry into the peritoneal cavity such as bowel injury and vessel laceration. In addition, there are the risks of bladder injury when opening the parietal peritoneum to access the space of Retzius. In patients who have had many previous operations, there may be extensive adhesions barring access to the space of Retzius. Lastly, there is the small but real risk of herniation of intra-abdominal organs through the port wounds.

THE EXTRAPERITONEAL APPROACH

The extraperitoneal approach (transumbilical) has appeal because the space of Retzius itself is an extraperitoneal space, so why invade the peritoneal space to start with? The main advantage of the extraperitoneal approach is therefore the avoidance of invading the peritoneal space with its inherent risks of injury to the intra-abdominal organs. Preperitoneal scarring secondary to previous abdominal surgery is detrimental to the preperitoneal approach as much as to the transperitoneal route, if not more so. The two intrinsic disadvantages to the preperitoneal approach are the inability to access the cul-de-sac and rectovaginal space and the reduced operating field. The secondary ports for insertion of the needle holder and other accessory instruments need to be placed closer to the midline, making it technically more difficult to approach the intended site at an appropriate angle. One may conceive to open the preperitoneal space more widely, as is done for preperitoneal hernia repair. However, this is not routinely done for surgery of the space of Retzius.

Technically, there are differences between classic transperitoneal laparoscopy and preperitoneal laparoscopy. Although apparently minor, they are important. For preperitoneal laparoscopy, the incision is made lateral to the umbilicus rather than in the middle of the umbilicus because the peritoneum is more loosely attached to the anterior wall structures the further one goes from the umbilicus. The choice of the umbilicus as the site of incision is mainly to remain in the middle for optimal approach to both the left and right side. Insufflation with carbon dioxide (CO_2) may be made before or after a space has been developed. Entry into the preperitoneal space is best confirmed by digital palpation. Development of the space can be achieved using commercially available balloon devices or by digital dissection. The balloon technique has the advantage that pressure can be maintained for several minutes until some degree of hemostasis is achieved. The disadvantage of the balloon technology is its cost. Once the preperitoneal space has been developed, one can insert the ancillary trocars under direct visualization. As pointed out earlier, the site of insertion of the ancillary trocars is more medial than for conventional laparoscopy.

THE 'RETZIUSSCOPY' APPROACH

With this approach, the surgeon intends to enter the space of Retzius through the shortest possible access route (i.e. suprapubically). It does seem to be a logical reasoning. However, the angle of approach of the optic and the ancillary instruments becomes awkward. Techniques based on gasless laparoscopy combined with Retziusscopy are being favored by some. This does away with the rigid trocar and thus increases maneuverability of the instruments. We do not have enough experience with this technique to enable us to voice a fair critique of the method. However, we fail to grasp any apparent advantage of Retziusscopy over transumbilical preperitoneal laparoscopy.

General Principles of Dissection

Regardless of the technique of access to the space of Retzius, the surgeon will first aim to reach the upper edge of the pubic bone, close to the midline. The pubic bone represents the upper limit of the anterior aspect of the space of Retzius. In patients with previous surgery in the area, this part of the dissection may prove to be very difficult. Digital palpation of the pubic bone while performing the dissection is sometimes helpful. Once the pubic bone is reached, it is recommended to extend the dissection until both ligaments of Cooper are clearly identified. The next step consists of developing the actual space of Retzius. In our experience, the dissection is done bluntly with progressive careful pressure along the pubic arch laterally and downwards to unveil the obturator fascia on both sides. The areolar tissue of the space of Retzius is left attached to the anterior aspect of the bladder.

At this stage of the dissection, it should be possible for the surgeon to visually monitor vaginal manipulation of the urethra and bladder neck, which is a great help for further progress of the intervention. Vaginal examination helps in orientation as much as the presence of a Foley bulb in the bladder. Manual identification of the ischial spine helps in identifying the arcus tendineus crossing the obturator fascia. This represents the general dissection of the space of Retzius: the space is dissected until both arcus are visualized in their entire length. Further dissection will vary depending upon the technique favored by the surgeon.

Mobilization of the Periurethral Fascia

For the Burch-type procedure, mobilization of the periurethral fascia is necessary in order to optimize approximation between the endopelvic fascia and the ipsilateral ligament of Cooper. First the vaginal fascia (or pubocervical fascia or endopelvic fascia) is properly identified by palpation and inspection. The site where sutures or staples are to be placed is chosen. Then a pledget attached to a grasper and firmly secured with a suture, is introduced through one of the suprapubic ports. Disposable pledgets are available. The surgeon ideally places his or her own finger in the vagina to guide the dissection by the pledget. The pledget can be pushed over a firmly held finger or vice versa. Some colleagues will ask an assistant to place a finger guarded with a thimble in the vagina and to mobilize the fascia from below against a firmly held pledget. This maneuver is performed on both sides and is sometimes the cause of some significant bleeding. When performing a paravaginal type repair this mobilization is not absolutely necessary because less distance is to be bridged between the endopelvic fascia and the lateral pelvic wall. The impact of this dissection on subsequent bladder function has to our knowledge not been studied.

Fixation of the Periurethral Fascia

There are many ways to achieve fixation of the periurethral fascia. There is no agreement on any aspect of this critical part of the procedure and we suspect that most surgeons who perform this type of surgery under laparoscopic control or not have their own convictions and dogmas regarding where and how tight these sutures should be. We, for one, believe in using sutures and not staples or mesh or any combination of sutures, staples or mesh. We believe that laparoscopic suturing can be learned. In a Burch-type approach, two or more sutures are placed on each side of the bladder neck. A straight needle attached to a suture of choice is used because it is easier to handle. When placing the first suture on either side, two bites are taken through the fascia. A Roeder knot is tied extracorporeally and pushed down while an assistant is elevating the vaginal wall toward the ipsilateral ligament. It is not always possible to attain direct approximation of the fascia to the ligament for all four sutures, particularly when an anterior vaginal repair has been performed previously.

One of the authors (AS) estimates that the main difference between open and laparoscopic Burch colposuspension lies in the distance between the two sutures applied on either side. It seems that the sutures are closer together when the procedure is performed laparoscopically. This difference can, however, not be identified during vaginal examination. One should also mention that most surgeons

performing an open Burch will place all sutures before tying them in order to optimize approximation between the vaginal fascia and the pubic bone. This is not routinely the case for laparoscopic procedures, although it could be done theoretically.

When performing a paravaginal-type repair, the endopelvic fascia is attached to the arcus tendineus on both sides. This requires more maneuverability of the needle and needle holder. A curved needle is preferred, especially when passing the suture through the sidewall at the level of the arcus tendineus. The number of sutures on one side is not necessarily the same as the number of sutures of the other side, but 2–4 sutures are applied on both sides.

One of the authors (TV) favors the paravaginal approach and modifies the procedure slightly by connecting the most anterior suture – which is passed through the so-called pubo-urethral ligament (a thickening of the pubocervical fascia) – to the ipsilateral Cooper's ligament. This maneuver plicates the pubo-urethral ligament and causes elevation of the pubocervical fascia, but significantly less than that achieved with a Burch-type procedure.

Numerous variations and combinations exist, but it is important to recognize the anatomic structures and to perform a procedure that will stabilize the hypermobile bladder neck.

Peritoneal and Skin Closure

Postoperative care after laparoscopy as a rule is characterized by early patient mobilization after the procedure. This is generally seen to be an advantage. When a patient is actually discharged from the hospital depends more upon health care policy issues than on her clinical condition.

The procedure-specific postoperative issue is catheterization. There are numerous schemes. Generally patients require some assistance in voiding for up to 3–4 days on average. This may be in the form of an indwelling catheter or intermittent self-catheterization. Dr Smith favors a suprapubic 'Bonnano' catheter, which is inserted at the end of the laparoscopic procedure under direct visualization and remains in place until the patient is able to void with a residual of less than 150 ml. Dr Vancaillie prefers to leave the Foley in place, unclamped, until the patient is ambulating. The Foley is then removed. Residual urine is measured after spontaneous voiding and intermittent self-catheterization started if the residual is over 150 ml. Alternatively, if the patient refuses self-catheterization, the Foley is replaced for another three days. Figures 33.1–33.5 relate to the procedures described in this chapter. An alternative procedure is illustrated in Figures 33.6–33.14.

330

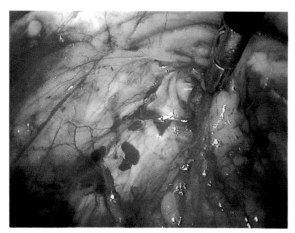

Figure 33.1 View of the space of Retzius after initial dissection. The laparoscopic instrument is pointing at the urethra, which runs anterior to posterior. To the left of the urethra is the pubocervical fascia (endopelvic fascia) followed by the arcus tendineus and the obturator fascia. In the left upper corner of the image the lower border of the pubic bone can be seen. The left pubo-urethral ligament is clearly visible on the left of the laparoscopic grasper.

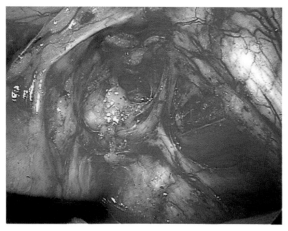

Figure 33.3 Close-up view of the right pubo-urethral ligament of the same patient as in Figure 33.2. A similar situs is seen. In this illustration two other structures are clearly visible, namely Cooper's ligament in the upper right corner and the arcus tendineus, running from approximately the center of the image to the right lower corner. Again the pubo-urethral ligament is reduced to a few strands, which insert onto the lower edge of the pubic bone to the right of the symphysis.

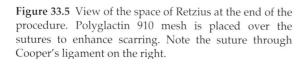

Figure 33.5 View of the space of Retzius at the end of the procedure. Polyglactin 910 mesh is placed over the sutures to enhance scarring. Note the suture through Cooper's ligament on the right.

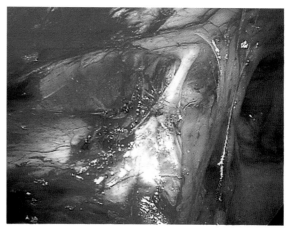

Figure 33.2 Close-up view of the left pubo-urethral ligament of a different patient. It can be clearly seen how the obturator fascia at the level of the insertion of the pubo-urethral ligament is torn off the muscle and the pubic bone, exposing bare muscle fibers. The insertion of the pubo-urethral ligament is reduced to a few fibers attached lateral to the symphysis.

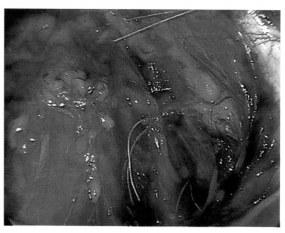

Figure 33.4 View of the right paravaginal space after placement of three sutures, which plicate the pubocervical fascia. The most anterior of these sutures is placed through the pubo-urethral ligament and is attached to the ipsilateral Cooper's ligament. The most distal of these sutures is placed in front of the ischial spine through or slightly above the arcus tendineus.

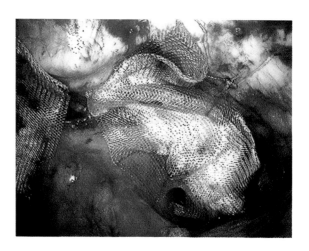

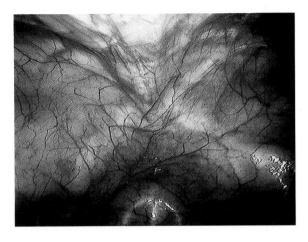

Figure 33.6 Anterior abdominal wall down to the pelvis. Outline of bladder and Foley catheter just visible

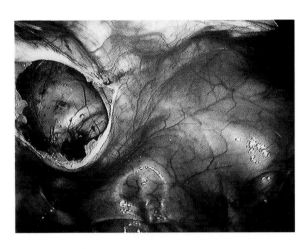

Figure 33.7 Anterior peritoneum opened on left side. Left superior pubic ramus visible.

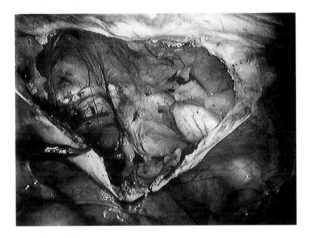

Figure 33.8 Pubic symphysis, pubic rami and bladder visible through peritoneal incision.

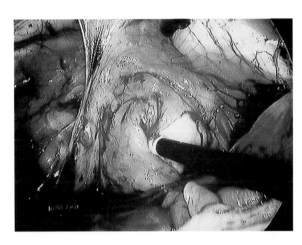

Figure 33.9 Endopelvic fascia lateral to the urethra is mobilized with the surgeon's finger in the vagina and a pledget.

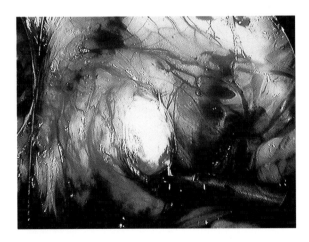

Figure 33.10 Needle is passed through the endopelvic fascia lateral to the urethra on the right side.

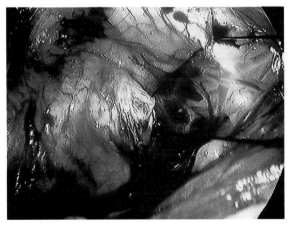

Figure 33.11 Suture material is seen passing through endopelvic fascia on the right and Cooper's ligament on the right side.

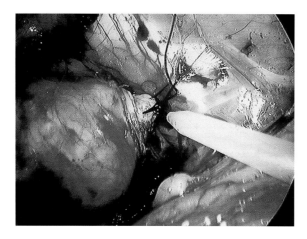

Figure 33.12 Roeder knot is tightened down bringing end of pelvic fascia up to Cooper's ligament.

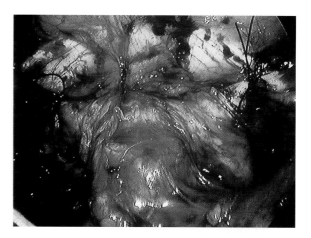

Figure 33.13 View of retropubic space with both sets of sutures in place.

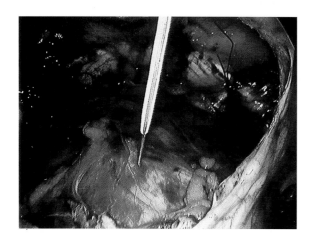

Figure 33.14 Suprapubic catheter inserted after bladder has been filled.

Complications of Laparoscopic Bladder Neck Suspension

Complications due to placement of trocars, CO_2 insufflation and the Trendelenburg position obviously apply here, as do the general intraoperative risks such as bleeding and postoperative morbidity of fever. Procedure-specific complications are the long-term problems previously discussed such as the occurrence of enterocele and *de novo* urgency symptoms.

A short-term complication, which does not seem to be as frequent during open procedures, is the bladder injury. As published, two bladder injuries occurred within the first four procedures performed by one of the authors (TV). Subsequently, two more injuries happened, one during the twenty-second intervention and the fourth more than 100 proce-

dures later. There is some improvement over time, but the overall incidence is still around 2%. Opponents to the laparoscopic approach have used this relatively high incidence as an argument against laparoscopic interventions within the space of Retzius.

Results of Laparoscopic Bladder Neck Suspension

The authors each perform, in essence, a different type of laparoscopic retropubic bladder neck surgery. The results will therefore be presented separately and not pooled. Dr Smith's results are as follows:

- 116 laparoscopic colposuspensions were performed between February 1993 and June 1995.
- 71 (61%) had genuine stress incontinence (GSI) on urodynamic testing preoperatively; 16 (14%) had GSI and detrusor instability, and 29 (25%) had other diagnoses in addition to GSI.
- 73 (63%) had a colposuspension alone performed, while 42 (37%) had another procedure including 18 sacrocolpopexies, eight hysterectomies and various other reconstructive procedures.
- During the colposuspensions there were six bladder injuries, four of which were repaired laparoscopically.
- Four patients required laparotomy, two for bladder repair and two because of difficulty gaining access to the retropubic space.
- The time taken in theater (which includes recovery from anesthesia, but not induction of anesthesia) changed from an average of 116

minutes for the first ten cases to 62 minutes for cases 40–50. This time change highlights the learning curve for both the surgeon and the theater team.

- Postoperatively, 15 of the 115 women had significant pyrexia (temperature over 38°C). Four cases were attributed to urinary tract infections, one to respiratory tract infection and two to wound hematomas. In the remaining nine cases no cause was found.

- The average length of catheterization was four days ranging from 2–12 days. One patient has needed to self-catheterize intermittently for longer than three months.

- At six months review of 89 cases with urodynamics assessment and clinical examination, nine cases of *de novo* detrusor instability have been demonstrated (10%). Of the seven cases in this group with preoperative detrusor instability, four cases were found to have resolved, one case successfully retrained and two cases were unchanged on postoperative urodynamics.

- Examination of these patients revealed four cystoceles, one uterine prolapse, one enterocele, two enteroceles with rectoceles and five rectoceles, representing an incidence of new prolapse of 15%.

- 63 of 74 women with GSI or mixed incontinence undergoing primary surgery were cured at six months follow-up (85%) compared with nine of 15 women undergoing secondary surgery, giving a combined overall cure rate of 77%.

- The cure rate in women with GSI, undergoing primary surgery was 94%.

The results obtained by Dr Vancaillie are in most aspects similar, although data collection has been significantly less sophisticated. Between June 1991 and December 1992, 42 patients underwent laparoscopic bladder neck suspension. When interviewed over the phone by an independent investigator, 40 patients reported that they were satisfied and 24% experienced either continued or *de novo* urgency symptoms.

Conclusion

The early results from laparoscopic colposuspension can lead to cautious optimism for a role in bladder neck surgery. The procedure is more demanding than open colposuspension on the surgeon and the theater team, but is accompanied by the same advantages for the patient as for all other procedures that have been adapted to laparoscopy, namely reduced postoperative pain and faster recuperation.

References

Alcalay M, Monga A, Stanton SL (1994) Burch colposuspension – how long does it cure stress incontinence? *Neurology and Urodynamics* **13(4)**: 495–496.

Burch JC (1961) Urethrovaginal fixation to Cooper's ligament for correction of stress incontinence, cystocele and prolapse. *American Journal of Obstetrics and Gynecology* **81**: 281–290.

Burton G (1997) A three prospective randomised urodynamic study comparing open and laparoscopic colposuspension. *Neurology and Urodynamics* **16(5)**: 353–354.

Cardozo LD, Stanton SL, Williams JB (1979) Detrusor instability following surgery for genuine stress incontinence. *British Journal of Urology* **51**: 204–207.

Elia G, Bergman A (1994) Prospective randomised comparison of three surgical procedures for stress urinary incontinence: five year follow-up. *Neurology and Urodynamics* **13(4)**: 498–500.

Harewood JM (1993) Laparoscopic needle colposuspension for genuine stress incontinence. *Journal of Endourology* **7(4)**: 319–322.

Kiilholma P, Makinen J, Chancellor MB, Pitkanen Y, Hirvonen T (1993) Modified Burch colposuspension for stress urinary incontinence in females. *Surgery, Gynecology and Obstetrics* **176(2)**: 111–115.

Liu CY (1993) Laparoscopic retropubic colposuspension (Burch procedure). A review of 58 cases. *Journal of Reproductive Medicine* **38(7)**: 526–530.

Marshall VF, Marchetti AA, Krantz KE (1949) The correction of stress incontinence by simple vesico-urethral suspension. *Surgery, Gynecology and Obstetrics* **88**: 509–518.

McDougall EM, Klutke CG, Cornell T (1995) Comparison of transvaginal versus laparoscopic bladder neck suspension for stress urinary incontinence. *Urology* **45**: 641–646.

Moschowitz AV (1912) The pathogenesis, anatomy and cure of prolapse of the rectum. *Surgery, Gynecology and Obstetrics* **15**: 7–21.

Ou CS, Presthus J, Beadle E (1993) Laparoscopic bladder neck suspension using hernia mesh and surgical staples. *Journal of Laparoendoscopic Surgery* **3(6)**: 563–566.

Pereyra AJ (1959) A simplified surgical procedure for the correction of stress urinary incontinence in women. *Western Journal of Surgery, Obstetrics and Gynecology* **67**: 223–226.

Polascik TJ, Moore RG, Rosenberg MT, Kavoussi LR (1995) Comparison of laparoscopic and open retropubic urethropexy for treatment of stress urinary incontinence. *Urology* **45(4)**: 647–652.

Shull BL, Baden WF (1989) A six year experience with paravaginal defect repair. *American Journal of Obstetrics and Gynecology* **160**: 1432–1440.

Stamey TA (1973) Endoscopic suspension of the vesical neck for urinary incontinence. *Surgery, Gynecology and Obstetrics* **36**: 547–554.

Vancaillie TG, Schuessler WW (1991) Laparoscopic bladder neck suspension. *Journal of Laparoendoscopic Surgery* **1(3)**: 169–173.

34

Laparoscopic Repair of Enteroceles and Pelvic Floor Support Procedures

C.Y. LIU* AND S. NAIR†

*Chattanooga Women's Laser Center, Tennessee, USA
†Kandang Kerbau Hospital, Singapore

Introduction

As the life expectancy of women in many developed and developing countries has increased so has the prevalence of a variety of pelvic floor relaxation disorders. Our understanding of the pathophysiology of this geriatric degenerative disease that mainly occurs in elderly women is still evolving. Basic vaginal supportive anatomy remains unchanged, but we have, in recent times, realized that there are two concepts pivotal to the understanding and management of pelvic support disorders.

The first is to appreciate the dynamic rather than static nature of the support system embodied in the pelvic floor. The levator ani muscle in the main, and its similarly striated counterparts, when functioning appropriately maintain a constant tone (i.e. active support). In instances of increased intra-abdominal pressure, it contracts as a reflex to increase the resistance and support of the pelvic floor. However, when there is denervation or direct injury to the levator ani muscle during childbirth or due to the constant onslaught of chronic excessive intra-abdominal pressure (e.g. in chronic pulmonary disease or due to frequent lifting and straining activities) the burden of the pelvic support function is laid upon the endopelvic fascia and ligaments that attach the pelvic organs to the pelvic sidewalls (passive support).

The tensile strength of the primarily fibromuscular endopelvic fascia is limited and hence it tends to strain and eventually rupture. This in turn produces defects in the pelvic floor, resulting in the often distressful clinical manifestation of pelvic organ prolapse and urinary and/or fecal incontinence.

This brings us to the second concept – that of the multiple defect approach. It must be understood that the above sequence of events occurs in a global fashion rather than restricted to being only the clinically evident defective component of the pelvic floor. The multiple defect concept has two major implications. In the perioperative evaluation of the patient, the entire pelvic floor must be thoroughly assessed and all defects must be rectified. Isolated repairs result in due course in non-reinforced segments of the pelvic floor being exposed to the inordinate stress of gravity upon the pelvic organs and the repeated episodes of increased intra-abdominal pressure such that further anatomic disruptions occur in the future, requiring additional surgery. A classic example of this is the development of enteroceles, rectoceles and vaginal prolapses after a Burch colposuspension, which are reported to occur in as many as 28% of such patients (Wiskind et al., 1992).

Hence, it appears that if the goal of reconstructive pelvic support surgery is to restore normal function by correcting or, in certain instances, overcorrecting the defects, then it must be a systematic repair of each of these individual defects. A careful assessment of these multiple defects must be carried out preoperatively followed by intraoperative confirmation. In order to do this in an orderly and reproducible manner, the pelvic floor defects can be conveniently divided into three compartments, namely:

- The anterior compartment comprising the urethrocele and cystocele.

- The middle compartment, which manifests as the uterovaginal prolapse.
- The posterior compartment, the defects being the enterocele and rectocele.

Applied Anatomy of Pelvic Floor Support

The pelvic viscera are attached to the pelvic side-walls via the endopelvic fascia. During episodes of increased intra-abdominal pressures the lumbo-sacral lordosis reflects the force vector anteriorly towards the lower abdominal wall and the anterior pelvic wall (i.e. symphysis pubis, pubic bone, obturator internus muscle and arcus tendineus fascia) – the ultimate support of all pelvic organs.

The endopelvic fascia is the fibromuscular continuum of connective tissue that encompasses the vagina and fans out to its peripheral bony and ligamentous attachments. It can be described in thirds by the level of the vaginal canal it supports (Figure 34.1):

- Superiorly it suspends the upper vagina and cervix through the cardinouterosacral ligaments forming the pericervical ring.

- The mid-portion of the vagina attaches to the arcus tendineus fascia of the pelvis anteriorly through the pubocervical fascia and to the medial fascia of the levator ani (iliococcygeus muscles) posteriorly through the rectovaginal septum.
- Inferiorly, the pubocervical fascia blends with the urogenital diaphragm anteriorly and rectovaginal septum fuses with the perineal body and levator ani (puborectalis muscles) posteriorly.

The urogenital diaphragm forms the peripheral attachment of the lateral wall of the vagina and the perineal body to the ischial pubic rami. It is the rectovaginal septum with its attachment to the cardinouterosacral ligaments superiorly and fusing with the perineal body and levator ani inferiorly that supports the cul-de-sac and posterior vagina, preventing enterocele, rectocele and vaginal prolapse.

The levator ani muscle comprises the pronounced pubococcygeus muscle sling and the iliococcygeus muscle that attaches as a sheet to the arcus tendineus fascia of the obturator internus muscle. The levator ani muscle is like a supportive platform for the pelvic viscera and the pubococcygeus 'sling' component compresses and obliterates the urethral,

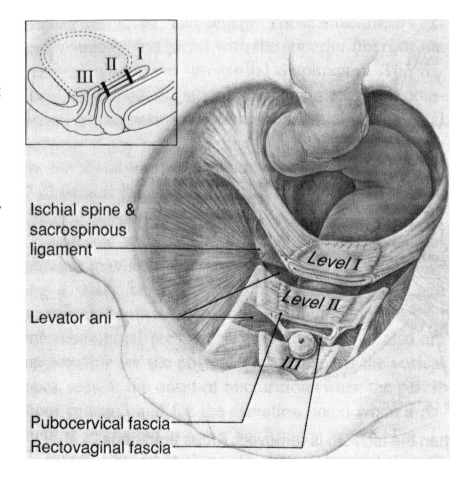

Figure 34.1 Levels of support of the vagina. In level I (suspension), endopelvic fascia suspends the vagina from the lateral pelvic walls. Fibers of level I extend both vertically and also posteriorly toward sacrum. In level II (attachment), the vagina is attached to arcus tendineus fascia pelvis and superior fascia of the levator ani muscles. In level III (fusion), the pubocervical fascia and rectovaginal septum fuse with the urogenital diaphragm anteriorly and perineal body and levator ani posteriorly. (From DeLancey (1992) *American Journal of Obstetrics and Gynecology* **166**: 1717, with permission.)

Ischial spine & sacrospinous ligament

Levator ani

Pubocervical fascia

Rectovaginal fascia

Level I

Level II

III

vaginal and rectal lumina by anterior displacement towards the immobile pubic bone. Hence, in the erect position, the vaginal axis comes to lie in almost a horizontal plane in its upper two-thirds, which rests upon the levator ani muscle.

Preoperative Patient Evaluation

Digital palpation and visual inspection of all pelvic floor defects when the patient is at rest and during straining are crucial for the accurate identification of the defects causing prolapse of pelvic contents through the pelvic floor.

The patient is best placed at a head-up recline of 45–60°, the lower limbs slightly abducted at the hips and flexed at least 90° at the knees in a semi-squatting position with the feet resting upon boot-like foot stirrups (Figure 34.2). A single-blade Sims' speculum is used to retract the anterior or posterior vaginal wall in turn to inspect the opposite wall respectively.

Anterior Compartment Defects

These are assessed by retraction of the posterior wall and noting the location of the urethrovaginal crease and rugosity of the vaginal mucosa. The cystocele can result from three specific anterior wall defects (i.e. the central, lateral and transverse defects).

The central defect is recognized by the loss of vaginal rugosity as the bladder herniates through a tear in the pubocervical fascial hammock. This 'distention' cystocele, as it is sometimes called, leaves only vaginal mucosa and bladder wall or urethral

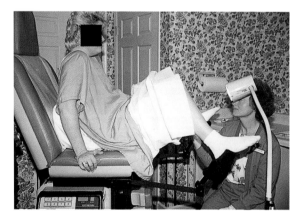

Figure 34.2 Patient's position in the examination room. Patient is in sitting, almost in semi-squat position. An electric-powered examination table is helpful.

mucosa interspersed between the examining finger and a catheter passed through the urethra and placed upon the bladder base.

With the lateral or paravaginal defect, there is detachment of the pubocervical fascia from the pelvic sidewall, resulting in a 'displacement' cystocele. When a patient with a paravaginal defect 'squeezes' her vagina and rectum, there is either slight or absent superolateral movement of the lateral vaginal sulcus, which in normal circumstances is drawn upwards and laterally. An open sponge ring forceps can be used to elevate the lateral vaginal walls, hence mimicking the lateral vaginal support needed to overcome this defect.

The transverse defect does not alter the mobility of the bladder neck, but causes the bladder base to herniate through the point of disruption of the pubocervical fascia from the pericervical ring. Hence, instead of causing urinary stress incontinence, it produces a sense of incomplete voiding.

A distention cystocele can be corrected by a traditional anterior colporrhaphy, but this would be ineffective for a displacement cystocele. Hence, in planning the appropriate reconstructive surgery, these three defects must be differentiated during the preliminary clinical examination.

Posterior Compartment Defects

These comprise the enterocele and the rectocele, which are best assessed by retracting the anterior vaginal wall. The posterior vaginal wall is supported by the rectovaginal septum (Denonvilliers' fascia) and its peripheral attachments.

An enterocele is a hernia through the cul-de-sac that descends between the vagina and rectum. By definition, an enterocele exists when peritoneum of the pelvis contacts the vaginal mucosa directly without an intervening fascial layer. In all true vaginal enteroceles, the primary defect is a break between the upper edge of the rectovaginal septum and the cervix (or vaginal vault) where it normally fuses with the pericervical ring of the fascia and uterosacral ligaments. The upper edge of the rectovaginal septum retracts downward, allowing the enterocele to dissect beneath the vaginal mucosa. As the enterocele descends it may ride over the rectovaginal septum or it may simply push the edge of the rectovaginal septum downward towards the introitus. If the edge is pushed downward, the rectovaginal septum will tear laterally from its attachments to the fascia overlying the iliococcygeus muscle.

An enterocele may or may not be associated with some vaginal vault or uterine prolapse, most often in the post-hysterectomy patient. In vaginal vault prolapse, the vault has separated from the uterosacral ligaments, and when there is an accompanying enterocele there has also been a separation of the upper edge of the rectovaginal septum from the pubocervical fascia of the anterior vaginal wall as well as from the uterosacral ligaments. Although rare, there are instances in which there is vaginal vault prolapse with essentially no associated enterocele.

A defect further down along the recto-vaginal septum manifests itself as the rectocele.

Two-hands rectovaginal examination is mandatory in demonstrating enteroceles and rectoceles. The enterocele occurs as a distinct bulge superior to the rectocele and is accentuated if the patient performs Valsalva's maneuver. By replacing the cervix using a tenaculum or the vaginal apex post-hysterectomy to its normal position, the enterocele can be more clearly demonstrated.

Waters (1946) described a technique by which an enterocele could be differentiated from a rectocele using a bivalve speculum. By drawing the speculum gradually out of the introitus the enterocele is shown to bulge into the vagina. If a finger in the rectum maintains contact with the rectal mucosa throughout the passage of the speculum out of the vagina then there is no rectocele. If, however, the rectal mucosa falls forward into the vagina, and the finger has to be flexed anteriorly to maintain contact, then the finger is at the site of a rectocele. However, in the later sections of this chapter it will be shown that distinction between an enterocele and rectocele is important only in so far as the surgeon must ensure that they are repaired concomitantly. A deficiency of the perineal body allowing normal rectum to bulge into the vagina is a pseudorectocele.

Middle Compartment Defects

These are determined by the location of the cervix or post-hysterectomy, the vaginal apex. Descent of the vaginal apex will often recur after isolated anterior and posterior defect repairs because it is frequently missed when there are voluminous anteroposterior defects.

When there are associated symptoms of urinary leakage, a meticulous history is needed, paying particular attention to the voiding symptoms (urgency, frequency, urge incontinence, nocturnal enuresis and dysuria) and systemic medical or neurologic disorder and medication history. In our practice we have found that urinary incontinence questionnaires and voiding diary are invaluable tools for us to obtain patient's information. The component of

detrusor instability and overflow incontinence must be detected before surgery.

Simple office tests include urinalysis, urine culture, stress and Q-tip test, simple cystometry and residual urine measurement. Formal urodynamics are necessary only if there are deviations in these office tests, if the patient has had failed incontinence surgery or if the patient is elderly (i.e. over 60 years of age) and frail (Liu, 1996a).

Furthermore, during physical examination, particular attention should be paid to determining the integrity of the sensory and motor functions of the S2, S3 and S4 dermatomes, especially if there is total vaginal vault prolapse. The existence of concomitant urinary stress incontinence must be elucidated after reduction of the vault prolapse.

Hence, the rational approach towards the repair of pelvic floor defects is meticulous confirmation of the multi-compartment deficiencies pre- and intra-operatively and then adoption of a surgical strategy that restores each of these individual defects concomitantly. It is incumbent upon gynecologists to realize that the adoption of this strategy to the repair of pelvic floor defects is the rule and not the exception if one is to avoid an epidemic of recurrent vault prolapses after gynecological procedures such as hysterectomies, colposuspensions and pelvic floor defect repairs (Liu, 1996a).

Symptomatology

Other than the appearance of a 'mass' at the introitus causing discomfort and involuntary loss of urine in instances of genuine stress incontinence, the other common symptom, especially with enteroceles is a sensation of 'fullness' within the vaginal area.

Pelvic floor support disorders can inhibit and even prevent normal sexual function. This is a distressing symptom that many women suffer silently and often intentionally omit when seeing the doctor.

The goal of the gynecologist must be to enable the patient to discuss her symptoms and the impact they make on her quality of life openly and comfortably. The physician's task is to elucidate these symptoms in the hope that he or she can relieve the patient's suffering and discomfort.

However, with pelvic floor support disorders, the presence of symptoms alone are an insufficient indication for surgery. As the extent of the defect may not necessarily correlate with the subjective severity of the symptoms, the decision to undergo surgery must originate from the patient and not from the surgeon. Furthermore, the gynecological surgeon must be explicit in outlining the objectives of surgery and dispel any unrealistic expectation of the surgical outcome (Liu, 1996a).

It behoves every gynecologist to acquire the necessary understanding and skills required to effectively correct this albeit non-life-threatening condition that is nearly always profoundly incapacitating and diminishes quality of life.

Laparoscopic Approach

The laparoscopic approach provides many advantages to the surgeon during the intraoperative delineation and repair of pelvic floor deficiencies. The increased intraabdominal pressure of the pnemoperitoneum helps in the intraoperative accentuation and display of all defects, both overt and suspected, during the initial clinical evaluation. There is a magnified and high-resolution image transmitted onto the video screen providing good exposure and heightened visibility, thus enabling accurate dissection and precise preventive hemostasis. It also ensures exact strategic placement of sutures, approximation of tissues without undue tension and avoidance of injury to vital structures such as the large vessels, ureters, rectum and the bladder. Finally, laparoscopy can provide abdominal access without the morbidity of a large incision, enabling the patient more rapid mobility, allowing her to return sooner to her normal life style.

Contraindications

These include contraindications to any form of surgery such as systemic conditions causing low cardiac output or severe emphysema. Hazards more specific to laparoscopy are those related to carbon dioxide (CO_2) gas insufflation. CO_2 is easily absorbed through the peritoneum and patients with poor lung function are less able to exhale excess CO_2, resulting in hypercapnia and acid–base imbalance.

Surgical contraindications include severe concomitant pathology such as extensive adhesions, severe endometriosis or large pelvic masses. However, these situations are relative and depend upon the surgeon's dexterity in handling these pathologies laparoscopically.

Operative Technique

Preliminary Preparation

The patient is placed in a modified lithotomy position with the hips abducted and leveled at 180° to the abdomen so that the thighs do not obstruct the movement of laparoscopic instruments at the lower lateral posts. The knees are flexed to about 90° with the foot resting on boot-like (Allen Medical System, Cleveland, Ohio, USA) stirrups and not supported at the popliteal fossae, as there is a predilection to peroneal nerve pressure injury.

A steep Trendelenburg position is necessary, particularly during enterocele and total vaginal vault prolapse repairs. The bladder is catheterized and when retropubic colposuspension and paravaginal repair are contemplated, about 30 ml of indigo carmine is introduced so that any breach of the bladder wall is recognized by the efflux of blue dye.

An intraumbilical 10 mm trocar is introduced either directly or after initial establishment of a pnemoperitoneum using a Veress needle. If there have been previous laparotomies, access can be gained at Palmer's point along the lower left subcostal margin at the mid-clavicular line via the Veress needle to establish the pneumoperitoneum. Introduction of a 5 mm trocar at the same point through which the laparoscope is passed provides visual access to take down anterior abdominal wall adhesions and facilitate placement of the umbilical trocar.

Secondary trocars could be either a 10 mm suprapubic port (enables introduction of suture needles) and two lower lateral ports at the level of the iliac crests, lateral to the inferior epigastric vessels (Vancaillie and Butler 1993). Alternatively, four secondary ports, two lower ones as above and two other lateral and higher ports, at the level of the umbilicus and along the outer border of the rectus abdominis muscle can also be used (Liu, 1993). It is mandatory that the gynecological surgeon who performs laparoscopic pelvic floor repair is skillful in laparoscopic suturing both extracorporeally using the knot pusher (e.g. Clark–Reich, Marlow Medical, Chicago, Illinois, USA) and intracorporeally with laparoscopic instruments. These procedures are described in Chapter 6.

All visible pathologies such as adhesions and endometriosis can be tackled laparoscopically as can procedures such as adnexectomy and hysterectomy where indicated. The entire pelvic floor is then carefully surveyed through the laparoscope, with assessment by concomitant digital vaginal palpation to determine the extent and laxity of the tissue defects.

Posterior defects such as an enterocele and vaginal vault prolapse are repaired laparoscopically before anterior defect repairs (i.e. retropubic colposuspension and paravaginal repairs) as the former are difficult to perform once the anterior defects are repaired. The low rectocele repair and perineorraphy is best performed vaginally. We believe that ureteral identification and dissection are important in preventing ureteral injury in this form of surgery and should be routinely carried out before the start of any extensive pelvic reconstructive procedure (Figure 34.3).

Laparoscopic Enterocele Repair

This procedure is often indicated as a prelude to retropubic colposuspension where the cul-de-sac is prophylactically obliterated to prevent the future occurrence of an enterocele.

Moschcowitz (1912) proposed to obliterate the cul-de-sac to repair and/or prevent enteroceles by placing purse-string sutures through the peritoneum of the cul-de-sac. However, this procedure proved to be ineffective for either preventing or repairing enteroceles as peritoneum does not provide any supporting role and can be stretched endlessly. Laparoscopically; for the prevention of an enterocele before retropubic colposuspension, we use the modified Moschcowitz procedure by placing nonabsorbable permanent sutures deep into the wall of the cul-de-sac to include the medial fascia of the levator ani (iliococcygeus muscle) on both pelvic sidewalls and rectovaginal septum on the posterior vaginal wall. These sutures should also include the peritoneum on both channels of the rectosigmoid colon, but avoid the serosal layer of the rectosigmoid colon. These sutures begin at the lowermost extent of the pouch of Douglas and continue cephalad until the entire cul-de-sac is obliterated. The uppermost sutures must also include the uterosacrocardinal ligaments and the rectovaginal septum. Special care must be paid to avoid injuring or kinking the ureters during the placement of these last sutures.

For laparoscopical enterocele repair, the apex of the vagina must be pushed upward with the vaginal probe. Dissection is carried downward from the vaginal apex along both the anterior and posterior vaginal walls until the edges of the pubocervical fascia anteriorly and the rectovaginal septum posteriorly are accurately identified. The enterocele sac of the peritoneum is dissected free and excised. The excess vaginal mucosa has to be trimmed if the enterocele is large. The rectovaginal septum is reattached to the uterosacral ligaments and, in the post-hysterectomy patient, to the pubocervical fascia. Traditional standard operations such as Moschcowitz, Halban and McCall culdoplasty will sometimes indirectly accomplish repair of a small enterocele. However, it is far better to identify the anatomic defects and repair them with either concentric purse-strings or interrupted anteroposterior closure stitches. It should be emphasized that the use of permanent suture material is desirable.

The operative maneuvers described so far for enterocele repair are almost never performed in isolation from the repair of other pelvic floor defects. Enteroceles, especially of the pulsion type, may coexist with a vaginal vault prolapse. The correction of such massive eversion of the vagina involves some form of vaginal vault suspension, which is

Figure 34.3 Ureteral identification and dissection before extensive pelvic floor reconstruction is crucial in preventing ureteral injury.

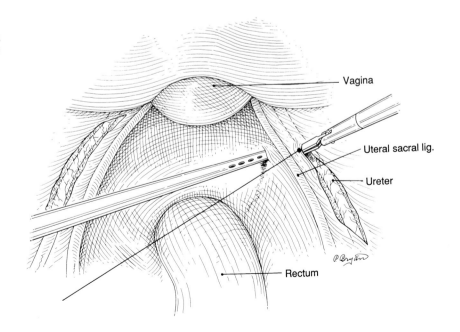

just part of the total reconstruction of the pelvic floor necessary for restoring the normal vaginal anatomy and function. The procedures that are described below for vaginal vault suspension must be preceded by an enterocele repair. The enterocele repair itself facilitates the natural progression to the surgery of vaginal vault suspension.

Laparoscopic Vaginal Vault Suspension

In order to understand the mechanics of laparoscopic vaginal vault suspension (Figure 34.4), the surgeon has to grasp the concept that the supports of the vaginal vault can be described as three tiers, each supporting one-third segments of the vaginal tube (DeLancey, 1992). The components of each level are described earlier in this chapter in the discussion on the applied anatomy of pelvic support.

The description of the surgery for vaginal vault suspension would logically conform to the three natural levels of vaginal support. The support of the upper third of the vagina can be reconstituted by either of three alternatives:

- High McCall vaginal vault suspension.
- Sacrospinous vaginal fixation.
- Sacrocolpopexy.

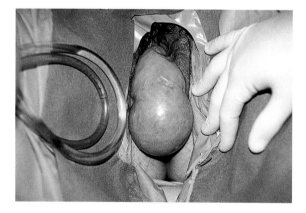

Figure 34.4 Total genital procidentia with complete vaginal eversion.

LAPAROSCOPIC HIGH McCALL VAGINAL VAULT SUSPENSION

In this procedure, the disrupted ends of the uterosacral ligaments are identified by applying cephalad traction to the rectosigmoid. Using a vaginal probe to gently displace the vagina toward the sacrum, the level along the uterosacral ligament to which the vagina vault apex extends is identified. Both ureters must be clearly displayed from the pelvic brim to the deep pelvis hence, isolating the uterosacral ligaments and keeping the ureters out of the way.

Using a number 2 Gortex suture on a CV-0 needle (WL Gore & Associates, Phoenix, AZ, USA) or other permanent suture, the uterosacral ligaments are consecutively plicated, the first purse-string suture being applied 2 cm caudad to the existing enterocele suture. The plication includes the rectovaginal septum and the peritoneum of both pararectal fossae. Similarly a second and a third such purse-string sutures are passed through the uterosacral ligaments about 1.5–2 cm above the first suture (Figure 34.5). The last suture, which is most proximal to the sacral insertion of the uterosacral ligaments, must be applied without undue tension upon the vagina nor constriction over the sigmoid colon. This type of reconstruction provides the most physiological suspension of the vaginal vault.

LAPAROSCOPIC SACROSPINOSUS VAGINAL FIXATION

This technique is essentially a laparovaginal procedure (Figure 34.6). The surgeon palpates the ischial spines and the sacrospinosus ligaments transvaginally, thus identifying laparoscopically the location of these landmarks. The peritoneum overlying the right sacrospinosus ligament is opened and loose areolar tissue lying between the peritoneum and sacrospinosus ligament is dissected down toward the sacrospinosus ligament. The sacrospinosus ligament can be readily identified. Using a number 2 Gortex or equivalent permanent suture, the needle is driven into the sacrospinosus ligaments 2–3 cm medial to the ischial spine so as not to injure the pudendal neurovascular bundle. Two throws of the sutures are applied both to the sacrospinosus ligaments and the superolateral posterior aspect of the vaginal vault, which includes the rectovaginal septum, but not yet breaching the vaginal mucosa. Extracorporeal ligatures are passed down using the Clark–Reich (Marlow Medical, Chicago, Illinois, USA) knot pusher while the assisting surgeon tends to gently approximate the vagina flush with the sacrospinosus ligament. A rectal probe is essential to displace the rectum laterally off to the left side and out of the way during contralateral pararectal dissection to expose the ischial spine and sacrospinosus ligaments for safe suture placement.

LAPAROSCOPIC SACROCOLPOPEXY

This procedure is associated with significant morbidity even when done abdominally, the most alarming complication being life-threatening hemorrhage due to injury of the presacral vessels when applying sutures to anchor the suspensory graft (autologous or synthetic) to the presacral ligaments

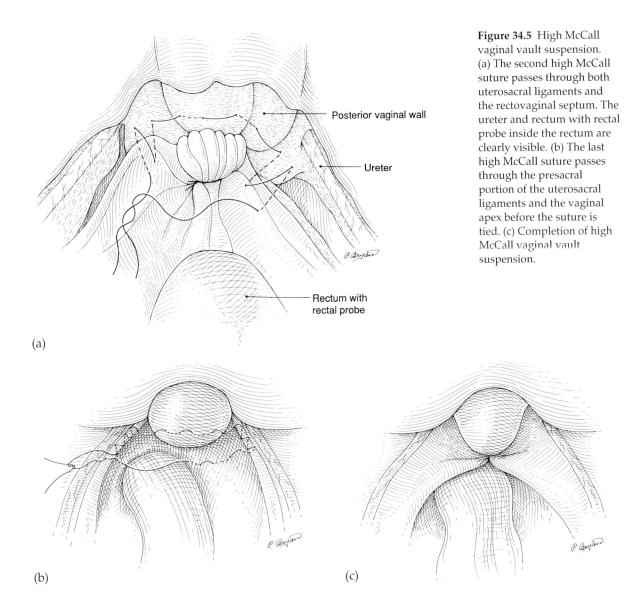

Posterior vaginal wall

Ureter

Rectum with
rectal probe

(a)

(b)

(c)

Figure 34.5 High McCall vaginal vault suspension. (a) The second high McCall suture passes through both uterosacral ligaments and the rectovaginal septum. The ureter and rectum with rectal probe inside the rectum are clearly visible. (b) The last high McCall suture passes through the presacral portion of the uterosacral ligaments and the vaginal apex before the suture is tied. (c) Completion of high McCall vaginal vault suspension.

(Sutton *et al.*, 1981). Furthermore, there have been reports of graft rejection and extrusion through the vagina, detachment of the graft from the vagina and rupture of the posterior vaginal wall distal to the attachment of the graft to the vagina (Addison *et al.*, 1989). There is also a higher risk of infection especially because of the more extensive dissection required and the presence of a foreign body.

Nevertheless, sacrocolpopexy is useful when the vagina is too short to be brought to the ischial spine. A probe in the vagina is used to reduce the prolapse and put limited tension on the vaginal apex so that the peritoneal investments can be reflected off to expose the pubocervical fascia and the rectovaginal septum. The bladder is dissected off from the pubocervical fascia, as is the rectum from the rectovaginal septum, thus denuding a 3–4 cm length of vagina. The sigmoid colon is then deflected to the left exposing the hollow of the sacrum just below the promontory. The presacral peritoneum is incised sagittally down towards the vagina with a

rightward extension to avoid the sigmoid colon. Dissection of the areolar tissue over the presacral space exposes the longitudinal presacral ligaments. Extreme caution must be exercised during this stage of the procedure where meticulous avoidance and/or hemostasis of the presacral vessels and delineation of the right ureter averts possible injury to these structures.

Recently, it has become customary to use synthetic materials such as Mercilene or Gortex mesh (2.5 cm by 10 cm) (W.L. Gore, Flagstaff, Arizona) introduced intra-abdominally through a 10 mm trocar. Multiple and substantial vaginal sutures to anchor one end of the mesh to the anterior and posterior aspects of the vagina vault is mandatory to produce a secure graft-to-vagina attachment. The other end of the graft is sutured in a similar fashion to the longitudinal ligaments of the sacrum, extreme care being taken to clearly visualize and avoid the presacral vessels. The vaginal probe is adjusted so that the vaginal apex is directed towards the hollow of the sacrum without

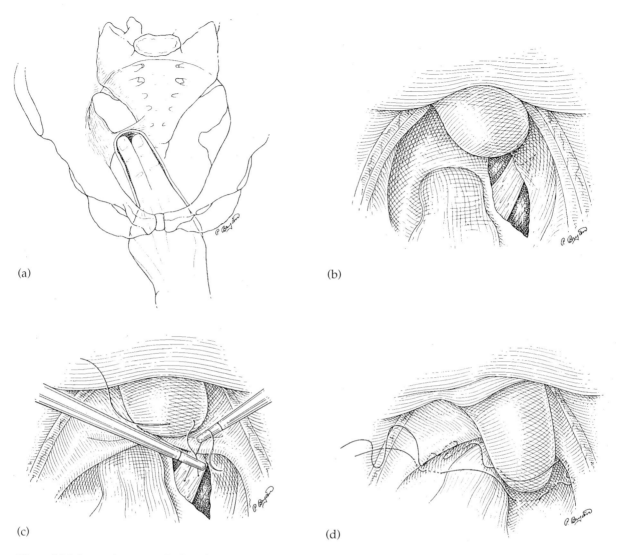

(a)

(b)

(c)

(d)

Figure 34.6 Sacrospinosus vaginal vault suspension. (a) Surgeon's fingers inside the vagina palpate the ischial spine and sacrospinosus ligament while viewing the examining fingers through the laparoscope. (b) The peritoneum overlying the sacrospinosus ligament is opened either transversely or longitudinally and the loose areolar tissue is dissected out towards the sacrospinosus ligament. (c) Sutures are placed through the posterior wall of the vagina just below the apex and pass through the sacrospinosus ligament away from the ischial spine. (d) The apex of the vagina is pushed against the sacrospinosus ligament while the surgeon ties the sutures to prevent any gap between the vagina and sacrospinosus ligament.

undue tension. Meticulous reperitonealization is achieved, taking care to conceal the entire graft to avoid dense adhesion formation between it and loops of intestine.

COMPARISON OF THE THREE TECHNIQUES FOR REPAIRING UPPER THIRD VAGINAL VAULT SUSPENSION

In comparing the above three techniques, the laparoscopic sacrocolpopexy is the most technically demanding and carries the highest risk of serious morbidity. The limitation of sacrospinous fixation, however, is its inadequacy to suspend the vagina in an android or anthropoid pelvis. Here, the sacrospinous to introitus distance is short, hence,

causing shortening of the vagina. It also carries the risk of pudendal neurovascular injury during suture placement. It appears therefore that the high McCall is the least complex yet most physiological in retaining the vagina in a midline and horizontal position (which is not quite obtainable even with sacrospinous fixation) with the added benefit of a satisfactory vaginal depth (Liu, 1996d).

Technique for Repairing the Middle Third of the Vagina Support

The supports of the middle third of the vagina comprise the pubocervical fascia anteriorly and the rectovaginal septum posteriorly.

When the pubocervical fascia is separated from its lateral attachment to the arcus tendineus fascia of the pelvis, a paravaginal defect occurs. This type of defect is the primary etiology of the cystourethrocele accounting for more than 80% of all such cases. The other types of defects (central and transverse) have been described earlier. When a paravaginal defect causes urethral hypermobility the patient will exhibit stress urinary incontinence (SUI). About 90% of patients with paravaginal defects also present with urinary stress incontinence (Liu, 1996). The paravaginal repair will be described later along with the retropubic colposuspension.

Posteriorly, the rectovaginal septum may be detached from the medial fascia of iliococcygeus muscle of the pelvic sidewall or has a midline tear secondary to poor healing of an old episiotomy wound. Such lateral and midline defects would result in a rectocele. It is possible to repair these pararectal and midline defects of the rectovaginal septum laparoscopically, but accessibility into the depths of the pelvis require expert laparoscopic suturing skill. Repair of the rectovaginal septum for the more caudad defects near the perineal body is best tackled vaginally.

Technique for Repairing the Lower Third Vaginal Suspension

Anteriorly, the laparoscopic paravaginal repair (see below) enables the periphery of the lower vagina to be secured onto the most caudal margin of the arcus tendineus fascia of the pelvis. Posteriorly, the rectovaginal septum is reconstituted into the medical fasciae of the puborectalis muscles and the perineal body along with a perineorrhaphy where necessary.

It should be emphasized that normally puborectalis muscles are about 2 cm apart at this level and midline plication of these muscles in the traditional posterior colporrhaphy is unphysiological and may cause discomfort and even dyspareunia for the patient postoperatively.

The recent evidence obtained from defecographic and magnetic resonance imaging (MRI) studies of patients with rectoceles seems to indicate that the vast majority of rectoceles are of low rectoceles with a transverse defect (the rectovaginal septum detaches from the perineal body). Therefore, the logical way to repair rectoceles is vaginally.

LAPAROSCOPIC PARAVAGINAL SUSPENSION

The anterior wall of the middle third of the vagina gains its support through the peripheral attachment of the pubocervical fascia to the arcus tendineus fascia of pelvis of the obturator interae muscles on the lateral pelvic walls. The pubocervical fascia acts as a hammock or backstop that enables the bladder neck and proximal urethra to be compressed close anteroposteriorly during increased intra-abdominal pressure. As described earlier in this chapter, pubocervical fascial defects that cause cystourethroceles can be divided into four different types: namely, paravaginal, transverse, midline and distal defects (Richardson, 1990).

The pubocervical fascia can rupture within itself producing a central defect in the 'hammock'. This causes the bladder to balloon out through this breach. If it occurs at the bladder neck, this also manifests as stress incontinence. To repair this defect, the peripheral edges of the tear must be carefully isolated by undermining the pubocervical fascia from the vagina to obtain accurate approximation of the defect. The traditional method of anterior colporrhaphy can produce a secure repair of this defect.

Yet another central but more cephalad defect occurs when the pubocervical fascia separates from the pericervical ring that spans into the cardinal and uterosacral ligaments. Here the base of the bladder herniates into the anterior vaginal fornix and forms a pure cystocele without displacing the urethral or urethrovesical junction. Hence, these patients do not experience urinary stress incontinence, but have problems completely emptying the bladder. Transverse defects can occur with the paravaginal defect, which is the separation of the pubocervical fascia from the arcus tendineus fascia of the pelvis of the lateral pelvic wall, particularly in cases of total vaginal prolapse. Paravaginal defects can occur unilaterally or bilaterally and are frequently associated with the clinical symptoms of urinary stress incontinence.

To perform a laparoscopic paravaginal suspension, the patient is prepared as described earlier. An 18–20 French Foley catheter with a 30 ml balloon tip is then inserted into the bladder. The bladder is then emptied and approximately 30 ml of concentrated indigo carmine dye is instilled into the bladder and the catheter is clamped. This is done so that inadvertent perforation of the bladder can be easily recognized through the efflux of the blue dye. A transverse incision is made across the parietal peritoneum about 2 cm above the symphysis pubis and is then extended laterally to just within the two lateral umbilical ligaments. Careful dissection with meticulous hemostasis of the parietal peritoneum away from the anterior abdominal wall towards the pubic bone enables the surgeon to enter the retropubic space without undue 'blood staining' of the tissues. Dissection is carried out in the areolar tissue plane to display the symphysis pubis, the obturator foramen and the obturator neurovascular bundle, and more laterally the vaginal sulci as it detaches from the arcus tendineus fascia of the pelvis and all the way to the ischial spine. Fastidious removal of the paravaginal fat is desirable as it promotes fibrosis and scar formation in the paravaginal area for ultimate adherence of the vagina to the lateral pelvic wall.

The shining gleam of the pubocervical fascia, exposed as a vaginal 'cone', is formed by external digital elevation of the vagina lateral to the bladder. The bladder is reflected medially and permanent sutures such as 2 '0' prolene are used to suture the superior lateral sulci of the vagina to the arcus tendineus fascia of the pelvis. In order to avoid the prominent vasculature of the periurethral plexus, a full thickness stitch in a figure of '8' can be applied, not only to get a good anchoring point onto the vagina, but also as a hemostatic maneuver. These interrupted sutures are applied as a longitudinal array. With the operator's finger inside the vagina as a guide to the vaginal suture placement, the first suture anchors the upper lateral vaginal sulcus to the arcus tendineus fascia of the pelvis, beginning close to the ischial spine, and thereafter, consecutively ventral towards the symphysis pubis. Although it is ideal to apply the first suture through the arcus tendineus fascia as close to the level of the ischial spine as possible, a safety distance of at least 1 cm ventral to the ischial spine must be maintained to avoid injuring the pudendal neurovascular bundle as it passes through the pudendal canal. (Figure 34.7)

After meticulous hemostasis by either bipolar coagulation or application of sutures, the entire retropubic space is thoroughly irrigated with copious amounts of Ringer's lactate solution. The peri-

toneal defect is closed with an absorbable suture and cystoscopy is performed to ensure that no suture has traversed through the bladder wall. Intravenous administration of indigo carmine dye results in its efflux through the ureteric orifices, hence confirming that there has not been any kinking or obstruction of the ureters.

Careful vaginal examination should be performed at the completion of the paravaginal repair. If the surgeon feels that additional support is needed to the urethro-vesical (U-V) junction and proximal urethra or there is coexisting severe stress urinary incontinence, a retropubic Burch-type colposuspension should be performed as well.

Laparoscopic Retropubic Colposuspension

It has been shown that in comparison to the needle bladder neck suspension, Burch colposuspension and vaginal anterior colporraphies for the treatment of stress urinary incontinence, the Burch procedure was superior and had the most impressive long-term results (Bergman and Elia, 1995).

The operation is begun in the similar way as described for the paravaginal suspension. However, the critical landmarks such as the iliopectineal or Cooper's ligament, the obturator canal and the aberrant obturator vessels along with the obturator neurovascular bundle should be clearly identified. Subsequent dissection of the paravaginal fat is undertaken as described for the paravaginal suspension. The bladder is mobilized medially and shining white pubocervical fascia is identified. Sutures are applied at the level of the midurethral and the urethrovesical junction, 2 cm lateral to these structures in order to avoid

Figure 34.7 Paravaginal repair. The first suture is placed approximately 1–1.5 cm caudad to the ischial spine to avoid injury to the pudendal neurovascular bundle; 5–6 interrupted figure of eight sutures are usually required in each side of the pelvis.

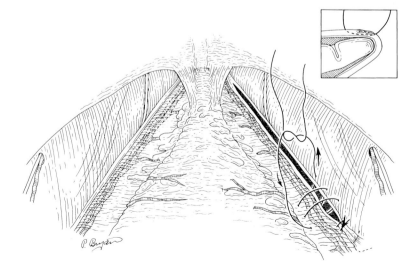

compromising the urethral sphincteric mechanism. Double bites of vaginal tissue are taken for more secure anchorage either using 1 '0' Ethibond (Ethicon, Somerville, NJ, USA) or 2 '0' Gortex (W.L. Gore, Flagstaff, Arizona) followed by the passage of the needle and sutures through a point in the ileopectineal ligament directly adjacent to the vaginal anchor point. The anterior vaginal wall is tented to produce a vaginal core bilaterally, thus elevating the vagina towards the ileopectineal ligaments, but without undue tension because it is unnecessary to have surface approximation of these two points of anchorage. Ethibond or Gortex sutures are applied on each side of the mid-urethra and bladder neck with the ligatures passed down using a Clark-Reich knot pusher (Figure 34.8). Hemostasis is secured using further sutures and/or bipolar coagulation. The operative site is irrigated with Ringer's lactate and a suprapubic catheter is inserted under direct vision into the bladder. Cystoscopy is useful in ensuring that no sutures have traversed the bladder and the efflux of intravenously administered indigo carmine dye through the ureteric orifices ensures the surgeon that no ureteric obstruction or kinking has occurred. Reperitonealization is performed as described earlier for the paravaginal suspension.

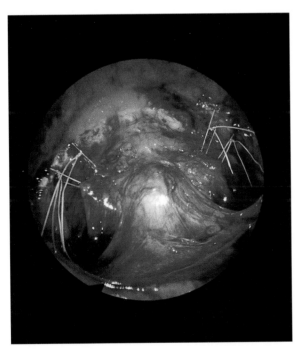

Figure 34.8 Burch colposuspension. Two sutures with permanent material, double looped into the anterior vaginal wall and passed through the ipsilateral side of Cooper's ligament on each side of urethra, creating a hammock like support for the U-V junction and proximal urethra.

Another laparoscopic approach to the retropubic suspension is the use of a strip of polypropylene and surgical staples (Ou *et al.*, 1993). Polypropylene mesh promotes tissue ingrowth and adds strength and support for long-term results. It is less technically demanding than suturing and hence makes it a more reproducible procedure for the majority of gynecologists. A prospective study of 69 women randomly assigned to two groups, namely the suture group or the mesh–staple group showed that at least in the first year, both methods were equally effective in curing the stress incontinence (Ross, 1996). However, a longer follow-up period is required before there can be wide-scale adoption of the mesh–staple technique.

Postoperative Care

The great advantage of the laparoscopic approach in performing pelvic floor reconstruction, whether a retropubic Burch colposuspension or a total vaginal suspension, is that the patient requires very little analgesia and becomes mobile very quickly after the operation, so can be discharged within 1–2 days of surgery. In cases where a Burch colposuspension has been performed, patients can be discharged with a suprapubic catheter, which is removed once the residual urine measurements are less than 50 ml. Patients who have undergone this kind of surgery tend to be well enough to resume their routine activities quite quickly. However, for this reason, the surgeon must instruct the patients to limit their activities to less strenuous activities for at least three months following surgery to allow time for fibrosis and scar tissue formation to provide the necessary strengthening of the reconstructed pelvic support. It is also important for the gynecologist to counsel the patient to avoid sexual intercourse for a customary six-week period in order to allow preliminary healing.

Conclusion

The laparoscopic approach has been shown to be eminently successful, at least in the short term, in enabling gynecologists to efficiently repair nearly all pelvic floor defects (Liu, 1993, 1996; Vancaillie 1993). The complication rates in these initial series has not been shown to be greater than that expected for the open approaches.

Aside from providing excellent laparoscopic visualization of the pelvic floor defects, the heightened positive intra-abdominal pressure created by the pneumoperitoneum makes the less obvious pelvic defects more prominent. Along with digital vaginal examination the surgeon is not only able to confirm the preoperative findings, but also systematically repair all existing but covert defects. At the conclusion of the entire procedure, laparoscopic visualization with digital vaginal confirmation ensures the surgeon that all defects have been repaired.

The repair of pelvic floor defects is one of the most intriguing areas in laparoscopic surgery and we are at present in the phase of evolution, allowing great latitude for innovation in this new territory. Pelvic surgeons would readily admit that our perception of the dynamic support of the pelvic floor is as yet in its embryonic phase. The future is therefore in understanding the neurophysiology and the biophysics of the pelvic floor and its supporting structures and to derive efficient strategies to prevent or rejuvenate pelvic support functions.

The ultimate answer to the prevention and if possible the reversal of the destructive changes that take its toll on the pelvic floor support mechanisms lie in understanding the genetics of this neuro-muscular connective tissue 'disease'. This aspect is unfortunately lacking in our present understanding of degenerative diseases. Until there are genetic and/or biochemical interventions to counter these support disorders gynecological surgeons interested and committed in relieving the symptoms of women with these disorders must endeavor to understand the principles of and acquire the surgical skills necessary for the management of pelvic support disorders. There must be a total rethink of the traditional concepts governing pelvic relaxation and its surgical correction. We must attempt to reassess the way in which we perform a vaginal hysterectomy, abdominal hysterectomy and pelvic relaxation surgery and objectively scrutinize the outcomes of our surgery to ascertain whether or not some of the later sequelae of unnoticed and untreated pelvic floor defects can be avoided by preventive surgical maneuvers.

References

Addison WA, Timmons MC, Wall LL *et al.* (1989) Failed abdominal sacral colpopexy: observations and recommendations. *Obstetrics and Gynecology* 74: 480.

Bergman A, Elia G (1995) Three surgical procedures for genuine stress incontinence: Five-year follow-up of a prospective randomized study. *American Journal of Obstetrics and Gynecology* 173: 66–71.

Bergman A, Ballard CA, Koonings PV (1989) Primary stress urinary incontinence and pelvic relaxation: prospective randomised comparison of three different operations. *American Journal of Obstetrics and Gynecology* 161: 97–101.

DeLancey JOL (1992) Anatomic causes of vaginal prolapse after hysterectomy. *American Journal of Obstetrics and Gynecology* 166: 1717–1728.

Holly RL (1994) Enterocele: A review. *Obstetrical and Gynecological Survey* 49(4): 284–293.

Liu CY (1993) Laparoscopic retropubic colposuspension: A review of 58 cases. *Journal of Reproductive Medicine* 38: 526–530.

Liu CY (1996a) Anatomy and clinical evaluation of pelvic floor defects. In Liu CY (ed.) *Laparoscopic Hysterectomy and Pelvic Floor Construction*. pp. 299–312. Massachusetts: Blackwell Science.

Liu CY (1996b) Laparoscopic cystocele repair: paravaginal suspension. In Liu CY (ed.) *Laparoscopic Hysterectomy and Pelvic Floor Construction*. pp. 330–340. Massachusetts: Blackwell Science.

Liu CY (1996c) Laparoscopic retropubic colposuspension. In Liu CY (ed.) *Laparoscopic Hysterectomy and Pelvic Floor Construction*. pp. 313–329. Massachusetts: Blackwell Science.

Liu CY (1996d) Laparoscopic vaginal vault suspension. In Liu CY (ed.) *Laparoscopic Hysterectomy and Pelvic Floor Construction*. pp. 349–365. Massachusetts: Blackwell Science.

Liu CY, Paek WS (1993) Laparoscopic retropubic colposuspension (Burch procedure). *Journal of the American Association of Gynecologic Laparoscopists* 1: 31–35.

Moschcowitz AV (1912) The pathogenesis, anatomy and care of prolapse of the rectum. *Surgery, Gynecology and Obstetrics* 15: 7.

Nichols DH, Randall CL (1989) *Vaginal Surgery*, 3rd edition. pp. 313–317. Baltimore: William and Wilkins.

Ou CS, Presthus J, Beadle E (1993) Laparoscopic bladder neck suspension using hernia mesh and surgical staples. *Journal of Laparoendoscopic Surgery* 3: 563–556.

Richardson AC (1990) How to correct prolapse paravaginally. *Contemporary Obstetrics and Gynecology* 35: 100–114.

Ross J (1996) Two techniques of laparoscopic Burch repair for stress incontinence: A prospective, randomised study. Presented at the 25th Annual Scientific Meeting, American Association of Gynecological Laparoscopists, Chicago, Illinois. October, 1996.

Sutton GP, Addison WA, Livengood CH, Hammond CB (1981) Life-threatening hemorrhage complicating sacral colpopexy. *American Journal of Obstetrics and Gynecology* 140: 836.

Vancaillie TG, Butler DJ (1993) Laparoscopic enterocele repair – description of a new technique. *Gynecological Endoscopy* 2: 211–216.

Waters EG (1946) A diagnostic technique for the detection of enterocele. *American Journal of Obstetrics and Gynecology* 53: 810.

Wiskind AK, Creighton SM, Stanton SL (1992) The incidence of prolapse after the Burch colposuspension. *American Journal of Obstetrics and Gynecology* 167: 399–405.

Zacharin RF (1992) Use of vaginal skin graft in posterior colporrhaphia. *Australian and New Zealand Journal of Obstetrics and Gynaecology* 32: 146.

Laparoscopic Surgery for Endometriosis and Adhesions

35

Diagnosis of Endometriosis: Laparoscopic Appearances

JOHN A. ROCK and SUJATHA REDDY

Emory University School of Medicine, Atlanta, USA

Introduction

Endometriosis is a condition affecting women in the reproductive age group. Signs of endometriosis may be evident on physical examination. Rectovaginal examination is essential to identify tender nodularity of the uterosacral ligaments. If endometriosis infiltrates the rectovaginal septum, patients may present with dyschezia or cyclic rectal bleeding. Endometriosis has been identified on the vulva, at the umbilicus, and in episiotomy scars. Complete ureteral obstruction has been reported. This can be temporarily reversed by the administration of danazol or gonadotropin releasing hormone (GnRH) agonists (Rivlin, 1990). Lesions involving the diaphragm can lead to chronic and recurrent pneumothorax at the time of menstruation. Lesions have been found in the upper and lower extremities, the pericardium and the lung.

The correlation between endometriosis and both infertility and pain is well documented, but several aspects of this disease, including the pathophysiology and the most effective treatment, are not well understood. Current treatment modalities are based upon the premise that removal of endometriotic lesions will increase a patient's fecundity (Adamson *et al.*, 1993) or decrease her pain (Sutton *et al.*, 1994). The importance of a comprehensive understanding of the various appearances of endometriosis cannot be understated, for effective surgical treatment cannot be achieved if the presence of the disease is not appreciated.

A non-invasive method to diagnose endometriosis is not currently available. CA-125, a complex membrane glycoprotein, has been shown to be elevated in some patients with endometriosis. Unfortunately it is neither sensitive enough nor specific enough to be used for screening or diagnosis. CA-125 in conjunction with painful nodularity on pelvic examination (done during menstruation) has been shown to have a specificity of 80–90%, but its sensitivity is about 40% (Koninckx *et al.*, 1996).

The skill of the surgeon is crucial to the accurate recognition of endometriosis. Use of the laparoscope has dramatically increased over the last couple of decades. Virtually all gynecologists use laparoscopic surgery if only to perform tubal sterilization.

Removal of ectopic endometriotic tissue is essential for the successful treatment of endometriosis. The natural history of endometriosis remains unclear. The disease, if untreated, is thought to progress. Pregnancy has been thought to induce a 'remission' of endometriosis. McArthur and Ulfelder (1965) reported a variable effect of pregnancy on endometriosis. In the 24 patients they studied, more patients experienced disease persistence than permanent regression. Treatment of endometriosis involves two steps:

- Visualization of endometriosis.
- Subsequent removal of the lesion.

The surgeon who does not routinely perform laparoscopic surgery will certainly diagnose typical endometriotic lesions, but risks missing a substantial amount of subtle endometriosis. Even an experienced laparoscopic surgeon who has treated hundreds of patients with endometriosis can miss (7%) or underdiagnose (50%) a substantial number of patients (Martin *et al.*, 1989). This level of diagnostic accuracy may reflect the diagnostic ability of a small group of physicians with a special interest in the laparoscopic diagnosis and treatment of endometriosis. The diagnostic sensitivity of all groups of physicians using laparoscopic surgery correlates with the number of procedures performed. The physicians with the least number of cases, correctly identified endometriosis by visual identification in only 41% of the cases while physicians with the greatest caseload displayed a sensitivity of 86% (Martin *et al.*, 1990).

Analysis of normal-appearing peritoneum with the scanning electron microscope has demonstrated endometriosis in up to 25% of cases (Murphy *et al.*, 1986). Histologically, endometriosis has been shown in 13% of normal-appearing peritoneum samples from patients with endometriosis and in 6% of normal appearing peritoneum samples taken from patients without endometriosis (Nisolle *et al.*, 1990).

Systematic Approach to Evaluation of the Pelvis

The laparoscopic surgeon should adhere to a systematic and meticulous method of evaluating the pelvis to assure complete diagnosis of endometriosis. Small endometriotic lesions may become more visible just before or during menses. Similarly, laparoscopy performed during suppression of ovarian steroidogenesis by danazol or GnRH agonists may lead to an inaccurate assessment of disease extent (Evers, 1987). Before initiation of laparoscopy, a single-tooth tenaculum is attached to the anterior lip of the cervix and an intrauterine cannula is placed into the uterus to allow the uterine displacement needed to visualize the posterior uterus and the uterosacral ligaments. Alternatively, a Humi cannula (Unimer, Wilton, Connecticut, USA) may be inserted. Following placement of the laparoscope and a suprapubic 5 mm probe, the surgeon should be careful not to rub the peritoneum with the probe while manipulating the pelvic organs. This can traumatize the peritoneum and cause micro-bleeding, which is easily confused with atypical endometriosis. An aggressive bimanual examination should be avoided for the same reason.

The laparoscope affords the surgeon the capability of minifying or magnifying the field of view, depending upon the proximity of the laparoscope to the tissue. Murphy (1992) details the correlation of the operating distance and the degree of magnification for several of the commonly used laparoscopes (Table 35.1). An increased operating distance

results in minification and a panoramic view, which provides an excellent overview of the pelvis, but is not appropriate for diagnostic purposes. Near-contact laparoscopy with the resulting magnification has been suggested as the method of choice for meticulous analysis of the peritoneum for subtle abnormalities (Redwine, 1987a).

The development of high-resolution monitors and video cameras allows the surgeon to perform operative laparoscopy while standing up and viewing the monitor rather than bending over for the entire case peering directly through the laparoscope. There is some compromise in resolution, even with the best camera and monitor, in comparison with direct vision. Thus, evaluation of peritoneal abnormalities should be verified by direct visualization with the surgeon's eye to increase the sensitivity in detecting subtle lesions.

The upper abdomen including the right paracolic gutter, the liver, gallbladder, left paracolic gutter and the appendix should be assessed to rule out significant pathology before focusing on the pelvis. A panoramic view provides a general assessment of the pelvis. A detailed inspection of the pelvis is achieved under magnification with the laparoscope in close proximity to the peritoneum. Occasionally the surgeon may find an adherent mass in the posterior cul-de-sac or attached to the posterior uterus. Release of the adhesions that make up this mass can result in the release of dark red or chocolate-colored fluid. Adhesions should be removed to allow an optimal view of the peritoneal surfaces. The anterior compartment is evaluated with the assistant elevating the intrauterine cannula, displacing the uterus posteriorly. The anterior uterus, bladder flap, abdominal wall, appendix and both round ligaments are visually inspected. Adhesions are more likely to involve the left adnexa than the right as a result of the position of the sigmoid colon. The right fallopian tube, and ovary are inspected for the pres-

Table 35.1 Hopkins' laparoscope: 10 mm with 3 mm operating channel. (Reproduced with permission from Murphy, 1992).

Working Distance	Magnification		
	Wolf*	Olympus*	Storz*
3 mm	–	8.2	10
5 mm	–	5.7	6
10 mm	3.19	3.2	3
15 mm	–	2.2	2
20 mm	1.71	1.7	1.5
30 mm	–	1.2	1
50 mm	0.73	0.7	0.6

*Personal communication

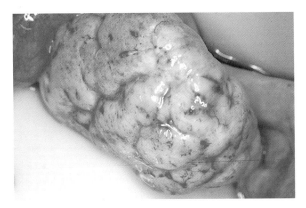

Figure 35.1 Red lesions and adhesions on ovarian surface.

ence of endometriosis and adhesions as adhesions may also represent endometriosis (Figure 35.1). The fallopian tubes are generally free of gross disease and are patent. An increase in the size of the ovary should alert the surgeon to the possibility of the presence of an endometrioma. These are rarely larger than 10 cm, and develop over several months as a result of intracystic hemorrhage. Care must be taken during elevation of the ovary to avoid traumatizing the peritoneum overlying the broad ligament with the blunt probe. Alternatively, atraumatic forceps may be used to grasp the ovarian ligament and elevate the ovary. The broad ligament underlying the left ovary, the uterosacral ligaments and the posterior cul-de-sac are inspected. A survey of the left adnexa and broad ligament completes the diagnostic portion of the laparoscopic surgery. If visually a diagnosis cannot be assigned with certainty, excision of the peritoneal abnormality or a representative biopsy should be taken for histologic analysis.

Anatomic Distribution of Endometriosis

Knowledge of the anatomic distribution of endometriosis will help the surgeon to focus on these areas of importance. The areas most commonly involved with endometriosis include:

- The anterior and posterior cul-de-sac.
- Ovaries.
- Posterior broad ligaments.
- The uterosacral ligaments (Jenkins et al., 1986).

Endometriosis involves the left side of bilateral pelvic structures more frequently than the right. The area of pelvic adhesions roughly correlates with the locations of endometriosis. The specific incidence of involvement by location of 182 patients evaluated laparoscopically is shown in Table 35.2.

The anatomic distribution of endometriosis is influenced by both uterine position and age. An

Table 35.2 Implants and adhesions by anatomic location. (Reprinted with permission from the American College of Obstetricians and Gynecologists, *Obstetrics and Gynecology*, 1986, **67**: 335–338.)

Location	Implants		Adhesions	
	Number of patients	%	Number of patients	%
Anterior cul-de-sac	63	34.6	4	2.2
Posterior cul-de-sac	62	34.0	20	11.0
Right ovary	57	31.3	26	14.3
Left ovary	81	44.0	45	24.7
Right anterior broad ligament	2	1.1	2	1.1
Left anterior broad ligament	0	0	3	1.6
Right round ligament	1	0.5	2	1.1
Left round ligament	1	0.5	2	1.1
Right fallopian tube	3	1.6	20	11.0
Left fallopian tube	8	4.3	28	15.4
Right posterior broad ligament	39	21.4	30	16.5
Left posterior broad ligament	46	25.2	50	27.5
Right uterosacral ligament	28	15.3	5	2.7
Left uterosacral ligament	38	20.8	8	4.4
Uterus	21	11.5	6	3.3
Sigmoid	7	3.8	22	12.1
Right ureter	3	1.6	0	0
Left ureter	2	1.1	3	1.6
Anterior bladder flap	1	0.5	1	0.5
Small bowel	1	0.5	4	2.2
Anterior abdominal wall	0	0	3	1.6
Omentum	0	0	4	2.2

anteverted uterus is more commonly associated with anterior compartment endometriosis than a retroverted uterus (*P* < 0.0005) (Jenkins *et al.*, 1986). Posterior compartment disease is seen most commonly in patients with a posterior uterus, but is observed regardless of uterine position in the majority of patients. Redwine (1987b) observed an age-related change in the anatomic distribution of endometriosis. The frequency of endometriosis involving the posterior cul-de-sac, uterosacral and broad ligaments decreased with age while involvement of the ovaries increased with age. The severity of endometriosis, as determined by the revised American Fertility Classification system (1995), does not correlate with the amount of pain a patient experiences (Fedele *et al.*, 1990). Several recent studies have shown a correlation between the depth of infiltration and pelvic pain (Cornillie *et al.*, 1990; Koninckx *et al.*, 1991) as well as a relationship between the number of implants and dysmenorrhea (Perper *et al.*, 1995).

Laparoscopic Appearance of Endometriosis

Sampson (1921, 1924, 1927) used descriptive terms such as red raspberries, purple raspberries, blueberries, blebs and peritoneal pockets in his original series of articles. Subsequent articles primarily emphasized the pigmented, blue or black 'powderburn' appearance of endometriosis. The concept of endometriosis as a uniform-appearing pigmented lesion has permeated the psyche of the average gynecologist to the point that this type of lesion is still referred to as typical endometriosis. In fact, the subtle or nonpigmented form of endometriosis truly represents the majority of lesions (Redwine, 1987b).

Histologically, endometriosis is comprised of both endometrial glands and stroma. Visually, endometriosis presents a vast array of appearances. The gross appearance of endometriosis is a result of several factors, including the relative proportion of glands and stroma, amount of scarring, intralesional bleeding and quantity of hemosiderin. While the relative contribution of the above factors results in a continuum of visual appearances, the most commonly described types of endometriosis include scarred white lesions, strawberry-like reddish lesions, red flame-like lesions, reddish polyps, clear vesicular lesions, adhesions, peritoneal defects, yellow–brown patches and black puckered lesions.

Goldstein *et al.* (1980) described petechial and bleb-like endometriosis in adolescent patients.

Jansen and Russell published a study in 1986 in which they performed 137 biopsies of abnormal-appearing non-pigmented peritoneum in 77 patients. The idea that endometriosis could be found in lesions devoid of pigmentation 'typical of this disease' was a departure from the contemporary thinking of the time. Endometriosis was histologically present in 53% of the biopsies, which was significantly different from biopsies of normal-appearing peritoneum, which failed to detect endometriosis (*P* = 0.005) (Jansen and Russell, 1986).

White opacified and red flame-like lesions most commonly (81%) represented endometriosis (Figure 35.2). Characteristically, white opacified peritoneum is peritoneal scarring, which may be raised or thickened. Red flame-like lesions may be elevated (Figure 35.3). These red lesions have been shown to be biologically active. Glandular lesions contained endometriosis in 67% of the cases. Glandular lesions grossly appear the same as normal endometrium (e.g. at hysteroscopy). Subovarian adhesions without peritubal adhesions typical of an infectious etiology represented endometriosis in two of four cases. Other lesions that also contained endometriosis included yellow–brown peritoneal patches (47%), circular peritoneal defects (45%) and rarely, cribriform peritoneum (9%). Figure 35.4 depicts superficial yellow–brown endometriosis. Vesicular excrescences, which are loosely attached to the

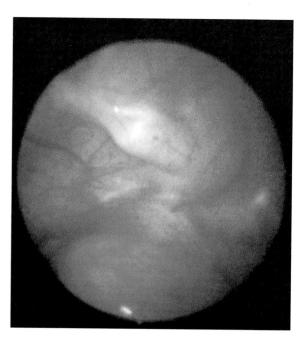

Figure 35.2 Fibrotic endometriosis in bladder peritoneum.

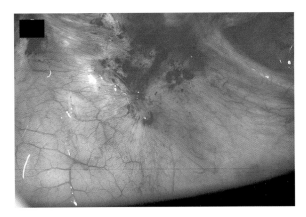

Figure 35.3 Red raised lesions.

peritoneum, represent a reaction to oil-based contrast medium.

Non-pigmented endometriosis progresses to pigmented endometriosis over time (Jansen and Russell, 1986). Second-look laparoscopy in untreated patients 6–24 months following the initial surgery documented pigmented lesions in areas that previously contained non-pigmented, but abnormal peritoneum. Redwine's report suggested a progression of the visual appearance of endometriosis from clear to red to white to black with increasing age of the patient (Redwine, 1987a). Increasing age is associated with a decreasing incidence of subtle or atypical endometriosis and an increased incidence of 'typical' endometriosis, endometrioma and deeply infiltrating endometriosis (Koninckx *et al.*, 1991).

Martin *et al.* pioneered the excisional techniques for the treatment of abnormal-appearing peritoneum (Stripling *et al.*, 1988; Martin *et al.*, 1989). This provided the basis for extensive histologic study of abnormal peritoneum and the delineation of a wide array of appearances of endometriosis. The initial study described five different types of endometriotic lesions (puckered black, white, red, clear and pink lesions) in 109 patients (Stripling *et al.*, 1988). Superficial clear papules of endometriosis are seen in Figure 35.5. Atypical endometriosis was noted in 55% of patients and was an isolated finding in 13% of the patients.

The puckered black lesion ('typical' endometriosis) is comprised of stroma, glands, fibromuscular scarring and intraluminal debris (Stripling *et al.*, 1988) (Figure 35.6). White endometriosis must be differentiated from postoperative scarring and from fibrotic adhesions resulting from inflammatory disease. Histologically, white endometriosis contains sparse glands and stroma embedded in fibromuscular scar tissue. The red polypoid lesion is composed primarily of native-appearing glands and stroma while flat red lesions are hypervascular. Deep endometriotic lesions may be associated with strawberry-like reddish areas. White scarred areas of endometriosis are frequently associated with strawberry-like reddish areas. The strawberry-like lesion may actually represent extension of deeper invasive lesions to the surface (Adamson, 1990). The amount of debris and intraluminal hemosiderin determines the intensity of coloration of brown and black lesions. In a subsequent study Martin *et al.* (1989) used up to 20 descriptive terms to characterize the appearance of endometriosis.

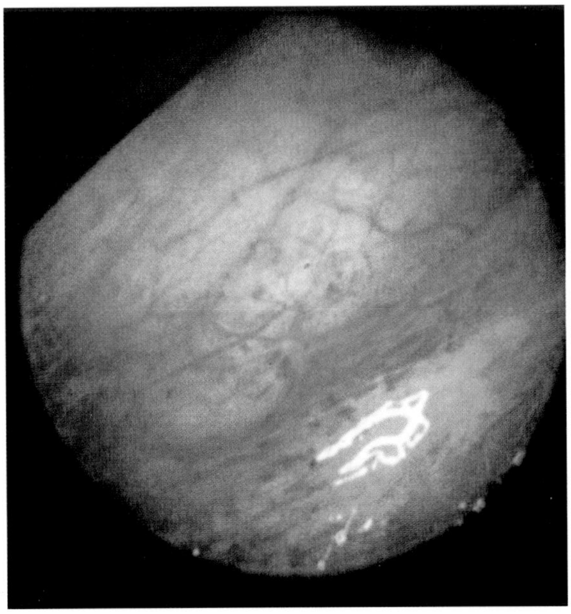

Figure 35.4 Superficial early confluent yellow–brown endometriosis.

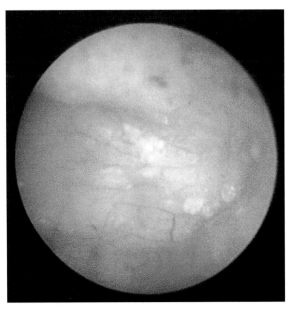

Figure 35.5 Superficial clear papules of endometriosis.

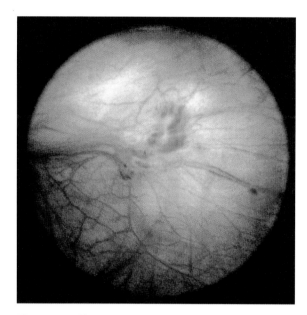

Figure 35.6 Classic powderburn endometriosis.

Allen and Masters (1955) described the presence of a peritoneal defect on the posterior aspect of the broad ligament in patients with pelvic pain. They postulated that the peritoneal defect was a result of trauma secondary to excessive motility of the uterus. It was not until later that the causal relationship between endometriosis and peritoneal defects was described (Chatman, 1981). Peritoneal defects frequently occur in areas of the pelvis that overlie loose connective tissue. The anatomic distribution of peritoneal defects is outlined in Table 35.3. Approximately 80% of peritoneal defects are associated with endometriosis, either on the border of the defect or in the defect itself (Chatman and Zbella, 1986).

Among patients with endometriosis 28% have peritoneal defects, which is significantly greater ($P < 0.005$) than the 7% of patients with peritoneal defects in the general population (Chatman and Zbella, 1986). There is no correlation between the presence of peritoneal defects and the severity of endometriosis.

A three-year prospective study of 643 consecutive laparoscopies demonstrated a highly significant correlation between pain and deeply infiltrating endometriosis (Koninckx *et al.*, 1991). When the depth of the endometriotic implant is taken into account, pelvic pain does not significantly correlate with the pelvic area or volume of endometriosis nor with the presence or size of endometriomas. Deeply infiltrating endometriosis is found primarily in the rectovaginal septum and the uterosacral ligaments (Figure 35.7) and occasionally in the uterovesical fold. Visually these lesions appear as white plaques with puckered black spots or isolated puckered black spots (Figures 35.8, 35.9). In some patients, particularly those with bowel involvement, deep endometriosis may present with retraction only. The diagnosis of deep endometriosis and evaluation of the extent of endometriosis is determined by palpation with the blunt probe and intraoperative rectovaginal examination (Reich *et al.*, 1991). Endometriosis may be hard and sclerotic, which when retracted with a blunt probe causes movement of the surrounding tissue en bloc. The lesion should be resected and/or vaporized until soft supple tissue is encountered. The tissue cannot be directly palpated, but with experience subtle differences in the consistency of the tissue can be appreciated visually. Surgical estimation of the depth of the lesion correlates well with histologic findings (Cornillie *et al.*, 1990).

Koninckx and Martin (1992) have described three types of infiltrating endometriosis.

Table 35.3 Anatomic distribution of peritoneal defects. (Reproduced with permission of the publisher, The American Fertility Society, from Chatman and Zbella, 1986.)

Location	Number of patients	%
Posterior cul-de-sac	19	31
Right broad ligament	18	29
Left broad ligament	18	29
Left uterosacral ligament	3	4
Right uterosacral ligament	2	3
Anterior cul-de-sac	2	3

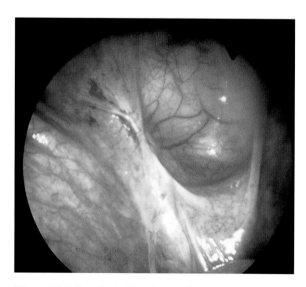

Figure 35.7 Deeply infiltrating endometriosis involving the uterosacral ligaments causing scarring.

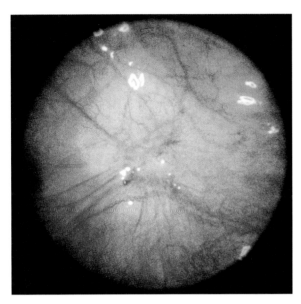

Figure 35.8 Invasive endometriosis with 'classical' lesions and fibrosis causing peritoneal contraction.

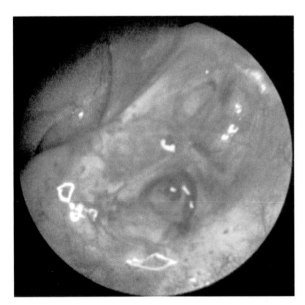

Figure 35.9 Deeply invasive fibrotic endometriosis causing marked peritoneal distortion.

- Type I lesions are large pelvic areas of typical or subtle lesions surrounded by white sclerotic tissue. When excised the deep disease grows progressively smaller with deeper sectioning – the infiltrating disease takes on a conical distribution.
- Type II lesions are formed by retraction of the bowel and are recognized clinically as small classic lesions associated with retraction. In some women induration is associated with the retraction even if no lesion is visible. Excision usually reveals the presence of a nodule.

- Type III endometriosis is nodular and associated with the rectovaginal septum. This type of endometriosis is clinically suspected if nodularity of the septum is felt during rectovaginal examination or if dark blue lesions are seen at the vaginal fornix at the time of speculum examination. Type III disease is the most severe form and often spreads laterally to involve the ureter.

Not all abnormalities of the peritoneum represent endometriosis. Other lesions that may mimic endometriosis include old suture, residual carbon from laser surgery, splenosis, reaction to oil-based contrast medium, epithelial inclusion, Walthard's rests, adrenal rests, secondary breast and ovarian cancer and inflammatory cystic inclusions (Jansen and Russell, 1986). Differentiation between atypical endometriosis and other lesions may be impossible visually, but may be achieved histologically through excision or biopsy. An abnormality of the peritoneum, no matter what its size, shape or appearance should suggest the possibility of endometriosis. Biopsy of these atypical lesions often confirms the presence of disease. Occasionally a biopsy specimen is interpreted histologically as fibrotic tissue, but in the appropriate clinical setting this is probably a sequel of endometriosis and suggests the presence of endometriosis.

Summary

The appearance of endometriosis is quite diverse, ranging from very subtle lesions, which are difficult to visualize grossly, to the typical black puckered 'powderburn' lesions. The subtle or atypical lesions probably represent a more active form of endometriosis. With increasing age, there is a progression to the less active 'typical' form. Retraction of the peritoneum may be the only sign of deeply infiltrating endometriosis. A combination of laparoscopy, palpation with the blunt probe and intraoperative rectovaginal examination may be needed to make a diagnosis of endometriosis. The ability to diagnose atypical and subtle appearances of endometriosis is directly related to the experience and skill of the surgeon.

References

Adamson GD (1990) Diagnosis and clinical presentation of endometriosis. *American Journal of Obstetrics and Gynecology* **162**: 568–569.
Adamson GD, Hurd SJ, Pasts DJ, Rodriguez BD (1993) Laparoscopic endometriosis treatment: is it better? *Fertility and Sterility* **59**: 35–44.

Allen WM, Masters WH (1995) Traumatic laceration of uterine support. *American Journal of Obstetrics and Gynecology* **70**: 500–513.

American Fertility Society (1995) Revised American Fertility Society classification of endometriosis. *Fertility and Sterility* **43**: 351.

Chatman DL (1981) Pelvic peritoneal defects and endometriosis: Allen–Masters syndrome revisited. *Fertility and Sterility* **36**: 751.

Chatman DL, Zbella EA (1986) Pelvic peritoneal defects and endometriosis: future observations. *Fertility and Sterility* **46**: 711–714.

Cornillie FJ, Oosterlynck D, Lauweryns JM, Konninckx PR (1990) Deeply infiltrating pelvic endometriosis: histology and clinical significance. *Fertility and Sterility* **53**: 978–983.

Evers JL II (1987) The second-look laparoscopy for evaluation of the result of medical treatment of endometriosis should not be performed during ovarian suppression. *Fertility and Sterility* **47**: 502–504

Fedele L, Parazzini F, Bianchi S, Areaini L, Candiani GB (1990) Stage and localization of pelvic endometriosis and pain. *Fertility and Sterility* **53**: 155–158.

Goldstein DP, DeCholnoky C, Eman J (1980) Adolescent endometriosis. *Journal of Adolescent Health Care* **1**: 37.

Hesla JS, Rock JA (1996) Endometriosis. In Thompson JD, Rock JA (eds) *TeLinde's Operative Gynecology*. pp. 585–624. Baltimore: JB Lippincott Co.

Jansen RPS, Russell P (1986) Nonpigmented endometriosis: clinical, laparoscopic, and pathologic definition. *American Journal of Obstetrics and Gynecology* **155**: 1154–1159.

Jenkins S, Olive DL, Haney AF (1986) Endometriosis: pathogenetic implications of the anatomic distribution. *Obstetrics and Gynecology* **67**: 335–338.

Koninckx PR, Martin DC (1992) Deep endometriosis: a consequence of infiltration or retraction or possibly adenomyosis externa? *Fertility and Sterility* **58**: 924.

Koninckx PR, Meuleman C, Demeyere S, Lesaffre E, Cornillie FJ (1991) Suggestive evidence that pelvic endometriosis is a progressive disease, whereas deeply infiltrating endometriosis is associated with pelvic pain. *Fertility and Sterility* **55**: 759–765.

Koninckx PR, Meulman C, Oosterlynck D, Cornillie FJ (1996) Diagnosis of deep endometriosis by clinical examination during menstruation and plasma CA-125 concentration. *Fertility and Sterility* **65**: 280–287.

Martin DC, Hubert GD, Vander Zwaag R, El-Zeky FA (1989) Laparoscopic appearances of peritoneal endometriosis. *Fertility and Sterility* **51**: 63–67.

Martin DC, Ahmic R, El-Zeky FA *et al.* (1990) Increased histologic confirmation of endometriosis. *Journal of Gynecologic Surgery* **6**: 275–279.

McArthur JW, Ulfelder H (1965) The effect of pregnancy upon endometriosis. *Obstetrical and Gynecological Survey* **20**: 709.

Murphy AA (1992) Diagnostic and operative laparoscopy. In Thompson JD, Rock JA (eds) *TeLinde's Operative Gynecology*. pp. 361–384. Baltimore: JB Lippincott Co.

Murphy AA, Green WR, Bobbie D, dela Cruz ZC, Rock JA (1986) Unsuspected endometriosis documented by scanning electron microscopy in visually normal peritoneum. *Fertility and Sterility* **46**: 522–524.

Nisolle M, Paindaveine B, Boudon A *et al.* (1990) Histologic study of peritoneal endometriosis in infertile women. *Fertility and Sterility* **53**: 984–988.

Perper MM, Nezhat F, Goldstein H, Nezhat CH, Nezhat C (1995) Dysmenorrhea is related to the number of implants in endometriosis patients. *Fertility and Sterility* **63**: 500–503.

Redwine DB (1987a) Age-related evolution in color appearance of endometriosis. *Fertility and Sterility* **48**: 1062–1063.

Redwine DB (1987b) The distribution of endometriosis in the pelvis by age groups and fertility. *Fertility and Sterility* **47**: 173–175.

Reich H, McGlynn F, Salvat J (1991) Laparoscopic treatment of culdesac obliteration secondary to retrocervical deep fibrotic endometriosis. *Journal of Reproductive Medicine* **36**: 516–522.

Rivlin ME, Miller JD, Krueger RP, Patel RD, Bower JD (1990) Leuprolid acetate in the management of ureteral obstruction caused by endometeriosis. *Obstetrics and Gynecology* **75**: 532–536.

Sampson JA (1921) Perforating hemorrhagic (chocolate) cysts of the ovary. *Archives of Surgery* **3**: 245.

Sampson JA (1924) Benign and malignant endometrial implants in the peritoneal cavity and their relationship to certain ovarian tumors. *Surgery, Obstetrics and Gynecology* **38**: 287.

Sampson JA (1927) Peritoneal endometriosis due to dissemination of endometrial tissue into the peritoneal cavity. *American Journal of Obstetrics and Gynecology* **14**: 422.

Stripling MC, Martin DC, Chatman DL, Vander Zwaag R, Poston WM (1988) Subtle appearance of pelvic endometriosis. *Fertility and Sterility* **49**: 427–431.

Sutton CJG, Ewen SP, Whitelaw N, Haines P (1994) Prospective randomized, double-blind, controlled trial of laser laparoscopy in the treatment of pelvic pain associated with minimal, mild, and moderate endometriosis. *Fertility and Sterility* **62**: 696–700.

36

Rectovaginal Septum Adenomyotic Nodule: A Distinct Entity. A Series of 460 Cases

JACQUES DONNEZ, MICHELLE NISOLLE, MIREILLE SMETS, SALIM BASSIL AND FRANÇOISE CASANAS-ROUX

Department of Gynecology, Catholic University of Louvain, Brussels, Belgium

Introduction

In the pelvis, three different forms of endometriosis must be considered (Donnez et al., 1992):

- Peritoneal endometriosis.
- Ovarian endometriosis.
- Rectovaginal septum endometrosis.

Recently, Nisolle (1996) has demonstrated that the three entities are distinct and have a different histopathogenesis.

Red lesions (red vesicles, polypoid lesions, red flame-like lesions, hypervascularized areas or even petechial peritoneum) (Donnez and Nisolle, 1988; Nisolle et al., 1990; Donnez et al., 1992) have recently been proved to be a very active form of the disease (Nisolle et al., 1993). Our hypothesis is that red lesions are more aggressive and progress to the so-called typical or black lesions, which must be considered as an enclosed implant surrounded by fibrosis.

Ovarian chocolate-colored fluid cysts are according to the hypothesis of Hughesdon (1957) the consequence of the invagination of superficial implants into the ovary. Our hypothesis (Donnez et al., 1996; Nisolle, 1996) claims that the endometrioma is the consequence of metaplasia of invaginated mesothelium. Endometriomas can also develop within the ovaries and this type of cystic ovarian endometriosis must be considered as another severe form of endometriosis, often related to infertility.

A third form of the disease is deep-infiltrating endometriosis of the rectovaginal septum. Sampson (1922) defined cul-de-sac obliteration as 'extensive adhesions in the cul-de-sac, obliterating its lower portion and uniting the cervix or the lower portion of the uterus to the rectum; with adenoma of the endometrial type invading the cervical and the uterine tissue and probably also (but to a lesser degree) the anterior wall of the rectum'. For us, rectovaginal septum endometriosis is in fact an 'adenomyotic nodule'.

Treatment options for pain or infertility secondary to cul-de-sac obliteration include ovarian suppression therapy with danazol or gonadotropin releasing hormone (GnRH) agonists or surgery (Donnez et al., 1990; Reich et al., 1991; Koninckx, 1993). Recently, some gynecologists (Reich et al., 1991; Nezhat et al., 1992; Canis et al., 1993; Donnez et al., 1993) have developed the endoscopic technique.

Patients

Our series of 460 cases of rectovaginal septum endometriosis is presented here. In the majority of cases, the main symptom was severe pelvic pain, and 25% of patients had pelvic pain and infertility. All patients with infertility underwent an evaluation of ovulation, cervical mucus–sperm interaction (postcoital test) and male factor (defined as < 15 million sperm ml^{-1} using a Makler counting chamber).

Preoperative radiography of the colon was carried out in order to evaluate the involvement of the rectal surface. Profile radiography of an air contrast barium enema offers the best evaluation of the infiltration of the rectal anterior wall (Figure 36.1).

The surgical techniques have evolved gradually, but all of them involve separation of the anterior rectum from the posterior vagina and the excision or ablation of the endometriosis in that area. Aquadissection, scissor dissection and electrosurgery with an unmodulated (cutting) current are used by some authors (Reich *et al.*, 1991), while others (Nezhat *et al.*, 1992; Donnez *et al.*, 1994) prefer to use the carbon dioxide (CO_2) laser. A mechanical bowel preparation was administered orally on the afternoon before surgery to induce brisk self-limiting diarrhea, which rapidly cleanses the bowel without disrupting the electrolyte balance. All the laparoscopic procedures were performed using general anesthesia. A 12 mm operative laparoscope was inserted through a vertical intraumbilical incision. Three other puncture sites were made 2–3 cm above the pubis, in the midline and in the areas adjacent to the deep inferior epigastric vessels, which were visualized directly.

Clinical and Laparoscopic Aspects (Table 36.1)

The examination with a speculum reveals either a normal vaginal mucosa or a protruded endometriotic nodule in the posterior fornix. By palpation, the diameter of the lesion can be evaluated. Palpation is often painful; the presence of the nodule accounts

Table 36.1 Rectovaginal endometriosis: technical aspects ($n = 460$).

Duration	69 min (40–132 min)
Hospitalization	2.8 days (2–5 days)
Laparoscopic bowel resection	0

for symptoms like deep dyspareunia and dysmenorrhea. To determine the cul-de-sac obliteration, a sponge on a ring forceps was inserted into the posterior vaginal fornix. A dilatator (Hegar 25) was systematically inserted into the rectum (Figure 36.2). Complete obliteration was diagnosed when the outline of the posterior fornix could not be seen through the laparoscope. Cul-de-sac obliteration was partial when rectal tenting was visible, but the sponge in the posterior vaginal fornix protruded between the rectum and the inverted U of the uterosacral ligaments. However, sometimes a deep infiltrating lesion of the rectovaginal septum is only barely visible by laparoscopy.

Surgical Technique

Deep fibrotic nodular endometriosis involving the cul-de-sac (Figure 36.3(a)) requires excision of the nodular fibrotic tissue from the posterior vagina, rectum, posterior cervix and uterosacral ligaments. As described by Reich *et al.* (1991), attention was first directed towards a complete dissection of the anterior rectum throughout its area of involvement until the loose tissue of the rectovaginal space was reached. A sponge on a ring forceps was inserted into the

Figure 36.1 Profile radiography of an air contrast barium enema offers the best evaluation of the infiltration of the rectal anterior wall. Typical 'endometriotic' infiltration of the rectal anterior wall (arrows).

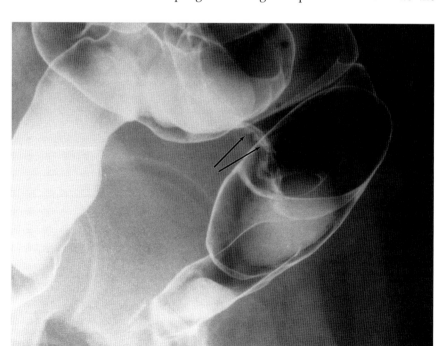

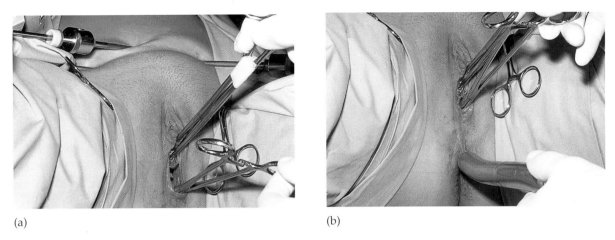

(a) (b)

Figure 36.2 Determination of cul-de-sac obliteration. (a) A sponge on a ring forceps was inserted into the posterior vaginal fornix. An intrauterine manipulator fixed with a Pozzi forceps is also used. (b) A dilatator (Hegar 25) is inserted into the rectum.

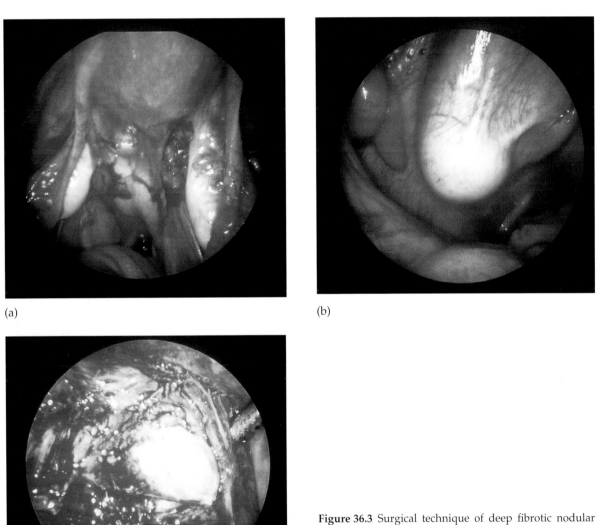

(a) (b)

(c)

Figure 36.3 Surgical technique of deep fibrotic nodular adenomyosis removal. (a) The rectum is adherent to the posterior part of the cervix. (b) Laparoscopic view of the dilatator inserted into the rectum. (c) After dissection of the anterior part of the rectum, the posterior vaginal fornix is incised. The vaginal sponge is visible.

posterior vaginal fornix and a dilatator (Hegar 25) was placed in the rectum (Figure 36.3(b)). In addition, a cannula was inserted into the endometrial cavity to markedly antevert the uterus. The peritoneum covering the cul-de-sac of Douglas was opened between the 'adenomyotic' lesion and the rectum.

We use a technique of first freeing the anterior rectum from the loose areolar tissue of the rectovaginal septum before excising and/or vaporizing visible and palpable deep fibrotic endometriosis. This approach is possible even when anterior rectal muscularis infiltration is present. Careful dissection is then carried out using the aquadissector for aquadissection and the CO_2 laser for sharp dissection until the rectum is completely freed and identifiable below the lesion. Excision of the fibrotic tissue on the side of the rectum is attempted only after the rectal dissection is complete (Figure 36.3(c)). A partial rectal resection was never performed in our series. In cases of deep infiltrating lesions, the vaginal wall is more or less penetrated by the adenomyosis and excision of a part of the vagina is essential.

Dissection is performed accordingly, not only with the removal of all visible endometriotic lesions, but also the vaginal mucosa with at least a

0.5 cm disease-free margin. Lesions extending totally through the vagina were treated with *en bloc* laparoscopic resection from the cul-de-sac to the posterior vaginal wall; the pneumoperitoneum was maintained and the posterior vaginal wall was closed vaginally. The anterior rectum can be reperitonealized by plicating the uterosacral ligaments and lateral rectal peritoneum across the midline using 4–0 Polydioxanone (Reich *et al.*, 1991) or Tissucol or Interceed (Johnson and Johnson, Ascot, UK) (Donnez and Nisolle, 1995) (Figure 36.4).

In our series of 460 cases, laparoscopic rectal perforation occurred in four cases (Table 36.2). Perforation was diagnosed at the time of the laparoscopy. In two cases, the rectum was repaired by laparotomy and in the two other cases by colpotomy. Laparoscopic dissection was successfully performed in all cases, even when the radiography of the colon showed bowel involvement. During the same period, five cases of rectal endometriosis and eight cases of sigmoid colon endometriosis were diagnosed. All 13 patients had no nodules of the septum, but bowel wall endometriosis which provoked menstrual rectorragia. In the 13 cases, laparotomy and bowel resection were performed. In all cases, histology proved the histologic involvement of mucosa by endometriotic tissue.

Histology

Deep vaginal endometriosis associated with pelvic endometriosis can take the form of nodular or polypoid masses involving the posterior vaginal fornix. It has been called 'adenomyotic nodule of the rectovaginal septum' (Donnez and Nisolle, 1995; Donnez *et al.*, 1995). Adenomyosis exhibits a varied functional response to ovarian hormones. Proliferative glands

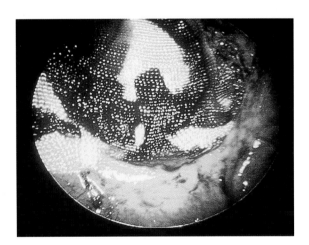

Figure 36.4 Final view after rectovaginal nodule resection and application of Interceed (Johnson and Johnson).

Table 36.2 Rectovaginal endometriosis: complications ($n = 460$).

Rectal perforation*	4 (0.9%)
Delayed hemorrhage	
(<24 h postoperatively)	2 (0.4%)
Urinary retention	3 (0.6%)
Ureteral injury	0
Bladder injury	0

*The perforation was recognized during the procedure and the defect was repaired either by colpotomy ($n = 2$) or by minilaparotomy ($n = 2$).

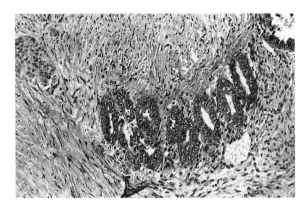

Figure 36.5 Rectovaginal adenomyosis. Scanty endometrial type stroma and glandular epithelium are disseminated in muscular tissue. (Gomori's trichrome × 110.)

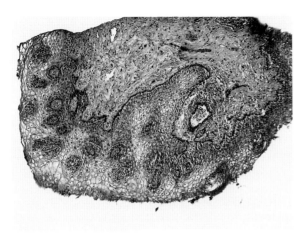

Figure 36.6 Endometrial glands and stroma are found up to the vaginal mucosa (Gomori's trichrome × 80).

and stroma are generally observed in the first half of the menstrual cycle. An adenomyoma is a circumscribed nodular aggregate of smooth muscle and endometrial glands, and usually, endometrial stroma (Figures 36.5 and 36.6). This type of lesion is not actually endometriosis, but a specific disease called adenomyosis characterized by the presence of abundant muscular tissue invaded by glandular epithelium covered with a scanty stroma. Adenomyosis may not respond to physiologic levels of progesterone, and secretory changes are frequently absent or incomplete during the second half of the cycle (Donnez et al., 1995). Often endometriotic glands and stroma were found by serial section up to the vaginal mucosa, which was sometimes replaced by endometrial epithelium. Sometimes, 'invasion' of the muscle by a very active glandular epithelium proved that the stroma is not necessary for invasion in this particular type of pathology called adenomyosis.

Cytokeratin and Vimentin Staining

The evaluation of intermediate filaments by cytokeratin staining showed a similar pattern throughout the menstrual cycle when compared to eutopic endometrium, the cytokeratin H-score in glandular epithelium during the luteal phase being significantly lower in the nodules than in the other tissue.

Vimentin was never expressed during the follicular phase in glandular epithelium and stroma of nodules. During the luteal phase, the vimentin H-score in the stroma was similar to that of eutopic endometrium, but significantly lower in the glandular epithelium.

The presence of a lower expression of cytokeratin in glandular epithelium could be interpreted as a lower degree of differentiation or as a delay in differentiation. The very low vimentin reactivity, and

the absence of any decrease throughout the cycle in the glandular epithelium of nodules would account for both the low degree of differentiation and the unresponsiveness to endogenous hormonal variations.

Estrogen Receptor (ER) and Progesterone Receptor (PR) Content

The pattern of ER content of the nodule glandular epithelium was similar to that observed in eutopic endometrium throughout the cycle, a significant decrease occurring during the luteal phase in both tissues. However, at the stromal level, a significant increase of ER was observed in the nodules throughout the cycle whereas a significant decrease occurred in eutopic endometrium. The progesterone receptor (PR) content pattern throughout the menstrual cycle was different in the two tissues. Indeed, although a significant decrease was observed in eutopic endometrium, a significant increase was noted in the nodules throughout the cycle, in the glandular epithelium as well as in the stroma.

The variations of ER and PR content in the nodules throughout the cycle suggest that they are probably not regulated by steroids. The absence of response to serum progesterone levels also suggests different regulatory mechanisms for endometriotic steroid receptors.

Discussion

In the pelvis, three different forms of endometriosis (Donnez et al., 1992) must be considered: peritoneal, ovarian and rectovaginal septum. By evaluating the mitotic activity and stromal vascularization, we have recently proved (Nisolle et al., 1993) that peritoneal red lesions are the most aggressive form of the disease and progress to the so-called typical or black lesion, which must be considered as an enclosed implant surrounded by fibrosis. This type of infiltration must be clearly differentiated from the rectovaginal endometriotic nodule.

Koninckx (1993) recently described three types of deep-infiltrating endometriosis:

- Deep infiltrating endometriosis of type I is a rather large lesion in the peritoneal cavity and infiltrating conically with the deeper parts becoming progressively smaller. It has been suggested that this type of endometriosis is caused by infiltration.
- In type II lesions, the main feature is that bowel is retracted over the lesion, the latter becoming deeply situated in the rectovaginal

septum although not really infiltrating it.

- Type III lesions are the deepest and most severe. They are spherically shaped, situated deep in the rectovaginal septum, and often only visible as a small typical lesion at laparoscopy. This lesion is often more palpable than visible, originates from the rectovaginal septum tissue and consists essentially of smooth muscle with active glandular epithelium and scanty stroma.

In our study, the rectovaginal nodule was histologically similar to an adenomyoma (Zaloudek and Norris, 1987). Indeed it was a circumscribed nodular aggregate of smooth muscle, endometrial glands and endometrial stroma. As in the 'adenomyoma', secretory changes were frequently absent in 'endometriotic' rectovaginal nodule. Sometimes, the invasion of the muscle by a very active glandular epithelium without stroma proved that the stroma is not mandatory for invasion with this particular type of pathology called adenomyosis. In some instances, it could be seen that the vaginal pluristratified epithelium was replaced by a glandular epithelium. The fact that ciliated cells were present and the coexpression of both vimentin and cytokeratin (Donnez et al., 1996) proved the müllerian origin of the nodule, certain histologic characteristics of which were completely different from those observed in peritoneal lesions (Nisolle et al., 1990). In our series, deep fibrotic tissue assumed to contain endometriosis was excised or vaporized from the anterior rectum with the aid of multiple rectovaginal examinations. Cul-de-sac dissection was followed by excision of deep fibrotic endometriosis without cul-de-sac reconstruction. In four cases, the bowel lumen was entered. A comprehensive laparoscopic procedure, while not eradicating all of the endometriosis, may result in considerable pain relief or a desired pregnancy. While we recognize that bowel resection may be necessary in rare cases, it seems prudent to curtail, rather than encourage, the widespread use of such an aggressive, potentially morbid procedure.

In conclusion, deep infiltrating endometriosis should be considered as a specific disease that differs from mild or minimal endometriosis and ovarian cystic endometriosis. We suggest that this disease entity should be called 'rectovaginal adenomyosis'.

References

Canis M, Wattiez A, Pouly JL et al. (1993) Laparoscopic treatment of endometriosis. In Brosens I, Donnez J (eds) Endometriosis: Research and Management. pp. 407–417. Parthenon Publishing.

Donnez J, Nisolle M (1988) Appearances of peritoneal endometriosis. In Proceedings of the IIIrd International Laser Surgery Symposium, Brussels.

Donnez J, Nisolle M (1995) Advanced laparoscopic surgery for the removal of rectovaginal septum endometriotic or adenomyotic nodules. Baillière's Clinical Obstetrics and Gynecology 9: 769–774.

Donnez J, Nisolle M, Casanas-Roux F (1990) Endometriosis-associated infertility: Evaluation of preoperative use of danazol, gestrinone and buserelin. International Journal of Fertility 35: 297–301.

Donnez J, Nisolle M, Casanas-Roux F (1992) Three-dimensional architectures of peritoneal endometriosis. Fertility and Sterility 57: 980–983.

Donnez J, Nisolle M, Casanas-Roux F, Clerckx F (1993) Endometriosis: rationale for surgery. In Brosens I, Donnez J (eds) Endometriosis: Research and Management. pp. 385–395. Parthenon Publishing.

Donnez J, Nisolle M, Casanas-Roux F, Anaf V, Smets M (1994) Laparoscopic treatment of rectovaginal septum endometriosis. In Donnez J, Nisolle M (eds) An Atlas of Laser Operative Laparoscopy and Hysteroscopy. pp. 75–85. Parthenon Publishing.

Donnez J, Nisolle M, Casanas-Roux F, Bassil S, Anaf V (1995) Rectovaginal septum endometriosis or adenomyosis: laparoscopic management in a series of 231 patients. Human Reproduction 10: 630–635.

Donnez J, Nisolle M, Gillet N, Smets M, Bassil S, Casanas-Roux F (1996) Large ovarian endometriomas. Human Reproduction 11: 641–646.

Hughesdon PE (1957) The structure of endometrial cysts of the ovary. Journal of Obstetrics and Gynaecology of the British Empire 64: 481–487.

Koninckx PD (1993) Deeply infiltrating endometriosis. In Brosens I, Donnez J (eds) Endometriosis: Research and Management. pp. 437–446. Parthenon Publishing.

Nezhat C, Nezhat F, Pennington E (1992) Laparoscopic treatment of lower colorectal and infiltrative rectovaginal septum endometriosis by the technique of video laparoscopy. British Journal of Obstetrics and Gynaecology 99: 664–667.

Nisolle M (1996) Peritoneal, ovarian and rectovaginal endometriosis are three distinct entities. Thèse d'Agrégation, Université Catholique de Louvain

Nisolle M, Casanas-Roux F, Donnez J (1988) Histologic study of ovarian endometriosis after hormonal therapy. Fertility and Sterility 49: 423–426.

Nisolle M, Paindaveine B, Bourdon A, Berliere M, Casanas-Roux F, Donnez J (1990) Histologic study of peritoneal endometriosis in infertile women. Fertility and Sterility 53: 984–988.

Nisolle M, Casanas-Roux F, Anaf V, Mine JM, Donnez J (1993) Morphometric study of the stromal vascularization in peritoneal endometriosis. Fertility and Sterility 59: 681–684.

Reich H, McGlynn F, Salvat J (1991) Laparoscopic treatment of cul-de-sac obliteration secondary to retrocervical deep fibrotic endometriosis. Reproductive Medicine 36: 516.

Sampson JA (1922) Intestinal adenomas of endometrial type. Archives of Surgery 5: 217.

Zaloudek C, Norris HJ (1987) Mesenchymal tumors of the uterus. In Kurman R (ed.) Blaustein's Pathology of the Female Genital Tract. p. 373. Springer-Verlag.

37

Laser Vaporization of Endometriosis

JOSEPH R. FESTE

Ob/Gyn Associates, Houston, Texas, USA

Introduction

One of the most common diseases amenable to treatment by a laser delivered through a laparoscope is pelvic endometriosis. Endometriosis is basically a disease of the peritoneal surface and is therefore readily treated with laser energy. At first a surgeon's use of the laser through the laparoscope should be limited to treating only minimal and mild cases of endometriosis (Stages I and II). With experience, the laser laparoscopist can safely and successfully treat moderate (Stage III) and severe (Stage IV) endometriosis laparoscopically except when colon resection is required. Eventually, with careful use of either the operative laparoscope or the second-puncture probe, one can safely and adequately vaporize most visible endometriotic implants. Ideally, if endometriosis is diagnosed at laparoscopy performed for the evaluation of infertility or pelvic pain, it can be vaporized at the time and the need for long-term medical therapy or subsequent major surgery is reduced.

General Considerations

Vaporization with laser energy offers several advantages over bipolar cautery, endocoagulation of endometriotic implants or ultrasonic energy. With unipolar or bipolar cauterization it is not possible to control the 'star burst' effect. Neither bipolar cautery, ultrasound energy nor endocoagulation provides a way to gauge the depth of removal of the endometriotic implant. Therefore there is little, if any, way to know at the time of the procedure whether the lesion has been completely destroyed. However, with the carbon dioxide (CO_2) laser, but a little less with the argon or potassium titanyl phosphate (KTP) lasers, the process of vaporization allows visualization of the three-dimensional boundaries of the lesion, thereby permitting its complete destruction and removal. Since endometriosis can exist microscopically adjacent to an obvious lesion, a margin of 2–3 mm should be treated around each lesion. In general, especially for the beginner, power densities of 2500–5000 W cm^{-2} are used. Debulking endometriotic implants is best performed by using a continuous firing mode. This setting will provide additional hemostasis over a superpulse mode. However, for lesions overlying a vital structure, the ureter, urinary bladder, colon or larger blood vessels, single or repeat pulse modes or lower power continuous modes provide safer vaporization. Single or repeat pulse modes allow a 100–200 µm depth of vaporization, and thus substantially limit the depth of penetration. In addition, the intermittent blast of the laser decreases heat transfer, prevents damage to the underlying tissue, and prevents injury to vital structures. Single or repeat pulse modes are generally the safest modality for the beginning CO_2 laser laparoscopist. Recently, use of high power density superpulses has been advocated to vaporize peritoneal endometriosis. However, the potential depth of penetration dictates the need for extreme care when these settings are used. In most instances, the surgeon rapidly pulses the laser with the foot pedal in order to keep the depth of penetration under control, but this technique should only be used by experienced surgeons.

The lesions of endometriosis are basically avascular. Therefore, hemostasis is a concern only in the underlying or adjacent normal tissues. When an endometriotic implant is vaporized, the bubbling of old blood is seen first, followed by a curdy white material representing vaporization of the stromal layer. After the entire endometriotic lesion has been vaporized, retroperitoneal fat is encountered, and the appearance of the 'bubbling of water' confirms complete vaporization of the lesion. The absorption of the CO_2 laser by water prevents deeper penetration of the laser beam for a few seconds after the endometriotic implant is vaporized. However, this phenomenon may not be appreciated over the uterosacral ligaments when the implants are extremely dense and deep.

Although they share some characteristics, such as avascularity, endometriotic lesions vary considerably in appearance. The various forms of endometriosis are noted in Chapters 35 and 36. Whether the lesion presents as a white scar, a hemosiderin deposit, a bullous lesion or a raised red or port wine-colored lesion, all of the peritoneal disease must be completely vaporized or excised. The diffuse hemosiderin deposits and clear vesicular lesions are the most active and produce significant pain and infertility. The tendency is to overlook these areas and look more intently for the textbook-type of lesions. However, even the areas that appear to be only old scar tissue, especially after therapy with either danazol or a gonadotropin releasing hormone (GnRH) agonist for several months, should be completely vaporized. If left alone, these lesions are very likely to be activated in time by the influence of estrogen and to again become symptomatic. If the areas of vaporization are extensive, the biodegradable graft, Interceed (Johnson & Johnson, Arlington, Texas, USA), can be used to minimize the development of adhesions postoperatively (Adhesion Barrier Study Group, 1989). When this barrier is used there must be extreme hemostasis in the area to which it is applied. Fortunately, the laser energy will provide this effect most of the time.

Techniques

Peritoneum and Soft Tissue

Usually small implants can be excised, vaporized or coagulated. However, the deep infiltrating lesions over 3 mm in depth have been reported in about 60% of patients in some series (Martin *et al.*, 1989) must be treated carefully. For these deeper lesions, vaporization or excision should be taken down to

the level of healthy tissue. The tissue distortion that occurs with vaporization techniques can be confusing and deep lesions can be missed. In some instances, it may be preferable to excise rather then vaporize the lesion (Martin and Vander Zwaag, 1987). This is particularly true when there are many lesions in the same area. Not only is excision easier but it is safer if the point of dissection is over vital structures (Figure 37.1).

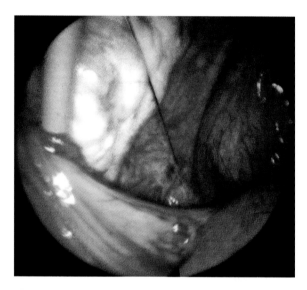

Figure 37.1 Excision of endometriosis implants over ureter.

For excision, the lesion is outlined by cutting through the peritoneum and into the loose connective tissue with the laser. The underlying loose connective tissue and fat are injected below the peritoneum with irrigating solution to dissect through these layers. This technique is call 'hydrodissection' (or aquadissection) (Nezhat and Nezhat, 1989). Dissection with an irrigating solution is used in vascular areas to avoid inadvertently cutting across large vessels and is used in the broad ligament to push the ureter away from the peritoneum (Figure 37.2). The fluid acts as a backstop to the CO_2 laser, preventing injury to the tissue beneath the peritoneal lesion. Once tissue has been excised it is removed through the laparoscope. Tissue too large for removal through the trocar sheath is cut into smaller sections with scissors or removed by mini-laparotomy or colpotomy.

The advantages and disadvantages of excision are listed in Table 37.1. The method of removal of peritoneal implants should depend upon the surgeon's own experience and skills. A superpulse or ultrapulse laser can be used to decrease carbonization by facilitating rapid vaporization and reduction of the amount of lateral tissue desiccated

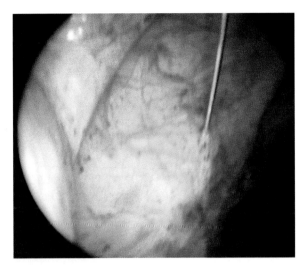

Figure 37.2 Hydrodissection with irrigating solution to lift the lesion off the ureter.

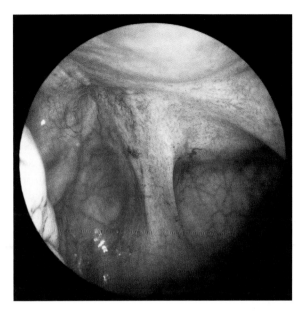

Figure 37.3 Carbon particles from residual vaporization of endometriosis.

Table 37.1 Advantages and disadvantages of excisional method.

Advantages
  Creates less smoke
  Leaves less carbon than vaporization
  Provides tissue for diagnosis
  More likely to remove all deep lesions
Disadvantages
  Removes unnecessary peritoneum
  Technically can be more difficult
  Slightly more time consuming

or coagulated. Some authors recommend removal of the carbon by using pusher sponges (Taylor *et al.*, 1986). However, one of the reasons for using the laser is that it coagulates while it cuts; removing the carbon with a sponge defeats the purpose by wiping off the clots as well as creating microscopic bleeding. Instead, a strong stream of heparinized Ringer's lactate may be introduced through an irrigation probe to wash the carbon from the tissue. Even though carbon is inadvertently left behind, it will have no impact on the patient's well-being. There are no data to support an adverse effect of the carbon left at the time of surgical therapy because the carbon deposits are covered by the healing peritoneum. It is interesting that after laser photovaporization of the cervix the carbon deposits are removed by the body's scavenging system. However, the skilled surgeon must learn to recognize residual carbon at a subsequent laparoscopy. Typically, it appears as a discrete black speck that

appears to have embedded in the peritoneum. There are no areas of scarring around the lesion and no signs of glandular tissue (Figure 37.3). Unless this distinction is made, the patient may be classified as having recurrent endometriosis rather than carbon particles from previous laser surgery.

Bladder Lesions

Bladder lesions can be handled in much the same way as peritoneal disease if the lesions are on the surface of the peritoneum. If a patient has hematuria or irritable bladder symptoms without a definite bladder infection, cystoscopy should be performed. If the lesion involves the bladder mucosa or muscularis, excision may be necessary at laparotomy. All of the peritoneum overlying the bladder can be completely removed. Over a period of 1–2 weeks, reperitonealization will take place and the peritoneum will be completely restored. However, the likelihood of development of extensive adhesions between the bladder and uterus is so great that it is necessary to take every precaution to prevent this from happening. I have used Interceed, the biodegradable cellulose made by Johnson and Johnson to prevent formation of adhesions in this area (Adhesion Barrier Study Group, 1989). If adhesions are allowed to form, irritative bladder symptoms may follow.

Ureter and Uterine Vessels

It is imperative that the ureter and uterine vessels are identified before vaporization of endometrial implants in close proximity to their known location. In the case of a ureter, the peritoneum can be opened above the ureter in an area distal or proximal to the lesion. The path of the ureter can be traced simply by incising the peritoneum with a pair of microscissors or laser until the lesion is identified. With a blunt probe or hydrodissection, the ureter can be easily moved to the side before the lesion is vaporized. If the ureter or large vessel cannot be moved because of significant attachment to the peritoneum or invasion into the ureter itself, laparoscopic removal should not be attempted. Laparotomy should be performed instead. Laparoscopic resection of a segment of ureter has been performed with a laparoscopic ureteral anastomosis (Nezhat and Nezhat, 1989). However, this approach cannot be recommended until there is more clinical evidence to show that the technique is safe and effective.

Cul-de-sac Disease

Most deep cul-de-sac dissections have been performed in the past by laparotomy. With the recent development of new instrumentation, it is now feasible to dissect the cul-de-sac by laparoscopy in most cases. It is extremely important for the lower colon of the patient who has any significant bowel symptoms such as bleeding, pain with defecation, or rectal pressure, to be evaluated by barium enema and colonoscopy. If there is involvement of the mucosa or muscularis, laparoscopic treatment should not be attempted. If the evaluation is negative, then the dissection can be performed.

For proper identification of the rectum and vagina, plastic probes should be inserted into each orifice and the cul-de-sac identified (Figure 37.4). Partial obliteration of the cul-de-sac may be even more difficult to deal with than complete obliteration, caused occasionally by 'tenting up' of the serosa of the colon attached to the back of the vagina. Careful dissection with the laser will gradually separate the two structures. The probes will facilitate identification of the exact location of the vaginal and rectal mucosa (Figure 37.5). In cases of complete obliteration of the cul-de-sac, the probes are invaluable in preventing perforation of the colon. However, it is highly recommended that all patients with colon endometriosis have a thorough bowel preparation such as a clear liquid diet for 48 h and Fleet Phospho-Soda the night before surgery and Fleet enemas in the morning.

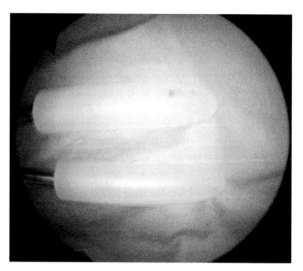

Figure 37.4 Rectal and vaginal probes used in identifying these cavities at laparoscopy.

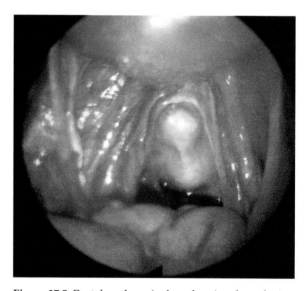

Figure 37.5 Rectal and vaginal probes in place during dissection of the cul-de-sac.

The selection of power density and wavelength most often depends upon the surgeon's experience. At first one should use low power densities in the range of 2500–7000 W cm^{-2} and repeat pulses may be preferable when the laser is first used. Once one is more familiar with the system and the effects on tissue, superpulses or ultrapulses with an average power or 10–30 W can be used. Care must be taken at these higher pulses to avoid entering the muscularis of the rectum. As noted, use of the rectal and vaginal probes will help to prevent such an accident.

Colon

A more extensive discussion of the treatment of colon disease can be found in Chapter 38. However, a few comments are in order regarding superficial disease of the colon. In all patients who are suspected of having some bowel involvement, bowel preparation is mandatory. Whether this is a simple or complete bowel preparation depends upon the surgeon's own preference. Inadvertent entry into the colon would not necessitate a colostomy when a bowel preparation has been used. A superficial lesion, involving the serosal surface only, can be easily removed with a superpulse laser beam of 5–10 W moved rapidly across the colon. As long as the muscularis is not entered, there is no need to close the defect. However, if the muscularis is entered, a 4 0 or 5–0 permanent suture should be used to close the defect. Defects in the mucosa should be closed with absorbable sutures. A physician who lacks the skill to place these small sutures by laparoscopy should resort to laparotomy. Obstructing or concentric lesions generally should be approached by laparotomy. As noted in Chapter 38, instrumentation is available for laparoscopic segmental bowel resections. However, this procedure should only be attempted by an expert laparoscopic surgeon.

Other Areas

During the diagnostic portion of the laparoscopic procedure, care should be taken to look for endometriosis in unusual places such as in the canal of Nuck, pelvic brim, Allen–Masters windows (Allen and Masters, 1955), serosal surface of the small bowel, liver, diaphragm and fallopian tube. In most areas, except the diaphragm, the disease can be easily vaporized with a continuous mode at 8–10 W. When dealing with the round ligament as it enters the canal of Nuck, one must be certain to remove all of the disease. In some instances, endometriosis has been noted deep in the canal and is occasionally found under the inguinal ligament, preventing approach by laparoscopy but requiring direct access through the inguinal ligament itself. Endometriosis on the diaphragm must be carefully vaporized with a low power continuous mode (3–4 W). This area should only be approached by skilled laparoscopic surgeons.

The peritoneal defects commonly known as Allen–Master defects or windows are frequently associated with endometriosis at their base (Figure 37.6). It is important in these cases to open the window and vaporize all the endometriosis within the defect. As these defects can cause pelvic pain or serve as an area for collection of reflux menstrual blood, it is necessary to open the defects even if endometriosis cannot be seen. Should Sampson's theory be correct (Sampson, 1927), then this

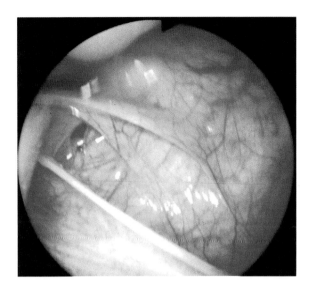

Figure 37.6 Allen–Masters windows seen at laparoscopy to contain endometriosis.

procedure would theoretically prevent recurrence of endometriosis in these areas.

Summary

The treatment of peritoneal endometriosis with laser energy is the most suitable method available. The precision and accuracy of the laser beam and especially the 'what you see is what you get' effect of CO_2 laser, makes the wavelength described in this chapter ideal for surgically treating peritoneal endometriosis. Although this chapter is limited to peritoneal disease, the use of laser energy is obviously very important in removing endometriosis of the ovary and deep endometrial implants involving the cul-de-sac and colon. The value of the laser is limited only by the skill and efficiency of the surgeon.

References

Adhesion Barrier Study Group (1989) Prevention of postsurgical adhesions by INTERCEED (TC7), an absorbable adhesion barrier: a prospective, randomized multicenter clinical study. *Fertility and Sterility* **51**: 933–938.

Allen WM, Masters WH (1955) Traumatic laceration of uterine support. *American Journal of Obstetrics and Gynecology* **70**: 500.

Martin DC, Vander Zwaag R (1987) Excisional techniques with the CO₂ laser laparoscope. *Journal of Reproductive Medicine* **32**: 753.

Martin DC, Hubert GD, Levy BS (1989) Depth of infiltration of endometriosis. *Journal of Gynecologic Surgery* **5**: 55.

Nezhat C, Nezhat FR (1989) Safe laser endoscopic excision or vaporization of endometriosis. *Fertility and Sterility* **52(1)**: 149–151.

Sampson J (1927) Peritoneal endometriosis due to menstrual dissemination of endometrial tissue into peritoneal cavity. *American Journal of Obstetrics and Gynecology* **14**: 422.

Taylor MV, Martin DC, Poston W, Dean DL, Vander Zwaag R (1986) Effect of power density and carbonization on residual tissue coagulation using the continuous wave carbon dioxide laser. *Colposcopy and Gynecologic Laser Surgery* **2**: 169.

38

Monopolar Electroexcision of Endometriosis

DAVID B. REDWINE

2190 NE Professional Court, Bend, Oregon, USA

Introduction

Pain is a more common and more specific symptom of endometriosis than infertility, but not all pelvic pain is due to endometriosis. The clinician treating a patient with endometriosis seeks one of two distinct therapeutic endpoints:

- The successful treatment of symptoms.
- The successful treatment of the disease.

Successful treatment of symptoms may result from any of several nonspecific treatments, which may not have any effect on the disease, while successful treatment of endometriosis requires that something physically destructive is done to the disease, which may not have any effect on symptoms. Although these endpoints seem separate enough, the distinction blurs in clinical practice and even research on the disease is hampered by this lack of focus. The clinician must ask: am I really treating the disease or just its symptoms?

Symptoms of Endometriosis

Patients with pelvic pain due to endometriosis may describe a sharp, stabbing, burning, knifelike pain, which is unrelated to the menses, but can be aggravated by the menstrual flow. Since the cul-de-sac, uterosacral ligaments and medial broad ligaments are the areas of the pelvis most commonly involved by the disease (Table 38.1), physical events that

Table 38.1 Anatomic distribution of endometriosis in 1532 patients treated surgically by the author as of June 5, 1996.*

Site	Number of patients	(%)
Pelvis		
Cul-de-sac	1093	(71.34)
Left broad ligament	798	(52.09)
Right broad ligament	671	(43.80)
Left uterosacral ligament	662	(43.21)
Right uterosacral ligament	611	(39.88)
Bladder	493	(32.18)
Left ovary	276	(18.02)
Right ovary	259	(16.91)
Fundus	241	(15.73)
Left fallopian tube	131	(8.55)
Right fallopian tube	90	(5.87)
Left round ligament	51	(3.33)
Right abdominal wall	44	(2.87)
Left abdominal wall	34	(2.22)
Right round ligament	21	(1.37)
Intestine		
Sigmoid	274	(17.89)
Rectal nodule	183	(11.95)
Ileum	62	(4.05)
Cecum	28	(1.83)
Appendix**	40	(2.61)

*164 endometriosis patients with previous hysterectomy or previous hysterectomy and bilateral salpingo-oophorectomy are excluded from this tabulation.

**Some patients had previous appendectomy.

impact on these areas will frequently produce pain. Therefore, dyspareunia is common, as is pain with defecation during menses. Menstrual aggravation of this pre-existing pelvic pain may be misinterpreted by the clinician as uterine cramping or dysmenorrhea, and it is important to attempt to distinguish between pain due to endometriosis and pain from uterine or ovarian origins.

Obliteration of the cul-de-sac due to invasive disease of the pelvic floor and anterior wall of the rectum may produce pain with defecation throughout the month, and the clinician will do well to note this distinction. Additionally, involvement of the anterior rectal wall may produce constipation which worsens around the menses.

Signs of Endometriosis

The cardinal sign of endometriosis is tenderness of the cul-de-sac or uterosacral ligaments elicited by gentle palpation with the internal examining fingers. It is helpful to avoid the use of the external examining hand, since this will give a clearer indication of true pelvic tenderness. Patients with endometriosis will usually respond to palpation of the posterior pelvis with at least a facial grimace, if not arching of the back and moving up on the couch away from the examining hand. Tender nodularity is almost pathognomonic for endometriosis, while examination during menses may reveal tender nodularity, which is absent at other times of the menstrual cycle (Fallon *et al.*, 1946). Cyclic rectal bleeding is uncommon in patients with intestinal endometriosis (Redwine, 1992a).

Imaging Tests

Imaging tests are not particularly helpful in managing patients with pelvic pain due to endometriosis. Any test result will be either normal or abnormal, and no test will relieve a patient's pain. An abnormal test may prompt more timely surgery, although a normal test should not cause a clinician to dismiss a patient's complaint of pain or the finding of tenderness or nodularity on examination. Intestinal endometriosis almost never penetrates through to the bowel lumen, and intestinal radiographs or colonoscopy examinations are usually negative in the majority of cases of intestinal endometriosis. A decision to proceed with a surgical diagnosis of endometriosis is best made on the basis of suggestive symptoms and signs of disease rather than any test result. Pelvic ultrasound may occasionally be helpful in obese patients or in patients with uterine symptoms that might be due to fibroids missed on pelvic examination.

Advantages of Monopolar Electroexcision of Endometriosis Over Medical Therapy

Medical therapy results in profound temporary relief of hormonally-responsive pain of any origin, including uterine adenomyosis, uterine leiomyomas, primary dysmenorrhea, ovulation pain and endometriosis. This relief of pain does not prove that all the pain that is relieved is due to endometriosis. The nonspecificity of medical therapy results in a factitious magnification of the apparent therapeutic effect, which has led a generation of gynecologists to believe in error that endometriosis might be eradicated by medical therapy. Similarly, relief of symptoms does not prove that endometriosis is being effectively eradicated by medical therapy. Indeed, the perception of improvement of endometriosis following medical therapy has been based both on nonspecific response of symptoms and on the visual assessment at surgery done at the conclusion of therapy. A literature review of studies of medical therapy (Redwine 1992b) indicates a high persistence of biopsy-proven disease at the end of therapy, even in patients with minimal disease. Since all medical therapy is based on the belief that pregnancy and the menopause physically destroy endometriosis, and since these beliefs were never scientifically validated, the limitations of medical therapy come as no surprise.

In contrast, surgeons have been removing diseased tissue from the body for thousands of years. Surgery is eminently understandable to physicians as well as to patients in its mechanical effects. Surgery eradicates the disease, and if the clinician believes that the disease causes symptoms, surgery will eradicate those as well.

Advantages of Monopolar Electroexcision or Laser Excision of Endometriosis Over Superficial Laser Vaporization, Electrocoagulation or Endocoagulation

While laser vaporization, electrocoagulation, or endocoagulation are popular forms of laparoscopic treatment and have the ability to destroy endometriosis, these forms of ablation may not burn deeply enough to destroy invasive disease. Indeed, the likelihood of failure of electrocoagulation is increased when more substantial disease of the uterosacral ligaments exists (Hasson, 1979). Additionally, none of the influential papers on electrocoagulation supply all the information needed to allow a clinician to duplicate this technique, such as the type of electrosurgical generator used, the power setting in watts, the waveform used, the type of active electrode, and the surgical technique employed. None of these forms of therapy returns a pathology report, so the surgeon is the sole judge of what is being treated and how completely it is destroyed. A surgeon employs the senses of sight and touch to ply his trade, and these forms of treatment may compromise both these senses. None of these three forms of treatment has been validated by long-term follow-up as being effective in eradication of endometriosis.

Laparoscopic excision of endometriosis provides a pathology report, allows treatment of deeply invasive disease, and can be done by monopolar electroexcision, laser excision, or sharp dissection. With either monopolar electroexcision or laser excision, high power densities are used to result in a quick clean cut, which can augment blunt dissection for removal of endometriosis. It is important for clinicians to understand that laser vaporization of endometriosis is not the same as laser excision of endometriosis. The author's technique of monopolar electroexcision of endometriosis will be described below, but in skilled hands, laser excision can be equivalent to this method. Palpation and handling of the tissue with scissors and graspers results in tactile feedback, which enhances surgery. Every surgical technique normally used at laparotomy to treat endometriosis can be duplicated endoscopically with simple, inexpensive tools and using excisional techniques familiar to all gynecological surgeons at laparotomy. Finally, laparoscopic excision of endometriosis has a long-term record of efficacy, which has been shown by lifetable analysis to result in effective treatment of endometriosis, even in patients resistant to other forms of therapy (Redwine, 1991). Studies of laser vaporization, electrocoagulation and endocoagulation have focused on symptom outcomes rather than long-term validation of disease destruction, reoperation, and rates of recurrence or persistence. This focus on symptom response rather than disease response makes it difficult to interpret the true efficacy of these modalities in the eradication of endometriosis, particularly since most studies are combined with perioperative medical therapy.

Monopolar Electroexcision of Endometriosis

Does the Patient Need Preoperative Preparation of the Large Bowel?

Certain symptoms and signs suggest the possibility of intestinal endometriosis, and these patients should receive a bowel preparation before surgery. Rectal pain and rectal pain with defecation through-out the month suggest the presence of a rectal nodule of endometriosis. Previous surgery revealing bowel disease or obliteration of the cul-de-sac as well as tender nodularity of the cul-de-sac or uterosacral ligaments are signs associated with the presence of intestinal involvement. Obliteration of the cul-de-sac is sometimes identified in operative reports as 'severe cul-de-sac adhesions' or as 'adherence of the rectosigmoid colon to the uterus'. Thus, although a previous surgeon may have given a passing description of the morphologic findings, the likely presence of a rectal nodule frequently escapes cognition. The presence of a rectal nodule increases the likelihood of disease of the mid-sigmoid, terminal ileum, appendix or cecum.

The bowel preparation I use is NuLytely (generic name: polyethylene glycol 3350), which is composed of polyethylene glycol 31.3 mmol l^{-1}, sodium 65 mmol l^{-1}, chloride, 53 mmol l^{-1} and bicarbonate 17 mmol l^{-1}, (Braintree Laboratories, Braintree, Massachusetts, USA) – 4 l are given orally the afternoon before surgery (8 oz po q 10 minutes) followed by two enemas the evening before surgery results in a superb bowel preparation.

Patient Positioning for Surgery

The patient is placed in a low lithotomy position with a retention catheter in the bladder. Positioning of the legs is particularly important to avoid nerve injury. If knee stirrups are used, extra thick padding under the knees is needed to avoid peroneal nerve paresis. To avoid patient hypothermia, a warming blanket can be placed under the patient, and blankets are placed around the upper torso, head and arms. The arms are ideally tucked along the side of the patient to allow full mobility by the surgeon and the assistant. The irrigation fluid is warmed in a microwave oven to approximately 36°C before it is placed in the pressurized irrigation system. An intrauterine manipulator is placed for intraoperative manipulation, and the table is placed in a steep Trendelenburg position.

Instrumentation

Monopolar electroexcision of endometriosis requires the simplest of tools. After placing an intrauterine manipulator, a 10 mm operating laparoscope with a 3 mm operating channel accepting 3 mm scissors is placed through an all-metal umbilical sheath. Laser laparoscopes are to be avoided since they have a 5 mm air channel, which reduces optical resolution and allows bothersome play in the shaft of the scissors during surgery

(Figure 38.1). If 5 mm scissors are used through the 5 mm channel of a laser laparoscope, the surgical field of view will be obscured by the size of the scissors, and the current density delivered to the tissue will be proportionally reduced because of the larger electrical footprint of the 5 mm instrument. Two 5.5 mm trocars are placed lateral to the inferior epigastric vessels near the top of the pubic hair line with a suction/irrigator passing through the right lower quadrant sheath and a 5 mm atraumatic grasper passed through the left lower quadrant sheath. Intraoperative irrigation is performed with heparinized lactated Ringer's solution. The author uses a ValleyLab (Boulder, Colarado, USA) Force 2 or Force 4 electrosurgical generator. A bipolar coagulator, endoloop sutures and sutures of 3–0 chromic and 3–0 silk will allow almost any presentation of endometriosis to be treated laparoscopically. A high-flow insufflator is helpful, but a video camera and monitor may slow the pace of surgery compared to direct vision down the laparoscope.

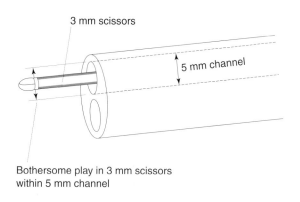

Figure 38.1 There is bothersome play of 3 mm scissors within a 5 mm channel.

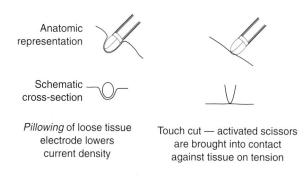

Figure 38.2 Electrical activation of the scissors before touching the tissue helps avoid pillowing of the tissue around the active electrode.

The monopolar electrosurgical generator is set at 90 W of pure cutting (non-modulated) or 50 W of coagulating (modulated) current. Either of these two waveforms can be used for either cutting or coagulation. Pure cutting current is most useful for peritoneal incisions, while the greater voltage potential of coagulation current makes it the current of choice for retroperitoneal or parenchymal cutting. Monopolar scissors are the most versatile tool for resection of endometriosis, allowing various cutting or coagulating surfaces, sharp or blunt dissection, retraction, coagulation or fulguration of bleeders, the ability to grasp and rearrange tissue, and tactile feedback. Instrument exchanges are decreased, and dissection is very fast and virtually bloodless. Cutting tissue is independent of the mechanical sharpness of the scissors. It is important to realize that during laparoscopic electroexcision of endometriosis, the tissue to be cut is held on strong tension and the scissors are electrically activated before touching the tissue. This helps avoid 'pillowing' of the tissue around the active electrode (Figure 38.2), which will reduce the current density under the active electrode. Reduction of current density will result in messy coagulation rather than a clean cut. Finally and importantly, reusable monopolar scissors are inexpensive and lasting.

Identification of Disease

Effective surgical treatment of endometriosis begins with accurate identification of disease. Inaccurate disease identification results in incomplete surgical treatment and confusion about the disease (Redwine, 1990). Some endometriotic lesions can change in appearance with advancing age (Redwine 1987b; Koninckx *et al.*, 1991). Laparoscopy (Vasquez *et al.*, 1984; Redwine, 1988, 1989; Redwine and Yocom, 1990; Nisolle *et al.*, 1990) combined with a knowledge of the morphologic characteristics of normal peritoneum (Redwine, 1988) appears to be more effective than laparotomy (Murphy *et al.*, 1986) in identifying small lesions of endometriosis due to its magnifying effect in near-contact mode. Basic science studies of microscopic endometriosis predict that accurate identification of disease will allow complete destruction of all disease in 75–100% of patients (Redwine, 1988; Redwine and Yocom, 1990). Most patients have disease that is non-hemorrhagic (Figure 38.3).

The general gynecologist will more frequently encounter endometriosis patients with pain than with infertility (Redwine, 1987a). Since invasive disease is strongly associated with the presence of pain (Koninckx *et al.*, 1991), special attention must be paid to its appearance. Invasive disease is more

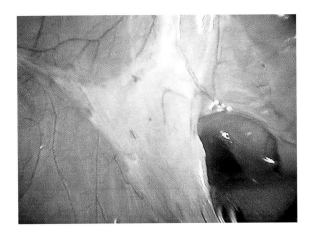

Figure 38.3 The 5 mm suction/irrigator is inserted in a peritoneal pocket of the right cul-de-sac. The whitish fibrosis to the left of the pocket is positive for endometriosis. The individual glands of endometriosis can be seen as small islands of translucency surrounded by rings of white stroma.

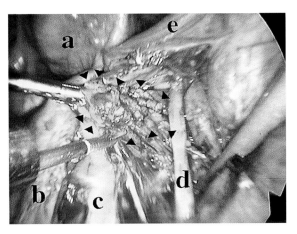

Figure 38.5 The nodule of endometriosis shown in Figure 38.3 is surrounded by arrowheads and has been dissected off the right obturator nerve (d) and lies attached to the adjacent underlying peritoneum. The right infundibulopelvic ligament (b) and the right internal iliac artery (c) have been skeletonized by retroperitoneal dissection. The uterine fundus (a) and the right round ligament (e) are seen in the background. A suction/irrigator is seen on the right edge of the frame and is laterally retracting the right external iliac artery and vein. It is necessary to excise all retroperitoneal fibrosis in order to ensure complete removal of all endometriosis. Surgical techniques that do not result in skeletonization of structures encased in fibrosis will leave invasive endometriosis behind.

likely to be undertreated than superficial disease and frequently has a yellowish-white cast due to overlying fibrosis. Ironically, disease with such an appearance has been trivialized in the past as being 'burned out', when actually it represents highly active 'burned in' disease. Excision of endometriosis ensures that the surgeon will encounter any invasive retroperitoneal fibrotic disease that may be present and increases the likelihood of complete removal. Some innocuous-appearing lesions may at first appear to be superficial, but may invade well beyond the retroperitoneal fatty areolar tissue to involve major pelvic nerves (Figures 38.4, 38.5) or even the periosteum of the ilium (Redwine and Sharpe, 1990).

Techniques of Monopolar Electroexcision of Endometriosis

Laparoscopic electroexcision of endometriosis consists of perhaps 80% blunt dissection to prepare the surgical field and 20% electrosurgery to sever abnormal tissue from healthy tissue. When electrosurgery is used, coagulation current is more versatile than pure cutting current, so it is used more frequently. Monopolar electrosurgery is used in short bursts after the plane of separation between diseased tissue and healthy tissue has been developed. Short bursts of electrosurgery applied to surgical fields where normal tissue has been separated from diseased tissue results in increased surgical safety. When coagulating bleeding vessels, the vessel is specifically grasped first with the scissors, and then 50 W of coagulation current is applied briefly to stop the bleeding.

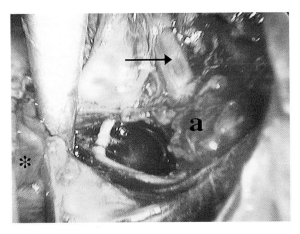

Figure 38.4 Retroperitoneal dissection of the right pelvic sidewall shows a fibrotic nodule of endometriosis (a), wrapped around the right obturator nerve (arrow). The fimbriated end of the right fallopian tube is demarcated by the asterisk.

Superficial Peritoneal Resection

Since most patients do not have severely invasive disease, this is a technique that is very commonly used. During palpation with the graspers, small superficial lesions will be seen to slide easily over retroperitoneal vessels. Normal peritoneum adjacent to diseased peritoneum is grasped, elevated away from underlying vital structures and pulled strongly toward the opposite side of the pelvis. The peritoneum is nicked with the scissors using 90 W of pure cutting current and then the unactivated scissors are used to bluntly dissect the abnormal peritoneum away from underlying structures. The abnormal peritoneum is then grasped and put on strong traction (Figures 38.6, 38.7), so that pure cutting current can then be used to circumscribe the abnormal peritoneum, which is then removed.

Deep Peritoneal Resection

When a lesion is larger, has fibrosis, or retroperitoneal invasion is suspected because vessels or the ureter cannot be seen, the peritoneum adjacent to the lesion should be nicked with cutting current, and the hole grasped and elevated medially so that the scissors can bluntly dissect the lesion away from

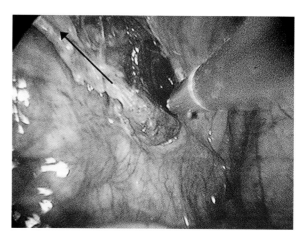

Figure 38.7 After the abnormal peritoneum has been surrounded with a line of incision with pure cutting current, the abnormal peritoneum is placed on further stretch, exposing retroperitoneal fatty tissue. This retroperitoneal fat is being pulled in the direction of the black arrow, and the tissue on traction will be transected with a short burst of 50 W of coagulation current. Since only tissue on traction and in full vision will be transected with electrosurgery, damage to underlying vital structures is unlikely to occur.

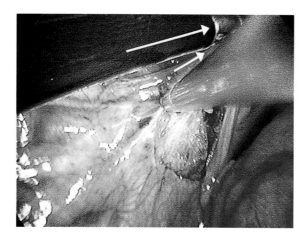

Figure 38.6 This view down an operating laparoscope shows 3 mm scissors entering the surgical field diagonally from the upper right corner of the frame. The shaft of a 5 mm atraumatic grasper is seen across the top of the frame. The larger white arrow along the shaft of the grasper indicates the direction the surgeon is pushing the grasper jaws, which are holding abnormal peritoneum involved by endometriosis. This results in tissue tension along the line indicated by the smaller arrow. This peritoneum on stretch will be transected with electrosurgery applied through the tip of the 3 mm scissors.

underlying structures. Then, grasping either the lesion or the adjacent normal peritoneum as required, the line of incision can be extended around the lesion, with retroperitoneal blunt dissection working towards the center of the bottom of the lesion. It is only during retroperitoneal dissection that the invasiveness of endometriosis will be appreciated. As the more deeply invasive lesion is elevated away from underlying vital structures, retroperitoneal dissection leaves tendrils of somewhat fibrotic tissue, which can be severed with 50 W of coagulation current.

Resection of the Uterosacral Ligament

Either uterosacral ligament may be involved by invasive endometriosis with a volume of 15 cc, with fibrotic extension down to the sacrum. Resection of the entire uterosacral ligament is the only treatment that will ensure complete removal. To resect the uterosacral ligament, incise the peritoneum lateral and parallel to it with 90 W of cutting current. This incision of the adjacent broad ligament results in automatic retraction of the peritoneum with resultant visualization of the retroperitoneal structures. The ureter and uterine vessels can now be dissected bluntly laterally to ensure that they are not near the uterosacral ligament. The ligament can actually be bluntly undermined along much of its lateral length, and this will define much of the ensuing dissection. With bulky invasive disease, fibrosis will extend laterally to involve the ureter, branches of the hypogastric vessels, or the obturator nerve descending along the lateral pelvic wall. In this case the dissection must begin in uninvolved peritoneum more posteriorly along the broad ligament with the dissection working around the ureter inferiorly towards the uterosacral ligament. Just medial to the point where the uterine vessels cross the ureter are the inferior branches of the uterine vessels, which join with vessels ascending from the posterior vaginal wall. Blunt dissection alternating with meticulous use of brief bursts of monopolar current is necessary to separate the uterosacral ligament from these vessels. If bleeding is encountered, it can be safely controlled with monopolar coagulation because the dissection at this point is well medial to the previously identified ureter. Once the lateral margin of the uterosacral ligament has been dissected away from these branches of the uterine vessels, a peritoneal incision is made with cutting current medial and parallel to the ligament. Next, the insertion of the uterosacral ligament into the posterior cervix is divided with unipolar coagulating current at 50 W. The uterosacral ligament is grasped and dissected away from the pelvic floor using a combination of sharp, blunt and electroexcision. As the dissection retreats from the area of the cervix and the endometriotic invasion is completely undermined, it will be seen that the uterosacral ligament becomes less dense and spreads out into the surrounding perirectal connective tissue. At this distal point the ligament is transected and removed.

Ureterolysis, Angiolysis and Neurolysis

Retroperitoneal fibrosis associated with invasive endometriosis will commonly invest the ureters and occasionally the internal iliac vessels and their branches and rarely major pelvic nerves. In these situations, gentle mechanical dissection is required in order to ensure complete removal of disease. An uninvolved area of normal peritoneum is chosen adjacent to the visible peritoneal lesion, then grasped and elevated. The graspers allow just the outer layers of peritoneum to be grasped so the ureter will not tent up into the area of surgery. The elevated peritoneum is then nicked with the pure cutting current. The scissors are inserted retroperitoneally and undermine the peritoneum, bluntly separating it from the underlying vital structures. The peritoneal incision can then be extended along the lesion. This further exposes the retroperitoneal space, and the ureter must be identified. In thin patients, the peristalsis may be quite obvious, while further gentle blunt dissection may be required to identify the ureter in more obese patients. Although it is taught at laparotomy that the ureter is commonly found attached to the peritoneum that is dissected medially away from the pelvic sidewall, the laparoscopic perspective is different. With laparoscopic surgery, the peritoneum anterior to the ureter is commonly incised first, and the ureter will often be seen to lie directly beneath the area of dissection in the visual axis of observation. The graspers can now alternately grasp either the peritoneum or the ureter as the scissors bluntly dissect the ureter out of the fibrosis. Occasional short bursts of monopolar coagulating current will bloodlessly transect peritoneal vessels or tendrils of fibrosis attached to the ureter. It is occasionally necessary to lay the ureter completely bare from the pelvic brim to the uterine vessels. In rare instances the uterine vessels must be sacrificed with bipolar coagulation or endoloops in order to dissect the ureter completely out of investing fibrosis, which may extend towards the base of the bladder.

Retroperitoneal fibrosis resulting from invasive endometriosis can pass beyond the ureter to involve the large pelvic blood vessels, most commonly the branches of the internal iliac artery. The thinner-walled veins lie deeper along the pelvic sidewall and it is rarely necessary to operate around them. The rigidity of the arteries and the fact that they are less commonly involved with severe fibrosis than the ureter makes the dissection easier, since an artery is a more stable structure than the ureter. Still, it is necessary to proceed with caution in this area. The use of monopolar coagulation current along the sidewall will occasionally result in stimulation of the muscles controlled by the unseen obturator or femoral nerves. Although this does not seem to result in any deficit, it is prudent to switch to sharp or blunt dissection or bipolar coagulation if this recurs often.

Involvement of major pelvic nerves by endometriosis is rare, but can be treated by laparoscopic excision using careful blunt and sharp dissection.

Ovarian Endometriosis

Small areas of superficial ovarian endometriosis can be excised by cutting the cortex around the lesion with pure cutting current or sharp dissection and then undermining the cortex with the scissors. This results in removal of more normal ovarian tissue than with laser vaporization or electrocoagulation, although an occasional intraovarian accumulation of bloody fluid may be encountered that was not visually apparent initially. To preserve ovarian tissue, it is more prudent to fulgurate or vaporize larger superficial lesions and probe the interior of the ovary with a needle to search for underlying chocolate cysts (Candiani *et al.*, 1990). Many red superficial lesions are just hemorrhagic adhesions, while not all chocolate cysts are endometriotic (Sampson, 1921) (see Chapter 22).

Endometriotic cysts are frequently adherent to the pelvic sidewall, uterus or sigmoid colon at points of previous rupture and contiguous endometriosis. Therefore an ovary adherent to the pelvic sidewall should bring to mind the possible presence of an underlying endometrioma cyst. When dealing with such cysts, the likelihood of endometriosis in the opposing structure should be considered and dealt with by deep peritoneal resection techniques. Endometriotic cysts usually rupture during surgical treatment. After irrigation and suction of the cyst fluid from the peritoneal cavity, the edge of the cyst wall is grasped and the scissors are used bluntly to dissect away the normal ovarian cortex. If the edge of the cyst wall is indistinct and cannot be grasped easily, the scissors can be used to cut along the normal ovarian cortex adjacent and parallel to the open edge of the cyst cavity. This incision is carried just to the fibrotic capsule of the cyst. The graspers now may grasp a small 'handle' of ovarian cortex attached to the edge of the cyst, allowing a more positive purchase and facilitating the dissection. The endometriotic cyst is then dissected out of the ovarian stroma using blunt dissection. It is occasionally necessary to coagulate bleeders at the base of the cyst. Suture of the cyst wall is not recommended since this may result in increased adhesions. However, suture of an ovary is rarely necessary if the ovarian bleeding cannot be controlled with monopolar electrocoagulation or if the anatomy of the ovary is grossly distorted.

Endometriosis of the Large Bowel

In descending order, the most common sites of intestinal involvement by endometriosis are the sigmoid, rectum, ileum, cecum and appendix (see Table 38.1). The large bowel is composed of four layers: the serosa, outer longitudinal muscularis, inner circular muscularis and mucosa. The serosa does not extend below the peritoneal reflection. Endometriosis almost never penetrates into the bowel lumen, and intestinal diagnostic studies will fail to detect most cases of intestinal disease. Many invasive bowel lesions have a yellowish fibrotic appearance, which blends well with the bowel wall, while other lesions may have associated hemor-

rhage (Figure 38.8). For ease of identification, it is helpful to palpate the bowel wall with the graspers or to slide a ring forceps up and down the bowel to identify a mass effect, which may snap off the end of the ring forceps. If laparoscopic bowel surgery is anticipated, antibiotic prophylaxis and preoperative osmotic bowel evacuation are prudent in case the lumen is entered. My antibiotic regimen is 3 g Unasyn (ampicillin sodium 2 g plus sulbactam sodium 1 g; Roerig, New York, USA) intravenously preoperatively or intraoperatively followed by three more doses every six hours postoperatively.

For penicillin-allergic patients, 1 g Ancef (cefazolin sodium, Smith Kline Beecham, Philadelphia, Pennsylvania, USA) is given intravenously preoperatively or intraoperatively followed by three more doses every six hours postoperatively. Small superficial lesions may be excised by serosal resection and suturing the bowel wall may not be necessary.

The layers of the bowel wall allow partial thickness resection of more invasive lesions. The scissors cut sharply or with short bursts of electrosurgery through the serosa and muscularis to a depth sufficient to allow the lesion to be undermined. This will occasionally require exposure of the mucosa. In many cases, the lesion can then be dissected away from the mucosa without penetration of the lumen (Figure 38.9). The dissection planes offered by the layers of the bowel wall result in a clean, almost bloodless dissection, but the surgeon can easily dissect too far past the lesion, so a two-dimensional awareness of the extent of the lesion along the bowel wall is necessary at all times. The seromuscular defect in the bowel wall is closed with interrupted 3–0 silk sutures.

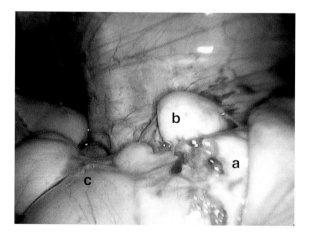

Figure 38.8 Endometriosis of the cecum (a), appendix (b) and ileum (c). Hemorrhagic lesions frequently occur on top of more deeply fibrotic lesions.

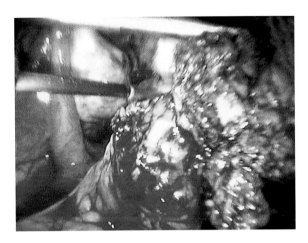

Figure 38.9 A large nodule of endometriosis has been dissected off the mucosa of the sigmoid colon. The nodule is held by graspers seen at the top of the frame. 3 mm scissors are seen below the graspers and have bluntly separated the nodule from the bowel wall without penetrating the adjacent light pink mucosa. The nodule is cyanotic since it is almost completely separated from the bowel.

If the disease and its accompanying fibrosis extend to the submucosa, the dissection will frequently enter the bowel lumen. This allows the extent of the lesion to be palpated through the mucosa under direct visualization. A ring forceps in the bowel creates a dependent space within the bowel where the remaining bowel preparation fluid can collect. As a result, spillage of bowel contents into the pelvis is uncommon. If spillage occurs, copious irrigation and suction is used after closure of the bowel. Full thickness defects can be repaired with a mucosal stitch of running 3–0 chromic followed by interrupted 3–0 silk to close the muscularis and serosal layers. If multiple full thickness resections are anticipated, each defect should be closed before the next is created to limit bowel spillage.

Although not emphasized in the literature, obliteration of the cul-de-sac is highly predictive of the presence of disease invading the anterior wall of the rectum as well as invasive disease of the uterosacral ligaments and the hidden cul-de-sac. Many clinicians may observe 'dense cul-de-sac adhesions' or 'the rectum adherent to the posterior cervix' without realizing that their next thought should be that the anterior wall of the rectum is probably involved with endometriosis. Surgical treatment of the obliterated cul-de-sac involves more than an attempt at mechanical separation of the rectum from the cervix. It includes the appreciation and recognition of the need to remove all invasive endometriosis.

This will frequently require an *en bloc* resection of the uterosacral ligaments, posterior cervix and cul-de-sac, as well as the rectal nodule. If the ovaries are involved by large endometriomas adherent to the pelvic sidewalls, consideration should be given to proceeding with a laparotomy rather than continuing with laparoscopy. This is because ovarian and pelvic sidewall involvement by endometriosis combined with treatment of the obliterated cul-de-sac will result in lengthy surgery, which may be beyond the physical and mental capabilities of the gynecologist.

Laparoscopic surgical treatment of the obliterated cul-de-sac involves specific steps, which are consistently reproducible and will allow an experienced laparoscopist to complete this surgery successfully. These surgical steps include:

- Lateral isolation of the uterosacral ligaments.
- Transverse incision across the cervix above the adherent bowel.
- Intrafascial dissection down the cervix toward the rectovaginal septum.
- Medial isolation of the uterosacral ligaments by development of the rectovaginal septum.
- Transection of the uterosacral ligaments at their insertion into the posterior cervix.
- Mobilization of the rectum by transection of the lateral rectal attachments and *en bloc* resection of the mobilized mass.

These steps can be most efficiently accomplished by use of coagulation current. This may result in partial thickness, full thickness or segmental resection and end to end anastomosis of the bowel. Deep partial and full thickness resections are repaired as discussed above.

Segmental bowel resection with end to end anastomosis is occasionally required for large nodules or multiple nodules along a length of bowel. This can be accomplished intracorporeally laparoscopically (Redwine and Sharpe, 1991; Sharpe and Redwine, 1992), or by transanal (Nezhat *et al.*, 1992) or transvaginal techniques (Redwine *et al.*, 1996). In any laparoscopic technique for segmental bowel resection, it is helpful to separate the mesentery from the bowel segment to be removed by operating directly against the bowel wall where the vessels are smaller and easily controlled with short bursts of coagulation current. A ring forceps in the bowel allows intraoperative manipulation and also results in evacuation of residual liquid bowel preparation material. Once the segment has been sufficiently isolated from its mesentery, it can be delivered transvaginally for segmental resection and anastomosis. If more length is required, the peritoneum alongside the bowel can be incised rostrally. After completion of the anastomosis, the pelvis can be filled with fluid and air injected rectally with a urological syringe to check for leaks.

Complications

The potential complications of laparoscopic surgery include those specific to laparoscopy (injuries caused by trocar insertion, insufflation of carbon dioxide or patient positioning) and those common to laparotomy treatment (bleeding, infection, damage to internal organs and resulting reoperation). Among 359 patients undergoing laparoscopic excision of endometriosis by sharp dissection, only two significant complications were noted, both in association with management of severe adhesions (Redwine, 1991). Among 66 patients undergoing full thickness laparoscopic bowel resection (including 14 undergoing intracorporeal or transvaginal segmental resection and end to end anastomosis), there have been two (3%) serious complications. One patient undergoing transvaginal segmental bowel resection developed a symptomatic rectal stricture, which may require reoperation. Another patient undergoing full thickness anterior rectal wall resection developed a leak of the suture line, which became apparent within three days after surgery. The integrity of the suture line in this patient had been proven intraoperatively by underwater air examination and by injection of povidone iodine. Since a sigmoidoscopy was also performed after these two tests, it is possible that the suture line was disrupted by mechanical trauma. This patient required a temporary colostomy, which has since been reversed. As with laparotomy, intraoperative recognition of unanticipated injury to adjacent vital structures allows them to be repaired primarily at that time, with little serious consequence (Gomel and James, 1991). Unrecognized surgical injury, however, can lead to postoperative morbidity or mortality soon after the completion of surgery.

If a small hole is created in the unprepared bowel, colostomy should not necessarily be performed. Instead, a small defect should be closed laparoscopically with interrupted 3–0 silk and the resulting integrity of the bowel should be checked by underwater air pressure examination. Copious intraoperative irrigation should be performed and postoperative prophylactic antibiotics should be given for approximately 24 hours. If laparotomy and colostomy were to be summarily performed, this would usurp the highly likely probability that the patient would do well with a simple laparo-

scopic repair as well as lead to a later laparotomy for closure of the colostomy.

Among over 569 patients undergoing aggressive monopolar electroexcision of endometriosis by the author since April 1991 there has not been a single incident of unintended injury due to monopolar electrosurgery.

Perioperative Patient Management

Modern laparoscopic surgery is major surgery that bears little resemblance to the ten-minute diagnostic laparoscopy that might have been performed in 1970. The notion that most laparoscopic surgery can be performed on an outpatient basis is unreasonable. Unanticipated admission to the hospital following outpatient surgery has been found to be most strongly associated with the use of general anesthesia and the performance of laparoscopy (Gold et al., 1989). Hospital surgical committees should require minimal recovery criteria to have been met before discharging patients from outpatient surgical centers. These should include cessation of vomiting, demonstrated ability to retain both liquids and pain medication by mouth, and the ability to ambulate to the bathroom with minimal assistance. Patients are frequently discharged too early with unrelenting nausea and vomiting and are unable to retain oral fluids and pain medications. Advanced laparoscopic surgery most commonly results in a hospitalization of 24 hours or less, although laparoscopic segmental bowel resection may require hospitalization of up to five days.

Most patients can resume full activities by three weeks, while intercourse should be delayed for five weeks, especially in patients with cul-de-sac or uterosacral ligament resections. The first two menstrual flows may be unusually painful, and fatigue is common for up to six weeks. Some patients may require four months to appreciate the full extent of pain relief.

Patient Outcome

Lifetable analysis of long-term rates of reoperation and recurrent diagnosis of endometriosis after non-laser resection indicate a maximum occurrence of new disease of 19%, achieved in the fifth postoperative year (Redwine, 1991). Most reoperated patients had no endometriosis, and when disease was present, it was always superficial and minimal in amount. Adhesion formation was more likely to occur following surgery on or around the ovaries, or where adhesions existed at the time of laparoscopic excision. The low rate of recurrence is identical to that found following laparotomy (Wheeler and Malinak, 1987) and is apparently a consequence of the non-spreading nature of endometriosis, which has been demonstrated by three studies (Redwine, 1987a; Koninckx *et al.*, 1991; Marana *et al.*, 1991). Pain relief following excision of endometriosis at laparoscopy or laparotomy has been documented in several publications (Redwine, 1994a, 1994b, 1995).

Complete surgical eradication of endometriosis is possible and will result in pain relief in patients whose pain is due to endometriosis. If pain persists, this does not necessarily indicate a failure of surgical therapy to eradicate endometriosis. Instead, persistent pain indicates the need for more specificity in determining preoperatively which types of pain are more likely to be due to endometriosis.

References

Candiani GB, Vercellini P, Fedele L (1990) Laparoscopic ovarian puncture for correct staging of endometriosis. *Fertility and Sterility* **53**: 994–997.

Fallon J, Brosnan JT, Moran WG (1946) Endometriosis. Two hundred cases considered from the viewpoint of the practitioner. *New England Journal of Medicine* **235**: 669–673.

Gold BS, Kitz DS, Lecky JH *et al.* (1989) Unanticipated admission to the hospital following ambulatory surgery. *Journal of the American Medical Association* **262**: 3008–3010.

Gomel V, James C (1991) Intraoperative management of ureteral injury during operative laparoscopy. *Fertility and Sterility* **55**: 416–419.

Hasson HM (1979) Electrocoagulation of pelvic endometriotic lesions with laparoscopic control. *American Journal of Obstetrics and Gynecology* **135**: 115–119.

Koninckx PR, Meuleman C, Demeyere S, Lesaffre E, Cornillie FJ (1991) Suggestive evidence that pelvic endometriosis is a progressive disease, whereas deeply infiltrating endometriosis is associated with pelvic pain. *Fertility and Sterility* **55**: 759–765.

Marana R, Muzii L, Caruana P *et al.* (1991) Evaluation of the correlation between endometriosis extent, age of the patients and associated symptomatology. *Acta Europaea Fertilitatis* **22**: 209–212

Murphy AA, Green WR, Bobbie D *et al.* (1986) Unsuspected endometriosis documented by scanning electron microscopy in visually normal peritoneum. *Fertility and Sterility* **46**: 522–524.

Nezhat F, Nezhat C, Pennington E (1992) Laparoscopic proctectomy for infiltrating endometriosis of the rectum. *Fertility and Sterility* **57**: 1129–1132.

Nisolle M, Paindaveine B, Bourdon A *et al.* (1990) Histologic study of peritoneal endometriosis in infertile women. *Fertility and Sterility* **53**: 984–988.

Redwine DB (1987a) The distribution of endometriosis in the pelvis by age groups and fertility. *Fertility and Sterility* **47**: 173–175.

Redwine DB (1987b) Age related evolution in color appearance of endometriosis. *Fertility and Sterility* **48**: 1062–1063.

Redwine DB (1988) Is 'microscopic' peritoneal endometriosis invisible? *Fertility and Sterility* **50**: 665–666.

Redwine DB (1989) Peritoneal blood painting: an aid in the diagnosis of endometriosis. *American Journal of Obstetrics and Gynecology* **161**: 865–866.

Redwine DB (1990) The visual appearance of endometriosis and its impact on our concepts of the disease. *Progress in Clinical Biologic Research* **323**: 393–412.

Redwine DB (1991) Conservative laparoscopic excision of endometriosis by sharp dissection: lifetable analysis of reoperation and persistent or recurrent disease. *Fertility and Sterility* **56**: 628–634.

Redwine DB (1992a). Laparoscopic *en bloc* resection for treatment of the obliterated cul de sac in endometriosis. *Journal of Reproductive Medicine* **37**: 695–698.

Redwine DB (1992b) Treatment of endometriosis-associated pain. In Olive DL (ed.) *Endometriosis: Infertility and Reproductive Medicine Clinics of North America.* pp. 697–720. Philadelphia: WB Saunders.

Redwine DB (1994a) Remote postoperative recollection of preoperative pain in patients undergoing excision of endometriosis. *Journal of the American Association of Gynecologic Laparoscopists* **1**: 140–145.

Redwine DB (1994b) Endometriosis persisting after castration: Clinical characteristics and results of surgical management. *Obstetrics and Gynecology* **83**: 405–413.

Redwine DB, Sharpe DR (1990) Endometriosis of the obturator nerve. *Journal of Reproductive Medicine* **35**: 434–435.

Redwine DB, Yocom LB (1990) A serial section study of visually normal pelvic peritoneum in patients with endometriosis. *Fertility and Sterility* **54**: 648–651.

Redwine DB, Sharpe DR (1991) Laparoscopic segmental resection of the sigmoid colon for endometriosis. *Journal of Laparoendoscopic Surgery* **1**: 217–220.

Redwine DB, Perez JJ (1995) Pelvic pain syndromes. In Arregui ME, Fitzgibbons RJ, Katkhouda N, McKernan JB, Reich H (eds) *Principles of Laparoscopic Surgery: Basic and Advanced Techniques.* pp. 545–558. New York: Springer-Verlag.

Redwine DB, Koning M, Sharpe DR (1996). Laparoscopically assisted transvaginal segmental bowel resection for endometriosis. *Fertility and Sterility* **65**: 193–197.

Sampson JA (1921) Perforating hemorrhagic (chocolate) cysts of the ovary. *Archives of Surgery* **3**: 245–323.

Sharpe DR, Redwine DB (1992) Laparoscopic segmental resection of the sigmoid and rectosigmoid colon for endometriosis. *Surgical Laparoscopy and Endoscopy* **2**: 120–124.

Vasquez G, Cornillie F, Brosens I (1984) Peritoneal endometriosis: scanning electron microscopy and histology of minimal pelvic endometriotic lesions. *Fertility and Sterility* **42**: 696–703.

Wheeler JM, Malinak LR (1987) *Contributions to Gynecology and Obstetrics* **16**: 13–21.

39

Laparoscopic Treatment of Advanced Endometriosis

DAN C. MARTIN

1717 Kirby Parkway, Memphis, Tennessee, USA

Introduction

Superficial endometriosis can be destroyed by coagulation while infiltrating lesions require dissection, vaporization or excision (Martin *et al.*, 1989a). Although the depth is related to the size for infiltrating lesions, endometriosis is flattened against the cyst wall in large ovarian endometriomas and does not infiltrate more than 1.5 mm. Thus, exploration, examination and coagulation of the inner lining of even large endometriomas are capable of destroying the endometriosis that lines these.

Although the surgical approach to advanced endometriosis is important, this cannot be used unless lesions are recognized. The difficulty in recognizing the many appearances of surface endometriosis are well known (Jansen and Russell, 1986; Semm, 1987; Redwine, 1987; Martin *et al.*, 1989b; Moen and Halvorsen, 1992). Deep and extensive disease can have a subtle presentation. Stage 0, Score 0 endometriosis can be found with significant bowel and ureteral damage (Moore *et al.*, 1988). Unseen bowel lesions may require palpation for identification (Weed and Ray, 1987). In addition, intraovarian endometriosis (Russell, 1899) and tubal remnant endometriosis (Sampson, 1928) can escape detection.

Pelvic examination during menstruation is needed to find many deep nodules (Koninckx and Martin, 1994; Koninckx, 1996). Careful palpation and examination in the office in addition to examination during menses appear to be needed for preoperative evaluation.

As a separate concern, pelvic inflammatory disease with bilateral ovarian hemorrhagic corpus lutea has an appearance very similar to extensive endometriosis. Two almost identical cases were presented at the Fourth World Congress on Endometriosis in Bahia. One was inflammatory disease and hemorrhagic corpus lutea by histology; the other was said to be severe endometriosis with no histologic confirmation (unpublished data). Clarifying the differences between endometriosis and other similar lesions appears important both for minimal disease and for chocolate cysts (Martin and Berry, 1990; Martin *et al.*, 1994).

Equipment

Bipolar electrosurgery, thermal coagulation, laser coagulation and laser vaporization have all been used to destroy endometriotic lesions without sending the lesions for pathologic confirmation. However, excisional techniques have resulted in increased awareness and increased documentation of the various forms of endometriosis and increase the potential for complete removal of the disease (Martin and Vander Zwaag, 1987; Redwine, 1987; Martin *et al.*, 1989b; Redwine, 1991). Excisional technique can be performed using scissors, lasers or electrosurgical knives as cutting instruments and using bipolar coagulation or mechanical occlusive devices for hemostasis. Although each of these techniques has its own proponents, all appear to result in appropriate patient care. Continued investigation is needed to determine whether certain equipment is best for a given problem (Martin, 1991b). At present, it seems reasonable to conclude that the equipment that appears the most useful to the surgeon is the one that he or she should use.

Ovarian Endometriomas

Smaller ovarian endometriomas can be biopsied and then the base coagulated or vaporized. Endometriomas that are larger than 2 cm require more extensive preoperative preparation and discussion. The larger they are, the greater the chance of finding unexpected cancer (Maiman et al., 1991; Schwartz, 1991a). In addition, those greater than 5 cm are more technically difficult to control as the walls collapse and overlap in the operative field (Martin, 1990). Large endometriomas can take 2–5 hours to remove through a laparoscope. Treatment can consist of drainage, biopsy and coagulation or stripping (Semm and Friedrich, 1987). An intermediate approach is to stage it with limited treatment at first operation and then use postoperative medical suppression, monitoring by sonogram and being prepared to perform a subsequent operative laparoscopy to remove any residual endometriosis.

The easiest approach is to drain the ovarian cyst, take representative biopsies and then coagulate the remnant wall with bipolar coagulation or with laser (Martin and Diamond, 1986; Brosens and Puttemans, 1989). Once the cyst has been drained and lavaged, endometriomas generally have a red or red and brownish mottled appearance on a white fibrotic background. A more uniform brownish appearance is present when these are residual hemorrhagic corpus lutea. Both endometriomas and hemorrhagic corpus lutea contain a significant amount of hemosiderin and this cannot be used as part of the histologic differentiation (Martin and Berry, 1990). Biopsies are most commonly positive when they are taken from the red ridges. The brownish areas are commonly hemosiderin-laden and the cellular architecture is not recognizable.

The stripping technique (Semm and Friedrich, 1987) is begun by aspirating or by opening and draining the cystic ovary. Once it is opened and drained, the inner wall is inspected. If there are areas that suggest cancer, these can be biopsied and a frozen section performed. The opening is generally on the dependent or the broad ligament side to lessen the chance of midpelvic or bowel adhesions. The wall of the endometrioma is then grasped and slowly peeled out of the healthy ovary. A relaxing incision into the healthy ovary sometimes facilitates this stripping. In addition, dissection with water

solutions may help develop the plane of dissection. If the cyst is large and the capsule is adherent near the hilar vessels, the cyst wall can be amputated away from the hilar vessels and then the endometriosis coagulated over this area. Coagulation is effective as the depth of infiltration of endometriosis in the capsule has not been more than 1.5 mm with large endometriomas (Martin, 1990).

Staging the operation may be advantageous and may avoid unnecessary damage to the ovaries. When the ovarian endometriomas are stripped, the specimen commonly includes a thin wall of healthy ovary. Stripping a large endometrioma may remove so much healthy ovarian tissue that the ovary is destroyed. Drainage, biopsy and coagulation allows these endometriomas to shrink in size and potentially avoids further surgery. The disadvantage is that anything short of complete stripping of the internal wall may increase the chance of missing a small focal cancer. After the initial surgery, medical suppression is used and the patients followed by sonography. If there is no evidence of persistence, the medication is stopped and the patients are observed. If persistence occurs, a second laparoscopy is performed and the cyst is stripped or coagulated at that time.

Sutures are not used and adhesions have not been a problem (Martin, 1990, 1991a; Diamond et al., 1991). This is compatible with other studies (Brumsted et al., 1990; De Leon et al., 1990; Meyer et al., 1991; Nezhat et al., 1991a).

If there is great concern regarding the possibility of ovarian cancer on the basis of sonographic appearance or tumor markers (Schwartz, 1991b), then oophorectomy is indicated. If this is to be performed at laparoscopy, spill should be avoided. This can be accomplished by first dissecting the ovary away from its vessels (Figures 39.1–39.7) and off the lateral sidewall and then placing it in a bag. The neck of the bag is closed and pulled through a small incision. With the neck of the bag in an extra-abdominal position, the cyst is then drained. This will generally collapse the cyst so that it can be pulled through the previous trocar incision. Alternatively, a morcellator can be placed in the bag and the cyst morcellated while in the bag. This is based on the techniques used for nephrectomy by urologists.

Deep Infiltration

Although coagulation is effective on lesions less than 2 mm depth, deep lesions with infiltration

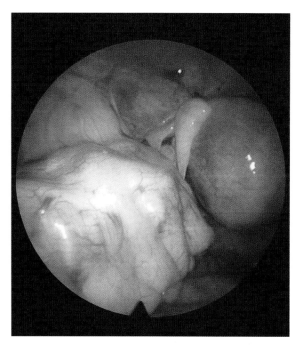

Figure 39.1 This first patient had persistent left adnexal pain and tenderness following a previous attempt at laparoscopic resection of left broad ligament endometriosis. At the first operation, the ureter was not recognized and the procedure was discontinued. The left tube and ovary are hidden behind the sigmoid colon, which is adherent to the left tube and ovary with what appear to be congenital bands and/or adhesions from her endometriosis.

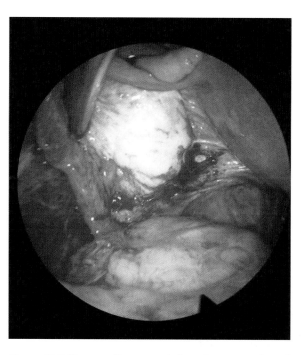

Figure 39.3 Dense adherence of the tube, ovary, broad ligament and uterosacral ligament are seen in the area overlying the ureter.

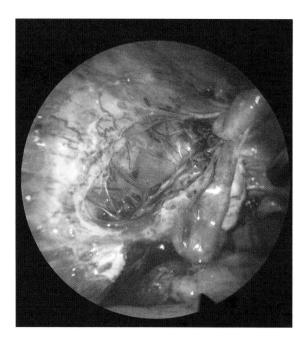

Figure 39.2 The sigmoid colon has been freed from the left tube and ovary and an initial incision made into the left broad ligament lateral to the tube. This portion of the dissection of the infundibulopelvic ligament and ovarian vessels has been done with the carbon dioxide (CO_2) laser in a superpulse mode.

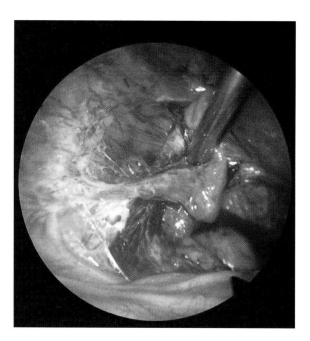

Figure 39.4 Both the lateral and medial leaves of the broad ligaments have been dissected in order to visualize the infundibulopelvic ligament with the ovarian vein and artery. The ureter has been identified in the lower portion of the field. To this point, all dissection has been performed with the CO_2 laser. Bipolar coagulation and endoloops will be used for hemostasis from the ovarian vessels while bipolar coagulation alone will be used to remove the pedicles from the uterus.

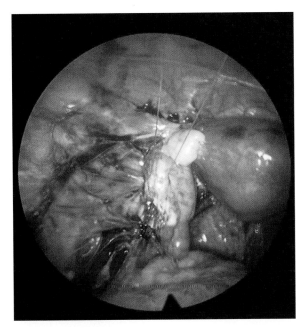

Figure 39.5 The infundibulopelvic ligament has been coagulated at three points and then cut. An endoloop tie has been placed over the ovarian vascular pedicle.

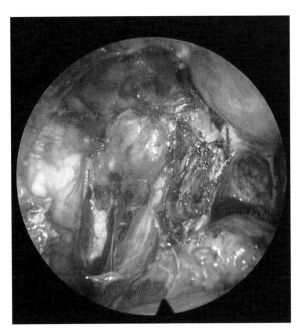

Figure 39.7 Once the ureter was dissected out of the area of the surgical resection, bipolar coagulation and scissors were used for hemostasis before resecting the tube and ovary from the uterus. Compare the tissue distortion of the utero-sacral ligament in this photograph with the lack of tissue distortion following CO_2 laser lysis and initial dissection in Figure 39.2.

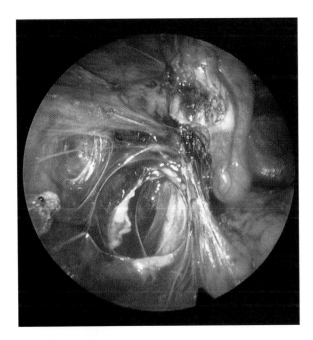

Figure 39.6 The ureter, uterosacral ligament, broad ligament and ovary are densely adherent in the middle of the picture. This area was dissected using a blunt probe and hydrodissection.

≥3 mm were seen in 61% of patients (Martin *et al.*, 1989a) and greater than 6 mm in 9–38% of patients (Koninckx *et al.*, 1991). These deeper lesions require techniques designed for this depth. Although vaporization can be used to remove them, vaporization of larger lesions creates a significant amount of smoke. With deep lesions and when carbon accu-

mulates, residual endometriosis is found in association with carbon or tissue residual following previous vaporization (Martin and Diamond, 1986; Martin, 1990).

Excision has been more reliable for removing these lesions (Figures 39.8–39.11). This has been performed with bipolar coagulation and scissors (Redwine, 1990) and with lasers (Martin and Vander Zwaag, 1987; Nezhat *et al.*, 1989; Cornillie *et al.*, 1990; Koninckx *et al.*, 1991). In addition to scissors or laser as an incising instrument, fluid solutions and blunt probes are used for mechanical dissection. A combination of various mechanical, electrosurgical and laser techniques provides a more comprehensive approach than relying on only one of these techniques.

Mid cul-de-sac endometriosis may be in the rectovaginal septum or involving the rectosigmoid colon. Stage I and II endometriosis are contained within the septum in a position behind the cervix or the posterior upper vault (Adamyan, 1993). This location is one that generally avoids the bowel. This position allows complete resection of full thickness penetration as a combined laparoscopic and vaginal surgery (Martin, 1988; Maher *et al.*, 1995), a laparoscopic operation or a vaginal operation. In Stage I and II there is an intact cul-de-sac with no gross distortion. On the other hand, in Stage III and IV there is distortion of the cul-de-sac with the rectum

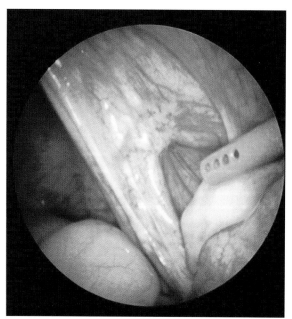

Figure 39.8 In this second patient, peritoneal involvement of the broad ligament overlying the ureter is seen on the right.

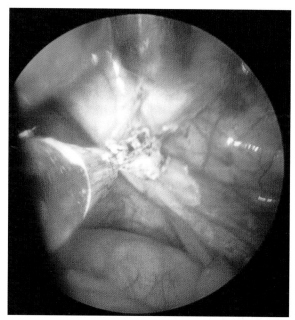

Figure 39.10 The lesion is grasped and pulled medially and then the CO_2 laser is used to dissect through loose connective tissue. If the lesion is pulled further to the midline, fluid solutions will be placed to use as a backstop.

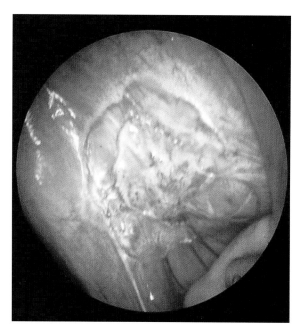

Figure 39.9 The initial part of the dissection is to outline the lesion using the CO_2 laser in superpulse.

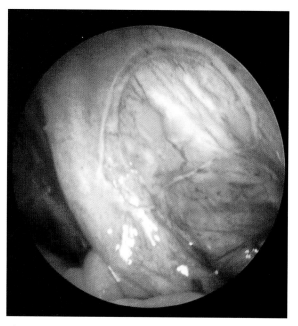

Figure 39.11 The appearance after this resection shows a very thin white rim of coagulation at the perimeter, but the rest of the tissue is healthy with no evidence of damage to the underlying structures.

pulled forward towards the cervix. These are discussed later in the section on rectosigmoid infiltration.

Of academic and theoretic interest, Stage I and II endometriosis (Adamyan, 1993) have similarities to types I and III deep endometriosis (Koninckx and

Martin, 1994). On the other hand, Stage III and IV are compatible with type II disease. One interpretation of this is that Stages I and II are congenital and rise from metaplastic changes occurring in müllerian rests in the rectovaginal septum and are histologically similar to adenomyosis (Donnez *et al.*,

1996). This theory holds that true bowel endometriosis is more likely to be a form of peritoneal endometriosis. This hypothesis is supported by certain embryologic considerations of the rectovaginal septum (Nichols and Randall, 1996) as a remnant of the fetal peritoneum (Gruenwald, 1942), but not supported by gravity distribution mapping (Fallon, 1951).

Bladder and Ureteral Involvement

The majority of lesions overlying the ureter and bladder are in the peritoneum and loose connective tissue and are not adherent to the urinary structures. Sharp dissection with laser, electrosurgery or scissors combined with blunt dissection using probes or hydrodissection (Nezhat and Nezhat, 1989) is used to separate the endometriosis from the underlying structures. If the bladder or ureter does not push away easily, dissection can result in immediate opening or delayed perforation. Avoid difficult dissection unless prepared to manage the possibility of this type of damage.

Unintended ureteral injury has been corrected laparoscopically (Gomel and James, 1991). Ureterolysis and uretero-neocystostomy has been performed by laparoscopic surgery (Nezhat *et al.*, 1991b, 1996). Furthermore, urologists have performed lymph node dissections and radical prostatic resections under laparoscopic control.

Rectosigmoid Infiltration

Infiltration of the rectosigmoid is suggested by a palpable mass on rectal examination, rectal bleeding at the time of menses, persistent pain following laparoscopic removal of recognized lesions, and pain on defecation. Palpation of this area requires close attention to the presence of tenderness, particularly when extending laterally to the bowel and towards the sacral margins. With the deep uterosacral margins involved, lesions can extend around, behind or infiltrate into the rectosigmoidcolon. As this type of surgery has a distinct chance of rectosigmoid resection and anastomosis, a gynecologist or general surgeon familiar with deep bowel surgery is needed. Although this chapter will discuss laparoscopic management of these lesions, they are more commonly managed by laparotomy. This is particularly true for those where the infiltration is lateral to the bowel and is more palpable than visual.

As long as the lesions can be delineated by visualization and by mechanical palpation, they can be resected laparoscopically. However, large lesions can be missed at laparoscopy, but palpated at laparotomy. In addition, the three mesenteric nodules and approximately 50% of the appendiceal involvements in my series were missed at laparoscopy but picked up by palpation at laparotomy. The technical aspects of laparoscopic resection and suturing are easier to overcome than the lack of palpation and manual control.

In preparation for deep resection, a combination of mechanical and antibiotic bowel preparation is used. For those gynecologists who do their own bowel surgery, this will be their routine bowel preparation. If the gynecologist is using a general surgeon as a consultant, the bowel preparation should be that of the general surgeon. Self blood-banking is encouraged as these procedures can last 3–5 hours and if deep vessels are encountered, blood loss can be slow, but substantial.

In controlling these deep resections, the use of intrauterine, intravaginal and rectal manipulators is helpful (Reich *et al.*, 1991). Reich uses a combination of a Sims' curette in the uterus, a sponge on ring forceps in the vagina and a rectal probe in the rectosigmoid area. The rectal probe is a modified 81 French probe. The use of a 25 mm rectal dilator as a probe for distention is discussed later in this chapter.

The initial dissection is to resect the posterior uterine, cervical and uterosacral margins down to the level of the rectovaginal septum. If the rectovaginal septum is free of disease, healthy fat and loose connective tissue will be entered and then the mass is developed laterally and towards the rectal margin. If there is vaginal involvement, laparoscopic colpotomy (Davis and Brooks, 1988; Martin, 1988) is used to remove the vaginal component and to reach the healthy rectovaginal septum.

The posterior cervix is hard to distinguish from the infiltrating endometriosis and careful palpation of this area is needed to limit the amount of healthy cervix removed. Frequent palpation, both vaginal and rectal, can help maintain the orientation, which is frequently lost during these deep dissections. If the vagina is entered, two wet 4 × 4 sponges are placed in the vagina to stop the gas from escaping and to maintain the pneumoperitoneum for the laparoscopy.

An initial series of five patients had anterior rectal wall resection with removal of as much of the component as could be recognized laparoscopically but without full thickness resection. All five of these have subsequently had exploratory laparotomy for residual disease. The largest area that had been missed was a linear area along the anterior wall of approximately 2 cm in length and 1 cm in diameter. These techniques are currently used on small lesions with preparation for full thickness resection and/or laparotomy if needed (Figures 39.12–39.19). Rectal probes are used to help identify residual endometriosis as demonstrated in Figures 39.13–39.17.

For those surgeons who plan to do full thickness resections, Reich reports that using the surgeon's or assistant's finger in the rectum helps identify the extent. Three of Reich's first 236 patients have had full thickness resection with laparoscopic suturing (Reich *et al.*, 1991). I have used an alternative approach for suturing these areas. When there has been full thickness muscularis involvement by small (less than or equal to 1 cm) lesions in the

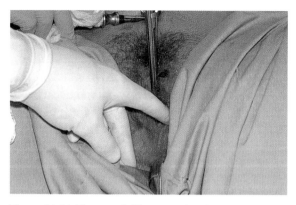

Figure 39.14 The rectal dilator is placed into the rectum and then the gloves are changed.

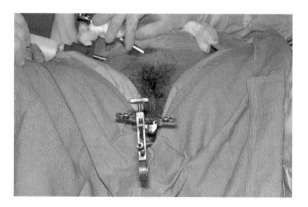

Figure 39.15 The rectal probe is then draped separately to avoid contaminating the rest of the operating field.

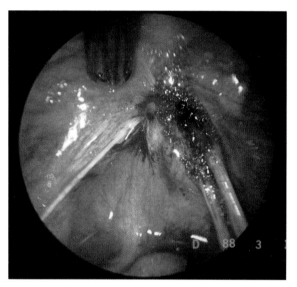

Figure 39.12 In this third patient, a large lesion of the right uterosacral and mid cul-de-sac has pulled the rectum into the cervix.

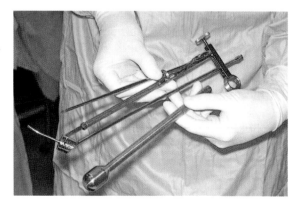

Figure 39.13 The equipment used for this type of dissection includes the Valtchev (Conkin Surgical Instruments) uterine mobilizer to flex the uterus and the 25 mm EEA (end-to-end anastomotic) dilator to distend and define the rectal wall.

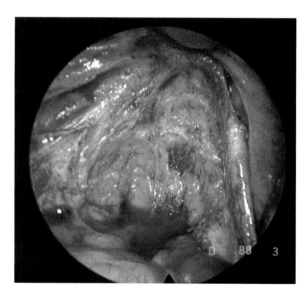

Figure 39.16 Once the resection is complete, the pelvis appears to be free of disease and the rectosigmoid has been freed into a posterior position. This picture is taken with the rectal probe out of position so that there is no distention of the rectum. The location of the rectum becomes easier when the rectal probe is placed as seen in Figure 39.17.

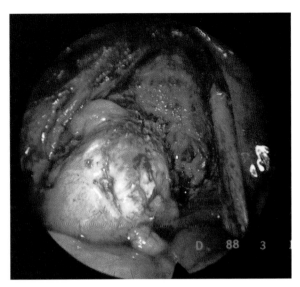

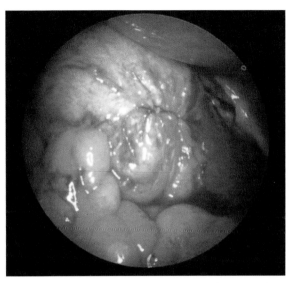

Figure 39.17 With pressure from the rectal probe, residual disease is seen on the right outer margin of the rectosigmoid. Further dissection was needed to remove this part of the lesion. At the end of this dissection, the rectal probe showed no evidence of full thickness perforation. Air can also be injected into the rectum with the rectum under water to check for air leak. However, in spite of testing for perforation, it can still occur as a delayed effect if there is significant compromise to the rectal wall or rectal vasculature.

Figure 39.19 At the end of the suturing, the muscularis layers are closed and healthy non-damaged tissue is noted at the margin.

scopic control for suturing. These have been performed in one patient with a 1 cm rectosigmoid nodule and two additional patients in whom the bowel was densely adherent to the ovary and was entered in the process of freeing bowel from the ovary. In these three patients, an attempt at dissection and resection had been abandoned at a first operation followed by subsequent informed consent and preparation for bowel surgery.

Using cul-de-sac resection techniques, Reich has reported a 76% pregnancy rate for patients with partial cul-de-sac obliteration and a 72% pregnancy rate for patients with complete cul-de-sac obliteration. When broken down by staging, he reported a 100% pregnancy rate for Stage II, 75% for Stage III and 70% for Stage IV (Reich *et al.*, 1991).

Using similar techniques, resections have included rectal and sigmoid anastomosis (Nezhat *et al.*, 1991a; Lyons, 1996). Redwine concluded that if the patient continued to be symptomatic despite meticulous removal of all endometriosis, other causes should be considered. In addition, repeat operations were unproductive and patients with persistent pain appeared to benefit from radical surgery (Redwine, 1991; Redwine and Sharpe, 1991). Nezhat has adapted these techniques to perform deep rectal resection and anastomosis.

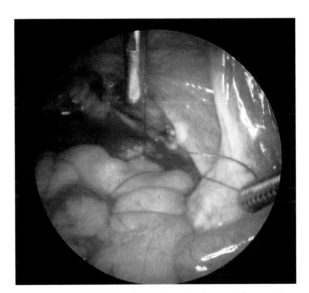

Figure 39.18 This fourth patient had partial resection of the muscularis. Intracorporeal suturing technique was used to oversew this area.

rectosigmoid or low sigmoid, I have pulled these through a colpotomy incision and sutured these vaginally. When the entrance has been at the mid or high sigmoid, a mini-laparotomy has been used, with the bowel moved into this area under laparo-

Laparotomy

Laparotomy is still the standard for surgical therapy of deep and bowel endometriosis. At laparotomy, palpation, delicate handling of deep tissue and multilayered closures are enhanced. Open surgery is used when these characteristics are needed. This appears most useful when patients have deep rectal involvement palpated in the office, deep extension lateral to the rectum extending towards the sacrum and/or persistent pain following initial laparoscopic resection.

In my hands, laparotomy continues to allow better identification of bowel, appendiceal and mesenteric endometriosis. Approximately 50% of appendiceal lesions and all three of my patient's mesenteric lesions were identified at laparotomy, but missed at laparoscopy. This agrees with conclusions that many bowel lesions are like icebergs, with the majority hidden within the muscle (Weed, 1987).

Complications

The major difficulty with deep infiltration involves determining the depth and involvement of other structures such as the ureter, bowel and bladder. Complications have included ureteral lacerations corrected at laparoscopy, bowel lacerations corrected at laparoscopy, bowel lacerations with laparotomy and colostomy, bladder peritoneal fistulas, ureteroperitoneal fistulas and delayed rectal perforation (Martin and Diamond, 1986; Gomel and James, 1991).

The frequency of complications increases if there is deep nodular endometriosis. Examination during menses appears to be mandatory for adequate identification of these lesions. When recognized, preoperative suppression with gonadotropin releasing hormone (GnRH) analogs is associated with decreased complication and reoperation rates (Koninckx, 1996).

Conclusions

The laparoscopic treatment of endometriosis is not limited by the stage or size of the disease. However, extensive laparoscopic treatment can require significantly more time than the same procedure at laparotomy and laparoscopy compromises palpation and delicate handling. These factors and a patient's desires regarding surgery must be balanced in order to come to a reasonable plan of approach for a given clinical situation.

Major complications of the treatment of advanced endometriosis.

- Incomplete procedure due to deep infiltration.
- Recognized ureteral laceration or transection.
- Recognized bowel perforation.
- Leg paralysis or foot drop due to long procedures in stirrups.
- Delayed ureteral perforation.
- Delayed or unrecognized bowel perforation with peritonitis.
- Death secondary to peritonitis.

References

Adamyan L (1993) Additional international perspectives. In Nichols DH (ed.) *Gynecologic and Obstetric Surgery.* pp. 1167–1182. St Louis: Mosby Year Book.

Brosens IA, Puttemans PJ (1989) Double-optic laparoscopy. Salpingoscopy, ovarian cystoscopy and endo-ovarian surgery with the argon laser. *Baillière's Clinical Obstetrics and Gynaecology* **3**: 595–608.

Brumsted JR, Deaton J, Lavigne E, Riddick DH (1990) Postoperative adhesion formation after ovarian wedge resection with and without ovarian reconstruction in the rabbit. *Fertility and Sterility* **53**: 723–726.

Cornillie FJ, Oosterlynck D, Lauweryns JM, Koninckx PR (1990) Deeply infiltrating pelvic endometriosis: histology and clinical significance. *Fertility and Sterility* **53**: 978–983.

Davis GD, Brooks RA (1988) Excision of pelvic endometriosis with the carbon dioxide laser laparoscope. *Obstetrics and Gynecology* **72**: 816–819.

De Leon FD, Edwards M, Heine MW (1990) A comparison of microsurgery and laser surgery for ovarian wedge resections. *International Journal of Fertility* **35**: 177–179.

Diamond MP, Daniell JF, Johns DA *et al.* (1991) Postoperative adhesion development after operative laparoscopy: Evaluation at early second-look procedures. *Fertility and Sterility* **55**: 700–704.

Donnez J, Nisolle M, Smoes P, Gillet N, Beguin S, Casanas-Roux F (1996) Peritoneal endometriosis and endometriotic nodules of the rectovaginal septum are two different entities. *Fertility and Sterility* **66**: 362–368.

Fallon J (1951) Endometriosis. Evidence of tubal origin in the distribution of lesions. *Archives of Surgery* **62**: 412–419.

Gomel V, James C (1991) Intraoperative management of ureteral injury during operative laparoscopy. *Fertility and Sterility* **55**: 416–419.

Gruenwald P (1942). Origin of endometriosis from the mesenchyme of the celomic walls. *Americal Journal of Obstetrics and Gynecology* **44**: 470–474.

Jansen RPS, Russell P (1986) Nonpigmented endometriosis: clinical, laparoscopic, and pathologic definition. *American Journal of Obstetrics and Gynecology* **155**: 1154–1159.

Konincks PR (1996) Complications of CO_2 laser endoscopic excision of deep endometriosis. *Human Reproduction* **11**: 2263–2268.

Konincks PR, Martin DC (1994) Treatment of deeply infiltrating endometriosis. *Current Opinion in Obstetrics and Gynecology* **6**: 231–241.

Konincks PR, Meuleman C, Demeyere S, Lesaffre E, Cornillie FJ (1991) Suggestive evidence that pelvic endometriosis is a progressive disease, whereas deeply infiltrating endometriosis is associated with pelvic pain. *Fertility and Sterility* **55**: 759–765.

Lyons TL (1996). Laparoscopic resection of rectovaginal endometriosis using the contact ND:YAG laser and primary closure with suturing techniques. *Journal of Pelvic Surgery* **2**: 8–11.

Maher P, Wood C, Hill D (1995) Excision of endometriosis in the pouch of Douglas by combined laparovaginal surgery using the Maher abdominal elevator. *Journal of the American Association of Gynecologic Laparoscopists* **2**: 199–202.

Maiman M, Seltzer V, Boyce J (1991) Laparoscopic excision of ovarian neoplasms subsequently found to be malignant. *Obstetrics and Gynecology* **77**: 563–565.

Martin DC (1988) Laparoscopic and vaginal colpotomy for the excision of infiltrating cul-de-sac endometriosis. *Journal of Reproductive Medicine* **33**: 806–808.

Martin DC (1990) Therapeutic laparoscopy. In Martin DC (ed.) *Laparoscopic Appearance of Endometriosis* 2nd Edition. Vol. I, pp. 21–29. Memphis: Resurge Press.

Martin DC (1991a) Laparoscopic appearance of ovarian endometriomas. In Pitkin RM, Scott JR (eds) *Clinical Obstetrics and Gynecology*. pp. 452–459. Philadelphia: JB Lippincott.

Martin DC (1991b) Tissue effects of lasers. *Seminars in Reproductive Endocrinology* **9(2)**: 127–137.

Martin DC, Berry JD (1990) Histology of chocolate cysts. *Journal of Gynecologic Surgery* **6**: 43–46.

Martin DC, Diamond MP (1986) Operative laparoscopy: Comparison of lasers with other techniques. *Current Problems in Obstetrics, Gynecology, and Fertility* **9**: 563–601.

Martin DC, Vander Zwaag R (1987) Excisional techniques for endometriosis with the CO_2 laser laparoscope. *Journal of Reproductive Medicine* **32**: 753–758.

Martin DC, Hubert GD, Levy BS (1989a) Depth of infiltration of endometriosis. *Journal of Gynecologic Surgery* **5**: 55–60.

Martin DC, Hubert GD, Vander Zwaag R, El–Zeky FA (1989b) Laparoscopic appearance of endometriosis. *Fertility and Sterility* **51**: 63–67.

Martin DC, Khare, VK, Parker L (1994) Clear and opaque vesicles: endometriosis, psammoma bodies, endosalpingiosis or cancer. In Coutinho, Elsimar M, Spinola, Paulo and de Moura, Hanson L (eds). *Progress in the Management of Endometriosis*. New York: Parthenon Publishing.

Meyer WR, Gainger DA, DeCherney AH, Lachs MS, Diamond MP (1991) Ovarian surgery on the rabbit: Effect of cortex closure on adhesion formation and ovarian function. *Journal of Reproductive Medicine* **36**: 639–643.

Moen MH, Halvorsen TB (1992). Histologic confirmation of endometriosis in different peritoneal lesions. *Acta Obstetricia et Gynecologica Scandinavica* **71**: 337–342.

Moore JG, Binstock MA, Growdon WA (1988) The clinical implications of retroperitoneal endometriosis. *American Journal of Obstetics and Gynecology* **158**: 1291–1298.

Nezhat C, Nezhat FR (1989) Safe laser endoscopic excision or vaporization of peritoneal endometriosis. *Fertility and Sterility* **52**: 149–151.

Nezhat C, Crowgey SR, Nezhat F (1989) Videolaseroscopy for the treatment of endometriosis associated with infertility. *Fertility and Sterility* **51**: 237–240.

Nezhat C, Silfen S, Nezhat F, Martin D (1991a) Surgery for endometriosis. *Current Opinion in Obstetrics and Gynecology* **3**: 385–393.

Nezhat C, Pennington E, Nezhat F, Silfen SL (1991b) Laparoscopically assisted anterior rectal wall resection and reanastomosis for deeply infiltrating endometriosis. *Surgical Laparoscopic Endoscopy* **1**: 106–108

Nezhat C, Nezhat F, Nezhat C, Nasserbakht F, Rosati M, Seidman DS (1996) Urinary tract endometriosis treated by laparoscopy. *Fertility and Sterility* **66**: 920–924.

Nichols D, Randall CL (1996) *Vaginal Surgery*. Baltimore: Williams and Wilkins.

Redwine DB (1987) Age-related evolution in color appearance of endometriosis. *Fertility and Sterility* **48**: 1062–1063.

Redwine DB (1990) Laparoscopic excision of endometriosis (LAPEX) by sharp dissection. In Martin DC (ed.) *Laparoscopic Appearance of Endometriosis*, 2nd edition. Vol. I, pp. 9–19. Memphis: Resurge Press.

Redwine DB (1991) Conservative laparoscopic excision of endometriosis by sharp dissection: Lifetable analysis of reoperation and persistent or recurrent disease. *Fertility and Sterility* **56**: 628–634.

Redwine DB, Sharpe DR (1991) Laparoscopic segmental resection of the sigmoid colon for endometriosis. *Journal of Laparoendoscopic Surgery* **1**: 217–220.

Reich H, McGlynn F, Salvat J (1991) Laparoscopic treatment of cul-de-sac obliteration secondary to retrocervical deep fibrotic endometriosis. *Journal of Reproductive Medicine* **36**: 516–522.

Russell WW (1899) Aberrant portions of the Müllerian duct found in an ovary. *Johns Hopkins Hospital Bulletin* **94–96**: 8–10.

Sampson JA (1928) Endometriosis following salpingectomy. *American Journal of Obstetrics and Gynecology* **16**: 461–99.

Schwartz PE (1991a) An oncologic view of when to do endoscopic surgery. *Clinical Obstetrics and Gynecology* **34**: 467–472.

Schwartz PE (1991b) Ovarian masses: Serologic markers. *Clinical Obstetrics and Gynecology* **34**: 423–432.

Semm K, Friedrich ER (1987) *Operative Manual for Endoscopic Abdominal Surgery*. Chicago: Year Book Medical Publishers.

Weed JC, Ray JE (1987) Endometriosis of the bowel. *Obstetrics and Gynecology* **69**: 727–730.

40

Laparoscopic Treatment of Bowel Adhesions (Enterolysis)

JAMES F. DANIELL* AND RICHARD W. DOVER[†]

*2222 State Street, Nashville, Tennessee, USA
[†]Royal Surrey County Hospital, Guildford, UK

Introduction

Bowel adhesions that form following intraperitoneal trauma of many causes can be associated with obstruction, intermittent ileus or chronic abdominal pain (Weibel and Majno, 1973; Alexander-Williams, 1987; Keltz et al., 1995). In the past bowel adhesions were usually only lysed when producing severe symptoms or bowel obstruction. In addition, it was considered ill advised to attempt laparoscopy in patients with a history of previous bowel obstruction or suspected omental or bowel adhesions (Cook, 1977). Now, with the greater interest in operative laparoscopy, better equipment and excellent training, both general surgeons and gynecologists are aggressively exploring methods to lyse bowel adhesions via laparoscopy. This chapter will review our experiences, techniques and results for treating bowel adhesions via the laparoscopic approach.

History

A few general surgeons have been active in laparoscopy for over a decade, performing appendectomy (De Kok, 1977; Semm, 1983; Schreiber, 1987) and enterolysis (Kjer, 1987) with good reported results. However, only with the advent of laparoscopic cholecystectomy have North American general surgeons widely accepted laparoscopy (Reddick et al., 1989). As general surgeons embrace laparoscopy, they are also beginning to consider that bowel adhesions may cause chronic pain in addition to obstructive symptoms. Finally, some of these general surgeons are starting to recommend and perform laparoscopic enterolysis for patients with adhesions and abdominal pain.

Gynecologists have long noted that post-surgical adhesions are a common finding at laparoscopy (Daniell and Pittaway, 1983; DeCherney and Mezer, 1984; Diamond et al., 1984). Often these patients are asymptomatic, but certain patients have pain localized in areas overlying known intra-abdominal adhesions. Laparoscopic enterolysis has been reported, specifically following appendectomy (Kleinhaus, 1984), open pelvic surgery in females with post-surgical adhesions and lower abdominal pain (Goldstein et al., 1979; Kresch and Seifer, 1984; Rapkin, 1986; Kjer, 1987; Fayez and Clark, 1994; Tschudi et al., 1993), and in the treatment of acute small bowel obstruction (Adams et al., 1993). Initially, techniques for managing bowel adhesions laparoscopically were simple blunt lysis, electrosurgery or sharp dissection. More recently, lasers, including the carbon dioxide (CO_2) laser (Sutton and MacDonald, 1990) and fiberoptic lasers (Daniell, 1989) have been reported to successfully accomplish enterolysis at laparoscopy.

Armamentarium Available for Laparoscopic Enterolysis

All of the standard methods for adhesiolysis used at laparotomy can now be applied laparoscopically. Initially these included sharp and blunt dissection in combination with traction. More recently, the use of irrigation fluids under pressure has proved to effectively separate tissue planes and to allow lasers or electrosurgical energy to be safely applied laparoscopically for adhesiolysis (Daniell, 1989). Both unipolar and bipolar cautery can be used laparoscopically to deal with adhesions. However, electrosurgical energy is dangerous when used contiguous to the bowel. It is now possible using fine needle electrodes to dissect laparoscopically closer to the bowel than was possible in the past. The CO_2 laser, which has been investigated for laparoscopic use for over a decade, allows vaporization close to the bowel with minimal lateral thermal effect (Sutton and MacDonald, 1990). However, the CO_2 laser can be associated with significant bleeding, generates intraperitoneal smoke, and cannot be used under fluids. More recently, fiberoptic lasers such as the potassium titanyl phosphate (KTP) have been used laparoscopically for many procedures, including enterolysis (Daniell, 1989). Because of its deep thermal effects, the neodymium:yttrum-aluminum-garnet (Nd:YAG) laser is probably not appropriate for enterolysis except if used with expensive synthetic sapphire tips. Fiberoptic laser energy can be delivered under fluids, which effectively eliminates lateral heat transfer from the areas of planned impact to the adjacent bowel. This reduces the risk of thermal damage to the bowel and allows work in a wet field without smoke generation during aquadissection.

Even more recently, titanium clips, which can be placed directly on the bowel serosa without damage (except for direct pressure), have become available for laparoscopy. Special microtipped scissors for laparoscopy now allow fine sharp dissection close to bowel serosa. Finally, the argon beam coagulator (ABC), which allows a non-touch mode of electrosurgical energy, is undergoing clinical investigations for laparoscopic use (Daniell et al., 1993). The ABC allows almost instantaneous hemostasis and can be used in a wet field with no smoke production. It can penetrate tissues 2–3 mm (Bard Electro Medical Systems, 1988), so it must be used judiciously on the bowel serosa. It can be very effective for accomplishing hemostasis during laparoscopic dissection for enterolysis.

It should be emphasized that laparoscopic enterolysis is an advanced operative laparoscopic procedure and should only be attempted by persons comfortable with multiple punctures and skilled in using multiple systems of laparoscopic surgery.

Patient Evaluation and Selection for Laparoscopic Enterolysis

The relationship of chronic abdominal pain to adhesions is very difficult to evaluate scientifically. There are many patients who have extensive abdominal adhesions and no symptoms. There are also patients with marked localized pain that appears to be related to intra-abdominal adhesion formation. Exactly why some patients have pain secondary to adhesions while others do not remains an enigma. Thus, it is important to practice extensive preoperative evaluation and counselling before undertaking attempts at laparoscopic enterolysis.

Most patients referred for an attempt at laparoscopic enterolysis give a history of multiple previous laparotomies with previous adhesiolysis having already been performed by laparotomy, with persistence of symptoms. The patients have often been evaluated by multiple physicians, including internists, gastroenterologists, general surgeons, and psychologists or psychiatrists. As no specific diagnostic tests available to physicians can confirm or rule out abdominal adhesions, accurate diagnosis can only be made by direct intraperitoneal visualization. It is common for patients referred to us to have had extensive work-ups, including magnetic resonance imaging (MRI), computerized tomography (CT), upper gastrointestinal investigations, barium enema, and colonoscopy, with the final conclusion by their physicians that there is no pathology. The patient is then referred to a pain center or psychologist or psychiatrist for chronic pain management. Many of these patients have functional overlay and/or psychologic problems, but the majority of symptomatic patients with a history of adhesions at previous laparotomy will be found to have abdominal adhesions at laparoscopy.

These patients with chronic pain are usually very frustrated with their previous medical care and require careful preoperative counselling and consultation. It is important to warn patients that undertaking a laparoscopy with a history of probable bowel adhesions is risky and may lead to immediate laparotomy because of bowel damage, intraperitoneal bleeding or inability to correct the pathology encountered. It is important to stress to patients and their families that clinical results of laparoscopic enterolysis are not good in all cases. The patient must make the final decision whether to accept the risks associated with attempted operative laparoscopy in these situations or alternatively to cope with chronic pain, intermittent obstruction or other symptoms.

As general surgeons more widely accept the value

of laparoscopy, many patients who in the past have suffered with undiagnosed chronic abdominal pain will be correctly diagnosed as having post-surgical adhesions. These patients can then be given the opportunity to consider laparoscopy as an alternative to no treatment, chronic narcotic use, or repeated laparotomies. Conventional wisdom among surgeons in the past was to offer enterolysis only if the patient was obstructed. In our opinion, this leaves many symptomatic patients in a very difficult medical situation. Certainly there are many data to confirm that any abdominal surgical procedure can result in postoperative adhesions following open or laparoscopic surgery (Diamond *et al.*, 1991). Thus, physicians should always consider abdominal adhesions when evaluating abdominal pain in patients with previous abdominal surgery of any type.

Preoperative Preparation of the Patient for Surgery

We believe that laparoscopic enterolysis is always risky and should only be performed with a general surgeon as co-surgeon or available for immediate assistance if needed. Preferably the patient should consult with this general surgeon preoperatively so that rapport can be established and the patient can be clearly aware of the potential for open bowel surgery, including possible resection and/or temporary diversion. Our method of preoperative bowel preparation consists mainly of 24 hours of clear liquids, with an enema at home the night before surgery. Occasionally, preoperative antibiotics will be given orally by the consulting general surgeon, but usually we only give them intravenously immediately before surgery. All patients must give preoperative consent for possible immediate laparotomy, including all potential procedures that might occur. Ideally, blood should be available, with self-donation preferable.

Operating Room Preparation for Laparoscopic Enterolysis

Since every laparoscopy performed for enterolysis may end up as a laparotomy, it is mandatory that the operating room personnel are prepared for possible laparotomy. Equipment for video monitoring, for open laparoscopy, and a full complement of operative instruments, including aquadissection systems and lasers (if used by the surgeon), should be available. These procedures often involve more

than three punctures. Thus, the surgeon should always request skilled assistants experienced at operative laparoscopy for these difficult operations. To attempt this type of operative procedure without video control is very difficult because the assistant must have adequate visibility to provide the delicate traction, countertraction and exposure that is necessary during dissection. The anesthesiologist should be aware that this may be a long procedure and plan accordingly. The supine position is usually best, since the patient's thighs may hinder laparoscopic manipulations in the dorsal lithotomy position. In females, a uterine elevator or sponge stick in the vagina will aid manipulation during surgery. If necessary, the urinary bladder can be distended with methylene blue dye and/or fiberoptic ureteral stents can be placed if dissection involves the ureters or bladder.

Technique of Establishing Entry into the Abdomen for Laparoscopic Enterolysis

Establishing pneumoperitoneum for initial visualization of the peritoneal cavity is particularly dangerous in patients who have multiple scars from previous laparotomies and thus may have intestine adherent to the abdominal wall. The three methods for accomplishing this are:

- open laparoscopy;
- preliminary insertion of a Veress needle to accomplish pneumoperitoneum; or
- direct trocar insertion with insufflation of gas after initial visualization with the laparoscope.

We believe that the latter option has no place in cases of laparoscopic enterolysis because of the high risk of impaling adherent loops of bowel with the larger trocar, this belief having been substantiated in animal models (Elhage *et al.* 1996). Open laparoscopy can certainly be performed and has been described extensively in the past (Hasson, 1971) but even with this technique perforations are not unknown (Soderstrom, 1993). A recent development has been the transparent ended cannula with a mid-line cutting blade (Visiport, Autosuture Company, Connecticut, USA). This allows direct laparoscopic visualization of the abdominal wall perforation process layer by layer and may well aid the safety of primary trocar entry in patients with adhesive disease. The use of the left upper quadrant as the site of initial entry has been suggested as the most appropriate for patients who have undergone a previous laparotomy (Palmer, 1974; Lang *et al.*, 1993) as it is unusual for adhesions to be present in this area unless a previous splenectomy or gastrectomy has been performed. Although the initial description relates to insertion under the left costal margin, the use of the ninth intercostal space also has its advocates. Our preference is to attempt Veress needle placement at least 5 mm away from any skin incision. The Veress needle is inserted using standard methods and CO_2 is infused at pressures under 20 mmHg. If satisfactory pneumoperitoneum can be established, a 5 mm trocar is inserted and a 5 mm diagnostic laparoscope passed through this initial trocar for initial inspection of the peritoneal cavity. If successful pneumoperitoneum cannot be established, so-called 'finger laparoscopy' can be attempted. With this technique, a mini-laparotomy incision is made and the index finger is inserted and used to bluntly dissect away any structures adherent to the parietal peritoneum in the area of the small incision. Once this area is dissected, a trocar can be placed and the laparoscope introduced.

Each case of laparoscopic enterolysis is different, and thus placement of extra trocars varies, depending upon the fixation of adhesions and/or bowel to the abdominal wall and the patterns in which this fixation occurs. Enterolysis and adhesiolysis are basically the same, the difference being to be careful to distinguish fatty omentum from actual bowel serosa. Omentum or bowel fat is most often adherent to the parietal peritoneum, but occasionally loops of intestinal serosa may be directly attached to this region.

The basic dissection principle is the same as for laparotomy, the difference being that one must work through fixed locations and from a distance. Once the initial visualization of the bowel and its distortion is assessed, a decision is made for the placement of extra trocars. There is no standard location for the extra trocars. This depends upon the location of adhesions and the surgeon's plan for lysis. For instance, if the transverse colon is adherent to the umbilicus, but a free space is seen in the right lower quadrant, a second 5 mm trocar could be placed there and instruments passed for initial manipulation and dissection. It is rarely possible to accomplish enterolysis effectively with only two probes. Thus, safe enterolysis usually requires at least four trocar sites. This allows one for visualization, one for retraction, one for countertraction, and one for dissection. Most of the dissection can be done using 5 mm ports, particularly if a low light video camera with good resolution is used (Circon ACMI, Santa Barbara, California, USA). If necessary, a 5 mm trocar site can be enlarged to 10 mm to introduce an operating scope, which allows instruments to pass down the line of sight, thus allowing dissection without introducing another trocar.

It will be necessary to change the view of the operator to successfully visualize all areas of adhesions. This can be easily accomplished by placing the 5 mm laparoscope through the different ports, and thus interchangeably operating from a different angle. Initially this can be difficult with the video monitor, since most physicians are accustomed to working from one location. The surgeon may find it necessary to change his position around the operating table to maintain orientation and good hand–eye coordination. For instance, for dealing with adhesions beneath the umbilicus, placing the laparoscope suprapubically and looking upwards will give a good view of those adhesions. Accessory probes through each lateral trocar mid-abdomen would then allow effective access for safe dissection.

Method for Enterolysis

Our basic technique for enterolysis is to identify the bowel and omentum and carefully dissect these from the peritoneum, trying to occlude large vessels as they are encountered. This may require the use of laparoscopic clips or electrosurgical or laser energy. Pretied suture loops can be used for hemostasis in larger pieces of omentum, but it is better to occlude each vessel hemostatically before it is separated as the layers of fat are initially dissected from the abdominal walls.

In females, particularly after hysterectomy, adhesions may adhere to the vaginal cuff and bladder peritoneum and along the lateral pelvic sidewalls. A most difficult problem in females is the ovarian remnant syndrome (Utian et al., 1978), in which a residual portion of ovary is often buried retroperitoneally, with the colon adherent to it encompassing the entire area in a mass. Recurrent ovarian function in this fixed area often causes lower abdominal pain in many of these cases. Dissection in this area is particularly tedious and requires an understanding of the anatomy, a willingness to dissect the ureter and vessels retroperitoneally, as well as patience, adequate experience, and the proper equipment.

Our primary method for enterolysis is to use 5 mm atraumatic alligator grasping forceps to grab either bowel or omentum and then attempt blunt dissection and aquadissection with a disposable 5 mm suction/irrigation probe through which we pass a 600 μm KTP/YAG fiber (Figure 40.1). KTP laser energy is used to vaporize thicker bands and the blunt probe through which it passes is used for aquadissection via a disposable suction/irrigation system (Pump Vac Plus, Marlow Medical,

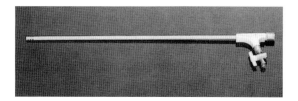

Figure 40.1 The 5 mm disposable suction/irrigation probe used for aquadissection, smoke and fluid suction and blunt dissection is shown here. A 600 μm fiberoptic laser fiber can be passed through the inner channel for tissue vaporization during irrigation.

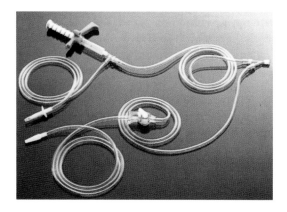

Figure 40.2 This disposable suction/irrigation system for laparoscopic enterolysis has many advantages. The vacuum syringe allows the scrub nurse to vary the volume and pressure of fluid used for aquadissection instantaneously. The valve allows venting of smoke or fluids simultaneously via wall suction. The inflow tubing attaches to a bag of heparinized Ringer's solution (5000 units of heparin per liter), which can be attached to the operating table since pressure or gravity is not needed to accomplish irrigation via the vacuum syringe.

Willoughby, Ohio, USA) (Figure 40.2). This is accomplished while maintaining traction and countertraction with atraumatic graspers. If bleeding cannot be controlled with the KTP laser, endoloop sutures can be placed or laparoscopic clips can be placed using a disposable 10 mm clip applier (US Surgical, Norwalk, Connecticut, USA). Since March 1991 we have used the ABC with a setting of 40–80 W to coagulate bleeding omental vessels in a smokeless non-touch technique using a disposable laparoscopic probe (Birtcher Medical Systems, Irvine, California, USA). Copious volumes of warmed heparinized Ringer's solution (5000 units heparin per liter) are used during the procedure, for both aquadissection and irrigation.

Complications of laparoscopic enterolysis

There are obvious risks associated with attempting laparoscopic enterolysis. These include immediate bowel perforation, bleeding that cannot be controlled laparoscopically, injury to the bowel that results in delayed perforation, ileus, peritonitis, or failure of resolution of the patient's symptoms.

All these patients have a high risk of having adhesions between the abdominal wall and underlying omentum and bowel, making perforation at the time of insertion of the primary trocar a real possibility. Various techniques have been described that aim to reduce the incidence of this complication. It is possible that the use of the left upper quadrant site may be the most prudent option when dealing with a patient with a previous mid-line incision, since these have been shown to be associated with significantly more abdominal wall adhesions than a Pfannenstiel incision (Brill *et al.*, 1995).

Should a bowel perforation be noted, the perforating instrument should not be removed since its presence acts as a marker for the injury. Removal often causes the damaged area to disappear into the multiple loops of small bowel, making its retrieval and subsequent evaluation more difficult and time consuming. Although oversewing a small perforation may be well within the capabilities of most gynecologists, it would seem prudent in these increasingly litigious times, to obtain the opinion and/or assistance of a gastrointestinal surgeon if one is not already present in theater if a perforation is noted.

The one lesson that must be learnt is that all perforations are not recognized immediately, and many take several days to become apparent. Traumatic perforations may present up to nine days later, while perforations secondary to electrical injury may not become apparent for up to 15 days (Soderstrom, 1993). It is salient to note that 51 of 60 patients suffering a traumatic perforation developed increasing abdominal pain within the first three postoperative days. The development of increasing pain or even a failure to improve following laparoscopic surgery of any variety should raise concerns over the possibility of an unrecognized perforation and prompt swift action since delay can be fatal. Of the 13 patients surgically explored 72 hours after the onset of symptoms, three eventually died.

Methods to Reduce Postsurgical Adhesion Formation at Laparoscopic Enterolysis

There are many data in the gynecological literature addressing postsurgical adhesion formation after laparotomy. Recent data suggest that laparoscopic surgery also has a high risk of producing postsurgical adhesions, including both recurrence of old adhesions and *de novo* adhesions, no matter what type of surgical techniques are used (Diamond *et al.*, 1991). Thus we should expect that adhesions may reform after laparoscopic enterolysis. Methods that hope to reduce this re-adhesion formation include the use of heparinized Ringer's solution (5000 units of heparin per liter), careful placement of Interceed (Ethicon, Somerville, New Jersey, USA) intraperitoneally over raw areas, and consideration for early second-look laparoscopy after laparoscopic enterolysis.

There is a large body of literature addressing prevention or reduction of postsurgical adhesions in gynecology, but at present nothing has proved to be clinically effective. The natural history and evolution of adhesion formation after abdominal surgery are still poorly understood in humans. Careful surgical techniques that limit tissue trauma and bleeding and minimize the raw tissue left intraperitoneally are probably the most important factors in reducing postsurgical adhesion formation. At present it seems overly aggressive to routinely recommend early second-look laparoscopy for all patients who have undergone laparoscopic enterolysis. However, in those patients who do not report improvement in their abdominal pain six weeks after extensive enterolysis via laparoscopy, discussion with the patient about a possible second-look laparoscopy should be considered.

Presently, sodium hyaluronate, which is the natural lubricant found in body joints, is being evaluated for its potential to reduce postsurgical adhesions. Whether this substance will be found to be of benefit is unknown at this time as randomized prospective clinical trials using early second-look laparoscopy are just beginning to evaluate its effectiveness for reducing postsurgical adhesions.

Results of Laparoscopic Enterolysis

The actual results of laparoscopic enterolysis are difficult to evaluate scientifically because it requires direct subsequent intraperitoneal observation or alternatively accepting patients' subjective opinions of their clinical improvement. Our initial report retrospectively questioned 42 patients who had undergone at least three previous laparotomies and underwent subsequent laparoscopic enterolysis with fiberoptic laser energy (Daniel, 1989). In this series, 67% of the patients stated that their symptoms were improved when they responded to a questionnaire sent at least six months after their

laparoscopic enterolysis. Fourteen patients were not improved, and ten of those subsequently underwent laparotomy because of persistence of pain, known intraperitoneal adhesions, and inability to cope with their pain non-surgically.

Sutton and MacDonald (1990) in a subsequent report of laparoscopic adhesiolysis using the CO_2 laser as the primary method of dissection, reported 84% improvement in 65 patients with abdominal pain and adhesions without endometriosis. They concluded that laparoscopic adhesiolysis was effective therapy and not a mere placebo effect. A more recent study, also using the CO_2 laser, has produced remarkably similar results with 88% of patients having complete relief of pain (Fayez, 1994). The remaining 12% all derived benefit from the surgery, but were left with some residual discomfort. However, this was not sufficiently severe to impair their daily activities.

North American general surgeons have not yet published data on their experience with laparoscopic enterolysis because of the short time over which they have been attempting these procedures. However, personal communication with general surgeons practicing laparoscopic enterolysis in our area reveals that approximately two-thirds of their patients obtain satisfactory results with this therapy for abdominal pain related to postsurgical bowel adhesions.

The Future of Laparoscopic Enterolysis

As more general surgeons become skilled at laparoscopy, more patients who have bowel adhesions will probably be offered laparoscopic treatment if they are symptomatic. Concomitantly, gynecologists who are also becoming more aggressive at laparoscopy, will find it easier to recruit general surgeons to assist them with laparoscopic enterolysis. One of our problems several years ago was to recruit a general surgeon to assist us at attempts at laparoscopic enterolysis. The difficulties in finding a general surgeon willing to assist at laparoscopy are thankfully now gone for gynecologists. In the future, both gynecologists and general surgeons will treat bowel and other intra-abdominal adhesions more aggressively laparoscopically as they are encountered. Thus, more data will hopefully come forth from both gynecologists and general surgeons based on their experiences dealing with bowel adhesions at laparoscopy.

Animal work in various models will also hopefully be reported from both general surgical and gynecological investigators. This should lead to better instrumentation and techniques for successfully dealing with bowel adhesions laparoscopically, as well as better training for trainee laparoscopists. Patients should benefit from this 'minimally invasive surgery' as treatment for symptomatic bowel adhesions compared to the previously required major open abdominal laparotomy. It does however remain to be seen whether the long-term benefits of laparoscopic enterolysis enjoyed by the vast majority, outweigh the increasing numbers of patients who have to undergo laparotomy to repair the damage caused at attempted laparoscopic treatment of their adhesions.

All laparoscopists should carefully explore the potential for incorporating laparoscopic enterolysis into their practises. Only those laparoscopists who feel very comfortable with aggressive laparoscopic surgery, take the time to acquire the proper training and skills, and practice good patient selection and counselling, should attempt these potentially risky procedures. Much work is needed in carefully controlled animal studies, and both prospective and retrospective analysis of clinical data before firm conclusions can be drawn concerning the efficacy of laparoscopic enterolysis. We encourage all interested endoscopists to join us in evaluating this complicated and difficult medical problem, exploring the role that laparoscopy plays in the management of intra-abdominal adhesions.

Enterolysis

- Provide careful preoperative counselling.
- Discuss and document fully the potential complications especially bowel perforation, colostomy and need for a laparotomy.
- Beware of perforation at the time of insertion of the primary trocar. Consider alternative techniques and sites.
- Insert sufficient accessory ports to allow a safe procedure.
- Be completely familiar with the different depth of thermal effects produced by different energy sources.
- Electrosurgery is potentially very dangerous when used on the bowel. Keep its use to a minimum and beware of thermal injury from other instruments.
- Consider bowel perforation in cases of increasing pain postoperatively.
- Develop a close working relationship with a gastrointestinal surgeon, and look to involve him or her in these cases.
- Do not attempt what your training and experience has not prepared you for.
- In case of difficulties, have a very low threshold for conversion to a laparotomy.

ABC

- Understand the principles and practices of electrosurgery.
- Only fire the ABC when the point of impact is clearly visible and it is safe to do so.
- Be aware of the possibility of a sudden rise in intra-abdominal pressure and the development of a gas embolism.
- Remember that the tissue effect achieved is dependent upon the power setting, distance from the impact site, argon flow rate and the characteristics of the underlying tissue.

Procedure-specific complications (courtesy of I.C. Jourdan and M.E. Bailey, Laparoscopic General Surgeons, Royal Surrey County Hospital, Guildford, UK)

- Adhesions to anterior abdominal wall may cause perforation of attached viscera during entry of Veress needle. Bowel at greatest risk.
- Adhesions may limit positions for trocar insertion, which may compromise technique.
- Adhesions may obscure view and distort anatomy increasing risk of injury.
- Mechanical dissection of adhesions may result in tearing of attached viscera and vasculature. Spleen is particularly vulnerable.
- Adhesions may act as conduits for electrical current resulting in distant burns. Burns to bowel serosa may present as delayed perforation.

References

Adams S, Wilson T, Brown AR (1993) Laparoscopic management of acute small bowel obstruction. *Australian and New Zealand Journal of Surgery* **63**: 39–41.

Alexander-Williams J (1987) Do adhesions cause pain? *British Medical Journal* **294**: 659.

Bard Electro Medical Systems (1988) *System 6000 Argon Beam Coagulator Tissue Effects.* Technical document. Englewood, Colorado: Bard Electro Medical Systems, Inc.

Brill AI, Nezhat F, Nezhat C, Nezhat C (1995) The incidence of adhesions after prior laparotomy: a laparoscopic appraisal. *Obstetrics and Gynecology* **85**: 269–272.

Cook WA (1977) Needle laparoscopy in patients with suspected bowel adhesions. *Obstetrics and Gynecology* **49**: 105–106.

Daniell JF (1989) Laparoscopic enterolysis for chronic abdominal pain. *Journal of Gynecologic Surgery* **5**: 61.

Daniell JF, Pittaway DE (1983) The role of laparoscopic adhesiolysis in an *in vitro* fertilization program. *Fertility and Sterility* **40**: 49.

Daniell JF, Fisher B, Alexander W (1993) Laparoscopic evaluation of the argon beam coagulator – initial report. *Journal of Reproductive Medicine* **38(2)**: 121–125.

DeCherney AH, Mezer HC (1984) The nature of posttuboplasty pelvic adhesions as determined by early and late laparoscopy. *Fertility and Sterility* **41**: 643.

De Kok H (1977) A new technique for resecting the non-inflamed not-adhesive appendix through a mini-laparotomy with the aid of the laparoscope. *Archivum Chirurgicum Neerlandicum* **29**: 195–197.

Diamond MP, Daniell JF, Feste J, McLaughlin D, Martin DC (1984) Pelvic adhesions at early second-look laparoscopy following carbon dioxide laser surgery procedures. *Infertility* **7**: 39–44.

Diamond MP, Daniell JF, Feste J, Martin DC (1991) Postoperative adhesion development after operative laparoscopy: evaluation at early second-look procedures. *Fertility and Sterility* **55**: 700–704.

Elhage A, Lanvin D, Qafli M, Querleu D (1996) Le benefice de la micro-laparotomie ombilicale 'open laparoscopy' pour l'abord coelioscopique. Etude experimentale. *Journal de Gynécologie, Obstétrique et Biologie de la Reproduction* **25(4)**: 373–377.

Fayez JA, Clark RR (1994) Operative laparoscopy for the treatment of localized chronic pelvic-abdominal pain caused by postoperative adhesions. *Journal of Gynecologic Surgery* **10**: 79.

Goldstein DP, DeCholnoky C, Leventhal JM, Emans SJ (1979) New insights into the old problem of chronic pelvic pain. *Journal of Pediatric Surgery* **14**: 675.

Hasson HM (1971) Modified instrument and method for laparoscopy. *American Journal of Obstetrics and Gynecology* **110**: 886–887.

Keltz MD, Peck L, Liu S, Kim AH, Arici A, Olive DL (1995) Large bowel-to-pelvic sidewall adhesions associated with chronic pelvic pain. *Journal of the American Association of Gynecologic Laparoscopists* **3(1)**: 55–59.

Kjer JJ (1987) Laparoscopy after previous abdominal surgery. *Acta Obstetricia et Gynecologica Scandinavica* **66**: 159.

Kleinhaus S (1984) Laparoscopic lysis of adhesions for postappendectomy pain. *Gastrointestinal Endoscopy* **5**: 304.

Kresch AJ, Seifer DB (1984) Laparoscopy in 100 women with chronic pelvic pain. *Obstetrics and Gynecology* **64**: 672.

Lang PFJ, Tamussino K, Honigl W (1993) Palmer's point: an alternative site for inserting the operative laparoscope in patients with intra-abdominal adhesions. *Gynaecological Endoscopy* **2**: 35–37.

Palmer R (1974) Safety in laparoscopy. *Journal of Reproductive Medicine* **13**: 1–5.

Rapkin AJ (1986) Adhesions and pelvic pain: a retrospective study (1986). *Obstetrics and Gynecology* **68**: 13.

Reddick EJ, Olsen D, Daniell J *et al.* (1989) Laparoscopic laser cholecystectomy. *Laser Medicine and Surgery News and Advances* 38–40.

Schreiber J (1987) Early experience with laparoscopic appendectomy in women. *Surgical Endoscopy* **1**: 211–216.

Semm K (1983) Endoscopic appendectomy. *Endoscopy* **15**: 59–64.

Soderstrom R (1993) Bowel injury litigation after laparoscopy. *Journal of the American Association of Gynecologic Laparoscopists* **1(1)**: 74–77.

Sutton C, MacDonald R (1990) Laser laparoscopic adhesiolysis. *Journal of Gynecologic Surgery* **6**: 155.

Tschudi J, Mueller M, Klaiber C (1993) Ist Die laparoskopische Adhasiolyse sinnvoll? *Schweizerische Medizinische Wochenschrift* **123(21)**: 1128–1130.

Utian WH, Katz M, Davey DA, Carr PJ (1978) Effect of premenopausal castration and incremental doses of conjugated equine estrogens on plasma follicle-stimulating hormone, luteinizing hormone, and estradiol. *American Journal of Obstetrics and Gynecology* **132**: 297–302.

Weibel MA, Majno G (1973) Peritoneal adhesions and their relation to abdominal surgery. *American Journal of Surgery* **126**: 345.

41

Prevention of Adhesion Development

MICHAEL P. DIAMOND* AND LISA BARRIE SCHWARTZ†

*Wayne State University, Detroit, USA
†New York University, New York, USA

Introduction

Treatment of adhesions is estimated to cost over 1.2 billion dollars in the USA in one year alone, not including expenses due to loss of work and decreased productivity. For this reason alone, adhesion reduction (and hopefully one day, prevention) should be a major goal of surgical procedures. Obviously, the elimination of postoperative adhesion development would also reduce suffering from infertility, pelvic pain and small bowel obstruction, and the difficulty of reoperative surgery. The etiology of adhesive disease, in addition to surgical trauma, includes pelvic infections, hemorrhage, other types of peritoneal irritation such as foreign body reactions (e.g. talcum powder from surgical gloves, fluff from gauze pads, fibers from torn paper drapes, and reactive suture materials) and endometriosis. The combination of blood with tissue injury is also likely to lead to adhesion formation.

The mechanism of adhesion development has been described as a variation of the normal peritoneal healing process, is currently considered to be independent of the inciting etiology, and is likely to stem from suppressed endogenous fibrinolytic activity due to inhibition of plasminogen activator activity (PAA). Thus, fibrin deposits formed as part of the inflammatory response to peritoneal injury persist (instead of being resorbed due to the function of PAA) and subsequently become infiltrated by fibroblasts forming fibrous adhesions. Factors known to inhibit PAA include tissue ischemia (caused by crushing, ligating or stripping peri-

toneum), surgical trauma (i.e. devascularization, necrosis), and grafting or suturing tissue or other materials to peritoneal defects. Thus, it is not surprising that these factors are thought to stimulate postoperative adhesion development. Of course, this is an overly simplified representation of the healing process. For example, we are just beginning to realize the role of modulators of PAA such as plasminogen activator inhibitors 1 and 2 (PAI-1 and PAI-2), metalloproteases, tissue metalloprotease inhibitors (TIMPs), growth factors (e.g. transforming growth factor (TGF)-β and tumor necrosis factor (TNF)-α), cytokines (e.g. interleukin (IL)-1, IL-6), and integrins, which have been implicated in adhesion development.

Adhesion Reformation versus *De Novo* Adhesion Formation

Adhesion reformation refers to postoperative adhesions located at the same site as the adhesions that were lysed at the initial operative procedure, whereas *de novo* adhesion formation refers to newly formed adhesions present at a location that did not have adhesions at the time of the initial surgical procedure. Each of these categorizations can be further segregated according to whether surgical procedures other than adhesiolysis were performed at that site. Although current data suggest that adhesion formation and reformation differ, the pathophysiology of reformation and *de novo* formation has not yet been well elucidated. However, adhesion reformation is considered to be more difficult to prevent.

In a multicenter study (Diamond et al., 1991), the frequency and severity of adhesion reformation and de novo adhesion formation following laparoscopic surgery was assessed in 68 women. Although the mean adhesion score had decreased by 50% ± 4% as assessed at second-look laparoscopy (SLL) within 12 weeks of the initial operative laparoscopy procedure, 96% of women still had pelvic adhesions. Adhesion reformation was noted in all these women (41% of adhesions were filmy and avascular, while 61% were dense and vascular). De novo adhesion formation occurred in only 16% of women. Likewise, another group (Nezhat et al., 1990) evaluated 157 women at SLL after laparoscopic surgery and noted the occurrence of adhesion reformation, but no de novo adhesion formation. Thus, there remains a high incidence of adhesion development following operative laparoscopy, but de novo adhesion formation is probably less of a problem. Therefore, the focus of this review will be on the methods currently available to prevent adhesion reformation following gynecological endoscopy.

Laparoscopy versus Laparotomy

In a series of reports in which SLL was employed after reproductive pelvic surgery performed at laparotomy, pelvic adhesions were noted in 56–100% of women (Raj and Hulka, 1982; Surrey and Friedman, 1982; Daniell and Pittaway, 1983; DeCherney and Mezer, 1984; Diamond et al., 1984a; McLaughlin, 1984; Pittaway et al., 1985; Trimbos-Kemper et al., 1985; Diamond et al., 1987).

To assess whether the method of entry into the abdominal cavity would alter postoperative adhesion development, Filar et al. in 1987 compared postoperative adhesion formation following standard uterine injury at laparoscopy versus laparotomy in the rat model, and reported no significant difference between the two groups. In contrast, in 1989 Luciano et al. reported fewer adhesions following laparoscopy compared with laparotomy in the rabbit uterine horn model. Thus, the animal literature contains conflicting reports on whether endoscopic surgery will reduce postoperative adhesions.

The question of whether laparoscopic procedures are less likely than laparotomy to lead to postoperative pelvic adhesions has not been adequately studied clinically, probably because of difficulties with proper randomization and control. Postulations as to the reduction of adhesion such as less tissue drying, tissue manipulations, foreign bodies and lack of trauma from packing the bowel at laparoscopy need to be further investigated as potential incremental improvements from laparotomy, although as noted above adhesive development in patients as a whole after laporoscopic adhesiolysis is nearly ubiquitous. In fact, in theory, it is difficult to suggest a mechanism by which adhesion reformation following adhesiolysis using equivalent techniques should be any different based on the manner of entry into the abdominal cavity.

Microsurgery

The backbone of the tenets of gynecological microsurgery rests on the use of appropriate precise surgical techniques aimed at minimizing adverse factors that suppress endogenous PAA and lead to a reduction in adhesion development. In addition to using the microscope, loupes, or laparoscope when appropriate for magnification (which allows the use of fine microsurgical instruments and fine suture of low tissue reactivity), this also involves minimizing tissue handling and trauma, meticulous hemostasis with pinpoint electrocautery, frequent irrigation to prevent tissue drying, elimination of foreign bodies, avoidance of tissue devitalization, and excising rather than incising adhesions. General surgical principles should also include avoiding crushing instruments, irrigating rather than sponging, and eliminating the application of devascularized tissue grafts. When possible, the use of a small fine-caliber tapered atraumatic needle is recommended. Smooth-tipped forceps should be used whenever possible to avoid crushing tissue. A suction apparatus that does not allow delicate tissue to be sucked into the lumen should be used. Woven material should be avoided since it has been shown to cause adhesions due to serosal abrasion. Moist packs are preferable to dry ones. One additional tenet of gynecologic microsurgery, which is often stated, is precise approximation of tissue planes. Based on animal and clinical studies (Diamond and DeCherney, 1987), this premise is now questionable. It has repeatedly been demonstrated in animal studies that closure of ovarian defects after uniform lesioning results in greater, not less, adhesion formation. In humans, the study design has been less than ideal, but also suggests that cortex closure will result in a greater likelihood of adhesion development. While it is not yet appropriate to advocate avoidance of tissue plane closure, these observations do suggest the need to pay particular attention to the method, manner, and circumstances in which non-vital structures are approximated.

These issues about the surgical technique used in the performance of a surgical procedure and the extent to which surgical trauma can be minimized are of utmost importance for reducing postoperative adhesion development.

Careful attention to the choice of suture material is necessary. Catgut sutures are classically the most reactive and should be avoided intraperitoneally when performing reproductive gynecological surgery. Polyglycolic acid (Dexon, Davis and Creeks, Dunbury, Connecticut, USA) and polyglactin (Vicryl, Ethicon, Somerville, New Jersey, USA) reportedly produce much milder foreign body reactions. Multi filament suture reportedly causes more inflammation than monofilament suture. Polydioxanone (PDS), a synthetic absorbable monofilament suture, has been shown by some investigators to cause fewer adhesions than multi filament suture (DeCherney and Laufer, 1983), although others were unable to confirm this difference (Neff et al., 1985).

Meticulous microsurgical technique does not, however, appear to be the sole panacea, since use of these principles in six different studies still resulted in postoperative adhesions at SLL in 56–100% of patients (Raj and Hulka, 1982; Surrey and Friedman, 1982; Daniell and Pittaway, 1983; McLaughlin, 1984; Pittaway et al., 1985; Trimbos-Kemper et al., 1985), although one study reported improved postoperative pregnancy rates after lysis of adhesions using microsurgical (57%) versus macrosurgical (25%) techniques (Diamond, 1979).

Laser Surgery

Use of the laser during reproductive pelvic surgery hypothetically enables more precise incisions, reduced tissue handling and bleeding, and shorter operating time, which have been suggested as causing less tissue trauma and therefore reduced adhesion formation. The carbon dioxide (CO_2) laser is currently most frequently used, but the argon, potassium titanyl phosphate (KTP 532), and neodymium:yttrium-aluminum-garnet (Nd:YAG) lasers are becoming more popular.

However, like microsurgery, results from laser surgery have also been disappointing with regard to eliminating postoperative adhesion formation, with 57–86% of patients having postoperative adhesions at the time of SLL, despite the initial use of the laser in the pelvic surgical procedure (Diamond et al., 1984a; McLaughlin, 1984; Diamond and DeCherney, 1987). In another study, there was no difference in adhesion reformation following laser surgery versus electrosurgery (Talent, 1987). Thus at this time, while the choice of lasers or another surgical modality may be a surgeon's choice based on his or her own experience and expertise, there are no clinical data to prove the benefit of one modality as compared to another either with regard to reduction of postoperative adhesion development, improved chance of pregnancy or reduction in postoperative pelvic pain or bowel obstruction.

Second-look Laparoscopy

The use of SLL following pelvic surgery to assess the pelvis and treat postoperative adhesions has not been thoroughly investigated. Hypothetical potential benefits of SLL include providing postsurgical pelvic assessment, evaluating operative techniques and perioperative therapies, and enhancing initial surgery with the implementation of operative laparoscopic techniques. Several investigators have reported adhesions at early SLL to be predominantly fine, filmy, avascular, and easy to lyse, with less blood loss than the adhesions found at late SLL, which are thick, dense and more vascular (Surrey and Friedman, 1982; Daniell and Pittaway, 1983; DeCherney and Mezer, 1984; Diamond et al., 1984a; McLaughlin, 1984; Trimbos-Kemper et al., 1985; Diamond and DeCherney, 1987).

Pregnancy rates following SLL were found to be 52% at early SLL versus 17% at late SLL by one group (Surrey and Friedman, 1982), but in contrast equal rates were found in both groups in other studies (Raj and Hulka, 1982; DeCherney and Mezer, 1984).

Morbidity, inconvenience, discomfort and expense have been arguments against the use of SLL to evaluate and treat postoperative adhesive disease. While it has been demonstrated by two reports that SLL reduces the extent of adhesions as assessed at third-look laparoscopy, the most important question with regard to early SLL has yet to be resolved; namely whether performance of this procedure improves efficacy (e.g. pregnancy rate, pain reduction).

Adjuvants

Adjuvants have been widely used in attempts at postoperative adhesion reduction. There are numerous uncontrolled non-uniform studies reported in the literature with conflicting results, and the efficacy of adjuvant usage remains inconclusive. Adhesions can be reduced by adjuvants that intervene at various steps in the adhesion formation cascade to decrease the initial inflammation, prevent coagulation, stimulate PA, mechanically separate injured peritoneal surfaces or inhibit fibroblastic proliferation.

Reduction in the inflammatory response is achieved with glucocorticosteroids, non-steroidal anti-inflammatory drugs (NSAIDs) and antihistamines such as promethazine. Glucocorticosteroid use can be complicated by immunosuppression causing infections and wound dehiscence. Progestins also have immunosuppressive effects, causing decreased antibody production and vascular permeability and increased degradation of granulation tissue. Anticoagulants and fibrinolytic agents have been used to prevent persistence of the fibrinous mass, but require high doses with hemorrhagic complications. Perioperative prophylactic antibiotics are commonly used despite a lack of studies. Intravenous doxycycline to empirically treat *Chlamydia* and other infectious organisms is currently a popular regimen. There are promising reports on pentoxifylline, a methylxanthine derivative, for reducing postoperative adhesion reformation in animal models by interfering with multiple steps of the adhesion development process (Steinleitner *et al.*, 1990); currently clinical continuation is lacking.

Use of intra-abdominal instillates and barriers to mechanically separate adjoining raw peritoneal surfaces during the healing process has been extensively studied in both animals and humans. Instillates are thought to prevent early fibrinous adhesion formation by separating raw surfaces by the mechanisms of hydroflotation (increasing intraperitoneal volume by third spacing of fluid into the abdominal cavity) and siliconization (coating tissue surfaces, which reduces direct apposition of traumatized structure). Hyskon (Pharmacia, Piscataway, New Jersey, USA), consisting of 32% dextran 70 (200 ml) has been the most widely used intra-abdominal instillate during pelvic laparotomy or laparoscopy, although studies present inconsistent results. Although shown to be beneficial in most animal models, results of human trials have been variable. Of the four clinical trials, Hyskon was beneficial in two (Adhesion Study Group, 1983; Rosenberg and Board, 1984) and non-beneficial in two (Jansen, 1985; Larsson *et al.*, 1985). Risks, although rare, include fluid imbalance with its sequelae, pseudopulmonary embolus (symptoms due to diaphragmatic irritation), and anaphylaxis. A wide variety of other types of intra-abdominal

instillates have also been used including saline, mineral oil, silicone, povidone, vaseline and crystalloid solutions without consistent efficacy in animal studies. In animal studies hyaluronic acid solutions have variably been reported as being ineffective or effective in reducing postoperative adhesion development when applied at the completion of a surgical procedure. However, when applied as a precoat upon opening the abdominal cavity and intermittently during surgery, it successfully reduces *de novo* adhesion formation in both animal studies (Burns *et al.*, 1995) and a human clinical trial (Diamond *et al.*, 1996).

An additional solution that has shown efficacy is carboxymethylcellulose (CMC), a viscous hydroscopic fluid, which has been shown to reduce adhesion formation and adhesion reformation scores in a rabbit uterine horn model (Diamond *et al.*, 1988a). These observations are consistent with observations of efficacy of CMC in animal studies by other groups. Recently, a film composed of modified hyaluronic acid and carboxymethylcellulose (Seprafilm, Genzyme Cambridge, Massachusetts, USA) has been shown to reduce postoperative adhesion development in general surgery (Becker *et al.*, 1996) and gynecologic studies (Diamond *et al.*, 1996b). In the general surgery study patients underwent colectomy at laparotomy and were randomized to placement or no placement of Seprafilm beneath the midline abdominal incision. Patients subsequently underwent a second surgical procedure to take down the ileostomy and view the underside of the midline incision. Among control subjects, 96% had adhesions in contrast to 51% of the Seprafilm treated subjects (Becker *et al.*, 1996). In the gynecology trials, women were randomized to have their uterus wrapped with Seprafilm after performance of myomectomy. At the time of SLL it was shown that Seprafilm treated patients had fewer sites adherent to the uterus as well as reduced adhesion severity and extent (Diamond *et al.*, 1996b) Recently, a gel formulation of modified hyaluronic acid and carboxymethlycellulose has been successfully used in animal models in two species to reduce postoperative adhesion development (Burns *et al.*, 1996).

In other recent studies, poloxamer 407 (a biocompatible) polymer, which manifests the property of reverse thermal gelation, existing as a liquid at room temperature and a solid at body temperature, has been shown to reduce adhesion development in an animal model (Leach, 1994).

Both endogenous tissues and exogenous materials have been used as barriers to adhesion formation. Devascularized tissue grafts are no longer used since they increase postoperative adhesion formation. Use of material barriers (e.g. metal, plastic, rubber) has also been abandoned since a second procedure is usually necessary to remove them. In addition, foreign body reactions can be precipitated by synthetic materials. The hemostatic agents Surgicel, Gelfoam, and Gelfilm have been used as barriers with efficacy. Interceed (TC7; Ethicon, Somerville, New Jersey, USA), an absorbable barrier, is a 'distant cousin' of Surgicel. Specifically designed for adhesion reduction, Interceed is an oxidized regenerated cellulose material in a knitted weave, differing from Surgicel in the degree of oxidation, porosity, density, and weave. Interceed gelates on raw peritoneum to form a continuous surface within eight hours, preventing fibrin band formation and subsequent fibroblast invasion. Other possible biochemical effects have not yet been explored. Hemostasis must be meticulous before applying Interceed since the presence of blood significantly reduces its ability to minimize subsequent adhesion formation. The efficaciousness of Interceed has now been demonstrated in repeated clinical trials involving parietal peritoneum, ovaries, and fallopian tubes (Wiseman et al., 1994).

A recent prospective multicenter trial showed that Interceed can be safely and easily applied at laparoscopy (Azziz et al., 1991). An average of two pieces were placed per patient with an average time required per piece of 2 minutes 40 seconds. The material was successfully placed through either the umbilical sleeve (using a grasper) or the suprapubic sleeve (using either a grasper or an endoloop applicator). Efficacy of Interceed following laparoscopic application in women has been suggested (Mais et al., 1995).

One additional product available for clinical use is Preclude (formerly Gore-tex Surgical Membrane, W.L. Gore, Flaggstaff, Arizona, USA), an inert, non-reactive material composed of polytetrafluoroethylene. This material has been used by cardiothoracic surgeons as a synthetic pericardial membrane for over ten years. In clinical trials it has been shown to significantly reduce uterine adhesions after myomectomy.

Summary

The reproductive pelvic surgeon continues to face the persistent problem of adhesion reformation interfering with the postoperative results of reproductive pelvic surgery. Prevention is of paramount importance, and should be strived for by carefully applying the combined armamentarium of microsurgical principles, surgical instrumentation and equipment, and adjuvants.

Although adhesion reformation is reduced when these approaches are used, elimination has not yet been achieved. Thus, there remains room for further improvement in therapy. A better understanding of the pathophysiology, especially at the molecular level, may lead to future opportunities, which may be able to be individualized based on unique characteristics of the patient.

References

Adhesion Study Group (1983) Reduction of postoperative pelvic adhesions with intraperitoneal 32% dextran 70: a prospective randomized clinical trial. *Fertility and Sterility* **40**: 612–619.

Azziz R, Murphy AA, Rosenbery SM et al. (1991) Use of an oxidized regenerated cellulose absorbable adhesion barrier at laparoscopy. *Journal of Reproductive Medicine* **36**: 479–482.

Becker JM, Dayton, MT, Faxio VW et al. (1996) Prevention of postoperative adhesions by a sodium hyaluronate-based bioresorbable membrane: a prospective, randomized double-blind multicenter study. *JACS* (In press).

Boyers SP, Diamond MP, DeCherney AH (1988) Reduction of postoperative pelvic adhesions in the rabbit with Gore-tex surgical membrane. *Fertility and Sterility* **49**: 1066–1070.

Burns JW, Skinner K, Colt MJ (1995) Prevention of tissue injury and post surgical adhesions by precoating tissue with hyaluronic acid solutions. *Journal of Surgical Research* **59**: 644–652.

Burns JW, Skinner K, Colt MJ et al. (1996) A hyaluronate based gel for the prevention of post-surgical adhesions. Evaluation in two animal species. *Fertility and Sterility* **66**: 814–821.

Daniell JF, Pittaway DE (1983) Short-interval second-look laparoscopy after infertility surgery. A preliminary report. *Journal of Reproductive Medicine* **28**: 281–283.

DeCherney A, Laufer N (1983) The use of a new synthetic monofilament suture, polydioxanone (PDS), for surgery. *Fertility and Sterility* (abstract) **39**: 401.

DeCherney AH, Mezer HC (1984) The nature of post-tuboplasty pelvic adhesions as determined by early and late laparoscopy. *Fertility and Sterility* **41**: 643–646.

Diamond EE (1979) Lysis of postoperative pelvic adhesions in infertility. *Fertility and Sterility* **31**: 287–295.

Diamond MP (1995) Surgical aspects of infertility. In Sciarra JW (ed.) *Gynecology and Obstetrics*. pp. 1–23. Philadelphia: Harper and Row.

Diamond MP, DeCherney AH (1987) Pathogenesis of adhesion formation/reformation: application to reproductive pelvic surgery. *Microsurgery* **8**: 103–108.

Diamond MP, Daniell JF, Feste J et al. (1984a) Pelvic adhesions at early second look laparoscopy following carbon dioxide laser surgical procedures. *Infertility* **7**: 39–44.

Diamond MP, Daniell JF, Martin DC et al. (1984b) Tubal patency and pelvic adhesions at early second-look laparoscopy following intraabdominal use of the carbon dioxide laser: initial report of the intraabdominal laser study group. *Fertility and Sterility* **42**: 717–723.

Diamond MP, Daniell JF, Feste J *et al.* (1987) Adhesion reformation and *de novo* adhesion formation after reproductive pelvic surgery. *Fertility and Sterility* **47**: 864–866.

Diamond MP, DeCherney AH, Linsky CB *et al.* (1988) Assessment of carboxymethylcellulose and 32% dextran 70 for retention of adhesion in a rabbit uterine horn model. *International Journal of Fertility* **33**: 278–282.

Diamond MP, Daniell JF, Johns DA *et al.* (1991) Adhesion formation and reformation after operative laparoscopy: assessment at early second look procedures. *Fertility and Sterility* **55**: 700–704.

Diamond MP, *et al.* (1996a) Precoating with Sepracoat™ [HAL-C™] reduces *de novo* adhesion formation in multicenter randomized, placebo-controlled gynecologic clinical trial. *43rd Annual Meeting of the Society for Gynecologic Investigation. Philadelphia, Pennsylvania, March 1996.*

Diamond MP *et al.* and the Seprafilm Adhesion Study Group (1996b) Reduction of adhesion after uterine myomectomy by Seprafilm membrane (HAL-F): A blinded, prospective, randomized, multicenter clinical study. *Fertility and Sterility* **66**: 904–910.

Filar S, Gomel V, McComb PF (1987) Operative laparoscopy versus open abdominal surgery: a comparative study on postoperative adhesion formation in the rat model. *Fertility and Sterility* **48**: 486–489.

Interceed (TC7) Adhesion Barrier Study Group (1989) Prevention of postsurgical adhesions by Interceed (TC7), an absorbable adhesion barrier: a prospective randomized multicenter clinical study. *Fertility and Sterility* **51**: 933–938.

Jansen RPS (1985) Failure of intraperitoneal adjuncts to improve the outcome of pelvic operations in young women. *American Journal of Obstetrics and Gynecology* **153**: 363–371.

Larsson B, Lalos O, Marsk L *et al.* (1985) Effect of intraperitoneal instillation of 32% dextran 70 on postoperative adhesion formation after tubal surgery. *Acta Obstetricia et Gynecologica Scandinavica* **64**: 437–441.

Leach RE (1994) Poloxamer 407: Application as a resorbable barrier in adhesion reduction. In Leach RE (ed.) *Infertility and Reproductive Medicine Clinics of North America* **5**: 539–550.

Luciano AA, Maier DB, Koch El *et al.* (1989) A comparative study of postoperative adhesions following laser surgery by laparoscopy versus laparotomy in the rabbit model. *Obstetrics and Gynecology* **74**: 220–224.

Mais V, Ajussa S, Marongiud *et al.* (1995) Reduction of adhesion reformation after laparoscopic endometriosis surgery: A randomized trial with oxidized regenerated cellulose absorbable barrier. *Obstetrics and Gynecology* **86**: 512–515.

McLaughlin DS (1984) Evaluation of adhesion reformation by early second-look following microlaser ovarian wedge resection. *Fertility and Sterility* **42**: 531–537.

Neff MR, Holtz GL, Betsill WL (1985) Adhesion formation and histologic reaction with polydioxanone and polyglactin suture. *American Journal of Obstetrics and Gynecology* **51**: 20–23.

Nezhat CR, Nezhat FR, Metzger DA *et al.* (1990) Adhesion reformation after reproductive surgery by video-laseroscopy. *Fertility and Sterility* **53**: 1008–1011.

Pittaway DE, Daniell JF, Maxson WS (1985) Ovarian surgery in an infertility patient as an indication for a short-interval second-look laparoscopy: a preliminary study. *Fertility and Sterility* **44**: 611–614.

Raj SG, Hulka JF (1982) Second-look laparoscopy in infertility surgery: therapeutic and prognostic value. *Fertility and Sterility* **38**: 325–329.

Rosenberg SM, Board JA (1984) High-molecular weight dextran in human infertility surgery. *American Journal of Obstetrics and Gynecology* **48**: 380–385.

Steinleitner A, Lambert H, Kazensky C *et al.* (1990) Pentoxifylline, a methylxanthine derivative, prevents postsurgical adhesion reformation in rabbits. *Obstetrics and Gynecology* **75**: 926–928.

Steinleitner A, Lambert H, Kazensky C *et al.* (1991) Poloxamer 407 as an intraperitoneal barrier material for the prevention of postsurgical adhesion formation and reformation in rodent models for reproductive surgery. *Obstetrics and Gynecology* **77**: 48–52.

Surrey MW, Friedman S (1982) Second-look laparoscopy after reconstructive pelvic surgery for infertility. *Journal of Reproductive Medicine* **27**: 658–660.

Trimbos-Kemper TCM, Trimbos JB, van Hall EV (1985) Adhesion formation after tubal surgery: results of the eight day laparoscopy in 188 patients. *Fertility and Sterility* **43**: 395–400.

Talent T (1987) Adhesion reformation after reproductive pelvic surgery with and without the carbon dioxide laser. *Fertility and Sterility* **47**: 704–706.

Wisemen DM (1994) Polymers for the prevention of surgical adhesion. In *Polymeric Site Specific Pharmacotherapy.* pp. 370–421. Chichester: Wiley and Sons.

Laparoscopic Oncologic Surgery

42

Laparoscopic Pelvic Lymphadenectomy

DENIS QUERLEU* AND ERIC LEBLANC†

*Hôpital Jeanne de Flandre, Lille, France
†Centre Oscar-Lambret, Lille, France

Current clinical methods of staging pelvic carcinomas are highly inaccurate in detecting metastases to the pelvic lymph nodes (Feigen *et al.*, 1987). The sensitivity of lymphangiography is less than 30%. This technique is unable to visualize internal iliac and other medial node groups. Computerized tomography (CT) and magnetic resonance imaging, with sensitivity ranging from 33–70% are insensitive if the nodes are not macroscopically enlarged. Lymphoscintigraphy is too unreliable for routine use.

As a consequence, lymph node biopsy remains the only reliable method for appraising the status of pelvic lymph nodes. However, the pathologic specimens are taken either during a presurgical staging laparotomy, adding a significant morbidity or during the surgical step of treatment, at a time when primary treatment decisions have already been taken.

Apart from tumor volume and stage, the presence of lymph node metastasis is the most relevant prognostic factor for most pelvic malignancies, particularly prostatic cancers in men and carcinoma of the cervix in women, and may influence treatment choice, especially for those patients with early-stage tumors.

Pelvic lymph node picking by a retroperitoneal endoscopic approach has been described (Wurtz *et al.*, 1987). Progress in laparoscopic surgery gives the opportunity to perform a surgically satisfactory pelvic lymphadenectomy, removing the obturator, external iliac and hypogastric lymph nodes. Dargent and Salvat (1989) have described a panoramic retroperitoneal approach. We have described the technique of pelvic lymphadenectomy by laparoscopy (Querleu, 1989; Querleu *et al.*, 1991). Our group (Querleu, 1992, 1993a, 1994), as well as the University of Arizona group (Childers *et al.*, 1993) later developed the technique of paraaortic lymphadenectomy up to the level of the left renal vein.

Surgical Technique

The technique is carried out on both sides. The patient is placed in the supine position without any flexion of the hips. No cervical tenaculae nor uterine cannulation is necessary. This point is particularly important in cases of carcinoma of the cervix, where trauma to the tumor is unwanted. Under general anesthesia with tracheal intubation a pneumoperitoneum is created and an 11 mm laparoscope (Karl Storz, Germany) is placed through a minimal umbilical incision. A video camera is attached. After observation of the liver surface, the appendix and the internal pelvic organs, two 5 mm incisions are made in the right and left inguinal areas, and trocars are introduced into the abdomen. Ancillary 4.5 mm scissors, atraumatic forceps and irrigation/aspiration aspiration devices are required to be available throughout the procedure. An additional incision is made in the midline above the symphysis pubis, and a 10–12 mm trocar is inserted so that the surgeon is ready at any time to use endoscopic clips and later to remove lymph nodes out of the abdomen with a three-arm retractable Dargent forceps (Lépine, Lyon, France) or any other grasper.

The surgical technique may be described in three parts, involving historical developments of the technique and different rationale:

- The interiliac lymphadenectomy is limited to the area located between the external and internal iliac arteries, including the obturator nodes, the internal iliac nodes and the middle external iliac nodes; its indications are endometrial and early cervical cancers.
- The common iliac lymphadenectomy is the necessary complement to interiliac dissection when full pelvic node dissection is required.
- The parametrial lymphadenectomy is the latest achievement of laparoscopic surgery in gynecologic cancer; it involves dissection of the distal part of the cardinal ligament, removing the parametrial nodes while sparing the vessels and nerves of the cardinal ligament; it may be used in the future as a complement to a laparoscopic or vaginal modified radical hysterectomy.

All these types of lymphadenectomy may be accomplished by a preperitoneal approach or by a transperitoneal approach.

Interiliac Lymphadenectomy

Interiliac lymphadenectomy is performed on each side as follows. The external iliac vessels, ureter, umbilical artery, and in lean patients, obturator nerve, are identified under the peritoneal surface. The operation begins with an incision with scissors of the pelvic peritoneum between the round and infundibulopelvic ligaments. The round ligament is grasped with the forceps. The peritoneum is cut near the round ligament and then easily torn to open the whole area between the round and infundibulopelvic ligaments (Figure 42.1). The incision is made parallel to the axis of the external iliac vessels.

The paravesical space is entered, then widened by blunt dissection between the umbilical artery medially and the external iliac vessels laterally. The instrument grasping the round ligament is freed, closed and placed in the paravesical space, pushing medially the umbilical artery. The pelvic floor is easily reached, either medially or laterally to the obturator pedicle, usually without any bleeding. The cellulolymphatic area below the external iliac vein is then clearly visible and safely dissected (Figure 42.2). The inferior aspect of the external iliac vein is separated by blunt dissection with a closed forceps (Figure 42.3). The obturator nerve is identified and dissected caudally to the point where it leaves the pelvis. The fatty tissue between the obturator nerve and the external iliac vein is then grasped, and thoroughly separated from the pelvic wall. At this point, the pubic bone and the internal obturator muscle are exposed (Figure 42.4). The caudal part of the connective tissue pedicle is then detached by gentle traction from the area of the obturator foramen and femoral canal. The tissue flap is then firmly grasped and moved cranially, then carefully dissected from the external iliac vein and artery laterally and the umbilical artery medially (Figure 42.5). The upper limit of this part of the dissection is the angle between the external iliac vein and the hypogastric vein. Care must be taken in this area to avoid injury to the hypogastric vein or to visceral or parietal veins. At this point, it is advised to free the external iliac vein, and if necessary the external iliac artery, from the pelvic wall by blunt dissection. This allows not only removal of the nodes located between the artery and vein, but also separation of the deep obturator nodes from the obturator muscle. The deep obturator nodes are then ready for removal by gentle traction on their medial aspect, medial to the external iliac vein.

In the next step, the interiliac artery and the branches of its anterior trunk have to be identified. This can be done by blunt dissection of the lateral aspect of the obliterated umbilical artery, which

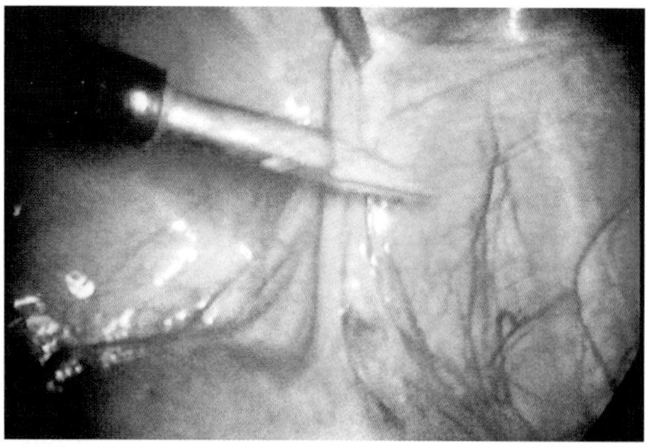

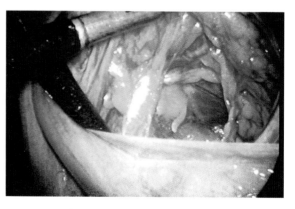

Figure 42.1 Incision of peritoneum between the round and infundibulopelvic ligaments.

Figure 42.2 Laparoscopic view after opening of the paravesical space.

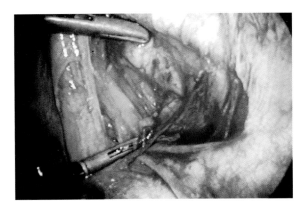

Figure 42.3 Identification and blunt dissection of the external iliac vein.

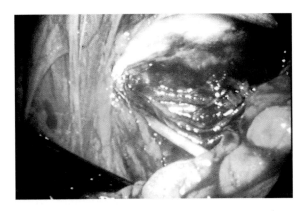

Figure 42.4 Exposition of the pubic bone, the obturator pedicle and the internal obturator muscle.

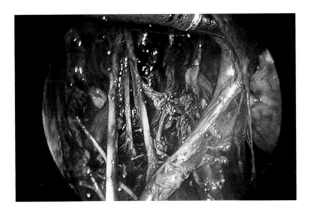

Figure 42.5 Final result.

leads to the origin of the uterine artery and then to the anterior trunk. Care must be taken to avoid injury to the obturator artery. Finally, the nodes located at the bifurcation of the common iliac artery are removed by further dissection of the internal and external iliac arteries. The infundibulopelvic ligament is moved by an ancillary instrument to open this upper part of the interiliac dissection. The first centimeters of the external or internal artery are identified first by gentle blunt dissection. The nodes are freed from the medial aspect of the external iliac vein.

As a rule, the cellulolymphatic tissue is gently separated by traction with a grasping forceps and blunt dissection with the closed tip of another instrument. Additional section of fibrous or lymphatic attachments is sometimes necessary. The tissue sample is thus dissected *en bloc* or in two or three parts, according to the anatomy and firmness of the areolar tissue. The sample has then to be extracted from the abdomen by means of the 10-mm trocar, avoiding any contamination of the abdominal wall by carcinomatous cells. Hemostasis is checked. A minimal amount of blood may have to be aspirated. At the end of the procedure, the peritoneum is left open to allow drainage of lymphatic fluid into the abdomen.

Full Pelvic Lymphadenectomy

In some instances, removal of the nodes located outside the interiliac area may be indicated. Removal of nodes lateral to the external iliac artery requires a blunt dissection between the psoas muscle and the external iliac artery, taking care not to injure the psoas muscle. Removal of common iliac and presacral nodes requires the placement of an incision in the parietal peritoneum above the infundibulopelvic ligament. The ureter must be identified and displaced. This step is usually included in the low paraaortic dissection. The technique currently employed may be summarized as follows. The video monitor is placed at the head of the operating table, and the surgeon stands between the legs of the patient. The surgeon holds the instruments introduced through the left and the lower portals. The assistant holds the endoscope and the instrument introduced through the right port. The operating table is placed in a 10° Trendelenburg position and tilted to the left. The bowel is gently retracted towards the left upper quadrant. The aorta is identified under the peritoneum, up to the level of the mesenteric root. The posterior peritoneum is incised over the lower centimeters of the aorta and the right common iliac artery. The left margin of the incision is grasped by the assistant with a forceps and retracted laterally to the left side of the patient, ensuring in most cases retraction of the bowel. The common iliac vessels are identified and freed by blunt dissection. Laterally, the psoas muscles and the ureters are easily reached. Throughout the operation, blunt dissection with the closed end of atraumatic forceps or with the tip of the aspiration device (used at the same time to clarify the operative field when necessary) seems to provide the safest way of freeing the cellulolymphatic flaps. Electrosurgery with monopolar scissors may also be used. As soon as part of a flap is freed from the great vessels, it may be firmly grasped with forceps and elevated to show its posterior aspect overlying the vessels or the prevertebral plane. Care must be taken during dissection from the great vessels (Figure 42.6), particularly the left common iliac vein, and from the presacral and low lumbar veins.

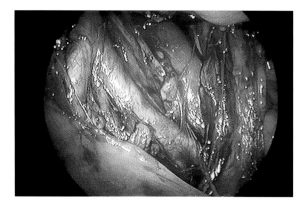

Figure 42.6 Dissection of the right common iliac artery.

Parametrial Lymphadenectomy

The removal of the parietal lymph nodes related to the uterus is generally referred to as 'pelvic' lymphadenectomy. However, these nodes are not the only ones involved in the natural history of cervical carcinomas.

Some lymphatic channels occasionally interrupted by one or rarely several nodes may be found running along the uterine artery. They may be selectively removed by laparoscopy by blunt separation from the uterine artery, or their removal may be included in the removal of the entire uterine artery during radical hysterectomy. This step of the operation is quite feasible by laparoscopy as part of a full laparoscopic hysterectomy or as part of a laparoscopically assisted radical vaginal hysterectomy (Querleu, 1993b).

Much more frequently, lymph nodes are found in the cardinal ligament (paracervix). They are anatomically spread either in the proximal part of the ligament, close to the uterus, or in the distal part of the ligament, closer to the pelvic wall. The proximal part of the ligament cannot be sampled without performing a radical hysterectomy at the same time, and cannot be included in a staging procedure. On the other hand, the cellulolymphatic component of the distal part of the ligament may be removed separately from the uterus. We have labeled this part of the staging procedure 'parametrial lymphadenectomy'. When the cardinal ligament is not macroscopically involved, cancer may spread by lymphatic channel and node involvement. The rationale of removal of the cardinal ligament is then

the removal of the lymphatic tissue along with the surrounding fatty tissue of the ligament. There is no support for the transection of vessels and nerves that may lead to ischemic fistula formation and to long-term voiding difficulty secondary to bladder denervation. The magnified laparoscopic view, the usually clean operative field, and a direct access with the tip of the laparoscope and of the laparoscopic instruments to the deep pelvic structures gives us an opportunity to carefully dissect the distal part of the cardinal ligament without unnecessary surgical trauma to the vessels and nerves.

The approach for parametrial lymphadenectomy is essentially the same as for parietal interiliac lymphadenectomy. An instrument is placed in the paravesical space, pushing the bladder medially when the senior surgeon works on the anterolateral side of the cardinal ligament, or placed in the pararectal space, pushing the rectum medially, when the senior surgeon works on the posteromedial side of the cardinal ligament. As a consequence, the surgeon can work with two hands without any interference from other instruments. When dissecting on the right side, for example, the surgeon is standing on the right side of the patient with the instruments placed in the middle line and in the right lower quadrant. The assistant holds the camera in his right hand and a retractor in his left hand, pushing the bladder or rectum towards the left side of the patient.

As the general direction of the cardinal ligament is posterolateral, this ligament has two visible faces, an anterolateral and a posteromedial one. The edge of the ligament is formed by the anterior branch of the internal iliac artery. To start this step of the operation, it is advised to complete first the parietal lymphadenectomy. As a consequence, the paravesical space is already opened. If necessary, this opening has to be enlarged. Additional blunt dissection is carried out to identify the levator ani. It is usually easy to identify, deeper than the obturator nerve, the arcus tendineus leaving the ischial spine. In this area, care must be taken to identify and as a consequence not to injure large obturator and parietal veins, as well as the obturator artery, which may be quite small. It is then necessary to further develop the medial part of the paravesical space, to move the lateral wall of the bladder, and to free the whole anterolateral aspect of the cardinal ligament as medial as possible. The superior vesical artery is the first landmark. If forms the upper edge of the vesical ligament ('lateral bladder pillar'), the lateral aspect of which can be entirely freed down to the level of the pelvic floor by blunt dissection (Figure 42.7).

After this step, the lateral part of the cardinal ligament, between the pelvic wall and the insertion of

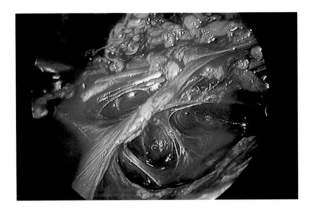

Figure 42.7 Skeletonization of the vessels and nerves of the right parametrium.

the vesical ligament, is clearly identified. Its antero-lateral aspect is made of arteries, veins and cellulo-lymphatic tissue. The vessels include vaginal and inferior vesical arteries, deep uterine veins, and vaginal and vesical veins. These veins usually join the deep obturator vein to form the hypogastric vein, but one must be aware of the numerous possible anatomic variants. The main part of the cellulolymphatic tissue usually lies anterior to the vessels, at the medial part of the common visceral ligament. This part can usually been dissected *en bloc* by blunt dissection, allowing removal of a rectangular flap measuring approximately 2 cm in width and 1–1.5 cm in height. This flap corresponds to the part of the cardinal ligament removed in type 3–4 extended hysterectomies after the placement of a clamp at the root of the cardinal ligament. After the removal of this flap, the deep uterine vein is clearly identified. It is usually joined by vesical and vaginal veins coming from the vesical ligament.

In the distal part of the common visceral ligament near the pelvic wall (Figure 42.8), the cellular tissue is spread between the vessels and has to be carefully and gradually removed in small pieces. The vessels are identified, a small amount of fatty tissue is

elevated with a grasping forceps, and the vessels are separated from the specimen by gentle blunt dissection. This careful and gradual dissection leads to the identification and skeletonization of all the vessels of this part of the pelvic wall, including the internal pudendal and deep obturator veins, and some other landmarks, including the ischial spine and posterior to it, the lumbosacral trunk. It is not necessary to extend the dissection in the major ischiatic foramen where the fatty tissue becomes more abundant.

The dissection has then been completed on the posteromedial aspect of the cardinal ligament. The pararectal space is entered, medially to the internal iliac artery. It is further developed by blunt dissection, moving the rectum medially to identify the promontory and the presacral fascia. In some cases, the first sacral nerve is identified at the level of the first sacral foramen as well as the parasympathetic nerves leaving this nerve and running parallel to the pelvic wall. One of the goals of this dissection is to spare these nerves. The landmark to avoid dividing them are the rectal vessels. The rectal vessels are directed medially, overlying the pelvic autonomic nerves. The cellulolymphatic tissue of this part of the cardinal ligament is located medial to the rectal vessels and superficial to the nerves. It is usually less abundant, more dense and more firmly attached to the vessels and to the connective tissue of the ligament than it is on the anterior face of the ligament. Blunt dissection is again advised, but elective bipolar cautery followed by sharp dissection may be necessary.

Ovarian Transposition

In premenopausal patients, a laparoscopic transposition of the ovaries may be added in order to avoid ovarian irradiation. This operation can be completed in the same way as it is done by laparotomy: section of the utero-ovarian pedicles after hemostasis by electrocautery, extra- or intracorporeal knots or endo-GIA staplers, section of the peritoneum circumscribing the adnexa, freeing of the ovarian ligament, placement of the adnexa in the paracolic gutters. The ovaries may be attached to the lateral peritoneum using sutures or clips or maintained in a high position by creating a peritoneal tunnel in the paracolic gutter. An incision is made as high as possible in the paracolic gutter, then the retroperitoneal space is developed between this incision and the incision of the broad ligament in order to create a peritoneal bridge. The adnexa are passed under the bridge and placed in the paracolic gutter. They are maintained by the bridge, and no suture or further fixation is necessary. Care must be taken to

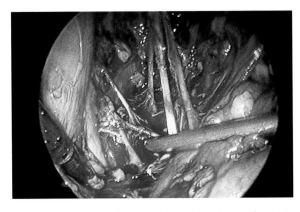

Figure 42.8 Right pelvic wall. Ischial spine and sciatic nerve.

avoid torsion of the infundibulopelvic ligament. Endoscopic metallic clips are placed at the lower pole of the ovary for later radiologic localization.

Results

In our series, 283 patients underwent laparoscopic pelvic lymphadenectomy, combined with aortic dissection in 49. Of these patients, 200 presented with Fédération Internationale de Gynécologie-Obstétrique (FIGO) IA2 ($n = 25$), IB ($n = 127$), IIA ($n = 17$), proximal IIB ($n = 31$) carcinoma of the cervix. The other patients presented with carcinoma of the endometrium ($n = 38$), ovarian borderline or invasive adnexal cancers ($n = 24$), urologic malignancy ($n = 21$). Selection of patients was based upon the absence of cytologically positive nodes visible on CT scans. The average duration of the operation was 63 minutes in the last 50 cases; 3–22 nodes were available for pathologic examination. The numbers of nodes retrieved increased with experience, reaching an average of 10.1 nodes in 1996 in the interiliac area on each side. For cervical carcinomas, the positivity rate was 0 for stage IA2 patients, 24% for stage IB patients and 36% for stage IIA and IIB. In a series of 153 node-negative patients with up to seven-year follow-up, five lateropelvic recurrences occurred. This 3.2% false negative rate is similar to the rate observed with earlier series of patients managed with open lymphadenectomy.

The survival curve of our cervical cancer patients with up to 90 months of follow-up is similar to the survival curve of a historical control group of early cervical cancers matched for stage, age and nodal status managed with a standard laparotomy approach (data submitted for publication).

Observed Complications

Four intraoperative complications were observed. One patient did not tolerate the prolonged pneumoperitoneum and we had to abandon the procedure after removal of only three nodes. In another case, bleeding from the umbilical artery necessitated bipolar coagulation of the vessel. In a third case, injury to an epigastric artery at a second-puncture entry required elective hemostasis. In one patient venous bleeding in the left paravesical space was controlled by compression with the endoscopic forceps. No emergency laparotomy was necessary during the period of study.

When laparoscopic lymphadenectomy was performed as the only procedure, the postoperative period was uneventful and the patients were discharged the following day. A pelvic hematoma was observed five days after laparoscopic pelvic lymphadenectomy and radium application, but it resolved spontaneously. Four lymphocysts were observed. No bowel adhesions were noticed at further laparotomy, and spontaneous healing of the peritoneum always occurred without intraperitoneal sequelae (Figure 42.9). However, dense fibrosis of the retroperitoneal tissue was noticed in five cases.

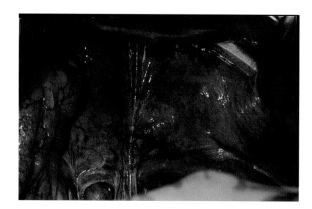

Figure 42.9 Peritoneal healing after pelvic lymphadenectomy.

Potential Morbidity: Prevention and Management

Selection of patients is based on general contraindications to prolonged pneumoperitoneum: morbidly obese patients and patients with advanced coronary or respiratory disease are excluded. However, these concerns may be overcome by the use of a low abdominal pressure, less than 10 mm Hg (1.33 kPa).

Many potential complications may occur during laparoscopic pelvic lymphadenectomy. Although many of them have not yet been observed in our experience, advice concerning their management will be given. Only specific complications will be addressed, and divided into three categories: intraoperative, early and late complications.

Intraoperative Complications

VASCULAR INJURY

This is the major potential risk of laparoscopic pelvic lymphadenectomy, but is much less frequent than one would expect.

Diffuse oozing is comparatively rare, even in moderately obese patients, even when preventive hemostasis by clips is not used. In our experience, hemostasis of capillary vessels is either not necessary or obtained after irrigation with warm saline solution. This low incidence of bleeding is likely to be due to the pressure of the pneumoperitoneum.

Injury of large vessels is even rarer as the magnification provided by the laparoscope allows a precise dissection of the paravesical fossae. Significant bleeding may, however, occur by injury to pelvic arteries or veins. Injury to the branches of the hypogastric artery (particularly uterine artery, superior vesical artery or umbilical artery) is managed by direct hemostasis of the vessel: clips (7 mm clips are preferable) or bipolar hemostasis should be instantly available. In the same way, laceration of pelvic veins (particularly aberrant obturator veins and less commonly obturator, uterine or epigastric veins) may be managed laparoscopically – unless the bleeding stops after two minutes of compression of the injured vessel, clips or coagulation should be used.

Injury of the external iliac or hypogastric artery is very unlikely. Experience of the laparotomy approach is that it is usually due to bleeding from an aberrant minor branch, and may be managed by application of a clip. Injury of the external iliac vein or of a main branch of internal iliac veins is the most serious potential risk of pelvic lymphadenectomy. It may occur during node sampling, and is usually due to a lateral laceration of the vessel. Two areas must be dissected with special care:

- The inferior aspect of the external iliac vein, near the obturator foramen, where inappropriate traction may lead to tearing of aberrant obturator veins at their junction with the external iliac vein.
- The area below the hypogastric artery bifurcation.

In this respect, beginners are strongly advised against attempts at dissection of fixed lymph nodes. When such unresectable nodes are encountered, the diagnosis of metastasis is possible by cytologic examination of fine needle aspirates, but debulking is also feasible in experienced hands, with careful dissection of the large vessels. The nodes measuring more than 1 cm in diameter have to be removed using endoscopic bags. If bleeding of the external iliac vein occurs, compression may again be successful: a closed forceps may be pushed strongly, thus compressing the vessel against the pelvic sidewall. If hemorrhage persists, the use of clips or coagulation is not advised as it may worsen the laceration. Introduction of vascular sutures through second-puncture trocars is theoretically possible, and we

have repaired a 2 mm injury of the external iliac vein laparoscopically; clips may also be used to fix small lateral openings of large veins. Larger laceration of a large vessel may have to be managed by laparotomy, but no such case occurred in our series.

Bleeding from the ovarian ligament is prevented by gentle handling and retraction of this ligament. If it occurs, management includes placement of clips, staples or bipolar coagulation. If laparoscopic transposition of the ovary is indicated, the surgical technique follows the same principles as that employed at laparotomy: section of the utero-ovarian anastomosis and dissection of the ovarian ligament in order to move the ovary above the pelvic brim. Bleeding may occur predominantly at the level of the uterine cornua, from the uterine artery or veins, and is usually prevented by primary coagulation or application of clips or staples. Coagulation of bleeders is possible in this area.

NERVE INJURY

The risk of nerve injury is limited to accidental section of the obturator nerve. This accident is very unlikely, and is prevented by careful dissection of the paravesical fossa, facilitated by the laparoscopic magnification. As section of the obturator nerve has minor motor and sensitive consequences, no repair is warranted.

URETERAL INJURY

This is unlikely if only interiliac node sampling has been carried out. The ureter is not in the operative field and is usually retracted along with the ovarian ligament, even during dissection of the hypogastric bifurcation. However, the upper area of the dissection must always be managed carefully, avoiding unnecessary grasping of tissues or blind coagulation. If necessary, the ureter may be identified under the peritoneum and dissected free from the pelvic brim to the parameter. Ureteral repair is obviously necessary in case of surgical injury.

MISSING LYMPH NODES

This is not a complication, but leads to a loss of accuracy of the method, and to inadequate care to unsuspected node-positive patients. The first concern is the risk of missing obturator or external iliac nodes, which may be prevented by careful identification of nerve and vessels up to the hypogastric bifurcation and thorough ablation of the cellulolymphatic tissue. In this respect, the learning curve is a problem: beginners are advised to check the quality of node sampling at subsequent laparotomies, by counting the average number of sampled nodes, or by comparing the observed incidence of lymph node metastasis in the cases they manage to that observed in the literature for cervical cancers of the same stage (Averette *et al.*, 1987). An experimental study, yet unpublished, has been carried out in our laboratory to assess the learning curve and then to compare the safety and accuracy of the laparoscopic approach for pelvic and paraaortic lymphadenectomy versus laparotomy. The results may be summarized as follows:

- The learning curve reaches a plateau after ten cases for pelvic lymphadenectomy and 20 cases for paraaortic lymphadenectomy.
- The number of retrieved nodes is identical for the two techniques.
- The operative time is similar for pelvic lymphadenectomy in the two arms.
- The adhesion formation rate is significantly lower after laparoscopic dissection.

Missing distant nodes are another problem. The risk of skip metastasis in the periaortic area must be addressed. As far as early cervical or endometrial cancer is concerned, the incidence of aortic nodes in the absence of pelvic nodes is very low, presumably less than 2%. However, if the technique is applied to cases of advanced cervical carcinoma, periaortic sampling is considered.

Early Postoperative Complications

The postoperative period is usually quite uneventful. Many potential complications are possible, but are nonspecific. General complications of laparoscopy such as undiagnosed bowel injury or complications of a radical hysterectomy performed at the same time will not be discussed in this chapter.

Early postoperative hemorrhage has never occurred in our experience. Acute anemia and clinical signs of hemoperitoneum clearly indicate emergency reoperation. If the patient's condition is relatively stable, it is possible to repeat the laparoscopy. Laparoscopic aspiration of blood and clots is cumbersome but possible, and allows precise localization of the bleeding. The problem can be solved by coagulation or clip application. Otherwise, a laparotomy may be needed.

In cases of moderate bleeding, the patient may develop a pelvic hematoma. Surgical drainage is usually not necessary, as many pelvic hematomas do not require any treatment or may be managed by aspiration under ultrasound monitoring.

Lymphocyst formation is a peculiar complication of lymph node biopsy. Some operators believe that this complication may be prevented by liberal use of surgical clips before division of lymphatic vessels and by closed suction drainage of the retroperitoneum. This technique may be applied laparoscopically. Although we do not place preventive clips for lymphostasis nor any drain in the dissection area, we have seen only a few cases of significant lymphocyst in our experience, probably because we leave the peritoneum opened. Drainage of lymph fluid into the peritoneal cavity is followed by resorption until the leakage of lymph fluid spontaneously stops. If a lymphocyst develops, aspiration under ultrasound monitoring is a safe and efficient management.

Ileus may be caused by the adhesion of the small bowel to the operative field. We advise an early second look laparoscopy when such a complication is suspected: recent adhesions are usually quite easy to free laparoscopically.

Late Complications

Leg lymphedema is rare after pelvic lymphadenectomy and its incidence should be lowered by avoiding removal of the lymphatic area external to the external iliac artery.

Tissue scarring after laparoscopic lymphadenectomy may involve peritoneal or retroperitoneal repair. The peritoneum usually heals with minimal scarring and no or minimal adhesions. If adhesions develop, there is a risk of late bowel occlusion or of radiation injury. The areolar tissue in the retroperitoneal space heals with a dense fibrosis, making subsequent dissections uneasy and risky. For this reason, it is advisable to perform the radical hysterectomy, if indicated, the same day or not later than seven days after laparoscopic lymphadenectomy.

Indications

Laparoscopic pelvic lymphadenectomy may become an indispensable tool in gynecologic or urologic oncology whenever pathologic examination of the pelvic lymph nodes is necessary and adequate in the pretherapeutic staging of pelvic malignancies. Laparoscopic or extraperitoneal paraaortic lymphadenectomy may extend the indications for laparoscopic staging of pelvic tumors. On the other hand, laparoscopic, as well as surgical, staging is useless when the presence of metastatic cells has been documented by fine needle aspiration of suspicious nodes shown by CT scanning.

The first indication in gynecologic oncology is the staging of early operable carcinoma of the cervix (Querleu *et al.*, 1991). The risk of 'skip' metastases to the paraaortic nodes without pelvic node involvement is very low (less than 1%) in these cases, and occurs almost only in patients with large tumors (over 4 cm). As a consequence, stage IB 1 with negative pathologic staging may be cured by local therapy (brachytherapy, radical vaginal surgery or radical trachelectomy in selected cases). On the other hand, radical hysterectomy does not seem justified when metastatic nodes are present (Potter *et al.*, 1990). In addition, some stage IA2 cervical carcinomas without pelvic node metastasis can be treated by cervical conization alone. Laparoscopic staging may thus reduce the cost and effects on fertility of the treatment of early carcinomas of the cervix.

The role of laparoscopic lymphadenectomy may in the future be investigated in the staging of advanced carcinomas of the cervix. However, the poor outcome of patients with paraaortic nodal metastasis regardless of treatment (Stehman *et al.*, 1991) and the necessity of external irradiation regardless of pelvic node involvement, limits the role of pathologic staging of such tumors to investigational settings.

Laparoscopic pretherapeutic staging of stage I endometrial carcinomas is not very useful for the patient, insofar as surgery is indicated, whatever the node status. Furthermore, the prevalence of lymph node metastasis is low in this condition. However, laparoscopic lymphadenectomy may be included in the surgical step of treatment in association with vaginal surgery. In the same way, laparoscopic lymphadenectomy and oophorectomy may be an adequate management of unsuspected endometrial adenocarcinomas found in hysterectomy specimens.

Ovarian carcinomas are best treated by laparotomy. However, thanks to progress in laparoscopic surgery, the laparoscopic surgeon may meet the criteria for adequate staging and therapy for some cases of early ovarian carcinoma.

Laparoscopic staging may become popular among urologic oncologists in the near future. The prognostic value of lymph node involvement is important in cases of bladder or prostate carcinoma as patients without node metastasis may be treated by surgery, while surgery is not indicated for those with metastatic disease.

Conclusion

As far as major laparoscopic surgery is concerned, it should first be stressed that laparoscopic lymph-adenectomy is a feasible operation, but only in experienced hands. Thorough knowledge of oncologic surgery, including the anatomy of the pelvic extraperitoneal spaces and management of vascular injuries, and, of course, of laparoscopic surgery techniques, is mandatory. Complete instrumentation, including a full set of scissors, forceps, irrigation and suction devices, clip applicators and bipolar coagulation, is necessary not only to perform the standard operation, but also to manage potential minor and even major complications. The patient must be informed that an emergency laparotomy may unexpectedly be performed. Therefore, only surgeons experienced in gynecologic oncology and operative laparoscopy should undertake this operation. However, potential severe complications are infrequent in clinical practice. Laparoscopic lymphadenectomy may therefore be considered as a safe procedure and helps to reduce the cost and risks of management of carcinoma of the cervix, as well as other pelvic malignancies.

This technique was the first application of endoscopy in gynecologic or urologic oncology, and has paved the way to further progress. Laparoscopic radical hysterectomy (Canis *et al.*, 1990) or laparoscopically assisted radical vaginal hysterectomy (Querleu *et al.*, 1991), with full ureter dissection from the iliac area to the bladder, has been performed and paraaortic dissection by laparoscopy has been introduced into clinical practice. As late results confirm the safety and efficiency of these new techniques, laparoscopy has become a major tool in pelvic oncology.

The detail of complications is available in our series. One case had to be interrupted due to preoperative coronary ischemia. Significant hemorrhage occurred in 5 cases, but these were managed laparoscopically in every case. No bowel or urinary complication occurred. As a result, no unintended laparotomy had to be performed in this large series. Postoperative blood collection occurred in three cases, and symptomatic lymphocyst in four. As postoperative complications were managed conservatively or under radiologic guidance, no secondary laparotomy for complication was performed. As mentioned earlier, we missed 3.2% positive nodes which developed later as pure lateropelvic recurrences and were the cause of treatment failure.

Summary

Pelvic lymphadenectomy is feasible by transperitoneal laparoscopy. An incision of the peritoneum between the round and infundibulopelvic ligament on each side gives access to the retroperitoneal space. Subsequently, laparoscopic surgery allows precise dissection of external and internal iliac vessels, umbilical artery and obturator nerve. The peritoneum is left open, and the lymph drains into the peritoneal cavity. Between November 1988 and June 1997, 283 patients underwent laparoscopic pelvic lymphadenectomy, 200 of them with stage I or II carcinoma of the cervix. An average of 20 inter-iliac nodes were removed during the last two years, and there was no significant morbidity. The average duration of the operation was 63 minutes in the last 50 cases. The positivity rate was consistent, stage for stage, with the expected rate. In a series of 153 node negative patients with up to 7 year follow-up, 5 pure lateropelvic recurrences occurred. This 3.2% false negative rate is similar to the rate observed in earlier series of patients managed with open lymphadenectomy.

Laparoscopic staging of gynecologic or urologic pelvic malignancies may reduce the incidence of laparotomy in these cases. Node-negative early cervical carcinomas may be managed by a vaginal surgical approach. Node-positive patients are managed by radiation therapy in our group. Endometrial cancer patients may benefit from the comfort of the combination of laparoscopic staging and vaginal or laparoscopically-assisted vaginal simple hysterectomy.

Potential surgical complications specific to laparoscopic lymphadenectomy. Damage may occur to the following structures. (List compiled by Mr Anthony Weekes, Consultant Gynaecologist, Romford Hospital, Essex.)

- Vascular:
  — Iliac vessels.
  — Lumbar vessels.
  — Accessory obturator vessels.
  — Inferior mesenteric artery.
  — Inferior vena cava.
  — Aorta.
  — Ovarian vessels.
  — Aberrant renal vessel.

- Nerves:
  — Genitofemoral nerve.
  — Obturator nerve.

- Urinary:
  — Ureter.
  — Bladder.

- Long term:
  — Lymphocyst formation.
  — Leg edema.

The risk of injury is increased in node positive patients, particularly if the involved lymph nodes are densely adherent to blood vessels and may tear the vessel wall during attempts to remove them.

References

Averette HE, Donato DM, Lovecchio JL, Sevin BU (1987) Surgical staging of gynecologic malignancies. *Cancer* **60**: 2010–2020.

Canis M, Mage G, Wattiez A *et al.* (1990) La chirurgie endoscopique a-t-elle une place dans la chirurgie radicale du cancer du col utérin? *Journal de Gynécologie, Obstétrique et Biologie de la Reproduction* **19**: 921.

Childers JM, Hatch KD, Tran AN, Surwit EA (1993) Laparoscopic para-aortic lymphadenectomy in gynecologic malignancies. *Obstetrics and Gynecology* **82**: 741–747.

Dargent D, Salvat J (1989) *L'Envahissement Ganglionnaire Pelvien.* Paris: Medsci-McGraw-Hill.

Feigen M, Crocker EF, Read J, Crandon AJ (1987) The value of lymphoscintigraphy, lymphangiography and computed tomography scanning in the preoperative assessment of lymph nodes involved by pelvic malignant conditions. *Surgery, Gynecology and Obstetrics* **65**: 107–110.

Potter ME, Alvarez RD, Shingleton HM, Soong SJ, Hatch KD (1990) Early invasive cervical cancer with pelvic lymph node involvement: to complete or not to complete radical hysterectomy? *Gynecologic Oncology* **37**: 78–81.

Querleu D (1989) Lymphadénectomie pelvienne sous contrôle coelioscopique. *Deuxième Congrès Mondial d'Endoscopie Gynécologique, Clermont-Ferrand, France.*

Querleu D (1991) Hystérectomies de Schauta-Amreich et Schauta-Stoeckel assistées par coelioscopie. *Journal de Gynécologie Obstétrique et Biologie de la Reproduction* **20**: 747–748.

Querleu D (1992) Laparoscopic paraaortic lymphadenectomy in the staging of advanced carcinoma of the cervix. *International Congress of Gynecologic Endoscopy, AAGL 21st Meeting.* Chicago, 25 September.

Querleu D (1993a) Laparoscopic paraaortic lymphadenectomy. A preliminary experience. *Gynecologic Oncology* **49**: 24–29.

Querleu D (1993b) Laparoscopically-assisted radical vaginal hysterectomy. *Gynecologic Oncology* **51**: 248–254.

Querleu D, Leblanc E (1994) Laparoscopic infrarenal node dissection for restaging of carcinomas of the ovary or fallopian tube. *Cancer* **73:** 1467–1471.

Querleu D, Leblanc E, Castelain B (1991) Laparoscopic pelvic lymphadenectomy in the staging of early carcinoma of the cervix. *American Journal of Obstetrics and Gynecology* **164**: 579–581.

Stehman FB, Bundy BN, Di Saia P *et al.* (1991) Carcinoma of the cervix treated with radiation therapy I. A multivariate analysis of prognostic variables in the gynecologic oncology group. *Cancer* **67**: 2776–2785.

Wurtz A, Mazeman E, Gosselin B *et al.* (1987) Bilan anatomique des adénopathies rétropéritonéales par endoscopie chirurgicale. *Annales de Chirurgie* **41**: 258–263.

43

Laparoscopic Aortic Lymphadenectomy

NICHOLAS KADAR

Seton Hall University, and The New Margaret Hague Women's Health Institute, Secaucus and Englewood Hospital and Medical Center, Englewood, New Jersey, USA

Laparoscopic aortic lymphadenectomy, like all operations used to treat malignant disease, has raised both technical and oncological issues, and, as with most laparoscopic cancer operations, technical considerations have been at the forefront of the debate. There are a number of reasons for this.

- First, the oncologic aspects of cancer treatment remain the same regardless of the route by which the operative component of therapy is carried out. For example, questions about the indications for lymphadenectomy, the type of lymphadenectomy to perform, and the place, if any, of adjuvant pelvic radiation that have dogged the management of stage I endometrial and cervical cancer are not altered in any way just because the lymphadenectomy is carried out laparoscopically.
- Second, *prima facie* the limitations of laparoscopic surgery are likely to be technical, related to such factors as obesity, exposure, the inability to palpate tissues, rupture of cysts or lymph node capsules, and extraction of the resected tissue from the peritoneal cavity.
- Third, the quality of a cancer operation, be it a lymphadenectomy, radical hysterectomy or colectomy, has always been judged by well accepted surgico-anatomic and pathologic criteria such as node counts, frequency of positive nodes, quality of surgical planes, tumor margins, tumor handling, tumor spill, and so on. Not surprisingly, therefore, the same criteria have been used to assess laparoscopic cancer operations, and it has been tacitly assumed

that if by these criteria a laparoscopic operation met the same standards as its open counterpart then its effectiveness as cancer treatment should also be the same.

In other words, questions about laparoscopic cancer operations have been couched in technical terms not because their effectiveness in treating cancer was ignored, but simply because it was assumed that any reduction in that efficacy would be most likely to have a technical basis. This assumption has now been questioned by numerous reports of abdominal wall recurrences at trocar sites (port-site recurrences) following laparoscopic resection of colon and other cancers, as well as diagnostic laparoscopy in ovarian cancer, and will be considered later in this chapter.

It is important to bear in mind, however, that a laparoscopic cancer operation cannot be expected to deliver therapeutically more, so to speak, than its open counterpart. All one is aiming at with a laparoscopic approach is to achieve the same surgical result as with a laparotomy, but with less morbidity to the patient. It follows, therefore, that the indications for a particular laparoscopic operation should be the same as those for its open counterpart, and if these indications are controversial, they will be just as controversial if the operation is performed laparoscopically. The controversy surrounding the routine use of surgical staging in cervix cancer, for example, is no argument against performing aortic lymphadenectomy laparoscopically.

This perhaps obvious point deserves emphasis

here because aortic lymphadenectomy has arguably been the gynecologic oncologist's most controversial operation ever since it was first used in the management of cervix cancer by my former Chief, Dr James Nelson, in the 1970s (Nelson *et al.*, 1977). The wide acceptance of this procedure in the USA and, to a lesser extent, in Europe, as reflected by its incorporation into the International Federation of Gynecology and Obstetrics (FIGO) staging for endometrial and ovarian carcinoma and its use in the management of both early and advanced stage cervical cancer has been far more a product of rationalization and habit than clear evidence of its clinical value, and has created great scope for controversy. The reasons for performing this operation have continued to change since it was first used to 'stage' advanced cervix cancer by Nelson, and vastly different operations in terms of radicality continue to masquerade under the same name. Given the great scope for disagreement over many aspects of this operation in general, there is a very real danger that these will obfuscate questions specific to the laparoscopic procedure.

In as much as the goal of laparoscopic surgery is to reduce morbidity, and morbidity is generally higher after radical surgery than after operations for benign disease, laparoscopic surgery is potentially used to greatest advantage in our discipline in the treatment of gynecologic malignancies. Quality of life issues have been neglected for far too long by oncologists and its objective study is still in its infancy. Nonetheless, it seems that newly diagnosed cancer patients will generally accept highly toxic treatments for even only a 1% chance of cure (Slevin *et al.*, 1990). Although much needs to be learned about the variables that affect such decisions, the message is clear: reduction in morbidity cannot be at the expense of survival. At the same time, the chance of cure, however small, must be real, not putative, and we must be sure it is real before subjecting patients to treatments that are associated with high rates of real complications and a real risk of death.

History of the Open Operation

Many factors have influenced the surgical evolution of aortic lymphadenectomy and its use in the management of gynecologic malignancies. The operation initially performed by most gynecologic oncologists not only lacked the sound theoretic and empirical basis that underlay its use in the treatment of testicular cancer, but was technically a pale shadow of its urologic counterpart. It began as a pre-caval fat pad biopsy, and has largely remained a limited operation consisting of removal of fatty nodal tissue from in front of the aorta and vena cava below the inferior mesenteric artery (Nelson *et al.*, 1977). Few gynecologic oncologists carry the dissection above the inferior mesenteric artery, much less mobilize and dissect behind the great vessels as urologic oncologists do. Indeed, the Gynecologic Oncology Group (GOG), who by incorporating aortic lymphadenectomy into almost all of its surgical protocols, has been most influential in promoting the use of this operation in the USA, requires only removal of pre- and peri-aortocaval, inframesenteric lymphatic tissue for an aortic lymphadenectomy.

Lymphadenectomy Versus Lymph Node Sampling

The justification for the widespread use of such a limited operation, which quite rightly came to be called lymph node 'sampling', was to be found in the changing purpose for which lymphadenectomies in general were ostensibly being carried out, namely diagnosis rather than therapy. The finding that in breast cancer axillary lymph node metastases were markers for distant spread that signalled the need for systemic treatment called into question the concept of a therapeutic lymphadenectomy, and engendered the assumption, for reasons that have yet to be clearly articulated, that diagnostic lymphadenectomies need not be as radical as therapeutic ones. But, the term 'diagnostic' in this context was meant simply to connote that the function of the lymphadenectomy was to identify patients who needed systemic therapy and not that a less radical operation was needed.

Clearly, even if we accept that lymphadenectomy serves only a diagnostic purpose and contributes to survival only by identifying the need for adjunctive therapy, it does not follow that a diagnostic lymphadenectomy should in principle be surgically less radical than a therapeutic one because a selective operation might miss nodal metastases in some patients who would thereby be denied potentially curative therapy. The proper corollary as regards how extensive a lymphadenectomy should be is that once a positive lymph node is discovered and the need for systemic therapy identified further resection of lymphatic tissue serves no useful diagnostic purpose. Of course, this presumes that the removal of residual enlarged nodes has no survival advantage and does not enhance adjuvant therapy, which is untrue (see below) and that adjuvant therapy is more effective than surgery or surgery plus adjuvant therapy for occult disease that might be present in the remaining lymph nodes, for which again there is no evidence. If the purpose of lymphadenectomy is believed to be entirely diagnostic and prognostic, however, it is an equally obvious corollary that if the adjuvant therapy in question is indicated irrespective of whether lymph node metastases are present or not, then any type of a lymphadenectomy becomes totally superfluous. However, most gynecologic oncologists have not been deterred from sampling pelvic nodes in patients with endometrial carcinoma even if the patient has a poorly differentiated or deeply invasive tumor and is going to receive pelvic radiation postoperatively regardless of whether the lymph nodes are positive or not.

The term lymph node sampling, engendered by the concept of a diagnostic lymphadenectomy, meant different things to different people, but in general, it liberalized the gynecologic indications for lymphadenectomy and extended the anatomic boundaries of the procedure, even as resection of nodal tissue from each anatomic region was becoming less complete. Thus, for many years, lymphadenectomy essentially meant a pelvic lymphadenectomy to the gynecologist, used mainly to treat early invasive carcinoma of the cervix and patients with vulvar carcinoma metastatic to the inguinofemoral lymph nodes, and by pelvic lymphadenectomy was meant complete excision of the external, internal and common iliac and obturator nodes. From the early 1970s onwards, however, not only were the indications for lymphadenectomy broadened to include endometrial and ovarian carcinoma (and sarcomas and fallopian tube carcinomas as well), but the limits of the lymphadenectomy were extended to encompass the 'para-aortic' lymph nodes to varying degrees. Aortic lymphadenectomy, for example, was not only incorporated into the classic Meigs–Bonney radical hysterectomy for carcinoma of the cervix, but also became a routine part of a 'staging' operation for endometrial cancer.

Purpose of Aortic Lymphadenectomy

DIAGNOSIS AND RESECTION OF ENLARGED NODES

When applied to the selective removal of clinically enlarged lymph nodes, as practiced, for example, by Wertheim, the term lymph node sampling was not only accurate and descriptive, but, as Downey *et al.* (1989) were later to show, it had therapeutic value, at least as far as pelvic lymph nodes were concerned. There were no five-year survivors among surgically staged women with cervical cancer and macroscopically enlarged positive pelvic nodes, if the malignant nodes were not resected before radiation, whereas the survival of women who had a lymphadenectomy before radiation therapy was 51% and approached the 57% survival of women who had only microscopic nodal metastases. The survival value of removing clinically enlarged aortic lymph nodes in cervix cancer has been demonstrated only anecdotally. Piver *et al.* (1981) found that patients with clinically enlarged aortic nodes could be salvaged only if one node was affected; Podczaski *et al.* (1990) reported that three of nine women with aortic lymph node metastasis who were long-term survivors had palpably enlarged para-aortic nodes at staging laparotomy.

From its dose–response relationship in head and neck cancer and the radiotolerance of normal tissues we know that the probability of sterilizing enlarged lymph nodes in the pelvic and para-aortic region by radiation therapy alone is very low, making excision of large nodal metastases at least in principle logical. For example, to control tumors up to 2 cm in size requires a radiation dose of 6000 cGy delivered over six weeks, and the aortic region simply does not tolerate such doses (Fletcher and Shukovsky, 1975). Therefore, the uncertainty about the value of resecting clinically enlarged aortic nodes notwithstanding, clinically enlarged aortic nodes have to be resected if the patient is to have any chance of being cured by extended field radiation.

In the setting of advanced cervical cancer for which Nelson intended it to be used, there was considerable rationale for a limited para-aortic 'lymphadenectomy' to identify disease spread to the aortic region and the need for extended field irradiation. Nodal spread in this disease was known to be an orderly affair and skip lesions rare. Spread to the high common and 'low' para-aortic nodes occurred in 30–60% of women with advanced stage disease. Nodes targeted for removal were outside the conventional radiation portals and would remain untreated by what were then conventional treatment fields. Thus, removing the most easily accessible nodes made sense both from a clinical and a statistical viewpoint. However, the use of the same operation for endometrial and ovarian cancer, as promoted by the GOG, made no anatomic sense at all because the lymphatics draining the uterine fundus and ovaries can reach the para-aortic region directly via the infundibulopelvic ligaments and drain into lymph nodes situated above the origin of the inferior mesenteric artery; nor did it make sense to try to detect lymph node metastases by merely sampling clinically normally appearing nodes.

CURATIVE TREATMENT

Early experience even with aortic lymph node sampling was catastrophic because the radiation doses delivered to the aortic region were far too excessive (6000 cGy). For example, in a series of 102 surgically staged cases of advanced cervical cancer treated with extended field radiation at the MD Anderson Cancer Center, the operative mortality was 3%, the bowel complication rate was 30% and mortality from bowel complications was 10% (Wharton et al., 1977). Although the toxicity was drastically decreased by reducing the radiation dose to the aortic region to a tolerable level (about 4500 cGy), only subclinical disease can be controlled by these doses of radiation (Fletcher and Shukovsky, 1975), and higher doses may be required to sterilize tumor cells in an operative bed.

Although five-year survival rates as high as 40% were reported from some centers after surgical staging and extended field radiation (Potish et al., 1985), this has been the exception rather than the rule, and it is far less obvious than has been generally (and tacitly) assumed that this result is attributable to the radiation rather that resection of the malignant nodes during surgical staging. It is well recognized that postoperative pelvic radiation does not generally improve the survival of women with carcinoma of the cervix and pelvic lymph node metastases who are treated with radical hysterectomy and pelvic lymphadenectomy (Morrow et al., 1991), and there is no reason to expect postoperative radiation to be more effective at a site where it is less well tolerated. The tacit assumption that extended field radiation is required after resection of positive aortic nodes is probably attributable to the fact that aortic 'lymphadenectomy' involves a much less thorough removal of lymphatic tissue than a pelvic lymphadenectomy. However, the GOG data reported by Morrow et al. (1991) clearly show that some women with aortic lymph node metastases can remain disease free for extended periods after resection of the involved nodes without extended field radiation and without a systematic radical aortic lymphadenectomy.

It was these considerations that prompted Professor Burghardt to launch the elegant series of surgico-anatomic studies in Graz in the late 1970s that have been continued by both his successor, Professor Winter, as well as by Pierluigi Benedetti-Panici and colleagues in Rome (Winter et al., 1988; Winter, 1993; Girardi et al., 1989, 1993a, 1993b; Benedetti-Panici et al., 1991, 1992, 1993, 1996; Petru et al., 1994) and other Italian oncologists (Ferraris et al., 1988; Di Re et al., 1989; Scarabelli et al., 1995). The intention of these groups was:

- To test the feasibility of a systemic lymphadenectomy aimed at removing all nodal tissue from the pelvis and para-aortic region.
- To determine the number of lymph nodes that could be recovered from each anatomic area.
- To establish the pattern and frequency of lymph node metastases in various gynecologic malignancies.
- Finally, to determine if lymphadenectomy had curative value.

The salient findings with respect to the aortic region were as follows.

The lymph nodes in the aortic region can be divided into eight distinct groups designated pre-, para- and retro-caval, pre-, para- and retro-aortic, and, superficial and deep intercavo-aortic (Benedetti-Panici et al., 1992), although the distinction between the last two groups may be redundant. The primary sites of spread in cervical cancer were the paracaval, para-aortic and aortocaval groups of nodes (Benedetti-Panici et al., 1996), and spread to these second echelon of nodes did not occur in the absence of pelvic nodal disease (Winter et al., 1988; Benedetti-Panici et al., 1996). The primary nodal sites of spread from ovarian cancer were the pre- and para-aortic and pre- and para-caval groups of nodes (Benedetti-Panici et al., 1993). Metastases to the aortic region occurred in about 10% of stage I cases and 70% of more advanced stage disease (Benedetti-Panici et al., 1993; Petru et al., 1994; Burghardt et al., 1991). In at least 70% of cases both the pelvic and 'para-aortic' nodes were involved, and isolated aortic lymph node metastases occurred in no more than 10–15% of cases, even in advanced stage disease, and not at all in some studies (Scarabelli et al., 1995). In 80% of cases the metastases were less than 1 cm in size (Benedetti-Panici et al., 1993), and in over 50% of stage I cases they were less than 2 mm (Petru et al., 1994). Retrocaval and retro-aortic nodes were not primarily involved in cancer of the ovary or cervix. The pattern of spread to the aortic nodes in endometrial cancer has yet to be reported.

Investigators in both Graz and Rome recovered more lymph nodes and a higher frequency of positive nodes than had been generally reported from other centers and attributed this finding to their more extensive technique for systemic lymphadenectomy. However, both groups also serial sectioned their lymph nodes and prepared multiple rather than the conventional number (Slevin et al., 1990) of blocks from each node. They also examined the surgical specimens for clinically non-palpable lymph nodes using special embedding techniques. Therefore, the extent to which their more extensive surgical dissection actually increased the lymph node harvest and the frequency of positive nodes remains uncertain, for they also made a more meticulous pathologic search for lymph nodes and lymph node metastases in their surgical specimens.

These data can also be interpreted as showing that great variability exists in the number of lymph nodes recoverable by essentially identical surgical techniques, and that the correlation between the average number of lymph nodes recovered and the proportion of positive nodes is rather poor. For example, in women with stage I ovarian cancer, the mean node count recovered by the Graz group was 13, and 10% (2/21) of the patients had aortic lymph node metastases (Petru *et al.*, 1994). By contrast, the mean number of nodes detected in an identical group of women by the Rome group using identical surgical and pathologic techniques was 29, yet only 6% of the women had positive aortic nodes (Benedetti-Panici *et al.*, 1993). In women with ovarian cancer, 80% of the metastases were less than 1 cm in size (Benedetti-Panici *et al.*, 1993).

The radical systematic aortic lymphadenectomy advocated by oncologists in Graz and Rome requires an abdominal incision that extends from the xiphisternum to the pubis and exteriorization of the bowel. It is associated with a serious complication rate of at least 10% and a 16–18 day hospitalization. The operation is limited to women less than 70 years of age and the mean age of the reported series has been less than 50. It is also limited to non-obese women, although obesity has not been objectively defined. The therapeutic value of aortic lymphadenectomy has not been demonstrated nor is there any evidence that a higher survival rate is obtained with this more radical operation than with a more limited operation or indeed elective aortic radiation alone (i.e. without aortic lymphadenectomy) in women with positive pelvic nodes. A randomized trial comparing whole pelvic radiation with or without elective aortic radiation in patients with stage IIB carcinoma of the cervix showed a strong trend towards improved survival of patients receiving elective aortic radiation (*P* = 0.043) (Rotman *et al.*, 1990).

History of Laparoscopic Aortic Lymphadenectomy

The evolution of laparoscopic aortic lymphadenectomy has been just as fitful as that of its open counterpart and its history compounded by considerable jockeying as to who performed what type of aortic lymphadenectomy first. Childers claimed to be the first to perform this operation, but Nezhat *et al.*

(1992) in fact removed lymphatic tissue from the 'para-aortic' region two years before Childers, although their operation was totally unindicated and performed inappropriately for stage IA2 carcinoma of the cervix. Querleu (1993), in a report on only four cases, claimed to be the first to perform a 'supramesenteric' aortic lymphadenectomy (although it is unclear when this was), which is perhaps ironic for he had earlier noted that 'it is impossible at this time to explore para-aortic nodes by laparoscopy' (Querleu *et al.*, 1991). Interestingly, no-one has claimed to be the first to perform a left-sided aortic lymphadenectomy, possibly because the nature of these early 'lymphadenectomies' was at first obscure. The removal of fixed and/or enlarged malignant para-aortic nodes, both right and left sided, was first performed by Kadar in 1992 (Kadar, 1993; Kadar and Pelosi, 1994), who performed supramesenteric and bilateral laparoscopic aortic lymphadenectomies in that year and who continues to have the largest series of positive aortic lymph nodes to date.

Childers and Surwit (1992) were certainly the first to perform an indicated 'aortic lymphadenectomy' in 1991, and were tireless in promoting this operation. However, the majority of their procedures were precaval fat pad biopsies with which they recovered less than three nodes from most patients and a very low proportion of positive nodes and were not acceptable staging lymphadenectomies, even by the rather conservative standards of radicality of the GOG. Thus, although aortic lymphadenectomy continues to be associated with the Arizona group, who subsequently extended the radicality of their operation, they also embroiled the operation in controversy by their failure to define the exact radicality of their original 'aortic lymphadenectomy' and the number of nodes they recovered with it, and by their inability to dissect the left side of the aorta initially and to perform the operation in obese women. By 1993, Childers *et al.* (1993) had amassed an impressive series of 61 attempted laparoscopic aortic lymphadenectomies of which 57 (93%) were successfully completed, and wrote that 'the feasibility of transperitoneal laparoscopic para-aortic lymphadenectomy is clearly demonstrated in our series', but the validity of this claim has been questioned (Spirtos *et al.*, 1995a) because only 12 of these lymphadenectomies were bilateral and only four supramesenteric. The operation could not be performed in women who weighed over 180 pounds and only three (5%) patients had positive aortic nodes. These statistics were unacceptable to European gynecologic oncologists who have continued to condemn the laparoscopic management of gynecologic malignancies to this day largely on the basis of the inadequacy of the lymphadenectomy.

Some of this criticism is, however, disingenuous for several reasons. First, regardless of the route by which it is carried out, the therapeutic value of aortic lymphadenectomy has not been convincingly demonstrated, and its requisite radicality is, therefore, far from established, for there is no evidence to link increased radicality with increased survival. There are data purporting to show a survival advantage from systematic pelvic and aortic lymphadenectomy in advanced, optimally debulked ovarian cancer associated with residual disease (< 2 cm) (Burghardt *et al.*, 1991). However, these data are unconvincing to this author because the two-year survival of optimally debulked women who did not have a lymphadenectomy (16%) was far less than has been generally reported from other centers for similarly treated women. There are also unpublished data by Knapstein purporting to show that the proportion of positive nodes increases with the number of lymph nodes recovered, but these are at variance with data reported by the Miami group (Koechli *et al.*, 1993). Thus, even if the same degree of radicality could not be achieved laparoscopically as with an open operation, there is no evidence that this has any detrimental clinical consequences.

Second, there is in fact considerable evidence that by conventional anatomic and pathologic criteria lymphadenectomy can be carried out just as adequately laparoscopically as by laparotomy. That this is the case for the limited 'inframesenteric' aortic lymphadenectomy required for all GOG surgical protocols and used by almost all American gynecologic oncologists is beyond dispute. The node counts recovered and the frequency of positive nodes are just as high; fixed enlarged nodes can be resected just as effectively (Figure 43.1), the anatomic extent of the operation is comparable and morbidity and hospital stay are much reduced (see below). In fact, by the same presumptive criteria of adequacy that have been applied to the open procedure – number of nodes recovered, frequency of nodal metastases – there is evidence that laparoscopic aortic lymphadenectomy produces similar results as its more radical open counterpart. For example, for cervical cancer (stages IIB–IVA and stage IB with positive pelvic nodes) this author obtained an average node count of 12.8 and a 66% frequency of positive nodes, even in his first cases (Kadar and Pelosi, 1994). These values match those reported by Winter and colleagues (Petru *et al.*,1994), who recovered an average of only 13 para-aortic nodes even in ovarian cancer and with an operation that extended to the renal vessels and included a retrocavo-aortic dissection.

Third, the laparoscopic operation has been held to an entirely different standard from the open one. This is perhaps best reflected in the fact that the GOG requires reporting of node counts only for laparoscopic surgical protocols and not for surgical protocols involving laparotomy. Also, although 'obesity', for example, is a well recognized contraindication to conventional aortic lymphadenectomy, and was an exclusion criterion specifically cited by Winter and Benedetti-Panici in their staging studies, the inability to perform laparoscopic aortic lymphadenectomy in women over 180

Figure 43.1 Bilateral, inframesenteric laparoscopic aortic lymphadenectomy and resection of a 5 cm lymph node fixed to the left lower aorta.

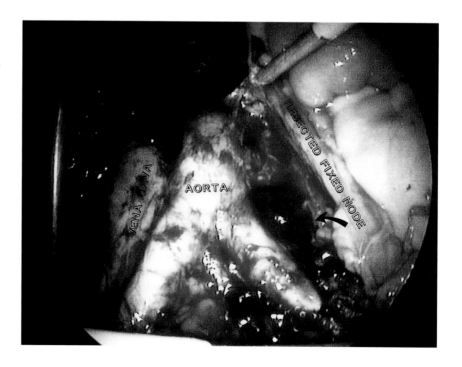

pounds by the Arizona group has been repeatedly cited as a limitation of the operation (Childers *et al.*, 1993). In fact, many patients weighing more than 180 pounds or with body mass indexes greater that 30 and 35 have undergone successful laparoscopic aortic lymphadenectomy (five of the author's cases weighed over 180 pounds and two weighed over 250 pounds), and there is no evidence that open aortic lymphadenectomy can be carried out successfully in a higher proportion of obese patients (however defined) than with laparoscopic aortic lymphadenectomy.

The same observation applies to age. Women aged 70 years or more were excluded from the surgical staging studies of Winter and Benedetti-Panici, yet many women, particularly with endometrial cancer, are older than this. We have shown the general feasibility of laparoscopic surgery in women aged 65 or more (mean age 72 years) (Kadar, 1995a). Although we have only two patients aged over 70 years who have had an aortic lymphadenectomy we have performed laparoscopic pelvic lymphadenectomy in ten women aged over 70 to date (Kadar, unpublished observations).

In summary, the type of aortic lymphadenectomy performed by the vast majority of gynecologic oncologists (inframesenteric, pre- and peri-aortocaval) can be carried out just as effectively laparoscopically as by a laparotomy. As we shall see, there is considerably less morbidity and a shorter hospital stay with the laparoscopic approach, and the restrictions on the laparoscopic operation with respect to the type of patient or the type of aortic nodal pathology that can be treated are no greater than with the conventional one. The same is almost certainly true of a supramesenteric, pre- and peri-aortocaval lymphadenectomy, although there is much less published information on this more extended type of lymphadenectomy, performed either laparoscopically or conventionally.

It cannot yet be claimed in absolute terms that an aortic lymphadenectomy can be carried out as radically laparoscopically as by the conventional approach because experience with retrocaval and retro-aortic laparoscopic dissections is still limited, and what little there is remains unpublished. However, this may be clinically irrelevant because there is little evidence that survival is improved by the more radical operation. The more radical operation has been combined with non-standard methods of evaluating the specimen pathologically, so the extent to which the higher lymph node harvest and frequency of lymph node metastases are actually attributable to the increased radicality of the operation remains entirely unclear and open to debate. The recent attacks on laparoscopic lymph-

adenectomy from Germany that have been based on these arguments should be assessed in the light of these considerations.

Author's Indications for Aortic Lymphadenectomy

In my opinion aortic lymphadenectomy is greatly overused today, particularly by American gynecologic oncologists, who now carry out so-called aortic lymph node sampling in almost all women with gynecologic malignancies with the exception of grade I stage I endometrial cancer that invades less than half of the myometrium. Yet, a rationale for making aortic lymphadenectomy a routine part of the surgical treatment of early invasive cancer of the cervix or endometrium cannot be found in the frequency of aortic lymph node metastases in these malignancies because this has been consistently reported to be less that 5%. For example, in a recent study by Spirtos *et al.* (1995a) only one of 40 (2.5%) patients undergoing laparoscopic aortic lymphadenectomy had aortic lymph node metastases (and the patient had pelvic lymph node metastases as well), and a similarly low frequency was reported by Childers *et al.* (1993), even though many more women had advanced malignancies in their series.

I restrict primary aortic lymphadenectomy to women with:

- Advanced cervix cancer.
- Early stage ovarian cancer.
- Cases of stage I endometrial and cervical cancer in which the pelvic lymph nodes are clinically suspicious and metastatic disease confirmed by frozen section (Kadar *et al.*, 1995).

In other words, I do not routinely send completely normal appearing nodes for frozen section because as processed in a general pathology laboratory frozen section is unreliable in these cases (Bjornsson *et al.*, 1993). In the vast majority of patients with early stage endometrial and cervical cancer the operation will not be required, but most cases of laparoscopic aortic lymphadenectomy have been performed in just such cases. If pelvic lymph node metastases are found on permanent section, patients are offered the option of aortic lymphadenectomy as a second operation (Bjornsson *et al.*, 1993) or extended field irradiation and no further surgery (Photopulos *et al.*, 1992).

A relatively recent if uncommon indication for aortic lymphadenectomy has been advanced ovarian cancer in which all clinical disease is resected at surgery. The usual situation is one in which a patient has a large pelvic mass and omental metastases, but only one or two flecks of tumor on the peritoneum, usually under the right hemidiaphragm. Burghardt first suggested that extensive lymphadenectomy is warranted in such cases because a high proportion of these patients have retroperitoneal disease in the lymph nodes, and these may be less sensitive to chemotherapy than peritoneal disease (Burghardt *et al.*, 1986). Evidence for such a differential sensitivity to chemotherapy is based entirely on the finding that the frequency of nodal disease at second-look laparotomy is similar to that found at primary surgery, but it is a line of reasoning that disregards the possibility that women with lymph node metastases may have less chemosensitive tumors, which almost always fail intraperitoneally as well. Moreover, the finding that pelvic lymphadenectomy increased the five-year survival of women with advanced ovarian cancer from 13% to 53% (Burghardt *et al.*, 1986) is inconsistent with subsequent data indicating that 65% of women with advanced ovarian cancer had involvement of the aortic nodes (Burghardt *et al.*, 1991), which were not resected in the earlier study. We now offer neoadjuvant chemotherapy and interval laparoscopic surgery to women with advanced ovarian cancer (Kadar 1995a, 1997b), and if there is no residual disease or only minimal peritoneal disease present at interval surgery we perform a primary aortic lymphadenectomy after hysterectomy, omentectomy and pelvic lymphadenectomy.

Our highly selective approach to aortic lymphadenectomy has meant that we have performed far fewer aortic lymphadenectomies to date than many of our colleagues, but the frequency of positive nodes in our specimens (50%) has been much higher. Moreover, our lymphadenectomies also seem to be more complete and/or more extensive because our lymph node harvest has been consistently higher than that reported by others. For example, the mean number of 12.8 lymph nodes recovered even in our first six cases was almost double the mean number of 7.9 lymph nodes recovered by Spirtos *et al.* (1995a) with a mature technique in 40 women, unselected with respect to pathology, but highly selected with respect to body mass index.

One final point is that I do not routinely perform a pelvic lymphadenectomy in patients with advanced cervical cancer unless they have enlarged pelvic lymph nodes on computerized tomography (CT). There is no evidence that surgery plus radiation therapy improves control of microscopic pelvic nodal disease and it has the potential of increasing complications. Indeed, much of the early toxicity from surgical staging of advanced cervical cancer was from the pelvic

component of therapy (Nelson *et al.*, 1977). If the lymph nodes are enlarged, however, they are resected, as this may have a survival advantage (Downey *et al.*, 1989).

Review of Anatomy

Aortic or para-aortic lymphadenectomy are unfortunate misnomers for the operative removal of the lumbar lymphatic nodal chain that lies in the retroperitoneum along the course of the great vessels and serves as the primary lymphatic drainage for the ovaries and kidneys, and the secondary drainage site for the pelvic organs and the perineum. Urologists divide the lumbar lymphatic chain of lymph nodes into three areas (left para-aortic, right para-caval, and inter-aortocaval), but Winter and Benedetti-Panici have divided them into at least seven (pre-, para- and retrocaval, pre-, para- and retro-aortic, and superficial and deep intercavo-aortic). These ascending lymphatic channels eventually coalesce to form the thoracic duct behind the aorta and right renal artery in front of L1, and lateral lymph flow between these channels is from right to left.

The small bowel mesentery is about 15 cm long and attaches the small bowel (jejunum and ileum) to the posterior abdominal wall along a line extending obliquely downwards from the ligament of Treitz, which lies on the left side of L2, to in front of the right sacroiliac joint (Figure 43.2a). The inferior leaf of the mesentery crosses the aorta just below the third (horizontal) part of the duodenum, which crosses retroperitoneally in front of the great vessels below the origin of the superior mesenteric artery. The third part of the duodenum covers the left renal vein, and below it the ovarian arteries where they arise laterally from the front of the aorta. The lower border of the duodenum may also cover the origin of the inferior mesenteric artery from the left side of the front of the aorta. The posterior parietal peritoneum is reflected off the posterior abdominal wall to form the lower leaf of the small bowel mesentery at about this level (see Figure 43.2a). The bifurcation of the aorta is about 4 cm below this point cephalad to the sacral promontory.

The inferior mesenteric artery runs obliquely downwards and to the left in the mesentery of the descending colon, and after giving off the left colic and sigmoid arteries, it crosses the pelvic brim in the base of the rectosigmoid mesentery, medial to the left ureter, as the superior rectal artery. The left ovarian vessels cross the left ureter just below the origin of the inferior mesenteric artery, which

Figure 43.2a Anatomy of the posterior parietal peritoneum. (Reproduced with permission from Kadar N (1995b) *Atlas of Laparoscopic Pelvic Surgery*. Boston, MA: Blackwell Science.)

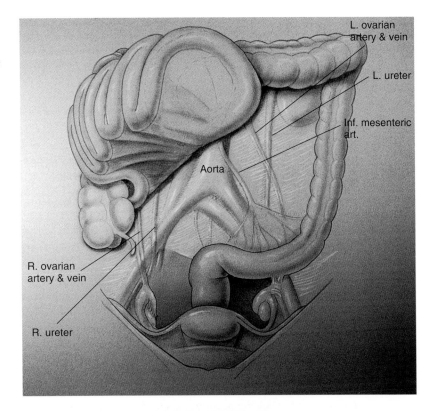

Figure 43.2b Retroperitoneal anatomy of 'para-aortic' region. (Reproduced with permission from Kadar N (1995b) *Atlas of Laparoscopic Pelvic Surgery*. Boston, MA: Blackwell Science.)

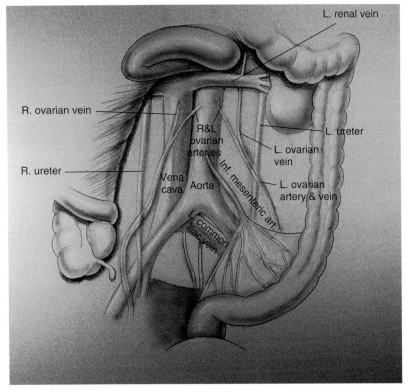

lies medial to the ureter throughout its course. Therefore, above the mesenteric artery the ovarian vessels will be found medial to the ureter (Figure 43.2b).

The left renal vein crosses in front of the aorta on its way from the left kidney to the inferior vena cava, which lies just to the right of the aorta. The left ovarian vein drains at right angles into the lower wall of the left renal vein, approximately 2 cm to the left of the aorta, and the left ureter lies lateral and at a point deep (dorsal) to the ovarian vein. The left adrenal vein drains into the superior wall of the left renal vein directly above its junction with the left ovarian vein (see Figure 43.2b). It can easily be avulsed if ill-conceived attempts are made to elevate the left renal vein. The left renal vein covers the left renal artery, which is therefore usually not seen during aortic lymphadenectomy.

The second lumbar artery can usually be seen arising from the left inferolateral border of the aorta just below where the left renal vein crosses in front of the aorta (see Figure 43.2b). Rarely, an accessory renal artery can arise at this point, but its origin will be much more anterior. It is important to distinguish this anomaly from the lumbar artery because if it is divided it can lead to infarction of the lower pole of the kidney. The next lumbar artery arises just below the origin of the ovarian artery, and the last one is just above the bifurcation of the aorta. The four lumbar arteries correspond to the first four lumbar vertebrae and are paired. The medial member of each pair arises from the right posterolateral wall of the aorta, and can be injured as the deep lying nodes between the aorta and vena cava (aortocaval) are resected.

To the right of the aorta lies the inferior vena cava. Apart from the lumbar veins, which join its inferoposterior border, the only tributary of the inferior vena cava is the right ovarian vein, which joins it at the level of the origin of the ovarian arteries (see Figure 43.2b). The right renal vein is very short and together with the left renal vein and the vena cava itself, covers the right renal artery. Both the right renal artery and vein are covered by the third part of the duodenum and usually need not be exposed during supramesenteric laparoscopic aortic lymphadenectomy for gynecologic malignancies.

Surgical Technique

The most important principle underlying our techniques for retroperitoneal dissection, be it pelvic or para-aortic, is that the peritoneum is the best bowel retractor. Peritoneal incisions are kept small, and in our pelvic dissection no structure or ligament is divided until dissection of the retroperitoneum is complete.

Positions of the Patient, Trocars, Surgeon and Camera

We place patients in Allen-type stirrups with the knees flexed and thighs abducted, but not flexed at the hips, even if only a para-aortic lymphadenectomy is planned because we have found that the sigmoid colon can be very usefully retracted laterally with a rectal mobilizer (Reznick). We use a steep Trendelenburg position and usually rotate the patient slightly to her left. Four trocars are placed in the standard position (Figure 43.3), but the lateral trocars are placed somewhat higher than for a pelvic operation, as for an enlarged uterus. An additional 5 mm trocar is placed in the left or right upper quadrant through which a long atraumatic grasping forceps is introduced and used to elevate the small bowel mesentery and posterior parietal peritoneum after the retroperitoneum has been entered.

After the trocars have been placed and the peritoneal cavity inspected, the laparoscope is switched to the suprapubic port and the video monitors are positioned on either side of the head

Figure 43.3 The standard four-trocar technique used for laparoscopic pelvic surgery. (Reproduced with permission from Kadar N (1995b) *Atlas of Laparoscopic Pelvic Surgery.* Boston, MA: Blackwell Science.)

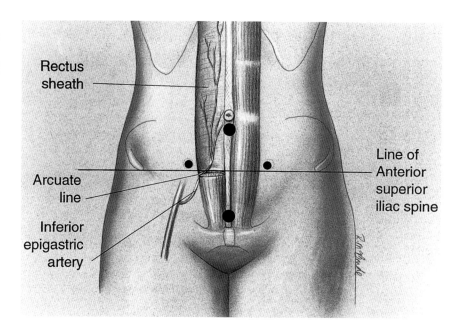

of the table, cephalad to the surgeon and the surgeon's assistant, at 10 and 2 o'clock, as for a cholecystectomy. The surgeon stands on the patient's right and views the monitor just above (i.e. to the right of) the assistant. I have tried standing between the patient's legs, which gives a very natural anatomic view of the retroperitoneum, but it makes camera manipulation awkward. The sigmoid colon is displaced laterally with the rectal probe, and the surgeon dissects with instruments (scissors, spoon forceps, suction/irrigator, bipolar forceps) placed through the right lateral and umbilical ports. The ports on the left side are for the assistant. The one in the upper abdomen is usually used to elevate the small bowel mesentery and posterior parietal peritoneum, and the left lower port is used to provide general assistance.

The Peritoneal Incision

We have tried incising the posterior peritoneum in several ways. Mobilization of the colon by division of its peritoneal attachments in the paracolic gutter, as in the open operation, does not work well laparoscopically. The incision has to be extended too far cephalad, and small bowel invariably falls into the operative field through the apex of these laterally placed incisions.

Anatomically, the easiest and most natural peritoneal incision is one made over the right common iliac artery, parallel to the root of the small bowel mesentery from the cecum to the ligament of Treitz,

again as in the open operation. Most oncologists who perform this operation use this approach. It works well enough in thin patients and anatomic structures are easy to identify, but it makes for too large a peritoneal incision and difficulties can arise if the small bowel cannot be kept in the upper abdomen as frequently happens in obese patients (Figure 43.4).

We prefer to enter the retroperitoneum through a small incision in the posterior parietal peritoneum placed directly in front of the aorta (i.e. using preaortic incision), although it is more difficult to identify the retroperitoneal structures at first with this approach.

Small bowel is first displaced out of the pelvis using the suction/irrigator as a probe, and the root of the mesentery is elevated with the upper bowel grasper (Figure 43.5a). If the small bowel will not stay in the upper abdomen, the surgeon 'walks' along the root of the small bowel mesentery with two atraumatic forceps placed successively one above the other, as one would explore the cervix for a postpartum tear, except proceeding obliquely upwards rather than circumferentially. The posterior parietal peritoneum is opened in front of the aorta about 1 cm below the reflection of the small bowel mesentery onto the posterior abdominal wall as the posterior parietal peritoneum (Figure 43.5b). If there is a lot of difficulty keeping the small bowel out of the way, a more distal site just above the sacral promontory medial to the sigmoid mesentery is selected. Once the peritoneum has been incised it can then be elevated and used to keep bowel out of the way (Figure 43.5c).

Figure 43.4 The aorta has been approached by extending a pelvic peritoneal incision along the right common iliac artery. Notice the large size of the opening in the posterior parietal peritoneum and bowel encroaching on the operative field.

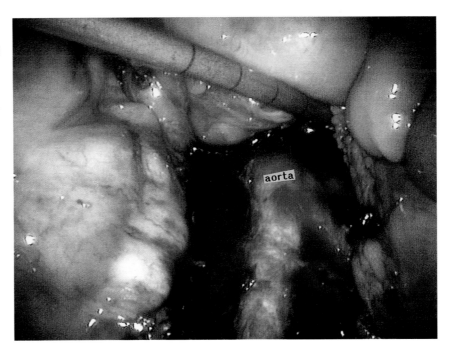

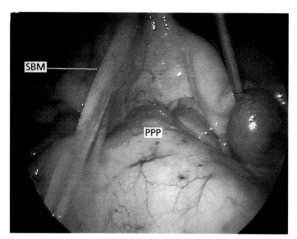

Figure 43.5a The root of the small bowel mesentery is elevated with grasping forceps. SBM, small bowel mesentery; PPP, posterior parietal peritoneum.

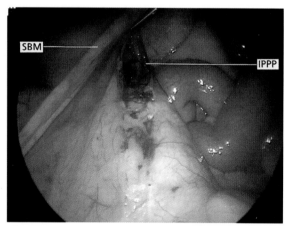

Figure 43.5b Posterior parietal peritoneum is incised just below the root of the small bowel mesentery. SBM, small bowel mesentery; IPPP, incision in posterior parietal peritoneum.

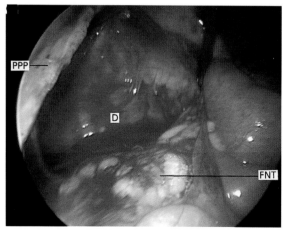

Figure 43.5c The posterior parietal peritoneum is elevated to keep the small bowel out of the operative field. PPP, posterior parietal peritoneum. (Figures 43.5a,b and c reproduced with permission from Kadar N (1995b) *Atlas of Laparoscopic Pelvic Surgery*. Boston, MA: Blackwell Science.)

Planes of Dissection

The peritoneum is picked up with dissecting forceps, desiccated with bipolar forceps and incised with scissors; the incision is extended proximally to the root of the small bowel mesentery and distally to a variable point in front of or cephalad to the sacral promontory. The incision is not extended all at once, but stepwise, gauging the length required as the dissection proceeds. Using mostly blunt dissection, a plane is developed between the peritoneum and the node bearing fatty areolar tissue overlying the great vessels. The plane is extended laterally on each side to the ureters, which are elevated with the peritoneum and not mobilized from it (Figure 43.6). On the left, the dissection is carried under the inferior mesenteric artery which is elevated with the mesentery of the descending colon (Figure 43.7). It is important to develop this plane properly and widely before carrying the dissection down to the adventitia of the aorta otherwise bleeding will occur and some nodal tissue may also be elevated with the peritoneum, bowel mesentery and retroperitoneal fat during retraction, and the tissue will not be removed. Once the correct plane has been developed, the duodenum is elevated by blunt dissection with the suction/irrigator or a probe.

The node bearing areolar tissue in front of the aorta is then incised and the incision is carried down to the adventitia of the aorta. It is not always easy to know where to make this incision because the great vessels are covered by node bearing tissue and the aorta can usually only be seen clearly at this stage in thin patients without retroperitoneal pathology. The duodenum and the origin of the

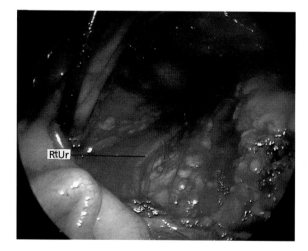

Figure 43.6 The right ureter is elevated on the peritoneum and defines the lateral limit of the dissection. RtUr, right ureter. (Reproduced with permission from Kadar N (1995b) *Atlas of Laparoscopic Pelvic Surgery*. Boston, MA: Blackwell Science.)

Figure 43.7 The inferior mesenteric artery and sigmoid mesentery are elevated to allow dissection of the left distal aortic and high common iliac nodes.

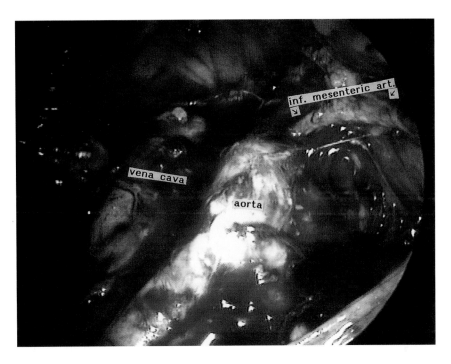

inferior mesenteric artery are also usually ill-defined at this point, and the root of the mesentery is elevated to retract the bowel, and is not in its anatomic position. Thus, there may be no certain landmarks to orientate the surgeon in the superior–inferior plane. It is usually possible to 'feel' the sacrum with a dissecting probe, which serves as a useful guide to the midline, and the pulsations of the aorta can often be 'felt' if it is gently pressed with a probe, but much less clearly than one might imagine.

The nodal tissue is incised higher rather than lower (which is the natural tendency) just below the inferior mesenteric artery and below the inferior leaf of the small bowel mesentery. There are no important structures in front of the aorta at this point, although the origin of the inferior mesenteric artery may be more medial than usual, and may also not be clearly seen in an obese patient. If it is injured it should be clipped close to the aorta to maintain the collateral circulation to the distal large bowel via the left colic artery and the artery of Drummond. Division of the inferior mesenteric artery facilitates the dissection considerably, and is well tolerated, but I have not adopted this routinely for fear that it might affect oxygenation of pelvic tumors, as well as increase the complication rate from postoperative radiation. If the dissection is started too low there is a danger of injuring the left common iliac vein as it crosses the midline below the bifurcation of the aorta, just above the sacral promontory (Figure 43.8). Once the plane between the aorta and the overlying nodal tissue has been

developed, however, and the glistening surface of the aorta is seen, the dissection is very straightforward, provided one takes time to coagulate all small vessels that are encountered. The biggest challenge is to keep bowel out of the way. This is done by elevating the posterior parietal peritoneum, and the incision in it must not therefore be made too large.

Removal of the Fatty Nodal Tissue; Lymphadenectomy Proper

The limits of the dissection are the bifurcation of the aorta inferiorly and the ureters laterally. The superior extent of the dissection is either the third part of the duodenum or the renal vein, in which case the duodenum must be mobilized. The nodal tissue is removed in a systematic fashion as far as possible, but the plan of attack often needs to be varied if there is either very little or a great deal of tissue in the area.

We usually start with the left sided dissection. It is puzzling to this author why the left sided dissection has been considered to be more difficult than the right by some oncologists (Spirtos *et al.*, 1995a). It is in fact no more difficult and much safer because there are no large veins to contend with. The inferior mesenteric artery does, however, need to be dissected free (Figure 43.9), and if its origin is lower than usual, this can make exposure more difficult.

Working in a broad plane, the nodal tissue is mobilized *en bloc* from the front of the aorta and

Figure 43.8 The sacral promontory and left common iliac vein crossing the midline can be seen after removal of presacral nodes.

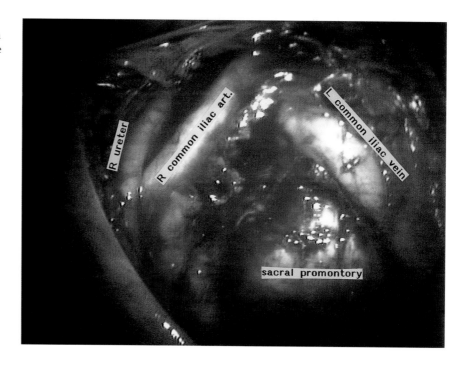

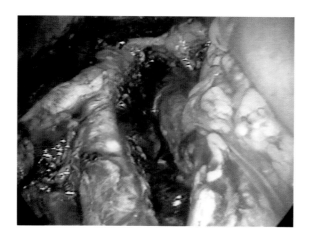

Figure 43.9 Inframesenteric portion of left-sided aortic lymphadenectomy. Inferior mesenteric artery has been dissected free. The lateral limit of the dissection is the left ureter, which is greatly dilated in this patient.

upper part of the left common iliac artery, and extended as far laterally as possible. The tissue is frequently stuck posteriorly by the left edge of the aorta, and it is often advantageous to 'skip' to a more lateral point, identify the left ureter, elevate it on the peritoneum, and dissect the tissue in front of the psoas muscle from lateral to medial to the point of fixity of the tissues by the side of the aorta. The nodal bundle is then transected either proximally or distally, wherever it is most free (usually in front of the common iliac artery), and the tissue teased off the psoas, pushing the wall of the aorta somewhat medially as one goes. One

needs to take care not to injure the vertebral arteries, and on no account pull hard if resistance to the dissection is encountered. If these are injured and retract into the vertebral foramina, laparotomy will be necessary, and even then hemostasis may be difficult to secure.

The problem on the right side stems from the inability to see the wall of the inferior vena cava clearly until the areolar sheath investing it has been incised. The wall of the vein merges imperceptibly with the investing tissue placing it at risk of injury during the initial incision into the sheath. The dissection is in fact easier if there is more rather than less tissue in the area because the nodal tissue can then be grasped very superficially and elevated. Cautious dissection below the elevated tissue will allow one to enter the caval sheath, and once the glistening surface of the cava is seen the incision is extended proximally to the duodenum and inferiorly to the level of the right common iliac artery. Working again in a broad plane, a combination of sharp and blunt dissection is used to clean the cava of fatty areolar tissue, continuing laterally along the psoas muscle as far as the right ureter. There are usually some small branches from the lower part of the vena cava, which should be clipped or coagulated before division, although avulsion rather than division of the uncoagulated vessels is the major risk to guard against.

It is a simple matter to extend the dissection to the left renal vein. Blunt dissection is used almost exclusively, and the duodenum elevated towards the right using the bowel graspers in the left upper and

Figure 43.10 The duodenum is elevated to expose the left renal vein.

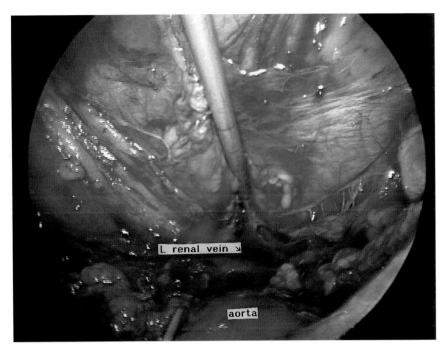

left lower trocars (Figure 43.10). The plane of dissection above the inferior mesenteric artery continues along the front of the aorta towards the renal vein. The ovarian artery is the first structure to be encountered and has to be ligated, and as the dissection continues to the left of the aorta and nodal tissue is cleared from the front of the psoas muscle, the left ovarian vein is seen medial to the left ureter, but does not need to be ligated (Figure 43.11). On the right side, the right ovarian artery that crosses in front of the vena cava, and the right ovarian vein that drains into the front (or sometimes the side) of the vena cava have to be divided as node bearing tissue lying lateral to and in front of the vena cava is removed. Nodal tissue between the aorta and vena cava is only removed after the adventitia of both the aorta and vena cava have been identified and are clearly visible (Figure 43.12). The planes of dissection are extended up as far as the left renal vein, which is cleared of fatty areolar tissue, but is not elevated. The right renal vein does not usually need to be dissected out and identified. The completed dissection is shown in Figure 43.13a and diagrammatically in Figure 43.13b.

Figure 43.11 Left-sided supramesenteric dissection has been completed and left ovarian vein is seen draining into the left renal vein.

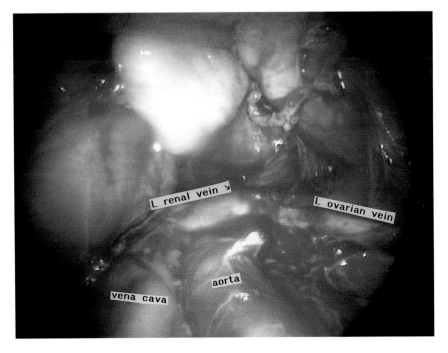

Figure 43.12 Intercavo-aortic nodes are being removed. Notice that the right ovarian artery and vein have not been divided as yet, and that in this patient the vein drains into the lateral side of the vena cava.

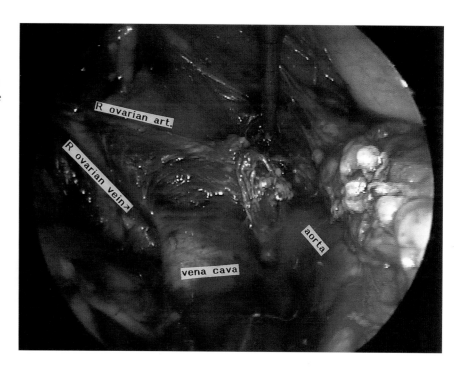

Complications

The author's reservations about aortic lymphadenectomy notwithstanding, it has to be said that if this operation is to be performed at all, the advantages of performing aortic lymphadenectomy laparoscopically are arguably greater than for any other gynecologic operation. Of our 12 cases of pure aortic lymphadenectomies (i.e. those not combined with a hysterectomy), only two patients stayed in hospital for more than one day, one to control severe pain from advanced cervical carcinoma, and the other to manage postoperative exacerbation of severe chronic obstructive airways disease (COAD) in a four pack-a-day smoker. There were no complications except for this exacerbation of severe COAD in a very heavy smoker, and only two patients required transfusions. In the patient with severe COAD, it was recognized that removal of the extensive, fixed pre- and paracaval nodal disease would necessarily cause laceration of the vena cava, and so after preparing the operative field and mobilizing the specimen laparoscopically this fixed chain

Figure 43.13a The completed dissection in a patient with stage IIIB carcinoma of the cervix. Notice that the inferior mesenteric artery was clipped and divided in this patient.

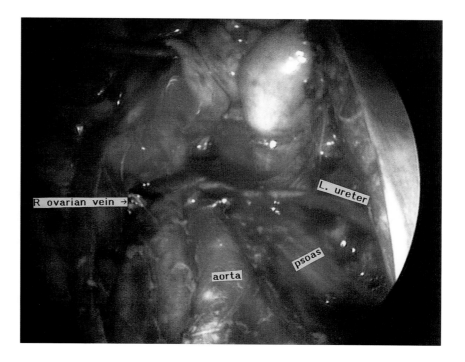

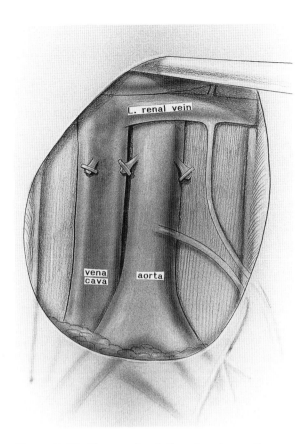

Figure 43.13b The completed dissection shown diagrammatically. (Reproduced with permission from Kadar N (1995b) *Atlas of Laparoscopic Pelvic Surgery*. Boston, MA: Blackwell Science.)

of nodes was resected and the cava sutured through a small 3–4 cm paraumbilical incision under laparoscopic guidance, using what amounted to a gasless laparoscopic technique.

There were no failures or conversions to a laparotomy among these or any other patients who have had an aortic lymphadenectomy by the author, and six of the 12 women had positive aortic nodes. All but one of the lymphadenectomies (11 of 22 overall) were bilateral, and all but three were extended to above the inferior mesenteric artery. This compares favorably with a mean hospital stay of eight days and a serious acute complication rate of 10–15% (injuries to the great vessels or ureters, postoperative bowel obstruction) following extraperitoneal aortic lymphadenectomy (Weiser *et al.*, 1989; Gallup *et al.*, 1993).

The author had to convert a case of laparoscopic aortic lymphadenectomy he performed as a guest surgeon abroad due to bleeding from a small laceration in the inferior mesenteric artery. Ordinarily such bleeding is very easy to control by clipping the

artery close to the aorta, but it does require suction apparatus that can keep up with the rate of bleeding otherwise the site of bleeding cannot be properly exposed. Moreover, if conversion for bleeding is deemed necessary, one should first try to tamponade the bleeding through a minilaparotomy incision before proceeding with the laparotomy because sudden release of the pneumoperitoneum will exacerbate the bleeding and cause unnecessary blood loss.

Childers *et al.* (1993) also reported very few complications among 57 women with aortic lymphadenectomies, although 45 of these were unilateral lymphadenectomies only. There was only one caval injury requiring laparotomy. Ignoring incisional hernias at 12 mm port sites, which were not closed in the early cases, Boike *et al.* (1994) reported one delayed thermal injury to the abdominal part of the left ureter, but the overall complication rate was significantly lower among women with endometrial cancer who were managed laparoscopically than among those who were managed with laparotomy, and hospital stay was almost halved by the laparoscopic approach. On the other hand, Spirtos *et al.* (1995a) reported a rather high complication rate even for a mature surgical technique in a highly select group of women, although all their laparoscopic aortic lymphadenectomies were bilateral and supramesenteric. Nonetheless, they had a 12.5% laparotomy rate and 5% delayed complication rate even after excluding two port-site hernias. The mean number of aortic nodes recovered was also rather low (7.9), as was the frequency of positive nodes (2.5%). Although the node count was equivalent to what has been reported for the open inframesenteric operation in the American literature (Buchsbaum, 1979), it was much lower than that recovered by the authors with a supramesenteric aortic lymphadenectomy at laparotomy (Spirtos *et al.*, 1995b).

Port-Site Recurrences

Many of the uncertainties that surround the clinical value of aortic lymphadenectomy in the treatment of gynecologic malignancies have nothing to do with the route by which the operation is carried out, but the questions raised by port-site recurrences are uniquely 'laparoscopic'. There are many published cases of port-site recurrences after laparoscopic treatment of malignant disease and recent animal studies show that a pneumoperitoneum may facilitate intra-abdominal dissemination of tumor cell lines in experimental animals. These findings have raised the most disturbing possibility that laparoscopic operations by traditional surgico-anatomic and pathologic criteria allow satisfactory removal of malignant tumors, that may nonetheless compromise the survival of patients with malignant disease because the surgical environment created promotes tumor growth and dissemination. What are we to make of these reports? This question has been addressed in detail elsewhere (Kadar, 1997), and only the most pertinent clinical conclusions will be summarized here.

Port-site recurrences in humans are almost certainly the result of direct inoculation of tumor cells into the subcutaneous tissues during surgery, and facilitation of their growth by the healing process in small skin incisions. There is considerable evidence in animals that healing wounds enhance the growth of tumor cells more than unwounded tissues, and circumstantial evidence in humans suggests that small wounds may do so more than large ones. For example, ovarian cancer almost never recurs in a laparotomy incision even if it is exposed to malignant cells for an extended period during a prolonged operation for bulky disease and ascites, yet clinical tumor can develop in a paracentesis needle track within days. Also, if an abdominal wall recurrence develops after laparotomy for colon cancer in patients who recently had laparoscopic operations for benign disease it is almost always at the trocar sites used for the previous laparoscopy, not the laparotomy incision. Moreover, traumatized subcutaneous tissues do not support the growth of intravenously injected tumor cells even though trauma increases tumor uptake by these tissues, but if tumor cells are inoculated directly, the greater the size of the tumor inoculum the greater the enhancement of tumor growth in a skin incision (Kadar, 1997).

A pneumoperitoneum may increase the risk of port-site recurrences by increasing the size of the tumor inoculum in subcutaneous tissues, although this is far from certain. In a recent study of patients with advanced ovarian cancer, for example, abdominal wall recurrence rates were similar in women subjected to paracentesis and diagnostic laparoscopy, suggesting no laparoscopic milieu effect. There is, in addition, no evidence that laparoscopy enhances generalized dissemination of tumors, and there is evidence that tumor growth at port-sites can be prevented by appropriate therapy.

The seeming paradox that port-site recurrences cannot be equated with impaired survival is reminiscent of the findings that in endometrial cancer radiation therapy reduces the frequency of vaginal vault recurrences without increasing survival. This is explained by the fact that either the vaginal vault is but one locus of disseminated recurrence or it is the site of an isolated recurrence that is amenable to secondary cure. By analogy, port-site recurrences after the laparoscopic treatment of malignant disease seem to fall into two distinct categories:

- Those that are isolated recurrences in small skin incisions, which can be prevented by therapy.
- Those that are but one manifestation of disseminated intraperitoneal disease.

Most port-site recurrences have occurred following laparoscopic colectomy for colon cancer or laparoscopic cholecystectomy involving gallbladders that contained occult malignancies, and there are two explanations for the higher propensity for port-site recurrences to develop in these malignancies than with gynecologic tumors (see below). First, the laparoscopic technique for both these operations, entailing as it does dragging cancerous tissue through a small incision, resembles the Paul–Mikulicz operation, which was abandoned early in this century because of the high rate of wound recurrences associated with it. Not surprisingly, therefore, 50% of the port-site recurrences reported have been at the tumor extraction site. Second, in all but one of the remaining true port-site recurrences reported, the patients had Dukes' B or C lesions (i.e. T3 or T4 lesions with or without lymph node metastases). In these lesions tumor cells extend to and are exfoliated from the bowel serosa, and the recurrence rate is 40–75%. Many cases also do not receive adjuvant therapy after surgery, and colon cancer is, in any case, much less sensitive to chemotherapy than ovarian cancer and less radiocurable than cervical or endometrial cancer. In other words, the high probability of tumor dissemination into the peritoneal cavity coupled with lack of effective therapy to the port-sites accounts for the predisposition to port-site recurrences of these patients. Only one Dukes' A lesion has been associated with a port-site recurrence; the other reported case recurred at the extraction site (Kadar, 1997).

Port-site recurrences associated with gynecologic malignancies have occurred almost exclusively following diagnostic laparoscopy for pelvic masses that subsequently proved to be malignant, and were always associated with disseminated intraperitoneal disease (Maiman *et al.*, 1991; Gleeson *et al.*, 1993; Kindermann *et al.*, 1995). In every case, the ovarian cyst was ruptured during surgery or disseminated disease was already present, proper histologic examination of the cyst was not carried out at the time of laparoscopy, and definitive treatment was delayed, usually by several weeks. Other than documented gross mismanagement and accelerated tumor growth at trocar sites, these studies shed no light whatsoever on the safety or efficacy of laparoscopic management of frank or suspected ovarian malignancies, much less on the laparoscopic management of gynecologic malignancies in general. Indeed, they do not even demonstrate that laparoscopic management entraps gynecologists, so to speak, into mismanaging adnexal masses that prove to be malignant because none of the surveys examined the fate of patients with malignant ovarian cysts who were managed by generalists with a laparotomy.

Port-site recurrences following appropriate laparoscopic surgical therapy of gynecologic malignancies are uncommon. In fact only one case has been reported to my knowledge for an incidence of 1% among women with metastatic (intraperitoneal or retroperitoneal) disease, mostly from ovarian cancer (Childers et al., 1994). (The patient with a port-site recurrence had a microscopically positive second-look laparoscopy and recurred before any further treatment.) This author has observed three port-site recurrences following laparoscopic lymphadenectomy for positive pelvic and/or aortic nodes, and one case associated with stage IV endometrial carcinoma. All recurrences occurred at untreated port-sites in association with disseminated disease (Kadar, 1997).

To sum up, the laparoscopic management of malignant disease predisposes patients to port-site recurrences by creating small abdominal incisions, which are conducive to tumor growth. Port-site recurrences result if the malignancy treated has a propensity to exfoliate cells into the peritoneal cavity and the trocar site remains untreated or the malignancy is refractory to adjuvant therapy (as is the case with colon and gallbladder cancer). Whether or not a pneumoperitoneum enhances significantly the inoculation of exfoliated tumor cells into the trocar incisions is unknown and speculative at this time. However, because gynecologic malignancies are sensitive to adjuvant therapy and women at increased risk of port-site recurrences can be reliably identified, these recurrences are preventable by appropriate postoperative therapy. However, it is important to be aware that the lower lateral ports and upper abdominal ports used for aortic lymphadenectomy are not within the standard radiation portals used for either pelvic or extended field radiation.

The laparoscopic management of gynecologic malignancies can also potentially predispose patients to port-site recurrences by enhancing tumor cell exfoliation into the peritoneal cavity by causing rupture of ovarian cysts in patients with stage IA and IB ovarian cancer, rupture of the capsule of lymph nodes containing metastatic disease, and perhaps also by manipulation of the uterus in patients with endometrial and cervical cancer. However, these problems can be potentially prevented in most cases by modifying specimen extraction techniques (use of specimen bags and vaginal tubes) and port-site recurrences in those at risk averted by appropriate postoperative therapy. Evidence that laparoscopic management of any malignancy impairs survival by promoting tumor dissemination within the peritoneal cavity or systemically is lacking at this time.

Conclusions

Aortic lymphadenectomy is indicated only in a minority of women with gynecologic malignancies, and a survival advantage from aortic lymphadenectomy has not been conclusively demonstrated, even in the subset of patients for whom it is believed to be indicated. Nonetheless, in a few cases of carcinoma of the endometrium and cervix extended survival after resection of aortic lymph nodes containing metastatic disease has been clearly documented. Although tolerable doses of aortic radiation can probably sterilize subclinical disease in this region, the value of postoperative aortic radiation after resection of positive aortic nodes has not been established, just as there is little convincing evidence that pelvic radiation after radical hysterectomy and pelvic lymphadenectomy is beneficial in patients with carcinoma of the cervix and positive pelvic nodes.

There is considerable evidence to show that aortic lymphadenectomy can be carried out laparoscopically just as effectively and safely as via a laparotomy and that the laparoscopic approach reduces hospital stay and postoperative morbidity. Fixed and enlarged lymph nodes that cannot be sterilized by radiation alone can also be resected laparoscopically, although there have been no survivors after the laparoscopic resection of fixed enlarged aortic nodes, and it is uncertain whether these women are curable by any means. It is also unclear how extensive an aortic lymphadenectomy needs to be, especially whether it is necessary to mobilize and remove nodal tissues from behind the aorta and vena cava. The extensiveness of laparoscopic and conventional aortic lymphadenectomy seem to be comparable. A more extensive lymphadenectomy can probably be carried out via a laparotomy in absolute terms, but whether this is necessary or indeed desirable is far from established.

References

Benedetti-Panici P, Scambia G, Baiocchi G, Greggi S, Mancuso S (1991) Technique and feasibility of radical para-aortic and pelvic lymphadenectomy for gynecologic malignancies. *International Journal of Gynecologic Cancer* **1**: 133–140.

Benedetti-Panici P, Scambia G, Baiocchi G, Matonti G, Capelli A, Mancuso S (1992) Anatomic study of para-aortic and pelvic lymph nodes in gynecologic malignancies. *Obstetrics and Gynecology* **79**: 498–502.

Benedetti-Panici P, Greggi S, Maneschi F *et al.* (1993) Anatomical and pathological study of retroperitoneal nodes in epithelial ovarian cancer. *Gynecologic Oncology* **51**: 150–154.

Benedetti-Panici P, Maneschi F, Scambia G *et al.* (1996) Lymphatic spread of cervical cancer; an anatomical and pathological study based on 225 radical hysterectomies with systematic pelvic and aortic lymphadenectomy. *Gynecologic Oncology* **62**: 19–24.

Bjornsson BL, Nelson BE, Reale FR, Rose PG (1993) Accuracy of frozen section for lymph node metastasis in patients undergoing radical hysterectomy for carcinoma of the cervix. *Gynecologic Oncology* **51**: 50–53.

Boike G, Lurain J, Burke J (1994) A comparison of laparoscopic management of endometrial cancer with traditional laparotomy. *Gynecologic Oncology* (Abstract) **52**: 105.

Buchsbaum HJ (1979) Extrapelvic lymph node metastases in cervical carcinoma. *American Journal of Obstetrics and Gynecology* **133**: 814–824.

Burghardt E, Pickel H, Labousen M, Stettner H (1986) Pelvic lymphadenectomy in operative treatment of ovarian cancer. *American Journal of Obstetrics and Gynecology* **155(2)**: 315–319.

Burghardt E, Girardi F, Lahousen M, Tamussino K, Stettner H (1991) Patterns of pelvic and paraaortic lymph node involvement in ovarian cancer. *Gynecologic Oncology* **40**: 103–106.

Childers JM, Surwit EA (1992) Combined laparoscopic and vaginal surgery for the management of two cases of stage I endometrial carcinoma. *Gynecologic Oncology* **45**: 46–51.

Childers JM, Hatch KD, Tran A-N, Surwit EA (1993) Laparoscopic para-aortic lymphadenectomy in gynecologic malignancies. *Obstetrics and Gynecology* **82**: 741–747.

Childers JM, Aqua KA, Surwit EA, Hallum AV, Hatch KD (1994) Abdominal wall tumor implantation after laparoscopy for malignant conditions. *Obstetrics and Gynecology* **84**: 765–769.

Di Re F, Fontanelli R, Raspagliesi F, Di Re E (1989) Pelvic and para-aortic lymphadenectomy in cancer of the ovary. In Burghardt E, Monaghan JM (eds) *Operative Treatment of Ovarian Cancer*. pp. 131–142. London: Baillière Tindall.

Downey GO, Potish RA, Adock LL, Prem KA, Twiggs LB (1989) Pre-treatment surgical staging in cervical carcinoma: therapeutic efficacy of pelvic lymph node resection. *American Journal of Obstetrics and Gynecology* **160**: 1056–1061.

Ferraris G, Lanza A, D'Addato F *et al.* (1988) Techniques of pelvic and para-aortic lymphadenectomy in the surgical treatment of cervix carcinoma. *European Journal of Gynaecological Oncology* **9**: 83–86.

Fletcher GH, Shukovsky LJ (1975) The interplay of radiocurability and tolerance in the irradiation of human cancers. *Journal of Radiation Oncology, Biology and Physics* **56**: 383–397.

Gallup DG, King LA, Messing MJ, Talledo OE (1993) Paraaortic lymph node sampling by means of an extraperitoneal approach with supraumbilical transverse 'sunrise' incision. *American Journal of Obstetrics and Gynecology* **169**: 307–312.

Girardi F, Lichtneger W, Tamussino K, Hass J (1989) The importance of parametrial lymph nodes in the treatment of cervical cancer. *Gynecologic Oncology* **34**: 206–211.

Girardi F, Pickel H, Winter R (1993a) Pelvic and parametrial lymph nodes in the quality control of the surgical treatment of cervical cancer. *Gynecologic Oncology* **50**: 330–333.

Girardi F, Petru E, Heydarfadai M, Haas J, Winter R (1993b) Pelvic lymphadenectomy in the surgical treatment of endometrial cancer. *Gynecologic Oncology* **49**: 177–180.

Gleeson NC, Nicosia SV, Mark JE, Hofman MS, Cavanagh D (1993) Abdominal wall metastases from ovarian cancer after laparoscopy. *American Journal of Obstetrics and Gynecology* **169**: 522–523.

Kadar N (1993) Laparoscopic resection of fixed and enlarged aortic lymph nodes in patients with advanced cervix cancer. *Gynaecological Endoscopy* **2**: 217–221.

Kadar N (1995a) Laparoscopic surgery for gynecologic malignancies in women aged 65 years or more. *Gynaecological Endoscopy* **4**: 173–176.

Kadar N (1995b) *Atlas of Laparoscopic Pelvic Surgery.* Chapter 14. Boston, MA: Blackwell Science.

Kadar N (1997a) Laparoscopic management of gynecologic malignancies – time to quit? *Gynaecological Endoscopy* **6**: 135–142.

Kadar N. (1997b) The laparoscopic management of ovarian carcinoma: preliminary observations and suggested protocols. *Gynaecological Endoscopy* (In press).

Kadar N (1998) Mechanism and prevention of port-site recurrences following laparoscopic treatment of gynecologic malignancies. *British Journal of Obstetrics and Gynaecology* (In press).

Kadar N, Pelosi MA (1994) Can cervix cancer be adequately staged by laparoscopic aortic lymphadenectomy? *Gynaecological Endoscopy* **3**: 213–216.

Kadar N, Homesley H, Malfetano J (1995) New perspectives on the indications for pelvic and aortic lymphadenectomy in the management of endometrial carcinoma and their relevance to surgical staging. *Gynaecological Endoscopy* **4**: 109–118.

Kindermann G, Massen V, Kuhn W (1995) Laparoskopisches 'Anoperieren' von ovariellen Malignomen. *Geburtshilfe und Frauenheilkunde* **55**: 687–694.

Kinney WK, Alvarez RD, Reid GC *et al.* (1989) Value of adjuvant whole pelvic irradiation after Wertheim hysterectomy for early stage squamous carcinoma of the cervix with pelvic nodal metastasis: A matched-control study. *Gynecologic Oncology* **34**: 258–262.

Koechli OR, Sevin B-U, Nadji M, Guerra L, Guerhardt R, Averette HE (1993) Relationship between extent of lymph node dissection and incidence of lymph node metastases in patients with cervical cancer treated by radical hysterectomy. *Gynecologic Oncology* (Abstract) **49**: 146.

Maiman M, Seltzer V, Boyce J (1991) Laparoscopic excision of ovarian neoplasms subsequently found to be malignant. *Obstetrics and Gynecology* **77**: 563–565.

Morrow CP, Bundy BB, Kurman RJ *et al.* (1991) Relationship between surgical–pathological risk factors and outcome in clinical stage I and II carcinoma of the endometrium. A Gynecologic Oncology Group study. *Gynecologic Oncology* **40**: 55–65.

Nelson JH Jr, Boyce J, Macasaet M *et al.* (1977) Incidence, significance and follow-up of para-aortic lymph node metastases in late invasive carcinoma of the cervix. *American Journal of Obstetrics and Gynecology* **128**: 336–340.

Nezhat CR, Burrell MO, Nezhat FR, Benigno BB, Welander CE (1992) Laparoscopic radical hysterectomy with paraaortic and pelvic lymphadenectomy. *American Journal of Obstetrics and Gynecology* **166**: 864–865.

Petru E, Lahousen M, Tamussino K *et al.* (1994) Lymphadenectomy in stage I ovarian cancer. *American Journal of Obstetrics and Gynecology* **170**: 656–662.

Photopulos G, Poston W, Simmons J, Sandles L, Bielski W (1992) High risk stage I and II endometrial cancer treated with pelvic lymphadenectomy to determine the need for pelvic radiation. *Gynecologic Oncology* (Abstract) **45**: 103.

Piver MS, Barlow JJ, Krishnamsetty R (1981) Five-year survival (with no evidence of disease) in patients with biopsy-confirmed aortic node metastasis from cervical carcinoma. *American Journal of Obstetrics and Gynecology* **139**: 575–578.

Podczaski ES, Stryker JA, Kaminski P *et al.* (1990) Extended-field radiation therapy for carcinoma of the cervix. *Cancer* **66**: 251–258.

Potish RA, Twiggs LB, Okagaki T, Prem KA, Adcock LL (1985) Therapeutic implications of the natural history of advanced cervix cancer as defined by pre-treatment surgical staging. *Cancer* **56**: 956–960.

Querleu D (1993) Laparoscopic para-aortic node sampling in gynecologic oncology: a preliminary experience. *Gynecologic Oncology* **49**: 24–29.

Querleu D, Leblanc E, Castelain B (1991) Laparoscopic lymphadenectomy in the staging of early carcinoma of the cervix. *American Journal of Obstetrics and Gynecology* **164**: 579–581.

Rotman M, Choi K, Guse C *et al.* (1990) Prophylactic irradiation of the para-aortic node chain in stage IIB and bulky stage IB carcinoma of the cervix: initial treatment results of RTOG 7920. *International Journal of Radiation Oncology, Biology, Physics* **19**: 513–521.

Scarabelli C, Gallo A, Zarrelli A, Visentin C, Campagnutta E (1995) Systematic pelvic and para-aortic lymphadenectomy during cytoreductive surgery in advanced ovarian cancer: potential benefit on survival. *Gynecologic Oncology* **56**: 328–337.

Slevin ML, Stubbs L, Plant HJ *et al.* (1990) Attitude to chemotherapy: comparing views of patients with those of doctors, nurses and general public. *British Medical Journal* **300**: 1458–1460.

Spirtos NM, Schlaerth JB, Spirtos TW, Schlaerth AC, Indman PD, Kimball RE (1995a) Laparoscopic bilateral pelvic and paraaortic lymph node sampling: an evolving technique. *American Journal of Obstetrics and Gynecology* **173**: 105–111.

Spirtos NM, Gross GM, Freddo JL, Ballon SC (1995b) Cytoreductive surgery in advanced epithelial cancer of the ovary: the impact of aortic and pelvic lymphadenectomy *Gynecologic Oncology* **56**: 345–352.

Weiser EB, Bundy BN, Hoskins WJ *et al.* (1989) Extraperitoneal versus transperitoneal selective paraaortic lymphadenectomy in the pretreatment surgical staging of advanced cervix cancer. (A Gynecologic Oncology Group Study). *Gynecologic Oncology* **33**: 283–289.

Wharton JT, Jones HW, Day TG, Rutledge FN, Fletcher GH (1977) Pre-irradiation celiotomy and extended-field irradiation for invasive carcinoma of the cervix. *Obstetrics and Gynecology* **49**: 333–338.

Winter R (1993) Lymphadenectomy. In Burghardt E (ed.) *Surgical Gynecologic Oncology*, pp. 281–289. Stuttgart: George Thieme.

Winter R, Petru E, Haas J (1988) Pelvic and para-aortic lymphadenectomy in cervical carcer. In Burghardt E, Monaghan JM (eds) *Operative Treatment of Cervical Cancer*. pp. 857–866. London: Ballière Tindall.

44

Laparoscopic Vaginal Radical Hysterectomy

D. DARGENT

Hôpital Edouard Herriot, Lyon, France

The use of laparoscopy in the field of gynecologic oncology is now very popular. The movement started at the end of the 1980s when we described laparoscopic pelvic lymphadenectomy. Our aim was to revive the use of vaginal surgery in the treatment of uterine cancer and especially vaginal radical surgery for uterine cervical cancer (Dargent, 1987). Our experience had taught us that vaginal radical hysterectomy (VRH) was as effective and less morbid than abdominal radical surgery. However, it necessitated a complementary pelvic lymphadenectomy, which we carried out using two inguinoiliac extraperitoneal incisions. The outcome for our patients was improved (postoperative casualties were 0.3% versus 0.9% for patients undergoing the Wertheim procedure), but the surgery was not 'patient friendly' resulting in three scars (two inguinoiliac and one perineal) instead of one. Using laparoscopy in order to perform the pelvic lymphadenectomy has overcome this drawback.

In the years following our first description laparoscopic lymphadenectomy developed rapidly. However, the real usefulness of this new approach was questionable. Most surgeons who performed laparoscopic lymph node dissection proceeded to laparotomy and just added the hazards of the new surgery to the hazards of the old one! In this context a new operation was described (Canis *et al.*, 1990) named laparoscopic radical hysterectomy (LRH), which is developing rapidly (Nezhat *et al.*, 1992; Sedlacek *et al.*, 1995; Spirtos *et al.*, 1996). Our aim, in this chapter, is not to enter the polemic between the supporters of this surgery and the supporters (Kadar and Reich, 1993; Schneider and Hatch, personal communication) of laparoscopically assisted vaginal radical hysterectomy (LAVRH). We just indicate that LRH is more time consuming and hazardous than LAVRH. However, LAVRH necessitates a thorough training in vaginal surgery – a training that is not easy to acquire.

The aim of this chapter is to describe the technique we have set up with Denis Querleu and which we have named laparoscopic vaginal radical hysterectomy (LVRH). Before describing this technique, in which the laparoscopic maneuvers really transform the vaginal operation making it easy to teach and learn, we recall the steps we made before arriving at the new surgery.

A prerequisite of the surgery we describe is defining the indications properly. Early infiltrative cervical cancer is the unique indication. Endometrial cancer is not an indication, neither are in situ IA1 cervical cancers. Infiltrative cervical cancer stage IA2, stage IB and early stage II are appropriate indications. Among these cases, experience has taught us (Dargent and Mathevet, 1996) that the most suitable indication is that the diameter of the tumor is less than 4 cm: a discriminative criterion that we now put at the top of our algorithm (see later).

Laparoscopic Lymphadenectomy and Schauta Operation

At first we used a simple addition of laparoscopic lymphadenectomy to the classic Schauta operation.

Laparoscopic Lymphadenectomy

The laparoscopic lymphadenectomy can be done either through the extraperitoneal (Dargent and Salvat, 1989) or transperitoneal approach (Querleu et al., 1991). We have always favored the extraperitoneal approach since the lymph nodes are extraperitoneal organs and it is better to treat them using the extraperitoneal route as there is no involvement with the bowel either during or after surgery. However, the use of the extraperitoneal approach does demand special training; gynecologists are not as familiar with it as urologists. In addition, taking the extraperitoneal route can be impossible even in the most skilled hands due to adhesions resulting from previous laparotomy. For these reasons, both the extraperitoneal and transperitoneal approaches have to be mastered by the laparoscopic surgeon.

The extent of lymph node dissection remains a disputed issue. We favor 'targeted lymphadenectomy' rather than 'systematic lymphadenectomy'. We know that, in cases where the pelvic lymph nodes are not involved, metastases in the common iliac and aortic lymph nodes may exist but are relatively rare (less than 2%). We therefore recommend limiting the dissection to the interiliac area, removing only the obturator and hypogastric lymph nodes. If these lymph nodes are uninvolved, continuing the dissection further is not worthwhile except in patients with adenocarcinoma or if there is an involvement of numerous capillary-like spaces: in both situations the lymphnodal 'skipping' is classically regarded as more frequent than usual.

Systemic pelvic and aortic dissection has, for us, limited and specific indications in the field of early infiltrative cervical cancer. In the cases where we perform an interiliac laparoscopic dissection for early cervical cancer the only circumstances where we extend the dissection are those where the interiliac

lymph nodes are positive (approximately 15% of cases). If the interiliac involvement is massive (5% of cases) we perform the upper dissection laparoscopically before referring the patient to the radiotherapist: pelvic or extended field radiotherapy depending on the state of the aortic nodes. In cases of limited interiliac involvement (one or two nodes involved; 10% of cases) we perform a systematic lymphadenectomy with a therapeutic perspective. This therapeutic systematic lymphadenectomy has to be exhaustive. It can be achieved by laparoscopic surgery. However, it is performed more quickly using a laparotomy and possibly more safely, so careful case selection is important (Figure 44.1).

The technique we used in our earlier experiences, and still use in some instances, is as follows. The laparoscope is introduced into the extraperitoneal space through a mini-laparotomy performed in the mid-line 3 cm above the pubic bone and followed by a digital preparation of the retroparietal space. We distend the operating field with carbon dioxide (CO_2) through the sheath of the laparoscope and then introduce two forceps through 5 mm trocars, the first one into the suprapubic area at the level of the pubic spine and the second one symmetric to it in relation to a horizontal line running at the level of the mini-laparotomy. The suprapubic forceps mobilizes the peritoneal sac medially. The upper forceps maintains the sac, the suprapubic forceps goes further, the upper forceps maintains the result and so on, until the pelvic wall has been entirely exposed, the upper level of the dissection being the bifurcation of the common iliac artery. Then the lymph nodes are detached while delicately dissecting the lymphatic channels and the connective fibers that attach them to the surrounding structures. Once the lymph nodes are prepared they are extracted using the celioextractor – a three-pronged forceps – which is introduced through a 10 mm trocar replacing the 5 mm suprapubic trocar.

Figure 44.1 Algorithm for the management of uterine cervical cancer.

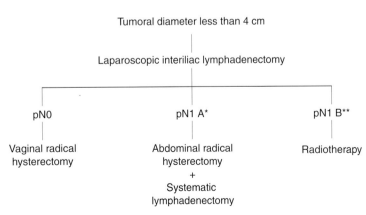

Cancer of the Cervix

Tumoral diameter less than 4 cm

Laparoscopic interiliac lymphadenectomy

pN0 → Vaginal radical hysterectomy

pN1 A* → Abdominal radical hysterectomy + Systematic lymphadenectomy

pN1 B** → Radiotherapy

* pN1A = 1 or 2 positive lymph nodes
** pN1B = 3 or more positive lymph nodes

Schauta Operation

There are two variants of the Schauta operation.

- The first variant was devised by Amreich and is more radical than the operation devised some decades previously by his Austrian compatriot Schauta.
- The second was devised by Stoeckel from Germany, who unlike Amreich, tried to make the operation less aggressive and therefore less radical than the Schauta operation.

The first variant is best for the larger tumors and the second for smaller tumors.

The Schauta–Amreich operation starts with a paravaginal incision. This Schuchardt incision enables us to open the pararectal space and thereafter the paravesical space, which is reached while turning around the caudal brim of the cardinal ligament (paracervix). The formation of the vaginal cuff is the next step of the operation. The incision is performed at the level of the junction between the middle and upper thirds of the vagina. Once the vaginal cuff has been fashioned it is then grasped using a series of Chroback forceps and the vesicovaginal space is opened in the mid-line. Next the bladder pillar is prepared. The lateral part of the bladder pillar is cut first and this incision exposes the 'knee' of the ureter. Once the ureter is defined the medial part of the bladder pillar can be divided. This division enables us to identify the arch of the uterine artery, which is dissected cephalad and then cut as high as possible. After completion of the left side the same preparation is carried out on the right side where the paravesical space has been opened as it is done in the Schautra–Stoeckel operation (see below). Then the pouch of Douglas is opened. The recto-uterine and uterosacral ligaments are divided. The paracervical ligaments can then be clamped and divided at their origin.

The Schauta–Stoeckel operation is performed without an initial paravaginal incision. The opening of the two paravisceral spaces (paravesical and pararectal) is achieved using forceps put on the outside lip of the circular wound created for separating the vaginal cuff from the vaginal sheath. In order to open the left paravesical space forceps are placed at one o'clock and three o'clock. We then pull them centrifugally and a depression becomes visible, which we only have to deepen in order to enter the paravesical space. We do the same with forceps placed at three o'clock and at five o'clock in order to open the pararectal space on the left side. The same procedure is done symmetrically and the following steps of the operation are carried out in the same way as in the Schauta–Amreich procedure. As the opening of the paravisceral spaces is not as large as

in the Schauta technique the extirpation of the paracervical tissues is less radical.

Celio–Schauta Operation

After six years of combining laparoscopic lymphadenectomy with the Schauta operation we changed, under the influence of Denis Querleu from Roubaix (Querleu, 1991) to a new operation we named the Celio–Schauta in order to keep alive the term of 'celioscopy', which was used by Raoul Palmer, who is the father of modern laparoscopy, and to celebrate the name of Schauta. In fact the operation we described in 1992 (Dargent and Mathevet, 1992) was a true combination of laparoscopic and vaginal surgery rather than an addition of two techniques. The main idea was to improve the radicality while taking advantage of the possibilities provided by the laparoscopic approach. In fact putting the clamps at the level of the origin of the cardinal ligaments is not easy arriving from below due to the funneled shape of the pelvis, but it is easy coming from above, especially if we use the laparoscopic approach.

Laparoscopic Part of the Celio–Schauta

The laparoscopic part of the Celio–Schauta can only be carried out with an umbilical approach. At first we used the classical transumbilical transperitoneal technique. After having observed one postoperative intestinal obstruction linked to the incarceration of bowel in one of the widely opened pararectal spaces, we moved back to the preperitoneal approach, opening it at the level of the umbilicus rather than in the suprapubic area. Such an approach is made feasible by the new optical trocars that have been developed (Visiport, Autosuture, Ascot, UK; US Surgical Corp, Newark, NJ, USA and Optiview, Ethicon Endo Surgery, Edinburgh, UK; Cincinatti, Ohio, USA), which has a dividing and transparent tip that can be introduced in the selected space under direct visual guidance. Once the preperitoneal space has been prepared the trocar is removed and the insufflation continued through the sheath, which is left in place. First a 5 mm trocar is introduced in the mid-line, which enables us to introduce an instrument. The posterior aspect of the abdominal wall is prepared widely. Two lateral ports are opened (10–12 mm). Then the peritoneal bag can be moved away. This preparation is made easier by cutting the two round ligaments at the level of their entry into the inguinal rings.

The lymphadenectomy generally starts at the level of the crossing of Cooper's ligament by the iliac vein. The tissues located along the caudal and medial aspects of the vein are detached from it proceeding from front to back. These tissues, which include the interiliac lymph nodes, are grasped and extracted using the celio-extractor. The lymph nodes located laterally to the iliac vein are extracted at the end.

The laparoscopic preparation for the Schauta operation continues by preparing the cardinal ligament (paracervix). In order to prepare this 'ligament' we have to open the paravesical and the pararectal spaces. Opening the first one is not a problem: it has been made while doing the infravenous lymphadenectomy and we merely have to push the dissection caudally to the level of the obturator nerve in order to find the levator muscle, which is the bottom of the paravesical space. Opening the pararectal space is a little more difficult. We do it while pushing the dorsal fold of the broad ligament medially after having located the retroligamental part of the ureter, which is attached to it. Following the ureter caudally we reach the point where it is crossed by the uterine artery. Once this ureteric tunnel is located we can enter the pararectal space, the entry of which is located dorsally and laterally to the crossing of the ureter by the uterine artery.

Section of the cardinal ligament is the final goal of the laparoscopic preparation for the Schauta operation. It is easy to do if the previous preparation has been properly carried out. This section can be performed using various techniques. The endostapler is the best choice. Two cartridges are enough for each side: one firing for the anterior branch of the internal iliac artery (common trunk of umbilical and uterine arteries), one firing for the underlying vessels (uterine veins, vaginal artery and vaginal veins).

Vaginal Part of the Celio–Schauta

After the laparoscopic preparation, the Schauta operation differs little from the classic operation. After making the vaginal cuff the first thing we do is open the pouch of Douglas and then cut the most caudal part of recto-uterine and sacro-uterine ligaments. Once the dorsal attachments of the uterus are cut we directly enter the pararectal spaces. The dorsal surfaces of the ligaments being free, we move to the ventral surfaces and open the vesico-vaginal space in the median line. The bladder pillars can be treated at this moment. Each of them is treated as it is during the classic procedure. Treatment of the bladder pillar ends with decross-ing of the uterine artery and the ureter (the classic 'deroofing' of the ureter as it is called in abdominal surgery). This is done very easily by pulling on the afferent branch of the arch of the artery and then cutting it as high as possible, but without doing a prophylactic hemostasis, which is unnecessary. Following this the specimen is extracted after cutting the remaining part of the recto-uterine and uterosacral ligaments at the same time as the posterior fold of the broad ligament, to which the retroligamental part of the ureter remains attached. The surgeon must be careful when cutting it.

LVRH or Celio–Schauta version 2

The LVRH we have designed jointly with Denis Querleu is a new development in the philosophy of the laparoscopic vaginal approach. The basic concept remains that of taking the best aspects of the two components of the surgery. The guiding concept is still improving the radicalness of this surgery in order to afford the best chances of cure. But the new concern is attempting to avoid the urologic problems following radical surgery, consequences which are generally regarded as inevitable. Bladder voiding difficulties (retention, dysuria and stress incontinence) are very common after radical surgery. These difficulties are initially due to spastic contraction of the urethral sphincter and then to sclerosis linked to infection and inflammation. The initial spastic phenomenon is linked with transection of the parasympathetic nerves running along the cardinal ligament and crossing the vagina to join the posterior part of the urethra. This transection is more frequent as the paracervical resection is large, especially if the colpectomy is also large.

In order to lessen these urologic complications an attempt is made to identify the parasympathetic nerves in their pelvic course and to preserve them before dividing the cardinal ligament. These nerves stem from the hypogastric plexus, which lies deep in the pararectal space at the border of the lateral aspect of the rectum. The nerves devoted to the uterus (nervus pelvicus) and to the bladder (nervus pelvicus accessorius) split at various levels. If the split takes place at the level where the plexus crosses the cardinal ligament the division of this ligament is not dangerous. If the split takes place before the crossing, the division of the cardinal ligament is dangerous.

Identification of the nervus pelvicus can theoretically be easy when operating under laparoscopic guidance thanks to the magnification provided by the endoscope. In fact, although it is rather easy to find alongside the pelvic floor (sacrospinous muscle and iliococcygeus muscle) nerves running from back to front and joining the dorsolateral root of the cardinal ligament, identifying the nerves and managing to preserve the branches devoted to the bladder is not enough to avoid urologic complications. This is the very disappointing observation we have made during the three years we have used the first Celio–Schauta technique.

Our disappointment concerning the 'nerve sparing' operation led us to modify our approach and to use the laparoscopic tool another way in order to improve the radicalness while not impairing the bladder function. We therefore conceived the LRVH, or Celio–Schauta version 2, which we have now used for the past 18 months. The rationale for this technique is simple: cleaning out of the lateral part of the cardinal ligament under laparoscopic guidance and halfway transection of the same using the transvaginal approach.

Division of the cardinal ligament at the level of its origin is carried out in radical hysterectomy to facilitate the removal of all cellular tissue included in the complex network of vessels and nerves, which serves as the skeleton of the ligament. This cellular tissue includes lymphatic vessels arranged in micro-nests or micro-cushions as well as lymph nodes of various size. Girardi et al. (1989) has demonstrated that such lymph nodes were present in 78% of his cases. They are randomly spread in the ligament. They can be involved by the cancer as soon as it reaches stage IA2. These lymph nodes have to be removed, but there is no need to divide the vascular and nervous skeleton of the ligament.

From the anatomicosurgical point of view the cardinal ligament can be divided into two parts, the lateral and the medial, the junction of which is located roughly at the point of origin of the ventrolateral expansion from the ligament to the lateral aspect of the bladder. The point where the two parts join is the point inside which one has to cut the ligament in the 'proximal radical hysterectomy' (Piver II). Cutting at this level does not give rise to urologic complications. One solution to the problem described here could be appealing systematically to the Piver II operation; a solution that seems to fit the IB tumors in the cases where the pelvic lymph nodes are negative. According to Girardi et al. the rate of paracervical involvement in such cases is only 3.6% and the involved nodes are located in the medial part of the ligament in three out of five listed cases.

Although the risk of lateropelvic recurrence is low it is not absolutely nil after a Piver II radical hysterectomy done for a stage IB pN0 cancer. Treating the distal (lateral) part of the ligament is the only way of avoiding such a failure. We can do

it quite easily under laparoscopic guidance. In fact the anatomy of the vascular skeleton of the ligament is more simple as we get closer to the pelvic wall. Dissecting it with laparoscopic instruments under the optical magnification provided by the endoscope is not really difficult or dangerous. The result we obtain after this microsurgical dissection is more radical than after the most radical (Piver IV) transection of the ligament.

Laparoscopic dissection of the proximal (medial) part of the cardinal ligament is difficult and dangerous as the vascular network is rich and plexoid. The surgeons who favour the LRH cut the medial part of the ligament laparoscopically and use energy sources such as argon beam coagulators or bipolar coagulation to minimize the bleeding, which is one of the disadvantages of the technique. Trying to dissect these vessels would be misguided as it is easy to clamp them at the appropriate level and remove the medial part of the ligament using the transvaginal route.

Laparoscopic Part of the LVRH

The laparoscopic part of the LVRH does not differ from the laparoscopic part of the Celio–Schauta in its first steps. We recommend the preperitoneal approach for all cases if it is suitable. After pelvic lymphadenectomy we open the paravesical and pararectal spaces widely. The specific part then starts.

Dissecting the lymph nodes lying between the paracervical vessels does require more caution than dissecting the pelvic lymph nodes. Sharp dissection has to be avoided. Blunt dissection is the gold standard. Using alternatively the so called crocodile and the so called cobra forceps (Micro-France, Bourbon l'Archambault, France) one pulls the lymph nodes at the same time one pushes the vessels. This procedure lessens the risk of injuring the nodes and the vessels (Figure 44.2).

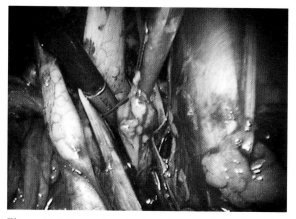

Figure 44.2 Removing the lymph nodes lying lateral to the right common iliac vein.

We recommend to start on the ventral aspect of the cardinal ligament. This aspect is the most accessible as the plane where the ligament is located describes a ventralwards curvature: the upper part (cervical part) is positioned along the umbilico-coccygeal axis, while the lower part (vaginal part) is positioned in a plane almost perpendicular to the first one. This disposition makes the lymph nodes more accessible, but it makes the vessels connected to the lymph nodes more vulnerable. Be careful when dissecting the network involving the collaterals of the internal iliac artery and vein.

The dissection of the dorsal aspect of the cardinal ligament starts at the point of contact with the inferior aspect of the common iliac vein. Then we move medially to the dorsal surface of the ligament. We generally meet more veins on this aspect just as we meet more arteries on the ventral aspect, but there is no rule: the axis of the internal iliac vein can be either dorsal or ventral. Either way the dissection, while being limited to the lateral part of the ligament, has to be driven up to the bottom of the pararectal space as it was pushed on the other aspect up to the bottom of the paravesical space (Figure 44.3). The sciatic spine and the insertion of the sacro-spinous ligament can be seen at the bottom of the space.

The following steps of the 'paracervical dissection' concern the spaces located laterally to the iliac vessels up to the level of the convergence of the internal iliac and the external iliac veins. One starts using the space located between the external iliac artery and the external iliac vein. Pushing medially the external iliac vein can be enough for opening largely the laterovenous place. But it can be insufficient, specially on the right side of the patient. In these cases one has to open the space located between the external iliac artery and the psoas muscle. In this way one gets access, while pushing

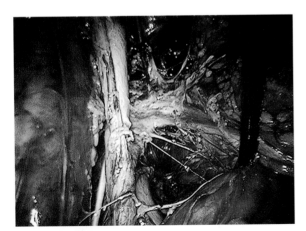

Figure 44.3 The lateral part of the left paracervical ligament as it is seen after laparoscopic clearing.

medially the external iliac artery and vein to the lymph nodes bearing tissues located lateral to the origin of the common iliac vein. Take care while cleaning out this area not to injure the obturator nerve, the first root of the sciatic plexus and the veins that cross the nerves perpendicularly (Figure 44.4).

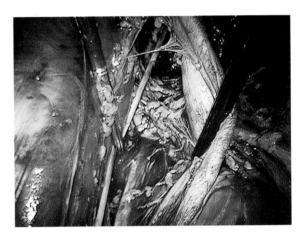

Figure 44.4 The retrovascular part of the lateral part of the left paracervical ligament – the obturator nerve and the lumbosacral nerves are seen; the superior gluteal vessels cross them perpendicularly.

The very last step of the laparoscopic part of the LVRH is to control and cut the uterine arteries. Their origins are found while following the internal iliac artery, going with the stream, or following the superior vesical artery, going against the stream. (If the preperitoneal approach is used one has to know that the bladder having been detached and pushed dorsalwards, the superior vesical arteries follow the same pathway which seems unusual for the surgeon familiar with the transperitoneal approach.) Clips, bipolar cauterization or both can be used to control the arteries. Then the arteries are cut and the medial stumps are pulled medialwards (Figure 44.5). The deroofing is initiated but not entirely carried out. This will be done during the vaginal part of the operation.

Vaginal Part of the LVRH

The vaginal part of the LVRH initially does not differ from the standard Schauta–Stoeckel operation (see above). The differences appear at the time the bladder pillars are attacked. The bleeding is much less (almost nil): that is the first and very enjoyable difference. The treatment of the uterine artery is much easier: that is the second and very interesting particularity. In fact once the knee of the ureter is

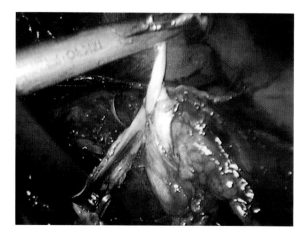

Figure 44.5 The medial stump of the left uterine artery is detached from the lateral and ventral aspects of the ureter.

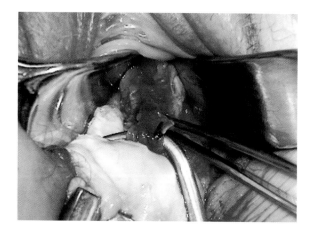

Figure 44.7 Demonstrating the clip placed on the left side at the origin of the uterine artery before it was cut at the end of the laparoscopic part of the operation.

pushed away laterally and the arch of the uterine artery identified, one only has to pull gently on the descending branch of this arch while working smoothly around it with an anatomical dissector (Figure 44.6); the origin of the artery (marked by a clip or a scar of cauterization) arrives quickly into the operative field (Figure 44.7). Afterwards one only has to open the pouch of Douglas and to cut the recto-uterine ligaments. Thereafter one pushes the lateral vaginal flap in order to make free the inferior brim of the cardinal ligament. Then the clamps can be put onto this ligament (Figures 44.8 and 44.9). After cutting it the operation is over.

The operative specimen is like a Schauta–Stoeckel specimen. That means that 2 cm only of paracervical tissue are attached to it. But the lateral part of the ligament which remains in the abdomen of the

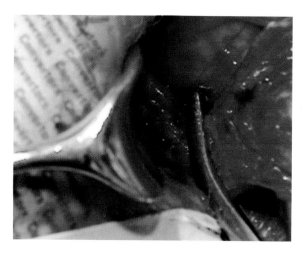

Figure 44.8 Clamping the right paracervical ligament. The medial stump of the uterine artery is drawn medially (upper right corner of the picture). The clamp is put just underneath the knee of the ureter (central part of the picture).

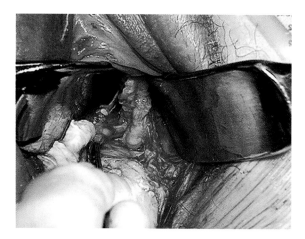

Figure 44.6 Pulling on the descending branch of the arch of the left uterine artery. The bladder pillar has been opened. The knee of the ureter appears as vertical (middle of figure). The uterine artery enters the operative field transversally inside the knee of the ureter.

patient has been completely cleaned out during the laparoscopic part of the operation (Figure 44.10). We do an operation with a radicality equal to that of the Schauta–Amreich procedure but which is no more dangerous than the Schauta–Stoeckel procedure.

A Variant of LVRH: the Radical Trachelectomy

The concept of a combined approach making the radical surgery equally or more radical at the same time as less mutilating can be pushed further in the cases where the cancer grows on only the external

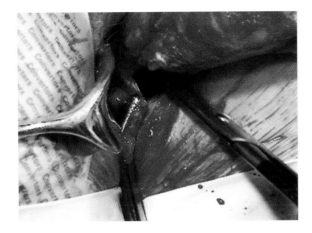

Figure 44.9 The lateral stump of the paracervical ligament on the right side. The hemostatic stitch will be made at the contact of the knee of the ureter.

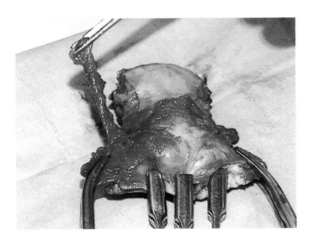

Figure 44.10 The operative specimen. The uterine artery is entirely removed. The lateral part of the paracervical ligament remains in the abdomen of the patient, but it has been cleared during the laparoscopic part of the surgery (see Figures 44.3, 44.4).

surface of the cervix. In these cases, the uterine body and the ovaries and tubes can be preserved and the uterine arteries can be maintained, so that the chance of pregnancy is preserved. That is the rationale for the radical trachelectomy which has been developed by us since 1987 (Dargent, 1994). The laparoscopic treatment of the lateral part of the paracervical ligament that we have performed since 1995 obviously increases considerably the radicalness (and safety) of the procedure.

There is no difference between the laparoscopic parts of LVRH and radical trachelectomy except

that the uterine artery is not cut. The lateral parts of the cardinal ligaments are thoroughly cleaned out, including the area located around the origin of the uterine arteries, but the arteries themselves remain untouched. As for the vaginal part of the operation, this starts the same way as the LVRH. When the knee of the ureter is pushed laterally the arch of the uterine artery is exposed and the descending branch of it is cleaned as much as possible lateralwards, but neither dissected, clamped or cut. If lymph nodes are seen at the level of the crossing between the uterine artery and ureter they are dissected out and sent to the laboratory. The artery itself is preserved. Afterwards the operation continues as for LVRH. The cardinal ligament is cut at 2 cm from its insertion into the cervicovaginal junction and then the isthmus is divided. A prophylactic cerclage is inserted and finally an isthmovaginal anastomosis is carried out.

References

Canis M, Mage G, Wattiez A *et al.* (1990) La chirurgie endoscopique a-t-elle une place dans la chirurgie radicale du cancer du col utérin? *Journal de Gynécologie Obstétrique et Biologie de la Reproduction* **19**: 221.

Dargent D (1987) A new future for Schauta's operation through pre-surgical retroperitoneal pelviscopy. *European Journal of Gynecology and Oncology* **8**: 292–296.

Dargent D (1994) Pregnancies following radical trachelectomy for invasive cervical cancer. *Gynecologic Oncology* (Abstract 14, SGO Twenty fifth Annual Meeting) **52**(1): 105.

Dargent D, Salvat J (1989) *Envahissement Ganglionnaire Pelvien. Place de la Pelviscopie Retro-péritonéale.* Paris: Medsi McGraw–Hill.

Dargent D, Mathevet P (1992) Hystérectomie élargie laparoscopico-vaginale. *Journal de Gynécologie Obstétrique et Biologie de la Reproduction* **21**: 709–710.

Dargent D, Mathevet P (1996) Laparoscopic assisted vaginal radical hysterectomy. In Cusumagno PG, Deprest JA (eds) *Advanced Gynecologic Laparoscopy.* pp. 219–229. New York: Parthenon Publishing Group.

Girardi F, Lichtenegger W, Tamussino K *et al.,* (1989) The importance of parametrial lymph nodes in the treatment of cervical cancer. *Gynecologic Oncology* **34**: 206–211.

Kadar N, Reich H (1993) Laparoscopically assisted radical Schauta hysterectomy and bilateral laparoscopic pelvic lymphadenectomy for the treatment of bulky Stage IB carcinoma of the cervix. *Gynaecological Endoscopy* **II**: 135–142.

Nezhat C, Burell M, Nezhat F *et al.* (1992) Laparoscopic radical hysterectomy with para-aortic and pelvic node dissection. *American Journal of Obstetrics and Gynecology* **166**: 864–865.

Querleu D (1989) Laparoscopic lymphadenectomy.

Second World Congress of Gynecologic Endoscopy. Clermont-Ferrand, 5–9 June.

Querleu D (1991) Hystérectomies de Schauta Amreich et Schauta Stoeckel assistées par coelioscopie. *Journal de Gynécologie Obstétrique et Biologie de la Reproduction* **20**: 747–748.

Querleu D, Leblanc E, Castlelain B (1991) Laparoscopic pelvic lymphadenectomy in the staging of early carcinoma of the cervix. *American Journal of Obstetrics and Gynecology* **164**: 579–581.

Sedlacek TV, Campion MJ, Reich H *et al.* (1995) Laparoscopic radical hysterectomy: a feasibility study. *Gynecologic Oncology* (Abstract) **56**: 126.

Spirtos NM, Schlaerth JB, Kimball RE *et al.* (1996) Laparoscopic radical hysterectomy (Type III) with aortic and pelvic lymphadenectomy. *American Journal of Obstetrics and Gynecology* **6**: 1763–1768.

45

Laparoscopic Radical Hysterectomy for Cervical Cancer

M. CANIS, A. WATTIEZ, G. MAGE, P. MILLE, J.L. POULY AND M.A. BRUHAT

Department of Obstetrics, Gynecology and Reproductive Medicine, Centre Hospitalier Universitaire, Clermont-Ferrand, France

Laparoscopic hysterectomy was first reported in 1989 (Reich et al., 1989) and laparoscopic pelvic lymphadenectomy in 1991 (Querleu et al., 1991). Since that time several laparoscopic techniques of radical hysterectomy combined with a vaginal approach have been reported (Canis et al., 1990; Querleu, 1991; Dargent and Mathevet, 1992; Nezhat et al., 1992; Dargent, 1993; Kadar and Reich, 1993; Spirtos et al., 1996). Our first case was a carefully selected patient with stage IA2 squamous carcinoma of the cervix, who received preoperative cesium radiotherapy. This cautious approach was necessary at first with such a controversial laparoscopic procedure (Canis et al., 1990). In 1992, Dargent performed the first proximal laparoscopic transection of the cardinal ligament with an endostapler (Dargent and Mathevet, 1992). Following this report and with increased experience, our technique became more radical, enabling treatment of our patients by surgery alone (Piver et al., 1974). Should all the previously reported advantages of laparoscopic surgery be confirmed in patients treated surgically for cervical carcinoma, this laparoscopic approach will appear very attractive. However, the series published so far have included only a small number of cases with a short follow-up (Nezhat et al., 1993; Querleu, 1993), and so this laparoscopic radical hysterectomy procedure cannot be considered as a standard.

As one may have anticipated, the development of laparoscopic radical hysterectomy confirmed that 'the term radical hysterectomy connotes many different operations' (Piver et al., 1974). In the present report we will describe two techniques and preliminary results. The first technique includes section of the cardinal ligament at the pelvic sidewall; in the second technique the excision of the cardinal ligament is less radical as it is cut below the ureter after proximal section of the uterine artery.

Patient Set-up and Initial Steps

The preoperative work-up includes an intravenous pyelogram, a chest radiograph and magnetic resonance imaging (MRI) to measure the volume of the tumor and to assess the pelvic and para-aortic nodes, and a complete pre-anesthetic assessment. A mechanical bowel preparation is administered on the day before surgery so that the bowel can be easily pushed away from the pelvis, thus minimizing the Trendelenburg to 10° or less, which is essential during long laparoscopic procedures.

The procedure is performed in a low lithotomy position under general anesthesia with endotracheal intubation. To perform the vaginal steps of the operation easily, it should be possible to increase thigh flexion and abduction. A Foley catheter is placed. The uterus is mobilized with a Valtchev mobilizer without cervical dilatation. Compared to the curet we used to use, this device improves the uterine anteversion facilitating exposure for the posterior steps of the operation. It also allows a better exposure of the cervicovaginal area due to the direct mobilization of the cervix, which was only mobilized by an instrument applied on the uterine fundus.

Vaginal and rectal probes may be necessary to facilitate dissection of the rectovaginal space. A complete set of laparoscopic instruments should be available including three curved laparoscopic scissors, three 3 mm large bipolar forceps, three atraumatic grasping forceps, two atraumatic hemostatic forceps, endoclips, two needle holders, one Clark knot pusher, a high flow electronic insufflator (9 l min^{-1}) and a powerful suction/irrigation apparatus (Bruhat *et al.*, 1992). A second operating table with all the instruments required for a laparotomy is prepared to allow an immediate repair of a large vessel injury. Vaginal retractors and Krawback forceps are necessary to perform the vaginal part of the procedure (Dargent and Mathevet, 1995).

A 10 mm 0° laparoscope is inserted intraumbilically. According to the uterine size and mobility, the ancillary trocars are inserted high enough to ensure that all the instruments can be used during every step of the operation. Whenever possible the trocar entry sites are chosen to ensure that the instruments will be perpendicular to the tissue during key steps of the operation such as the hemostasis of the cardinal ligaments and dissection of the ureters. Usually two 5.5 mm trocars are inserted laterally to the rectus muscle, thus avoiding the epigastric vessels. A 10 mm trocar is placed in the midline or lateral to the umbilicus in small patients. This 10 mm trocar allows immediate insertion of endoclips and of sutures with curved needles. Moreover this diameter is required for easy extraction of lymph nodes. In difficult cases, a fourth ancillary trocar may be necessary to dissect the distal part of the ureter.

The surgeon stands on the patient's left, usually operating with the instruments inserted in the left and the median suprapubic ports. The first assistant is on the patient's right, holding the videocamera and working with the instruments inserted through the right trocar. The second assistant is standing between the patient's legs, and mobilizes the uterine cannula. One nurse stands on the patient's left making the instruments immediately available to the surgeon; occasionlly she works as a third assistant holding the left instrument when the surgeon is working with the median and the right instruments. One or two circulating nurses are in the room. The anesthesiologist monitors the patient's pulse rate, blood pressure and blood carbon dioxide concentration, he/she should be trained in extensive laparoscopic procedures.

Two video monitors are necessary. One is placed at the patient's right foot for the surgeon, the second assistant and the nurse, and the other at the patient's left foot for the first assistant. Although we are working with only two monitors, a third screen located over the patient's head would be useful for the second assistant and for the surgeon when he stands between the legs to dissect the para-aortic nodes.

Whenever possible, three rules should be followed:

- First the peritoneum should be incised without coagulation and while it is elevated with atraumatic forceps. In this way the intra-abdominal pressure and the carbon dioxide will enter the retroperitoneal space and facilitate the dissection. If both peritoneal leaves are stuck together by previous coagulation, the opening of the retroperitoneal space is more difficult.
- Second, all bleeding, however minimal, should be stopped immediately to maintain optimal visibility. Indeed a little bleeding stains the retroperitoneal tissues making the operation more difficult. To achieve this meticulous hemostasis, the retroperitoneal spaces are dissected with two instruments, always including bipolar forceps. As palpation is impossible, vision is essential for the endoscopic surgeon.
- Third, large vessels such as the uterine artery or the infundibulopelvic ligament should be skeletonized and stretched when applying bipolar coagulation. In this way the diameter of the vessels is decreased and the coagulation is more effective since the electric current is applied on the vessel itself and not on the surrounding tissue.

Aspiration of the peritoneal fluid for cytologic examination and inspection of the entire peritoneal cavity are performed first. This evaluation establishes whether the laparoscopic approach is feasible. Poor local conditions, such as extensive adhesions or a very large uterus may lead to conversion to laparotomy. To allow satisfactory dissection of the left pelvic nodes, the sigmoid colon is mobilized. The round ligaments are coagulated and cut above the external iliac vein allowing easy access to the pelvic lymph nodes and to the paravesical fossa. The lateral end of the round ligament is then elevated and the peritoneum is incised above the external iliac vessels.

The adnexa are managed according to:

- The patient's age.
- The volume of the tumor.
- The pathologic diagnosis.

In patients ≤ 40 years of age with a well-differentiated squamous cell carcinoma ≤ 3 cm, the ovaries are preserved. The adnexal vessels are stretched, pushing the uterus towards the opposite pelvic sidewall and pulling the adnexa laterally. In this

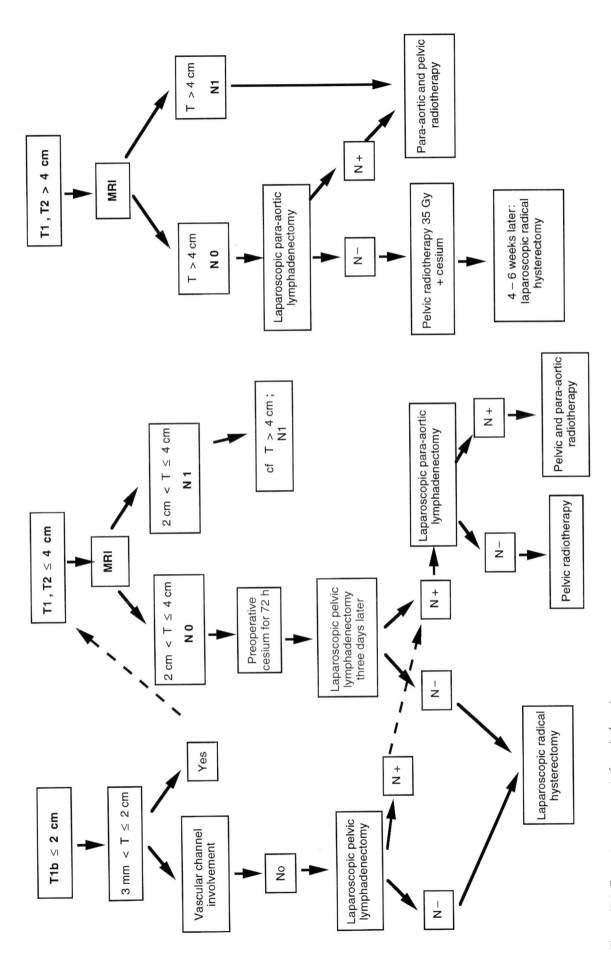

Figure 45.1 Current management of cervical carcinoma.

way the adnexal vessels are easily coagulated with bipolar forceps and cut with scissors. Then the adnexa are elevated and pulled laterally; the medial peritoneum is incised parallel to the ovarian vessels, allowing free mobilization of the adnexa, which will be sutured in the paracolic gutter with non-absorbable sutures. The right lateral peritoneal incision is extended up the paracolic gutter; this is not necessary on the left side where the sigmoid colon has been mobilized. Traction on the ovarian vessels is minimized; twisting should be carefully avoided.

The approach is different when the ovaries are removed. While pulling both the adnexa and the uterus towards the opposite pelvic sidewall, the lateral peritoneal incision is extended up to the infundibulopelvic ligament. The ureter is identified by inspection or by dissection and the infundibulo-pelvic ligament is coagulated and cut.

The Lymphadenectomy

The umbilical artery is identified and dissected up to the internal iliac artery to ensure complete dissection of the pelvic nodes and easier identification of the internal iliac artery, which will be the main landmark for the dissection of the pararectal fossa. Then, while pulling the umbilical artery medially, the paravesical fossa is opened bluntly using scissors and bipolar forceps or an atraumatic probe such as the aspiration lavage cannula. The dissection of the paravesical fossa can be stopped when the obturator nerve has been identified. The lymph nodes are separated from the external iliac vein, the obturator internus muscle, the iliopubic bone and the obturator nerve as previously described (Wattiez et al., 1993). At the end of the dissection, the external iliac vessels are separated from the lateral pelvic sidewall to complete or to check the excision of the obturator nodes. The lymph nodes are immediately removed from the abdomen. While extracting the nodes, the abdominal wall is protected using an endobag or the 10 mm trocar with a 5 mm forceps and a 5 mm external reducer.

If indicated (Figure 45.1) the para-aortic lymph nodes located below the inferior mesenteric artery are removed. The technique has been described by others (Childers et al., 1993; Querleu and Leblanc, 1994; Pomel et al., 1995). In our experience, we have found that to achieve a satisfactory dissection of the nodes located below the left renal vein, the ancillary trocars should be inserted closer to the umbilicus than to the pubic symphysis; higher than usual for a pelvic procedure such as radical hysterectomy. Dissection of the nodes located below the level of the inferior mesenteric artery is much easier than dissection of the upper para-aortic area below the left renal vein. When necessary the laparoscope is introduced through the median 10 mm suprapubic trocar or in the left suprapubic area to dissect the left side of the aorta as recommended by Pomel et al. (1995).

The Radical Hysterectomy

Anatomy (Figure 45.2)

The cardinal ligament should be represented as a parallelepiped oblique anteriorly and medially. The limits of this volume are identified as follows:

- The upper limit is the uterine artery.
- The posterior surface is identified while dissecting the pararectal fossa.
- The inferior surface is freed from the levator muscle.
- The anterior surface is more complex: laterally it is identified when dissecting the paravesical space whereas medially it is connected to the bladder.
- The lateral surface is the origin of this cardinal ligament and of the vessels along the pelvic sidewall.
- The medial surface is connected to the uterus.

The cardinal ligament is connected to the bladder by two vesicouterine ligaments, one is medial to the ureter and the second lateral to it (Frobert, 1981). To free the ureter, this external ligament is coagulated and cut in two steps: one above and one below the ureter. One should understand that the obliquity of the ureter differs from that of the cardinal ligament. Posteriorly the ureter enters the ligament just under its upper limit (i.e. the uterine artery), so the ureter can be freed only by cutting the uterine artery. Whereas in the anterior part of the parallelepiped the ureter enters the bladder and is located more deeply. Dissection of this distal part requires several steps.

To excise the parametrium five of the six surfaces of the parallelepiped should be dissected and cut, while freeing the ureter from the parametrium.

Dissection of the Paravesical and of the Pararectal Spaces

This essential step, which exposes the cardinal ligament is usually bloodless. However, if necessary, hemostasis should be meticulous. While pulling the

Figure 45.2 Anatomy of the cardinal ligament. (1, internal part of the vesicouterine ligament; 2, external part of the vesicouterine ligament; 3, space between the lateral and the anterior part (external part of the vesicouterine ligament) of the cardinal ligament; 4, space between the paravesical and the pararectal space; 5, ureter; 6, umbilicouterine artery; 7, cardinal ligament; 8, levator muscle; 9, pararectal fossa.) (Adapted from Frobert, 1981.)

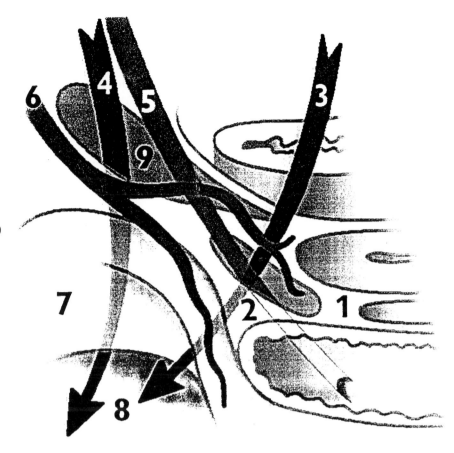

umbilical artery, the paravesical space is easily identified. The loose connective tissue is dissected bluntly with scissors and bipolar forceps. It is sometimes necessary to push the uterus towards the contralateral infundibulopelvic ligament and/or to pull the peritoneum medially. Once the space has been identified, the paravesical fossa is developed up to the levator muscle while moving the bipolar forceps and the scissors in opposite directions. When developing the posterior part of this space, identifying the anterior surface of the parametrium, one should be cautious to avoid traumatizing the uterine veins as hemostasis of bleeding uterine veins would be difficult at this time.

To dissect the pararectal space, the posterior peritoneum is grasped and pulled medially. Thereafter, posterior to the internal iliac artery, the fossa is opened bluntly, taking into account the direction of the vessels of the cardinal ligament, which are not perpendicular to the pelvic sidewall, but oblique anteriorly and medially. To facilitate the dissection of the lower part of the fossa up to the levator muscle, an aspiration/lavage cannula is placed inside the fossa to retract the peritoneum and the ureter and to improve the view with short aspirations whenever the operating field is obscured by blood or lymph. Three working instruments are necessary

to expose and to dissect this posterior fossa. At the bottom of this space the pelvic splanchnic nerve (Kobayashi, 1967; Sakamoto, 1986) is identified and preserved whenever possible.

As the treatment of bleeding is more difficult at laparoscopy, the technique used to open the pelvic fossae may differ from that used at laparotomy. Indeed at laparotomy, the fossae were always opened up to the levator muscle in one step, but a more progressive approach may be preferred at laparoscopy, the deepest part of the fossae being dissected only after section of the upper part of the lateral surface of the cardinal ligament (i.e. the uterine vessels). When these vessels are coagulated and cut, better retraction can be achieved, the deeper part of the fossae are more easily exposed, and the bleeding encountered during the dissection more easily controlled. In contrast, bleeding in the deeper part of the posterior fossae would be difficult to control if it occurred at the beginning of the dissection.

Dissection of the Rectovaginal Space and the Uterosacral Ligaments

In our opinion the posterior step should be one of the first steps of the procedure. Section of the posterior uterine ligaments aids mobilization of the uterus and facilitates the dissection of the parametrium and of the ureters. Furthermore these steps are easier when there is no bleeding from the anterior steps of the operation. When incising the posterior peritoneum, one decides how large the excision of the peritoneum and of the uterosacral ligaments will be, and where the ureter will be freed from the peritoneum and the periureteral plane opened. This point is essential as blood supply brought to the ureter by the peritoneum is important to prevent postoperative ureteral complications.

The posterior peritoneum is grasped under the infundibulopelvic ligament and pulled medially. Then the peritoneum is dissected from the underlying tissue and incised towards the uterosacral ligament. During this step the ureter is identified and separated from the peritoneum. Extending this incision below the ureter up to the posterior cul-de-sac requires coagulation of the upper part of the uterosacral ligament. Then the peritoneum that will be excised is pulled anteriorly and medially to free the ureter from the peritoneum and from the uterosacral ligament.

To dissect the rectovaginal space, the uterus is anteverted and anteflexed if possible according to the tumor anatomy. The rectum is elevated and pulled posteriorly. The rectovaginal space is developed with scissors and bipolar coagulation. A vaginal probe may be used to identify the plane and to improve the exposure of the lower part of the dissection. This plane may be difficult to identify. However, an avascular space can be found in most patients. If many vessels are encountered, the correct plane has not been identified and one will almost always find it closer to the vagina. A similar technique is used to separate the rectum from the uterosacral ligaments.

The ureter is checked and further separated from the uterosacral ligaments, which can then be safely coagulated as their lateral aspect has been identified when opening the pararectal fossa.

Section of the Cardinal Ligament

The hemostasis of the vessels along the pelvic sidewall is the treatment of the lateral surface of the cardinal ligament. Several techniques including endoclips and endo staplers have been proposed for the hemostasis of these vessels (Dargent and Mathevet, 1992). We have used bipolar coagulation in most cases and found it safe, since we have had no postoperative hemorrhage among 17 patients. Preventive hemostasis is the key to an effective and quick hemostasis. Indeed coagulation of bleeding

areas induces carbonization, which prevents the efficacy of bipolar coagulation. The vessels of the cardinal ligament are dissected, coagulated and cut. Generally four vessels are identified during this dissection. If the paravesical space is developed laterally to the umbilical artery, the umbilicouterine artery is cut before its bifurcation, whereas when it has been dissected medially to the umbilical artery, this artery and its bladder branch will be preserved. This second technique should be preferred to avoid urologic complications.

Both cardinal ligaments should be coagulated and cut before dissection of the ureters. Hemostasis of all uterine vessels makes dissection of the ureters much easier.

Dissection of the Ureter and Vesicouterine Ligaments

Dissection of the vesicovaginal plane is the first step – it should be large enough to allow the dissection of the vesicouterine ligaments and to identify the inferior margin of the vaginal cuff.

To dissect the bladder, the uterus is pushed medially and posteriorly toward the promontorium (Masson et al., 1996). The anterior peritoneum is elevated and incised starting from the round ligament. The plane is developed with curved scissors and bipolar coagulation. To achieve this dissection several steps are often necessary. The lower part of the vesicovaginal plane is exposed only when grasping and carefully elevating the posterior surface of the bladder. This movement should be carried out slowly and carefully to avoid bladder injuries, which may be easily induced by an atraumatic forceps since the longer part of the instrument is outside of the abdomen. When the dissection is difficult, one should:

- First, avoid bleeding.
- Second, improve the exposure checking the uterine position and the bladder elevation.
- Third, fill the bladder with methylene blue.
- Fourth, elevate the bladder with two grasping forceps, thus exposing the space by pulling in two directions, the frontal and the sagittal planes.
- Fifth, use a probe in the anterior vaginal cul-de-sac.

The dissection of the ureter includes two steps:

- The section of the uterine artery.
- The dissection of the internal part of the vesicouterine ligament.

The ureter is freed from the uterine artery with a dissector working on its medial side. Adequate exposure is obtained by pulling posteriorly the posterior peritoneum still adherent to the ureter. Coagulation of the uterine artery is achieved with bipolar forceps; this hemostasis is easy as the vessel has already been cut laterally. This second section of the uterine artery is required only to free the ureter. Both parts of the uterine artery will be removed. The lateral part is excised when freeing the lateral part of the cardinal ligament from the pelvic floor, whereas the medial part is removed with the uterus.

The ureter then is dissected up to its entry into the bladder. A perfect exposure of this distal part of the ureteric tunnel is often difficult to obtain. A fourth suprapubic instrument may be necessary:

- First, the uterus is pushed laterally and posteriorly towards the opposite pelvic sidewall without any anteversion or anteflexion.
- Second, the bladder is elevated with atraumatic forceps placed close to the estimated site of the ureteral extremity.
- Third, the ureter is pulled back and laterally to allow dissection of its medial surface. Grasping of the ureter is avoided whenever possible either by pulling on the posterior peritoneum or using Babcock forceps. The ureteric tunnel is developed using a 5 mm curved dissector. As with laparotomy, the correct plane is in contact with the ureter. Hemostasis and section of the internal vesicouterine ligament should avoid ureteral trauma. When possible the hemostasis is achieved with endoclips.

At this point, the cardinal ligament has to be freed from its lateral connections to the bladder. This is achieved in two steps: one above and one below the ureter so that all of the tissues located between the vesicovaginal and the paravesical spaces will be coagulated and cut. The upper part is dissected with a curved forceps inserted through one lateral trocar and then coagulated and cut. Exposure is essential. The installation of the instruments and of the anatomic structures are similar to that described above, except for the ureter, which is pulled medially.

The ureter is then freed from its inferior attachments to the cardinal ligament. The vesicovaginal space is further dissected, allowing section of the lateral part of the vesicouterine ligament, which is essential for a radical excision of the cardinal ligament (Frobert, 1981). To expose this ligament, the bladder and the uterus are retracted as above. The ligament is sequentially coagulated with bipolar coagulation and cut. Then the dissection of the bladder is completed. Throughout these steps care should be taken to avoid dissection of the lateral surface of the distal end of the ureter from the bladder.

Finally, while elevating the cardinal ligament with atraumatic grasping forceps, its inferior surface is freed from the levator muscle. This step is completed when the vagina is identified. A probe may facilitate identification of the vagina.

The procedure is finished vaginally. In this way an adequate vaginal resection, 3 cm from the tumor margins, is easier. As in a Schauta operation (Schauta, 1908), several long Kocher claw forceps are used to identify the vaginal incision. Then the vagina is incised and dissected for 1 cm, allowing the anterior and posterior vaginal edges to be held together with three or four Kroback forceps. When necessary, the dissection of the vesicovaginal and rectovaginal spaces is completed up to the planes identified at laparoscopy. Similarly the paravesical and pararectal spaces are identified. When a complete excision of the cardinal ligament has not been achieved laparoscopically, strong hemostatic forceps such as angled Rodgers forceps are used to grasp the lower part of the parametrium laterally and of the uterosacral ligaments posteriorly. With increased experience in the laparoscopic approach, this vaginal step is shorter, including the vaginal excision and suture. Frozen sections are requested to check the vaginal margins. Hemostasis is achieved with Vicryl no. 1; the vagina is closed with polyglactin 910.

The pneumoperitoneum is then re-established, and hemostasis and ureteral peristalsis are checked. A thorough peritoneal lavage is carried out. The pelvic peritoneum is left open.

More Limited Laparoscopic Radical Hysterectomy

In patients with small tumors who receive preoperative radiotherapy, the operation is less radical. The uterine arteries are coagulated and cut proximally after the bifurcation from the umbilical artery, which is always preserved. The uterine vessels are then pulled medially, separated from the ureter and from the lower lateral part of the cardinal ligament. The dissection of the distal ureter and the posterior steps are achieved as described above. However, the cardinal ligament is not excised laterally along the pelvic sidewall, but is cut below the ureter. The hemostasis of the cardinal ligaments was often achieved vaginally at the beginning of our experience, but it is now achieved laparoscopically to facilitate the dissection of the ureter.

Postoperative Course

We used to leave the bladder catheter in for six days, but now it is removed on the third day. Antibiotic therapy is initiated peroperatively and continued until the bladder catheter is removed. The patients are discharged 48 hours later, once satisfactory micturition has been achieved. An intravenous pyelogram is performed on the twelfth day.

Results

Our preliminary results reported previously are not discussed. Of 15 cases carried out laparoscopically (Table 45.1):

- Some cases were converted to laparotomy because of extensive pelvic adhesions and/or the uterus was too big.
- The average operating time was about five hours, excluding the first case performed in 1989, but it was generally about four hours for the last cases performed.
- There were three complications. In one case bipolar coagulation induced blanching of the ureter, which prompted us to insert a double J catheter and this was left in place for one month. The follow-up intravenous pyelogram was normal. The second complication was a bladder laceration during the vaginal step. It was sutured vaginally. Healing took place with no fistula; however, the 65-year-old patient had severe postoperative urinary incontinence. (The length of the vagina was less than 2 cm in this patient.) The third patient was referred to our department for acute pelvic pain 40 days after the procedure. A vaginal vault evisceration was found. Under general anesthesia the prolapsed part of the omentum was excised and the edges of the vaginal cuff closed with interrupted sutures. At laparoscopy we found no sign of small bowel ischemia or trauma; some bowel adhesions were freed from the pelvic fossae.

To date all of the patients are alive without any sign of recurrence (survival time 4–52 months).

Discussion

Our experience in laparoscopic radical hysterectomy seems promising. With increasing experience, the operating time has become acceptable. We observed no postoperative hemorrhage, confirming that bipolar coagulation is reliable for sealing large vessels (Masson *et al.*, 1996). The intraoperative complications have resolved with minimal sequelae and the postoperative complications are acceptable. The magnification provided by the laparoscope is an advantage for minimizing trauma to the ureters and to the bladder. As meticulous hemostasis is required to avoid staining of the retroperitoneal tissue, the laparoscopic approach should be atraumatic and has even been described as a microsurgical approach (Nezhat *et al.*, 1993). Despite the longer operating time, laparoscopic radical hysterectomy led to most of the well-known advantages of laparoscopic surgery, such as decreased stress and hospital stay, making surgical treatment of cervical cancer more acceptable than open surgery.

Other groups have reported their experience in the laparoscopic management of cervical cancer. A major step forward came from Dargent and Mathevet (1992), who described a technique combining laparoscopic proximal hemostasis of the cardinal ligament and a Schauta operation. Knowledge of the Schauta operation is helpful when using a laparoscopic approach, since dissection of the distal part of the ureter is the most difficult and longest laparoscopic step. Several groups are using this technique. In contrast, we have developed a complete laparoscopic approach (Canis *et al.*, 1995). Spirtos *et al.* (1996) recently reported a similar technique. A complete laparoscopic procedure is in our opinion less traumatic and allows a more logical surgical technique as it is not always easy to find the same planes and anatomic spaces using a different surgical access to the pelvis. The longer operating time is the main disadvantage of the laparoscopic approach. Several years and prospective studies will be necessary to compare these two surgical techniques. Whatever the technique used, the vaginal way is the best choice for incising the vagina as it allows visual control of the vaginal resection, ensuring satisfactory tumor margins. In contrast, we are convinced from our experience with laparoscopic hysterectomy that it is necessary to check the peritoneum by laparoscopy after the vaginal step. This allows us to remove the blood clots (which are always found after the removal of the uterus), to perform a careful peritoneal lavage, and to check hemostasis using the magnification provided by the laparoscope. Meticulous hemostasis is a major advantage of laparoscopic surgery; it probably decreases the incidence of postoperative hematoma and *de novo* adhesion formation. Until now, we have never closed the peritoneum and have had no postoperative bowel occlusion. In contrast, Dargent and Mathevet (1992) reported one case of bowel

Table 45.1 Results of 15 cases carried out laparoscopically.

Case	1	2	3	4	5	6	7	8	9	10	11	12	13	14	15
Age (years)	30	34	36	63	43	43	43	35	35	58	65	48	33	75	44
Stage	IA2	IB	IA2	IA2*	IA2	IB	IB	IA2**	IA2	IIA	IB*	IB	IB	IB	IB*
Tumor volume		1 cm				1 cm	1 cm			3 cm	1 cm	4 cm	3 cm	1 cm	2 cm
Operation time	8 h	5 h 30	6 h	4 h 30	5 h	4 h 30	4 h 30	5 h 20	5 h	4 h 10	6 h	5 h	4 h 30	6 h	4 h
Associated procedures															
Preoperative lymphadenectomy		×					×			×	×		×		
Preoperative cesium		×				refused	×			×	×	xx†			
Ovaries retained		×	×						×						
Peroperative lymphadenectomy	×	×	×	×	×	×		×					×	×	×
Complications															
Peroperative					coagulation close to ureter double J						bladder injury V.V.				
Postoperative															
Bladder catheter removed on day	6	6	6	6	6	6	4	4	3	3	12	10	4	4	4
Postop hospital stay (days)	9	9	9	8	9	8	6	6	5	5	15	12	5	8	8
Follow-up (months)	61	57	55	45	33	33	21	17	15	15	15	12	7	5	3

* Cervix remaining
** Adenocarcinoma
† Cesium and external radiotherapy
V.V., Vesicovaginal

occlusion due to the incarceration of a bowel loop in the pararectal fossa and recommended a careful closure of the peritoneum combining a vaginal and a laparoscopic approach. Our case of vaginal vault evisceration can be explained by necrosis of the vagina, not by the non-closure of the pelvic peritoneum.

Other instruments have been proposed to achieve hemostasis of the cardinal ligament at the pelvic sidewall. Dargent (1993), Dargent and Mathevet (1992, 1995) and Spirtos et al. (1996) used an endostapler. This instrument requires two lateral suprapubic trocars of 10 mm or 12 mm in diameter. Moreover from our experience in the hemostasis of the adnexal vessels, this instrument is less reliable than bipolar coagulation, which is much slower. Dargent and Mathevet (1995) reported postoperative bleeding in a patient whose vessels were treated with endoclips. We have used endoclips to treat some of the vessels and found it to be safe. However, before the application of an endoclip, the vessel should be completely skeletonized and this may be difficult. The thermal damage induced by bipolar coagulation did not appear to be a major problem in our experience, and this technique is always our first choice. We sometimes use endoclips to treat the proximal part of the vessels, but they should not be used on the distal part because they are generally removed by the grasping forceps during the following surgical steps.

Until now there has been no recurrence in our experience. The value of a new technique cannot be established from a limited number of selected cases with a short follow-up. Similar results have been reported by other groups (Nezhat et al., 1993; Querleu, 1993; Dargent and Mathevet, 1995), but much larger and longer series will be necessary to demonstrate that the laparoscopic technique is safe and can be proposed as a valuable alternative to the conventional approach by laparotomy. We are convinced that the extent of the excision is not compromised by the laparoscopic approach and is similar to that achieved previously by laparotomy. This result has been recently confirmed by Spirtos et al. (1996) who routinely measured the parametrial width and the vaginal margin in ten cases.

Laparoscopic radical hysterectomy is still investigational and should be reserved for use by gynecologic oncologic surgeons trained in extensive laparoscopic procedures. These cautious conclusions are justified by the following arguments:

- First, many of our cases were performed by two senior surgeons with a wide experience of laparoscopic surgery, in an environment where endoscopic surgery has been used extensively for many years (Bruhat et al., 1992).

- Second, the surgical environment of laparoscopy and of laparotomy are different (Canis et al. 1994). For instance, at laparoscopy the intra-abdominal pH is lower (Greenwald et al., 1988). Sahakian et al. (1993) demonstrated that peritoneal lavage with a buffered solution (Ringer's lactate) in the rabbit decreased postoperative adhesion formation after an endoscopic procedure performed with a pneumoperitoneum created with carbon dioxide and this difference seems to be important when considering postoperative healing. The intra-abdominal pressure minimizes small vessel bleeding, but may appear to be a disadvantage when considering intraoperative dissemination of malignant cells. This has been demonstrated by experimental and clinical studies about trocar site metastasis (Pastner and Damien, 1992; Nduka et al., 1994; Mathew et al., 1996). One case occurred in a patient treated for a cervical cancer who had a laparoscopy before the treatment of the cancer. This patient had a recurrence less than six months after completion of the postoperative radiotherapy, suggesting that the tumor had an unusual and very poor biologic behavior (Pastner and Damien, 1992). At laparoscopy intra-abdominal packing is impossible, implying that trauma to the peritoneum is decreased and that protection of the upper abdomen is impossible. However, some data have suggested that laparoscopy may be beneficial for cancer patients. Indeed Allendorf et al. (1995) demonstrated in a murine model that intradermal tumor is more easily established and grows more aggressively after a laparotomy than after a laparoscopy. In the same way Mathew et al. (1996) reported a significantly increased incidence of abdominal wall metastasis after laparoscopic manipulation of an intraperitoneal tumor in a rat model, and also noticed that tumor growth was more important after a laparotomy than after a laparoscopy. In contrast Volz et al. (1996) clearly established that tumor growth in a nude mouse model after intraperitoneal injection of cancer cells is significantly improved by a pneumoperitoneum. However, there was no laparotomy control group in this study. When the results of clinical studies are so rare and experimental data are so conflicting, it seems logical to wait for more information before proposing the new technique as a gold standard.

From the technical point of view, the uterine cannulation appears to be the main disadvantage of the laparoscopic approach. The trauma to the tumor should be minimized: the instrument applied on the external cervical surface should be smooth, cervical dilatation should be avoided, and uterine manipulations should be minimal and gentle. We noticed that many steps could be achieved without or with only minimal uterine retraction. As the vaginal excision is performed from below, palpation of the tumor is less common at laparoscopy than at laparotomy, so surgical trauma to the tumor may not be much more important using this approach than the trauma induced by other surgical approaches. During the preoperative evaluation we decide, depending upon the tumor anatomy, whether uterine cannulation and the laparoscopic approach are reasonable. Thereafter the technique is adapted to these possibilities. Anteflexion should be avoided if the posterior vaginal cul-de-sac is involved, so the posterior steps are probably achieved more safely vaginally. Moreover, it can be seen from the therapeutic protocol presented in Figure 45.1, that most patients who are surgically treated for a large tumor receive preoperative radiotherapy, so the consequences of uterine manipulation are minimized.

As stated before '. . . any surgical procedure can be achieved endoscopically by experienced surgeons; therefore the main question is not to know whether or not the procedure is possible but if it is valuable and safe. These questions are to be answered using large prospective clinical trials, not wonderful pictures or beautiful videotapes' (Canis et al., 1992).

What are our indications for laparoscopic radical hysterectomy? When developing this technique, prudence prompted us to select small tumors and to operate on them after preoperative cesium and when the nodes had proved negative. This approach is still reserved for patients with negative nodes. Our current management is presented in Figure 45.1. This management includes laparoscopic lymphadenectomy as a staging procedure to improve the treatment of some groups of patients, whereas others are managed using protocols similar to those used before the development of this major staging tool. However, the benefits should outweigh the fact that some patients will have two surgical procedures. Involvement of the lymph nodes is such an important prognostic factor that benefits are very likely because we will improve the treatment of patients with positive nodes and avoid useless radiotherapy in patients with negative nodes. However, we still have to confirm that the five-year survival rate and complication rate are improved.

References

Allendorf JDF, Bessler M, Kayton MI et al. (1995) Increased tumor establishment and growth after laparotomy vs laparoscopy in a murine model. Archives of Surgery 130: 649–653.

Bruhat MA, Mage G, Pouly JL, Manhes H, Canis M, Wattiez A (1992) Operative Laparoscopy. New York: McGraw Hill, INC Health Professions Division.

Canis M, Mage G, Wattiez A, Pouly JL, Manhes H, Bruhat MA (1990) La chirurgie endoscopique a-t-elle une place dans la chirurgie radicale du cancer du col utérin? Journal de Gynécologie Obstétrique et Biologie de la Reproduction 19: 921.

Canis M, Mage G, Wattiez A, Pouly JL, Manhes H, Bruhat MA (1992) Vaginally assisted laparoscopic radical hysterectomy. Journal of Gynecologic Surgery 8: 103–106.

Canis M, Mage G, Wattiez A et al. (1994) The role of laparoscopic surgery in gynecologic oncology. Current Opinion in Obstetrics and Gynecology 6: 210–214.

Canis M, Mage G, Pomel C et al. (1995) Laparoscopic radical hysterectomy for cervical cancer. Baillière's Clinical Obstetrics and Gynaecology 9: 675–689.

Childers JM, Hatch KD, Tran AN, Surwitt EA (1993) Laparoscopic para-aortic lymphadenectomy in gynecologic malignancies. Obstetrics and Gynecology 82: 741–747.

Dargent D (1993) Laparoscopic surgery and gynecologic cancer. Current Opinion in Obstetrics and Gynecology 5: 294–300.

Dargent D, Mathevet P (1992) Hystérectomie élargie laparoscopico-vaginale. Journal dé Gynécologie Obstétrique et Biologie de la Reproduction 21: 709–710.

Dargent D, Mathevet P (1995) Schauta's vaginal hysterectomy combined with laparoscopic lymphadenectomy. Baillière's Clinical Obstetrics and Gynaecology 9: 691–705.

Frobert JL (1981) L'hysterectomie élargie dans le traitement du cancer du col utérin. MD Thesis University of Lyon.

Greenwald D, Nakamura R, DiZerega G (1988) Determination of pH and pKa in human peritoneal fluid. Current Surgery 45: 217–218.

Kadar N, Reich H (1993) Laparoscopically assisted radical Schauta hysterectomy and bilateral laparoscopic pelvic lymphadenectomy for the treatment of bulky stage IB carcinoma of the cervix. Gynaecological Endoscopy 2: 135–142.

Kobayashi T (1967) Presentation of the pelvic parasympathetic nerves in radical hysterectomy for cancer of the cervix. In Congress Edition of the 5th World Congress of Gynecology and Obstetrics, Scandinavia: 32.

Masson F, Pouly JL, Canis M et al. (1996) Hysterectomie per-coelioscopique. Une série continue de 318 cas. Journal de Gynécologie Obstétrique et Biologie de la Reproduction 25: 340–352.

Mathew G, Watson DI, Rofe AM, Baigrie CF, Ellis T, Jamieson GG (1996) Wound metastases following laparoscopic and open surgery for abdominal cancer in a rat model. British Journal of Surgery 83: 1087–1090.

Nduka CC, Monson JRT, Menzies-Gow N, Darzi A (1994) Abdominal wall metastases following laparoscopy. British Journal of Surgery 81: 648–652.

Nezhat CR, Burrell MO, Nezhat F, Benigno BB, Welander

E (1992) Laparoscopic radical hysterectomy with paraaortic and pelvic node dissection. *American Journal of Obstetrics and Gynecology* **166**: 864–865.

Nezhat CR, Nezhat FR, Burrell MO *et al.* (1993) Laparoscopic radical hysterectomy and laparoscopically assisted vaginal radical hysterectomy with pelvic and paraaortic node dissection. *Journal of Gynecologic Surgery* **9**: 105–120.

Pastner B, Damien M (1992) Umbilical metastases from a stage IB cervical cancer after laparoscopy: a case report. *Fertility and Sterility* **58**: 1248–1249.

Piver MS, Rutledge F, Smith JP (1974) Five classes of extended hysterectomy for women with cervical cancer. *Obstetrics and Gynecology* **44**: 265–272.

Pomel C, Provencher D, Dauplat J *et al.* (1995) Laparoscopic staging of early ovarian cancer. *Gynecologic Oncology* **58**: 301–306.

Querleu D (1991) Hystérectomies élargies de Schauta–Amreich et Schauta–Stoeckel assistées par coelioscopie. *Journal de Gynécologie Obstétrique et Biologie de la Reproduction* **20**: 747–748.

Querleu D (1993) Case report: laparoscopically assisted radical vaginal hysterectomy. *Gynecologic Oncology* **51**: 248–254.

Querleu D, Leblanc E (1994) Laparoscopic infrarenal paraaortic lymph node dissection for restaging of carcinoma of the ovary and of the tube. *Cancer* **73**: 1467–1471.

Querleu D, Leblanc E, Castelain B (1991) Laparoscopic lymphadenectomy in the staging of early carcinoma of the cervix. *American Journal of Obstetrics and Gynecology* **164**: 579–581.

Reich H, De Caprio J, McGlynn F (1989) Laparoscopic hysterectomy. *Journal of Gynecologic Surgery* **5**: 213–216.

Sahakian V, Rogers RG, Halme J, Hulka J (1993) Effects of carbon dioxide-saturated normal saline and Ringer's lactate on postsurgical adhesion formation in the rabbit. *Obstetrics and Gynecology* **82**: 851–853.

Sakamoto S (1986) Radical hysterectomy with pelvic lymphadenectomy. The Tokyo method. In Coppleson M (ed.) *Gynecologic Oncology.* pp. 877–886. Churchill Livingstone.

Schauta F (1908) *Die erweiterte vaginale totalexstirpation des uterus beim collumcarcinom.* Wien: J Safar.

Spirtos NM, Schlaerth JB, Kimball RE, Leiphart VM, Ballon SC (1996) Laparoscopic radical hysterectomy (Type III) with aortic and pelvic lymphadenectomy. *American Journal of Obstetrics and Gynecology* **174**: 1763–1768.

Volz J, Köster S, Weiß M *et al.* (1996) Pathophysiology of a pneumoperitoneum in laparoscopy. A swine model. *American Journal of Obstetrics and Gynecology* **174**: 132–140.

Wattiez A, Raymond F, Canis M *et al.* (1993) Lymphadenectomie iliaque externe par coelioscopie. *Annales de Chirurgie* **47**: 523–528.

46

Laparoscopic Management of Gynecologic Malignancy

JOHN M. MONAGHAN

Univeristy of Newcastle Upon Tyne, Newcastle Upon Tyne and Queen Elizabeth Hospital, Gateshead, UK

Introduction

Since the late 1980s there have been an increasing number of reports of the role of laparoscopic surgery in gynecologic oncology; however, this role still has to be fully defined. During the last seven years as laparoscopic minimal access surgery has developed we have seen a marked expansion in applications. A number of leading clinicians including Dargent, Querleu, Bruhat and Childers have shown, using highly skilled techniques, that laparoscopic minimal access surgery can be very successfully applied to a wide range of gynecologic oncology.

Gynecologic oncology is primarily a surgical subject. The management of the vast majority of cancer patients remains surgical and it is inevitable that with the development in minimal access surgery attempts should be made to transfer as much as possible of these skills into oncology. The significant advantages of minimal access surgery are obvious. Until recently the main principles of good surgical practice (i.e. wide exposure and good access) have been looked upon as contraindications to the use of laparoscopic techniques. However, the rapid developments of video camera technology combined with the use of multiport access have demonstrated the ease of performing complex procedures with minimal traumatic impact upon the patient. The extensive anatomic dissections that are traditionally part of oncology surgery are now seen to be feasible and successful in the hands of surgeons trained in both gynecologic oncology and minimal access surgery.

The author has enthusiastically taken up the challenge of laparoscopic surgery during the last five years beginning with an interest in laparoscopic assisted vaginal hysterectomy (LAVH), and then developing the full panoply of laparoscopic oncologic procedures, ranging from lymph node dissections as an adjunct to LAVH for cancer of the corpus through to radical vaginal hysterectomy (Schauta), coupled with laparoscopic lymphadenectomy for early invasive cancer of the cervix. The potential role of the laparoscope has also been explored in managing the complications of gynecologic oncology including lymphocysts and in assessing recurrent disease in ovarian cancer.

In spite of considerable interest and a large series of meetings, publications and training courses, the uptake and current practise of laparoscopic surgery for both benign and malignant disease is surprisingly low. It is not clear why this should be, except that the performance of oncologic procedures does require new skills, a major investment in training, new technology and a significant increase in operating time. At the present time laparoscopic surgical techniques do not form part of the subspecialty training program curriculum in either USA or in Britain, although this has been advocated (Edraki and Schwartz, 1995) and is currently being taught in at least two subspecialty programs in Britain.

Cervical Intraepithelial Neoplasia

In modern practice most patients found to have cervical intraepithelial neoplasia (CIN) will be treated using outpatient conservative therapy such as laser vaporization or loop diathermy excision; however, there will always remain a small percentage (3–5%) who have persistent cytologic or colposcopic abnormalities and will require definitive therapy. Associated gynecologic problems such as fibroids or menorrhagia will also push the clinician towards using hysterectomy as the treatment of choice.

Where hysterectomy is decided upon there is little doubt that the optimal therapy in terms of short hospitalization and speed of recovery is to use a minimal access surgical technique – that is LAVH, particularly if the ovaries are to be removed as part of the therapy. If the ovaries are to be conserved a vaginal hysterectomy will give excellent results. Using either of these techniques the surgeon can accurately identify and delineate any colposcopically abnormal areas on the cervix or vaginal fornices thereby reducing the risk of leaving a residue of pre-cancer behind. This is of particular value for the patient who has a lesion that extends from the cervix onto the fornices of the vagina (2.4%; Nwabinelli and Monaghan, 1991). The treatment of patients with persistent cytologic abnormalities using standard abdominal procedures is marred by a significant risk of leaving behind slivers of the cervix and vagina harboring areas of CIN, which may go on to develop into invasive lesions at a later date.

Probably the single most important advantage of the LAVH is the freedom given to the surgeon to remove the ovaries in those patients where it is appropriate to do so.

The Place of Laparoscopic Surgery in the Management of Microinvasive Disease of the Cervix

Over the years there have been confusing minor changes in the definition of microinvasive disease of the cervix. The condition is simply part of the spectrum of disease that flows from CIN through to late stage invasive cancer of the cervix. The problems that have arisen in defining the entity of microinvasive cancer have simply revolved around the drawing of lines that will most closely relate to the prognosis of the disease. As of late 1994, the International Federation of Gynecology and Obstetrics (FIGO) has recommended that the terms microinvasive carcinoma and early stromal invasion are abandoned and the following two new stages used in their place:

- In stage IA1 invasion from the basement membrane extends down to no more than 3 mm into the stroma and the lateral extension extends to no further than 7 mm.

- In stage IA2 the depth of invasion is 3–5 mm. Again the lateral extension should be no more than 7 mm.

FIGO has requested that pathologists should comment about lymphatic channel involvement, lymphocytic reaction and degree of differentiation of the tumor. These separate comments should be recorded for future assessment and possible modification of the staging criteria.

These definitions more closely relate to the oncologist's experience of prognosis and have allowed a more logical application of therapies. It is the author's view that laparoscopic surgery has a major role to play.

Techniques of Management

For stage IA1 (less than 3 mm of invasion) the risks of lymph node metastases are close to zero. Thus for these patients it is usually found that if the diagnostic procedure (e.g. loop diathermy, cone biopsy) has completely resected the lesion then no further therapy is necessary. However, if the patient has other gynecologic problems suggesting that a hysterectomy is appropriate then a laparoscopic procedure is optimal. Where excision of the stage IA1 lesion is incomplete then further assessment is necessary. This may take the form of further colposcopic assessment with endocervical curettage or brush cytology. However, the definitive assessment must be by loop diathermy biopsy or cone so that any incompletely resected margins can be reviewed. Often the margins reported to be involved have in fact been effectively dealt with by the diathermy used in the initial procedure. However, it is vital to eliminate the risk of a larger invasive cancer lying beyond the initial diagnostic biopsy – the tip of the iceberg phenomenon.

If the lesion has invaded 3–5 mm the risk of lymph node metastases increases to low single figure percentages. If the lesion has been reported as being completely excised then LAVH with laparoscopic assessment of the pelvic lymph nodes will provide considerable information and will effectively deal with the early invasive carcinoma of the cervix. In addition the procedure allows accurate delineation of any extension of disease onto the outer cervix or vagina, thus decreasing the risk of persistent abnormal smears.

Early invasive cancer spreads by lymphatic channel embolization rather than by permeation, thus preserving tissue between the primary tumor and the pelvic sidewall lymph nodes does not jeopardize the patient's prognosis. It is therefore recommended that for the patient requiring hysterectomy with stage IA1 cancer an LAVH, with or without ovarian removal, depending upon the wishes of the patient is the recommended course of action.

For stage IA2 an LAVH with or without removal of the ovaries as appropriate and node sampling or lymphadenectomy is recommended. The vexed question of whether node sampling or attempts at a comprehensive lymphadenectomy should be made remains unresolved. This dilemma was present long before the arrival of minimal access surgery and remains controversial.

Adenocarcinoma *in situ* and Early Invasive Adenocarcinoma of the Cervix

These conditions, once thought to be relatively rare, now present with marked frequency in large colposcopy clinics, particularly since the return to the widespread use of excisional methods of assessment and management (e.g. loop diathermy cone and excision biopsy).

The recommended role of minimal access surgery in these conditions is very similar to that for microinvasive squamous cancer.

The role of conservative therapy has been shown by Cullimore *et al.* (1992) for adenocarcinoma *in situ*. Most patients will be effectively treated by the loop diathermy cone biopsy that has made the diagnosis. The only caveat to this recommendation is the potentially more disparate nature of the condition when compared to the confluent nature of CIN. In spite of these reservations it is now generally recommended that adenocarcinoma *in situ* is managed as for CIN. Similarly the conditions when an LAVH would be appropriate are the same as for CIN (i.e. there are other additional reasons for performing a hysterectomy).

Early invasive adenocarcinoma of the cervix presents difficult management problems. We do not have a clear definition of a microinvasive disease for this type of cancer. Many clinicians are uncomfortable about the disparate nature of the condition and its tendency to develop deep in the substance of the cervix, resulting in large tumors before clinical diagnosis can be made. If a deep diagnostic cone is not performed then there is a significant danger of underdiagnosis of the true extent of the disease with a consequent undertreatment with a simple hysterectomy or LAVH.

There has been some uncertainty about the true risk of metastases to the ovaries, making the question of ovarian conservation rather vexed. Recently Shingleton and Orr (1995) noted that the risk of metastases to the ovaries for adenocarcinoma differs little from that for squamous carcinoma, being of the order of 1–1.5%. Conversely apprehension about the use of hormone replacement therapy (HRT) following treatment of adenocarcinomas, which includes oophorectomy, is unfounded, thus assisting the decision to remove ovaries as part of the definitive management.

Stage IB Cancer of the Cervix

For stage IB disease there is a higher risk of local spread and lymph node metastases (15–25%), and so a more comprehensive local radical therapy is necessary together with a full lymphadenectomy. As has been demonstrated in other cancer systems, most notably in urology (Schuessler *et al.*, 1991), pelvic lymphadenectomy can be carried out using minimal access techniques. Daniel Dargent (Dargent *et al.*, 1993) has demonstrated the feasibility of the combination of a Schauta radical vaginal hysterectomy together with either a transperitoneal or extraperitoneal dissection of the lymph nodes, as have others (Kadar and Reich, 1993). Querleu (1991), Bruhat (1994) and Spirtos *et al.* (1995) have also shown that the performance of a laparoscopic radical hysterectomy combined with true laparoscopic pelvic and para-aortic lymph node dissection can be performed comprehensively and satisfactorily. Nezhat *et al.* (1992) showed the feasibility of a true laparoscopic radical hysterectomy with pelvic and para-aortic lymphadenectomy. Childers *et al.* (1992) have shown the elegant use of monopolar diathermy for removing all pelvic and para-aortic lymph nodes. Criticisms of excess theater time and material costs have to some extent been countered by the marked reduction in inpatient time associated with these procedures. Twiggs *et al.* (1996) have carried out a sophisticated assessment of resource utilization where laparoscopic pelvic lymphadenectomy has been used before radical hysterectomy and concluded that 'the implementation of new technology in selected patients . . . does not invariably increase cost in this health care system'.

It is fascinating to see how reintroducing radical vaginal surgery such as the Schauta and adding modern minimal access surgery in the form of laparoscopic lymphadenectomy has countered many of the old arguments about the limited value of radical vaginal surgery in cancer care.

Delgado *et al.* (1994) have shown that using the Mitra approach to the pelvic nodes carried deep into the pelvis to allow the lateral parts of the cardinal ligaments to be stapled, the Schauta procedure can be simplified and significantly limits intraperitoneal contamination.

The author has now built up a significant experience of the Celio–Schauta procedure as Professor Dargent calls this combination therapy. The relative ease in obtaining good paracervical and paracolpos margins is impressive as is the ease of performing satisfactorily comprehensive lymphadenectomies.

Radical Trachelectomy

Professor Dargent has shown that in a highly selected group of patients who present with small stage IB cancer of the cervix and are anxious to preserve fertility, there is a real possibility of treating the cancer effectively and having successful pregnancies subsequently (Dargent *et al.*, 1994). The procedure involves careful selection and counselling; however, in spite of this a surprising number of the early series of patients requested termination of subsequent pregnancies.

The operation involves a wide excision of the cervix and the lateral support structures with a generous cuff of vagina as described for the Schauta operation. This vaginal element is combined with a laparoscopic lymphadenectomy. Recovery is rapid and pregnancies have been reported.

More Advanced Cancer of the Cervix

The ability to assess the lymph node status before definitive radiotherapeutic treatment is of enormous value. The significant limitations of lymphangiography, ultrasound, computerized tomography (CT) and magnetic resonance imaging (MRI) have demonstrated very frequently that although these techniques have a place where there is massive enlargement of the nodes, their accuracy is far from certain when there is smaller volume disease. The use of retroperitoneal and more recently transperitoneal minimal access techniques to assess and remove pelvic and para-aortic lymph nodes adds considerably to the information available before the planning of radiation therapy. Of patients with stage IIIB disease 30–40% will have involved pelvic and para-aortic lymph nodes. If these involved lymph nodes are not brought within the radiation field the therapy is worthless. At the present time the coordination between radiotherapists and minimal access surgeons still has to be improved.

Cancer of the Uterine Corpus

Cancer of the corpus is becoming more common than cancer of the cervix in the Western population. It is a disease that predominantly affects peri- and postmenopausal women, many of whom are a poor surgical risk due to obesity, diabetes mellitus, or hypertension. The advantages of minimal access surgery in this group of higher risk patients are obvious. Although operating times may be extended, postoperative recovery with the reduction in short and long-term morbidity is markedly reduced. The majority of cancers of the corpus are well differentiated stage I tumors, and for these patients laparoscopic vaginal hysterectomy with peritoneal washings and assessment of lymph nodes is a perfect technique, which should become standard (Phipps and Monaghan, 1993).

Vault recurrence will occur in a tiny minority (< 2%) of patients with well-differentiated cancer of the corpus. This precentage increases with poorer differentiation. It has been demonstrated that removal of a small cuff of vagina will reduce this low but significant risk of vaginal vault recurrence in cancer of the corpus. This technique can readily be applied in combination with minimal access surgery, thus improving the long-term prognosis of these patients. Childers *et al.* (1994) have shown the role of laparoscopic restaging in patients who have had inadequate primary procedures.

Unfortunately the vast majority of cancer of the corpus in developed countries is dealt with by the first gynecologist who sees the patient. As a consequence the transfer of surgical management from the general gynecologist with limited interest or skill in the area of minimal access surgery to the gynecologic oncologist with surgical skills in this area has been slow to develop. It is also somewhat surprising that after an initial rush of enthusiasm for minimal access surgery there has developed a marked polarization in its use. The skilled and very enthusiastic see more and more applications for minimal access procedures whereas the majority of gynecologists (in Britain) have not taken up the techniques very enthusiastically.

Cancer of the Ovary

The role of minimal access surgery in cancer of the ovary at the present time remains controversial. There has been considerable concern expressed about the risk of managing ovarian cysts, which although thought to be benign may later prove to be malignant. The risk of spillage, inadequate removal and tumor implantation in port sites has been stressed on a number of occasions. It is difficult to be categoric about the level of risk as only a small number of centers have any significant experience of the management of ovarian cysts using minimal access techniques.

The chances of inadequate removal of an ovarian invasive lesion arise when the clinician's judgement has proved flawed or where an apparently benign cystic lesion is found to contain a focus of malignancy. Because of the size of ovarian cysts measures have to be taken to reduce them for removal either via the ports or the vagina.

Following conventional management of ovarian carcinoma implantation of tumor will commonly occur in drain tracks and paracentesis tracks, resulting in the development of worrying masses in the abdominal wall. It is therefore considered important that repeated small volume paracentesis and the use of abdominal drains are avoided. It is because of this experience that oncologic surgeons are concerned about removing ovarian structures, whether complete or morcellated, through the ports. Efforts to reduce contamination using 'bags' appear to help, but no large studies have shown their value in oncology. Although there remains no convincing evidence that the spillage of contents of malignant cyst alters survival, aesthetically spillage is undesirable and every effort must be made to avoid it. Berek (1995) in a commentary in the *Lancet* reviewed the risk to the patient of both spillage and laparoscopic interventions and concluded that there did not seem to be any adverse effects in either of these situations and considered further discussion of these matters as unwarranted.

Assessment of Lymph Node Metastases

Lymph node metastases occur with alarming frequency in ovarian cancer: in stage I involvement has been reported in 10–20% of patients whereas for the most common stage of presentation (stage III), node positivity is noted in 60–80% of patients. Clearly the primary management of such patients with invasive cancer of the ovary will involve a standard laparotomy with removal of all visible tumor where possible. The advantage of removing the lymph nodes in terms of survival awaits the results of trials, but initial results of treatment protocols outwith a trial have suggested advantages to patients.

Unfortunately the vast majority of patients with ovarian cancer are operated upon by general gynecologists or surgeons. As a result very few of these patients have lymphadenectomies performed, resulting in a clear risk of leaving significant volumes of tumor behind in the lymph nodes. Querleu and LeBlanc (1995) have shown the value of laparoscopic infrarenal para-aortic lymph node dissection for restaging of ovarian and fallopian tube cancer. Pomel *et al.* (1995) have also shown the use of laparoscopic techniques to complete lymphadenectomies in such circumstances.

Following chemotherapy it is not infrequently found that patients still have evidence of tumor presence, as shown by persistently elevated tumor markers. In recent times considerable doubts have been expressed about the pivotal role of tumor markers and thoughts have turned to the possible role of laparoscopic techniques for the further assessment of such patients.

Role of Minimal Access Surgery in Second-Look Procedures

Second-look procedures were used very extensively in the 1970s for the assessment of progress during prolonged chemotherapy courses, but fell into disuse with the advent of platinum drugs in the 1980s. Indeed it became generally accepted that 'second-look procedures' should only be performed as part of a trial protocol. During this time there was also considerable doubt expressed about the role of interval debulking, which was occasionally performed if the persistent disease was resectable.

Tumor Marker Elevation

For the patient with persistently elevated or new elevations of tumor markers without any clinical or radiologic evidence of disease the clinician is faced with the following options:

- Should the patient be retreated with chemotherapy?
- Should a laparotomy be performed?
- Should the clinician await clinical or radiologic evidence of recurrence before taking action?

There may be a useful alternative using minimal invasive surgical techniques. The major concern in using laparoscopic techniques is the knowledge that the patient has had major disease with a previous laparotomy. The surgery involved has often been extensive with large abdominal scars and a high risk of adhesion formation. Standard techniques for achieving a pneumoperitoneum and for trocar placement are therefore fraught with danger and are thought by many clinicians to be unacceptably dangerous.

The use of open laparoscopic techniques whereby a tiny incision is made in the abdominal wall, usually periumbilically, allows visual access to the abdominal cavity. Such a technique has been described by Hassan. In recent times the introduction of direct visualization techniques has also been suggested as a means of reducing the risk of inadvertent entry into an intra-abdominal viscus. One example is the simple trocar with a curved shallow cutting blade, which can be used under direct vision by the operator allowing progressive safe entry into the abdominal cavity for:

- Fluid and solid tissue sampling.
- Release of adhesions.
- If appropriate, removal of pelvic and para-aortic lymph nodes for both diagnosis and therapy.

The Reassessment of Patients

There may be a place for laparoscopic techniques for a selected subgroup of patients who are known to have received incomplete surgical resection, which has been followed by an apparently successful course of chemotherapy (e.g. if the uterus or omentum has been left behind or lymph nodes have not been assessed). A preliminary laparoscopic approach with the patient consented for a full laparotomy may reveal the possibility of completing the surgery using minimal access techniques without jeopardizing the completeness of resection.

For a patient who has had a stage I cancer of the ovary diagnosed inadvertently as part of a procedure for 'benign' disease, laparoscopic reassessment may be valuable to obtain information such as the status of peritoneal washings, to allow correct staging.

Laparoscopic Techniques in Ovarian Screening

There has developed worldwide a patient-driven demand for ovarian cancer screening. At the present time there is little accurate screening available for the general population, but high-risk families are investigated. Unfortunately transvaginal ultrasound and CA125 estimation have the potential of generating equivocal results. This problem coupled with a highly anxious population has on occasions generated the need for a closer assessment of the ovaries or even their removal. These activities are best performed using laparoscopic techniques (Menczer *et al.*, 1993)

Cancer of the Vulva

The role of laparoscopy in vulvar cancer would appear initially to be minuscule; however, for those patients with large tumors a laparoscopic assessment of the pelvic lymph nodes and possible removal may be of enormous value. At the present time the general recommendation is that where two or more groin nodes are involved or a single node is completely replaced or there is nodal capsular rupture (Palidini *et al.*, 1994) then postoperative adjuvant radiotherapy should be performed to the groins and the external iliac lymph nodes. It is, however, likely that a large proportion of these patients will in fact have negative pelvic lymph nodes and therefore do not need to be treated in this way. If a laparoscopic assessment could be performed then the opportunity to reduce therapy further would be increased. Because of the rarity of cancer of the vulva and the difficulty of centralizing treatment it is not feasible to establish a prospective trial for this tiny subgroup of patients, but it is likely that it may be attempted as a treatment method in the near future (Monaghan), (Dargent, personal communication).

General Assessment of the Gynecologic Oncology Patients

For the gynecologic oncologists who use minimal access techniques it will be found that the laparoscope is often used for the pre-laparotomy or pre-definitive therapy assessment of tumor masses. In recent times the author has assessed a tumor lying in the paracolpos in a 13-year-old girl. The laparoscopic assessment before was very helpful in planning the definitive therapy which was conservative, maintaining the uterus, tubes and ovaries and a significant part of the vagina. This patient had a rare tumor of the paracolpos, probably arising in the Wolffian duct remnant.

The Management of Lymphocysts

Lymphocysts are an occasional problem for patients who have had radical pelvic surgery. They are most commonly encountered in urological practise, but are also commonly seen following radical gynecologic oncologic procedures, particularly radical hysterectomy (Ilancheran and

Monaghan, 1988). They most commonly occur when attempts to close the pelvic peritoneum leave a retroperitoneal space, which can close off. This fills with lymphatic fluid causing discomfort and pressure symptoms or severe malaise if the lymphocyst becomes infected. Attempts to reduce the risk of lymphocyst development have been made by draining the pelvis in a variety of ways. It was believed until recently that a combination of suction drainage and leaving the pelvic peritoneum open would be the most effective way of reducing lymphocyst development. Lopes *et al.* (1995) working in this department has shown in a randomized study of patients in whom the pelvic peritoneum was left open that whether drained or not the clinical identification of lymphocysts was identical and minimal (3%). However, lymphocysts were identified by pelvic ultrasound six weeks postoperatively in 15.6% of patients.

Treatment of Lymphocysts

The standard therapy for lymphocysts has been conservative, with observation of asymptomatic lymphocysts after diagnostic ultrasound to confirm no evidence of recurrence. If the lymphocyst had become infected antibiotics with an expectant policy was recommended. If the lymphocyst was causing pressure or obstructive symptoms laparotomy with marsupialization of the cyst was usually carried out.

Minimal access surgery allows the same marsupialization without the need for laparotomy. The cysts generally lie close to the pelvic brim and are easily accessed for drainage and deroofing; sometimes omentum can be sewn into the defect to improve drainage (Ancona *et al.*, 1991). It is important to remember that the cyst wall is often extremely thick and strong, being up to 1 cm in thickness in extreme cases.

Formation of Colostomy

Although the formation of colostomy falls mostly in the area of expertise of the gastrointestinal surgeon, not uncommonly the gynecologic oncologist needs to perform such a procedure. This can be performed relatively simply with minimal access techniques, eliminating the large scar and risk of soiling of the peritoneal cavity associated with laparotomy.

References

Ancona E, Rigotti P, Zaninotto G, Comandella M, Morpurgo E, Constantini M (1991) Treatment of lymphocele following renal transplantation by laparoscopic surgery. *International Surgery* **76**: 261–263.

Berek JS (1995) Ovarian cancer spread: Is laparoscopy to blame? *Lancet* **346**: 200.

Bruhat MA (1994) Laparoscopic radical hysterectomy and node dissection. Video presentation. Royal College of Obstetricians and Gynaecologists: London.

Childers JM, Hatch K, Surwit EA (1992) The role of laparoscopic lymphadenectomy in the management of cervical carcinoma. *Gynecologic Oncology* **47**: 38–43.

Childers JM, Spirtos NM, Brainard P, Surwit EA (1994) Laparoscopic staging of the patient with incompletely staged early adenocarcinoma of the endometrium. *Obstetrics and Gynecology* **83**: 597–600.

Cullimore J, Luesley D, Rollason T *et al.* (1992) A prospective study of conization of the cervix in the management of cervical intraepithelial glandular neoplasia – a preliminary report. *British Journal Of Obstetrics and Gynaecology* **99**: 314–318.

Dargent D, Roy M, Keita N, Mathevet P, Adeleine P (1993) The Schauta operation – its place in the management of cervical cancer. *Gynecologic Oncology* (Abstract) **49**: 109–110.

Dargent D, Brun JL, Roy M *et al.* (1994) La trachelectomie elargie. Une alternative a l'hysterectomie elargie radicale dans le traitment des cancers infitrants developpes sur la face externe du col uterine. *JOBGYN* **4**: 285–292.

Delgado G, Potkul RK, Dolan JR (1994) Retroperitoneal radical hysterectomy. *Gynecologic Oncology* **56**: 191–194.

Edraki B, Schwartz PE (1995) Operative laparoscopy and the gynecological oncologist. *Cancer* **76**: 1987–1991.

Ilancheran A, Monaghan J (1988) Pelvic lymphocyst – a 10 year experience. *Gynecologic Oncology* **29**: 333–336.

Kadar N, Reich H (1993) Laparoscopically assisted radical Schauta hysterectomy and bilateral pelvic lymphadenectomy for the treatment of bulky stage IB carcinoma of the cervix. *Gynaecological Endoscopy* **2**: 135–142.

Lopes A de B, Hall JR, Monaghan JM (1995) Drainage following radical hysterectomy and pelvic lymphadenectomy: Dogma or need. *Obstetrics and Gynecology* **86**: 960–963.

Menczer J, Dan U, Oelsner G (1993) Laparoscopic prophylactic oophorectomy in women belonging to ovarian cancer-prone families. *European Journal of Gynaecological Oncology* **41**: 105–107.

Nezhat C, Nezhat F, Welander C (1992) Laparoscopic radical hysterectomy and pelvic and para-aortic lymphadenectomy in the treatment of carcinoma of the cervix. *American Journal of Obstetrics and Gynecology* **166**: 864–865.

Nwabinelli J, Monaghan J (1991) Vaginal epithelial abnormalities in patients with CIN: clinical and pathological features and management. *British Journal of Obstetrics and Gynaecology* **98**: 25–29.

Paladini D, Cross P, Lopes T, Monaghan J (1994) Prognostic significance of lymph node variables in squamous cell carcinoma of the vulva. *Cancer* **74**: 2491–2496.

Phipps J, Monaghan JM (1993) Laparoscopic hysterectomy and cancer. *Surgical Oncology* **2 (Suppl.1)**: **1**: 67–72.

Pomel C, Provencher D, Dauplat J *et al.* (1995) Laparoscopic staging of early ovarian cancer. *Gynecologic Oncology* **58**: 301–306.

Querleu D (1991) Hysterectomies enlargies de Schauta–Amreich et Schauta–Stoekel assistees par coelioscopie. *Journal de Gynécologie, Obstétrique et Biologie de la Reproduction* **20**: 747–748.

Querleu D, LeBlanc E (1995) Laparoscopic infrarenal paraaortic lymph node dissection for restaging of carcinoma of the ovary and Fallopian tube. *Cancer* **73**: 1467–1471.

Schuessler WW, Vancaillie TG, Reich H, Griffith DP (1991) Transperitoneal endosurgical lymphadectomy in patients with localised prostate cancer. *Journal of Urology* **145**: 988–991.

Shingleton HM, Orr JW (1995) *Cancer of the Cervix.* p. 72. Philadelphia: Lippincott Co.

Spirtos NM, Schlaerth JB, Spirtos TW, Schlaerth AC, Indman PD, Kimball RE (1995) Laparoscopic bilateral pelvic and paraaortic lymph node sampling: An evolving technique. *American Journal of Obstetrics and Gynecology* **173**: 105–111.

Twiggs LB, Carter JR, Fowler JM *et al.* (1996) An estimation of resource utilization with the introduction of laparoscopic pelvic lymphadenectomy prior to radical hysterectomy in early cervical carcinoma: a progress report from the Laparoscopic Study Group at the Women's Cancer Center at the University of Minnesota Health Science Center. *International Journal of Gynecologic Cancer* **6**: 267–272.

47

Laparoscopic Management of Ovarian Malignancy and the Suspicious Adnexal Mass

LISELOTTE METTLER

Department of Obstetrics and Gynecology, University of Kiel, Kiel, Germany

Although initial reports on the role of laparoscopy in gynecologic malignancies center around staging procedures, laparoscopic lymphadenectomy (both pelvic and para-aortic) appears to be both feasible and adequate. Already laparoscopy plays an important role in a revival of radical vaginal hysterectomy for patients with early cervical cancer joined by laparoscopic lymphadenectomy. Also in early endometrial carcinomas the abdominal incision can be avoided by applying laparoscopic staging with vaginal hysterectomy or in combination with a laparoscopic lymphadenectomy according to the depth of infiltration in stage I patients. The role of laparoscopy in ovarian cancer, however, still has to be defined and we must be very cautious in using it for this group of patients.

Ovarian tumors arise in all stages of female life:

- During childhood, mostly as dysgermino-mas.
- After menarche as functional cysts.
- Around menopause as carcinomas, although carcinomas also occur during reproductive age.

The histologic picture of ovarian tumors is multifaceted, but an exact histologic classification is often difficult as ovarian tumors often grow very rapidly. So far an effective method for early diagnosis is not available.

The spectrum of therapy in ovarian cancer has changed during the last years, using more radical operations for the early stages of this disease, new chemotherapeutic strategies such as paclitaxel and even stem cell transplantation during high-dose chemotherapy; however, the general prognosis remains poor. Only women with an early ovarian cancer, stage I, which is often not discovered, have a higher percentage of survival compared to advanced stages. In order to maximize the survival potential, the surgical treatment of ovarian malignances has to be done with great care. The oncologic principles of ovarian surgery have to be closely observed during laparoscopic surgery. Unfortunately rupture of an ovarian stage Ia during cancer laparoscopy, as in laparotomy, can sometimes not be avoided. Since the beginning of the 1980s the use of laparoscopic procedures has increased worldwide and the question of tumor dissemination, especially with ovarian cancer, has became a subject for discussion.

However, for those gynecologic oncologists employing second-look procedures, it appears that an initial laparoscopy may preclude laparotomy in a majority of patients. Comparative survival data for patients with gynecologic malignancies managed by laparoscopy or laparotomy are still scarce.

In this chapter we aim to address the following points:

- Is staging laparoscopy an accepted technique?
- Is laparoscopy of any benefit as a second-look procedure?
- Is laparoscopic staging together with histologic tissue sampling the appropriate surgical technique for inoperable ovarian cancer with ascites and peritoneal carcinosis?
- Does endoscopic biopsy of ovarian cancer stage Ia change the destiny of a patient into ovarian cancer Ic?

Historical Background

Despite the recent advances in modern operative laparoscopy with many verified publications, very little has been published about the role of laparoscopy for patients with invasive ovarian carcinoma. In the late 1970s and early 1980s, laparoscopy was used for pre-treatment evaluation of patients whose initial staging laparotomy was felt to be inadequate to replace a staging laparotomy for patients with presumed stage III and IV disease. The laparoscopic recognition of diaphragmatic cancer metastases is significantly higher than at a laparotomic screening because of the magnification of at least 1:4 (Semm, 1984). In suspected cases of ovarian cancer, metastases were discovered in 62.5% of patients (10 of 16) who were originally thought to have stage I or stage II ovarian cancer (Bagley et al., 1973).

We suggested laparoscopy as a second-look procedure in ovarian cancer (Semm, 1984) together with other authors (Ozols et al., 1981; Berek et al., 1992). Although the identification of persistent disease in these early reports was lower than expected on the basis of reports with second-look laparotomies, the technique is advised if the whole abdomen is visible. If the entire abdomen is not visible one can always convert to a laparotomy. Although none of the early investigators sampled pelvic or para-aortic lymph nodes, we have always suggested routine blind biopsies and abdominal washings. The importance of washings for cytologic evaluation has been reported by several investigators (Mettler et al., 1993).

Basic Principles

In postmenopausal women an adnexectomy is the procedure of choice to minimize the possibility of rupturing an ovarian tumor. For women of reproductive age we primarily treat cystic ovarian structures by preserving the ovaries and attempt to exclude cancer preoperatively. In the early 1990s laparoscopic ovarian surgery reported an incidence of about 2–4% of ovarian cancer, which was biopsied and later treated surgically. As a result of discussions between the different laparoscopic societies and the warning finger of oncologists, this number can be diminished to 0.2–0.6%. Imaging should be strongly considered for each ovarian tumor preoperatively and laparoscopy for functional cysts must be avoided.

Preoperative Diagnosis

Before therapy an extensive clinical investigation is necessary to establish a differential diagnosis. Endometriotic cysts are differentiated from carcinomas by careful ultrasound diagnosis transvaginally, and if available, with Doppler and three-dimensional ultrasound. Special consideration has to be given to factors such as tumor size, the presence of unilocular or bilateral ovarian cysts, the existence of septa, the existence of solid particles, papillomatous structures and hematologic hints of malignancy. The result of ultrasound is put together as sonomorphology with a diagnosis that suggests benignity or malignancy.

Tumor markers, especially CA-125, have a special predictive value in premenopausal patients. False positive values are expected in cases of endometriosis and uterine fibromas.

During the postmenopausal period endometriosis and uterine fibromas often have an appearance consistent with that of malignancy.

Prerequisites for planned ovarian surgery of benign cysts are listed in Table 47.1.

Table 47.1 Prerequisites for investigation of ovarian cysts before laparoscopic surgery.

Investigation	Comment

Ultrasound
  Vaginal
  Adominal
  Doppler
  Three dimensional
	No solid echodense structures (exception dermoid cyst)

Tumor markers CA-125	Always in patients >40 years
Size of cyst	Larger than 15 cm in diameter
Hematologic parameters	
Magnetic resonance imaging (MRI), computerized tomography (CT) in some cases	

Intraoperative Diagnosis

Intraoperatively with the first view in the abdomen the situation is assessed again. The surgical procedure is converted into a laparotomy for cases of suspected malignancy. Intraoperatively a fluid sample can be taken from the pouch of Douglas for cytologic examination and peritoneal or other metastases can be looked for. Opening of cysts for diagnostic purposes is obsolete because in cases of malignancy this could provoke cell dispersion. Before manipulating an ovarian tumor the result of the cytologic examination of the fluid from the pouch of Douglas should be available if the surgeon has any suspicion of malignancy. If the surface of the ovary shows increased vascularization, lesions that cannot be assessed, papillary lesions, or possible malignancy, the procedure should be converted to a laparotomy even if the histology does not show a malignancy.

In the case of a minor suspect lesion on the surface of the ovary, a biopsy should be taken and a histologic diagnosis obtained intraoperatively. The frozen section can, however, present difficulties for the pathologist. If a clearcut diagnosis cannot be given or if the diagnosis does not fit the anatomic situation, it is better to stop the surgery and to wait for the final histology. Once the histology is clear, laparoscopic adnexectomy or a laparotomy are performed during the same operation. In cases of malignancy the extended laparotomy surgery must be performed within at least one week of the primary diagnosis if not performed at the same intervention. Any further delay carries the risk of waiting too long increasing the bad prognosis of the disease.

If there is no sign of malignancy, the ovarian tumor is tackled according to the age and life situation of the patient. During an adnexectomy, an oophorectomy, a partial oophorectomy or a cystectomy the ovarian tumors should be completely excised. Such a procedure carries an identical difficulty to that of laparotomy, and has to be considered if one wishes to preserve the organ. The ovarian tumor can be extracted using an appropriate bag, which is carried through a working channel through the abdominal layers. As bags are now available, some consider that extraction of an ovarian tumor through the trocar is no longer appropriate. After such an ovarian operation, hemostasis is obtained by coagulation, sutures or clips followed by an adequate rinsing and aspiration procedure to leave clean wound conditions.

Functional Cysts

To avoid unnecessary operations on functional cystic ovarian tumors, some doctors treat patients with an estrogen-suppressive regimen. Prerequisites are the existence of a one- or two-chamber cyst smaller than 5 cm in diameter and causing no pain. To monitor persistence vaginal ultrasound is used at intervals of no longer than four weeks. Usually we check these patients after four weeks. If the cyst increases in size, changes shape or does not diminish in size, the patient should be treated surgically according to the criteria by laparoscopy or laparotomy. An increase in size or an increase in abdominal pain calls for immediate surgical intervention.

Treatment of Ovarian Tumors at the Department of Obstetrics and Gynecology, University of Kiel 1992–1995

Between 1992 and 1995 at the Department of Obstetrics and Gynecology, University of Kiel, 165 new patients with ovarian cancer stage I to IV were treated according to appropriate criteria with operative radical laparotomy debulking and lymphadenectomy, omentectomy, and if necessary consecutive chemotherapy or radiotherapy. Endoscopic surgical procedures were performed in 1225 patients who presented with cystic ovarian tumors. The operative procedure in our hospital requires a direct laparotomy in cases of possible malignancy. In the cases presented over these four years none of the endoscopically performed biopsies and frozen sections indicated ovarian cancer. In such a case we would have performed the appropriate radical operation during the same surgical procedure after conversion to a laparotomy. We converted more cases to laparotomy than necessary in order to take a biopsy. Transabdominal extraction of the specimen was always performed in an endobag whether an adnexectomy, ovariectomy or ovarian cyst resection.

Figures 47.1–47.3 demonstrate ovarian cyst resection and adnexal bag extraction via laparoscopy (pelviscopy) in line drawings and in a series of endoscopic pictures. Oophorectomies (Figure 47.4) or adnexectomies (Figures 47.5, 47.6) were performed with the three loop ligation technique with sutures or stapling devices or after bipolar coagulation of the ovarian ligament. All these techniques facilitate adnexectomy, which was predominantly performed in postmenopausal patients.

Figure 47.7 gives details of the patients treated according to ages, the size of the ovarian cysts,

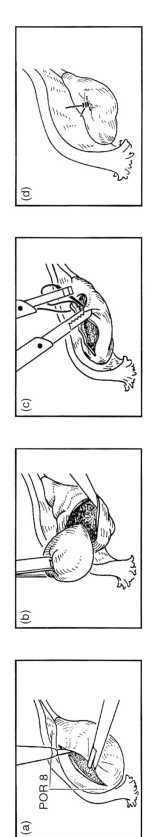

Figure 47.1 Pelviscopic enucleation of an ovarian cyst and suture of the ovarian lining. (a) Capsular incision. (b) Cyst resection. (c) Ovarian suture. (d) Final aspect after endoscopic ovarian cyst resection.

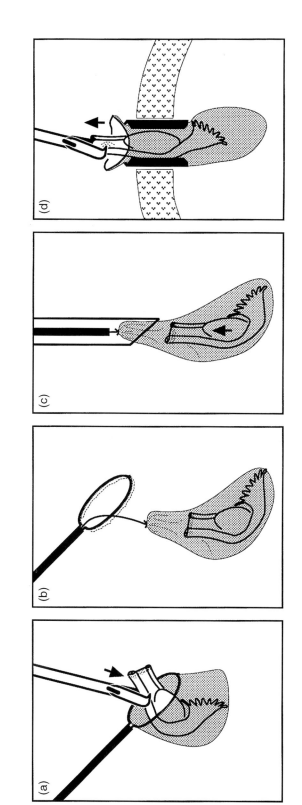

Figure 47.2 Bag extraction of endoscopically resected adnexa. (a) Positioning of adnexa into an endobag. (b) Closing the bag by pulling the string; (c) Insertion of the bag into the trocar. (d) Bag extraction.

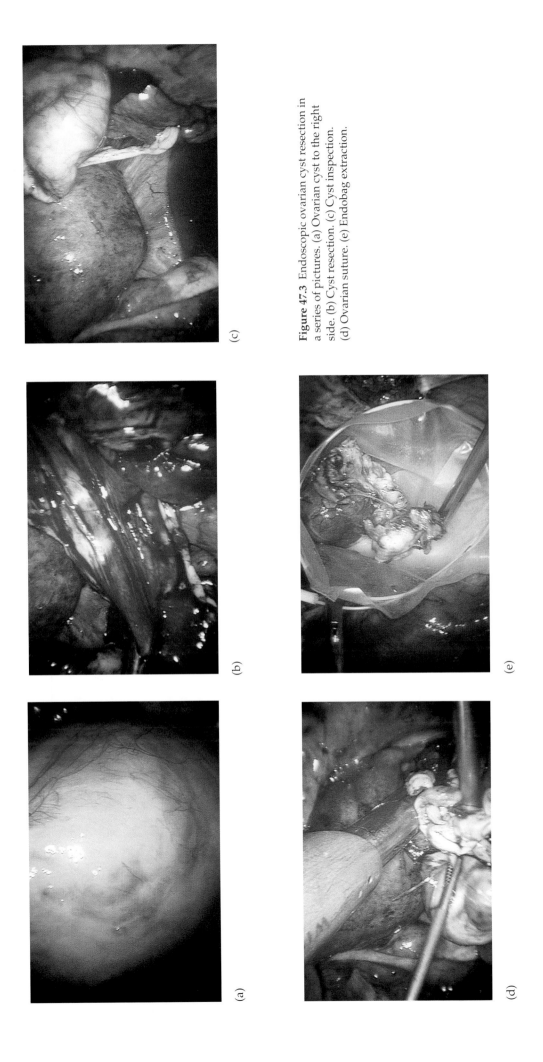

Figure 47.3 Endoscopic ovarian cyst resection in a series of pictures. (a) Ovarian cyst to the right side. (b) Cyst resection. (c) Cyst inspection. (d) Ovarian suture. (e) Endobag extraction.

(a)

(b)

(c)

(d)

(e)

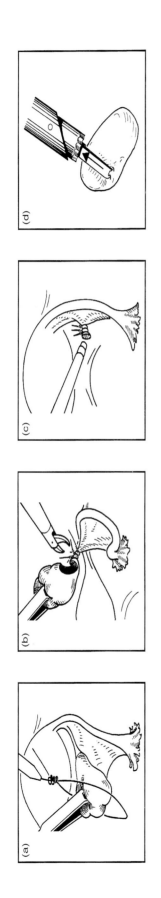

Figure 47.4 Endoscopic oophorectomy using the three loop ligation technique in four steps. (a) Positioning the first Roeder loop. (b) Ovarian resection after placement of three loops. (c) Endocoagulation of the ovarian stump. (d) Ovarian morcellation using 15 mm or 20 mm trocars.

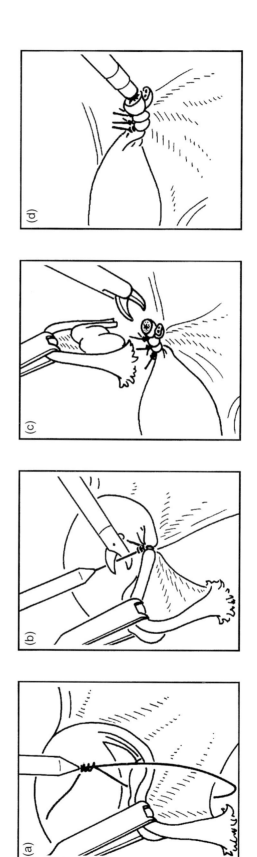

Figure 47.5 Endoscopic adnexectomy using the three loop ligation technique in four steps. (a) Placement of the first loop. (b) Cutting the loop. (c) Adnexal resection after positioning of three loops. (d) Endocoagulation of the stump.

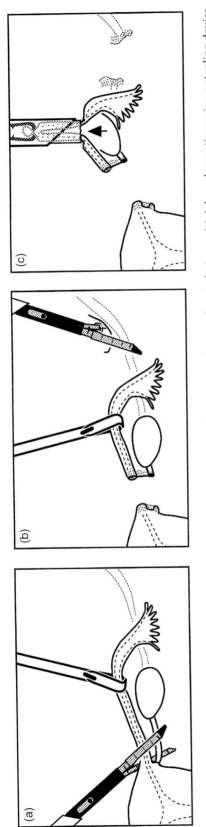

Figure 47.6 Endoscopic adnexectomy using the three loop ligation technique in three steps using stapling techniques. (a) Adnexal resection using a stapling device at the ovarian ligament. (b) Dissection of the infundibulopelvic ligament. (c) Adnexal resection.

Figure 47.7 Statistical evaluation of 1225 patients treated by endoscopic ovarian surgery according to their ages, size of ovarian cyst, color of cyst fluid and uni- or bilateral localization.

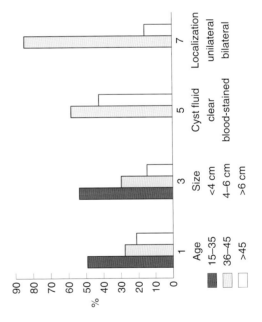

whether the cysts were septated or contained clear or bloodstained fluid, and whether the cysts were unilateral or bilateral. Histologic results revealed the broad spectrum of diagnosis, including the functional cysts referred to us as persistent ovarian cysts. Carcinomas were detected in 2.4% (Figure 47.8). Figure 47.9 specifies the patients in 1992, 1993, 1994 and 1995 for whom we converted the operation into a laparotomy. However, of these patients only two in 1992, five in 1993, two in 1994 and four

in 1995 had a malignancy. Figure 47.10 details outcome of those patients considered to have 'suspect' lesions at the first-look staging laparoscopy. Figure 47.11 gives the histologic results of the 13 patients who did have malignancies after conversion to laparotomy. These cancers were not recognized preoperatively, but during surgery and were managed by conversion to laparotomy. In one case we biopsied the ovary laparoscopically after receiving a diagnosis of borderline ovarian lesion and later

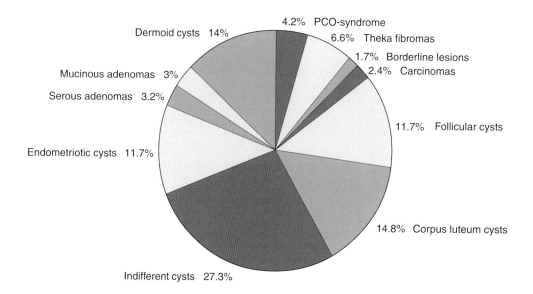

Figure 47.8 Pathologic distribution pattern of 1225 ovarian cysts treated endoscopically. (PCO-syndrome, polycystic ovary syndrome).

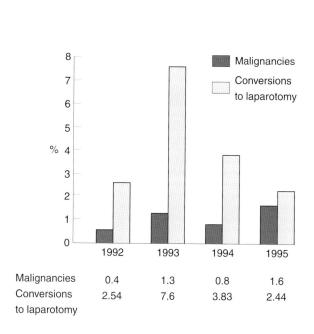

Figure 47.9 Conversion rate of pelviscopy to laparotomy 1992–1995 at ovarian endoscopic surgery.

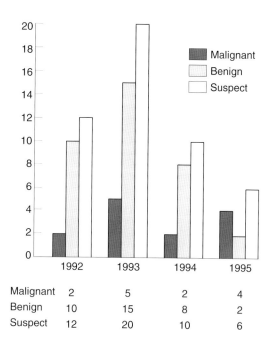

Figure 47.10 Diagnosis of possibly malignant (suspect) lesions at pelviscopic screening for ovarian surgery.

Specification of ovarian malignancies 1992–1995			
1992	**1993**	**1994**	**1995**
1 adenocarcinoma	3 adenocarcinomas	1 adenocarcinoma	4 adenocarcinomas
1 granulosa cell tumor with sarcoma	1 Krukenberg tumor	1 Krukenberg tumor	
	1 metastasis of non-Hodgkin lymphoma		

Figure 47.11 Specification of ovarian malignancies screened endoscopically but treated surgically by laparotomy.

the histopathologic evaluation of the paraffin section revealed a non-Hodgkin's lymphoma.

Rarely a biopsy performed laparoscopically will reveal malignancy and it can be interesting to reflect on the diagnosis and the appropriate therapy. Laparotomy and genital extraction in a patient with a metastasis of a non-Hodgkin's lymphoma in whom the diagnosis was not made at frozen section, but two days later, would not have been appropriate. Following the diagnosis, we performed a laparotomy and treated the patient appropriately for non-Hodgkin's lymphoma.

The standards of oncologic surgery must be observed when treating patients endoscopically. The tumors should be taken out in as many cases as possible without rupturing the capsule and without contamination. Considering these regulations, staging endoscopic surgery with the possibility of converting to laparotomy for the few cases found to be ovarian cancer does not present a higher risk for the patient than primary laparotomy. Any consecutive radical operation has to be done immediately or within the first week of diagnosis of all malignant adnexal tumors, ovarian cancer, tubal cancers, dsygerminomas, malignant teratomas and borderline cancers of the ovary. According to oncologic criteria an endoscopic biopsy of malignant adnexal tumors has to be avoided. In patients with non-suspect lesions preoperatively a laparoscopic biopsy may sometimes be indicated. The consecutive operation has to follow within the time limit of one week maximum. The question arises whether in a 25-year-old patient undergoing infertility treatment one should biopsy a pea-sized abnormal looking lesion on the ovary or take out the whole ovary at a laparotomy. However, in such a young patient one would hesitate to do more than a biopsy at the primary intervention even at a laparotomy. For these cases we would like to propose the following points for discussion:

- For every suspected non-benign lesion of the ovary, a fluid sample from the pouch of Douglas should be investigated before and after laparoscopy.
- An unexpected sudden malignant suspicious tissue appearance in an ovarian cyst is an indication for a frozen section.
- If there are unexpected malignant lesions the patient should be treated surgically by laparotomy with resection of the ovaries, adnexa, uterus, lymph nodes and omentum during the same intervention or within five days.
- Every patient with an ovarian cyst should be informed before the operation that the discovery of malignant change may result in a laparotomy with hysterectomy, bilateral adnexectomy and omental resection and possibly lymphadenectomy.
- If there are unexpected suspect lesions and the patient has given informed consent, a diagnostic biopsy is performed and a laparotomy within five days.
- Endoscopic organ extraction of an adnexal tumor should be performed with an endobag.

If in spite of the described precautions an ovarian cancer is biopsied, it has to be treated surgically as quickly as possible and be followed by immediate chemotherapy. This has to be done within one week of the first procedure.

The Role of Laparascopy in Stage I Ovarian Carcinoma

The role of laparascopy in stage I ovarian carcinoma has been addressed by different authors. Some surgeons have incorporated routine washings and blind biopsies in their staging procedures. The magnifying capability of videolaparoscopy and the ability to perform pelvic and para-aortic lymphadenectomy potentially make laparoscopic staging a useful technique. At present there are only a few case reports available describing laparoscopic staging of estimated stage I invasive carcinoma of the ovary.

Reich *et al.* (1990) were the first with their report of a 56-year-old woman with a 5 cm left ovarian neoplasm. After removing the adnexa through a colpotomy incision and confirming malignancy by a frozen section, they performed a laparoscopic assisted vaginal hysterectomy and right salpingo-oophorectomy along with a trans-vaginal infracolic omentectomy, a left pelvic lymphadenectomy and biopsy of the left pelvic sidewall. The histologic examination showed that both ovaries contained grade II serous papillary adenocarcinoma, but the eleven pelvic nodes and pelvic sidewall biopsies were all negative for malignancy. This group has been criticized for puncturing a malignant cyst, not obtaining intraperitoneal washings for cytology or multiple blind biopsies, especially of the right hemi-diaphragm, and not sampling para-aortic lymph nodes. However, they should also be congratulated for their innovation in using this technique in a patient who refused laparotomy.

In 1992 Nezhat *et al.* reported on four ovarian cancers diagnosed during laparoscopic management of 1011 women with adnexal masses. In this group they described a 6 cm right ovarian cyst that was opened and biopsied for papillary growth and revealed necrotic tissue with atypical glands. They performed a right salpingo-oophorectomy, appendectomy and peritoneal and omental biopsies laparoscopically.

Querleu (1993) described what is today considered an adequate laparoscopic surgical staging procedure for ovarian carcinoma for a 39-year-old woman with a serous tumor of low malignant potential. He successfully staged this patient laparoscopically by oncologic standards and performed washings, multiple biopsies, omentectomy and a pelvic and paraaortic lymphadenectomy. The 12 pelvic lymph nodes, the nine para-aortic lymph nodes and all biopsies were negative for metastatic disease.

In 1994 Querleu and LeBlanc reported on laparoscopic infrarenal para-aortic node dissection for staging of carcinoma of the ovary or fallopian tube. Four patients with presumed stage Ia ovarian cancer of low malignant potential were restaged following inadequate staging procedures. Three other patients had invasive cancer and were staged laparoscopically for presumed stage I disease. Endometrioid cancer of the ovary was found in two patients and one patient had a fallopian tube carcinoma. They described an adequate staging procedure including pelvic and para-aortic lymphadenectomy up to the renal veins removing an average of ten para-aortic lymph nodes.

Many staging laparotomies performed (e.g. at our department) do not include such a detailed field. Childers and colleagues in 1993 described para-aortic lymphadenectomies and gynecologic malignancies in 18 patients with ovarian cancer (Childers *et al.*, 1993a,b). In the majority of the patients these were second-look procedures for advanced disease, but in six patients they presumed stage I ovarian cancer. It is of great concern that laparoscopic staging of presumed stage I ovarian carcinoma misses extraovarian disease that would have been detected at laparotomy. However, as the screening capability during laparoscopy with the 4–8 times magnification in an adhesion-free abdomen is better than that at a laparotomy, this concern is unnecessary.

Laparoscopic Diagnosis and Surgery for Advanced Ovarian Cancer and Second-look Laparoscopies

We started to use videolaparoscopy 15 years ago, primarily for second-look procedures for advanced disease before or during chemotherapy. We investigated the effectiveness of laparoscopy in this combination.

Whenever possible advanced ovarian carcinoma should be treated with a primary debulking laparotomy. In cases of an ovarian cancer without tumor enlargement within the lower abdomen, laparoscopic diagnosis and histologic verification is justified. However, it must be possible to perform either a laparotomy with radical surgery including deperitonization, bowel resection, omentectomy, etc. or chemotherapy immediately after the diagnosis, especially for those cases with ascites. These interventions must be carried out in oncologic centers that have the infrastructure for radical operations and adequate medical therapy of ovarian carcinomas.

Our current experience of second-look laparoscopies has not been reported, but consists of 62 interventions performed on 48 patients with advanced ovarian carcinomas. All patients were primarily treated surgically with maximal surgical debulking and had received platinum based chemotherapy. They clinically showed no evidence of disease. Looking at tumor markers, we tested CEA and CA-125. Of CA-125, all were negative with the exception of four cases. If no obvious disease was noted immediately at laparoscopy, intraperitoneal washings were obtained and slices of adhesions and biopsies of many suspect and non-suspect areas were taken. Persistent disease was documented laparoscopically in 20 of our 62 procedures. We found metastatic disease with intraperitoneal metastases in seven patients. We had to convert the procedure to a laparotomy for five patients as the abdominal cavity, even after adhesiolysis, was not visible. Our results of second-look laparoscopies are therefore encouraging. We were able to avoid a laparotomy in over 90% of our patients. The positive rate was similar to that found at second-look laparoscopies and the patients had a shorter hospitalization time and less pain than with a repeat laparotomy. So far only two lymphadenectomies were performed among these patients. However, with increasing experience we will include this more often in our second-look laparoscopies. Childers in 1995 reported a series of 42 second-look laparoscopies performed in 38 patients with advanced ovarian or fallopian tube carcinoma – if there was no persistent disease by frozen section, they routinely performed multiple blind biopsies and laparoscopic lymphadenectomy. This combination of procedures at second-look laparoscopy revealed a 58% positive rate, which is similar if not higher than the reported rate for second-look laparotomy. Extrapolating these data they inferred that laparoscopic staging of presumed early ovarian carcinoma would disclose metastatic disease at a rate similar to that of laparotomy (Childers, 1995). Dargent in 1993 and Spirtos in 1993 described laparoscopic interventions in gynecologic cancer as clearcut alternatives to laparotomy.

Structural Prerequisites for Laparoscopic Operations of Ovarian Tumors

Ovarian tumors in which a malignancy has been almost excluded by preoperative diagnosis can be treated laparoscopically wherever the personal and apparative prerequisites (the surgeon's skill, and correct apparatus and instruments) for laparoscopic operations are met. However, if based on the preoperative investigations malignancy cannot be excluded and should be carried out at clinics where these prerequisites for an adequate and correct surgery for laparotomy are present.

Conclusion

Semm's (1984) indications for advanced laparoscopic surgery include possible diagnosis and

therapy of ovarian cancer. First reports on the role of laparoscopy for gynecologic malignancies have centered on staging procedures and second-look laparoscopies. Laparoscopic lymphadenectomy of both pelvic and para-aortic nodes is feasible and adequate. The number of lymph nodes to be resected for cure still needs to be defined.

We must be cautious about advocating laparoscopy for ovarian cancer treatment; however, it has been shown to be a useful staging procedure. Careful preoperative screening of the patient and precise definition of the cysts with imaging techniques allows us to frequently use laparoscopic surgery for ovarian cysts, leaving detectable cancer cases for laparotomy. Gynecologic oncologists employing staging and second-look procedures for ovarian cancer have to admit that an initial laparoscopy may preclude laparotomy for many patients. Survival data for patients with gynecologic malignancies managed by laparoscopy instead of laparotomy are of course lacking and this is the predominant question. In no way must survival be compromised by using a new surgical technique. According to the reports of Sevelda et al. (1990) and Dembo et al. (1990) the degree of differentiation and the existence of ascites are more relevant to decreasing the five-year survival rate after ovarian cancer stage I than rupture of capsule or penetration of the tumor. A dependency on these parameters was found by Dembo et al. (1990) and Sevelda et al. (1990).

As the question of endoscopic treatment of an adnexal mass is predominantly posed for the treatment of small ovarian tumors (ovarian tumors with solid particles in the cysts can be categorized as primary laparotomies) there remains a wide field of tissue alterations for laparoscopic treatment of adnexal masses and ovarian cysts with benign indications. For many young patients with non-malignant ovarian lesions such as endometriosis, benign

Table 47.2 Possible factors to assess during pelviscopy/ upper abdominal laparoscopy

Ovarian surface texture
Vascularization of tumor
Papillomatous or suspicious structures
Adhesions
Ascites
Cytology of rinsing fluid
Tumor sites of the peritoneum, intestine, liver, diaphragm
Size of primary tumor
Mobility of tumor
Amount of adhesions to intestines
Mobility of intestines
Indication for laparotomy with the possibility of 90% tumor reduction
Biopsy of primary tumor, peritoneum, omentum, intestines, liver, diaphragm

cysts, benign cystic proliferations and fibromas, a laparotomy can be avoided and the patient can be treated by laparoscopy. The laparoscopic therapeutic management of ovarian malignancy and suspicious adnexal masses cannot at present be recommended and has to be investigated with many careful studies before it can be debated. Factors to assess at pelviscopy, including upper abdominal laparoscopy, need to be included in any discussion (Table 47.2) on the laparoscopic treatment of ovarian cysts.

References

Bagley CM, Young RC, Schein PS, Chabner BA, DeVita VT (1973) Ovarian cancer metastatic to diaphragm frequently underdiagnosed at laparotomy, a preliminary report. *American Journal of Obstetrics and Gynecology* **116**: 397–400.

Berek JS, Griffiths CT, Levanthal JM (1992) Laparoscopy for second-look evaluation in ovarian carcinoma. *Obstetrics and Gynecology* **58**: 192–198.

Childers JM (1995) Operative laparoscopy in gynecologic oncology. In Cusumano PG, Deprest JA (eds) *Advanced Gynecologic Laparoscopy*. pp. 201–217. Brussels: Excerpta Medica.

Childers JM, Surwit EA, Hatch KD (1992) The role of laparoscopy in the management of cervical carcinoma. *Gynecologic Oncology* **47**: 38–43.

Childers JM, Brzechffa PR, Hatch KD, Surwit EA (1993a) Laparoscopicaly assisted surgical staging (L.A.S.S.) of endometrial cancer. *Gynecologic Oncology* **51**: 33–38.

Childers JM, Hatch KD, Tran AN, Surwit EA (1993b) Laparoscopic para-aortic lymphadenectomy in gynecologic malignancies. *Obstetrics and Gynecology* **82**: 741–747.

Dargent D (1993) Laparoscopic surgery in gynecologic cancer. *Current Opinion in Obstetrics and Gynecology* **5**: 294–300.

Dembo AJ, Davy M, Stenwig AE, Berle EJ, Bush RS, Kjorstad K (1990) Prognostic factors in patients with stage I epithelial ovarian cancer. *Obstetrics and Gynecology* **75**: 2.

Mettler L, Caesar G, Neunzling S, Semm K (1993) Stellenwert der endoskopischen Ovar-Chirurgie – kritische Analyse von 626 pelviskopisch operierten Ovarialzysten an der Universitätsfrauenklinik Kiel 1990–1991. *Geburtshilfe und Frauenheilkunde* **53**: 253–257.

Nezhat F, Nezhat C, Welander CE, Benigno B (1992) Four ovarian cancers diagnosed during laparoscopic management of 1011 women with adnexal masses. *American Journal of Obstetrics and Gynecology* **167**: 790–796.

Ozols RF, Fisher RI, Anderson T (1981) Peritoneoscopy in the management of ovarian carcinoma. *American Journal of Obstetrics and Gynecology* **140**: 611–623.

Querleu D (1993) Laparoscopic para-aortic lymph node sampling in gynecologic oncology: a preliminary experience. *Gynecologic Oncology* **49**: 24–29.

Querleu D, LeBlanc E (1994) Laparoscopic infrarenal para-aortic node dissection for restaging of carcinoma of the ovary or fallopian tube. *Cancer* **73**: 1467–1471.

Reich H, McGlynn F, Wilkie W (1990) Laparoscopic management of stage I ovarian carcinoma. A case report. *Journal of Reproductive Medicine* **35**: 601–604.

Semm K (1984) *Operative Manual for Endoscopic Abdominal Surgery*. pp. 339–340. Chicago: Yearbook Medical Publishers.

Sevelda P, Varra N, Schemper M, Salzer H (1990) Prognostic factors for survival in stage I epithelial ovarian carcinoma. *Cancer* **65**: 10.

Spirtos NM (1993) Laparoscopic radical hysterectomy with para-aortic and pelvic lymph node dissection. *American Journal of Obstetrics and Gynecology* **168**: 1643 (Letter).

Major Complications of Laparoscopic Surgery – Avoidance and Management

48

Bowel Complications of Laparoscopic Surgery

ANDREW POOLEY* AND R. SODERSTROM†

*Mayday Hospital, Thornton Heath, Surrey, UK
†1101 Madison Suite 580, Washington, USA

Bowel trauma is probably the most serious complication in gynecologic laparoscopic surgery, when the incidence is combined with the likelihood of severe or even fatal consequences. Laceration of a major blood vessel is more immediately life-threatening, but is more rare. In contrast, injury to the bowel frequently goes unnoticed during the procedure, leading to a delayed and insidious presentation with the infectious sequelae of perforation.

The true incidence of injury to the bowel is difficult to calculate and depends upon factors such as the expertise of the operators whose practice is being assessed and the complexity of the procedures attempted. In a survey published by the Royal College Of Obstetricians and Gynaecologists (RCOG) in 1978 (Chamberlain and Brown, 1978), the rate of bowel trauma during laparoscopic procedures was 1.8 per 1000 cases, with injury to the bowel mesentery in 1.1 per 1000 cases. In this survey of more than 50 000 cases there was one death, which was due to complications of bowel damage. The American Association of Gynecologic Laparoscopists (AAGL) have conducted two postal surveys of their members asking for details of complications of laparoscopic surgery in 1988 and 1991 (Peterson et al., 1990; Hulka et al., 1993). The rate of injury to the alimentary and urinary tracts combined was 2.8 per 1000 cases in the 1991 survey, which represented a 1.7-fold increase on the rate found in 1988. The RCOG and AAGL surveys were voluntary response postal questionnaires, with a low response rate (17% for the AAGL surveys), making it unlikely that the figures obtained represent the true incidences.

The most comprehensive review of complications of gynecologic laparoscopy is that published by Querleu et al. in 1993. This survey, which was retrospective for 1989–1990 and prospective for 1990–1991 documented any complications encountered during all laparoscopic surgical procedures performed in seven of the most active centers in France. A total of 17 521 cases were performed during the study period, with 27 cases of bowel trauma, a rate of 1.54 per 1000. The bowel trauma was sustained during adhesiolysis procedures in 20 (74%) of the 27 cases. The procedures performed were divided into four categories: diagnostic, minor, major and advanced, with unintended laparotomy rates for any cause being 1.1 per 1000 for diagnostic and minor procedures, 4.8 per 1000 for major cases, and 8.9 per 1000 for advanced cases. It must be remembered that this represents the practice of some of the world's most experienced gynecologic laparoscopic surgeons performing many of the most advanced procedures being undertaken at that time.

In a review of laparoscopic bowel trauma it is helpful to be systematic and discuss the various areas where problems might be encountered. Factors that ultimately lead to bowel injury can be identified at all stages in the operative process, including.

- Selection of the patient and the procedure.
- Preoperative preparation and anesthesia.
- Gaining entry to the abdomen.
- The operative procedure itself.
- Leaving the abdomen.

Inadequate postoperative surveillance and inappropriate subsequent management of bowel trauma contribute enormously to the impact of the complications encountered.

General and Preoperative Factors

There is no place in modern practice for an inexperienced surgeon to attempt any form of surgery in which he or she has not received appropriate training. Gone are the days when one could 'have a go' at something one has only read about, seen a videotape of, or witnessed once on a training course. Training and credentialling for endoscopic surgeons is currently the focus of attention of the governing bodies in many of the countries where this form of surgery is widely practiced. In the UK this has led to the inception of a nationally organized system of training centers in a joint venture between the Colleges of Gynaecology and Surgery. The amount and type of training needed to achieve various levels of competence has yet to be clarified and are the subject of many papers in the literature. Complications are likely when surgery is performed without the required skills and experience.

A second vital prerequisite for safe surgery is the selection of an appropriate procedure for the patient's condition and state of health. Situations such as obesity, scarring from previous surgery, sepsis in the abdominal wall or peritoneal cavity, and ileus do not necessarily constitute absolute contraindications to laparoscopy, but are likely to involve an increased risk of complications.

Opinions vary about the degree of patient preparation needed for various procedures. Some authors advocate the use of full bowel preparation with large volumes of iso-osmotic fluids such as polyethylene glycol, while others are content with a low residue diet and enemas or no preparation. One should remember that should a prepared bowel receive an injury that goes unnoticed, the normal flora will return within 24 hours. Thus, the value of a prepared bowel is in high-risk patients when the injury is discovered during the laparoscopic operation. The restricted space within which one has to operate at laparoscopy can be maximized by ensuring that the small and large bowel are relatively empty. Overdistension of the stomach will place it in a central position within the abdomen rendering it vulnerable to damage on gaining entry. Similarly, distension of the stomach pushes the transverse colon attached to its inferior border into a more caudad position beneath or even inferior to the umbilicus in the prone position. This can be avoided by preventing forced entry of gases during anesthetic induction and the passage of a nasogastric tube.

One cannot overemphasize the need to see what one is doing during any endoscopic procedure. If a problem that cannot be corrected is encountered with visual quality, consideration should be given to abandoning the procedure. Although not wishing to disappoint the patient, operating with a poor view invites a high risk of doing harm.

Specific safety aspects of some of the pieces of equipment used in laparoscopic surgery will be discussed below. Although it is apparently self-evident that one should not use equipment with which one is not familiar, devices such as diathermy are still used with no knowledge other than the one setting that has been used before.

Many of the more complex procedures can only be accomplished with the help of experienced and well-trained assistants. One must make allowance for the extra time needed to complete a procedure while having to instruct an inexperienced assistant. In any case one must allow sufficient time to perform each procedure without the need to rush. Operating at a faster than comfortable speed to finish the case or list on time at best invites the risk of incomplete treatment and at worst increases the risk that a complication may occur and possibly go unnoticed.

Entry to the Abdomen

There is probably more disagreement about the safest way to begin laparoscopy than any other single aspect. The promoters of the various techniques are firmly entrenched in their various camps, and there is little good research upon which to base a more scientific opinion. When one includes general surgical experience, injuries have been described to all regions of the alimentary tract and its mesenteries including the stomach, liver, spleen, small bowel, large bowel and omentum. In the study by Querleu et al. (1993) the need for a laparotomy to deal with any complication during diagnostic and minor procedures was 1.1 per 1000. It is reasonable to assume that most or all of these complications arose on gaining entry to the abdomen and that this figure approximates the incidence of complications that occur when establishing the laparoscopic approach.

The greatest dispute centers around whether to insufflate the peritoneal cavity before insertion of the primary trocar. The majority of gynecologists in the UK use a Veress needle to insufflate a variable amount of carbon dioxide (CO_2) in the belief that injury with the primary trocar will be less likely. Veress needle injury is not uncommon, and probably goes unnoticed in the majority of cases. When used, the needle should be checked for patency and to ensure that the springloaded obturator is working and of the correct length to guard the sharp tip. The various techniques for insertion of the Veress needle and confirmation of its position are described in Chapter 5, none of which have been shown to be reliable in all circumstances. It is logical to insufflate to a certain pressure rather than to a specific volume. The abdomen of a slim nulliparous women of short stature will distend to considerable pressure with 3 liters of CO_2, whereas such a volume in the abdomen of a tall overweight multiparous women will hardly lift the abdominal wall above the viscera beneath. The insufflation pressure should be sufficient to produce a firm 'bubble' to pierce with the primary trocar. For a trocar of given sharpness, the greater the tension of the abdominal wall, the less it will be indented by the tip before entry is gained (Figure 48.1).

The alternative approach is to insert the primary trocar directly without previous insufflation. This may be done after merely incising the skin and elevating the abdominal wall (Phipps, 1995) or with some dissection, even to the point of breaching the peritoneal cavity and the use of a purse-string suture to maintain a pneumoperitoneum. In general surgery the use of a blunt primary trocar as described by Hasson (1974) is widely practiced. This technique is not a guarantee of avoiding bowel injury (Soderstrom, 1993). There is one randomized trial in the literature comparing direct insertion of the primary trocar with insertion after Veress needle insufflation (Nezhat *et al.*, 1991). No major complications occurred, but minor complications of omental trauma and emphysema were more common in the insufflation group. In each group 20% required a second attempt at insertion of the instrument, and failure of insertion, with the need to switch to the alternative method was more common in the direct trocar insertion group.

In patients suspected of having subumbilical bowel adhesions, which might lead to injury even with the 'open' technique of Hasson, Soderstrom insufflates with the Veress needle placed in the left upper quadrant and after insufflation is accomplished, a 5 mm trocar and sleeve is inserted, again in the left upper quadrant. Through this trocar

sleeve, a cystoscope or hysteroscope lens is inserted to view the subumbilical area before placing the laparoscope trocar under direct vision.

Dispute also arises about the merits of disposable primary trocars with and without safety shields. It has been shown that the force needed to insert a new sharp disposable trocar is half that needed to insert a reusable trocar (Corson *et al.*, 1989). Complications are also more common if dull reusable trocars are used requiring greater force and multiple attempts at insertion (Baadsgaard *et al.*, 1989). Trocars with a so-called safety shield are no guarantee of avoiding bowel trauma (Soderstrom, 1993), and may even lead to a false sense of security. In September, 1996 the United States' Food and Drug Administration (FDA) gave notice to all trocar manufacturers that they were to remove the phrase 'safety shield' from their promotional materials and replace the phrase with 'shielded trocar'. One study in general surgical laparoscopy concluded that using an open approach was safer, quicker and cheaper than using disposable entry ports (Ballem and Rudomanski, 1993).

Special care is needed if it is suspected that adhesions are present beneath the umbilicus. Insufflation and insertion of a 5 mm trocar and endoscope at an alternative site will allow direct inspection of the underside of the abdominal wall. The main trocar can then be inserted under direct vision after division of adhesions if necessary. A technique has been described using percutaneous ultrasonography to identify adhesions of bowel to the abdominal wall based on the demonstration that the position of adherent viscera will not alter during deep inspiration (Marin *et al.*, 1987). The Visiport device (Autosuture, Ascot, UK) allows the presence of a laparoscope within the shaft of the perforating trocar, allowing direct observation of the path of entry. If bowel is morbidly adherent to the abdominal wall this device is unlikely to prevent injury, but it may improve detection of any damage caused.

Bowel trauma with the Veress needle or primary trocar often goes unnoticed at the time and during the rest of the procedure. Only the depressing site of the bowel lumen will immediately identify such a problem. Hints that injury may have occurred include fecal contamination on the tip of an instrument or in the abdomen, an intestinal odor at any time, and gradual distension of the bowel due to gas entering through the perforation.

Although it is reasonable to manage a case of bowel trauma with the Veress needle conservatively provided the defect is small and there is no contamination, larger punctures or lacerations caused by a trocar or instrument require primary

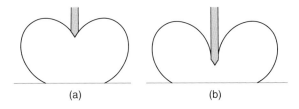

(a)   (b)

Figure 48.1 With a trocar of given sharpness a firmly distended abdominal wall (a) will be less indented before it gives way than a less well distended one (b), reducing the chance of injury to viscera with the trocar tip.

closure or resection. Some experienced operators are prepared to repair damage to the large bowel laparoscopically (Reich *et al.*, 1991), but most would advocate laparotomy. If a visceral injury is suspected, the offending instrument should be left in place to mark the site and also to prevent contamination with bowel contents. It is worth identifying a general surgical colleague who embraces the concepts of minimal access surgery to call upon in such circumstances. With small bowel injuries discovered during laparoscopy, a small or 'mini'-laparotomy may be sufficient to accomplish a direct repair followed by repeated liberal abdominal irrigation. The distress and anguish suffered by the patient on realizing that a laparotomy has been performed will be minimized if a large traditional incision and colostomy have been safely avoided.

Figure 48.2 shows the repair of a small hole in the terminal ileum sustained on insertion of the primary trocar. The enterotomy was recognized immediately on insertion of the laparoscope. The primary trocar was left *in situ*, and the affected portion of the bowel was exteriorized through a small enlargement of the umbilical incision, repaired and replaced.

If damage is suspected, it is important to examine the bowel thoroughly. One can cause through and through injuries, and damage multiple loops of bowel with concomitant vascular injury. It is essential to inspect the entire bowel in the affected region, its mesentery and the retroperitoneum in the vicinity.

In general terms repair of bowel trauma should only be performed by those with experience in bowel surgery who continue to perform such work. Should subsequent complications arise, as is often the case, or the bowel repair break down, the surgical credentials of the surgeon effecting the repair may be examined.

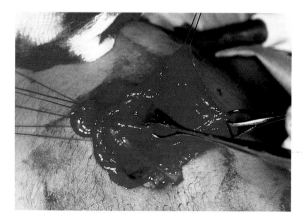

Figure 48.2 Repair of a small hole in the terminal ileum.

Secondary Portals

Having gained entry to the abdomen, it should be possible to insert all subsequent ports under direct vision. Adhesions tethering a portion of bowel to the underside of the abdominal wall can be readily identified, and an appropriate site free of adhesions can be selected for ancillary ports. Ensuring an adequate pressure of pneumoperitoneum should help avoid the bowel residing beneath the common sites for secondary ports. In modern practice visceral trauma sustained during secondary port placement is avoidable and consequently difficult to defend.

Energy Sources

Operator error accounts for more cases of bowel injury associated with the use of energy sources than equipment failure. In the recent past if a case of bowel injury was sustained during a laparoscopy in which electrosurgery was employed, the automatic assumption was made that the electrical energy was the cause of the damage. If legal action was started the use of electrosurgery would often be the main thrust of the plaintiff's case. In a survey of 66 cases of bowel trauma during gynecologic laparoscopy seven cases had already been settled on the basis of an electrical bowel injury, with this being the leading claim in all but one of the remainder (Soderstrom, 1993). The same author had previously published a description of the specific histologic appearances of various forms of injury on the intestine of rabbits (Levy and Soderstrom 1985). In electrical injuries there is an absence of the neovascularization seen in cases of trauma. Also, because of the coagulation necrosis and coaptation of the surrounding vascular bed, in electrosurgical injury there is a paucity of white cell infiltration; the opposite is found in traumatic injuries to the bowel.

With this knowledge the 66 cases in the later report were re-evaluated. On histologic slide review it was found that none of the three settled cases had in fact been cases of electrical injury, and only six of the remaining 59 were confirmed as such. Of the six confirmed cases, two were due to defective equipment, three were caused by operator error and one occurred as a 'calculated risk' during bowel adhesiolysis. Since that publication, Soderstrom has reviewed an additional 62 cases of delayed bowel injuries and only one was found to be caused by electrical desiccation.

Several excellent reviews have been published on the subject of laparoscopic electrosurgery with guidelines for safe practice and avoiding complications (Vancaillie, 1994; AAGL 1995).

In contrast to electrosurgery, the use of lasers during laparoscopy has a deserved reputation for a low incidence of visceral trauma (Ewen and Sutton, 1995). All operating theaters have one or more electrosurgical generators and junior surgeons quickly become familiar with their use at open surgery. This has in the past led to an overfamiliarity and failure to comprehend the added dangers of use at laparoscopy. In contrast, few centers have made much use of lasers, which tend to be treated with a greater respect. In the UK the use of lasers is tightly controlled, with a laser safety officer in each hospital, and rigid guidelines for their use and the credentialling of users.

One must be familiar with the properties of any energy source used. It has been demonstrated that tissue damage can be caused up to.

- 5 cm beyond the point of contact using monopolar electrosurgery (Wheeless, 1977),
- 5 mm for bipolar electrosurgery (Ryder and Hulka, 1993).
- 5 mm for endocoagulation (Semm and Friedrich, 1987).
- 2.7 mm for the CO_2 laser (Martin, 1991).

Laser energy and electrical energy can cause similar forms of injury to the bowel. The extent of damage extends beyond the confines of the visible serosal injury and the extent of the damage is related to the energy form used. Successful surgery on the bowel is closely related to the vascularity of the affected segment. With monopolar electrosurgery, the current will preferentially flow down vascular channels, leading to devascularization to a wider extent than the visible serosal injury. A non-contact laser injury causing a blanched area to appear on the bowel wall will be characterized by vascular damage to all of the blanched area. This means that local or excisional repair should involve wide margins of safety. In the review by Soderstrom (1993), two of the six electrical bowel burns were repaired immediately by minimal resection and oversewing, both of which broke down and needed further repair. It has been proposed that a similar thermal injury might be caused by leaving the laparoscope inside the abdomen during prolonged periods of loss of pneumoperitoneum: tissue lying against the tip of the laparoscope could become heated even with the use of modern 'cold' light sources. To date, there are no confirmed cases of bowel damage due to this cause.

Specific Procedures

Three operative procedures warrant special mention with respect to bowel trauma, namely:

- Adhesiolysis.
- Treatment for severe endometriosis.
- Posterior colpotomy.

The laparoscopic management of severe intestinal adhesions has been described as the 'Achilles heel' of minimal access gynecologic surgery (Garry, 1994), and should only be practiced within the confines of units with advanced experience and expertise. Even with great experience complications will be relatively frequent in such cases. In Querleu's report on complications in the seven most active units in this field in France (1993), 20 of the 27 cases of bowel trauma occurred during adhesiolysis. Added to this is the continuing doubt regarding the clinical significance of adhesions incidentally found at laparoscopy, and the possibility that divided adhesions may reform. One should have a clear outcome in mind when attempting such difficult surgery.

Advanced endometriosis with complete obliteration of the cul-de-sac is characterized by the morbid adherence of the small and large bowel, and the absence of identifiable tissue planes. It is not difficult to cause partial or full thickness damage to the bowel wall without being aware of one's proximity to the bowel lumen. If an injury to the sigmoid colon or upper rectum is suspected, the integrity of the bowel wall should be tested. This can be achieved quite simply by placing a Foley catheter with a 30 ml balloon in the lower rectum and infusing an antiseptic solution such as povidone–iodine above the balloon, while observing the bowel closely from above. Small tears and partial thickness damage are probably amenable to laparoscopic suture repair, but larger holes and cases of fecal contamination may be better dealt with by a bowel surgeon at laparotomy.

Tissue retrieval is often a tiresome part of a major laparoscopic operation. The desire to avoid extending one of the abdominal incisions has made posterior colpotomy a frequently used alternative. This is often performed using cutting monopolar diathermy with a wet swab in the posterior vaginal fornix. The danger comes when the pouch of Douglas is not deep in the anteroposterior diameter, with the anterior rectum in a more anterior position than suspected. Failure to direct the incision towards the back of the cervix increases the chance of damaging the rectum. The flexibility of long laparoscopic instruments can cause a whiplash effect with the monopolar electrode 'flicking' out of the end of the colpotomy incision and coming close to pelvic sidewall structures.

Leaving the Abdomen

Complications resulting from exiting the abdomen and closure of the incisions have received much attention in the literature in recent years. Numerous techniques and devices have been described to avoid the development of incisional hernias. The earliest reported case was described by Fear in 1968, when small bowel was seen to herniate through the umbilical incision on removal of the laparoscope. This group of complications has been under-reported in the past, with no cases recorded in the 1991 AAGL postal survey of 56 000 laparoscopic procedures (Hulka *et al.*, 1993). The increased incidence in recent years is due to a number of factors including:

- The increased use of larger portals.
- Longer procedures with greater manipulation and stretching of fascial defects.
- The use of anchoring fascial screws, which enlarge the size of the defect.
- Stretching of the incision when removing large surgical specimens.

Other implicated factors include pre-existing umbilical hernias, poor abdominal relaxation on removing the ports, and excessive coughing during reversal of anesthesia.

The chance that a hernia can occur is related to the size of the ports used. The incidence of herniation at extraumbilical sites has been calculated as 0.23% for 10 mm ports and 3.1% for 12 mm ports (Kadar *et al.*, 1993).

Attempts to close the fascial defect appear to reduce the chance of subsequent herniation, but do not eradicate it. In a report detailing 19 cases of incisional herniation, primary closure of the defect had been attempted in nine of the cases (Boike *et al.*, 1995).

The commonest finding within the hernia is small bowel, although the finding of cecum, colon and omentum has also been described (Boike *et al.*, 1995).

Frequently there is an insidious presentation with nausea, vomiting, and a swelling beneath the incision site. Classic signs of bowel obstruction may be absent if the hernia is of Richter's type, with only part of the antimesenteric circumference of the bowel wall within the hernia and incomplete occlusion of the lumen. In the absence of marked abdominal distension it is reasonable to perform a repeat laparoscopy if a hernia is suspected. In the series of

21 hernias in 19 patients described by Boike *et al.* (1995) three cases were successfully managed laparoscopically. Only two of the 19 patients had to undergo resection of the affected portion of bowel.

The incidence of such complications is reduced if all lateral ports are removed under direct vision, with closure of the fascia and peritoneum observed from below. This can be tiresome especially in an obese patient after a long demanding procedure, but patience and perseverance is recommended. No one device or closure technique is clearly superior and it is not important how it is done, provided the defect is closed securely and safely. Finally it is prudent to remove the umbilical trocar with the tip of the laparoscope slightly protruding to observe one's exit and hopefully detect any unnoticed through and through bowel injury (Figure 48.3) and to prevent bowel herniation into the umbilical site.

Postoperative Surveillance

The major compounding factor in many cases of bowel trauma at laparoscopy is the failure to appreciate the injury during the procedure. In only 60% of cases is the diagnosis made at the time of surgery, with the remaining 40% presenting over the next few days or even weeks, in varying states of ill health.

The most comprehensive review of cases of bowel trauma sustained during gynecologic laparoscopic surgery was published in 1993 (Soderstrom, 1993). This paper described the clinical findings in 66 cases that went to litigation. In six of the cases the injury was due to use of electrosurgery, two of which were diagnosed intraoperatively. In the remaining four cases the interval between the

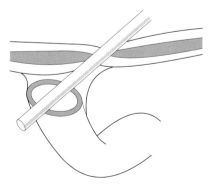

Figure 48.3 A through and through injury to a loop of bowel may be detected only by removing the laparoscope under direct vision to catch a glimpse of the bowel lumen.

original and reparative surgery was 5–15 days. Of the 60 cases of traumatic bowel injury, the range of time from surgery to onset of symptoms was 1–9 days. Among the patents, 65% were seen in their local emergency room, and 65% of this group were allowed home again. At presentation, 12 cases with a small bowel injury had a normal white blood cell count and normal temperature. All patients who had a raised white cell count and a pyrexia at presentation had a large bowel injury. Only 35% of cases X-rayed had free abdominal gas, and in 35% of cases with an intra-abdominal abscess who had an ultrasound scan, the abscess was not detected. This series included three deaths, all from septic shock, disseminated intravascular coagulation and adult respiratory distress syndrome. In each of these cases exploratory surgery was not performed for more than 72 hours after the onset of symptoms. In Soderstrom's most recent review of the subsequent 62 cases, there were four more deaths, each from similar causes. However, two patients died within 22 and 28 hours, respectively. These sobering cases remind us of how important it is to make a timely diagnosis and act promptly.

It is unfortunate that the first signs that all is not well and that bowel trauma may have occurred may not arise for days or even weeks after the original surgery. The trend towards ever earlier discharge of all surgical patients, most notably those having had major procedures through small incisions, increases the potential for misdiagnosis and delayed repair. The lesson is clear – patients should get progressively better after laparoscopic surgery and if a patient describes worsening or even just persistent abdominal pain, bowel trauma must be considered early and actively excluded. It is far better to explore a patient suspected of having a bowel injury and have an occasional negative finding, than to delay the diagnosis through procrastination. This places responsibility on the gynecologic laparoscopic surgeon to educate junior and senior colleagues, colleagues in general practice and in accident and emergency departments, and most importantly, the patients themselves.

Summary

The risk of injury to the bowel appears to be an inevitable part of all laparoscopic procedures. No device or surgical technique yet described claiming to avoid bowel injury has been shown to do so reliably. One must be aware of the potential contributing factors that exist at all parts of the surgical process. Constant vigilance and scrupulous adherence to recognized practices and techniques should serve to limit the danger to our patients. However, we, our colleagues, and our patients must be aware of the pitfalls as well as the benefits of this exciting surgical revolution.

References

American Association of Gynecologic Laparoscopists (1995) *Technical Bulletin. Electrosurgical Safety.* Santa Fe Springs: American Association of Gynecologic Laparoscopists.

Baadsgaard SE, Bille S, Egeblad K (1989) Major vascular injury during gynaecological laparoscopy. Report of a case and review of published cases. *Acta Obstetricia et Gynecologica Scandinavica* **68**: 283–285.

Ballem RV, Rudomanski J (1993) Techniques of pneumoperitoneum. *Surgical Laparoscopy and Endoscopy* **3**: 42–43.

Boike GM, Miller CE, Spirtos NM *et al.* (1995) Incisional bowel herniations after operative laparoscopy: A series of nineteen cases and review of the literature. *American Journal of Obstetrics and Gynecology* **172**: 1726–1733.

Chamberlain G, Brown JD (eds) (1978) *Gynaecological Laparoscopy. A Report of the Confidential Enquiry into Gynaecological Laparoscopy.* London: Royal College of Obstetricians and Gynaecologists.

Corson SL, Batzer FR, Gocial B *et al.* (1989) Measurement of the force necessary for laparoscopic trocar entry. *Journal of Reproductive Medicine* **34**: 282–284.

Ewen SP, Sutton CJG (1995) Complications of laser laparoscopy. Eleven years experience. *Minimally Invasive Therapy* **4**: 27–29.

Fear RE (1968) Laparoscopy: A valuable aid in gynecologic diagnosis. *American Journal of Obstetrics and Gynecology* **31**: 297–309.

Garry R (1994) The Achilles heel of minimal access surgery. *Gynaecological Endoscopy* **3**: 210–212.

Hasson HM (1974) Open laparoscopy: a report of 150 cases. *Journal of Reproductive Medicine* **12**: 234–238.

Hulka JF, Peterson HB, Phillips JM *et al.* (1991) Operative laparoscopy: American Association of Gynecologic Laparoscopists 1991 Membership Survey. *Journal of Reproductive Medicine* **28**: 569–571.

Kadar N, Reich H, Liu CY *et al.* (1993) Incisional hernias after major laparoscopic gynecological procedures. *American Journal of Obstetrics and Gynecology* **168**: 1493–1495.

Levy BS, Soderstrom RM, Dail DH (1985) Bowel injuries during laparoscopy: Gross anatomy and histology. *Journal of Reproductive Medicine* **30**: 168–179.

Marin G, Bergamo S, Miola E *et al.* (1987) Prelaparoscopic echography used to detect abdominal adhesions. *Endoscopy* **19**: 147–149.

Martin DC (1991) Tissue effects of lasers. *Seminars in Reproductive Endocrinology* **9(2)**: 127–137.

Nezhat FR, Silfen SL, Evans D *et al.* (1991) Comparison of direct insertion of disposable and standard reusable laparoscopic trocars and previous pneumoperitoneum with Veress needle. *Obstetrics and Gynecology* **78**: 148–151.

Peterson HB, Hulka JF, Phillips JM (1990) American Association of Gynecologic Laparoscopists 1988 Membership Survey on operative laparoscopy. *Journal of Reproductive Medicine* **35**: 587–589.

Phipps JH (1995) Avoidance of complications of laparoscopic hysterectomy. In Sutton CJG (ed.) *Baillière's Clinical Obstetrics and Gynaecology: Advanced Laparoscopic Surgery*, vol. 9, no. 4. London: Baillière Tindall.

Querleu D, Chevallier L, Chapron C, Bruhat M (1993) Complications of gynaecological endoscopic surgery. A French multicenter collaborative study. *Gynaecological Endoscopy* **2**: 3–6.

Reich H, McGlynn F, Budin R (1991) Laparoscopic repair of full thickness bowel injury. *Journal of Laparoendoscopic Surgery* **1**(2): 119–122.

Ryder RM, Hulka JF (1993) Bladder and bowel injury after electrodesiccation with Kleppinger bipolar forceps: A clinicopathological study. *Journal of Reproductive Medicine* **38**: 595–598.

Semm K, Freidrich ER (eds) (1987) *Operative Manual for Endoscopic Abdominal Surgery*. Chicago: Year Book.

Soderstrom RM (1993) Bowel injury litigation after laparoscopy. *Journal of the American Association of Gynecologic Laparoscopists* **1**: 74–77.

Vancaillie TG (1994) Electrosurgery at laparoscopy: guidelines to avoid complications. *Gynaecological Endoscopy* **3**: 143–150.

Wheeless CR (1977) Thermal gastrointestinal injuries. In Phillips JM (ed.) *Laparoscopy*. pp. 231–235. Baltimore: Williams & Wilkins.

49

Major Vessel Injuries

BARBARA S. LEVY

University of Washington School of Medicine, Washington, USA

Introduction

Laceration of a major abdominal blood vessel is one of the most devastating and immediately life-threatening complications of diagnostic and operative laparoscopy. Perforations of the aorta, vena cava, common, left and right iliac arteries and veins, superior mesenteric vessels, inferior and superficial epigastric, and patent umbilical veins have been reported. The true incidence of great vessel injury is unknown since the vast majority of these cases go unreported. The most recent survey sponsored by the American Association of Gynecologic Laparoscopists (AAGL) documents 14 major vessel injuries among 14 911 laparoscopic hysterectomies resulting in a rate of one per 1000 (Hulka *et al.*, 1997). If injuries to the abdominal wall vessels are included, the number increases to 382 in 14 911 (Hulka *et al.*, 1997; Hulka *et al.*, personal communication, 1996). Estimates of the incidence of major vessel injury in the published medical literature are based on anecdotal information. There have been few prospective studies published to date documenting complications of laparoscopic surgery. Retrospective surveys and anecdotal case reports are illustrative, but cannot give us a true picture of the incidence of these injuries. Undoubtedly, whatever the true incidence has been, as more complex intra-abdominal and retroperitoneal surgical procedures are performed endoscopically, all with multiple trocar insertions, the risk of major vessel injuries may increase.

Historically, patients at highest risk for vascular injury on initial trocar insertion have been young, thin, nulliparous women with well-developed abdominal musculature. In these women not only does the aorta lie less than one inch (2.5 cm) below the skin at the umbilicus, but the fascia and abdominal wall are tense and inelastic creating a tough barrier to insertion of instruments (Hulka, 1980; Kurzel and Edinger, 1983). Obesity may play a role as well in that identification of anatomic landmarks may be compromised and the surgeon, in an effort to avoid preperitoneal placement of the insufflating needle or trocar, may overzealously thrust the instrument in a perpendicular fashion and impale the retroperitoneal vessels against the sacral promontory. Elderly and chronically ill patients with poor tissue turgor or patients with multiple previous abdominal operations represent other groups with risk factors for vessel injury. Other risky situations may surface as older and more medically complex patients undergo laparoscopic procedures with increasing frequency.

Several technical factors have been identified as contributing to major vessel injury. Operator inexperience is clearly an important factor; most laparoscopic complications have been reported to occur in a surgeon's first 100 cases. Both blunt trocars and disposable sharp trocars have been implicated as predisposing to major vessel trauma (McDonald *et al.*, 1979; Shin, 1982). Hulka and Reich (1994) in their textbook of laparoscopic surgery remind us that 'The magic is in the magician and not in the wand'. Technical surgical errors may be associated with catastrophic injury in the retroperitoneum including:

- Failure to adequately stabilize the abdominal wall.
- Forceful thrusting motion for insertion.
- Perpendicular or lateral insertion of the needle or trocar.

- Failure to note anatomic landmarks.
- Abnormal or inappropriate patient positioning.

Each of these problems will be addressed in detail in this chapter and hopefully many vascular injuries will be avoided.

Anatomy

The anatomy of the retroperitoneal space with the corresponding abdominal wall landmarks must be recalled. The aortic bifurcation occurs at the level of L4 in 75% of people. The summits of the iliac crests are reliable landmarks for L4. The aortic bifurcation will be below L4–5 in 11% of people and above L4 in 9%. Even in massively obese patients the iliac crests are usually palpable. The bifurcation will be within 1.25 cm above or below the iliac crests in 80% of people (Gray, 1966). The position of the umbilicus is quite variable and should not be used to predict the location of the underlying great vessels. Placing patients in the Trendelenburg position before insertion of the insufflating needle or trocar increases the risk of retroperitoneal injury by rotating the sacral promontory into a position closer to the umbilicus (Lynn *et al.*, 1982). The angle of insertion must be adjusted to avoid the great vessels. With the diminished margin of safety both major vessel injury and preperitoneal insufflation will be more common with the patient in the Trendelenburg position.

It is important for the surgeon to be present in the operating room when the patient is positioned as well as when the sterile drapes are applied. Tucking an arm may significantly rotate the patient's hips and distort the symmetry of anatomic landmarks. This may be difficult to ascertain once the drapes have been applied. Many anesthesiologists, in an effort to expedite the procedure, will place the patient in a steep Trendelenburg position. It is the surgeon's responsibility to document for him or herself the position of the patient and the anatomic landmarks before needle, trocar or incision placement.

Abdominal Entry Techniques

After the patient has been properly positioned, the superior aspect of the iliac crest should be palpated and an effort made to trace the aorta and its bifurca-

tion by palpation. This allows the surgeon to assess the adequacy of anesthesia as well as the strength and tension of the abdominal wall before initiating insufflation. A superficial skin incision is then made. In thin, frail and multiparous patients an effort must be made to avoid penetration into the abdominal cavity. The author is aware of at least one death related to injury of the aorta at the time of the initial skin incision (Morrow, personal communication, 1995). One case of superior mesenteric vein laceration has been reported in the literature (Bartsich and Dillon, 1981). This injury occurred in a patient with a large rectus diastasis (separation of the rectus muscles at the midline) during the initial skin incision. The type of scalpel blade used during these cases is unknown; however, use of a number 12 blade may help avoid inadvertent peritoneal entry.

Before using any laparoscopic equipment, the surgeon should inspect and test it. On occasion the hospital personnel who sterilize and reassemble reusable instruments will leave out a spring or combine a long needle or trocar with a shorter sheath. Even with packaged disposable equipment, it is wise to test the device to assure its proper function.

During insertion of a Veress needle, be sure that the valve is open. This permits room air to enter the abdominal cavity immediately on entry into the peritoneum, thereby allowing the bowel and its mesentery to fall away from the needle tip. It will also allow immediate recognition of possible intravascular placement and prevent gas insufflation into the circulation.

Manual elevation of the abdominal wall may facilitate needle or trocar placement by stabilizing the tissues and increasing the distance to the retroperitoneum. Attempts to elevate the abdominal wall with towel clips, however, generally raise only the skin and fail to raise the fascia and peritoneum away from the intraperitoneal contents (Corson, 1980). This creates only the illusion of increased distance and safety. Elevation of the skin and subcutaneous space will increase the distance over which the needle or trocar must travel and may distort perception of the angle of entry by the surgeon. Vigorous bites with towel clips in an attempt to raise the full thickness of the abdomen may result in bowel perforation. With the abdominal wall manually stabilized or elevated the Veress needle or trocar should be firmly, but gently guided at 45° towards the hollow of the sacrum or towards the fundus of the elevated uterus if the anatomy has been difficult to palpate.

Correct intraperitoneal placement may be verified by placing a syringe with 10–20 ml of saline on the hub of the needle. The fluid should drop freely into the cavity. Re-aspiration will help to ascertain peritoneal or intravascular placement. Return of small bowel or stomach contents also demonstrates inappropriate placement. Blood return should prompt immediate suspicion of vascular injury unless there is a known pre-existing hemoperitoneum. No test is 100% accurate in determining the location of the instruments, however. If there appears to be difficulty or excess pressure during insufflation, the surgeon should suspect abnormal placement and consider another technique. If difficulty is encountered at the umbilicus or if there is a high likelihood of intra-abdominal adhesions in this region, the Veress needle may be positioned safely in the left upper quadrant under most circumstances. Avoid jostling the needle in an effort to improve insufflation or decrease insufflation pressure. Several reports indicate that further vascular injury has occurred when the Veress needle has been maneuvered after increased insufflation pressure had been noted. If the needle is just inside the retroperitoneal space, further manipulation of the needle could cause more great vessel injury.

Over 50% of the reported major vessel injuries have been caused by either the primary or ancillary trocars. Blunt trocars have been implicated in contributing to this complication. Blunt trocars require increased force to penetrate the fascia. Nicking the fascia with the scalpel will facilitate trocar insertion under these circumstances. Surgeons who are accustomed to reusable instruments may develop insertion techniques that prove hazardous if less forgiving razor-sharp disposables are substituted. With any trocar insertion, it is best to control the depth of penetration of the trocar tip with stabilizing guidance from the surgeon's nondominant hand. Marketing of disposable trocars with 'safety shields' has created a false sense of security among surgeons. In a recent letter to manufacturers the Food and Drug Administration has challenged all companies selling disposable trocars with shields to demonstrate safety before continuing to market and label the devices as 'safety shields' (FDA letter to trocar manufacturers, August 1996). The 'safety shield' is designed to lock in place covering the sharp trocar once the initial resistance has been decreased. Not infrequently it may not penetrate the peritoneum necessitating several passes with the trocar.

Most major vessel injuries occur with the use of large (10 mm or greater) disposable pyramidal trocars. To some extent these data may simply reflect the overall number of these types of trocars used rather than relative injury rates with distinct types and sizes of instruments. Hurd *et al.* (1993) studied the risk of vessel injury with different sizes of pyramidal and conical trocars in an animal model. When the vessel is directly punctured (0 mm between the tip of the trocar and the midportion of the vessel wall) these instruments are indistinguishable. However, as the placement of the trocar tip becomes distanced from the vessel, it is clear that large diameter pyramidal trocars are significantly more likely to lacerate a vessel wall, even at a distance of 4–5 mm. In the 1995 AAGL survey of complications at laparoscopic hysterectomy, the vast majority of vessel injuries related to trocars (145 of 178 reported lacerations) occurred with disposable trocars (Hulka *et al.*, 1997; Hulka, personal communication, 1996). Clearly sharp instruments and 'safety' shields do not preclude significant injuries to large vessels.

Some have argued that the 'Z' technique may lead to major vessel injury in the retroperitoneum by making the operator unaware of his or her actual angle of insertion (Katz *et al.*, 1979). In reality, burrowing 1–2 cm below the umbilicus should allow the trocar to begin its entry into the pelvic cavity well below the dangerous region of the sacral promontory in most patients with normal anatomy.

The surgeon should be familiar with multiple techniques for abdominal entry and insufflation. The open (Hasson) technique may be employed when difficulty is encountered penetrating the fascia or insufflating the abdomen. Mini-laparotomy may always be considered as well. Multiple passes with the needle or trocar should be avoided, and proceeding to an alternative technique early is advised in cases where difficulty is encountered.

All additional ports must be placed under direct vision. The inferior epigastric vessels may be identified by transillumination in thin patients and can generally be avoided. Strategies to reduce the risk of vessel injury in the abdominal wall include placement of the smallest possible trocars laterally with 10–12 mm trocars remaining in the midline as much as possible. In addition, the use of conical trocars in the lateral positions may be less traumatic to the abdominal wall vessels (Hurd *et al.*, 1993). Newer devices that are approximately the same diameter as a Veress needle and dilate the abdominal opening using a radially expanding system may prove even less likely to cause epigastric vessel damage.

The direction of secondary trocar insertion in the pelvis must be away from the sacral promontory and great vessels and towards the fundus of the uterus. Care must be taken to avoid lateral thrusting towards the pelvic sidewall. A small laceration of the uterine serosa is more easily controlled than a major vessel tear.

Damage to major vessels may also occur during the operative portion of the procedure after trocars have been safely placed. Dissection of the retroperitoneum for lymph node sampling, excision of endometriosis and extensive adhesiolysis place the pelvic sidewall vessels and the great vessels at risk. Sharp dissection, electrosurgery and lasers have all created unintended openings in major vessels. Extreme caution must be exercised when operating near the pelvic sidewall or in the vicinity of the great vessels.

Significant damage to retroperitoneal vessels may not be immediately apparent to the surgical team due to:

- Increased intra-abdominal pressure (pneumoperitoneum).
- Decreased venous pressure due to the Trendelenburg position.
- Retroperitoneal dissection and tamponade.

Recognizing Major Vessel Injury

Major vessel injury should be suspected whenever blood returns from the open insufflating needle. In addition, inspection of the abdomen directly underneath the area of trocar insertion immediately upon placement of the laparoscope may demonstrate a small amount of bleeding. If this is found, further investigation must be immediately undertaken to ensure that a retroperitoneal hematoma is not developing. These areas of injury may be difficult to appreciate if the surgeon is not aggressive in documenting the integrity of the retroperitoneal structures. This may require positioning the patient to displace the bowel in order to adequately visualize the great vessels. Sudden deterioration in vital signs (decrease in end-tidal carbon dioxide, decreased blood pressure and increased heart rate) in a previously stable patient after needle or trocar insertion should be considered to be due to a vascular accident until proven otherwise.

Peterson *et al.* (1982) reported a case in which a 38-year-old healthy woman died due to an unrecognized aortic injury. After initial insertion of the insufflating needle, the pressure was greater than 20 mm Hg. The needle was manipulated until a normal pressure reading was obtained, and the abdomen was insufflated with carbon dioxide. Four minutes after trocar insertion the patient's blood pressure was unobtainable. The surgeon searched the peritoneal cavity, but found no sign of bleeding. Resuscitation efforts were therefore geared for an anaphylactic reaction to anesthetic medication rather than exsanguination, and the patient died. Whenever any additional manipulation of the needle or multiple passes with the trocar are required and the patient becomes unstable, a

vascular injury must be suspected. A large hematoma may accumulate in the retroperitoneal space before any intraperitoneal sign of hemorrhage is apparent. The author is aware of several cases in which the anesthesiologist recognized rapid deterioration in a previously stable patient and made the erroneous assumption that gas embolism had occurred. This delayed definitive treatment by the surgeons. Whenever any catastrophic change in vital signs occurs during laparoscopic surgery, immediate laparotomy must be performed through a generous incision. If the patient is dying from a gas embolism the addition of a scar on her abdomen will not be problematic. However, if the etiology is a major vessel injury, delay in recognition and treatment may significantly increase morbidity. Control of large bleeding vessels can be obtained by digital pressure or with sponge packs until the patient is stabilized and appropriate surgical help has arrived. An additional anesthesiologist and a surgeon trained to manage vascular complications should be summoned immediately to the operating room. Once the patient has been stabilized, adequate visualization is obtained, and the peritoneum overlying the injured vessel is incised well above the area of injury. The vessels are isolated and all injuries identified and repaired with vascular sutures, clips or patches. Nezhat and colleagues (1995) have reported control of an iliac artery injury using bipolar electrodessication. This method risks total occlusion of the vessel and significant postoperative morbidity. Few sequelae have been reported when rapid and appropriate measures have been initiated after vascular injury.

Summary

In summary, major vessel injuries during laparoscopic surgery are, for the most part, avoidable. In the older literature, most reported injuries were related to Veress needle trauma. More recent papers (Nordestgaard, 1995) demonstrate an increasing incidence of major vessel injuries caused by trocars. In part this may be attributed to the increase in operative as opposed to diagnostic procedures where a larger number of trocars are inserted for each surgical case. The surgeon must palpate the abdomen and review the anatomy in each patient. The position of the patient should be verified and the equipment inspected. The Veress needle should be open to the air during insertion and directed at 45° towards the hollow of the sacrum. Each trocar must be inserted at the proper angle with careful controlled pressure. Finally, positive identification of abdominal wall vessels and insertion of all additional trocars under direct vision will prevent most major vessel perforations.

References

Bartsich EG, Dillon TF (1981) Injury of superior mesenteric vein: laparoscopic procedure with unusual complication. *New York State Journal of Medicine* **81**: 933.

Corson SL (1980) Major vessel injury during laparoscopy. *American Journal of Obstetrics and Gynecology* **138**: 589.

Gray H (1966) In Goss GM (ed.) *Anatomy of the Human Body*. 28th edition. pp. 646–647. Philadelphia: Lea and Febiger.

Hulka JF (1980) Major vessel injury during laparoscopy. *American Journal of Obstetrics and Gynecology* **138**: 138–590.

Hulka JF, Reich H (1994) *Textbook of Laparoscopy*. 2nd edition. p. 85. Philadelphia: WB Saunders.

Hulka JF, Levy BS, Parker WH *et al.* (1997) Laparoscopic-assisted vaginal hysterectomy: American Association of Gynecologic Laparoscopists 1995 Membership Survey. *Journal of the American Association of Gynecologic Laparoscopists* **4**: 167–171.

Hurd WW, Pearl ML, DeLancey JOL *et al.* (1993) Laparoscopic injury of abdominal wall blood vessels: a report of three cases. *Obstetrics and Gynecology* **82**: 673–676.

Katz M, Beck P, Tancer ML (1979) Major vessel injury during laparoscopy: anatomy of two cases. *American Journal of Obstetrics and Gynecology* **135**: 544–545.

Kurzel FB, Edinger DD (1983) Injury to the great vessels. A hazard of transabdominal endoscopy. *Southern Medical Journal* **76**: 656–657.

Lynn SC, Katz AR, Ross PJ (1982) Aortic perforation sustained at laparoscopy. *Journal of Reproductive Medicine* **27(2)**: 17–19.

McDonald PT, Rich NM, Collins CJ *et al.* (1979) Vascular trauma secondary to diagnostic and therapeutic procedures: laparoscopy. *American Journal of Surgery* **136**: 651–655.

Nezhat F, Brill A, Nezhat C *et al.* (1995) Traumatic hypogastric artery bleeding controlled with bipolar desiccation during operative laparoscopy. *Journal of the American Association of Gynecologic Laparoscopists* **2**: 171–173.

Nordestgaard AG, Bodily KC, Osborne RW *et al.* (1995) Major vascular injuries during laparoscopic procedures. *American Journal of Surgery* **169**: 543–545.

Peterson HB, Greenspan JR, Ory HW (1982) Death following puncture of the aorta during laparoscopic sterilization *Obstetrics and Gynecology* **59**: 133–134.

Shin CS. Vascular injury secondary to laparoscopy. *New York State Journal of Medicine* **82**: 935–936.

Yuzpe AA (1990) Pneumoperitoneum needle and trocar injuries in laparoscopy. A survey on possible contributing factors and prevention. *Journal of Reproductive Medicine* **35**: 485–490.

50

Genitourinary Complications

CEANA H. NEZHAT, FARR NEZHAT, DANIEL SEIDMAN AND
CAMRAN NEZHAT

Stanford University School of Medicine, California, USA

Ureter Injury

The development of the ureter is embryologically associated with the development of the female genital tract. This close association persists post-natally, predisposing women to ureteral injury.

Prevention of Ureteral Injury

Knowledge of the ureter's path through the pelvis and the vulnerable points are key to preventing injuries. The intrapelvic segment of the ureter is close to the broad ligament, ovaries and uterosacral ligaments, and injuries often occur in these areas. The surgeon should note the ureter's course through the peritoneum. Endometriosis and severe pelvic adhesions can thicken the peritoneum, obscuring the location of the ureter, especially near the uterosacral ligaments. If the ureter cannot be clearly identified through the peritoneum, it must be located by retroperitoneal dissection. Using hydrodissection, a horizontal incision is made in the peritoneum midway between the ovary and uterosacral ligament. The lower edge of the peri-toneum is grasped and pulled medially. Blunt dissection with the suction/irrigator probe helps locate the ureter lateral to the peritoneum. If the peritoneum is involved with endometriosis and there is retroperitoneal fibrosis, the ureter can be attached to the peritoneum. The horizontal incision

in the peritoneum is extended as necessary (Nezhat *et al.*, 1995a).

Until recently, most reported cases of ureteral injury during laparoscopic procedures involved electrocoagulation because it is the most reliable technique to arrest bleeding. As the use of other devices such as lasers or stapling devices increases, more injuries to the ureters are being reported (Granger *et al.*, 1990)

Ureteral injury can occur:

- During sharp dissection of an ovary adherent to the pelvic sidewall.
- In uterosacral transection.
- During ligation, transection or coagulation of the uterine arteries.
- When removing endometriotic implants or fibrosis from the ureter.
- While trying to control bleeding vessels.

Unrecognized anomalies in the location of the ureter may predispose the patient to injury. To avoid such injuries, the tissue being destroyed or removed and the location of the ureter must be identified before irreversible action is taken. Meticulous and continuous attention to the location of the ureter will reduce complications (Chaffkin and Luciano, 1993).

Methods to protect the ureter include hydro-dissection and resecting affected peritoneum. A small opening is made in the peritoneum and 50–100 ml of lactated Ringer's solution is injected along the course of the ureter. This displaces the ureter laterally, providing a plane for safe ablation of endometriotic implants, lysis of adhesions or resection of the involved peritoneum. Additionally, the fluid absorbs the laser energy, decreasing the risk of thermal damage to underlying tissue. This procedure is only applicable when the peritoneum is not densely adherent to the underlying ureter. During uterosacral transection, a backstop can be placed between the lateral aspect of the uterosacral ligament and ureter. Before using the bipolar forceps during adnexectomy, the infundibulopelvic ligament must be put under traction to identify the ureter and avoid thermal damage.

The routine use of preoperative intravenous pyelography is controversial and no prospective study confirms that this prevents ureteral injury. However, for selected patients, it may level ureteral obstruction or displacement and allow appropriate surgical planning. The routine use of ureteral catheters is not warranted, but we find a ureteral catheter useful in rare cases of severe endometriosis or adhesions with retroperitoneal fibrosis and displacement of the ureter.

Recognition of Ureteral Injury

It is reported that a favorite quote of Dr Thomas Green of Boston was 'The venial sin is injury to the ureter; the mortal sin is failure of recognition' (Green et al., 1962). Early recognition is critical to successful management (Nichols, 1988). Intraoperative ureteral damage is suspected when urine leakage or blood-tinged urine is noted, and indigo carmine dye is spilled intraperitoneally following intravenous administration. When surgical procedures involve the ureter, postoperative ureteral integrity can be ascertained by cystoscopy, ureteral catheterization or an intravenous retrograde pyelogram. Stenting of the ureter or repair by laparotomy is generally indicated, but laparoscopic repair of partial and full thickness injuries is an option for some laparoscopists.

Diagnosis of ureteral injury is usually made postoperatively by intravenous pyelography (IVP). Fever, flank pain, peritonitis, and abdominal distension 48–72 hours postoperatively should alert the clinician to possible ureteral injury. Leukocytosis and hematuria may be present. Since the patient's symptoms may be indistinguishable from those of ileus or bowel injury, IVP is indispensable in the differential diagnosis. A watery vaginal discharge, especially one with an odor of ammonia, should raise suspicion for a vesicovaginal or ureterovaginal fistula. A cystogram, in addition to IVP, is helpful in making the diagnosis.

Management of Ureteral Injury

Whether ureteral complications are discovered immediately or after a delay, consultation with a urologist should be considered. If the IVP indicates ureteral injury, initial therapy should involve attempts at either retrograde or antegrade stenting. Therapeutic options include ureteroureterostomy and ureteroneocystostomy. Both require stenting and drainage with a ureteral catheter. There have been several recent reports of conservative management of ureteral injuries, as well as laparoscopic management.

Following ureter injury re-anastomosis or implantation in the bladder can be managed laparoscopically. We have treated four such patients by laparoscopically (Nezhat et al., 1996a). The ureter is dissected and a 6 or 7-Fr ureteral catheter is passed through the ureterovesical junction under cystoscopic guidance. The catheter is advanced through the proximal portion of the ureter to the renal pelvis. The edges of the ureter are reapproximated using four interrupted 4–0 polydioxanone sutures (Figure 50.1). The postoperative course includes 4–6 weeks of stent placement and postoperative pyelography to confirm ureteral patency. If the bladder is not injured, the Foley catheter is removed. The ureteral stent is removed 6–8 weeks postoperatively. Periodic follow-up IVP or renal ultrasound are done to rule out stricture.

Bladder Injury

Prevention of Bladder Injury

Bladder injury is rare and usually occurs in patients who have had laparotomies or whose bladder is not emptied before surgery. Under these conditions, sharp instruments such as trocars and uterine manipulators can perforate or lacerate the bladder. Electricity and lasers can cause thermal injury and blunt instruments can cause a laceration. Certain laparoscopic procedures increase the risk of bladder injury:

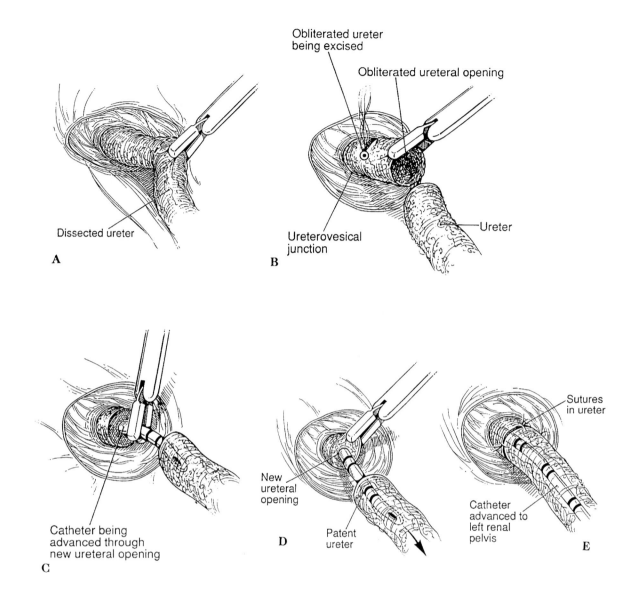

Figure 50.1 A: Ureterolysis is performed and the ureter involved with endometriosis and fibrosis is dissected and pulled medially. B: The obliterated portion of the ureter is excised with the CO_2 laser. C: Under cystoscopic guidance, a 7-Fr ureteral catheter is passed through the ureterovesical junction. D: The catheter is advanced through the proximal portion of the ureter to the renal pelvis. E: The edges of the ureter are approximated at 12, 3, 6, and 9 o'clock using four interrupted 4–0 polydioxanone sutures. (Reproduced, with permission, from Nezhat *et al.*, 1995a.)

- The Veress needle can perforate a distended bladder.
- A misplaced Rubin's cannula can perforate the vagina and bladder with upward pressure.
- Accessory trocar insertion can injure a full bladder, or one with distorted anatomy by previous pelvic surgery, endometriosis or adhesions, or if insertion is less than 4 cm above the symphysis pubis.

- Coagulation or laser ablation of endometriotic implants or adhesiolysis in the anterior cul-de-sac can predispose the patient to bladder injury. Hydrodissection or a backstop used with the carbon dioxide laser decreases this possibility.
- During a laparoscopic hysterectomy (LH) or laparoscopic assisted vaginal hysterectomy (LAVH) (Nezhat *et al.*, 1995b) the bladder

may be lacerated or torn, specifically if blunt dissection is used to free the bladder from the pubocervical fascia, particularly in women who have had a previous cesarean delivery, severe endometriosis (Nezhat *et al.*, 1996b) or lower segment myomas.

- Bladder injury can also occur while entering and dissecting the space of Retzius before laparoscopic bladder neck suspension.

To prevent injury, a Foley catheter is placed to drain the bladder. The position of the bladder should be assessed during the initial examination with the laparoscope. If the boundaries of the bladder are not clear, particularly when pelvic anatomy is distorted, the bladder should be filled with 350 ml of fluid to delineate its position. Care should be used when performing LH or LAVH and the assistant should push the uterus cephalad during bladder dissection.

Recognition of Bladder Injury

Intraoperative recognition of a bladder injury is important to prevent long-term sequelae. Signs of intraoperative bladder injury include:

- Air in the urinary catheter and bag during insufflation.
- Apparent pushing of the bladder by the accessory trocar as it is advanced through the abdominal wall.
- Blood in the urine.
- Urine drainage from the accessory trocar incision.
- Postoperative urinary retention, particularly if the amount of urine obtained during catheterization is less than anticipated.
- Postoperative signs of peritonitis.
- Leakage of indigo carmine from the injured site.
- Since trocar injury often involves both entry and exit punctures, locating both is important.

Some bladder complications become apparent postoperatively, particularly those caused by electrocoagulation. Signs and symptoms include decreased urine output, hematuria, suprapubic bruising, mass in the abdominal wall or pelvis, abdominal swelling, azotemia or peritonitis. If a bladder injury is suspected, a retrograde cystogram may demonstrate a bladder leak. An IVP may be necessary to differentiate the source and assess the possibility of multiple organ injuries.

Management of Bladder Injury

Small holes generally heal without sequelae. Trocar injuries to the bladder dome that are less than 1 cm do not require closure and can be managed by urinary drainage for 5–7 days. Drainage promotes healing, encourages spontaneous closure and minimizes further complications.

Lacerations may require a laparotomy, although some laparoscopists can repair the laceration laparoscopically. After identifying the injury, the location of the ureters and the distance between the injury and the ureters is determined. Then, any endometriosis, adhesions, or necrotic tissue is completely removed. The laceration is repaired in one layer using 0 polyglactin. The suture is placed through the serosa, muscularis and mucosa. A second layer may occasionally be necessary for reinforcement. Small injuries (less than 0.5 cm) that are away from the trigone and ureters may be repaired by placing one endoloop around the injury. Cystoscopy is performed to ensure that there is no damage to the ureteral orifices and the repair is watertight. A Foley catheter remains *in situ* for 4–10 days. Before removal of the Foley catheter, a cystogram is performed to ensure proper healing.

References

Chaffkin L, Luciano AA (1993) Ureteral injuries. In Corfman RS, Diamond MP, DeCherney AH (eds) *Complications of Laparoscopy and Hysteroscopy.* p. 134. Boston, MA: Blackwell Scientific Publications, Inc.

Granger DA, Soderstrom RM, Schiff SF *et al.* (1990) Ureteral injuries at laparoscopy: insights into diagnosis, management and prevention. *Obstetrics and Gynecology* **75**: 839.

Green TH Jr, Meigs JV, Ulfelder H, Curtin RR (1962) Urologic complications of radical Wertheim hysterectomy: incidence, etiology, management and prevention. *Obstetrics and Gynecology* **20**: 293.

Nezhat C, Nezhat F, Luciano AA, Siegler AM, Metzger DA, Nezhat CH (eds) (1995a) *Operative Gynecologic Laparoscopy: Principles and Techniques.* New York: McGraw-Hill.

Nezhat C, Nezhat F, Nezhat CH, Admon D, Nezhat A (1995b) Proposed classification of hysterectomies involving laparoscopy. *Journal of the American Association of Gynecologic Laparoscopists* **2**: 427–429.

Nezhat CH, Seidman DS, Nezhat F, Rottenberg H, Nezhat C (1996a) Laparoscopic management of intentional and unintentional cystotomy. *Journal of Urology* **156**: 1400–1402.

Nezhat C, Nezhat F, Nezhat CH, Nasserbakht F, Rosati M, Seidman DS (1996b) Urinary tract endometriosis treated by laparoscopy. *Fertility and Sterility* **66(6)**: 920–924.

Nichols DH (1988) *Clinical Problems, Injuries and Complications of Gynecologic Surgery*, 2nd edition. p. 181. Baltimore: Williams & Wilkins.

Hysteroscopic Surgery

51

Initiating a Hysteroscopic Program and Hysteroscopic Instrumentation

MICHAEL S. BAGGISH

Good Samaritan Hospital, Cincinnati, Ohio, USA

Introduction

Increasingly, direct visual examination of the uterine cavity has been taken up by gynecologists in place of blind or indirect evaluation methods. The advantages of seeing the pathology with one's own eyes are many:

- The most appropriate diagnosis is likely to be made.
- The pathology may be assessed accurately before treatment.
- A record of the examination can be obtained by still or video photography.
- The initial investigation can be completed quickly within the office or outpatient clinic setting.
- Capital expenditure of equipment is relatively small.

Many postgraduate courses are offered annually and are either completely or significantly dedicated to hysteroscopic techniques. Every residency program contains training in hysteroscopy as well as other endoscopic techniques. This trend began in the 1980s and was firmly ensconced in the 1990s.

A pattern for learning these techniques has emerged. The prospective student should plan to learn during a didactic conference the details of anatomy, pathology, optics, instrumentation, and principles of diagnostic and operative techniques. Practical 'hands on' experience is essential to learn how to manipulate the instruments and apply the lessons learned during the didactic sessions. I prefer to use heifer uteri in these laboratories, since they provide an accessible, reasonable model of the human uterus and are easily distended with water delivered by pump or syringe. Generally a two-day experience of combined didactics and laboratory sessions is sufficient to provide the practitioner with a suitable introduction to hysteroscopy. Clearly, as with any endoscopic technique, practice by doing simple, uncomplicated normal intrauterine assessment is the key to subsequent skillful operative hysteroscopic procedures. I recommend that the novice performs at least 25 diagnostic hysteroscopies before attempting the simplest operative procedure. Orientation within the uterus, particularly when doing hysteroscopy under direct video monitoring, is vitally important, since complications experienced during difficult operative procedures most frequently relate to loss of orientation within the uterus with resultant perforation and/or deep myometrial penetration.

The critical passage from a high level of confidence performing diagnostic hysteroscopy to skillful operative hysteroscopy must be attained gradually by planned steps, starting with the easiest intrauterine manipulations and advancing to difficult procedures. The greatest levels of skill are required for extraction of submucous myomas and treating extensive uterine adhesions. Simultaneous laparoscopy should be performed when operative hysteroscopy carries a risk of uterine perforation (e.g. septum resection). Again the beginner should never attempt to begin intrauterine surgery before gaining suitable diagnostic experience on many patients.

Initiation of a hysteroscopic program should therefore progress in a logical fashion. Suggested office and operating room plans are discussed below. As with other endoscopic techniques, familiarity with instruments and distending media as well as techniques is crucial to success.

Instrumentation

Any skilled craftsperson must acquire the best tools for the job. Although saving money where appropriate is meritorious, cutting corners with precision instruments will in the long run prove wasteful. The old adage 'you get what you pay for' holds true when selecting surgical instruments. The best rule is to buy the very best equipment that one can afford. It is infinitely better to purchase less equipment than to sacrifice quality.

Telescopes

The most important piece of equipment for hysteroscopy is the lens or telescope. The optics as well as the fiberoptic illumination bundles are packaged together in this single instrument. Most rigid telescopes range in diameter from 2 to 4 mm (o.d.). The best light shower and optical resolution are likely to be found in 4 mm (o.d.) instruments (Figure 51.1). However, for office hysteroscopy, as well as operative procedures, a 3 mm telescope can produce an acceptable video image particularly when magni-

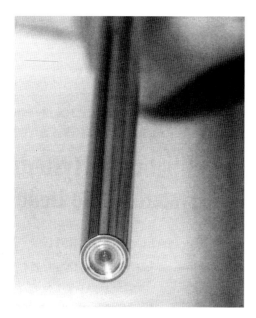

Figure 51.1 A 4 mm 0° telescope. The optics and fiberoptic light bundles are contained within the stainless steel skin.

fied by means of a zoom video camera. The smaller telescope permits the operator to employ a smaller sheath. Although flexible telescopes are now finding their way onto the market, they suffer from inferior resolution compared to that of the rigid equipment. The most convenient length for the hysteroscopic telescope is 35 cm. Shorter instruments offer no advantage and some distinct disadvantages when coupled to operative sheaths. The telescope (Figure 51.2) consists of three major parts:

- The magnifying eyepiece.
- The transmitting lens system.
- The objective lens.

The most commonly used terminal objective lenses provide a straight on view (0°) or offset view (30°). Selection of the lens is a matter of personal preference, but for the best panoramic operative view the 0° lens is recommended, particularly when using laser fibers or flexible or semirigid operating accessories. Rigid lenses are fragile and must be handled with due care to avoid injury. Rough handling, steam autoclaving, improper liquid disinfection and inadequate cleaning will shorten the life of the telescope and require expensive repairs as well as system down time. A properly cared for lens will last a lifetime and provide excellent service over and over again. I prefer to clean the telescope myself and to place it in its proper storage container after finishing each case. I am then assured that the instrument will function properly for the next procedure. Located just below the eyepiece is the fiberoptic coupling connection. At this location the fiberoptic cable joins the telescope. Each lens manufacturer has a unique coupling. Several companies supply attachments that permit a variety of cables to join their particular instrument. The latter is an advantage since any light generator and light cable can be used with a given telescope.

Fiberoptic Light Cable

Fiberoptic cables transmit intense cold light to the telescope (Figure 51.3) and form a conduit, which connects the high intensity (heat producing) generator to the telescope. The cable is filled with many incoherent drawn-out glass fibers capable of conducting light from the generator to the terminus of the cable. Obviously these cables are fragile and can be easily damaged if not handled carefully. Inspection of the end of the cable will readily determine whether fibers or groups of fibers have been broken. These are indicated by dark spots in an otherwise intense light shower. Inspection of the periphery of the cable in a darkened room can also

Figure 51.2 The lens consists of an objective lens, transmitting lens system and eyepiece.

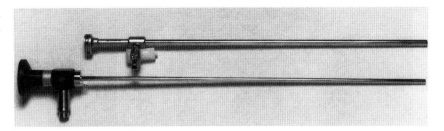

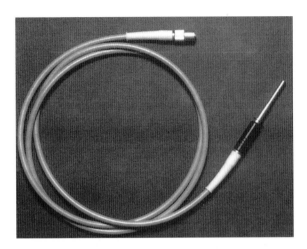

Figure 51.3 Flexible fiberoptic light cable transmits cold light from the generator to the lens.

reveal fiber disruption. This appears as light transmission through the sides of the cable. Poor light at the end of the telescope is almost always due to a damaged cable. The only alternative to substandard light is to replace the cable. Cables should be disinfected by soaking in Cidex (glutaraldehyde) for 15–20 minutes, followed by thorough washing in sterile water. At the end of the case, the fiber should be washed again, resoaked and cleansed again with water. The cable should then be stored dry in a protective container. Most hospitals and surgicenters have replaced liquid disinfection with gas sterilization. The only drawback to the latter is the long period required for aeration.

Light Generator

Several varieties of light generators are available on the market. These range from simple and inexpensive tungsten light generators (US $500–700) to costly xenon generators (US $2000–5000). For office use a simple apparatus will suffice; however, hysteroscopy performed in the operating room under video control demands intense light. Xenon (300 W) generators produce white light which is most favorable when coupled with endoscopic television

cameras (Baggish, 1997). Characteristically the simpler tungsten light generators produce an orange tinted light, which creates a rather poor color on the video monitor. Between these two types of generator are the 250 W metal halide generators. These produce intense light, which is adequate for video images, but characteristically give off a bluish tinge. The light bulbs in all these generators produce a lot of heat, so a fan is built into the cabinet to dissipate the heat and prolong bulb life. Should the fan become defective and not work properly, bulbs, which in fact cost $100 or more, will burn out prematurely.

Light generators and fiberoptic cables can be used interchangeably for hysteroscopy or laparoscopy. Obviously the more powerful generators are required for laparoscopy. All generators should be appropriately grounded and should be periodically inspected (and indexed) by biomedical engineering for low frequency electrical leakage.

Hysteroscopic Sheaths

Two general categories of sheaths are used for hysteroscopic procedures: diagnostic and operating. A sheath is required for panoramic hysteroscopy in order to serve as a conduit through which to instill the distending medium into the uterine cavity. The diagnostic sheath fulfils this singular requirement and measures approximately 4–5 mm in outer diameter (when coupled to a 3–4 mm telescope). The sheath is essentially a hollow stainless steel tube equipped with a proximal port through which the distending medium is injected. The telescope must couple tightly to the sheath with sufficient seal to prevent medium leakage at the telescope/sheath interface. The objective lens of the telescope should fit precisely, flush with the end of the sheath to produce an unobstructed view. Therefore each given manufacturer's lens must be matched correspondingly to the same manufacturer's sheath. The coupling mechanisms differ for different hysteroscopes, preventing the interchange of lenses and sheaths. A 5 mm sheath ordinarily will allow passage through nulliparous cervices without resorting to dilatation (Figure 51.4). A 4 mm sheath equipped

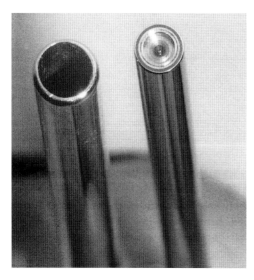

Figure 51.4 The 5 mm diagnostic sheath easily passes through the cervix and serves as a conduit for the distending medium.

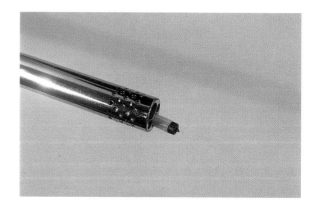

Figure 51.5 Isolated channel sheath. The large channel houses the telescope. The channels at 3 and 9 o'clock are for input of medium. The channel at 6 o'clock is 3 mm wide and serves as a conduit for operating instruments. The perforated outer sheath is used for fluid return.

with a 3 mm telescope can negotiate the endocervical canal more easily than the 5 mm sheath, and is ideal in the office setting. They are therefore ideally suited to office hysteroscopy. Hysteroscopic sheaths are sturdy and stand up to routine handling. They may be steam autoclaved. Obviously they should be thoroughly flushed and cleansed after usage and stored away clean. The stopcock mechanism should be disassembled, cleaned, lubricated and reassembled after each usage. The stopcock should be turned to the open position when stored. I prefer to clean the sheath with a long-handled wire brush, flush with sterile water and blow air through the sheath to dryness. From time to time the sheath as well as the shaft of the telescope should be polished with a high quality metal cleansing compound.

Three types of operative sheaths are currently manufactured – single-cavity and multichannel operating sheaths. Each type of operating sheath measures 7.5–8.5 mm in outer diameter and requires some mechanical dilatation of the cervix to gain entry into the uterine cavity.

SINGLE-CAVITY OPERATING SHEATHS

Single-channel sheaths share the cavity space between the telescope, operative accessory instruments (usually flexible or semi-rigid), and the distending medium (Figure 51.5). Two intake ports (opposite each other) are connected to the sheath and permit instillation of the medium from either side. These do not allow flushing of the uterine cavity. Recently some of these sheaths have been fitted

with a second sheath, which allows return of the medium (i.e. continuous flushing of the cavity), but this increases the diameter of the sheath. Some of the single-cavity sheaths are constructed with a terminal deflecting bridge, which allows some angulation of operating instruments. The bridge is controlled by two small wheel-like levers attached to the proximal portion of the sheath. Operating tools (e.g. scissors, graspers, biopsy forceps, fibers and electrodes) gain entrance to the sheath's interior by an operating port, again located at the proximal portion of the sheath, either at the 12 or 6 o'clock position. Rubber caps or nipples must be fitted onto this entry port to prevent leakage of the medium when an operating tool is in place. The greatest disadvantages of the single cavity sheath are:

- Inability to place instruments accurately into a given location within the uterine cavity, even when equipped with the rather cumbersome bridge device.
- Inability to routinely flush the cavity unless equipped with an oversheath.
- Limitation to the insertion of one operating tool.

MULTICHANNEL OPERATING SHEATHS

The multichannel operating sheath (Figure 51.6) was invented specifically to overcome the deficiencies cited above. The multichannel sheath has four isolated channels (Baggish, 1988). The large 4.5 mm channel accommodates the optics and light bundles (i.e. the telescope). Two separate channels serve for the instillation of the distending media. A single

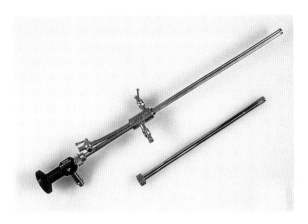

Figure 51.6 Panoramic view of multichannel operating sheath, 8.5 mm o.d. Note terminal perforations in outer sheath (return of medium).

3 mm operating channel is used for a variety of large operating devices including electrodes, scissors, grasping forceps, biopsy forceps and aspirating cannulas. A resecting loop may also be inserted for the purpose of shaving myomas or polyps. An oversheath permits constant flushing of the endometrial cavity by removing blood-tinged fluid and small debris. Obviously many different permutations of instrumentation may be selected. Of great advantage is the ability to flush the uterus continuously during the operation by attaching a suction to the outflow stopcock. The design of the multichannel sheath allows instruments to be placed anywhere within the uterine cavity. In its normal position the instruments are easily able to reach the posterior wall of the uterus, while rotation of the sheath 180° brings the instruments to the anterior wall. The author prefers the multichannel sheath for several intrauterine operations because of its cited advantages. Additionally, separate sheaths are specifically designed to accept 0° or 30° telescopes. Finally, the medium intake and outflow ports swivel to allow medium to be instilled equally easily from the operator's right or left side.

RESECTOSCOPE

A special adaption of the single-cavity sheath is the urologic sheath or gynecologic resectoscope. The modern version of this instrument employs constant-flow technology with inflow of medium entering the uterine cavity through the inner sheath and outflow of tinged fluid via the outer, terminally perforated, sheath.

The operating tools of the resectoscope consist of double-armed electrodes which are manipulated in and out by means of a spring-mechanism slide. The operator controls the apparatus with a trigger-like device through which the thumb and index (index and center) finger are inserted. The lens for the resectoscope is 2.8, 3 or 4 mm. The smaller telescope takes up less room in the channel, permitting better inflow of the distending medium. The ball electrode is currently the most popular method for ablation. The cutting loops (e.g. straight or angled) are excellent tools for resecting submucous myomas. These electrodes are all monopolar.

Operating Accessories

Operating tools are a vital part of hysteroscopy. Without them therapeutic measures would be impossible by the transcervical approach. Most of the mechanical instruments measure 2 mm in diameter and 35 cm in length. They are either flexible or semi-rigid (Figure 51.7) and by their very nature are somewhat delicate. The larger (i.e. 3 mm in diameter) flexible instruments are as sturdy as the rigid sheath variety of the past. The most common operative tool is scissors, which are used to cut lesions such as adhesions, septa, polyps or myomas. The flexible scissors are less likely to be broken by torque whereas the semi-rigid instruments provide greater stability for direction as well as sectioning of tissue. The semi-rigid instrument is susceptible to breakage at the point where the shaft joins the handle. Another useful conventional tool is the alligator grasping forceps (Figure 51.8) which are commonly used to hold onto and extract severed tissues. The biopsy forceps are really too small for obtaining suitable samples of tissue. Recently Cook OB/GYN Instrument Company marketed a series of very useful and disposable hysteroscopic accessories

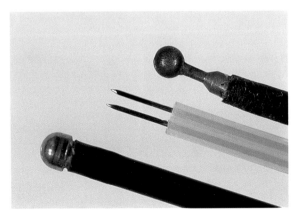

Figure 51.7 Three electrosurgical operating devices (electrodes). Bottom: button electrode; middle: 3 mm bipolar needle electrode; top: 3 mm ball electrode.

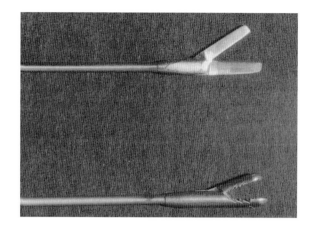

Figure 51.8 Close-up view of semi-rigid scissors and alligator grasping forceps.

(Figures 51.9, 51.10). The Cook 2–3 mm aspirating cannula is probably the single most valuable tool the surgeon has in his catalog of instruments. This simple aspirating device allows debris to be sucked out of the cavity, rendering a clear view of the field. This maneuver is essential for the performance of safe operative hysteroscopy. When combined with flushing sheaths (Figure 51.11), aspiration of larger particles may be carried out continuously in a fashion analogous to sponging or suctioning during a laparotomy. Hysteroscopic needles with varying sized tips may be used to manipulate intrauterine structures as well as to serve as a conduit for the injection of vasoconstrictive drugs.

Nipples and Plugs for the Operating Channel

In the past the only gasket available to cover the operating channel, preventing leakage of medium when operating tools were inserted was the simple urologic rubber nipple. Not uncommonly these nipples become dislodged during the operation, causing the medium to leak out and the uterine cavity to collapse around the operating device. Cook OB/GYN Instrument Company offers a Luer-lock type plastic cap, which locks onto the metal fitting of the operating channel (Baggish and Baltoyannis, 1988). This plug cannot become dislodged and does not leak (the urologic nipples do leak). Operating instruments can be conveniently moved in and out, similar to the action of a trombone slide. This permits operations to be performed relatively close to or distant from the objective end of the telescope (i.e. either highly magnified or in the panoramic view).

Figure 51.9 Cook OB/GYN Instrument Company hysteroscopic accessories: From above – hysteroscopic injection needles, aspirating cannula, medium injection tube, and leaf valve hysteroscopic plugs.

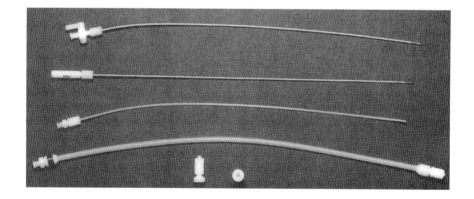

Figure 51.10 Close-up view of hysteroscopic injection needles 18 and 22 gauge.

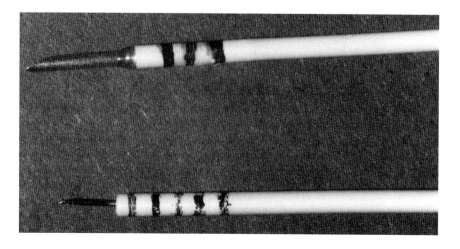

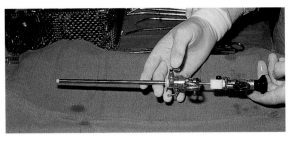

(a)

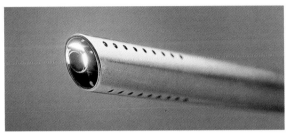

(b)

Figure 51.11 (a) Gynecologic resectoscope with monopolar cable attached. Note the telescope is locked into the sheath and the electrode is in the retracted position. (b) Close-up of the terminal portion of the resectoscope showing the cutting loop electrode in position.

Instruments for Medium Instillation

Several pieces of equipment are now available to facilitate the injection of distending media. These are discussed in detail in Chapter 53.

Hyskon Pump

Hyskon (32% dextran 70) is a highly viscid, crystal clear medium that does not mix with blood, is non-electrolytic and is well suited for both diagnostic and operative hysteroscopy. Although there is little difficulty injecting this material through operative sheaths, pressures of over 700 mm Hg are required to drive it through the narrow clearance of a 5 mm diagnostic sheath. For this reason a pump assist is very useful. The axiom of equating excellence with

simplicity holds in this instance. Cook OB/GYN Instrument Company produces a simple handheld screw device (Figure 51.12), which permits a substantial mechanical advantage for injecting Hyskon via a 60 ml syringe and through a diagnostic sheath. This device is simple to use and very safe. In contrast Hyskon pumps driven by carbon dioxide (CO_2) gas have proved to be complicated, expensive and unsafe in practice.

Low Viscosity Liquid Pumps

With the use of continuous flow resectoscopes and multichannel sheaths, pumps that deliver saline, lactated Ringer's solution and glycine at high flow rates facilitate surgery by constantly exchanging these blood-miscible solutions. Although a three litre plastic bag compressed with a blood pressure cuff can deliver the medium satisfactorily, the advent of variable pressure and flow pumps (Figure 51.14) has offered greater sophistication and flexibility to such a system. Several machines are now available on the market. The outflow from the pump is attached to the inflow port of the hysteroscopic sheath (i.e. in infusion). A suction pump withdraws the flushed uterine fluid via the outflow port, thereby completing a circuit and maintaining a clear operative field of view.

Video Equipment

Modern operative hysteroscopy is most beneficial when using a direct video camera hook-up to the eyepiece of the telescope. The advantages of this approach are multiple:

- Greater magnification for the surgeon.
- Elimination of optical risk for the surgeon when using a laser as the operative tool.
- Provision of visibility (operative field) for assistants and support personnel.
- Production of a permanent record of the operation.

Figure 51.12 Hand-operated Hyskon pump. This is ideal and 100% safe for office hysteroscopy.

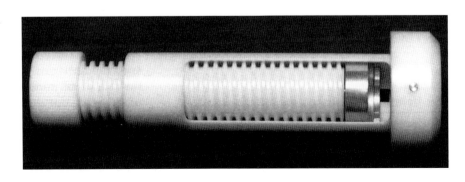

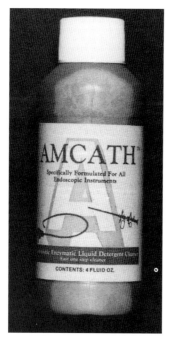

Figure 51.13 Proteolytic enzyme wash removes residual Hyskon from instruments.

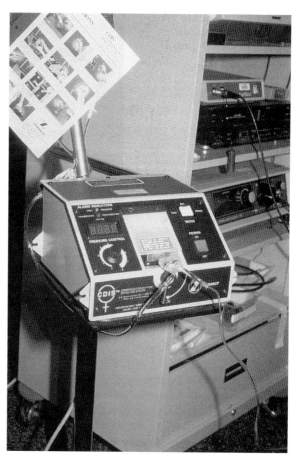

Figure 51.14 Electric low viscosity medium hysteroscopic pump. This type of pump maintains the flow rate and enough pressure to keep the uterine cavity distended for operative hysteroscopy.

The newer endoscopic video cameras offer high resolution as well as miniature composition. The better cameras provide the ability to change lens focal distance by zooming. This is an advantage particularly when a telescope with a diameter smaller than 4 mm is used. The 3 mm telescope produces a smaller image on the TV monitor. However, this image can be enlarged by the zoom mechanism such that it almost fills the monitor screen. Regardless of which video camera is selected, the prospective purchaser should be assured that the apparatus can be safely soaked in a cold sterilization liquid (e.g. Cidex) as well as gas sterilized. The video camera should be coupled to an appropriate high definition video monitor. These monitors range in size from 12–27 inches. Generally the smaller monitors (12–14 inch) produce a clearer picture overall.

Office Hysteroscopy

Diagnostic hysteroscopy is ideally suited to the office environment. Entry into the uterus can be accomplished with minimal discomfort by means of the 4 mm (o.d.) instrument. Here the organization of instrumentation is of prime importance to launch a successful program. I recommend securing a three-tier stainless steel cart mounted on wheels. The top shelf of the cart is reserved for the telescope, sheath, connecting tubing, tenaculum, syringes and solutions. The middle shelf is dedicated for the hysteroscopic CO_2 insufflator. The bottom shelf houses the fiberoptic light generator as well as fiberoptic cables. The advantage of the above set-up is that everything is located in one place and is always ready and accessible for use.

Various media can be used including Hyskon, saline or CO_2 gas. In order to carry out CO_2 hysteroscopy safely, a specially designed insufflator (i.e. one flowing at the rate of <100 ml min^{-1}) must be used. Contemporary units read out data digitally. Obviously the most important information is flow rate and intrauterine pressure. The former should never exceed 100 ml min^{-1} and the latter should never exceed 150 mm Hg. The advantages of CO_2 as a distending medium relate to its convenience, neatness and clarity. Although CO_2 is ideal for diagnostic hysteroscopy, it is inferior when compared to liquid media for operative hysteroscopy. However, one word of warning is necessary: CO_2 instilled into the uterus by means other than the type of insufflator mentioned above can result in disastrous embolism and death for the patient. If the proper equipment is not available hysteroscopy should not be carried out.

Special Instruments

Fiberoptic Laser

Lasers enjoy certain unique properties, which make them useful for hysteroscopic surgery (Baggish, 1983; 1989; Baggish and Baltoyannis, 1988). The laser that is currently most suitable for intrauterine procedures is the neodymium:yttrium-aluminum-garnet (Nd:YAG) laser. Nd:YAG lasers range in power outputs from 20–100 W. Most equipment suitable for hysteroscopic operations will put out approximately 60–100 W of power. The Nd:YAG laser operates in the near infrared (invisible) part of the spectrum at approximately 1064 nm and is conveniently transmitted by fine fibers to the operative site. These bare fibers range in diameter from 600 to 1200 μm. In no circumstances whatsoever should a coaxial or gas cooled fiber be used for operative hysteroscopy. Recently silicone extruded or sculpted fibers have appeared on the market. These fibers' terminal portions are available in several shapes (e.g. ball, conical, wedge) and tend to concentrate the Nd:YAG laser energy. Laser fibers may be used in the contact or non-contact position. Interestingly, penetration in the non-contact mode is deeper and less predictable than when the fiber touches the surface. Since the Nd:YAG laser acts by front scatter, the amount of coagulation injury to the tissue tends to be 4–5 times greater beneath the surface than the visible surface wound since laser energy is not conducted through tissue, unlike electricity. The lesions produced are more predictable. The 1064 nm wavelength is practically ideal since it penetrates all liquid media safely and instantaneously.

Electrosurgery Unit

The modern RF (radiofrequency) electrosurgical unit (ESU) is a very different piece of equipment to the older types of apparatus used during the 1970s and 1980s. The contemporary gold standard ESU is a computerized constant-output voltage machine operating at a frequency of 300–500 kHz.

The generator is equipped with monopolar and bipolar capabilities for both cutting and coagulation. Monopolar cutting may be performed at several settings with the degree of associated coagulation varying with the peak-to-peak voltage. The oscilloscopic picture of the waveform should be a pure sine wave. In contrast, older generators produced a blend of noisy waveforms, blending cutting and coagulation outputs.

Multiple safety features include isolated circuits, neutral electrode safety system, high and low current leakage alarms, and output errors.

The delivery system for electrosurgical energy is the electrode. Electrodes come in various sizes and types (e.g. ball, needle and loop electrodes). Additionally they may be either bipolar or monopolar in design. As with lasers, power (watts) is set on the generator. As a general rule the lowest power setting that will complete the job within a reasonable length of time is safest. The usual range of power settings for ablative or cutting hysteroscopic operations is 60–150 W.

The effects of flowing electrons and laser light in these circumstances is identical (i.e. thermal). At 100°C both types of apparatus will vaporize tissue (remove cells by explosive evaporation). Similarly at 60–70°C the tissue will be coagulated and desiccated.

Most accidents and complications associated with electrosurgery, other than perforation, are high-frequency leaks resulting in thermal burns.

Documenting Data and Servicing Instruments

A major component of learning a new technique is to record what one sees and does. This process is particularly important for obtaining proficiency with hysteroscopy. The video recorder is an excellent device to reach this end. A simple ½ inch recorder is satisfactory if there is to be no editing, whereas a ¾ inch recording is best if editing and future generations of tape are desired. Following a diagnostic or operative procedure, the tape should be reviewed:

- To evaluate the appearance of normal and abnormal structures.
- To see how manipulations of the hysteroscope exposed pathology.
- To determine the effectiveness of operative techniques.

If a video recording system is not available, documentation should be made in a diary for the operator's benefit. The color and contour of the endometrium should be noted and later correlated with the pathology; the various portions of the uterine body should be clearly identified on entrance and exiting. The configuration of the cornua and tubal ostia should be recorded. The central pillar-like structure formed by the fused müllerian ducts should be identified and variations noted; this is frequently confused with a septum (Baggish, 1990).

The recording should take place immediately after the operation in order to produce any benefit. Interestingly the compulsion to write down the hysteroscopic findings reinforces the visual experience and solidifies the learning process.

Finally, if equipment is to retain functionality with longevity, the gynecologist must learn to take apart and service his or her own hysteroscopic instruments.

Summary

In summary, a successful hysteroscopic program depends in order of importance upon:

- A well-trained endoscopist.
- Extensive diagnostic experience.
- Graded operative hysteroscopic experience.
- High-quality instrumentation.
- Organization and appropriate documentation.

Success demands persistence and repetition. As with all other things, short cuts frequently lead to retracing of steps already taken.

References

Baggish MS (1983) New instruments and techniques for hysteroscopy. *Contemporary Obstetrics and Gynecology* **22**: 67.

Baggish MS (1988) A new laser hysteroscope for Nd-YAG endometrial ablation. *Lasers in Surgery and Medicine* **8**: 99.

Baggish MS (1989) Update on hysteroscopes. *Contemporary Obstetrics and Gynecology* **34**: 125.

Baggish MS (1990) Endoscopic laser surgery. In Baggish MS (ed.) *Clinical Practice at Gynecology*, vol. 2. pp. 187–205. New York: Elsevier.

Baggish MS (1997) Hysteroscopy. In Thompson D, Rock J (eds) *Telinde's Operative Gynecology*, 8th edition. Philadelphia: Lippincott.

Baggish MS, Baltoyannis P (1988) New techniques for laser ablation of the endometrium in high risk patients. *American Journal of Obstetrics and Gynecology* **159**: 287.

Baggish MS, Sze HM (1996) Endometrial ablation: A series of 568 patients treated over an 11-year period. *American Journal of Obstetrics and Gynecology* **174**: 908–913.

De Cherney AH, Polan MI (1983) Hysteroscopic management of intrauterine lesions and intractable uterine bleeding. *Obstetrics and Gynecology* **61**: 392.

Garry R. Hasham F, Kokki MS *et al*. (1992) The effect of pressure on fluid absorption during endometrial ablation. *Journal of Gynecologic Surgery* **8**: 1.

Garry R, Shelley-Jones D, Mooney P, Phillips G (1995) Six hundred endometrial laser ablations. *Obstetrics and Gynecology* **85**: 24–29.

Neuwirth RS (1985) Hysteroscopic resection of submucous leiomyoma. *Contemporary Obstetrics and Gynecology* **25**: 103.

Neuwirth RS, Amin HK (1976) Excision of submucous fibroids with hysteroscopic control. *American Journal of Obstetrics and Gynecology* **126**: 95.

Valle RF (1990) Hysteroscopic removal of submucous leiomyomas. *Journal of Gynecologic Surgery* **6**: 89–96.

52

Diagnostic Hysteroscopy: Technique and Documentation

KEES WAMSTEKER AND SJOERD DE BLOK

Hysteroscopy Training Center, Haarlem, The Netherlands

Introduction

For many decades diagnosis of intrauterine disorders has been performed with dilatation and curettage (D and C) and hysterography. The relatively thick myometrial wall allows 'blind' sharp scraping of the endometrium from its substratum, apparently without permanent damage to the mucosa or the organ itself.

For the diagnosis or exclusion of endometrial cancer and hyperplasia D and C has appeared to be very effective as it is a good method to obtain adequate tissue samples for histologic examination from the uterine cavity. However, following the development of appropriate techniques for hysteroscopic visualization of the uterine cavity (Edström and Fernström, 1970; Lindemann, 1971), it has become apparent that D and C is unreliable for diagnosing other intrauterine pathology, especially benign tumors – direct visual inspection of the uterine cavity has revealed endometrial polyps, submucous fibroids and synechiae that D and C failed to reveal. In addition, hysteroscopic endosurgery has developed, enabling endosurgical treatment of almost all of these disorders with minimally invasive therapy, and requiring no or very short hospitalization.

Hysterosalpingography (HSG) is mainly used in infertility patients to detect intracavitary and tubal pathology. The reliability of the results depends upon the technique used. Comparison with hysteroscopic examination has demonstrated both false positive and false negative HSG uterine cavity findings. Hysterographic filling defects suggest intrauterine disorders and warrant further diagnosis. Hysteroscopy has appeared to be the most reliable method for determining the nature of intracavitary hysterographic abnormalities and defining the necessity for treatment. Hysterography is useful as a screening method, but it does not exclude intrauterine or (peri)tubal pathology.

More recently ultrasonography and especially transvaginal sonography (TVS) has developed into an effective tool for detecting (intra)uterine abnormalities:

- In postmenopausal bleeding a double layer thickness of the endometrium of 4 mm or less almost completely excludes intracavitary or endometrial pathology.
- In premenopausal women the method is less reliable, although intrauterine tumors like myomas and endometrial polyps will generally be detected or suspected.

The exact nature and localization of the pathology, however, can be rather difficult to determine with this indirect visual technique, which also lacks the facility for obtaining directed histologic specimens. As these aspects are of great importance in assessing the possibilities for successful transvaginal endosurgery, abnormal intrauterine findings with TVS should almost always lead to hysteroscopic direct visual and histologic diagnosis. TVS is the screening method while hysteroscopy is the diagnostic method – the techniques should be used together and not in competition.

Indications

Abnormal Uterine Bleeding

Abnormal uterine bleeding is the most common complaint of patients consulting the gynecologist and provides the most frequent indication for hysterectomy. D and C has been the diagnostic method of choice for many decades for these cases. However, for diagnosing non-malignant intrauterine pathology such as endometrial polyps (Figure 52.1) and intrauterine leiomyomas (Figure 52.2), which may cause uterine bleeding disorders, D and C appears to be unreliable (Wamsteker, 1977, 1984a; Gimpelson and Rappold, 1988; Loffer 1989; Motashaw and Dave, 1990).

Direct hysteroscopic inspection with adequate distention and visualization discloses almost every intrauterine abnormality with high accuracy. Additionally, it enables exact localization of the pathology and determination of its intracavitary extent. However, for the diagnosis of endometritis and adenomyosis, conclusive hysteroscopic criteria are still lacking.

For histologic examination selective samples of any abnormal tissue can be obtained by visually controlled biopsies. A significant percentage of benign intrauterine pathology disclosed by hysteroscopic diagnosis in patients with abnormal uterine bleeding can be treated with minimally invasive transcervical hysteroscopic endosurgery.

As the majority of intrauterine disorders resulting in abnormal uterine bleeding in the reproductive phase of life, the climacteric and the postmenopausal period, are benign types of pathology, D and C can no longer hold its position as the

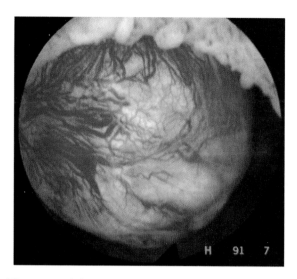

Figure 52.2 Submucous myoma with typical stretched and dilated capsular vessels.

primary diagnostic method for patients with abnormal uterine bleeding. Today ambulant or outpatient hysteroscopy with visually directed biopsies or directed curettage is to be recommended as the diagnostic method of choice for these cases.

With the more recently developed continuous flow (CF) technique the surface structure of the endometrium can be observed with very low intrauterine pressure, which prevents compression of the soft tissue of the mucosa and also reduces the transtubal flow of the distention medium.

Extensive studies have not indicated any negative effect of abdominal spill of the gas or liquid used for distention of the uterine cavity in panoramic hysteroscopy in cases of endometrial cancer (Wamsteker, 1977; Neis *et al.*, 1994).

Johnsson (1973) studied 764 patients with endometrial cancer stage I and II with a follow-up of 5–14 years. In all patients the diagnosis was made by curettage and in 606 patients hysterography had been performed before and sometimes during the treatment. In 158 patients no hysterography had been performed. The percentage of tumor recurrences and/or distant metastases was 30% in the non-hysterography group and 24% in the hysterography group. There was no significant difference in the localization of the recurrences in both groups. In the hysterography group abdominal spill of the contrast medium occurred in 72% and intravasation in 29% of the cases. The relation of tubal spill and recurrences or metastases could be studied in 592 patients. Tubal spill of the contrast medium occurred in 77% and intravasation in 28% of the patients who did not develop recurrences or metastases. In the patients with recurrences or metastases tubal spill occurred in 60% and intrava-

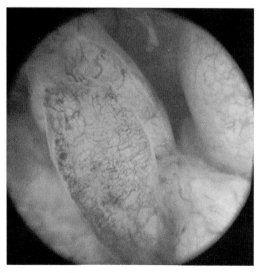

Figure 52.1 Endometrial polyp with atypical vessel structure.

sation in 31%. From this study the abdominal spill of fluid, applied under pressure in the uterine cavity in endometrial carcinoma, does not seem to have a negative effect on the prognosis.

In addition, intra-abdominal spread of intrauterine particles has been demonstrated during D and C (Barents and van der Kolk, 1975), but does not apparently increase the occurrence of recurrences or metastases in endometrial cancer. During curettage and even during bimanual palpation in patients with endometrial cancer tumor cells have been demonstrated in the inferior vena cava and the cubital vein (Roberts *et al.*, 1960).

Review of the literature does not indicate that hysteroscopy with abdominal spill of the distention medium should be considered more hazardous in cases of endometrial cancer than D and C used alone. Although D and C will seldom fail to disclose endometrial cancer (Figure 52.3) and hyperplasia, hysteroscopic investigation additionally enables the early detection of small endometrial cancers and determination of the localization, size and extent of the neoplasia and/or its precursors. Notwithstanding the above-mentioned considerations it seems to be sensible to recommend reducing transabdominal spill of distention medium as much as possible in these cases. This can be achieved by reducing the intrauterine working pressure during hysteroscopy in cases suspected of endometrial cancer.

Specific indications for hysteroscopic diagnosis in patients with abnormal uterine bleeding are:

- Hypermenorrhea or menorrhagia.
- Metrorrhagia.
- Intermenstrual bleeding.

- Postmenopausal bleeding.
- Intrauterine or endometrial abnormality on TVS or HSG.

In cases of cervical dysplasia or malignancy accurate *in vivo* diagnosis on a cellular level can be performed with contact microcolpohysteroscopy (Hamou, 1981). However, experience with determining cytologic pathology is a prerequisite for this technique.

Infertility

Hysteroscopic diagnosis and treatment appear to have been very important in patients with infertility or recurrent pregnancy loss. The method should be considered as complementary to TVS and HSG rather than competing with them in these patients.

Diagnostic hysteroscopy is always needed for intrauterine filling defects on HSG (Figure 52.4) to confirm or exclude pathology and to determine the nature of an abnormality and the possibilities for transcervical endosurgical treatment. If the filling defects are caused by intrauterine adhesions (IUAs, Figure 52.5), for which treatment by hysteroscopy is the method of choice, any other 'blind' intrauterine procedure can deteriorate the possibilities for hysteroscopic treatment by creating a false route or perforation and reducing the amount of residual normal endometrium, which is required for adequate regeneration after synechiolysis.

A diagnosis of IUAs can only be made with certainty by hysteroscopy (March, 1989) and the extent of the IUAs should be evaluated with hysteroscopy and HSG. To be able to compare the results of treatment and determine the therapeutic regimen, the adhesions should be classified from the hysteroscopic and HSG findings according to the IUA classification of the European Society for Gynaecologic

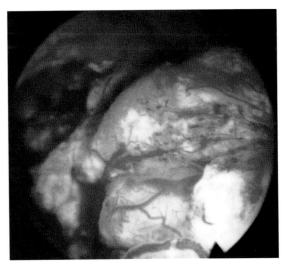

Figure 52.3 Adenocarcinoma of the endometrium with an irregular surface with necrosis and dilated tortuous vessels.

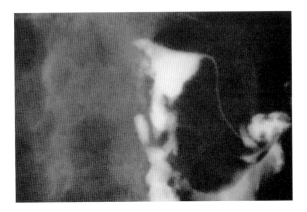

Figure 52.4 HSG with intrauterine filling defects caused by grade III IUAs (ESGE classification, see text).

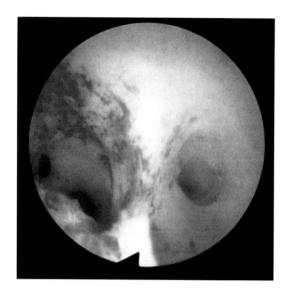

Figure 52.5 Grade III IUAs (ESGE classification, see text).

cavitary filling defects during HSG in infertility patients. In these cases hysteroscopic diagnosis will disclose the nature and extent of the pathology and the possibilities for endosurgical treatment (Figure 52.6). To be able to determine the (endo)surgical technique to use the classification for submucous

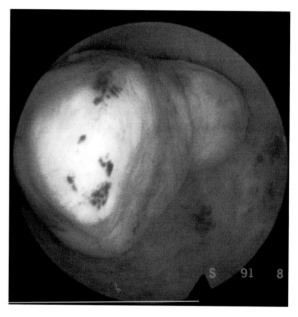

Figure 52.6 Submucous myoma without intramural extension (type 0, ESGE classification).

Endoscopy (ESGE) (Table 52.1) (Wamsteker, 1984b, 1997). In some cases the initial classification has to be changed during treatment.

Submucous myomas can be a reason for infertility or pregnancy loss (Kistner, 1971; Wallach, 1979). They generally cause abnormal uterine bleeding, but may be asymptomatic and only present as intra-

Table 52.1 ESGE classification of IUAs (1995 version). (Wamsteker, 1984b, 1997, Hysteroscopy Training Centre, Spaarne Hospital, Haarlem, The Netherlands.)

Grade	Extent of intrauterine adhesions*
I	Thin or filmy adhesions Easily ruptured by hysteroscope sheath alone Cornual areas normal
II	Singular dense adhesion Connecting separate areas of the uterine cavity Visualization of both tubal ostia possible Cannot be ruptured by hysteroscope sheath alone
IIa	Occluding adhesions only in the region of the internal cervical os† Upper uterine cavity normal
III	Multiple dense adhesions Connecting separate areas of the uterine cavity Unilateral obliteration of ostial areas of the tubes
IV	Extensive dense adhesions with (partial) occlusion of the uterine cavity Both tubal ostial areas (partially) occluded
Va	Extensive endometrial scarring and fibrosis in combination with grade I or grade II adhesions With amenorrhea or pronounced hypomenorrhea
Vb	Extensive endometrial scarring and fibrosis in combination with grade III or grade IV adhesions† With amenorrhea

*From findings at hysteroscopy and hysterography.
†Only to be classified during hysteroscopic treatment.

Table 52.2 ESGE classification of submucous myomas. (Wamsteker *et al.*, 1993, Hysteroscopy Training Centre, Spaarne Hospital, Haarlem, The Netherlands.)

Type	Degree of intramural extension
0	No intramural extension
I	Intramural extension < 50%
II	Intramural extension ≥ 50%

myomas of the European Society for Gynaecological Endoscopy according to their intramural extent (Wamsteker *et al.*, 1993; Emanuel and Wamsteker, 1997; Table 52.2) can be used. This classification should be part of the presurgical assessment of these intrauterine tumors in infertility patients. Submucous myomas without or with only limited intramural extension should be treated with endoresection as soon as the diagnosis has been made, as with increasing size, endoresection will become more difficult.

Other intrauterine disorders that may interfere with fertility and cause bleeding abnormalities are endometrial polyps, endometrial hyperplasia and endometritis. An abnormal uterine bleeding pattern in patients with infertility and ovulatory cycles always warrants diagnostic hysteroscopy or at least TVS. Hysteroscopy also offers the possibility of obtaining visually directed biopsies for studying the endometrial structure and cyclic development.

It is questionable whether diagnostic hysteroscopy should be performed early in the work-up of every infertility patient. The results do not seem to justify this policy as intrauterine disorders are seldom the primary cause of the infertility (Wamsteker, 1977; Surrey and Aronberg, 1984). However, hysteroscopy is indicated if there is a concomitant bleeding abnormality or a history of a complicated intrauterine procedure. Laparoscopy for infertility reasons should always be combined with hysteroscopy. This combination can be performed instead of HSG, providing a complete investigation of the anatomy of the internal genital organs in specific cases.

In cases of recurrent pregnancy loss hysteroscopy is indicated to exclude or diagnose intrauterine causes such as a congenital uterine malformation, intrauterine adhesions or submucous myomas, and to determine the possibilities for treatment with transcervical endosurgery.

Specific indications for diagnostic hysteroscopy in infertility patients are:

- Abnormal uterine bleeding.
- History of complicated intrauterine procedures or uterine surgery.

- History of recurrent pregnancy loss.
- Intrauterine abnormalities on TVS.
- Abnormalities of the uterine cavity or intrauterine filling defects with HSG.
- Together with laparoscopy if no hysteroscopy has been performed before.
- Infertility with unknown cause.
- Unsuccessful *in vitro* fertilization and embryo transfer (IVF–ET) if no hysteroscopy has been performed before.

Other Indications

SECONDARY DYSMENORRHEA

As secondary dysmenorrhea often appears to be due to intrauterine disorders such as submucous myomas, endometrial polyps or IUAs, hysteroscopic diagnosis should be performed in these cases as first diagnostic method.

'MISSING' INTRAUTERINE CONTRACEPTIVE DEVICE (IUCD)

If the retrieval threads of an IUCD are not visible, its location can be determined by ultrasonography. If ultrasonography indicates an abnormal position or if the IUCD has to be removed, hysteroscopy is the method of choice to visualize its complete or partial intrauterine position and to remove the IUCD safely under direct visual control.

COMPLICATED INTRAUTERINE MANIPULATIONS RELATED TO PREGNANCY

As most cases of intrauterine synechiae have their origin in instrumental intrauterine manipulations related to pregnancy, it may be worth performing diagnostic hysteroscopy six weeks or two months after such procedures. Grade I (Figure 52.7) or grade II IUAs (ESGE classification, see Table 52.1) have appeared to be rather frequently present and should be treated as soon as possible to prevent fibrotic extension. IUAs tend to extend and become tougher and more fibrotic with time. Early diagnosis and treatment appears to enhance fertility. Puerperal curettage for persisting bleeding or partially retained placenta and repeat evacuation after incomplete abortion curettage are especially notorious for the development of IUAs.

CONTROL OF INTRAUTERINE ENDOSURGERY

The results of intrauterine endosurgery should always be evaluated with a control hysteroscopy

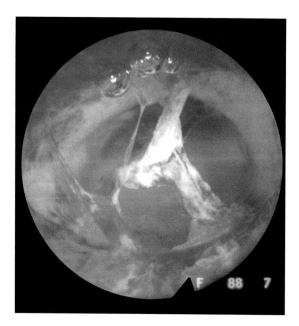

Figure 52.7 Fragile grade I IUAs (ESGE classification).

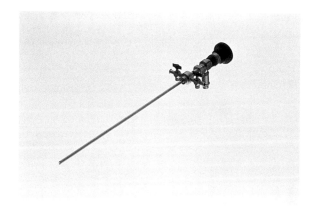

Figure 52.9 Single flow diagnostic hysteroscope with a 3 mm 30° foreoblique telescope and a 4 mm outer sheath (Olympus, Hamburg, Germany).

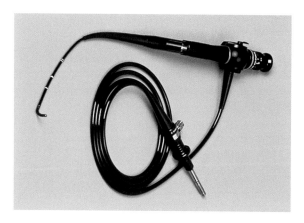

Figure 52.8 3.6 mm flexible fiberoptic hysteroscope (Olympus, Hamburg, Germany).

hysteroscopes – either a 3.6 mm flexible hysteroscope (single flow) or a 4 mm (single flow) or 4.5 mm (continuous flow) rigid hysteroscope with a 3 mm 30° foreoblique telescope (Figures 52.8–52.10).

For distension of the uterine cavity carbon dioxide (CO_2) or a low viscosity liquid can be used. CO_2 distention is especially suitable for office procedures as it is clean and requires only an insufflator (Figure 52.11). On the other hand gas distension will sometimes not provide adequate visualization due to mucus bubbles or blood in the uterine cavity. In these cases liquid distension with a continuous flow hysteroscope is to be preferred. To prevent having to repeat an inconclusive diagnostic procedure with CO_2 a 4.5 mm continuous flow hysteroscope with liquid distension should be available at the office.

two or three months after the procedure to assess endometrial healing, to exclude residual pathology and to remove adhesions, if present.

Hysteroscopy Settings and Instrumentation

Diagnostic hysteroscopy can be performed in the office, at an outpatient unit or in the operating theater.

Office Hysteroscopy

Hysteroscopy in the office is meant for pure diagnostic procedures, without anesthesia and without intervention. It should be performed with small size

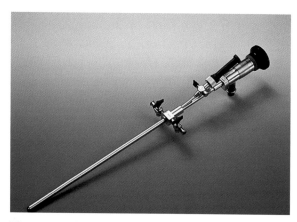

Figure 52.10 Design of 4.5 (3 mm telescope) and 5.5 mm (4 mm telescope) diagnostic continuous flow hysteroscope (Olympus, Hamburg, Germany); the in- and outflow channels are completely separate.

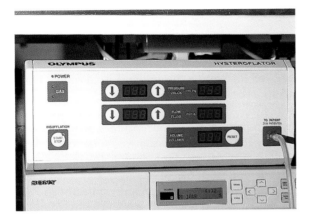

Figure 52.11 CO_2 insufflator for hysteroscopy with separately adjustable flow rate (max 100 ml min^{-1}) and intrauterine pressure (maximum 200 mm Hg) (Olympus, Hamburg, Germany).

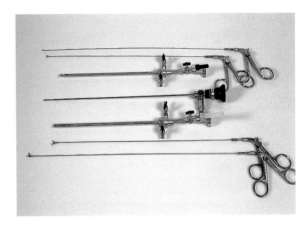

Figure 52.12 Operative 5.5 and 6.5 mm continuous flow hysteroscopes with 3 mm 30° telescope (Olympus, Hamburg, Germany) for minor interventions during diagnostic outpatient hysteroscopy.

The liquid used can be dextrose 5%, saline, lactated Ringer's, sorbitol 4 or 5%, glycine 1.5% or a sorbitol–mannitol solution. The liquid bag must be at least 1 m above the patient or an inflatable pressure cuff for 100–150 mm Hg infusion pressure should be available. In case of a very tight internal os it is useful to have a local anesthetic agent available.

Outpatient Unit

At the outpatient unit diagnostic hysteroscopic procedures can be combined with minor interventions. As additional assisting personnel are generally available the use of a rigid continuous flow hysteroscope with low viscosity liquid distension is preferred. For interventions pressurized liquid and local anesthesia must be available. In some cases the procedures may be performed under general anesthesia. The most appropriate instruments consist of a 3 mm 30° foreoblique wide angle telescope with 4.5, 5.5 and 6.5 mm continuous flow sheaths. Diagnostic procedures are performed with the 4.5 mm sheath and if interventions are required the outer sheath can be replaced with a 5.5 (for 5F instruments) or 6.5 (for 7F instruments) mm sheath (Figure 52.12). If high-frequency electrosurgical instruments are used saline should not be applied for uterine distension and only non-conductive liquids must be used.

With a 4.5 mm sheath the diagnostic procedure can be performed without anesthesia in 90% of the cases without significant discomfort to the patient. For interventions with the 5.5 or 6.5 mm sheath local anesthesia is required in approximately 50–75% of the cases depending upon the tightness of the internal os.

For diagnostic procedures at an outpatient unit flexible hysteroscopes can be used as well; however, they are not recommended as rigid continuous flow hysteroscopes perform much better. For the same reason the use of (pressurized) low viscosity liquid is preferred instead of CO_2.

Operating Theater

If an ambulatory outpatient unit is available diagnostic hysteroscopic procedures will only be performed in the operating theater for specific cases:

- Before an operative procedure to check the pathology.
- Combined with another procedure requiring regional or general anesthesia.
- In patients requiring general anesthesia.
- In patients who have already been admitted to the hospital.

Sometimes all diagnostic hysteroscopies are performed in the clinic at the operating theater.

As most diagnostic procedures at the operating theater will be performed with general anesthesia the diameter of the hysteroscope is not too important, which makes the 4 mm 30° telescope the most appropriate to use as it provides a larger and brighter image and is less fragile than a 3 mm telescope. For diagnostic procedures it is combined with a 5.5 mm continuous flow sheath and (preferably pressurized) liquid distension. In the operating theater saline should not be used as confusion may arise with resectoscopic procedures, which do not allow saline for uterine distension.

For interventions the 5.5 mm sheath can be replaced by a 7 or 8 mm continuous flow operating sheath with 5 or 7F semi-rigid instruments, electro-surgical probes or laser fibers.

Techniques

Some general rules concerning the technique are of great importance:

- A diagnostic hysteroscopic procedure should, if at all possible, be scheduled in the first half of the menstrual cycle.
- The hysteroscope should always be introduced into the uterine cavity under direct visual control.
- The technique should be a no-touch technique as far as possible.
- The hysteroscope should never be advanced towards the fundal area without adequate visualization or uterine distension as this can cause bleeding, endometrial damage, a false route and eventually perforation.
- To benefit from the advantages of the 30° telescope of rigid instruments the hysteroscope must be rotated in combination with horizontal and vertical movements.

During office or outpatient procedures vagal reactions can be prevented with 0.5 mg atropine administered intramuscularly 15 minutes before the procedure. Painful myometrial contractions during uterine distension can be prevented by the administration of a prostaglandin synthetase inhibitor orally two hours before the procedure.

The techniques for flexible and rigid hysteroscopy will be discussed separately.

Flexible Hysteroscopy

With the small diameter of 3.6 mm flexible hysteroscopes are especially suitable for diagnostic procedures in the office. The use of a tenaculum attached to the cervix is often not necessary. Many physicians prefer to use pressurized liquid distension medium such as saline or lactated Ringer's, others prefer CO_2. With liquids some fluid must be able to flow out through the cervix to enable flushing of the uterine cavity.

To pass the internal cervical os the endocervical canal should be in the middle of the image to prevent angling of the tip. This can be accomplished by moving the tip with the thumb manipulator, which is also used to bend the tip for complete visualization of the cornual areas. A flexible biopsy forceps can be used for tissue sampling for histologic examination.

Rigid Hysteroscopy

With the use of 4 or 5 mm single flow hysteroscopes CO_2 or a 32% dextran 70 (Hyskon ®) solution should be used for uterine distention. Visualization, however, can be hampered by mucus or blood, especially with CO_2. In this case a 4.5 or 5.5 mm continuous flow hysteroscope with a non-viscous liquid performs much better. For this reason we prefer to use these instruments as standard equipment for the outpatient unit and the operating room. The liquid should be infused under pressure either by gravity with the bag 1 m above the patient or by an inflatable pressure cuff. With a pressure cuff at 150 mm Hg visualization and cleaning of the uterine cavity is much faster than when using gravity pressures.

After insertion of the hysteroscope into the endocervix the endocervical canal must be visualized with rotating upwards, downwards, or lateral movements of the hysteroscope. Because the telescope has a 30° viewing angle a panoramic view will only be obtained if the hysteroscope is positioned at an angle towards the axis of the endocervical canal. The internal os must be passed with the 'blunt' angle of the tip of the hysteroscope just beneath the anterior wall. The posterior wall should not be visible in the image as this will result in detachment of the endometrium by the 'sharp' angle of the tip. Once in the uterine cavity the hysteroscope is advanced under visual control towards the fundal area and the cavity is flushed to clear it completely. Touching of the endometrium should be avoided as much as possible.

With continuous flow distension the outflow stopcock remains open all the time unless it has to be partially closed to accomplish adequate distension. With CO_2 distension the internal cervical os must fit closely round the sheath as considerable gas leakage through the cervix leads to failure. If there is a patulous cervix a vacuum adapter or a vertical tenaculum can be applied to prevent gas leakage. The hysteroscope should only be advanced through the uterine cavity when mucus bubbles have disappeared and adequate distension and visualization have been accomplished.

Minor Intrauterine Procedures

In a significant number of cases minor intrauterine diagnostic or therapeutic interventions can be performed during a diagnostic procedure, for example:

- Biopsies.
- Polypectomy.
- Synechiolysis.
- Focal coagulation.

An operating hysteroscope with working channel and operating instruments should therefore be available at a diagnostic hysteroscopy unit. Preferably this should be a continuous flow instrument (see Figure 52.10) because of the excellent performance with low viscosity liquid distension in difficult diagnostic procedures and minor endo-surgical interventions.

Documentation

The most frequently used methods for documenting endoscopic findings are handwritten reports with or without drawings. These reports can be made immediately after an endoscopic procedure and stored in the patient record file. However, describing endoscopic findings appears to be difficult and the descriptions are often unclear to others. Good quality drawings explain more than a careful description, but are time-consuming and strictly dependent upon the artistry of the endoscopist.

Hysteroscopic findings should be described schematically, mentioning both negative and positive findings at the different levels of the uterine cavity: the endocervical canal, the internal cervical ostium, the isthmus, the fundal and both cornual areas and the tubal ostia. Flow of the distention medium through the tubal ostium must be evaluated and reported. The appearance of the endocervical mucosa and the endometrium should be described. A preprinted diagram of the uterus with transections at different levels of the uterus can be used for immediate documentation in the patient's file.

It is beyond doubt that good quality pictures say much more than written reports or poor drawings. Modern technology and instruments have made imaging in endoscopy much easier with a constant quality. Visual image documentation with photography or video recording has become very important for teaching, education and evaluation of treatment.

Storage and retrieval of hard copy material has always been one of the main drawbacks in using these methods of documentation. Optical disc recorders coupled with computer systems solve these problems with a high storage capacity and instantaneous computerized retrieval possibilities. This equipment, however, is still expensive.

In hysteroscopic photography and video documentation the complete documentation system can be considered to be an 'imaging chain' from light source to film or videotape (Figure 52.13) (Wamsteker, 1989). The most important factor is the

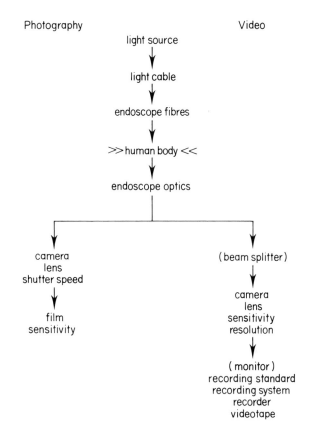

Figure 52.13 The 'imaging chain' in photographic and video documentation in endoscopy.

transmission of light into the human body and the quality of the endoscopic optics will be responsible for the final endoscopic image. The end result of the documentation relies upon the quality of each individual component of this chain. Each connection in this chain reduces the quality, with non-fitting connections being very detrimental to the process.

In photography five technical parts with five different connections (optical, magnetic and/or electronic) have to be in good order to complete the chain of documentation. Video recording requires six or even seven technical parts with seven or eight connections. Each part of the imaging chain needs to be compatible to obtain optimal end results. Equipment from one manufacturer does not usually fit with another manufacturer's connections. This aspect should be thoroughly investigated before buying equipment.

Since the uterus is a small dark red organ the light source and conduction of light are important contributors to the quality of the image. As hysteroscopy today is preferably performed with a video camera a high capacity light source becomes indispensable. For optimal documentation the capacity should be 300 W. Most of these light sources can be used for both photography and video recording. The light intensity and/or film speed as well as the exposure time in photography are generally automatically regulated by the light source. If not, an automatic camera is required, in which case the light intensity from the light source must be high enough to prevent long exposure times, which may result in blurred pictures.

The quality of the light cables is also important and should be the first thing checked if the quality of documentation is poor. Fiberoptic and fluid cables are available. Fluid cables are less flexible than fiber cables, but have increased light transmission. If there is fluid leakage they are worthless. Fiberglass cables should be checked regularly for ruptured fibers as this significantly reduces the light transmission. Olympus light guide cables (Olympus, Hamburg, Germany) have condenser lens systems at the tip to improve the focus at the light source–light cable and the light cable–hysteroscope connections, which produces a higher light intensity.

With the Olympus CLV-S light source (Olympus, Tokyo, Japan; Figure 52.14), which has a special 'high intensity' mode, special light guide cables have to be used with a filter. Normal standard light cables would burn immediately in the high-intensity mode. The performance of this light source in hysteroscopic imaging and documentation is excellent and fully automatic.

The condition of the telescope is another important factor in the 'imaging chain'. Damage of the light conduction fibers or of the optical lens system of the telescope will result in bad imaging and documentation quality. This can be brought about by lens fractures after dropping, fluid in the telescope due to leakage or steam sterilization of non-autoclavable telescopes.

A factor that is not directly equipment-related is the intrauterine environment. Atrophic endometrium is easy to image and document. In a uterine cavity with blood, the red color will absorb much of the light, significantly reducing the quality of photographs and video recordings. In these cases flushing the uterine cavity or the use of continuous flow hysteroscopes is advised before documentation.

Photography and video recording as the final parts of the 'imaging chain' will be discussed separately.

Photography

For hysteroscopic photography a 35 mm single-lens mirror reflex camera with 'through the lens' (TTL) exposure metering is preferred (Figure 52.15). This camera can only be used for endoscopic photography because the groundglass focusing screen has been replaced by a clear glass screen. Standardized adaptors between the telescope and the camera are available. For external flash generators only a non-automatic camera body can be used. Some automatic flash generators require an automatic camera body (light measurement in the camera body), while others will cope with a non-automatic body (light measurement in the lens) (Figure 52.16). Accessory equipment for cameras include:

- Motor drive winder for film advance.
- Record data-back for superimposition of different items of information.

Figure 52.14 High-power light source for video imaging and photography in hysteroscopy (Olympus, Tokyo, Japan); special light guide cables must be used in the high-intensity mode.

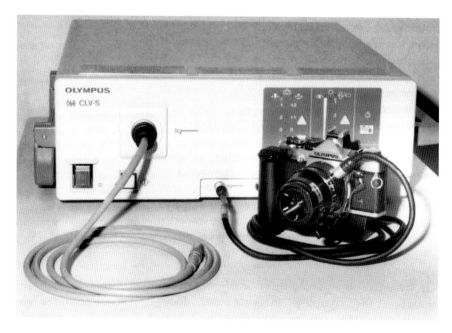

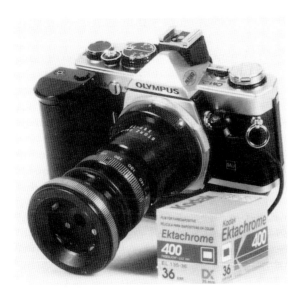

Figure 52.15 Automatic mirror reflex camera body with motor drive winder for film advance, record data-back and zoom lens (Olympus, Tokyo, Japan).

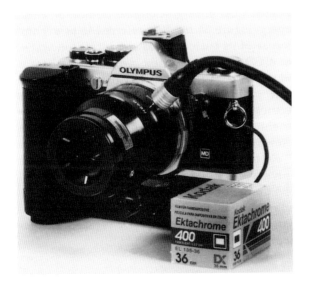

Figure 52.16 Automatic light adjustment with light measurement in the camera lens (Olympus, Tokyo, Japan); a non-automatic camera body can be used.

The quality of the lens of the camera is a very important feature in hysteroscopic photography. The aperture of the lens is calibrated in F- stops. The lower the F-number, the larger the lens opening (more light), but the less the depth of field. The focal length of the lens (f in mm) determines how much of the frame of the 35 mm film is exposed (Marlow, 1989). Some manufacturers provide zoom lenses with a focal length of 70–140 mm.

The film should be color-slide film balanced for electronic flash, the so-called 'daylight' film, emphasizing the blue light spectrum with temperatures between 5000–6100 K. The best results are obtained with professional films. However, these films must be stored at $\leq 13\,^{\circ}C$ and be removed from the refrigerator one hour before use. For good results, processing should be performed as soon as possible after use (Marlow, 1983).

Film sensitivity is designated by the ASA (American Standards Association), DIN (German equivalent) or ISO (comparable to ASA) number. For hysteroscopic photography ASA 400 provides the best results. Films with increased sensitivity may be used in situations with low light intensity, but will reduce the definition of the image. It is very important to take many pictures at different light intensities and shutter speeds and to choose only the best few for filing.

Video Documentation

The introduction of the miniature electronic chip cameras has increased the possibilities for video imaging in endoscopy. Both in hysteroscopy and laparoscopy direct viewing through the endoscope has largely been replaced by video endoscopy, in which the surgeon works directly from the video screen. Facilitated by this development video recording in specific cases has become a routine procedure.

VIDEO STANDARDS

Many different norm-standards exist all over the world (Wamsteker, 1989). The most important of these are:

- The PAL (phase alternating line) standard used in Western Europe (except for France), most countries in the Far East, most African countries, Australia and New Zealand.
- The NTSC (National Television Standard Committee) standard, also referred to as 'never the same color' because of its color instability, used in Northern America, Japan, some South American and Asian countries.
- The SECAM (Séquentiel Couleur a Mémoire) standard, used mainly in France and Eastern Europe and also in some African and some Asian countries.

Most professional equipment in Europe can be used for either PAL or SECAM and recently video players and monitors have become available that are also suitable for NTSC. For translation of videotapes from PAL to NTSC or vice versa, special norm-translation equipment is always necessary. The most important differences between PAL and NTSC are the differing color coding and number of image lines (PAL/SECAM 625 lines; NTSC 525 lines). PAL is more expensive, but has a higher stability and a true color reproduction, while NTSC has color instability due to atmospheric interferences and other disturbances. Using videotape recordings in different countries requires knowledge of the used video standard and, if applicable, norm-translation into the appropriate standard.

VIDEO SYSTEMS

The differing incompatible video standards complicate international video communication and exchange, and these complications are compounded by the various video recording systems and tape formats, which are also incompatible (Gisolf, 1987). Professional quality required two- or one-inch tape width for a long time, but more recently a 0.75 inch U-matic 'SP (superior performance) high-band' recording (also called BVU) with U-matic SP tapes is accepted as a professional (or broadcast) system. U-matic SP recordings are not compatible with U-matic low-band recorders (no color reproduction). The most recent Sony recorders (Sony Corporation, Tokyo, Japan), however, can accept both U-matic SP and low-band tapes (Sony VO-9600P recorder – Figure 52.17 – and the Sony VP-9000P player; Sony Corporation, Tokyo, Japan). Recording with 0.75 inch U-matic low-band is considered to be semiprofessional.

Another professional system is the Betacam or Betacam SP system, which takes a 0.5 inch Betamax cassette tape in special recording mode. A comparable professional 0.5 inch VHS counterpart is the M2 format. In 0.5 inch VHS a (semi)professional system

is also available – the Super VHS recorders and tapes with a higher horizontal resolution of 400 lines (standard VHS is approximately 250 lines).

For video recording in hysteroscopy of professional quality and at reasonable costs, 0.75 inch U-matic high-band is to be preferred. U-matic 0.75 inch low-band at least should be used for recordings to be edited. For routine use standard VHS or S-VHS is acceptable. If editing is required anyway, the VHS tape should be upgraded to U-matic SP high-band, Betacam SP or even one inch and edited at this format. After editing, the mastertape can be translated to VHS again. Editing in the normal VHS format will lead to too much loss of quality. At this moment not enough experience is available with the 8 mm format (V8) to comment on its use in hysteroscopic documentation and editing capabilities.

VIDEO CAMERA

An important breakthrough in the use of video in endoscopy has been the development of the so-called CCD (charge-coupled device) or 'chip' camera (Figure 52.18). It is referred to as a 'chip' because of its basic form as a silicon wafer. The CCD is an integrated circuit image sensor and depends upon the sensitivity of silicon to light. Light striking a silicone device decreases the electrical resistance of the silicon and generates current carriers. The photosensitive silicon elements store and transfer information as packets of electrical charge, which can be amplified. Individual picture elements are called 'pixels' and the number of pixels determines the sensitivity and resolution of the 'chip' (Sivak, 1986). The way the electrical charges are moved on the device is called 'charge-coupling'.

CCD video cameras are very small and light in weight, have a high sensitivity and relatively high resolution, and can be immersed in disinfecting

Figure 52.17 The Sony VO-9600P U-matic recorder (Sony Corporation, Tokyo, Japan) can be used for SP high- and low-band recordings.

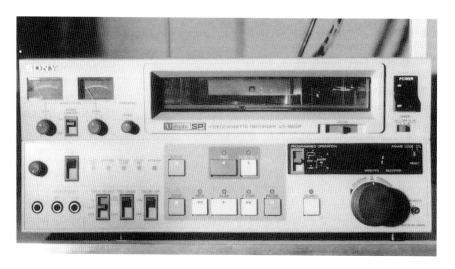

Figure 52.18 CCD video camera for endoscopy (Olympus, Tokyo, Japan).

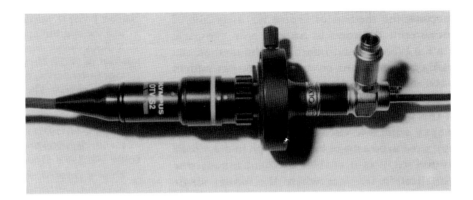

solutions. Recently autoclavable CCD cameras have been experimentally developed by Olympus. The cameras are connected with a cable to a camera control unit (CCU), which regulates light adjustment (via the light source) automatically or manually, color adjustment and (auto) white balance.

Most modern cameras have auto gain control (AGC), which can compensate for the reflections of very bright sites of the image. Most modern video light sources have an automatic brightness control function combined with the camera. The camera can be mounted directly on the ocular end of the hysteroscope (video endoscopy) or with a beam splitter, which also enables direct viewing through the hysteroscope.

Video endoscopy refers to a method, while the name video endoscope refers to an instrument. Electronic video endoscopes, with a CCD chip at the distal end of a flexible hysteroscope and mainly used in gastroenterology are not available for hysteroscopy and will not in the near future be competitive with the optical quality of the rigid telescopes due to the required limitation of the diameter.

MONITOR

High-quality professional RGB monitors should be used. They must be equipped with the same norm-standard as used in the video imaging system. Most modern professional monitors are multi-norm and can be used with PAL, SECAM and NTSC standards.

Most manufacturers recommend their own special monitors, which does not seem to provide specific advantages.

RECORDER

As stated before, a good quality recording system for hysteroscopy is the 0.75 inch U-matic low-band

system. For very high quality and professional recordings 0.75 inch U-matic SP high-band (BVU) should be used. The most widely used U-matic video recorders are the Sony VO-5600 (0.75 inch U-matic low-band) and the Sony VO-9600P (0.75 inch U-matic SP high- and low-band, see Figure 52.17). For routine use any good quality VHS recorder can be applied. The norm-standard again has to match the one used in the video imaging system.

VIDEO PRINTING

High quality video printers, like the Sony UP-5000P (Sony Corporation, Tokyo, Japan) with about 10–12 dots mm^{-2} provide an excellent alternative to hard copy photography. Printouts can be used for patient records and are of much better quality than the hard copies of presently available instant photography cameras. However, reproduction of slides from video prints is always lower quality than direct slide photography on good quality film.

HIGH-FREQUENCY INTERFERENCE

Several hysteroscopic surgical techniques are performed with high-frequency current. The frequency of the current has to exceed a lower frequency limit to avoid muscle and nerve stimmulation and is usually in the range of 300 kHz–2 MHz. As these frequencies are situated within the bandwidth of every video imaging system, this can cause electromagnetic interference to a video imaging system in use during electrosurgery (Flachenecker, 1987). The video system therefore has to be electromagnetically shielded or the high-frequency power of the electrosurgical unit must be reduced. Both techniques are applied in the most recently developed equipment.

Summary

Technological developments and new techniques have made hysteroscopy with visually directed biopsies the method of choice for the diagnosis of intrauterine disorders in patients with abnormal uterine bleeding and infertility. The method can easily be performed on an ambulant or outpatient basis and is, in combination with ultrasonography, almost completely replacing diagnostic D and C in these cases.

Flexible hysteroscopes are often used for office procedures. The performance of new small size continuous flow hysteroscopes with low viscosity fluid distension appears to be a major breakthrough in diagnostic hysteroscopy for office and outpatient procedures as it enables excellent intrauterine visualization in cases where the former single flow instruments failed. With this technique minor intrauterine endosurgical interventions have also become easy routine procedures.

Diagnostic hysteroscopy further opens the way to minimally invasive and uterus-preserving transcervical endosurgery.

Modern hysteroscopy is to be performed as video endoscopy with a CCD video camera directly coupled to the ocular of the hysteroscope. High-quality documentation with photography, video prints, video recording or optic disk storage has become an indispensable tool for communication, teaching and filing of endoscopic data.

References

Barents JW, van der Kolk G (1975) Iatrogene migratie van cellen en weefselelementen bij curettage. *Nederlands Tijdschrift voor Geneeskunde* **119**: 229–232.

Edström K, Fernström I (1970) The diagnostic possibilities of a modified hysteroscopic technique. *Acta Obstetricia et Gynecologica Scandinavica* **49**: 327–330.

Emanuel MH, Wamsteker K (1997) Uterine leiomyomas. In Brosens I, Wamsteker K (eds) *Diagnostic Imaging and Endoscopy in Gynecology*. pp. 185–198. London: WB Saunders.

Flachenecker G (1987) High frequency interference: Basic electrotechnical principles. In Wamsteker K, Jonas U, van der Veen G, van Waes PFGM (eds) *Imaging and Visual Documentation in Medicine*. pp. 85–94. Amsterdam: Excerpta Medica.

Gimpelson RJ, Rappold HO (1988) A comparative study between panoramic hysteroscopy with directed biopsies and dilatation and curettage. *American Journal of Obstetrics and Gynecology* **158**: 489–492.

Gisolf AC (1987) Video systems: Fighting the chaos. In Wamsteker K, Jonas U, van der Veen G, van Waes PFGM (eds) *Imaging and Visual Documentation in Medicine*. pp. 85–94. Amsterdam: Excerpta Medica.

Hamou J (1981) Microhysteroscopy: a new procedure and its original applications in gynecology. *Journal of Reproductive Medicine* **26**: 375.

Johnsson JE (1973) Hysterography and diagnostic curettage in carcinoma of the uterine body. *Acta Radiologica* **326** (Suppl): 1.

Kistner RW (1971) *Gynecology: Principles and Practice.* p. 476. Chicago: Year Book Medical Publishers.

Lindemann HJ (1971) Eine neue Untersuchungsmethode für die Hysteroskopie. *Endoscopy* **4**: 194.

Loffer FD (1989) Hysteroscopy with endometrial sampling compared with D&C for abnormal uterine bleeding. *Obstetrics and Gynecology* **73**: 16–20.

Marlow JL (1983) Endoscopic photography. *Clinical Obstetrics and Gynecology* **26**: 359–365.

Marlow JL (1989) Hysteroscopic photography. In Baggish MS, Barbot J, Valle RF (eds) *Diagnostic and Operative Hysteroscopy*. pp. 215–222. Chicago: Year Book Medical Publishers.

March CM (1989) Hysteroscopy for infertility. In Baggish MS, Barbot J, Valle RF (eds) *Diagnostic and Operative Hysteroscopy*. pp. 136–146. Chicago: Year Book Medical Publishers.

Motashaw ND, Dave S (1990) Diagnostic and therapeutic hysteroscopy in the management of abnormal uterine bleeding. *Journal of Reproductive Medicine* **35**: 616–620.

Neis KJ, Brandner P, Keppeler U (1994) Tumour cell spread via hysteroscopy? *Geburtshilfe und Frauenheilkunde* **54**: 651–655.

Roberts S, Long L, Jonasson O et al. (1960) The isolation of cancer cells from the bloodstream during uterine curettage. *Surgery, Gynecology and Obstetrics* **111**: 3.

Sivak MV (1986) Video endoscopy. *Cinics in Gastroenterology* **15**: 205–234.

Surrey MW, Aronberg S (1984) Hysteroscopic diagnosis of abnormal uterine bleeding: A clinical study. In Siegler AM, Lindemann HJ (eds) *Hysteroscopy, Principles and Practice*. pp. 121–122. Philadelphia: JB Lippincott.

Wallach EE (1979) Evaluation and management of uterine causes of infertility. *Clinical Obstetrics and Gynecology* **22**: 43–60.

Wamsteker K (1977) Hysteroscopie. PhD thesis. University of Leiden.

Wamsteker K (1984a) Hysteroscopy in the management of abnormal uterine bleeding in 199 patients. In Siegler AM, Lindemann HJ (eds) *Hysteroscopy, Principles and Practice*. pp. 128–131. Philadelphia: JB Lippincott.

Wamsteker K (1984b) Hysteroscopy in Asherman's syndrome. In Siegler AM, Lindemann HJ (eds) *Hysteroscopy, Principles and Practice*. pp. 198–203. Philadelphia: JB Lippincott.

Wamsteker K (1989) Documentation in laparoscopic surgery. *Baillière's Clinical Obstetrics and Gynaecology* **3**: 625–647.

Wamsteker K (1997) Intrauterine adhesions (synechiae). In Brosens I, Wamsteker K (eds) *Diagnostic Imaging and Endoscopy in Gynecology*. pp. 171–184. London: WB Saunders.

Wamsteker K, Emanuel MH, de Kruif JH (1993) Transcervical hysteroscopic resection of submucous fibroids for abnormal uterine bleeding: results regarding the degree of intramural extension. *Obstetrics and Gynecology* **82**: 736–740.

53

Distension Media and Fluid Systems

RAY GARRY

Women's Endoscopic Laser Foundation, South Cleveland Hospital, Middlesbrough, UK

Introduction

Continuous crystal clear vision is an essential prerequisite for safe and satisfactory hysteroscopy. The uterine walls are normally in apposition and to visualize the cavity, the walls must be separated by infusing a suitable medium under pressure.

Distension Media

Carbon Dioxide

The cavity may be distended with gas or fluid. For diagnostic hysteroscopy, particularly in the outpatient or office environment, gaseous distension media are usually preferred. The use of carbon dioxide (CO_2) was first described by Rubin (1925) and it is now the most frequently used gas. It is preferred because of its ready availability and convenience. It is the least messy of the available agents. CO_2 infused under pressure tends to flatten the endometrium and gives excellent visibility. It has virtually the same index of refraction as air and excellent photographs can be obtained with this medium.

A continuous flow is necessary to replace gas lost through the tubes, around the hysteroscope and absorbed into the uterus. The rate of flow must be carefully controlled for deaths have occurred from gas embolism. Intravasation can occur and bubbles of gas have been detected moving in the pelvic vessels during simultaneous hysteroscopy and laparoscopy (Donnez, 1989). The risk of gas embolism is proportional to the flow rate of the infused gas. Lindemann et al. (1976) demonstrated in a series of experiments in dogs that flow rates below 200 ml min^{-1} were associated with minimal changes in pulse rate and breathing. Flow rates above 400 ml min^{-1} were associated with tachypnea and arrhythmias and rates of 1000 ml min^{-1} were associated with death within 60 seconds. Physiologic mechanisms can cope with the transport of 150 ml min^{-1} of CO_2 without the risk of embolism or metabolic disturbance. Hulf et al. (1979) have shown no changes in electrocardiograms, PCO_2 or pH during CO_2 hysteroscopy with controlled rates of CO_2 flow. It is essential to use an infusion apparatus specifically designed for hysteroscopy. The maximum flow rate must be fixed at not more than 100 ml min^{-1} and a flow rate of 40 ml min^{-1} is usually adequate. Equipment designed for laparoscopy permits flow rates of 3000–4000 ml min^{-1} and must never be used for hysteroscopy.

The principal disadvantage of CO_2 as a distension medium is the tendency for troublesome gas bubbles to form. These are particularly likely to occur when the gas mixes with blood and can obscure vision. These bubbles can usually be avoided with good technique. Blood and mucus should be carefully cleansed from the cervical os with a dry swab and detergent skin cleansing agents should be avoided. The hysteroscope should be advanced slowly under direct vision after creating a series of microcavities just ahead of the tip of the hystero-scope. The instrument can, in this manner, be kept in the center of the canal and introduced into the uterine cavity without damaging the cervical mucosa, which is the usual source of bleeding.

Most workers use CO_2 hysteroscopy only for diagnostic purposes because bleeding and smoke can seriously impair vision during surgical manipulations. Gallinat *et al.* (1989), however, also use CO_2 during neodymium:yttrium-aluminum-garnet (Nd:YAG) laser ablation of the endometrium. They believe that this is safer than fluid distension of the uterus because CO_2 avoids the potentially serious risk of fluid overload. They have therefore designed a closed-circuit system to filter out smoke and plume produced during the ablation.

High-viscosity Fluids

Dextran 70 (Hyskon) has a molecular weight of 70 000 and is a mixture of 32% dextran in 10% dextrose. It is a thick viscous fluid and is electrolyte free, non-conductive and biodegradable. It was first used as a distension agent for diagnostic hysteroscopy by Edström and Fernström (1970) because it is optically clear and immiscible with blood. Baggish (1989) also considers it to be the best medium for operative hysteroscopic surgery because of its optical clarity and immiscibility with blood and because its consistency reduces the risk of extravasation into the uterine circulation. A pool of static dextran will remain optically clear for longer than a similar pool of a low molecular weight fluid and in such circumstances may be the preferred agent.

Dextran 70 is, however, a difficult medium to work with. Its high viscosity makes continuous infusion difficult, and a laborious and labour-intensive system of intermittent instillation and extraction with large syringes is required. Some force is required for this instillation and unless specially modified tubing is used, accidental disconnection of the tubing with consequent spraying of the sticky material is quite common. When dextran 70 dries it sets solid. If the equipment is not immediately and thoroughly washed in hot water, switches and taps will jam and expensive equipment can be readily ruined. When used with instruments producing high local temperatures, dextran 70 can caramelize and the dark brown color may impair vision.

Dextran 70 is hydrophilic and when infused into the circulation its high molecular weight pulls with it at least six times its own volume of fluid. Fluid overload and pulmonary edema may occur. Cases of non-cardiogenic pulmonary edema have also been described following the use of dextran 70 during hysteroscopy (Zbella *et al.*, 1985; Leake *et al.*, 1987). It is suggested that in such cases the dextran 70 may have a direct toxic effect on the pulmonary capillaries resulting in extravasation and interstitial pulmonary edema. Jedeikin *et al.* (1990) have described a case of disseminated intravascular coagulopathy and adult respiratory distress syndrome complicating dextran 70 hysteroscopy. Rare, but potentially fatal, anaphylactic reactions to dextran 70 have also been described (Borten *et al.*, 1983) and the incidence of such life-threatening complications is 0.069–0.008%.

Low-viscosity Fluids

A uterine cavity distended with a stagnant pool of low-viscosity fluid will initially be clear, but will soon become cloudy because of the accumulation of small particles of endometrial debris, which are dislodged during hysteroscopic manipulation. As such fluids are also readily miscible with blood any oozing will further cloud the fluid and impair vision. If the fluid is repeatedly replaced and a continuous flow of the fluid under pressure is established, bleeding will be prevented by a 'tamponade' effect and the endometrial debris will be flushed out, thereby maintaining continuous clear vision. Under these circumstances clear fluids are the simplest, most convenient and cheapest media for hysteroscopy.

5% DEXTROSE IN WATER

Goldrath *et al.* (1981) in his early cases of Nd:YAG laser ablation of the endometrium used 5% dextrose as the uterine distension medium, but in several cases he observed dilutional hyponatremia as an additional feature complicating fluid overload. As this substance has no clinical advantages over 0.9% sodium chloride solution, but has this significant additional risk of dilutional electrolyte disturbance its use can no longer be recommended.

1.5% GLYCINE

When electrical energy is used inside the uterine cavity it is essential to use a distension fluid that is electrolyte free. Glycine has been widely used for this purpose by urologists during transurethral resection of the prostate. It is optically clear and non-hemolytic and does not conduct electricity. Excessive absorption of such an electrolyte-free solution can be associated with hyponatremia and hemolysis. Magos *et al.* (1991) reported the systemic effects of the absorption of up to 4350 ml of glycine. A fall in serum sodium to 107 mmol l^{-1} (normal 140 mmol l^{-1}) was noted in one case and this was associated with a significant rise in lactate dehydrogenase, which is a marker of red cell breakdown. Glycine is metabolized in the liver and its breakdown can also be associated with an increase in ammonia radicals producing confusion, coma and death. Several deaths have occurred in Europe following intravasation of 1.5% glycine.

SORBITOL

Sorbitol is a non-conducting 3% sugar solution. It is optically clear and is being used as an alternative to glycine. It is hyperosmolar (165–180 mosmol) and excessive absorption can produce disturbances in blood glucose levels and diabetic features as well as overload and electrolyte disturbances.

0.9% SODIUM CHLORIDE

Normal saline is optically clear, cheap and readily available. The concentration of electrolytes in this fluid approximate to that in blood and it is metabolically inert. Excess intravasation is not associated with any major electrolyte or metabolic disturbances and any fluid overload can be rapidly reversed with diuretic therapy alone. Ringer's solution is even more physiologic with additional potassium radicals added, but is less freely available and in practice offers only theoretic advantages over normal saline.

Summary of Distension Media

CO_2 is the most convenient and least messy of the distension media to use. It is useful for diagnostic procedures and is particularly suitable for outpatient and office investigations. Operative manipulations provoking bleeding and the production of smoke and bubbles during ablation impair vision and make CO_2 less suitable for operative hysteroscopy. Dextran 70 is difficult to work with and is associated with rare, but serious complications. Sorbitol and glycine can both produce severe electrolyte and metabolic disturbances when absorbed in excess and are not recommended for routine use except when more physiologic fluids are contraindicated. In practice this means that such fluids should only be used when electrical energy is being used inside the cavity during electroresection or rollerball ablation. In all other circumstances 0.9%

sodium chloride infused in a continuous manner is the distension fluid of choice.

Infusion Systems

Hysteroscopes

When Goldrath first attempted Nd:YAG laser ablation he used a hysteroscope with an operating channel and a single channel, which he used for infusion of the distending fluid. There was no outflow channel available and fluid could only escape around the barrel of the hysteroscope. To ensure this occurred it was necessary to dilate the cervix widely. Many difficulties encountered during hysteroscopic surgery are caused by using inadequate or inappropriately designed equipment. It is now clear that good operating conditions require that the medium inside the cavity is frequently replaced and this can best be produced with a closed-circuit continuous flow system.

The uterine resectoscope is very closely modeled on the resectoscope used to perform transurethral resection of the prostate. Urologists have had many years in which to recognize the need for and to develop such a continuous flow system. Many resectoscopes have a continuous flow facility, usually in the form of an outer sheath, which surrounds the hysteroscope. With this arrangement fluid is infused into the cavity down the central barrel of the hysteroscope and leaves via the outer sheath. It is essential that the inflow and outflow channels are completely separate, communicating only at the distal end of the hysteroscope barrel.

Endometrial ablation using the Nd:YAG laser was first described in 1981. The early hysteroscopes used for this operation were slightly modified cystoscopes and were not specifically designed for the purpose. Many of the models still on the market are not suitable for laser hysteroscopy. Most operating hysteroscopes have at least two taps at the proximal end, but in many instances these taps communicate in the common barrel. In these circumstances irrigation of the cavity is impaired. Hysteroscopes with completely separate fluid inflow and outflow channels are to be preferred. Such a hysteroscope has been designed by Baggish and offers improved fluid circulation with consequent improved visibility (Figure 53.1). When a satisfactory continuous circuit is established inside the hysteroscope it is no longer necessary to dilate the cervix excessively; indeed it is better to restrict dilatation to that which will ensure a watertight fit between the canal and the hysteroscope. Such a fit is

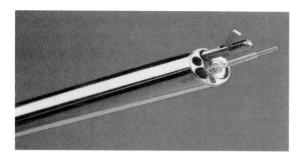

Figure 53.1 Weck–Baggish hysteroscope (Linvatec, North Carolina, USA) with an optic and three separate operating channels.

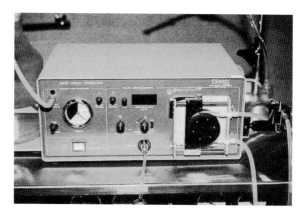

Figure 53.2 Hamou Hysteromat with a rotary pump connected to an integral pressure transducer.

facilitated if the outer barrel of the hysteroscope is round in cross-section. There seems little reason to continue to make hysteroscopes with an oval cross-section designed more to match the shape of the male urethra than the circular shape of both the cervical canal and the uterine dilators.

Fluid Instillation

The potential cavity inside the uterus requires the application of pressure to separate the walls. The minimum pressure required to produce a satisfactory degree of distension is usually about 40–50 mm Hg, but can vary considerably. This can be achieved with:

- Syringes. One or two large capacity syringes can be used to maintain uterine distension. Such a system is labor intensive and relatively uncontrolled as neither the flow rate nor the pressure inside the cavity is known.
- Hydrostatic pressure. A bag of infusion fluid suspended 60 cm above the uterus will enter the cavity with a pressure of about 45 mm Hg. Varying the height of the bag above the patient will clearly alter this infusion pressure. This is a simple and inexpensive system for controlling the inflow pressure.
- Pressure cuff. A suitably designed pressure cuff can be placed around the soft-walled infusion bag and the cuff inflated to a suitable level. Infusion rates can be varied by altering the pressure in the cuff.
- Simple pump. The tubing from the infusion bag can be led through a simple roller pump. The rate of infusion can be altered by varying the speed of rotation of the pump. A constant flow of fluid for a given pump rate will be produced regardless of the outflow resistance.
- Pressure-controlled pump. Various methods of limiting the pressure that a pump can produce have been devised. Quinones has described a compact regulating-compression

apparatus, which is favored by Magos and others. Hamou has developed a pressure-limited rotary pump (Hamou Hysteromat, K. Storz, Tuttlingen, Germany), which in a modified form is much favored by the author (Figure 53.2).

It was soon appreciated that an inherent problem of infusing fluid into the uterine cavity under pressure was that a proportion of the fluid could be absorbed from the cavity into the systemic circulation. Goldrath in his first paper on Nd:YAG laser ablation reported several cases of pulmonary edema and almost every subsequent worker has described similar complications. In a recent series of 859 cases of endometrial laser ablation, Garry *et al.* (1991) reported a mean fluid deficit of 1350 ml. In an earlier series Davis (1989) describes a case in whom more than 12 l of fluid entered the circulation.

Various approaches to minimizing such fluid absorption have been proposed (Table 53.1). Goldrath, because he only had a hysteroscope with a single channel available for fluid, found it necessary to recommend hyperdilatation of the cervix to allow fluid to escape from the cavity. This did provide the simplest form of safety valve to minimize the risk of excess intrauterine pressure. Lomano (1988) and Loffer (1987) both suggested that 'blanching' the surface of the endometrium rather than 'dragging' the laser fiber across and into the endometrium might minimize damage to the uterine vessels and hence reduce fluid absorption. Baggish and Baltoyannis (1988) advocated the use of the highly viscous dextran 70, which appeared to enter the circulation less easily. The author (Garry *et al.*, 1991) has suggested that the use of a Hamou Hysteromat pressure-controlled pump can be associated with a marked reduction in fluid absorption.

More recently Hamou *et al.* (1996) demonstrated that careful control of uterine pressure with an updated version of the hysteromat called an

Table 53.1 Suggested methods for reducing fluid absorption during endometrial laser ablation.

Year	Author	Cervical dilatation	Infusion	Outflow	Medium	Laser method
1981	Goldrath *et al.*	Wide	Syringe	Free	Saline	Dragging
1987	Loffer	Minimal	BP cuff	Free	Saline	Blanching
1988	Baggish and Baltoyannis	Minimal	Syringe	Syringe	Hyskon	Dragging
1988	Lomano	Wide	?	Free	Saline	Blanching
1989	Grochmal*	Minimal	BP cuff	Suction	Saline	Dragging
1989	Davis (a)	Wide	Pump	Free	Saline	Dragging
	(b)	Minimal	Gravity	Pump	Saline	Dragging
1991	Garry *et al.*	Minimal	Hamou pump	Free	Saline	Dragging

*Personal communication.

Endomat (Stortz) reduced the amount of fluid intravasated into patients undergoing hysteroscopic myomectomy. Procedures performed under Endomat control were shorter than those in which a gravity feed system had been used (10.5 min versus 24 min) and were associated with a lower risk of severe glycinemia (5.3% versus 16.6%). It was emphasized in this study that even under optimum pressure control fluid intravasation could and did occur, often rapidly and without warning. In these circumstances maintaining the intrauterine pressure just below the level of the mean arterial blood pressure permits early identification of major vessel bleeding.

Of the various systems for infusing fluid into the uterus, some deliver fluid at a constant rate of flow irrespective of the resistance inside the uterus. Syringes and simple roller pumps are examples of such a constant flow, variable pressure system. Other systems provide a fixed head of pressure, which results in a variable flow rate into the uterus depending upon the resistance in the infusion circuit. Gravity feed and pressure-limited pumps are examples of this constant pressure-variable flow rate system.

In general, the main advantage of a continuous flow system is that excellent vision will be continuously maintained. Providing that the outflow channel remains patent such a system ensures that there will always be adequate flow to wash out debris and adequate pressure to maintain a tamponade effect and prevent bleeding into the cavity. The disadvantage of such a system is that the flow continues irrespective of outflow resistance and in some circumstances the intrauterine pressure levels can rise in an uncontrolled way and may become unacceptably high. This may result in excessive absorption of the distending medium into the systemic circulation.

The advantage of a continuously limited fixed pressure system is that fluid absorption will be minimized. The disadvantage of this system is that as the present pressure level is approached the rate

of flow gradually slows and the flow stops completely when the limit is reached. This slow or stagnant fluid pool rapidly clouds and vision is soon impaired.

The ideal fluid distension system should be an amalgamation of both these systems. The pressure should be limited to prevent excess fluid absorption, but set at a level just below the threshold at which absorption occurs. By maintaining the pressure at this highest possible level the resultant flow of fluid should be maintained at a rate sufficient to flush out debris and maintain optimum visual conditions.

Factors Influencing Fluid Absorption

The first 105 patients on whom we performed endometrial laser ablation in South Cleveland Hospital had uterine distension produced with a simple continuous flow pump. The mean fluid absorption measured in this group was 1386 ml. In the next 92 cases the pump was replaced by a Hamou Hysteromat with a preset maximum pressure level. Using such a continuous pressure system the mean absorption fell to 209 ml, a reduction of 85% in mean volume absorbed. We therefore demonstrated that control of the intrauterine pressure profoundly influenced the amount of fluid absorbed.

To investigate in more detail the factors influencing fluid absorption we developed a system to measure intrauterine pressure directly. The pressure was measured by inserting a semi-rigid catheter down one channel of a Weck–Baggish hysteroscope. This hysteroscope has two operating channels angled only slightly from the midline and with a three-way tap one of these channels can accommodate both the path for fluid infusion and the fluid-filled catheter (Figure 53.3). The fluid in the recording catheter is maintained at a pressure of

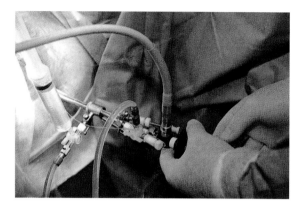

Figure 53.3 Weck–Baggish hysteroscope with a laser fiber in the left operating channel, a three-way tap for fluid inflow and a pressure-recording catheter in the right channel and a three-way tap for reverse flushing on the outflow channel.

300 mm Hg so there is no flow into this catheter. The end of the catheter was connected to a pressure transducer and a pressure monitoring system. Using this system we can observe the effects of varying intrauterine pressure on volume of fluid absorbed. We can also take X-ray hysterograms at specific intrauterine pressures and demonstrate visually the effect of such pressure changes.

In a prospective randomized trial we demonstrated in a group in whom the fluid was infused with a simple continuous flow pump that the mean volume of fluid absorbed was 1255 ml, and in the group in whom the intrauterine pressure was directly measured and carefully controlled the mean fluid volume absorbed was zero. The intrauterine pressure rose to a mean maximum value of 136 mm Hg in the simple pump group and to 70 mm Hg in the pressure-controlled group (Hasham *et al.*, 1992). We noted that fluid absorption appeared to occur in an 'all or nothing'

manner (i.e. if the intrauterine pressure remained below a critical level no fluid absorption occurred and if the pressure rose above that critical value absorption occurred, which then seemed to be unrelated to any further increases in pressure). This critical level appeared to be related to the mean arterial blood pressure (MAP). This conclusion based on our pressure studies was confirmed by our hystero-salpingogram observations. X-rays taken at any pressure level below the MAP at the completion of an ablation showed the radio-opaque dye confined to the uterine cavity (Figure 53.4). X-rays taken at any level above the mean arterial blood pressure showed dye freely entering the uterine capillaries and venous system, producing remarkably symmetrical veno-grams of the pelvic system (Figure 53.5).

We wondered if increasing the uterine muscle tone around the vessels would compress them and reduce the rate of fluid intravasation. Shelly-Jones *et al.* (1994) reported the apparently beneficial effect of infusing intravenous oxytocin in 5 cases who were experiencing rapid and severe fluid intravasation during endometrial ablation. In each case it was possible to measure the rate of fluid absorption before and after the administration of this medica-tion. There was a marked reduction in fluid absorp-tion in 4 of the 5 cases and oxytocin did seem to be of value in reducing excessive fluid absorption through its action in contracting the myometrium and thereby compressing the myometrial vessels.

We demonstrated that even small changes in uterine pressure would affect the passage of the radio-opaque dye. Pressures 5 mm Hg below the mean arterial pressure resulted in the dye staying in the cavity, and values 5 mm Hg above MAP resulted in the dye entering the venous system. The mean arterial pressure under anesthesia is usually

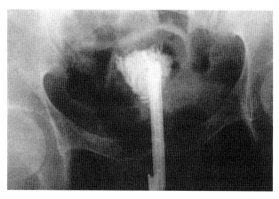

Figure 53.4 Radiograph of the uterine cavity at the end of endometrial laser ablation with the uterine pressure set at 80 mm Hg. Note the multiple irregularities caused by the laser furrows and that at this pressure all the dye is retained inside the uterine cavity.

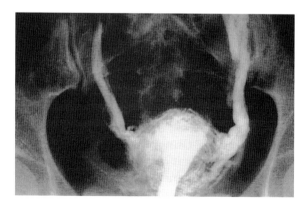

Figure 53.5 Radiograph of the uterine cavity at the end of endometrial ablation with the uterine pressure set at 160 mm Hg. Note that much of the radio-opaque material has left the cavity and is outlining the pelvic venous system, a typical finding in a 'high-pressure' absorption situation.

around 75–85 mm Hg and fluid absorption does not usually occur with intrauterine pressures of that level. We demonstrated, however, that in a patient with abnormally low MAP of 52 mm Hg an intrauterine pressure of 70 mm Hg provoked a fluid deficit of 850 ml, and conversely in two hypertensive patients with MAP respectively of 130 and 135 mm Hg intrauterine pressure levels of 120 mm Hg were associated with no fluid absorption. We conclude that the mean arterial pressure reflects the intrinsic resistance of the superficial layers of a given uterus to fluid intravasation. Maintaining intrauterine pressure below that level is usually associated with zero fluid absorption.

Once appropriate inflow and outflow rates are established the intrauterine pressure usually remains at a steady level. The levels of the intrauterine pressure and the MAP can be recorded at 5 min intervals, and in the normal situation the IUP should remain below the MAP. However, continuous pressure monitoring did on some occasions demonstrate a sudden, unexpected, and at times marked elevation in the intrauterine pressure levels. The almost invariable explanation for such rises in pressure was complete or partial obstruction of the outflow channel by particles of endometrial debris (Figure 53.6). Such obstructions produce a reduction in outflow with a subsequent build-up of intrauterine pressure. If recognized the obstruction can easily be freed by flushing with a syringe attached to the outflow channel. Such reverse flushing rapidly restores the uterine pressure to normal levels. We believe that in an otherwise steady state obstruction to the outflow channel is the principal cause of unexpected 'high-pressure' fluid absorption.

We believe that careful control of intrauterine pressure prevents most cases of excess fluid absorption. Using this system of direct pressure measurement and control in 23 consecutive cases of endometrial laser ablation we obtained zero fluid absorption in 21 cases. In one case with an unusually large cavity containing a pedunculated fibroid it was necessary to keep the intrauterine pressure above the mean arterial pressure deliberately to ensure adequate visualization and in this case a 1000 ml fluid deficit was noted. In the final case in this small series the procedure appeared to be technically uncomplicated and the intrauterine pressure remained below the MAP and indeed fell as the procedure progressed. In spite of this a fluid deficit of 1200 ml was observed. An X-ray hysterogram taken at the completion of this procedure gave a clue to the cause of this 'low-pressure' absorption – although the radiograph was taken at a pressure below the MAP dye entered the uterine veins. The hysterogram was not, however, the typical symmetric pattern and demonstrated only one side of the vascular tree (Figure 53.7). We have found that such asymmetric venograms are consistently associated with 'low-pressure' absorption and they seem to demonstrate a direct communication between the uterine cavity and a major uterine vessel.

This uncommon 'low-pressure' absorption occurred unpredictably and was difficult to study until we started to take endometrial laser biopsies. During the development of this technique to take full thickness endometrial biopsies with the YAG laser before endometrial laser ablation we noticed that every time we took such a biopsy we observed the same type of 'low-pressure' absorption. This occurred even when pressure control and fluid management were otherwise satisfactory. X-ray hysterograms demonstrated that these biopsies penetrate deep into the myometrium and can often be shown to enter major intrauterine vessels directly. As the pressure in the uterine veins is no more than 20 mm Hg and the pressure in the cavity inevitably in excess of 45 mm Hg, fluid will

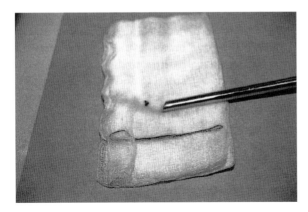

Figure 53.6 A particle of debris obstructing the outflow channel during an endometrial laser ablation.

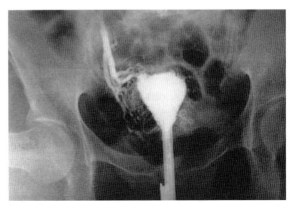

Figure 53.7 An X-ray hysterogram of a patient with 'low-pressure' absorption showing an asymmetric venogram demonstrated at an intrauterine pressure of 75 mm Hg.

inevitably be forced into the circulation from the cavity. We therefore suggest that this 'low-pressure' absorption is produced during endometrial ablation when the laser fiber or the resectoscope is taken too deeply into the myometrium, thereby producing a fistula between the large myometrial veins and the uterine cavity. It does not occur when tissue destruction is confined to the superficial layers of the uterine wall. Good technique, removing sufficient but not too much tissue, will minimize the risk of this type of fluid absorption.

In summary we believe that four main factors determine the amount of fluid absorbed from the uterine cavity during hysteroscopic surgery and they are:

- The intrauterine pressure.
- The mean arterial blood pressure.
- The patency of the outflow channel of the hysteroscope.
- The depth of penetration of the uterine instruments.

The superficial layers of the uterine cavity seem to prevent ingress of fluid into the systemic circulation until the pressure in the uterine cavity exceeds a value equal to the mean arterial pressure. When damage to the uterus is confined to the superficial layers absorption is dependent upon a simple pressure equation. If the mean arterial pressure exceeds the intrauterine pressure no absorption will occur. To ensure that this happens in practice it is necessary to ensure that the level of the intrauterine pressure is always less than the mean arterial pressure by limiting the infusion pressure. To avoid any resultant slowing and ultimate stagnation and consequent clouding of the fluid pool, it is necessary to ensure that the outflow channel remains patent at all times. To prevent direct entry into the major intramyometrial veins it is necessary to use correct techniques to restrict the depth of penetration of the laser fiber or resectoscope. With good control of the factors mentioned above other factors such as the size of the cavity, duration of the procedure and state of the endometrium do not seem to be important.

Summary

For optimal hysteroscopic surgery it is important to use an operating hysteroscope with separate channels for fluid inflow and outflow and to establish a closed continuous flow circuit with a watertight seal between the cervix and the hysteroscope. The intrauterine pressure should be measured and care-

fully controlled, complete patency of the outflow channel should be maintained, and a high fluid flow rate established. The laser fiber or the resectoscope wire should remove all the endometrium, but should not penetrate too deeply into the myometrium. If these principles are followed it is demonstrably possible to perform operative hysteroscopic surgery with continuous crystal clear vision and minimal fluid absorption.

References

Baggish MS (1989) Distending media for panoramic hysteroscopy. In Baggish MS, Bardot J, Valle RF (eds) *Diagnostic and Operative Hysteroscopy*. pp. 89–101. Chicago: Year Book Medical Publishers Inc.

Baggish MS, Baltoyannis P (1988) New techniques for laser ablation of the endometrium in high risk patients. *American Journal of Obstetrics and Gynecology* **159**: 287–292.

Borten M, Seibert CP, Taymor ML (1983) Recurrent anaphylactic reaction to intraperitoneal dextran-75 for the prevention of postsurgical adhesions. *Obstetrics and Gynecology* **61**: 755–757.

Davis JA (1989) Hysteroscopic endometrial ablation with the neodymium-YAG laser. *British Journal of Obstetrics and Gynaecology* **96**: 928–932.

Donnez J (1989) Instrumentation. In Donnez J (ed.) *Laser Operative Laparoscopy and Hysteroscopy*. pp. 207–221. Leuven: Nauwelaerts Printing.

Edström K, Fernström I (1970) The diagnostic possibilities of a modified hysteroscopic technique. *Acta Obstetricia et Gynecologica Scandanavica* **49**: 327–329.

Gallinat A, Lueken RR, Moller CP (1989) *The Use of the Nd:YAG Laser in Gynecological Endoscopy*. Laser Brief 14 Munich: MBB-Medizintechnik GmbH.

Garry R, Erian J, Grochmal S (1991) A multicentre collaborative study into the treatment of menorrhagia by Nd-YAG laser ablation of the endometrium. *British Journal of Obstetrics and Gynaecology* **98**: 357–362.

Goldrath MH, Fuller T, Segal S (1981) Laser photovaporization of the endometrium for the treatment of menorrhagia. *American Journal of Obstetrics and Gynecology* **140**: 14–19.

Hamou J, Fryman R, McLucas B, Garry R (1996). A uterine distension system to prevent fluid intravasation during hysteroscopic surgery. *Gynaecological Endoscopy* **5**: 131–136.

Hasham F, Garry R, Kokri MS *et al.* (1992) Fluid absorption during laser ablation of the endometrium in the treatment of menorrhagia. *British Journal of Anaesthesia* **68**: 151–154.

Hulf JA, Corall IM, Knights KM *et al.* (1979) Blood carbon dioxide changes during hysteroscopy. *Fertility and Sterility* **32**: 193–196.

Jedeikin R, Olsfanger D, Kessler I (1990) Disseminated intravascular coagulopathy and adult respiratory distress syndrome: life threatening complications. *American Journal of Obstetrics and Gynecology* **162**: 44–45.

Leake JF, Murphey AA, Zacur HA (1987) Noncardiogenic pulmonary edema: a complication of operative hysteroscopy. *Fertility and Sterility* **48**: 497–499.

Lindemann HJ, Mohr J, Gallinat A *et al.* (1976) Der Einluss von CO_2-gas während der Hysteroscopie. *Geburtshilfe und Frauenheilkunde* **36**: 153–156.

Loffer FD (1987) Hysteroscopic endometrial ablation with Nd-YAG laser using a non-contact technique. *Obstetrics and Gynecology* **69**: 6679–6689.

Lomano JM (1988) Photocoagulation of the endometrium with the Nd-YAG laser for the treatment of menorrhagia. *Journal of Reproductive Medicine* **31**: 148–150.

Magos AL, Baumann R, Lockwood GM *et al.* (1991) Experience with the first 250 endometrial resections for menorrhagia. *Lancet* **337**: 1074–1078.

Rubin IC (1925) Uterine endoscopy, endometroscopy with the aid of uterine insufflation. *American Journal of Obstetrics and Gynecology* **10**: 313–315.

Shelley-Jones DC, Garry R, Mooney P, Kumar CM, Kokri M (1994) The use of syntocinon in the management of excessive fluid absorption during endometrial ablation. *Australian and New Zealand Journal of Obstetrics and Gynaecology* **34**: 205–207.

Zbella EA, Moise J, Carson SA (1985) Noncardiogenic pulmonary edema secondary to intrauterine instillation of 32% dextran 70. *Fertility and Sterility* **43**: 479–480.

54

Laser Hysteroscopic Resection of Fibroids

J. DEQUESNE AND N. SCHMIDT

Lausanne Endoscopic Center (LEC), Lausanne, Switzerland

Uterine fibroids are one of the most commonly observed tumors in women of reproductive age. Problems associated with fibroids include bleeding, pain and infertility. Diagnostic and operative hysteroscopy allow visualization and treatment of uterine fibroids.

In 1985, Cornier presented the first European study on the hysteroscopic resection of submucous fibroids with the neodymium:yttrium-aluminum garnet (Nd:YAG) laser (Cornier, 1985). Since then, several studies have been carried out comparing different types of lasers and electrosurgical techniques for the hysteroscopic treatment of fibroids (Dequesne, 1986, 1990).

We have performed over 300 hysteroscopic interventions on uterine fibroids and have found little difference in cutting power between the laser and electrosurgical energy when treating the intracavitary portion of a fibroid. When treating the more difficult intramural portion, myolysis with the Nd:YAG laser is safer and more appropriate, although more costly. Techniques for fibroid resection must be adapted to depth of implantation in the uterine wall.

Classification, Diagnosis and Preparation

Preoperative hysteroscopy is extremely important for detecting certain malignant lesions and choosing the best operative procedure according to the type of fibroid. A basic hysteroscopic classification of uterine fibroids is illustrated in Figure 54.1 and includes:

- Type 1: pedunculated.
- Type 2: submucous.
- Type 3: small intramural.
- Type 4: large intramural.

Investigation of patients with fibroids will usually involve hysterosalpingography and ultrasonography including saline intrauterine sonography. If this has not already been done, diagnostic hysteroscopy is carried out in the office at the same time as endometrial biopsy and ultrasound. Occasionally, further biopsies may be obtained directly with the laser fiber during surgery.

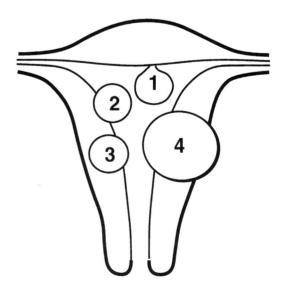

Figure 54.1 Classification of hysteroscopically observed uterine fibroids – pedunculated (1); submucous (2); small intramural (3); large intramural (4).

In this series, pretreatment was initially reserved for fibroids causing functional symptoms, but many infertility patients are now also referred and treated. Regardless of the type of fibroid, preoperative endometrial reduction allows greater precision when working with the laser and better recognition of low-profile fibroids, which may otherwise be hidden by the endometrium. Progestational agents and various estrogen–progestogen combinations are less effective than danazol, 400–600 mg daily for three weeks. However, weight gain and acne are frequently observed undesirable effects of danazol.

In recent series, researchers such as Donnez (Gillerot and Donnez, 1988; Donnez et al., 1989) and Maheux et al. (1985) have obtained endometrial reduction with gonadotrophin releasing hormone (GnRH) analogs (e.g. goserelin, 3.6 mg implant every four weeks), especially for patients presenting with type 3 fibroids (two-step surgery). This treatment is effective, because not only does it reduce the thickness of the endometrium, but it also reduces the volume of the fibroids (by about one-third in our series). Preoperative endometrial preparation also facilitates surgery by reducing vascularization and the associated risk of intravasation of the distention medium.

Equipment

The popular carbon dioxide (CO_2) laser used in gynecologic laparoscopy can not be transmitted through flexible optical fibers and through a liquid distending medium, thereby making its use in operative hysteroscopy impossible. The Nd:YAG, potassium titanyl phosphate (KTP) and holmium YAG (Ho:YAG) lasers do not have this limitation (Table 54.1) and have all been successfully used for the resection of uterine fibroids. The development of better sapphires and profiled fibers (Medilas, Munich, Germany) has also improved cutting power of these lasers over recent years. However, the Nd:YAG laser stands out as the laser of choice for myolysis of the intramural portion of uterine fibroids because it has the ability to penetrate tissue to a controlled depth of up to 7 mm, which is excellent for myolysis. It also has good hemostatic capabilities and is safe because energy from the laser beam is not transmitted to adjacent organs. The Nd:YAG laser is used at a power of 80–100 W, depending upon the fibroid, and the non-contact and contact techniques may be alternated for coagulation and cutting.

The first endoscope employed was a flexible hysteroscope, which was 5 mm in diameter including the operating channel. This instrument remains the hysteroscope of choice when cervical dilatation is to be avoided (infertility patients) or when access to the fibroid is difficult (cornual portion). In all other cases, the 8 mm rigid hysteroscope is more appropriate.

Low-viscosity fluids such as solutions of glycine, mannitol or sorbitol are safe, inexpensive and convenient, and provide excellent vision and distention of the uterine cavity. They may be used for either electrosurgical or laser resection of fibroids. The complication of media intravasation exists, but is rare when the intake is less than 1 liter. It is therefore critical to monitor fluid intake carefully. The distention medium we use is a 1.5% glycine solution. Originally a 3-liter container of solution was simply suspended above the patient during surgery. Currently, continuous irrigation fluid management systems such as the Hysteromat pump (Storz, Tuttingen, Germany) allow efficient monitoring of distention medium intake and output as well as precise control of the intrauterine pressure throughout the procedure.

Table 54.1 Physical and biological properties of lasers.

	CO_2	Nd:YAG	KTP	Ho:YAG
Wave length (μm)	10.6	1.064	0.532	2.1
Transmission by fiber	–	+	+	+
Absorbed by liquid medium	+	–	–	–
Effect on tissue				
Penetration depth (mm)	0.1–0.5	2–7	0.5–2	0.4–0.6
Thermal damage	+	++++	++	+
Coagulation	+	++++	++	+++
Vaporization	++++	+	++	++
Pigment sensitivity	no	yes	no	no
Cavitation	–	–	–	++++

Surgical Technique

Type 1 (Pedunculated) Fibroids

For pedunculated fibroids, the endometrium is reduced preoperatively with danazol for three weeks. The Nd:YAG laser is used in a non-contact technique to coagulate the base of insertion of the fibroid, and a contact technique is then used to cut the stalk of the fibroid (Figure 54.2). The fibroid is left in the uterine cavity unless it is small enough to be extracted at the end of the procedure.

Type 2 (Submucous) Fibroids

The endometrium is reduced preoperatively. If necessary, fibroid volume may also be reduced with pretreatment using GnRH analogues beginning at least 6–8 weeks before surgery. This allows sufficient time for vascular transformation and consequent volume reduction to take place.

Ablation involves passing the Nd:YAG fiber through the base of the fibroid using a contact technique to progressively remove points of insertion (Figure 54.3). Once the fibroid has been detached, it is left in the uterine cavity and will be expelled naturally. Large fibroids may be cut into smaller portions to facilitate expulsion.

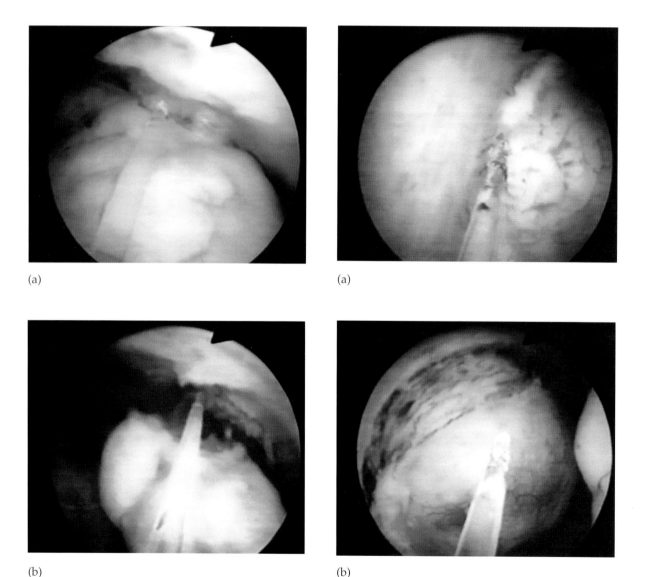

(a)

(a)

(b)

(b)

Figure 54.2 Resection of a type 1 (pedunculated) fibroid with the Nd:YAG laser.

Figure 54.3 Resection of a type 2 (submucous) fibroid with the Nd:YAG laser.

Type 3 (Small Intramural) Fibroids

In our early studies, the salient portion of the fibroid was cut and its intramural portion was myolysed during a single intervention (Table 54.2). Although this resulted in a normal menstrual cycle during initial follow-up and even a pregnancy rate of 51%, after 12 months a significant number of patients presented with recurrent abnormal bleeding as a result of new fibroid growth or migration of the intramural portion of the fibroid to the submucosa. To overcome this, patients presenting with type 3 uterine fibroids now receive GnRH analogs for 12 weeks and surgery takes place as a two-step procedure at weeks 4 and 12.

Table 54.2 Hysteroscopic myomectomy (first series) follow-up: 12 months.

	Number of patients	Good results
Type 1	20	20 (100%)
Type 2	27	25 (92%)
Type 3*	26	21 (80%)
Total	73	66 (90.4%)

*After 3 months, good results were observed in 96% (25/26) of patients treated for type 3 fibroids.

In the first procedure, resection of the salient dome using a contact technique is followed by myolysis with a non-contact technique to a depth of 5–7 mm. Myolysis reduces vascularization of the intramural portion, which often results in significant volume reduction and softening after 6–8 weeks and facilitates fibroid migration into the uterine cavity.

The second procedure at 12 weeks completely removes what essentially resembles a type 2 fibroid by the simple application of pressure or section with the laser.

Type 4 (Large Intramural) Fibroids

As with type 3 uterine fibroids, preoperative treatment with GnRH agonists is indicated.

If the patient has no desire for pregnancy, resection of type 4 fibroids by direct laparoscopy or laparotomy is the most appropriate procedure choice. However, in patients desiring pregnancy, these fibroids should be treated initially by submucous hysteroscopic resection as for type 3 fibroids, followed 8–12 weeks later by subserous enucleation of the remaining portion of the fibroid by laparoscopy or laparotomy.

We prefer complete laparoscopic resection with suture of the myometrium rather than myolysis with the Nd:YAG laser or with the bipolar needle electrode because in our experience bowel adhesion formation is less frequent with this method.

Postoperative Management

If large fibroids remained in the uterine cavity after the operation, second-look hysteroscopy, hysterosalpingography or ultrasound was systematically performed in our initial series of patients at eight weeks to confirm evacuation of the mass. However, since we have never observed a case where the fibroid has not been spontaneously evacuated, we currently reserve postoperative control only for infertility patients in whom it is important to confirm an empty uterine cavity and the absence of any intrauterine scarring. Scarring may be treated under paracervical anesthesia.

Outcome

In this study of over 300 hysteroscopic myomectomies, there has never been a case of uterine perforation with the Nd:YAG laser, nor any secondary postoperative bleeding. Two cases of postoperative endometritis were observed. There were also two cases in which more than 1 l of glycine was absorbed, but with no adverse effects on electrolyte concentrations. One case of hyponatremia at 125 mEq l^{-1} was seen.

Excellent results are achieved in most patients with type 1 and type 2 fibroids who undergo treatment with a single procedure (Tables 54.2, 54.3).

Table 54.3 Hysteroscopic myomectomy (second series) follow-up: 22 months.

	Number of patients	Good results
Type 1 and 2 (single procedure)	169	161 (95%)
Type 3 (two-step surgery*)	71	65 (91%)
Infertility (all types)	45	31 (68%)

*With the Ho:YAG laser, 9 of 12 fibroids of type 3 were successfully treated as a single-step procedure.

Type 3 fibroids treated in a single procedure had a good short-term outcome resulting from the hemostatic effect of the Nd:YAG laser, which coagulates blood vessels causing bleeding, and from aseptic necrosis of the salient portion of the fibroid. However, after one year the percentage of patients presenting recurrent abnormal bleeding was high as a result of new fibroid growth or migration of the intramural portion of the fibroid to the submucosa. Long-term outcome can be improved by treating patients with abnormal bleeding associated with type 3 fibroids with two successive interventions. Treatment of 52 fibroids of all three types in 45 infertility patients resulted in 31 term pregnancies and three miscarriages.

Discussion

Regardless of the instrumentation used for hysteroscopic surgery, endometrial reduction plays an important role and increases the precision of the surgery. Not only does reduction allow one to better distinguish the planes of cleavage, but it also reduces the thickness of the tissue 'chips', which can obscure the surgeon's view during the operation.

In our comparative series, danazol 400–600 mg daily was administered for three weeks, which seems sufficient for type 1 fibroids.

The cleavage technique for fibroids having their greatest diameter inside the uterine cavity does not change much with increased fibroid volume. When complete cleavage is not feasible, we still employ the Nd:YAG laser for hemostasis with better results for the treatment of anemia than GnRH agonists alone. In these cases, however, it is necessary to reoperate in order to remove the residual myolysed portion of the fibroid.

For the pretreatment of type 3 fibroids, we use GnRH agonists for three months because reduced volume and decreased vascularization are important for secondary myolysis and this certainly facilitates the second procedure.

Monopolar electrosurgical instruments such as the lasso and wire loop electrodes have a very attractive quality:price ratio and are favored by urologists. With such devices, there is a risk of transmitting current to adjacent organs (e.g. intestine, bladder) (Neuwirth, 1983; Hamou and Salat-Baroux, 1984; Baggish, 1988; McLucas, 1991; Nisolle et al., 1991). However, ablation of type 1 fibroids with the electrosurgical lasso requires only a few seconds and the removal of type 2 fibroids is some-

times faster with the resectoscope. In our recent comparative series, three times more glycine was used during procedures using the resectoscope compared to those using the Nd:YAG laser for fibroids of identical volume.

A major problem in the treatment of the intramural portion of type 3 fibroids with the resectoscope is the danger of hemorrhage and of opening large blood vessels, which sometimes causes both bleeding and intravasation of the distention medium. There is also the additional risk of perforation. A two-step procedure with the Nd:YAG laser is therefore likely to be safer for treating type 3 fibroids. When the laser is used in a non-contact technique, the penetration depth is 5–6 mm, resulting in myolysis and subsequent protrusion of the myolysed portion of the fibroid into the uterine cavity.

With the laser, there is a low risk of transmitting energy to adjacent organs, as can occur with monopolar electrosurgical instruments. Also, the non-contact technique, when properly performed, minimizes the risk of perforation. There have been no cases reported in the literature of uterine perforation with the Nd:YAG laser.

Future Developments

Considerable training is required to manage the technical aspects of the various laser parameters (power, timing, distance) in the treatment of type 3 fibroids, particularly for optimal myolysis to allow the second intervention to be short and effective. For this reason, over the past three years, we have investigated the treatment of type 3 fibroids in a single intervention by microfragmentation of the intramural portion with a Ho:YAG laser (Dequesne and Sumner, 1992). This is a pulsed laser that was first employed by orthopedic surgeons for arthroscopy and has a particular affinity for calcified and fibrotic tissue. It has the hemostatic properties of the Nd:YAG laser, but also results in excellent cavitation.

We initially used this laser at a power of 15 W and progressively increased this to 30 W to obtain better microfragmentation of the intramural portion of the fibroid to a depth of 1–2 mm. By alternating non-contact technique for the coagulation of blood vessels and contact technique for fragmentation, we have achieved complete treatment of type 3 fibroids in one operation. There is no problem of debris management with the Ho:YAG laser because the tissue fragments produced are extremely small. Also, the limited penetration and tissue damage produced by this laser reduce the risk of perforation.

Conclusion

We believe that the laser has an important role in the hysteroscopic treatment of intrauterine fibroids. The Nd:YAG laser has allowed us to successfully treat over 300 fibroids causing abnormal bleeding and infertility.

In the light of the cases discussed here and reports from the specialized literature, we consider laser myolysis of the intramural portion of fibroids to be a particularly effective technique with very few complications.

The inconvenience of treating type 3 fibroids as a two-step procedure with the Nd:YAG laser remains, but preliminary results with the Ho:YAG laser are encouraging. The Ho:YAG laser has the additional advantage of being safe and of not creating view blocking debris.

Potential major complications of operative hysteroscopy.

- Intravasation of distention medium.
- Hemorrhage.
- Uterine perforation (very rare with laser).
- Injury to bowel or bladder with electrical current.

References

Baggish MS (1988) New laser hysteroscope for Neodymium-YAG endometrial ablation. *Lasers in Surgery and Medicine* **8**: 99.

Cornier E (1985) Fibro-hystéroscopie au laser Nd:YAG dans le traitement des hémorragies rebelles. Presented at the *Journées Netter*. May 9, Paris, France.

Dequesne J (1990) Traitement hystéroscopique de l'infertilité au moyen du laser Nd:YAG. *Recherche et Gynécologie* **2** (7): 168.

Dequesne J, De Grandi P (1986) Focal treatment of uterine bleeding and infertility with Nd:YAG laser and flexible hysteroscope. *Journal of Gynecological Surgery* **5**: 177.

Dequesne J, Sumner D (1992) Use of holmium laser in gynecological endoscopic surgery. In Bastert G, Wallwiener D (eds) *Lasers in Gynecology*, p. 265. Berlin: Springer.

Donnez J, Clerckx F, Gillerot S, Bourgowon D, Nisolle M (1989) Traitement des fibromes utérins par implants d'agonistes de la LH-RH: évaluation par hystérographie. *Contraception Fertilité Sexualité* **17**: 569.

Gillerot S, Donnez J (1988) Les Agonistes de la LH-RH: une nouvelle approche dans le traitement de la myomatose utérine. *Journal of Reproductive Medicine* **29**: 575.

Hamou J, Salat-Baroux J (1984) Advanced hysteroscopy and micro-hysteroscopy. Our experience with 1000 cases. In Siegler AP, Lindemann HJ (eds) *Hysteroscopy. Principles and Practice*, p. 63. Lippincott.

Maheux R, Guilloteau C, Lemay A, Bastide A, Fazekas ATA (1985) Luteinizing hormone releasing hormone agonist and uterine leiomyomas: a pilot study. *American Journal of Obstetrics and Gynecology* **152**: 1034.

McLucas B (1991) Intrauterine applications of the resectoscope. *Surgery, Gynecology and Obstetrics* **172**: 425.

Neuwirth RS (1983) Hysteroscopic management of symptomatic submucous fibroids. *American Journal of Obstetrics and Gynecology* **62**: 509.

Nisolle M, Grandjean P, Gillerot S, Donnez J (1991) Endometrial ablation with the Nd:YAG laser in dysfunctional bleeding. *Minimally Invasive Therapy* **1**: 35.

55

Treatment of Dysfunctional Bleeding by Nd:YAG Laser

JACQUES DONNEZ, ROLAND POLET, MIREILLE SMETS, SALIM BASSIL, AUDE BELIARD and MICHELLE NISOLLE

Catholic University of Louvain, Brussels, Belgium

Summary

Both the electrical current of the resectoscope and the energy of the neodymium:yttrium-aluminum-garnet (Nd:YAG) laser have been effective tools in the destruction of endometrial tissue to a sufficient depth to avoid regeneration. Gonadotropin releasing hormone (GnRH) agonist therapy decreases the total uterine cavity area, which facilitates the surgical treatment and reduces the risk of fluid overload syndrome. The recurrence rate of menometrorrhagia is higher when the uterine cavity area is more than 10 cm^2.

The use of GnRH agonists is an adjunctive treatment for preoperative reduction of submucosal myomas so that a subsequent hysteroscopic myomectomy is possible. A two-step hysteroscopic therapy combined with GnRH agonist therapy is performed when the largest portion of the submucosal myoma is located in the uterine wall. A laparoscopic supracervical hysterectomy is performed for cases with numerous submucosal and intramural myomas because of a high risk of recurrence after the hysteroscopic procedure.

Endometrial Ablation in Dysfunctional Bleeding

Hysteroscopic surgical techniques have proved to be successful in the control of menorrhagia (Goldrath, 1985; Loffer, 1988). The hysteroscope allows destruction of the endometrium under direct vision. Both the electrical current (DeCherney and Polan, 1983; Vancaillie, 1989; Hamou, 1993) of the resectoscope and the energy of the Nd:YAG laser (Goldrath, 1985; Dequesne, 1989; Donnez and Nisolle, 1989, 1992; Gallinat et al., 1989; Nisolle et al., 1991) have been effective tools in the destruction of endometrial tissue to a sufficient depth to avoid regeneration.

The aim of this procedure is to decrease the menstrual flow sufficiently to allow patients to avoid hysterectomy. Indeed, amenorrhea and hypomenorrhea are recognized as sequelae of intrauterine adhesions; the laser ablation procedure is designed to create this condition. Other methods have been used in an attempt to create endometrial destruction and scarring including cryotherapy, superheated steam, intracavitary radium, rigorous curettage, quinocrine methylcyanoacrylate, oxalic acid, paraformaldehyde and silicone rubber. However, only the Nd:YAG laser (Goldrath, 1985; Loffer, 1988; Donnez and Nisolle, 1989; Garry et al., 1991) and the resectoscope (Vancaillie, 1989; Hamou, 1993) have produced acceptable results.

Patients who are considering this procedure must be aware that further childbearing is out of the question although there is an apparently minimal risk of pregnancy. Laser ablation is not a sterilization procedure and a concomitant sterilization could be proposed. Patients should undergo a diagnostic hysteroscopy with endometrial sampling prior to laser ablation. Patients with atypical endometrium should not be considered. The technique cannot be used for the treatment of abnormal endometrial conditions because some areas of the endometrium may not be destroyed.

The resectoscope has an advantage over the laser as its use does not require the major capital investment needed for a laser. However, the resectoscope is a unipolar electrical instrument and there is a risk of damaging the bowel or bladder with the current transmitted through the uterine wall or by actual penetration of the uterine wall with the cutting loop. There is also a risk of bleeding if major uterine vessels are transected by cutting too deeply into the uterine wall.

Laser energy, on the other hand, has some advantage in allowing a precision of tissue destruction that is not shared by the electrical energy used in the resectoscope. Unlike electricity, laser energy does not travel as extensively through tissue; its tissue effect depends upon the amount of power used and its effects are quite reproducible.

The three reasons for favoring the use of the Nd:YAG laser for endometrial ablation are:

- The use of a flexible quartz fiber.
- The ability to transmit laser energy to the tissue surface through a liquid distending medium (saline solution can be used).
- Its ability to penetrate tissue to a controlled depth.

Preoperative Therapy

Once the decision to proceed with surgery has been made, the endometrium is brought into a resting phase by treating with danazol (400 mg twice a day) beginning during the menses (Loffer, 1988) or by GnRH agonist therapy (Donnez *et al.* 1989a,b). Indeed, the use of GnRH analogs (Zoladex implant; Decapeptyl injection) has the advantage of reducing uterine size to facilitate the surgical procedure (Donnez and Nisolle 1989, 1992; Nisolle *et al.* 1991).

In our department, the implant was injected subcutaneously at the end of the luteal phase to curtail the initial gonadotropin stimulation phase always associated with a rise in estrogens. A significant shrinkage was found to occur after eight weeks of therapy. Indeed, as documented by hysterosalpingography imaging (using the short-line 'multipurpose test system' described by Weibel, 1979) (Donnez *et al.*, 1994a), the uterine cavity area decreased by an average of 35% (Donnez *et al.*, 1989a; Nisolle *et al.*, 1991, Donnez *et al.*, 1994a). The response was variable, however, ranging from 5–60%. The decrease in total uterine cavity area was greater in cases with a very enlarged uterine cavity (> 10 cm²) than in cases with an initial uterine cavity area less than 10 cm² (Figure 55.1).

The advantages of preoperative therapy are:

- Endometrial ablation is easier to perform (thin endometrium, small uterine cavity).
- There is a decreased risk of fluid overload (Donnez *et al.*, 1990a,b; Nisolle *et al.*, 1991).

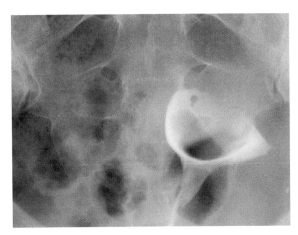

(a)

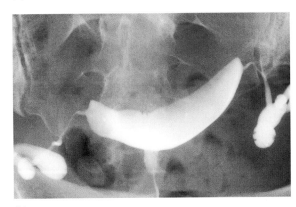

(b)

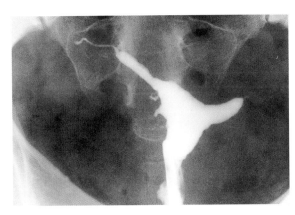

(c)

Figure 55.1 Classification of submucosal myomas (Donnez *et al.*, 1990; Donnez, 1993). (a) Submucosal fibroid whose greatest diameter is inside the uterine cavity. (b) Submucosal fibroid whose largest portion is located in the myometrium. (c) Multiple (> two) submucosal fibroids (myofibromatous uterus with submucosal fibroids and intramural fibroids) diagnosed by hysterography and hysteroscopy.

Endometrial Ablation Technique

Regional or general anesthesia is used, as local anesthesia is accompanied by considerable cramp. We prefer to perform all operative hysteroscopies with the uterine cavity well distended (the intrauterine pressure exceeding the venous pressure) to prevent bleeding from the endometrial surface.

The three techniques for applying laser energy to the endometrial cavity are:

- The touch technique (Goldrath et al., 1981; Goldrath, 1985).
- The non-touch technique (Loffer, 1988).
- A combination of both techniques.

Selection of Patients

In a series of more than 750 patients treated for menometrorrhagia by hysteroscopy, we tried to classify the uterine pathology in order to evaluate endometrial ablation in dysfunctional bleeding. Only women without intrauterine lesions were considered.

Two groups of patients were defined according to the size of the uterine cavity ($< 10 \text{ cm}^2$; $> 10 \text{ cm}^2$) before GnRH agonist therapy.

As stated earlier, patients contemplating this procedure were made aware that further childbearing could not be considered and had a diagnostic hysteroscopy with endometrial sampling before laser ablation.

Patients with an atypical endometrium were not considered.

Having decided to proceed with surgery, the endometrium was brought into a resting phase by GnRH agonist therapy (Donnez et al., 1989). The implant was injected subcutaneously at the end of the luteal phase to curtail the initial gonadotropin stimulation phase always associated with a rise in estrogens. One implant was systematically injected at weeks 0, 4 and 8. Today, we consider the ideal scheme of therapy to be:

- Preoperative GnRH agonist therapy by injection at weeks 0 and 4.
- Hysteroscopic surgery at week 5 or 6.

Indeed, a period of 4–5 weeks of very low estradiol levels (after the well-known flare-up effect) is sufficient to reduce the endometrium to a very thin postmenopausal state.

Results

Table 55.1 shows the results of our series of patients treated by a touch technique. In a first series of 50 patients (Donnez et al. 1989), the entire uterine cavity was subjected to endometrial ablation and this resulted in amenorrhea, meaning absolutely non-demonstrable vaginal bleeding, in 34% of cases.

Hypomenorrhea, indicating very light periods amounting to little more than several days of spotting, was observed in 60% of cases. Abnormal flow, meaning a bleeding similar to that which the patient experienced before developing menstrual problems, was observed in 4% of cases. Failure of treatment, with no significant decrease in the amount of the menstrual flow, was demonstrated in 2% of cases.

In a second series of 270 patients (Nisolle et al., 1991; Donnez et al., 1994a), endometrial ablation was carried out in the uterine cavity, except in an area 1 cm above the uterine isthmus, in order to

Table 55.1 Nd:YAG laser hysteroscopic endometrial ablation in two consecutive series of 50 patients who underwent endometrial laser ablation (ELA) and 270 patients who underwent partial endometrial laser ablation (PELA) for dysfunctional bleeding (myomas excluded).

	ELA	PELA	
		Uterine cavity area	
		$<10 \text{ cm}^2$	$>10 \text{ cm}^2$
Number of patients	($n = 50$)	($n = 200$)	($n = 70$)
Results			
Amenorrhea	17 (34%)	1 (0.5%)	1 (1.5%)
Hypomenorrhea	30 (60%)	189 (94.5%)	59 (84%)
Normal flow	2 (4%)	6 (3%)	6 (9%)
Failed	1 (2%)	2 (3%)	4 (6%)
Recurrence of menometrorrhagia (two-year follow-up)	2 (4%)	3/146 (2%)	6/49 (12%)
Total of failures (two years)	3/50 (6%)	5/146 (3%)	10/49 (20%)

avoid complete amenorrhea. In this group, the proposed goal was to obtain hypomenorrhea and not amenorrhea. In the first subgroup (uterine cavity area < 10 cm²) hypomenorrhea was achieved in 94.5% of cases. Amenorrhea occurred in only 1.5% of cases, and failures in 1% of cases (see Table 55.1). In the other subgroup (uterine cavity area > 10 cm²), the failure rate was higher (4/70; 6%). The operating time varied from 15–25 minutes. Blood loss was minimal. No uterine perforation occurred.

The follow-up of patients was long enough to prove that regeneration of endometrial tissue does not occur with the touch technique. The decrease in menstrual flow that occurred within the first 3–4 months did not vary over the ensuing years in our series of women with abnormal dysfunctional bleeding. When performed, hysterosalpingography revealed shrinkage of the uterine cavity. In the subgroup of women with a uterine cavity area over 10 cm², the recurrence rate of menometrorrhagia was significantly ($P < 0.01$) higher (20%) than that observed when the uterine cavity area was less than 10 cm² (3%) (see Table 55.1).

Since GnRH agonist therapy has been systematically administered and the continous flow hysteroscopic system used, fluid overload syndrome has not occurred.

Discussion

Numerous methods have been used in an attempt to create endometrial destruction and scarring and have included cryotherapy, superheated steam, intracavitary radium, rigorous curettage, quinacrine methylcyanoacrylate, oxalic acid, paraformaldehyde and silicone rubber. However, only the Nd:YAG laser and the resectoscope have provided acceptable results.

The resectoscope has an advantage over the laser as its use does not require the major capital investment needed for a laser. However, the resectoscope is a unipolar electrical instrument and there is a risk of damaging the bowel or bladder with the current transmitted through the uterine wall or by actual penetration of the uterine wall with the cutting loop. There is also a risk of bleeding if major uterine vessels are transected by cutting too deeply into the uterine wall.

In our second series of 270 women, 'partial' endometrial laser ablation was carried out to provoke hypomenorrhea so that a little bleeding could be observed at menstruation. Indeed, for psychologic reasons, hypomenorrhea could be preferable to amenorrhea. In theory this procedure could be proposed in the future to women in their forties in order to reduce menstrual flow even in the absence of dysfunctional bleeding.

In the literature, most authors have presented a high rate of 'immediate' good results (Table 55.2), but only a few (Nisolle et al., 1991) have published the long-term results. Indeed, significant differences have been observed according to the uterine cavity area. If the uterine cavity area is more than 10 cm², failure rates (6%) and recurrent menometrorrhagia rates (12%) are higher than those observed if the uterine cavity area is less than 10 cm² (respectively 3% and 2%). The significant differences related to the uterine cavity area account for some discrepancies in the results published and/or shown during the numerous congresses.

Postoperative bleeding and fluid overload leading to pulmonary edema never occurred in the second series. The problem is similar to that described for transurethral resection of the prostate (Van Boven et al., 1989). Fluid absorption could be influenced by the thickness of the endometrium and the vascularization of the chorion. These two parameters are in turn influenced by GnRH agonist therapy. In the last series of more than 700 cases, no fluid overload occurred since GnRH agonist therapy was systematically administered and the continuous flow hysteroscopic system used.

Table 55.2 'Immediate' good results (amenorrhea or hypomennorhea) after Nd:YAG laser ablation.

Author	Number of patients	Number of 'Good' results (%)
Goldrath (1985)	214	206 (96)
Loffer (1988)	55	38 (69)
Lomano (1988)	62	47 (76)
Baggish (1988)	14	10 (71)
Donnez and Nisolle (1989)	50	47 (94)
Nisolle et al. (1991)	270	250 (93)
Garry et al. (1991)	479	288 (60)
Gallinat and Lueken (1993)	145	136 (94)

In conclusion, GnRH agonist therapy decreases the total uterine cavity area, which facilitates surgical treatment and reduces the risk of fluid overload syndrome. Endometrial laser ablation is quickly performed by experienced gynecologists. The morbidity rate and hospitalization time are reduced in comparison with hysterectomy. Also, the primary advantage of this treatment is that hysterectomy can be avoided in young women with abnormal bleeding.

Submucous Myomas

Hysteroscopic Myomectomy

THE ROLE OF PREOPERATIVE GnRH AGONIST THERAPY

In our department, 376 women aged 23–43 years (mean 33 years) with symptomatic submucous uterine fibroids were treated with a biodegradable GnRH agonist (Zoladex implant, ICI, Cambridge, UK). The implant was injected subcutaneously at the end of the luteal phase to curtail the initial gonadotropin stimulation phase always associated with a rise in estrogen. One implant was systematically injected at weeks 0, 4 and 8. Hysteroscopic myomectomy was carried out at eight weeks.

Using the method previously described (Donnez *et al.*, 1989, 1990a), the reduction of very large submucous fibroid areas was calculated. When more than one fibroid was present, only the largest was evaluated. In all cases except four (Donnez, 1993), the fibroid area decreased by an average of 38%. However, the response was variable, ranging from 4–95%. The fibroid area was found to decrease significantly ($P < 0.01$) from the baseline area (7.2 ± 4.7 cm^2) to 4.4 ± 3.5 cm^2 by eight weeks of therapy. About 10% of myomas do not appear to respond well to GnRH agonist.

Classification of Myomas (Donnez, 1993, Donnez *et al.*, 1990a, 1994b,c (see Figure 55.1)

According to hysterosalpingography data, submucosal fibroids were classified as:

- Submucosal fibroid for which the greatest diameter was inside the uterine cavity.
- Submucosal fibroid for which the largest portion was located in the myometrium.
- Multiple (> two) submucosal fibroids (myofibromatous uterus with submucosal fibroids and intramural fibroids) diagnosed by hysterography and echography.

Techniques

SUBMUCOSAL FIBROID FOR WHICH THE GREATEST DIAMETER WAS INSIDE THE UTERINE CAVITY

All patients ($n = 233$) underwent myomectomy by hysteroscopy and Nd:YAG laser. In all cases except three, the operation was easily performed. The endometrium overlying the myoma was less vascular and the 'shrinkage' of the uterine cavity may have accounted for the relative ease of separating the myomas from the surrounding myometrium.

The myoma was left in the uterine cavity unless a decrease in myoma size was not observed after GnRH agonist therapy, because in this case histologic examination is required. No complications such as infection, bleeding or uterine contractions occurred. Office hysteroscopy, performed with carbon dioxide (CO_2) and carried out 2–3 months after myomectomy confirmed complete disappearance of the myoma, which was probably 'ejected' during the first menstruation after the procedure.

No hormonal therapy such as estrogen and progesterone was given. The operating time varied from 10–50 minutes (mean 24 ± 6 minutes).

LARGE SUBMUCOSAL FIBROID FOR WHICH THE LARGEST PORTION WAS LOCATED IN THE UTERINE WALL

A two-step operative hysteroscopy was proposed in cases of very large submucous fibroids for which the largest portion was not inside the uterine cavity, but inside the uterine wall ($n = 78$) (Donnez *et al.*, 1990a). After an eight-week preoperative GnRH agonist therapy, a partial myomectomy was carried out by resecting the protruded portion of the myoma. Thereafter, the laser fiber was directed as perpendicularly as possible at the remaining (intramural) fibroid portion and was introduced into the fibroid to a depth of 5–10 mm. During the application of laser energy, the fiber was slowly removed so that the deeper areas were coagulated. The endpoint of fibroid coagulation with this technique was identifiable by the observation of distinct 'craters' with brown borders on all fibroid areas. The depth of the intramural fibroid portion was already known as an echographic examination had been performed the day before surgery. The aim of this procedure was to decrease the size of the remaining myoma by decreasing the vascularity. This technique induces a myoma necrobiosis and can be called 'transhysteroscopic myolysis' (Donnez *et al.*, 1990a).

A GnRH agonist therapy was given for another eight weeks and a second-look hysteroscopy was then performed. In all cases, the myoma was found to protrude inside the uterine cavity and appeared very white and without any apparent vessels on its surface. The shrinkage of the uterine cavity allowed the residual myoma portion to be easily separated from the surrounding myometrium and dissected off. Myomectomy was then carried out. At the end of the procedure, the myoma can be left in the uterine cavity.

In all but five cases, the two-step therapy permitted completion of the myomectomy. In the five remaining cases, a 'third-look' hysteroscopy was necessary to achieve myomectomy. When performed, hysterography confirmed the normal appearance of the uterine cavity less than three months after the procedure.

FIBROMATOUS UTERUS

For cases of multiple submucosal fibroids, each myoma was either separated from the surrounding myometrium or totally photocoagulated. When only a small portion of the myoma was visible, the laser fiber was introduced into the intramural portion to a depth depending upon the myoma diameter (diagnosed by echography). While firing, the fiber was slowly removed. Each myoma was systematically destroyed. At the end of surgery, endometrial ablation with the Nd:YAG laser was carried out only in women over 35 years of age who did not wish to subsequently become pregnant to induce uterine shrinkage.

Results

Table 55.3 shows the long-term results according to the myoma classification of Donnez et al. (1994c).

In cases of large submucous fibroids for which the greatest diameter was inside the uterine cavity ($n = 233$), surgery was successfully carried out in 230 cases. In three cases, a stromal tumor was diagnosed. In one of these cases, dissection of the myoma from the myometrium was quite impossible because the plane of dissection could not be found. Thus, a frozen histology of the 'myoma' biopsy was carried out and revealed histologic characteristics of a stromal tumor. Vaginal hysterectomy was then carried out. The other two cases were diagnosed by the histologic examination of the removed myomas. Hysteroscopically, they appeared as benign myomas. Thus, the incidence of 'stromal tumors' in apparently benign myomas is 1.2% (3/233). It is important to note that all three cases were observed in the subgroups of myomas that did not respond well (< 10% decrease) to GnRH agonist therapy.

When successfully performed, myomectomy permits restoration of normal flow. Long-term result evaluation (Donnez, 1993) shows that recurrence of menorrhagia occurred more frequently (22%) in cases of multiple submucosal myomas than in cases of single submucosal myomas.

Recurrence of menorrhagia was provoked by the growth of myomas in other sites, as proved by hysterography and hysteroscopy.

Table 55.3 Surgical procedures and long-term results according to the site of myomas.

	Greatest diameter inside the uterine cavity	Largest portion located in the uterine wall	Multiple submucosal myomas (myomectomy and endometrial ablation)
Surgical procedures			
n patients	233	78	55
Successful	230	74	51
Failed	3*	4**	4†
Long-term results			
1-year follow-up			
n patients	132	42	39
Recurrence of menorrhagia	1 (1%)	1 (2%)	8 (20%)
2-year follow-up			
n patients	98	24	24
Recurrence of menorrhagia	2 (2%)	1 (4%)	6 (25%)

*Stromal tumor.
**A third-look hysteroscopy allowed the myoma to be removed.
†Myomectomy was not totally successful. (In two cases, second-look laser hysteroscopy was successfully performed. In the other two cases, vaginal hysterectomy was proposed and successfully performed.)

FERTILITY

A first evaluation of fertility in a series of 60 women was published in 1990 (Donnez *et al.*, 1990a). Among the 60 women, 24 wished to become pregnant and had no other fertility factors and of these 16 (66%) of them became pregnant during the first eight months after the return of menstruation. No miscarriages or premature labour occurred in this series; one cesarean section was necessary for fetal distress.

Discussion

Because most leiomyomas return to pretreatment size within four months of stopping GnRH agonist therapy, these agents cannot be used as definitive medical therapy (Healy *et al.*, 1984; Maheux *et al.*, 1985; Andreyko *et al.*, 1988; Friedman *et al.*, 1988). Several reports have demonstrated reductions in uterine and fibroid volumes of 52–77% after six months of GnRH agonist therapy, as assessed by ultrasound imaging. In our study, as documented by hysterographic imaging, there was an average decrease of 35% in the uterine cavity (Donnez *et al.*, 1989a,b). Another study (Donnez *et al.*, 1990) demonstrated reductions in fibroid area of 38% after eight weeks of GnRH agonist therapy. The response was variable, however, ranging from 2–95%. There was no difference in the extent of decrease according to the pretreatment fibroid area.

In cases of submucosal uterine fibroids, hysteroscopic myomectomy was carried out if the greatest diameter of the leiomyoma, as assessed by hysterography, was inside the uterine cavity. A treatment duration of eight weeks was advised before hysteroscopic myomectomy. Indeed, in a previous study, a significant uterine shrinkage was observed after eight weeks of therapy.

The preoperative blood loss was minimal, possibly because of the decreased vascularity of the myometrium, which was demonstrated by a significant reduction in the uterine arterial blood flow (Doppler) after treatment with a GnRH agonist (Matta *et al.*, 1988). In all cases (except when no decrease in myoma size was observed), the myoma was left in the uterine cavity and there were no complications. Probably, after a necrotic phase, the myoma was ejected with the menstrual blood.

For cases of very large fibroids where the largest diameter was not inside the uterine cavity, the myomectomy was carried out in two stages. During the first surgical procedure, the protruding portion was removed and the intramural portion was devascularized by introducing the laser fiber into the myoma to a depth of 5–10 mm, depending upon the depth of the remaining intramural portion. The distance beween the deepest portion of the myoma and the uterine serosa was evaluated by echography. A very interesting finding was that this intramural portion of the myoma became submucosal and protruded inside the uterine cavity, possibly because of the GnRH agonist induced uterine shrinkage, which provoked this protrusion of the remaining portion. In all cases, the largest diameter of the remaining portion of the myoma was inside the uterine cavity so that myomectomy was easily performed by separating it from the surrounding myometrium with the help of the Nd:YAG laser.

Conclusion

In conclusion, the use of a GnRH agonist represents an adjunct for preoperative reduction of tumor size to allow subsequent surgical treatment by hysteroscopy. In our series, even when the largest diameter was in the myometrium, the two-step hysteroscopic therapy combined with GnRH agonist therapy (Donnez *et al.*, 1990a; Donnez and Nisolle, 1992) was an ideal management of large submucous myomas, decreasing the need for myomectomy by laparotomy, which is often accompanied by increased operative blood loss and postoperative adhesion formation.

For cases of numerous submucosal and intramural myomas, there was a higher risk of recurrence compared with that for patients with only one submucosal myoma (Donnez, 1993). In view of this high rate of recurrence, we prefer to perform a laparoscopic supracervical hysterectomy (LASH) (Donnez and Nisolle, 1992, 1993) instead of the hysteroscopic procedure.

Because of the cessation of uterine bleeding, preoperative therapy resulted in restoration of a normal hemoglobin concentration, allowing the possibility of a later autologous transfusion (Donnez *et al.*, 1990a).

The hormonal endometrial status is one of the factors affecting fluid absorption. Endometrial vascularization may account for liquid resorption and this was reduced after preoperative GnRH agonist therapy. The amount of fluid absorbed was lower if the endometrium was atrophic. By reducing the amount of fluid absorbed, preoperative GnRH agonist therapy reduced the risk of fluid overload and this was another major advantage of this combined medical and surgical approach to therapy.

The advantages of preoperative use of a GnRH agonist are:

- Reduction of myoma size.
- Decreased risk of fluid overload.

- Restroation of a normal hemoglobin concentration.
- Detection of a stromal tumor.

Like Gallinat (1993), we believe that although YAG laser treatment requires experience and a thorough knowledge of the technique, it nevertheless has a lower complication rate than treatment with the resectoscope. For us, Nd:YAG laser treatment of large myomas must be considered as the safest method for the hysteroscopic surgical treatment of large myomas.

The Future of Endometrial Ablation

The ND:YAG Laser ITT Multifiber Device (The Donnez Device): Endometrial Ablation by Interstitial Hyperthermia

The recent development of new Nd:YAG optic fibers with lateral diffusion (ITT fibers) (E. Konwitz, personal communication), with the aim of simplifying the technical performance, has given rise to the idea of a multifiber Nd:YAG device (the Donnez device), which is conceptually close to the intrauterine contraceptive device (IUD). These new fibers act rather like an interstitial hyperthermic modality (Donnez *et al.* 1994d).

Before embarking on clinical trials with the device, an initial study of thermometric measurement on hysterectomy specimens was conducted to determine the appropriate power intensity and duration of treatment. As a second step, the device was tested on a first series of four patients.

MATERIALS AND METHODS

This new multifiber device (the Donnez device) is composed of three prototype ITT fibers designed for lateral diffusion (Figure 55.2); the two lateral segments have a diffusion length of 3 cm while the central segment measures 4 cm. The whole piece is contained inside a system of sliding sheaths. The ends of each fiber are cuffed by a semisupple Teflon bridge, giving the assembly some degree of rigidity. The device was developed in collaboration with Sharplan Laser Industry (Tel Aviv, Israel). Once the device has been inserted into the uterus, removal of the first sheath exposes the active segment of the fibers and pushing the two lateral fibers together gives the system an inverted triangular configuration, which conforms to the shape of the uterine cavity (see Figure 55.2).

In order to ensure a homogeneous distribution of

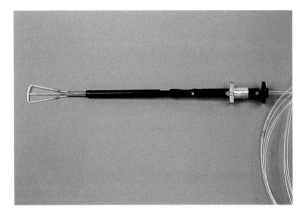

Figure 55.2 New multifiber device (the Donnez device).

power between the three fibers, the apparatus is equipped with an intermediate fiber fixed to a mirrored coupler to which the three fibers are connected.

In vitro thermometric study on hysterectomy specimens (Donnez *et al.*, 1994d)

Uteri of normal volume were obtained from patients undergoing vaginal hysterectomy for benign pathologies. Five thermocouples were inserted at the right uterine horn, fundus, left uterine horn, anterior wall and the isthmus. After immersion of the specimens in a thermostatic solution, an echoguided technique was used for precise measurement of the distance between the thermocouples and the fibers. The laser beam was then switched on for a total duration of 600 s, using a power of 30 W in continuous mode, with the specimens immersed in a thermostatic 37°C saline solution. The temperature inside the cavity reached 102–103°C after 4–5 minutes at a distance of 7 mm; it never exceeded 60°C within ten minutes of laser emission.

Macroscopically, a homogeneous and diffuse whitening of the endometrium was seen on opening the treated uterus. Fine superficial traces of carbonization were sometimes observed laterally on the supraisthmic portion, corresponding to pressure sites of the fibers on the tissue. On section, there was a tough 3 mm-deep white layer and beyond this the myometrium appeared softer and whitish at a depth of 4–5 mm. These features were related to an intense coagulation phenomenon.

Clinical thermometric study

The device was used in ten patients scheduled for various surgical procedures: eight were to undergo a routine hysteroscopic endometrial photocoagulation ablation for menorrhagia, together with a diagnostic laparoscopy for chronic pelvic pain, preceded by injection of one subcutaneous implant of a GnRH agonist four weeks earlier; the other two patients were to have their uterus removed (one LASH and one vaginal hysterectomy for uterine prolapse), providing pathologic data immediately following the interstitial hyperthermy procedure.

There was good access in all cases, allowing translaparoscopic insertion of the thermocouples into the serosa at the right uterine horn, fundus, left uterine horn, anterior uterine wall, anterior supraisthmus and posterior supraisthmus. Transvaginal insertion of thermocouples into the cervicovesical space and the rectovaginal space was also carried out. The uteri were of normal size.

Under general anesthesia and endotracheal intubation, the cervix was first dilated with Hegar probes up to number 10. The thermocouples were then fixed, either translaparoscopically or transvaginally. The device was finally inserted and opened, exposing the fibers. A power output of 30 W for a total duration of five minutes was selected. During the energy emission, the serosal temperatures were prospectively recorded and macroscopic changes were noted; the procedure would have been immediately discontinued if suspect temperatures had been observed or suspicious serosal blanching had appeared, indicating a possible uncontrolled localized hyperthermia. After five minutes, the device was removed, the intracavitary temperature was measured and a glycine medium hysteroscopy was performed.

Hysterectomy specimens were examined carefully to evaluate the histologic changes and, if possible, the depth of the thermal effect.

One patient undergoing endometrial ablation required vaginal hysterectomy six weeks later because conization (performed at the time of endometrial ablation) had revealed a cervical microinvasive carcinoma.

RESULTS

Figure 55.3 shows the typical temperature changes of the different serosal sites in one of the patients. Serosal temperatures never exceeded 41 °C; the temperature elevation curves evoked a saturation effect as initial temperatures rose quickly and soon stabilized. The intracavitary temperature was 102 °C during laser emission and 68 °C immediately following discontinuation of laser emission.

A glycine control hysteroscopy performed after photocoagulation showed a homogeneously and uniformly whitened cavity. The supraisthmic portion showed, in two cases, fine traces of superficial carbonization. Immediate histology was available on two hysterectomy specimens – in both, the endocervical canal showed congestion 2 mm in width, probably related to traumatic dilatation with Hegar probes. On the isthmic portion, the epithelium disappeared and an underlying 2 mm wide edematous zone was observed. At the cavity level, only the superficial layer of the endometrium was strikingly and diffusely ablated following treatment, with no serious damage to the myometrium.

One patient underwent a vaginal hysterectomy six weeks after the procedure as a punch biopsy of the cervix performed on the day of surgery revealed a microinvasive carcinoma. On macroscopic observation, the cavity appeared almost completely obliterated, leaving a 1.7 cm-long portion. Microscopically, complete disappearance of the endometrium was noted, together with myometrial damage estimated at about 4 mm in depth (Figure 55.4). Postoperative recovery was uneventful.

Discussion

Nd:YAG fibers used routinely for endometrial photocoagulation are of the 'bare' type; they diffuse the laser beam axially, forward, and precisely. For this reason, they need to be dragged along the cavity wall, using hysteroscopic control and glycine distending medium, according to a technique requiring previous training.

The advent of new optic fibers characterized by the ability to diffuse laterally along an active segment of 3–4 cm has initiated the idea of a multifiber device, inserted and retrieved as simply as an IUD, requiring no distending medium, no hysteroscopic control, no learning curve for the operator and possibly, ultimately, no general or locoregional anesthesia. The physical principle of this new technique is very different from the usual transhysteroscopic Nd:YAG fiber dragging technique. In the latter, photocoagulation of the tissue is obtained by a very short application of a very high power density beam; however, the new fibers need to be in contact with the tissue for a long period and then proceed rather like an interstitial hyperthermic modality.

The Nd:YAG laser delivers its energy to tissue in the form of heat through a mechanism of cellular protein absorption. When in contact with the tissue, the beam scatters and covers a vaguely hemispheric territory measuring 4–6 mm in radius. This measurement can be considered as the optic field of the laser. Beyond this limit, heat essentially diffuses by a simple gradient effect through the myometrium, which is a tissue of known poor thermal conductivity.

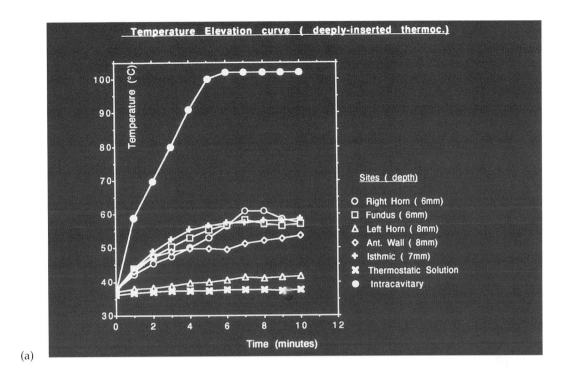

(a)

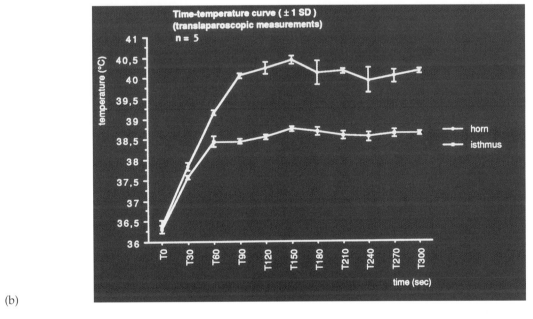

(b)

Figure 55.3 Temperatures during laser emission in different sites of the uterus. (a) In *vitro* study. (b) In *vivo* study.

Figure 55.4 Histologic view of hysterectomy specimen (hematoxylin and eosin × 25). Four weeks after laser emission, the endometrium has virtually disappeared. The myometrium shows signs of fibrosis to a depth of about 4 mm.

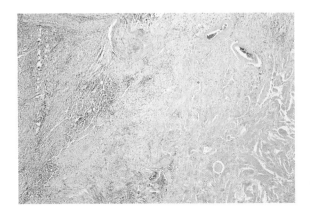

Cellular survival and macroscopic changes associated with short duration hyperthermia are well known. When tissue temperature reaches 60 °C, it suffers irreversible damage. Exposed to lower temperatures, its thermotolerance is time- and temperature-dependent – a living tissue can be expected to withstand one hour at 43 °C. Beyond this limit the resistance is halved for every 1 °C increase.

In vivo animal studies have to some extent confirmed this. When clinical application of hyperthermic sources is considered in a patient, this principle must be borne in mind.

Interstitial hyperthermia is a therapeutic concept used in oncology to treat primary and secondary malignant tumors; its effect is mediated by cytoskeletal and enzymatic protein denaturation. Nd:YAG laser is delivered alone or in combination with other treatments.

Before experimentation with the multifiber device, three successive generations of individual fibers were tested in order to determine the most suitable prototypes (Donnez *et al.*, 1994d). In laparotomized rabbits in which individual fibers inserted into uterine horns were tested under various energy protocols (ranging from 540–3600 J, 10 W for 54–360 s), macroscopic changes were noted at the time of the operation and four weeks later. Histologic examination was also performed in search of tubal occlusion, a condition compatible with an adequate and homogeneous lateral diffusion effect. This feature was found in 80% of cornua irradiated with third generation fibers only, at energy levels of at least 2700 J, together with homogeneously stenotic cornua. It was concluded that third generation fibers are the most homogeneous, the most capable of lateral diffusion and, consequently, the most suitable for clinical use. These results were particularly reproducible from experiment to experiment.

In our *in vitro* specimen study, the highest temperatures were reached at the isthmic portion and on the anterior wall respectively. These localizations both take advantage of a greater 'thermic concentration', related to the geometric positioning of the fibers: the power density would be expected to be higher in sites where the fibers are closer to one other. The close proximity of the bladder and the rectum at the level of the isthmus must be a constant consideration.

There is a risk of fiber breakage and in clinical use, this accident might be detected ultrasonographically by visualizing either fiber discontinuity or the abnormally rapid formation of an echographic thermal damage zone.

Our system is a completely new delivery system using laser emission to induce endometrial ablation by interstitial hyperthermia. It does not require hysteroscopy and could be used under local anesthesia. Recent publications confirm a growing interest in new modalities of endometrial ablation in order to make the procedure simpler and less hazardous. Phipps reported a series of menorrhagic patients treated by a microwave probe on whom a thermometric study was also conducted. *In vitro*, the multifiber device elevated the temperatures in the cavity rapidly up to 102 °C; at 6 mm, temperatures of 55 °C and 60 °C (58–67 °C according to the site) were found after five and ten minutes, respectively of laser emission. *In vivo*, the intracavitary temperature was 68 °C and serosal temperatures never exceeded 41 °C at any location after five minutes of laser emission. The discrepancy between *in vitro* and *in vivo* data is related to the cooling effect induced by the uterine arterial flow.

We conclude that the multifiber 'Donnez device' is an extremely simple modality based on interstitial hyperthermy used to perform endometrial ablation without a hysteroscope. The procedure can be performed under echographic control. Thermometric studies have shown correct temperature distribution, and early clinical experiments indicate favorable expectations regarding efficacy. While improvements are constantly being made with regard to the solidity of the system, further clinical investigations are being actively conducted.

References

Andreyko JL, Blumenfeld Z, Marschall LA, Monroe SE, Hricak H, Jaffe RB (1988) Use of an agonistic analog of gonadotropin-releasing hormone (nafarelin) to treat leiomyomas: assessment by magnetic resonance imaging. *American Journal of Obstetrics and Gynecology* **158**: 903.

DeCherney A, Polan ML (1983) Hysteroscopic management of intrauterine lesions and intractable uterine bleeding. *Obstetrics and Gynecology* **61**: 392.

Dequesne J (1989) Focal treatment of uterine bleeding and infertility with Nd:YAG laser and flexible hysteroscope. *Journal of Gynecologic Surgery* **5**: 177.

Donnez J (1993) Nd-YAG Laser hysteroscopic myomectomy. In Sutton C, Diamond M (eds) *Endoscopic Surgery.* p. 331. London: W.B. Saunders Company Ltd.

Donnez J, Nisolle M (1989) Laser hysteroscopy in uterine bleeding: endometrial ablation and polpectomy. In Donnez J (ed) *Laser Operative Laparoscopy and Hysteroscopy.* p. 277. Louvain: Nauwelaerts Printing.

Donnez J, Nisolle M (1992) Hysteroscopic surgery. *Current Opinion in Obstetrics and Gynecology* **4**: 439.

Donnez J, Nisolle M (1993) LASH: laparoscopic supracervical hysterectomy. *Journal of Gynecologic Surgery* **9**: 91–94.

Donnez J, Schrurs B, Gillerot S, Sandow J, Clerckx F (1989a) Treatment of uterine fibroids with implants of gonadotropin-releasing hormone agonist: assessment by hysterography. *Fertility and Sterility* **51**: 947.

Donnez J, Schrurs B, Clerckx F, Nisolle M (1989b) Les agonistes de la LH-RH une alternative dans le traitement de la myomatose utérine. *Contraception Fertilité Sexualité* **17**: 47.

Donnez J, Gillerot S, Bourgonjon D, Clerckx F, Nisolle M (1990a) Neodynium:YAG laser hysteroscopy in large submucous fibroids. *Fertility and Sterility* **54**: 999.

Donnez J, Malvaux V, Nisolle M, Casanas-Roux F (1990b) Hysteroscopic sterilization with the Nd-YAG laser. *Journal of Gynecologic Surgery* **6**: 149.

Donnez J, Nisolle M, Clerckx F, Casanas-Roux F, Saussoy P, Gillerot S (1994a) Advanced endoscopic techniques used in dysfunctional bleeding, fibroids and endometriosis, and the role of gonadotrophin-releasing hormone agonist treatment. *British Journal of Obstetrics and Gynaecology* **101**: 2.

Donnez J, Nisolle M, Gillerot S *et al.* (1994b) Endometrial ablation with the Nd-YAG laser in dysfunctional bleeding: evaluation of the results according to the size of the uterine cavity. In Donnez J, Nisolle M (eds) *An Atlas of Laser Operative Laparoscopy and Hysteroscopy.* pp. 313–322. London: The Parthenon Publishing Group.

Donnez J, Nisolle M, Clerckx F, Gillerot S, Saussoy P (1994c). Hysteroscopic myomectomy. In Donnez J, Nisolle M (eds) *An Atlas of Laser Operative Laparoscopy and Hysteroscopy.* pp. 323–335. London: The Parthenon Publishing Group.

Donnez J, Polet R, Mathieu PE, Konwitz E, Nisolle M, Casanas-Roux F (1994d) Nd-YAG laser ITT multifiber device (The Donnez device): a potential new modality for endometrial ablation by interstitial hyperthermia. In Donnez J, Nisolle M (eds) *An Atlas of Laser Operative Laparoscopy and Hysteroscopy.* pp. 353–359. London: The Parthenon Publishing Group.

Friedman AJ, Barbieri RL, Doubilet PM, Fine C, Schiff I (1988) A randomized, double-blind trial of gonadotropin releasing-hormone agonist (leuprolide) with or without medroxyprogesterone acetate in the treatment of leiomyomata uteri. *Fertility and Sterility* **49**: 404.

Gallinat A (1993a) Hysteroscopic treatment of submucous fibroids using the Nd:YAG laser and modern electrical equipment. In Lueken RP, Gallinat A (eds) *Endoscopic Surgery in Gynecology.* p. 72. Berlin: Demeter Verlag GmbH.

Gallinat A (1993b) Endometrial ablation using the Nd:YAG laser in CO_2 hysteroscopy. In Lueken RP, Gallinat A (eds) *Endoscopic Surgery in Gynecology.* p. 109. Berlin: Demeter Verlag GmbH.

Gallinat A, Lueken RP, Moller CP (1989) The use of the Nd:YAG laser in gynecological endoscopy. MBB Medizintecknik GmbH (ed.). *Laser Brief* **14**.

Garry R, Erian J, Grochmal S (1991) A multicentre collaborative study into the treatment of menorrhagia by Nd-YAG laser ablation of the endometrium. *British Journal of Obstetrics and Gynaecology* **48**: 357–362.

Goldrath MH (1985) Hysteroscopic laser surgery. In Baggish MS (ed.) *Basic and Advanced Laser Surgery in Gynecology.* p. 357. Norwalk, CT: Appleton-Century-Crofts.

Goldrath MH, Fuller TA, Segel S (1981) Laser photovaporization of endometrium for the treatment of menorrhagia. *Journal of Obstetrics and Gynaecology* **140**: 14.

Hallez JP, Netteer A, Cartier R (1987) Methodical intrauterine resection. *American Journal of Obstetrics and Gynecology* **156**: 1080.

Hamou J (1993) Electroresection of fibroids. In Sutton C, Diamond M (eds) *Endoscopic Surgery for Gynecologists.* pp. 327–330. London: WB Saunders Company.

Healy DL, Fraser HM, Lawson SL (1984) Shrinkage of a uterine fibroid after subcutaneous infusion of a LH-RH agonist. *British Medical Journal* **209**: 267.

Loffer FD (1988) Laser ablation of the endometrium. *Obstetrics and Gynecology Clinics of North America* **15**: 17.

Maheux R, Guilloteau C, Lemay A, Bastide A, Fazekas ATA (1985) Luteinizing hormone-releasing hormone agonist and uterine leiomyoma: pilot study. *American Journal of Obstetrics and Gynecology* **152**: 1034.

Matta WHM, Stabile I, Shaw RS, Campbell S (1988) Doppler assessment of uterine blood flow changes in patients with fibroids receiving the gonadotropin-releasing hormone agonist Buserelin. *Fertility and Sterility* **49**: 1083.

Neuwirth RS (1983) Hysteroscopic management of symptomatic submucous fibroids. *Obstetrics and Gynecology* **62**: 509.

Nisolle M, Grandjean P, Gillerot S, Donnez J (1991) Endometrial ablation with the Nd-YAG laser in dysfunctional bleeding. *Minimal Invasive Therapy* **1**: 35–39.

Van Boven M, Singelyn F, Donnez J, Gribomont B (1989) Dilution hyponatremia associated with intrauterine endoscopic laser surgery. *Anesthesiology* **3**: 71.

Vancaillie T (1989) Electrocoagulation of the endometrium with the ball-end resectoscope. *Obstetrics and Gynecology* **74**: 425.

Weibel ER (1979) Practical methods for biological morphometry. In Weibel ER (ed.) *Stereological Methods,* Vol 1. p. 101. Bern, Switzerland: Academic Press.

56

Hysteroscopic Metroplasty

RAFAEL F. VALLE

Northwestern University Medical School, Chicago, Illinois, USA

About 20–25% of women with septate uteri have reproductive problems, particularly abortions in the late first and early second trimester of pregnancy (Rock and Jones, 1977; Buttram and Gibbons, 1979; Rock and Zacur, 1983; Valle, 1985; Golan *et al.*, 1989; Carp *et al.*, 1990). In the past a laparotomy, to enter the uterine cavity, and a hysterotomy, which involves division of the uterine corpus, were required to treat a symptomatic septate uterus. Modern hysteroscopic surgery permits transcervical treatment via endoscopes, eliminating the need for entering the abdominal cavity and bisection of the uterus, which are both major surgical traumas to the patient.

In this chapter we will review the modern hysteroscopic treatment of the symptomatic septate uterus, but first we will discuss the etiology of this condition.

Embryology and Anatomy

The fallopian tubes and the uterus are of müllerian origin; in early embryologic development, the paramesonephric ducts fuse caudally and distally to form the upper vagina and the uterus, while the remaining upper segments result in the fallopian tubes. This process begins at 6–8 weeks of embryonic life and is usually completed at 12–14 weeks of gestational age. In the absence of müllerian inhibiting factor (MIF) produced by the testes, the paramesonephric or müllerian ducts progress to normal female development (Figure 56.1). The uterine septum usually completes its reabsorption by 19–20

weeks of fetal life. Failure to reabsorb results in a septate uterus with partial or complete septation (Moore, 1988) (Figure 56.2).

The anatomy resulting from arrest at fusion, canalization, or septal reabsorption depends upon the degree and the stage at which the arrest occurs. Because there is no failure of fusion with a septate uterus, the uterine body is uniform externally, differentiating this anomaly from the bicornuate uterus, in which there is lack of fusion, and an external uterine division. These two latter anomalies are usually symmetric (Buttram and Gibbons, 1979).

The septum of the uterine body can be various lengths and widths. Some septa are thin, while others are broad and produce thinner and smaller uterine cavities. Some septa only partially divide the uterine cavity, while others extend the entire length of the uterine corpus and occasionally the entire length of the uterine cervix. In 20–25% of patients, there is concomitant septation of the vagina; occasionally, bicornuate uteri have an additional septation of the uterus (Buttram and Gibbons, 1979; Valle, 1985).

Because of the close relationship of embryologic development with the urinary tract, uterine anomalies, particularly those involving one müllerian duct, may be associated with urinary tract anomalies, particularly of the ipsilateral kidney.

Indications for Surgical Treatment

The majority of women with septate uteri can have children; only 20–25% have spontaneous abortions, usually late first trimester or early second trimester

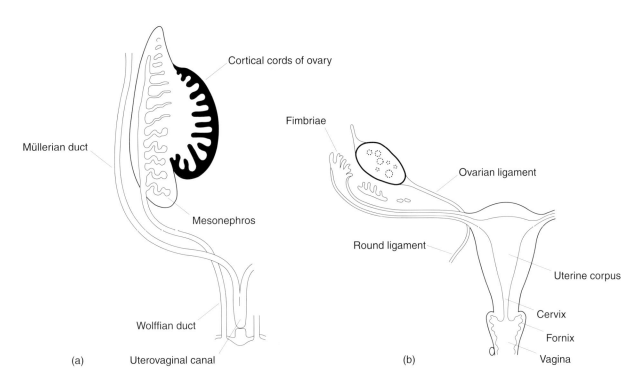

Figure 56.1 Diagram of female genital ducts at (a) eight weeks of development and (b) in the adult woman.

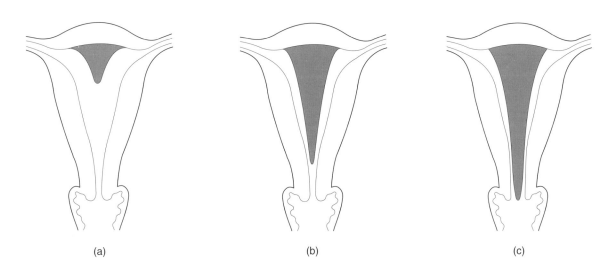

Figure 56.2 Septate uteri: (a) partial, (b) complete, (c) complete with septate cervix.

miscarriages initiated by mini-labors and bleeding. This problem seems to correlate with the length of the septum (Buttram and Gibbons, 1979). The more complete the septum, the higher the risk of reproductive failure. As the reproductive performance of the majority of women is not therefore affected by the septum it is important to rule out other possible causes when reproductive failure occurs, such as endocrine, genetic, metabolic and/or autoimmune

and alloimmune disorders. Other problems associated with this type of anomaly include fetal malpresentations, in about 20–30% of patients, and dysmenorrhea, in about 20% of patients (Golan *et al.*, 1989). If a termination of an early pregnancy fails, this may suggest a uterine anomaly, as may failure to remove products of conception and retained placental fragments.

Several theories have been offered to explain

repetitive abortions in patients with uterine septation, such as:

- Decreased uterine luminal space.
- Poor vascularization of the septum, which may impair implantation or nutrition of the blastocyst.
- Impaired development of the endometrium, which cannot therefore support the pregnancy.
- Decreased steroid and estrogen receptors.
- Decreased serum cystine aminopeptidase (CAP) decreasing neutralization of circulating oxytocin.
- Alteration of the cervical fibromuscular and connective tissue ratios with increased fibromuscular tissue and decreased connective tissue resulting in less resistance to cervical dilatation.

While all of these factors may have a synergistic role, the most generally accepted etiology has been that of decreased vascularization of the septal area as demonstrated during surgical division of these septa, thus affecting blastocyst implantation and nutrition of the implanted embryo (Fedele *et al.*, 1996).

The relationship between the septate uterus and infertility remains controversial; the general consensus is that this type of uterine anomaly does not cause infertility. Nonetheless, as the therapeutic approach to these anomalies has evolved, patients with primary infertility requiring assisted reproductive technologies or difficult treatments for infertility have lately been considered as candidates for treatment of the uterine septation (Heinonen *et al.*, 1982; Valle, 1995).

Preoperative Evaluation

Hysterosalpingography is the most accurate and effective method for diagnosing the septate uterus, particularly division of the uterine cavity. It is, however, difficult to consistently and accurately determine the presence of a uterine septum only by hysterosalpingography without confusing some of the anomalies with a bicornuate uterus; laparoscopy is therefore necessary to determine the exact external shape of the uterus to rule out this as a bicornuate uterus and to detect and treat any concomitant tuboperitoneal-associated pathology. Although sonography and magnetic resonance imaging (MRI) are useful for diagnosis, laparoscopy is most commonly used for guidance during treatment when the hysteroscopic approach is chosen. Finally, hysteroscopy can determine the actual

extent and thickness of the septum and provide a method of surgical treatment. It is important nonetheless, to evaluate other factors that may cause spontaneous abortions before deciding on surgical treatment of a uterine septum. A karyotype should be performed for both partners, and maturation of the endometrium should be evaluated with a mid-luteal phase serum progesterone and a late-luteal phase endometrial biopsy. Endocrine conditions such as hypothyroidism should be excluded with a thyroid stimulating hormone (TSH) assay.

Autoimmune and alloimmune conditions must be ruled out with a lupus anticoagulant factor study and a partial thromboplastin time (PTT) and by testing for anti-cardiolipin antibodies (ACA) and antinuclear antibodies (ANA). Because of their rarity alloimmune problems should only be evaluated in selected individuals with appropriate tissue typing for histocompatibility leukocyte antigens (HLA). Chronic endometritis is best excluded with an endometrial biopsy (Rock and Zacur, 1983; Carp *et al.*, 1990).

Finally, because of the close embryologic relationship of müllerian structures to the mesonephric ducts, renal anomalies should be ruled out. Although these urinary tract anomalies are not as marked and frequent with the septate uterus as with asymmetric uterine anomalies such as rudimentary horns or total absence of a unilateral uterine side, duplication of calyceal systems, renal ptosis, and other such anomalies have been described. Therefore, it is important to evaluate these patients with a screening intravenous pyelogram (IVP) (Buttram and Gibbons, 1979).

Methods of Treatment

Classic surgical treatments requiring laparotomy and hysterotomy were usually performed only in habitual aborters (i.e. women experiencing more than three spontaneous abortions in the early or late second trimester of pregnancy) due to their invasive nature. On many occasions, other adjunctive treatments were used, such as cerclage, bed rest, and tocolytics, to preserve the ongoing pregnancy, before surgical treatment was undertaken. With a new less invasive procedure such as hysteroscopic treatment, the indications have been liberalized to focus the attention on each individual patient and her unique reproductive failure.

The surgical treatment of the symptomatic septate uterus by abdominal metroplasty was performed by two different methods: the Johns metroplasty and the Bret–Tompkins-type metroplasty. These procedures are still performed in Europe and other parts of the world.

The Johns abdominal metroplasty involves transfundal excision of the uterine septum by removing a cuneiform portion of the fundal myometrium and septum with subsequent surgical repair (Jones and Jones, 1953) (Figure 56.3a). This technique has resulted in viable pregnancies in over 80% of patients and has been used as the gold standard to evaluate the success of newer procedures introduced to correct the symptomatic septate uterus. Disadvantages with this metroplastic procedure are the need for laparotomy, a hysterotomy and the possibility of postoperative adhesions, particularly at the tubal-ovarian regions, sometimes resulting in secondary infertility. When the patient has a hysterotomy, the waiting period before attempting pregnancy is prolonged (3–6 months), and should a pregnancy occur and be carried to term, a cesarean section is mandatory (see Figure 56.3a).

The Bret–Tompkins procedure involves bisection of the uterus in the anterior–posterior plane and transverse division of the uterine septum in the midline without excision of myometrial tissue (Bret and Guillet, 1959; Tompkins, 1962) (Figure 56.3b). This technique causes less bleeding than the Johns procedure and results in a more uniform uterine cavity, which is not reduced in size. The reproductive outcome following this procedure is similar to that obtained with the Jones method. For these reasons, most practitioners have preferred this second approach to treat the septate uterus. Nonetheless, the hysterotomy involved in both procedures carries the disadvantage of the need for a 3–6 month waiting period until pregnancy is permitted. A cesarean section is required when the pregnancy is carried to term (McShane *et al.*, 1983) to prevent possible uterine dehiscence and/or rupture. Furthermore, a significant number of women develop pelvic adhesions and secondary infertility following these procedures. Additionally, the hospitalization, disability, pain and inconvenience to the patient and associated cost are other major disadvantages.

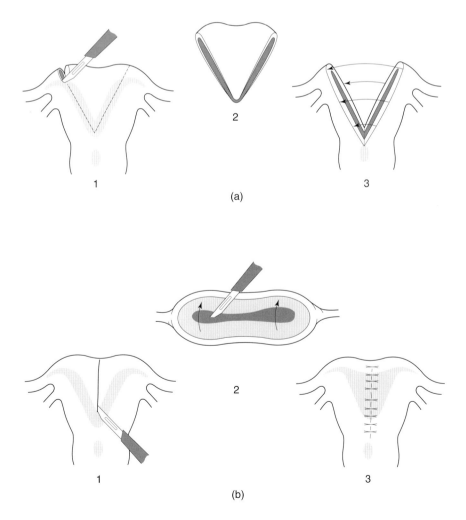

Figure 56.3 Diagrams of (a) Jones metroplasty (b) Bret–Tompkins metroplasty.

Modifications of these invasive techniques, such as El Mahgoub's technique (El Mahgoub, 1978) using small fundal transverse stab incisions and dividing the septum with long scissors transfundally, did not gain as much acceptance as the classic Jones and Bret–Tompkins techniques.

Hysteroscopic Metroplasty

The transcervical division of the uterine septum was attempted blindly by Ruge in 1884. However, the uncontrolled blind approach to the condition did not gain popularity among clinicians, and a direct approach was preferred, despite requiring a laparotomy and a hysterotomy. With abdominal metroplasty of the Bret–Tompkins type, the septum is incised at the midline and seldom bleeds upon incision. This observation helped in the initial approach of a visually directed incision of the septum using the hysteroscope. Following the introduction of modern hysteroscopy by Edstrom in 1970, the possibility of transcervical division of the uterine septum under visual control was initiated (Edstrom, 1974). This procedure began by gradually removing the septum with a hysteroscopic biopsy forceps, but when technological advances in operative hysteroscopes and instrumentation were introduced, the septum was approached by simple division with hysteroscopic scissors, and this method proved to be practical, relatively simple, and reproducible. The uterine septum is suitable for this approach because its fibrotic component is an embryologic remnant, it is poorly vascularized, particularly at the nadir of the septum and it can be visualized while division is performed. With the hysteroscopic transcervical endoscopic approach, the septum is divided under direct view and the avascular consistency of this embryonic remnant permits division without significant bleeding. The hysteroscopic approach also permits treatment in an ambulatory setting with minimal discomfort and morbidity to the patient. Because the uterine wall is not invaded, a cesarean section is required only for obstetric indications. The healing process with re-epithelization of the uterine cavity takes only 4–5 weeks, so patients are allowed to conceive sooner than with abdominal metroplasty. Hospitalization is not required, so expenses are markedly reduced (Fayez, 1986; Candiani et al., 1990). As there are no abdominal or uterine incisions, the pain and inconvenience to the patient are also decreased.

There are three different approaches to hysteroscopic metroplasty:

- Mechanical division of the septum with hysteroscopic scissors.
- Resectoscopic division with electrosurgery.
- Fiberoptic laser division of the uterine septum.

Whatever method is chosen, the best time for hysteroscopic surgery is in the early follicular phase to avoid the thick endometrium that follows ovulation. Although preparing the patient hormonally with danazol or GnRH analog is appealing, its cost may be impractical. Hormonal suppression provides a thin and atrophic endometrium that offers the best visual field for operative hysteroscopy.

Hysteroscopic Metroplasty with Scissors

An operative hysteroscope with a 7–8 mm outer diameter is required. A continuous flow system is most useful, not only to provide adequate visualization by a liquid distending medium's continuous washing of the uterine cavity, but also to help monitor fluids infused and fluids recovered.

The non-recovered fluids indicate the deficit, which should be controlled to prevent excessive intravasation. Hysteroscopic scissors can be flexible, semi-rigid or rigid. The flexible scissors are difficult to manipulate. Semi-rigid scissors are most commonly used because they permit targeted division of the tissue, they can be selectively directed to the area to be dissected, and they can be retrieved at will when a better unobstructed panoramic view is required. Semi-rigid scissors can be directed easily without much force or manipulation through the operative channel of the hysteroscope, facilitating hysteroscopic surgery, but they must be sharpened and tightened frequently. Scissors of the hook type are the most helpful to divide the uterine septum (Figure 56.4), particularly when reaching the broad fundal area where small superficial cuts must be made on the remaining septum to sculpture this fundal area (Figure 56.5) and avoid penetration into the juxtaposed myometrium (Halvorson et al., 1993).

The rigid scissors, often called optical scissors, are fixed to the end of the hysteroscope and can also be used to divide markedly fibrotic and broad septa. When using the fixed rigid instrument, it is important to have a perfect panoramic view while performing the septal division. The scissors should be introduced with utmost care to avoid uterine damage, as their sharp tips can easily perforate the uterus if force is exerted against the uterine wall (Howe, 1993).

With the use of mechanical tools in operative hysteroscopy, the best medium to distend the uterine cavity is one that contains electrolytes, particularly sodium, permitting a larger volume of unrecovered

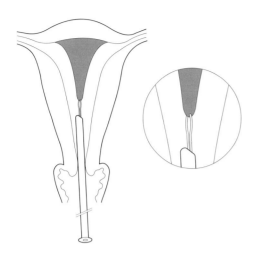

Figure 56.4 Hysteroscopic division of uterine septum with semi-rigid scissors. (Inset: closer view of septal division.)

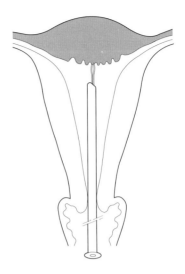

Figure 56.5 Completing division of the uterine septum at the uterine fundal area.

fluid to be used during the procedure. This advantage decreases the chances of water overload because the threshold for toxicity is increased as the added sodium acts as a diuretic and the patient will not be hyponatremic, therefore permitting more liberal use of diuretics if excessive fluid is not recovered. Normal saline (NaCl 0.9%), dextrose 5% in half normal saline (NaCl 0.45%), or Ringer's lactate, a balanced solution, can safely be used with good visualization. In general, no more than 1500 ml of fluid deficit should be permitted without establishing appropriate treatment with diuretics or even discontinuing the procedure.

The technique of uterine septal division with hysteroscopic scissors involves dividing the septum exactly at the midline where the tissue is more fibrotic and avascular. The novice approaching this operation tends to drift to the posterior uterine wall (Kazer *et al.*, 1992), where the vessels may reach the septum from the myometrial tissue causing unnecessary bleeding. The septal division is performed systematically beginning at the nadir from side to side, cutting small portions of the septum with each bite. Once the uterotubal cones are visualized, the cuts should become more shallow and the small vessels crossing the septum from the myometrium should be closely observed to avoid penetrating the myometrial tissue. With the laparoscope in place and its dimmed light, the assistant observes the translucency or diaphanoscopy of the hysteroscopic light through the uterine wall, warning the hysteroscopist of any increasing translucency as the division progresses in this fundal area. Once the septal division has been completed and before the instruments are removed, the uterine fundal area is observed hysteroscopically, decreas-

ing the intrauterine pressure to observe for significant bleeding. In the presence of arterial bleeding, selective coagulation is performed with a balltip electrode. If this is necessary, fluid for uterine distention should be switched to fluids devoid of electrolytes such as glycine, sorbitol or mannitol (Valle and Sciara, 1986; Daly *et al.*, 1987; March and Israel, 1987; Perino *et al.*, 1987a) (Figures 56.6–56.9).

As an alternative to laparoscopy, ultrasound may be used to monitor the hysteroscopic dissection and avoid penetration into the myometrium; however, it is important when using this sonographic aid to maintain the ultrasound transducer's beam in the plane where the scissors are operating.

The advantages of dividing the uterine septum with scissors are:

- The simple technique can be performed quickly.
- The technique is applicable to most septa.
- The scissors can be easily guided into the recessed areas of the septum.
- No electricity is used and so the media to distend the uterine cavity can contain electrolytes, giving a safety margin for use of fluids as a larger volume deficit can be permitted than if using fluid devoid of electrolytes.
- No additional expense and monitoring of energy sources is required.

Small hysteroscopic scissors can become easily dulled and loose and may not cut precisely, so they should be exchanged periodically and repaired. Also, division of the septum should be maintained in the midline to avoid bleeding. Sharp scissors can cause a perforation if not controlled, particularly in the uterine fundal and cornual regions.

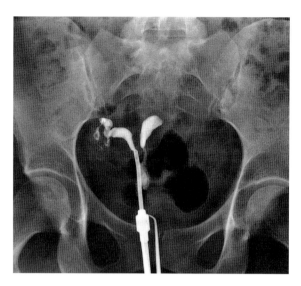

Figure 56.6 Hysterosalpingogram shows a midline division of uterine cavity.

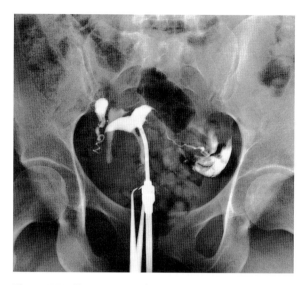

Figure 56.9 Postoperative hysterosalpingogram shows a unified uterine cavity.

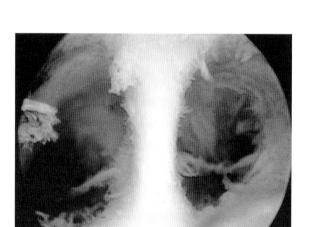

Figure 56.7 Hysteroscopic view of uterine septum.

Finally, not all hysteroscopes have a perfect continuous flow; therefore, a washing effect cannot be provided unless a double-channel hysteroscope or continuous flow hysteroscope is available (Table 56.1).

Resectoscopic Division of the Uterine Septum

A gynecologic resectoscope with an 8–9 mm outer diameter and a narrow and thin electrode (cutting loop, preferably pointed forward, knife electrode or wire electrode) can be used to divide the septum by contact electrosurgery (DeCherney *et al.*, 1986). Knife electrodes have been modified for this purpose and are available from the various manufacturing companies. Whether they are thinner or thicker depends upon the thickness of the tissue to

Table 56.1 Advantages and disadvantages of hysteroscopic metroplasty using scissors.

Advantages

    Relatively simple
    Quick
    More applicable to thin septa
    Media with electrolytes
    No energy sources required

Disadvantages

    Scissors get dull easily
    Bleeding if not in midline
    Possible perforation
    No washing effect unless double-channel hysteroscope used
    Thick septa are more difficult to divide

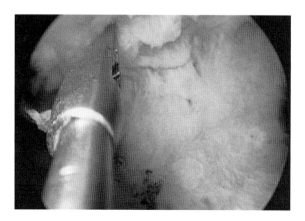

Figure 56.8 Hysteroscopic division of septum with semi-rigid scissors.

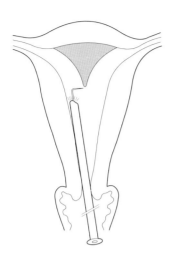

Figure 56.10 Resectoscopic metroplasty.

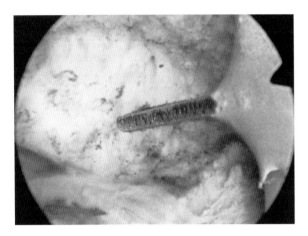

Figure 56.11 Resectoscopic division of uterine septum with a knife electrode.

be divided. The resectoscope allows an excellent continuous flow system that permits exact measurement of the volume of fluid infused and recovered, and provides continuous washing of the uterine cavity and a clear view, removing bubbles and debris produced during the procedure (Figures 56.10, 56.11).

If electricity is used with the resectoscope, only fluids devoid of electrolytes can be used – for example, sorbitol 3%, glycine 1.5% or mannitol 5%, offer clear visibility and permit the use of electrosurgery. Mannitol 5% has been recently recommended: as a good distending medium, decreasing the chances of hyponatremia in view of its osmotic diuretic effect. A specific and meticulous account of non-recovered fluid must be maintained during the procedure because excessive fluid intravasation can occur, causing water overload, which can be worsened by the lack of electrolytes. This lack can

trigger hyponatremia. When monitoring for fluid deficit, care must be taken not to permit more than 800 ml of deficit before determining the patient's serum sodium concentration and establish appropriate treatment if necessary and/or discontinue the procedure.

The uterine septum is divided, beginning at the apex or nadir by short and brief contacts of the loop or knife electrode with the septum. An unmodulated or pure cutting current at 90–100 W can be used; alternatively the current could be blended with 80% of unmodulated current delivery and 20% of modulated current. This is the only time the resectoscope is used cutting forward rather than with a shaving motion towards the operator, which is commonly used for polyps, myomas or endometrial resection. Extra care should be used in determining the exact depth of penetration and direction of the electrode. Laparoscopic or sonographic monitoring is mandatory for septal resection. It is important to observe the symmetry of both uterotubal cones and, with laparoscopy, the transillumination of the resectoscope's light through the uterine wall (Creinin and Chen, 1992; Yaron *et al.*, 1994). When using sonography as a monitoring aid, the thickness of the fundal uterine wall should be carefully observed. The resectoscopic electrodes will coagulate any vessel encountered, so upon reaching the uterine fundal area it is of utmost important to avoid resection into the myometrial tissue. The contact of the electrode should become even more superficial and the resectoscopic transillumination more clearly and meticulously observed by the assistant, with the laparoscope in place.

While dividing the uterine septum using electrosurgery, it is important to observe periodically from a distance the uterine cavity's symmetry at the level of the internal os. During the division of the septum, this symmetry may not be evident while working close to tissue.

With resectoscopic division of the uterine septum, bleeding is decreased compared with division with scissors due to the coagulating effect of the electrical energy, the cuts are easy and the uterine cavity is washed by the continuous flow of distending fluid through the resectoscope. Visualization is excellent and manipulation is relatively easy. The disadvantages are that monopolar electrical current is necessary and peripheral coagulation of the adjacent normal endometrium (which is a reservoir for future re-epithelialization of the area) may occur. Furthermore, at the juxtaposed myometrium, the landmarks are lost because the coagulating power of the electric energy may not allow for observation of the small arterial bleeders usually observed with mechanical division.

The fluids used for this procedure should not

contain electrolytes to permit electrosurgery, and care must be taken to avoid fluid overload if there is excessive intravasation. Broad septa, which tend to be more vascularized than thin ones, are best treated with the resectoscope (Table 56.2).

Table 56.2 Advantages and disadvantages of hystero-scopic metroplasty using the resectoscope.

Advantages

   No significant bleeding
   Cuts fast and easily
   Washing of uterine cavity
   Excellent visibility
   Advantageous for broad septa

Disadvantages

   Electrosurgery required (monopolar)
   Possible peripheral endometrial coagulation
   Landmarks of myometrium lost
   Need for fluids without electrolytes
   Needs proficiency with the resectoscope

Hysteroscopic Metroplasty with Fiberoptic Lasers

The septum can be divided with fiberoptic lasers, particularly the neodymium:yttrium-aluminum-garnet (Nd:YAG) laser with or without extruded or sculpted fibers of the sharp or conical type to permit cutting. The argon or the potassium titanyl phosphate-532 laser can also be used in this manner, although the lower power produced by these lasers makes cutting of the septum more tedious. Only sculpted or extruded fibers should be used in the uterus. Coaxal fibers fitted with sapphire tips need to be cooled continuously, either by fluids or by gases. Although fiberoptic lasers are not difficult to use with hysteroscopy, gases to cool sapphire tips should never be used in the uterus because of the high flow (about $1\,l\,min^{-1}$) required to cool the sapphire tips.

Because lasers are not conductive, electrolyte-containing fluids should be used to distend the uterine cavity. Normal saline, dextrose 5% in 1/2 normal saline, or Ringer's lactate are most useful for distending the uterine cavity and providing clear visualization. It is important to have some outflow channel in the hysteroscope when performing these hysteroscopic techniques to remove the debris and bubbles produced with the activated laser; a continuous flow hysteroscope or one with inflow and outflow channels is therefore most advantageous.

Division of the uterine septum should begin at the nadir of the septum in the midline, dividing the

septum from side to side. The fiber tip must be in the field of view at all times during activation of the laser. Care must be taken to move the fiber continuously to prevent boring into one hole. Because division of the septum with fiberoptic lasers can be tedious, the division should be systematic from side to side. The same precautions should be taken as with division of the septum with electrocoagulation. The operator must avoid invading the juxtaposed fundal myometrium as the coagulating power of the laser will also seal small arterial vessels at the fundal uterine wall. The uterine fundal area should keep a convex shape rather than a concave configuration to avoid inadvertently penetrating the muscular layer (Lobaugh *et al.*, 1994) (Figures 56.12, 56.13).

The advantages of hysteroscopic division with fiberoptic lasers are that:

● Bleeding is avoided in view of the coagulating power of the laser.
● Fiber lasers cut well and are easy to manipulate, perhaps even more easy to manipulate than the resectoscope.
● In view of the laser's lack of conductivity, fluids with electrolytes can be used.

The disadvantages are:

● The laser is an expensive energy source and needs maintenance and care.
● Special protective glasses or filters are necessary because the backscattering of this fiberoptic laser may damage the retina of the surgeon and other members of the operating team.
● The possibility of lateral scattering makes lasers theoretically problematic for the normal endometrium peripheral to the divided septum. Damage to this peripheral endometrium may slow epithelization of the newly denuded area.
● Lasers require special maintenance and assistance, including a laser safety officer for operating and calibrating the unit, and surveillance of appropriate protection for the assisting personnel.

As the procedure of dividing the uterine septum may be tedious, excessive amounts of fluid may be required. If the hysteroscope lacks a continuous flow system or double channel to collect the returning fluid after cleansing the cavity from bubbles and debris, excessive fluid may be absorbed by the patient. In the absence of a good monitoring system for measuring the inflow and outflow of the liquid medium, the deficit or unrecovered fluid may not be adequately measured, thereby subjecting the patient to the risk of developing pulmonary edema

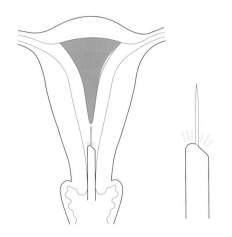

Figure 56.12 Hysteroscopic metroplasty with fiber laser.

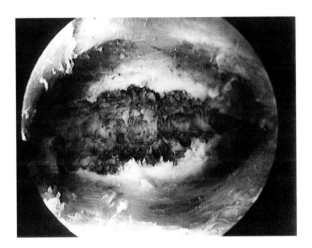

Figure 56.13 Hysteroscopic view of unified uterine cavity after laser metroplasty.

Table 56.3 Advantages and disadvantages of hysteroscopic metroplasty using fiberoptic laser.

Advantages

  No significant bleeding
  Cuts well
  Easy manipulation
  Can use fluids with electrolytes

Disadvantages

  Expensive
  Need special protective glasses
  Possible lateral scattering
  Requires special maintenance and assistance (laser
    safety officer)
  Continuous flow hysteroscope

sidered, including the use of diuretics, (Tables 56.3, 56.4).

Concomitant laparoscopy will warn the hysteroscopist of possible uterine perforation – the laparoscopist observes a uniform transillumination produced by the hysteroscope's light through the uterine wall and can warn the hysteroscopist of imminent perforation.

Hysteroscopic Treatment of Complete Uterine Septum

Division of partial or complete uterine septa dividing the uterine corpus is well established but hysteroscopic treatment of complete uterine septa including the cervix deserves special consideration. This type of anomaly produces two cervical openings. In patients with a complete uterine septum involving the cervix, the technique used is similar to that proposed by Daly *et al.* (1983). Once the laparoscope is in place, one of the cervices is grasped anteriorly with a tenaculum, and then the cervical canal is gradually dilated to 7–8 Hegar. The operative hysteroscope attached to its light source and irrigating solution is then introduced and

secondary to fluid overload despite the use of fluids containing electrolytes. It is therefore important to monitor the fluid infused and recovered, and to maintain the uterine pressure so that it does not exceed the mean arterial pressure of about 100 mm Hg. If more than 1500 ml of fluid is not recovered, therapeutic measures should be con-

Table 56.4 Comparison of hysteroscopic metroplasty using scissors, resectoscope or fiberoptic laser.

Feature	Scissors	Resectoscope	Fiberoptic laser
Simplicity	++	+	+
Speed	+++	++	+
Hemostasis	+	+++	+++
Applicable to all septa	+++	++	++
Evaluation of juxtaposed myometrium	+++	+	+
Expense	+	++	+++
possible perforation	+	+++	++
Required skill	+++	+++	+++
Fluid overload	+	++	++

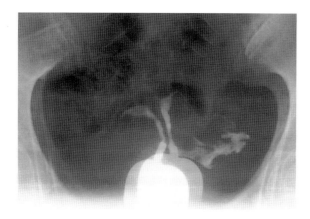

Figure 56.14 Hysterosalpingogram shows complete division of uterine cavity and cervix.

Despite the difficulty of the initial approach to the uterine septum involving the cervical canal, it is appropriate to divide only the corporeal portion of the septum without attempting removal of the cervical portion, particularly to avoid trauma to this area, which may produce untoward sequelae for future fertility. Traditionally it has been agreed to remove only the corporeal septum in these patients and not the cervical extension to avoid scarring or possible cervical incompetence. This type of treatment using traditional abdominal metroplasty has not caused problems with pregnancy and subsequent vaginal delivery (McShane *et al.*, 1983; Carp *et al.*, 1990, Valle, 1996). Because we now have a technique accomplishing the same objective hysteroscopically, the total uterine septum can be treated without removing the cervical extension. Embryologically, it is well known that reabsorption of the original complete septation of the uterus, cervix and vagina, begins at the lower portion of the uterus, close to the internal os (Moore, 1988). When reabsorption fails, this area is usually the thinnest of a persistent septum therefore, permitting the initial fenestration by hysteroscopy and then completion with a septal division, as if it were treatment of a complete uterine septum, therefore facilitating hysteroscopic metroplasty. Attempts to divide the cervical and corporal portion of the septum in one step have been described in some patients with apparently no untoward sequelae, but more experience and longer follow-up are necessary to perform this procedure routinely, particularly when dealing with broad cervical septa (Vercellini *et al.*, 1994). Therefore at present this treatment should be used as an alternative when the hysteroscopic treatment of the septum preserving the cervix fails, rather than to proceed with abdominal metroplasty. Nonetheless, these patients should be closely followed during their future gestations and if there are

observation begins at the level of the internal cervical os. A probe is then passed through the adjacent cervical canal and gentle indentation is performed just above the internal cervical os. Under hysteroscopic view, a small window is produced with hysteroscopic scissors or a thin knife electrode using the resectoscope. Once this is accomplished, the probe is inserted through this window. When sufficient space has been created to observe the opposed uterine cavity, the probe is withdrawn and the corresponding endocervical canal is occluded with a tenaculum. The hysteroscopic division of the remaining uterine septum is then begun at this level and it is progressively divided until there is symmetry of the fundal area, and both uterotubal cones and tubal openings are seen. The uterine cavity is observed systematically from the internal cervical os for symmetry and the operation is completed (Figures 56.14–56.19). Alternatively, the resectoscope fitted with a thin electrode or a fiber laser can also be used for this purpose (Rock *et al.*, 1987).

Figure 56.15 Diagramatic representation of septal indentation for initial hysteroscopic fenestration.

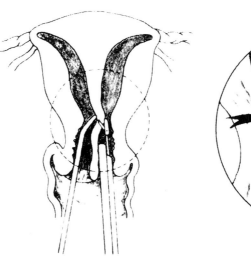
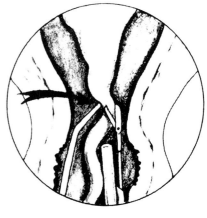

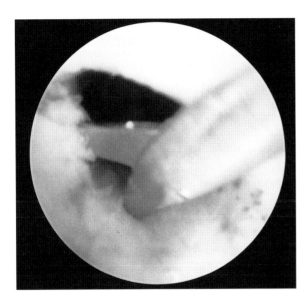

Figure 56.16 Beginning septal fenestration just above internal cervical os.

early signs of cervical incompetence a prophylactic cerclage should be performed.

Intraoperative and Postoperative Management

Prophylactic antibiotics are commonly used to prevent infection of the uterine cavity and specifically of the fallopian tubes when extensive intrauterine dissections are required. Intravenous cephalosporins can be used intraoperatively and continued for 3–4 days postoperatively orally. Cefazolin 1 g intravenous piggyback is used 30 minutes before surgery, followed by cefalexin 500 mg four times a day orally for 3–4 days following the procedure. While the use of high doses of conjugated natural estrogen such as conjugated estrogens is controversial, this medication may allow better and faster re-epithelization of the denuded area left by the division of the septum. High doses, such as conjugated estrogens 2.5 mg twice a day orally for 30 days can be used and terminal progesterone added in the form of medroxyprogesterone acetate 10 mg orally each day in the last ten days of this artificial cycle. When the patient completes withdrawal bleeding from hormonal therapy a hysterosalpingogram should be performed to assess the symmetry of the uterine cavity. Pregnancy can be attempted when a satisfactory result is obtained. The perpendicular axis and direction by which the uterine cavity is observed in hysterosalpingography means that this is an excellent method for assessing the surgical results. Hysteroscopy, which observes from the cervical axis, may not be as good for evaluating the symmetry of the uterine fundus. Either method can be used as long as the practitioner is aware of the drawbacks.

It is not unusual to see a small central fundal residual septal projection on hysterosalpingography following hysteroscopic division of the uterine septum. Nonetheless, when a small residual septum, less than 1 cm in length, is observed, no additional therapy is performed, as this residual septum has no clinical significance.

No stents are used postoperatively as formation of intrauterine adhesions following this treatment is practically non-existent based on experience with the Bret–Tompkins metroplasty and that obtained with hysteroscopic division of the septum (Valle, 1978; Vercellini *et al.*, 1989). Fundal adhesions observed postoperatively are usually due to an incomplete division of the septum.

Figure 56.17 Diagrammatic representation of completed septal fenestration.

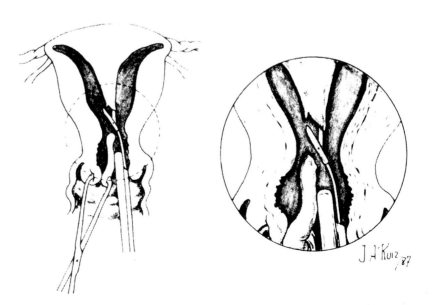

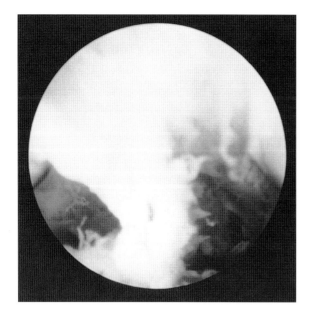

Figure 56.18 Hysteroscopic view of completed septal fenestration and residual corporeal septum.

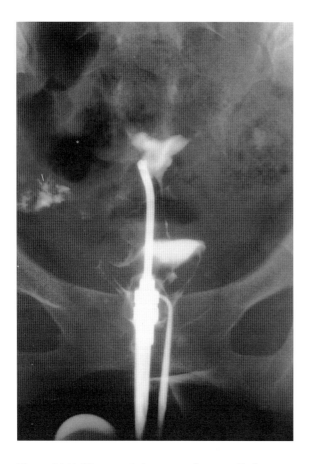

Figure 56.19 Hysterosalpingogram shows unified uterine cavity following hysteroscopic metroplasty of complete uterine septum with septate cervix.

Comparison of Results

The reproductive outcome following hysteroscopic treatment of a symptomatic septate uterus has surpassed that obtained with traditional abdominal metroplasty in patients who have previously had repetitive abortions, with over 85% of patients having a viable pregnancy (Siegler and Valle, 1988; Hassiakos and Zourlas, 1990; Siegler *et al.*, 1990). No cases of secondary infertility due to pelvic adhesions have occurred. Furthermore, the patient is spared a laparotomy and hysterotomy, eliminating the potential for pelvic adhesions as well as the associated pain, disability and expense. Patients treated hysteroscopically need to wait only four weeks to attempt conception and do not require a mandatory cesarean section. The procedure is performed on an ambulatory basis and patients are discharged 3–4 hours following endoscopic surgery.

Although there is more experience with hysteroscopic division of the uterine septum using hysteroscopic scissors, the reproductive outcome obtained using fiberoptic lasers, such as the argon, KTP-532, and the Nd:YAG laser fitted with sculptured fibers, seems to equal that obtained with hysteroscopic scissors (Daniell *et al.*, 1987; Daly *et al.*, 1989; Candiani *et al.*, 1991; Choe and Baggish, 1992; Fedele *et al.*, 1993). The original reporting on division of the uterine septum using the resectoscope with a cutting loop eliminated 30% of the patients because of inability to divide all septa, particularly broad ones (DeCherney *et al.*, 1986). This selective treatment may have had to do with the type of electrode used, particularly the 90° bent resecting loop. The new knife electrodes are thinner and better designed to reach these areas, and the feasibility rate seems to equal that obtained with hysteroscopic scissors and fiberoptic lasers. Although the choice of instruments depends in part upon the familiarity and experience of the operators with various modalities, the use of hysteroscopic scissors for division of the uterine septum has been favored by the majority of physicians performing this type of operation (Siegler and Valle, 1988; Hassiakos and Zourlas, 1990; Candiani *et al.*, 1991) (Table 56.5).

Other Concomitant Procedures

Pathology associated with a septate uterus requires the same treatment and preparations as that for lesions occurring alone. Polyps, submucosal myomas, and intrauterine adhesions can be associated with uterine septation and require treatment.

Table 56.5 Details and results of hysteroscopic metroplasty performed by different investigators. (Adapted from Siegler and Valle, 1988.)

Author	Number of patients	Medium	Technique	IUD	E/P	Antibiotics	Pregnancy			
							Term	Premature	Abortion	In Progress
Edstrom (1974)	2	Dextran 70, 32%	Rigid biopsy forceps	+	–	–	–	1 (19 wks)	–	–
Chervenak and Neuwirth (1981)	2	Dextran 70, 32%	Scissors adjacent to hysteroscope	+	+	+	1	–	–	–
Rosenberg et al. (1981)	1	Dextran 70, 32%	Flexible scissors	NA	NA	NA	NA	–	–	–
Daly et al. (1983)	25	Dextran 70, 32%	–	–	+	–	7	–	1	–
Perino et al. (1985)	11	CO_2	Flexible, semi-rigid scissors	+	–	–	NA	–	–	–
DeCherney et al. (1986)	72	Dextran 70,32%	Resectoscope	–	–	–	58	1	4	4
Corson and Batzer (1986)	18	Dextran 70, 32%, CO_2	Resectoscope and rigid scissors	–	–	–	10	1	2	2
Fayez (1986)	19	Dextran 70, 32%	Rigid scissors	Foley catheter	–	+	14	–	–	–
March and Israel (1987)	91	Dextran 70, 32%	Flexible scissors	+	+	–	44	4	7	7
Valle (1987)	59	D5W/Dextran 70, 32%	Flexible, semi-rigid	–	+	+	44	2	5	–
Choe and Baggish (1992)	19	Dextran 70, 32%	Nd:YAG with bare or sculptured fibers	Foley catheter (three patients)	+	+	10	1	1	3
Fedele et al. (1993)	102	Dextran 40, 10% in normal saline	Semi-rigid scissors (80) Argon laser (10) Resectoscope (12)	+ (21)	+ (39)	+	45	10	11	NA
Valle (1996)	124	D5 in 1/2 normal saline Glycine 1.5%	Semi-rigid scissors (98) Resectoscope (20) Nd:YAG laser (6)	–	+	+	84	7	12	–
Totals	545						317 (78.4)	26 (6.4%)	43 (10.6%)	16 (4.4%)

IUD, intrauterine device; E/P estrogens/progesterone; NA non-applicable

In general it is best to treat concomitant lesions before the uterine septum is divided to allow a better visualization of the symmetry of the divided uterine cavities. Occasionally, however, the septum has to be excised first to permit better visualization of the uterine cavity (Stillman and Asarkof, 1985).

The laparoscope is an excellent adjunct in monitoring the surgical treatment of the symptomatic septate uterus, revealing and aiding in the treatment of tubal-peritoneal pathology, and monitoring division of the uterine septum. Sonography has also been used for this purpose, but maintaining the transducer on the same plane with the operating hysteroscope is cumbersome. Maintaining appropriate uterine planes where the uterine wall, uterine septum, and operating instruments can be seen simultaneously is difficult, particularly when the uterus moves as the hysteroscopist proceeds with division of the septum. Nonetheless, concomitant sonography will increase the safety of performing these surgical procedures, if laparoscopy is contraindicated (Perino *et al.*, 1987b; Querleu *et al.*, 1990). No additional benefit can be added by sonography to visualize the pelvic structures and concomitant pathology such as adhesions, endometriosis or tubal distortions, except in observing enlargement of the ovaries and evaluating possible ovarian cysts (Valle, 1996).

Summary and Conclusions

A uterine septum may be the reason for reproductive failure, specifically repetitive spontaneous abortions, in 20–25% of women affected with this condition. When this occurs, the uterine septum requires surgical correction.

The treatment of the symptomatic septate uterus has been greatly facilitated by the hysteroscopic approach. The procedure that in the past required a laparotomy and hysterotomy with extensive hospitalization, disability, inconvenience and increased cost to the patient, can now be provided on an ambulatory basis with minimal invasive techniques. The preservation of the integrity of the uterine walls avoids unnecessary routine cesarean section for future viable pregnancies. The offending pathology is selectively treated without compromising normal structures and there are no untoward sequelae affecting future fertility with this approach. The endoscopic approach to treat the uterine septum therefore is one of the best applications of minimally invasive surgery.

The hysteroscopic treatment of the symptomatic septate uterus can be accomplished by three different techniques: scissors, resectoscope and fiberoptic laser. All three methods have advantages and disadvantages and must be used with knowledge of each particular technology and its drawbacks. Each technique should be tailored not only to the anatomy, embryology, and symptomatology of each process, but also to the experience and selective choice of the operator. The operator should select the appropriate method and technique for each patient. The goal of therapy should remain a successful viable pregnancy for those patients with impaired reproductive ability, keeping in mind the safety of the patient – the least morbidity possible, an absence of complications and untoward sequelae, overall effectiveness of the treatment and diminution of unnecessary cost. Based on the relative simplicity of the hysteroscopic method, its minimal invasion, the preservation of the uterine wall's integrity, and the excellent results achieved by this approach, hysteroscopic division of the symptomatic uterine septum should be accepted as the method of choice for the treatment of this uterine anomaly.

References

Bret AJ, Guillet B (1959) Hysteroplastie reconstructive sans resection musculaire dans les malformations uterines, cause d'avortaments a repetition. *Presse Medicale* **67**: 394–397.

Buttram VC, Gibbons WE (1979) Müllerian anomalies: A proposed classification (an analysis of 144 cases). *Fertility and Sterility* **32**: 40–46.

Candiani GB, Vercellini P, Fedele L, Carinelli SG, Merlo D, Arcaiini L (1990) Repair of the uterine cavity after hysteroscopic septal incision. *Fertility and Sterility* **54**: 991–994.

Candiani GB, Vercellini P, Fidele L, Garsia S, Brioschi D, Villa L (1991) Argon laser versus microscissors for hysteroscopic incision of uterine septa. *American Journal of Obstetrics and Gynecology* **164**: 87–90.

Carp HJA, Toder V, Mashiach S, Nebel L, Serr DM (1990) Recurrent miscarriage: a review of current concepts, immune mechanisms, and results of treatment. *Obstetrical and Gynecological Survey* **45**: 657–669.

Choe JK, Baggish MS (1992) Hysteroscopic treatment of septate uterus with Neodymium-YAG laser. *Fertility and Sterility* **57**: 81–84.

Creinin M, Chen M (1992) Uterine defect in a twin pregnancy with a history of hysteroscopic fundal perforation. *Obstetrics and Gynecology* **79**: 879–880.

Daly DC, Tohan N, Walters C, Riddick DH (1983) Hysteroscopic resection of the uterine septum in the presence of a septate cervix. *Fertility and Sterility* **39**: 560–563.

Daly DC, Walters CA, Soto-Albors CE, Riddick DH (1987) Hysteroscopic metroplasty: Surgical technique and obstetric outcome. *Fertility and Sterility* **48**: 623–628.

Daly DC, Maier D, Soto–Albors C (1989) Hysteroscopic metroplasty: Six years experience. *Obstetrics and Gynecology* **73**: 201–205.

Daniell JF, Osher S, Miller W (1987) Hysteroscopic resection of uterine septa with visible light laser energy. *Colposcopy and Gynecologic Laser Surgery* **3**: 217–220.

DeCherney AH, Russell JB, Graebe RA, Polan ML (1986) Resectoscopic management of Müllerian fusion defects. *Fertility and Sterility* **45**: 726–728.

Edstrom K (1974) Intrauterine surgical procedures during hysteroscopy. *Endoscopy* **6**: 175–181.

El Mahgoub, S (1978) Unification of a septate uterus: Mahgoub's operation. *International Journal of Gynecology and Obstetrics* **15**: 400–404.

Fayez JA (1986) Comparison between abdominal and hysteroscopic metroplasty. *Obstetrics and Gynecology* **68**: 399–403.

Fedele L, Arcaini L, Parazzini F, Verecellini P, Dinola, G (1993) Reproductive prognosis after hysteroscopic metroplasty in 102 women: life-table analysis. *Fertility and Sterility* **59**: 768–772.

Fedele L, Bianchi S, Marchini M, Frenchi D, Tozzi L, Dorta M (1996) Ultrastructural aspects of endometrium in infertile women with septate uterus. *Fertility and Sterility* **65**: 750–752.

Golan A, Langer R, Butovsky I, Caspi E (1989) Congenital anomalies of the müllerian system. *Fertility and Sterility* **51**: 747–855.

Halvorson LM, Aserkoff RD, Ozkowitz SP (1993) Spontaneous uterine rupture after hysteroscopic metroplasty with uterine perforation. A case report. *Journal of Reproductive Medicine* **38**: 236–238.

Hassiakos DK, Zourlas PA (1990) Transcervical division of the uterine septa. *Obstetrical and Gynecological Survey* **45**: 165–173.

Heinonen PK, Saarikaki S, Pystynen P (1982) Reproductive performance of women with uterine anomalies. *Acta Obstetricia et Gynecologica Scandinavica* **61**: 157–162.

Howe RS (1993) Third-trimester uterine rupture following hysteroscopic uterine perforation. *Obstetrics and Gynecology* **81**: 827–829.

Jones AW, Jones GES (1953) Double uterus as an etiologic factor in repeated abortions: Indications for surgical repair. *American Journal of Obstetrics and Gynecology* **65**: 325–339.

Kazer RR, Meyer K, Valle RF (1992) Late hemorrhage after transcervical division of a uterine septum: a report of two cases. *Fertility and Sterility* **57**: 930–932.

Lobaugh ML, Bammel BM, Duke D, Webster BW (1994) Uterine rupture during pregnancy in a patient with a history of hysteroscopic metroplasty. *Obstetrics and Gynecology* **83**: 838–840.

March CM, Israel R (1987) Hysteroscopic management of recurrent abortion caused by septate uterus. *American Journal of Obstetrics and Gynecology* **156**: 834–842.

McShane PM, Reilly RJ, Schiff I (1983) Pregnancy outcomes following Tompkins metroplasty. *Fertility and Sterility* 190–194.

Moore KL (1988) *The Developing Human. Clinically Oriented Embryology. The Urogenital System* 4th edition. pp. 246–285. Philadelphia: W.B. Saunders Company.

Perino A, Mencaglia L, Hamou J, Cittadini E (1987a) Hysteroscopy for metroplasty of uterine septa: report of 24 cases. *Fertility and Sterility* **48**: 321–323.

Perino A, Catinella E, Comparetto G *et al.* (1987b) Hysteroscopic metroplasty: The role of ultrasound in the diagnosis and monitoring of patients with uterine septa. *Acta Europaea Fertilitatis* **18**: 349–352.

Querleu P, Brasme TL, Parmentier D (1990) Ultrasound-guided transcervical metroplasty. *Fertility and Sterility* **54**: 995–998.

Rock JA, Jones HW (1977) The clinical management of the double uterus. *Fertility and Sterility* **28**: 708–806.

Rock JA, Zacur HA (1983) The clinical management of repeated early pregnancy wastage. *Fertility and Sterility* **39**: 123 140.

Rock JA, Murphy AA, Cooper WH (1987) Resectoscopic techniques for the lysis of a class V: Complete uterine septum. *Fertility and Sterility* **48**: 495–496.

Ruge P (1884) Einen Fall von Schwangerschaft bei uterus septus. *A. Geburtschilfe Gynakologie* **10**: 141–145.

Siegler AM, Valle RF (1988) Therapeutic hysteroscopic procedures. *Fertility and Sterility* **50**: 685–701.

Siegler AM, Valle RF, Lindemann HJ, Mencaglia L (1990) *Hysteroscopic Metroplasty. Therapeutic Hysteroscopy. Indications and Techniques.* pp. 62–81. The C.V. Mosby Company.

Stillman RJ, Asarkof N (1985) Association between Müllerian duct malformations and Asherman's syndrome in infertile women. *Obstetrics and Gynecology* **65**: 673–677.

Tompkins P (1962) Comments on the bicornuate uterus and twinning. *Surgical Clinics of North America* **42**: 1049–1062.

Valle RF (1978) Hysteroscopy: Diagnostic and therapeutic applications. *Journal of Reproductive Medicine* **20**: 115–118.

Valle RF (1985) Clinical management of uterine factors in infertile patients. In Speroff L (ed.) *Seminars in Reproductive Endocrinology*, vol. 3(3). pp. 149–167. New York Thieme–Stratton, Inc. Georg Thieme Verlag.

Valle RF (1995) Uterine septa. In Beiber EJ, Loffer FD (eds) *Gynecologic Resectoscopy*. pp. 128–152. Cambridge, MA: Blackwell Science.

Valle RF (1996) Hysteroscopic treatment of partial and complete uterine septa. *International Journal of Fertility* **41**: 310–315.

Valle RF, Sciarra JJ (1986) Hysteroscopic treatment of the septate uterus. *Obstetrics and Gynecology* **676**: 253–257.

Vercellini P, Fedele L, Arcaini L (1989) Value of intra-uterine device insertion and estrogen administration after hysteroscopic metroplasty. *Journal of Reproductive Medicine* **34**: 447–450.

Vercellini P, Ragni G, Trespide L, Oldani S, Panazza S, Crosignani PG (1994) A modified technique for correction of the complete septate uterus. *Acta Obstetricia et Gynecologica Scandinavica* **73**: 425–428.

Yaron Y, Shenhav M, Jaffa AJ, Lessing JB, Peyser MR (1994) Uterine rupture at 33 weeks' gestation subsequent to hysteroscopic uterine perforation. *American Journal of Obstetrics and Gynecology* **170**: 786–787.

57

Hysteroscopic Tubal Occlusion

FRANKLIN D. LOFFER

University of Arizona School of Medicine, Phoenix, Arizona, USA

The ease with which the tubal ostia can be seen hysteroscopically has challenged gynecologic endoscopists to find a transcervical method to occlude the fallopian tube for sterilization. Both blind and hysteroscopically controlled methods have been tried. These methods involve either:

- Injection of a sclerosing agent into the tube.
- Destruction of the interstitial portion of the tube.
- Occlusion of the tube with a plug.

Although the tubal ostia can be identified in virtually all patients it is difficult to achieve sterilization of the tube at its uterine junction. The primary reason for this difficulty lies in the inability to cause the tube to be consistently occluded by either an induced process of tissue scarring or by the tubal occluding devices.

This chapter will review:

- Hysteroscopic instrumentation and techniques for approaching the tubal ostia for sterilization procedures.
- The techniques and results of both the blind and hysteroscopic procedures involving injection of sclerosing agents, electrical destruction and the use of mechanical plugs.
- The reason for the difficulty and lack of success with each of these approaches.
- The formed in-place silicone plug, which is the only commercially available hysteroscopic tubal occlusion technique available at this time.

Although the success of transcervical sterilization procedures has been limited, it is the author's hope that a review of this chapter will provide historic and clinical information for those who attempt the currently available method or develop new ones.

Hysteroscopic Instrumentation and Techniques for Approaching the Uterine Tubal Ostia

The tubal ostia can be seen in virtually all patients if certain parameters in patient selection are chosen and appropriate hysteroscopic techniques employed. Among the author's 265 hysteroscopic tubal plug occlusion patients who underwent 310 procedures the tubal ostia were seen at the first procedure in 97.7% of women.

The optimal time for identification of the tubal ostia is in the immediate postmenstrual phase. Identification may be difficult if hysteroscopy is carried out late in the menstrual cycle since the endometrium will bleed easily on contact and the thick endometrium may obscure the tubal opening. It is unnecessary to suppress the endometrium for good visualization with danazol or gonadotropin releasing hormone (GnRH) analogs if the procedure is timed for the early proliferative phase.

Both rigid and flexible hysteroscopes can be used to identify and approach the tubal ostia during occlusion procedures. The rigid telescopes have the advantage of easier orientation since the optical view within the uterus has a fixed relationship to the light post in all telescopes. When a rigid hysteroscope is used, a 30° foreoblique lens provides the easiest-to-use optics for viewing the ostia. The hysteroscope can be introduced with the optics directed anteriorly in an anterior uterus and posteriorly in the posterior uterus. Once inside the cavity the corresponding tubal ostium will come into full view when the hysteroscope is rotated 90° in that direction.

Flexible hysteroscopes are slightly more difficult to orient when in the uterine cavity, but have the advantage that they can always be positioned to look directly into the ostia.

Introducing instruments and catheters into the tubal ostium is more difficult if a rigid hysteroscope is used. The deflecting arm of the Alberan bridge is helpful. It will allow the intrauterine position of the tip of flexible surgical instruments and catheters, which have been passed through the bridge's 7F operative channel, to be varied. A standard bridge without the deflecting arm can be used in the majority of cases, but limits the surgeon's ability to vary the direction at which the tubal ostium is approached. A continuous flow system will also improve results (deBlok et al., 1992).

Visualization of the tubal ostia can be compromised because of the presence of blood, mucus or endometrial debris, even when carbon dioxide (CO_2), 32% dextran 70 (Hyskon, Medisan Pharmaceuticals Inc., New Jersey, USA) or the low viscosity fluids are used to distend the uterus. Several methods are available for obtaining adequate visualization when the distending media alone is not providing adequate visualization (Loffer, 1990).

When visualization is a problem with CO_2 most surgeons would probably abandon it and choose one of the other media. Hyskon has the advantage that blood is not miscible with it. A clear view is obtained because any uterine bleeding is pushed aside by the distending media. Although the author used Hyston for all his tubal occlusion patients the ostia were still frequently obscured by mucus, debris or blood (Loffer, 1984). When this occurred the author used a 7F catheter (No. 104688–7, Karl Storz Endoscopy of America Inc., California, USA) with a syringe for suction. This was an indispensable part of visualizing the tubal ostium since a continuous flow system does not work optimally with Hyskon. When a low viscosity fluid is used and a continuous flow hysteroscopy is not available the same catheter described above can be used to 'vacuum' the cavity. The debris obscuring the tubal ostium is forced out of the uterus by the intrauterine pressure of the low viscosity fluid.

A Review of Techniques for Transcervical Tubal Occlusion

The appeal of a transcervical tubal occlusion technique lies in the fact that the tubes can be approached without a surgical incision. A blind method would allow greater application in both developed and developing countries than one that requires hysteroscopic equipment and skills.

Instrumentation for blind methods of injecting into the fallopian tube have been available for many years (Corfman and Taylor, 1966). The Femcet system was developed to inject methylcyanoacrylate into the fallopian tubes after occluding the uterine cavity with a balloon (Richart et al., 1987). A bilateral tubal occlusion rate was achieved in 71% after one application and 89% after a second application one month later. The patients experience a moderate degree of pain during the procedure. In addition there is the inconvenience and expense of a follow-up hysterosalpingogram. Although promising, this procedure is not available to clinicians at this time.

Ishikawa was reported to have achieved a 98% tubal closure in 136 cases using a blind thermal coagulation technique with the probe at a temperature of 135° for 30–35 s (Rimkus and Semm, 1974). Rimkus and Semm reported a similar technique, but did not publish results. These methods most likely carry the same disadvantage as the electrical methods, which will be discussed later in this chapter.

The injection of quinacrine as a nonspecific sclerosing agent has been reported by several authors. Blind injection into the uterine cavity yielded a bilateral closure rate of 88.2% and pregnancy rate of 1.2/100 women, but only after up to three instillations (Zipper et al., 1970). Direct instillation into the fallopian tube was also tried under hysteroscopic control (Alvarado et al., 1974). This technique is simple since it is easy to place catheters at each fallopian tube. A measured amount of quinacrine in saline was injected into each fallopian tube. The small amount of saline used prevented significant intraperitoneal spread in all but one of the 30 patients included in the report. Bilateral tubal closure rate was evaluated by hysterosalpingogram at three months post application in 16 of the 30 patients. Bilateral closure occurred in six, unilateral obstruction in six and no obstruction in four cases. Failure to occlude the fallopian tube did not appear to be related to the distending media washing the quinacrine out of the fallopian tube since two of the three unilateral closure failures occurred in the tube that was the second to be injected. Recanalization may eventually occur since only the tubal epithelium is destroyed, leaving a patent passage, which can be re-epithelialized.

More recently the insertion into the uterus of 252 mg of quinacrine pellets for two months produced a bilateral tubal closure rate of 73%, which increased to 94% after a third insertion. There were no side effects and no pregnancies after 24 months of follow-up (El Kady et al., 1993).

Electrical methods using high-frequency unipolar equipment initially appeared promising as a hysteroscopic tubal occlusion technique. It was assumed that it would carry a success rate similar to that of laparoscopic tubal coagulation. Numerous authors reported their early experience with this technique. The largest and most successful series involved 930 patients (Quinones et al., 1976). A bilateral tubal occlusion rate of 82.7% was achieved after the first electrocoagulation. An additional 15.5% of patients achieved bilateral tubal occlusion resulting in a total of 98.2% if a second electrocoagulation was done. The power used was 25 W for 8 s. No pregnancies were reported when bilateral tubal occlusion was demonstrated by hysterosalpingogram and the only complication was a perforation of the uterus with the hysteroscope.

Interest in electrical hysteroscopic tubal occlusion techniques essentially ceased after the publication of a collaborative study from ten institutions involving 773 cases (Darabi and Richart, 1977). Tubal patency was demonstrated by hysterosalpingogram or the occurrence of a pregnancy in 245 (31.7%) of cases. Major complications related to the procedure included acute peritonitis in seven patients (0.9%) and ectopic pregnancies in eight patients (1.0%). Bowel damage was documented as the cause of the peritonitis in three patients. One death occurred as a result of the bowel injury. Little interest in electrical hysteroscopic methods existed after this collaborative study because of the high failure rate and the reported complications. Factors relating to these results were studied in a later publication (Darabi et al., 1978).

The fact that a much higher bilateral closure rate and virtually no complications occurred in an equally large series performed by one operator (Quinones et al., 1976) suggests that the experience of the operating surgeon is critical in this procedure.

It is possible that instrumentation could have been developed that would have removed bowel injury as a possible complication. A bipolar probe with markings indicating the depth of cornual penetration may have been all that was needed. Variations in the length, amount, or type of current used may also have provided a higher closure rate.

However, it is the author's opinion that it is not the risk of bowel injury, but the high risk of ectopic pregnancies that makes destruction of the fallopian tube at the uterine junction an impractical method of sterilization. All tubal sterilization procedures carry with them a failure rate, of which a large number are ectopic pregnancies (Loffer and Pent, 1980). However, the risk of an ectopic pregnancy with the electrical hysteroscopic technique is unacceptably higher. Furthermore, when an ectopic pregnancy occurs, a disproportionate number are interstitial ectopic pregnancies. Of the six ectopic pregnancies in one series (Quinones et al., 1976), 50% were described as cornual; while 75% of the ectopic pregnancies in the collaborative study were cornual (Darabi and Richart, 1977). (The term cornual pregnancy denotes an ectopic pregnancy that develops in a rudimentary uterine horn (Hughes, 1977). Presumably the pregnancies described in these papers were interstitial pregnancies.)

The majority of the interstitial pregnancies reported were in tubes known not to be closed. However, the risk of ectopic and interstitial ectopic pregnancies may be even higher with long-term follow-up. Tubes that are apparently closed may recanalize or form fistulas resulting in pregnancies at long intervals after the sterilization procedure (Loffer and Pent, 1980). The length of follow-up in the collaborative study was less than one year in 83.4% of patients (Darabi and Richart, 1977).

The author believes that any method that relies on closure of the interstitial portion of the tube by scarring from necrosis will carry a high ectopic and interstitial ectopic pregnancy rate. The area may not scar closed, but rather slough out, leaving a ready site for recanalization and subsequent interstitial pregnancy. This problem is especially important since interstitial pregnancies carry a much higher risk to patients than other tubal pregnancies.

There are two reports of using the neodymium: yttrium-aluminum-garnet (Nd:YAG) laser to occlude the fallopian tubes hysteroscopically. The first series (Donnez et al., 1990) reported 30 patients in whom bilateral tubal occlusion was proven three months after surgery by hysterosalpingography. In this study a touch technique was used in which the laser energy was brought directly to the tissue via the quartz fiber. A power setting of 80 W was used and a total of 5000–8000 J were applied. The second series (Brumsted et al., 1991) was discontinued because of a bilateral closure in only four of 17 (24%) patients. This method differed in that a nontouch technique was used with a power setting of 50–60 W resulting in fewer total joules being applied to the tissue. Since the laser method, like the electrical method, depends upon the tubes scarring closed and preventing recanalization the author is concerned that a high interstitial pregnancy rate would also occur with this method.

Numerous mechanical plugs have been designed to occlude the tubal ostia. One only needs to view a picture of some of the many designs (Figure 57.1) to

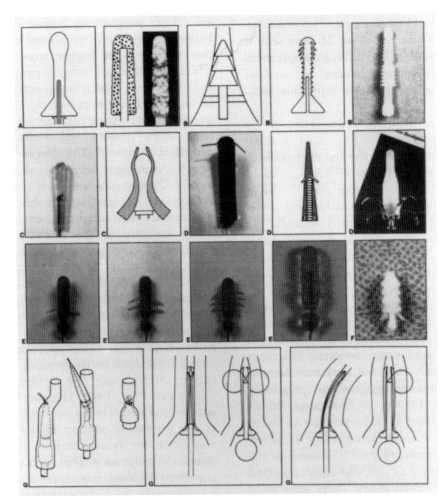

Figure 57.1 Intratubal devices and the principles of their fixation. (A) Insertion without any addition fixation, Bleier. (B) Corrugation of plug surface – left to right: Craft (porous); Sugimoto (Christmas tree pattern); Bleier (fishbone pattern). (C) Swelling after insertion – left to right: Brundin (hydratization); Popp (inflation). (D) Fixation with spines – left to right: Chargoy-Vera, Brueschke and colleagues; Hosseinian and colleagues. (E) Combination – Brundin (hydratization plus anchoring protrusions, the far right shows its swollen state). (F) Combination – Bleier (a solid pin is surrounded by a soft and corrugated cover with two spines). (G) Fixation by tubal wall penetration – left: Cimber (penetration and fixation through ligation; laparotomy is necessary); center and right: Popp (the wall penetrating 'claw' fixed the device; a dowel effect and a corrugated surface can also help the fixation). (Reproduced by permission from Siegler AM and Lindemann HJ (eds) (1984) *Hysteroscopy: Principles and Practice*. Philadelphia: JB Lippincott.)

realize that a simple method does not exist. Retention in the tubal ostium of most plugs was so poor that few underwent clinical trials.

Two tubal plugs have met with some success. One plug (Hamou *et al.*, 1984) is more appropriately defined as an intratubal device since it does not attempt to occlude the fallopian tube. Its expulsion is prevented by a single barb of thread projecting from the device. Long-term results are not available.

The other plug is the formed in-place silicone plug (The Ovabloc System, Advanced Medical Grade Silicones BV, PO Box 51-2810AB Reeuwijk, Kvk 29043456, The Netherlands). It avoids the high expulsion rate found with other plugs by virtue of its dumbbell shape. This plug is formed by the *in* *vivo* hardening of liquid silicone, which has been injected into the fallopian tube. This liquid silicone welds to a preformed intrauterine tip. The preformed tip and the larger ampullary portion of the plug effectively preclude it from being expelled into either the uterine or peritoneal cavity. This technique is the only transcervical tubal occlusion technique that is currently commercially available to clinicians.

The Ovabloc System

Patient selection is important when using the Ovabloc system since tubal occlusion is not achievable in all patients. The manufacturer of the Ovabloc system lists the following exclusion criteria:

- Acute or chronic cervicitis or vaginal infection – until gonorrhea and chlamydia infection have been ruled out.
- A recent history of pelvic inflammatory disease.
- Undiagnosed genital tract bleeding or the presence of a bleeding disorder.
- Congenital malformation of the genital tract or previous tubal surgery.
- Known or suspected genital tract malignancy.

Occlusion is more difficult in patients with a posterior uterus, especially if retroflexed, since the tubal ostia are not readily approached at an angle where silicone can be instilled. In addition, patients with a history of pelvic inflammatory disease have a high risk of having non-patent fallopian tubes and patency is necessary for silicone instillation.

The procedure is readily performed in an office setting using local anesthesia. As the procedure lasts 25–45 minutes the patient should be placed in a dorsal lithotomy position with the legs comfortably cradled. The vulva, vagina and cervix are prepared with 10% povidone–iodine or a similar solution. Draping is not necessary although the author places a sterile drape beneath the buttocks on which to place instrumentation. Anesthesia is provided by paracervical and intracervical block (Loffer, 1984).

Instrumentation needed for this procedure are:

- Paracervical/intracervical block tray.
- Sterile one-sided speculum.
- Tenaculum.
- Cervical dilators (should dilation be required).
- Light source and cable.
- 4 mm telescope and 8 mm continuous flow

sheath with an operative bridge with deflecting arm or a flexible hysteroscope with an operating channel.
- a method for uterine distention.

The metal instruments are sterilized by autoclaving. Only the hysteroscope and light cables are soaked in activated alkaline 2% glutaraldehyde for 20 minutes. The parts of the Ovabloc system that are purchased for indefinite use include:

- A mechanical fluid flow actuator (Figure 57.2).
- A mixing dish.
- A microsyringe to inject the silicone catalyst.
- Insulating cup to hold the syringe during mixing.

Items that are purchased for one-time use are:

- A frozen mixer – dispenser syringe containing raw silicone (Figure 57.3).
- A vial of catalyst to activate the silicone.
- Sterile coaxial catheters with soft tips (Figure 57.4).

The amounts of silicone and catalyst used, the times of mixing and injecting of materials, and the pressure needed to inject the silicone are standardized by the manufacturer. The variable factor, which is taken into account by the manufacturer, is the rapidity with which the silicone hardens after mixing the catalyst. This depends not only upon the silicone temperature, but the batch of silicone and the amount of catalyst injected.

After the silicone and catalyst are combined they are mixed by movements of the plunger of the silicone-containing syringe. This same syringe can then be converted by a spacer into a dispensing syringe (see Figure 57.3). After mixing, the syringe is placed in the fluid flow actuator (see Figure 57.2), which begins the injection of the hardening silicone through the catheter into the fallopian tube (see Figure 57.4). The initial pressure of 300 N is main-

Figure 57.2 Fluid flow actuator system (Advanced Medical Grade Silicones B.V., The Netherlands) used to drive the activated and hardening silicone out of the syringe and down the coaxial catheter and into the fallopian tubes. (Reproduced by permission of Siegler AM and Lindemann JH (eds) (1984) *Hysteroscopy: Principles and Practice*. Philadelphia: JB Lippincott.)

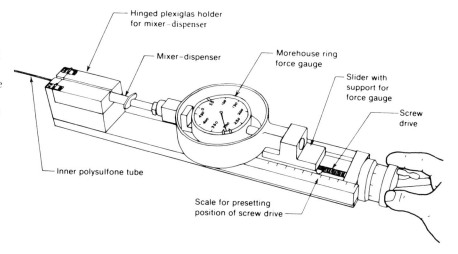

Figure 57.3 The mixer–dispenser syringe (Advanced Medical Grade Silicones B.V., The Netherlands) allows the catalyst to be injected with the silicone and mixed. A spacer converts it into an injection syringe, which is connected to the coaxial catheter and placed in the fluid flow actuator. (Reproduced by permission of Siegler AM and Lindemann HJ (eds) (1984) *Hysteroscopy: Principles and Practice.* Philadelphia: JB Lippincott.)

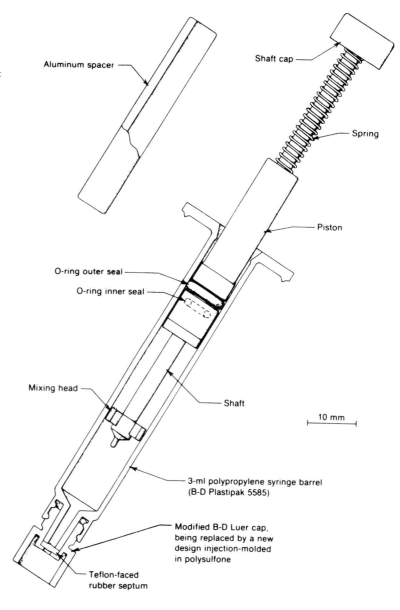

tained until the silicone is seen to enter the fallopian tube by the hysteroscopist. The pressure on the syringe by the fluid flow actuator is allowed to decrease as the syringe empties. The amount of silicone that flows into the fallopian tubes is therefore predetermined by the rapidity with which the silicone hardens, the timing of the onset of pressure on the syringe, and the pressure with which it is injected. Final curing of the silicone is determined on a test plate using silicone from the syringe dispenser before it is attached to the catheter. Once curing has occurred the inner part of the coaxial catheter is withdrawn. This breaks the column of cured silicone at the tubal plug tip.

The sequential steps in carrying out this procedure after preparing the patients and administering local anesthesia are as follows:

- The operative hysteroscope is inserted. (In the author's experience cervical dilatation has been necessary in only 30% of patients.)
- The uterine cavity is distended – CO_2, Hyskon or low viscosity fluid can be used.
- The cavity is cleared of blood, debris, etc. so that the tubal ostium can be identified.
- The prepackaged sterile coaxial catheter with a preformed soft silicone tip at the end is introduced through the hysteroscope operative channel into the uterine cavity. It is brought into contact with the tubal ostium. When Hyskon is used debris can be seen to pass with the Hyskon out through the fallopian tubes. This alerts the hysteroscopist to the direction of the intramural portion of the tube.
- Once the hysteroscopist feels that the tip has

Figure 57.4 Coaxial catheter with preformed soft obturator tip (Advanced Medical Grade Silicones B.V., The Netherlands). (Reproduced by permission of Siegler AM and Lindemann HJ (eds) (1984) *Hysteroscopy: Principles and Practice*. Philadelphia: JB Lippincott.)

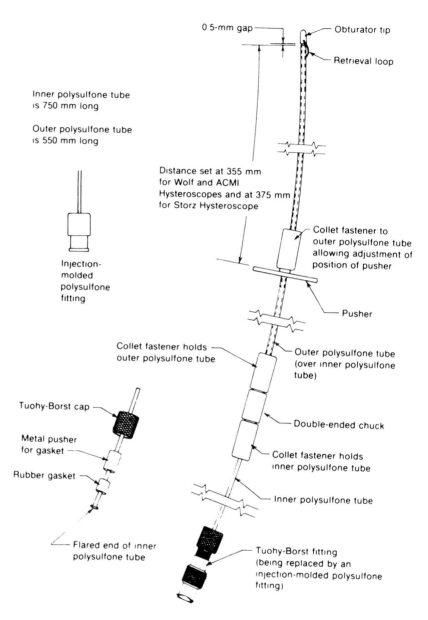

been appropriately applied to the ostium, the assistant is asked to inject a methylene blue dye solution through the coaxial catheter into the fallopian tube. This is done to demonstrate tubal patency and proper alignment of the catheter tip. The assistant should feel a free flow of the methylene blue solution. If the solution refluxes back into the uterine cavity a tight application of the catheter tip to the ostium has not been achieved. If a free flow is not detected there may be spasm of the fallopian tube or a blocked fallopian tube or the catheter tip may have been inappropriately applied and thus occluded. Tubal spasm is a frustrating problem for which there is no consistent method for obtaining relaxation (Cooper *et al.*, 1985). Time will only occasionally lead to relaxation so that the silicone can be injected.

- The procedure cannot be carried forward until there is a free flow of the methylene blue test. Once this has been detected the hysteroscopist holds the catheter in place without movement while the assistant removes the silicone syringe from the freezer and places it in the insulated holder. An insulator is necessary to avoid heat from the assistant's hand, which will raise the silicone temperature and alter its curing properties.
- A predetermined amount of catalyst is then injected into the silicone syringe and the mixer syringe handle is then pumped to mix the silicone and catalyst. Once a predetermined number of mixing strokes have been performed, a spacer converts the mixing syringe into a dispensing syringe. A small portion is injected onto a test plate before the syringe is attached to the coaxial catheter.

- At a predetermined time the fluid flow actuator is brought up to 300 N and the silicone is injected down the catheter. If curing is taking place appropriately the hysteroscopist will see the silicone appear at the end of the coaxial catheter and proceed on into the tube in a predetermined range of time (Figure 57.5a).
- The surgeon will see when the silicone has become so hardened that the pressure of the fluid flow actuator is insufficient to cause further infusion into the fallopian tube.
- Once the flow has stopped the assistant begins checking the curing of the silicone on the test plate.

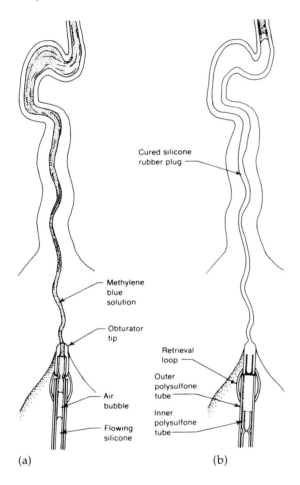

Figure 57.5 (a) When methylene blue and silicone (Advanced Medical Grade Silicones B.V., The Netherlands) are injected into the fallopian tube the obturator tip is held in place by the outer catheter. (b) When the silicone has hardened the inner part of the coaxial catheter is then withdrawn and breaks the silicone column (which has extended from the syringe to the ampullary part of the plug) at the junction of the preformed obturator tip. (Reproduced by permission of Siegler AM and Lindemann HJ (eds) (1984) *Hysteroscopy: Principles and Practice*. Philadelphia: JB Lippincott.)

- If curing occurs in a predetermined period of time the inner portion of the coaxial catheter is pulled back breaking the bond (Figure 57.5b). Then the whole catheter can be removed leaving an intact plug (Figure 57.6).

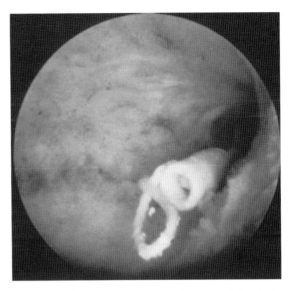

Figure 57.6 The larger preformed tip is seen lying in the uterine cavity attached to the thinner isthmic portion. Beyond and out of sight, in the isthmic part of the fallopian tube is a large distal portion.

- The procedure is carried out on the opposite side in this same fashion.
- Bilateral normal plugs can be determined by radiography (Dan and Goldstein, 1984; Fischer *et al.*, 1984). They appear as a tip with a narrow isthmic portion and enlarged ampullary portion (Figure 57.7a).

One of the problems that can occur during the instillation of silicone into the fallopian tube is reflux of silicone back into the uterine cavity. Slight additional pressure of the catheter against the tubal opening will usually solve this problem. If it does not, the procedure must be aborted since an undetermined amount of silicone will enter the fallopian tube and may result in a small distal enlargement (Figure 57.7b). In these cases the plug will eventually be lost into the uterus. There may also be inadequate silicone entering the fallopian tube if the curing time is too rapid.

If an inadequate plug is to be removed the preformed tip can be grasped and removed from the uterus. During this process the whole plug may be removed, but more likely it will break its connection with the formed in-place portion of the plug. The remaining part of the plug can often be flushed with the methylene blue test into the peritoneal cavity and another plug attempted.

If the tip does not bond appropriately to the formed in-place portion of the plug it will migrate into the peritoneal cavity (Figure 57.7c). A few plugs migrate intact into the peritoneal cavity because the interstitial portion of the tube is anatomically larger than normal (Figure 57.7d).

It is important that patients are not told that they are sterilized until bilateral normal plugs have been identified at the three-month radiograph. In one series four of six women who became pregnant had abnormal plugs. Two had plugs that had migrated into the peritoneal cavity and two had only one plug in place. In these two cases the other tube was believed to be closed because the methylene blue test and a subsequent hysterosalpingogram had shown blockage (van der Leij and Lammes, 1996).

The author enrolled 265 patients for his part of the formed in-place silicone plug study (Loffer and Loffer, 1992). Of these patients, 37 (14%) had two procedures and four patients had three procedures making a total of 310 procedures. Six patients were unable to have silicone injected and were dropped from the study. A successful procedure was defined

as the formation of bilaterally normal devices. Tip separation or tubal spasm were the primary reason why the initial procedure had to be repeated. Of the 259 patients who had silicone installed and were included in the study, 248 (96%) had normal devices and were believed to be occluded immediately following the final procedure. Before allowing a patient to rely on the Ovabloc device for contraception a radiograph was obtained at three months. At that time 225 (88%) of the 255 women who were seen still had normal devices. These women were then allowed to rely on the Ovabloc method as their only method of contraception.

Improved techniques and product modifications could significantly increase the number of plugs that remain normal from the immediate postoperative period to the three-month follow-up.

Of the 259 patients in the author's series who were studied, 208 patients are being followed-up and 190 rely on the formed in-place plugs as their only form of birth control. The 18 patients not relying on the plugs are not considered to be sterilized because their plugs were inadvertently damaged by

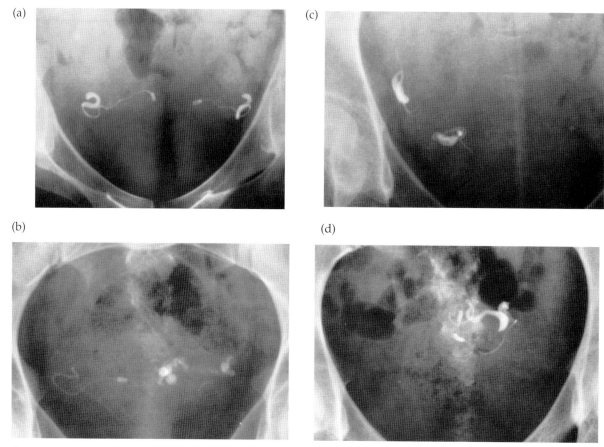

Figure 57.7 Types of formed in-place plugs as seen on radiography. (a) Bilateral normal dumbbell-shaped plugs. (b) On the left there is an inadequate distal tip resulting from premature hardening of the silicone. This may also occur with reflux into the uterine cavity. On the right there is intravasation of silicone into myometrium. (c) Bilateral tip separation resulting from inadequate bonding of the tip to the formed in-place portion of the plug. Both distal portions lie peritoneally. (d) Migrated intact plug lying free in the peritoneal cavity above a normal plug.

a dilatation and curettage or were removed at the patient's request. Of 51 patients who had silicone instilled who have been dropped from the study, for 31 the reason was failure to achieve bilateral devices, while 19 patients were lost to follow-up. One patient became pregnant while presumed sterilized.

The efficacy of the procedure is shown by the fact that only one patient became pregnant while presumed to be protected by the Ovabloc procedure. She had an ectopic pregnancy. Two other patients have become pregnant. One who had an ectopic pregnancy was never considered to be protected by the device and the other had the devices removed in order to become pregnant. She became pregnant, but only after a tuboplasty. Removal of plugs resulted in pregnancies in one series in only two of 16 patients (12.5%) (Reed, 1989). The tubes appear to scar closed in most patients.

There were 2501 patients entered into the Food and Drug Administration (FDA) clinical study by all investigators. Successful bilateral procedures were accomplished in 2054 (82%). Bilateral normal plugs remained at the last follow-up in 1858 (74.3%) of patients. This decline in normal plugs resulted from:

- A problem developing with the plug in 5.8% of patients (migration or expulsion in 2.9% and breakage or change in appearance in 2.9%)
- Disruption of the plugs by external factors in 1.9% (plug removal or intervening surgery).

Pregnancy occurred in 28 patients believed to have normal plugs, resulting in an annual pregnancy rate of 0.77% (Reed, 1989).

The Ovabloc procedure is an effective safe method of permanent contraception. Follow-up of the author's series in over 12 022 months of use has shown no serious side effects other than the one ectopic pregnancy. In 9915 women months of use the failure rate has shown a Pearl index of 0.12 and a life table pregnancy rate at five years of 0.0067 per 100 women. Other series have found similar results. The oldest series, which is based on 14 300 women months' exposure had a Pearl index of 0.84, and a life table pregnancy rate of 0.0093 per 100 women (Reed, 1991, personal communication). Similar results based on 8040 women months' exposure gave a life table rate exactly the same as the authors (0.0067) and a Pearl index of 0.30 (DeMaeyer, 1991, personal communication).

This Ovabloc method is well received by patients and provides an excellent office-based tubal occlusion procedure. It is commercially available in many areas of Europe. It has not completed the regulatory requirements of the FDA in the USA.

References

Alvarado A, Quinones R, Aznar R (1974) Tubal instillation of quinacrine under hysteroscopic control. In Sciarra JJ, Butler JC, Speidel JJ (eds) *Hysteroscopic Sterilization*. pp. 85–94. New York: Intercontinental Medical Book Corporation.

Brumsted JR, Shirk G, Soderling MJ, Reed T (1991) Attempted transcervical occlusion of the fallopian tube with the Nd:Yag laser. *Obstetrics and Gynecology* **77**: 327–328.

Cooper JM, Rigberg HS, Houck R, Acker M (1985) Incidence, significance and remission of tubal spasm during attempted hysteroscopic tubal sterilization. *Journal of Reproductive Medicine* **30**: 39–42.

Corfman PA, Taylor HC (1966) An instrument for transcervical treatment of the oviduct and uterine cornua. *Obstetrics and Gynecology* **27**: 880–883.

Dan SJ, Goldstein M (1984) Fallopian tube occlusion with silicone: radiographic appearance. *Radiology* **151**: 603–605.

Darabi KF, Richart RM (1977) Collaborative study on hysteroscopic sterilization procedures. A preliminary report. *Obstetrics and Gynecology* **49**: 48–54.

Darabi KF, Roy K, Richart RM (1978) Collaborative study on hysteroscopic sterilization procedures: Final report. In Sciarra JJ, Zatacuni GI, Speidel JJ (eds). *Risks, Benefits and Controversies in Fertility Control*. pp. 81–101. Hagerstown: Harper and Row.

deBlok S, Dijkman AB, Wamsteker (1992) Hysteroscopic tubal occlusion with Ovabloc ITD – results of 115 cases. *Gynaecological Endoscopy* **1**: 151–154.

Donnez J, Malvaux V, Nisolle M, Casanas F (1990) Hysteroscopic sterilization with the Nd:Yag laser. *Journal of Gynecologic Surgery* **6**: 149–153.

El Kady AA, Nogib HS, Kessel E (1993) Efficacy and safety of repeated transcervical quinacrine pellet insertion for female sterilization. *Fertility and Sterility* **59**: 301–304.

Fischer ME, Reed TP, Red DE (1984) Silicone devices for tubal occlusion: radiographic description and evaluation. *Radiology* **151**: 601–602.

Hamou J, Gasparri F, Scarselli GF *et al.* (1984) Hysteroscopic reversible tubal sterilization. *Acta Europaea Fertilitatis* **15**: 123–129.

Hughes EC (ed.) (1977) *Obstetric–Gynecologic Terminology*. pp. 418–419. Philadelphia: FA Davis Co.

Loffer FD (1984) Hysteroscopic sterilization with the use of the formed in-place silicone plugs. *American Journal of Obstetrics and Gynecology* **149**: 261–270.

Loffer FD (1990) Hysteroscopy. In Stangel JJ (ed.) *Infertility Surgery: A Multi Method Approach to Female Reproductive Surgery*. pp. 72–85. Norwalk: Appleton and Lange.

Loffer FD & Pent D (1980) Pregnancy after laparoscopic sterilizations. *Obstetrics and Gynecology* **55**: 643–648.

Loffer FD, Loffer PS (1992) Hysteroscopic tubal occlusion with the use of formed-in-place silicone devices: a long term follow up. *Gynaecological Endoscopy* **1**: 203–205.

Quinones R, Alvarado A, Ley E (1976) Hysteroscopic sterilization. *International Journal of Gynecology and Obstetrics* **14**: 27–34.

Reed TP (1989) Hysteroscopic sterilization with formed-in-place silicone rubber plugs. In Baggish MS, Barbot J, Valle RF (eds) *Diagnostic and Operative Hysteroscopy: A*

Text and Atlas. pp. 204–207. Chicago: Year Book Medical Publishers.

Richart RM, Neuwirth RS, Goldsmith A, Edelman DA (1987) Intrauterine administration of methyl cyano-acrylate as an outpatient method of permanent female sterilization. *American Journal of Obstetrics and Gynecology* **155**: 981–987.

Rimkus V, Semm K (1974) Sterilization by carbon dioxide hysteroscopy. In Sciarra JJ, Butler JC, Speidel JJ (eds)

Hysteroscopic Sterilization. pp. 75–84. New York: Intercontinental Medical Book Corporation.

van der Leij G, Lammes FB (1996) Office hysteroscopic tubal occlusion with siloxane intratubal device (The Ovabloc® method). *International Journal of Gynecology and Obstetrics* **53**: 253–260.

Zipper JA, Stachetti E, Medal M (1970) Human fertility control by transcervical application of quinacrine on the fallopian tube. *Fertility and Sterility* **21**: 581–589.

Endometrial Ablation Techniques

58

Transcervical Resection of the Endometrium (TCRE)

HUGH O'CONNOR*, ADAM L. MAGOS** AND J.A. MARK BROADBENT†

*The Coombe Women's Hospital, Dublin, Ireland
**University Department of Obstetrics and Gynaecology, The Royal Free Hospital, London, UK
†Department of Obstetrics and Gynaecology, Elizabeth Garrett Anderson Hospital, London, UK

Introduction

Menorrhagia accounts for approximately 35% of gynecologic consultations and 60% of these culminate in hysterectomy as a definitive treatment within five years of presentation (Coulter *et al.*, 1991). Medical treatment of this condition is often ineffective or poorly tolerated due to side effects and as a result hysterectomy has become the most frequently performed major surgery in women of reproductive age. The cost to the health service and to society is high and a less invasive cost-effective procedure would be a definite advantage.

Transcervical resection of the endometrium (TCRE) is one of the alternatives to hysterectomy, and like other techniques such as laser ablation of the endometrium, relies on the production of a therapeutic Asherman's syndrome (Asherman, 1950) within the uterine cavity, thereby ameliorating menstrual symptoms.

History

Neuwirth in 1978, described resection of submucous fibroids in women with abnormal uterine bleeding using a urologic resectoscope. He touched upon the idea of extending this local treatment to the entire uterine cavity, when in a review article, he discussed the possibility of systematically resecting the endometrium to the isthmus using a cutting loop fitted to an operating resectoscope (Amin and Neuwirth, 1983). In the same year DeCherney and Polan reported their experience with resectoscopic electrocoagulation of the endometrium as emergency treatment of intractable and life-threatening uterine hemorrhage in 11 women deemed unfit for hysterectomy who had not responded to conventional treatment. This series was updated four years later to include 21 women, all but three with either blood dyscrasias or other serious illnesses, who were treated with either endometrial diathermy or resection and followed for a maximum of six years (DeCherney *et al.*, 1987). The results were impressive: 18 of the 19 women who survived the underlying medical condition were amenorrhoeic and only one required further treatment.

Jaques Hamou introduced endometrial resection to Paris in 1985, using a modified technique. He suggested using non-viscous fluids such as glycine 1.5%, rather than dextran 70 and used the continuous flow resectoscope, as developed by Hallez *et al.* (1987), for easier and safer fluid control. He suggested that in otherwise healthy women with menorrhagia unresponsive to medical therapy, a partial endometrial resection should be performed instead of hysterectomy, aiming to reduce menstrual flow to an acceptable level without producing amenorrhea. Hamou justified leaving a rim of endometrium above the endocervix because of a fear that resection down to the endocervix would lead to cervical stenosis and because the Parisian women preferred to continue to menstruate, albeit lighter that before. Hamou demonstrated his new technique in Oxford, UK in 1988. Shortly after Magos *et al.* (1989) demonstrated a more extensive procedure of total resection of the endometrium. In effect, the gynecologist's version of transurethral resection of the prostate (TURP), and so the term 'transcervical resection of the endometrium' (TCRE) was coined.

Treatment Criteria

TCRE is not a definitive procedure and there is a definite failure rate. Patient selection and counselling are vital for a successful outcome. The ideal patient is over 45 years with regular heavy menses due to dysfunctional bleeding sufficient to warrant hysterectomy (Table 58.1). Irregular or prolonged menses and intermenstrual bleeding may not improve following TCRE unless the outcome is amenorrhea.

Table 58.1 Treatment criteria for TCRE.

Menstrual problems sufficient to warrant hysterectomy
Symptoms resistant to medical treatment
Family complete
Regular menstrual cycle
Benign endometrial histology
Normal cervical smear
Careful counselling

Relative contraindications
Uterine size greater than 12 weeks' pregnancy or cavity
   greater than 10 cm in length
Submucous fibroids less than 5 cm in diameter
Adnexal tenderness suggestive of pelvic inflammatory
   disease or endometriosis
Major uterovaginal prolapse or severe urinary symptoms

Rutherford *et al.* (1991) have estimated that up to 58% of women currently being treated by hysterectomy for menstrual abnormalities may be suitable for TCRE.

Careful counselling is mandatory before surgery. The likely outcomes in terms of amenorrhea rates, need for further surgery, need to use barrier methods of contraception if not sterilized and the fact that this is a relatively new procedure must be emphasized. It is important that the patients' expectations of surgery are in line with observed results, as a reduction in menstrual flow may not be a satisfactory outcome for the patient who desires amenorrhea.

Technique

A 26 F gauge continuous flow resectoscope fitted with a 4 mm forward-oblique telescope and a 24 F gauge cutting loop are generally used to perform TCRE. A 30° or a 12° telescope is used depending upon operator preference, but the 12° telescope does offer the advantage that the cutting loop remains in view when fully extended. Distention of the uterine cavity via the inner inflow sheath is required to allow access to the fundal and cornual regions. An intrauterine pressure of 80–120 mm Hg is usually needed; the uterine cavity will collapse if the pressure is too low and resection then becomes unsafe. The consequence of a high intrauterine pressure is excessive absorption of the irrigating fluid with the potential for intravascular volume overload. Uterine distention can be achieved by means of a simple gravity feed system and a sphygmomanometer cuff inflated around the bag of irrigant solution improves flow. Alternatively there are a number of commercially available irrigation pumps, such as the Quinones pump or Hamou Hysteromat (Storz, Tuttlingen, Germany). The pump controls fluid inflow by allowing for change in the pressure and rate of flow of fluid, outflow is achieved by continuous suction via the outer sheath of the resectoscope, usually with a negative pressure of −50 mm Hg. The effect of this continuous flow is to maintain a clear view of the uterine cavity. The pressure and rate of flow should be such as to maintain a clear view of the uterine cavity, but not so high as to promote excessive fluid absorption.

The resectoscope handle mechanism can be either active when the cutting loop is outside the resectoscope sheath at rest, or passive when the cutting loop is inside the resectoscope sheath at rest. We prefer the passive handle mechanism as the loop at rest does not interfere with inspection of the uterine cavity, and more importantly accidental trauma is less likely than when using a permanently exposed loop. The loop cuts to a depth of 3–4 mm.

Endometrial thickness varies throughout the menstrual cycle, being thinnest immediately following the menses and thickest in the luteal phase of the cycle. The loop has a limited depth of resection and although it is possible to resect the same area twice, this increases the chances of perforation. The postmenstrual endometrium is thin with little debris in the cavity and this is the ideal time to schedule TCRE. This is difficult from an administrative point of view, and therefore endometrial suppressants such as danazol or gonadotropin releasing hormone (GnRH) analogs can be used to thin the endometrium pharmacologically. We use either danazol 200 mg three times a day for six weeks before surgery or a GnRH analog such as goserlin for one month. Both regimens will produce a thin atrophic endometrium ideally suited for resection. Data submitted for publication from this unit show no difference in overall complication rates between those with pharmacologically prepared and unprepared endometrium, but there is a significant reduction in irrigant fluid deficit, operating time and blood loss in those patients who have a prepared endometrium (O'Connor and Magos, 1996). Primed endometrium is less 'fluffy' and consequently the outflow holes on the outer sheath of the resectoscope are less likely to be blocked.

Resection should include 2.5–3 mm of myometrium as endometrial glandular elements may extend this deeply (Reid and Sharpe, 1988). In practice 60–90% of the endometrial chip will consist of myometrium.

All procedures should be performed using video monitoring. This has advantages in terms of operator comfort, magnification of the operating field and theater staff interest and it facilitates teaching.

A blended (Blend 1) current set at 120 W cutting and 60 W coagulation is used to arm the cutting loop. The resection starts in the fundus of the uterus using a forward angled loop. The cornual and fundal endometrium is excised and the area widened forming a repository for endometrial chips. The resection then proceeds in a systematic fashion from 9 o'clock to the 3 o'clock position treating the posterior wall first, resecting just the amount of tissue that the loop traverses when extended. The chips are pushed into the fundus and the procedure is repeated on the anterior wall. The next segment of the uterus is now resected working all the time towards the cervix. Alternatively, long strips from fundus to cervix may be resected: these must be removed after each cut. The circular muscle fibers of the myometrium are used to judge the depth of cut. When performing partial endometrial resection a 0.5–1 cm rim of endometrium is left above the internal os, whereas the entire cavity is resected for total resection. The resected chips are removed using a flushing curet or polyp forceps and sent for histopathologic analysis. The cavity is then inspected, any residual endometrium is excised, and bleeding points coagulated. The cervix should now be dilated to Hegar 14–16, as this helps prevent later formation of hematometra.

Anesthesia

TCRE can be carried out under general anesthesia or combined local/sedo-analgesia (Magos *et al.*, 1991). The autonomic nerve supply of the uterus renders it relatively insensitive to touching, cutting or burning. Patient preference is usually the deciding factor as to which mode of anesthesia is used and approximately 35% choose to avoid a general anesthetic.

Occasionally local anesthesia will be preferred because of the medical condition of the patient.

Our current regimen involves admitting the patient starved one hour before surgery in time for premedication with oral temazepam 20 mg and rectal diclofenac 100 mg. Once in the operating theater, anxiolysis and light sedation are produced using small doses of intravenous midazolam, systemic analgesia with incremental doses of intravenous fentanyl, and finally local anesthesia with a combination of para- and intracervical and intrauterine lignocaine 1%/epinephrine 1:200 000 mixture, the latter injected under direct vision using the resectoscope. A maximum of 40 ml of local anesthetic can be given. Electrocardiogram and arterial oxygen saturation are monitored continuously, and facial oxygen is given routinely. Patients remain fully cooperative during surgery and some choose to watch their operation on the video monitor. The sedo-analgesia regimen is best managed by an anesthetist.

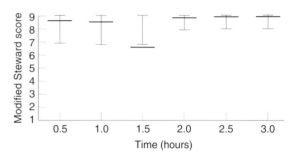

Figure 58.1 Recovery following endometrial resection performed under local anesthesia and sedation.

Postoperative recovery is rapid and within 3–4 hours most patients are ready for discharge (Figure 58.1). This regimen is well tolerated and most of those patients who require re-treatment choose to have it under sedo-analgesia. Approximately 1.6% of patients require conversion to general anesthesia (O'Connor and Magos, 1996). The combination of TCRE with local anesthesia avoids the major abdominal surgery and general anesthesia, and this is especially important for those patients with menorrhagia for whom hysterectomy is considered undesirable, dangerous or impossible (Lockwood *et al.*, 1992).

Results

Surgery

Most patients choose to undergo total rather than partial TCRE. Failure to complete the intended surgery is unusual – in our experience less than 5% (Magos *et al.*, 1991), even then the majority are satisfied with the improvement in menses. Surgery may be incomplete because of equipment failure or intra-operative complications.

Fluid Balance

Fluid dynamics during surgery depend upon factors such as endometrial preparation, tubal patency, concurrent hysteroscopic myomectomy, duration of surgery and intrauterine pressure.

Operating Time

Hysteroscopic experience is the greatest determinant of duration of surgery. Maher and Hill (1990) report operating times of 15–45 minutes, which compares well with our average time of 33 minutes (uncorrected for teaching). The presence of intrauterine pathology such as fibroids or lack of preoperative endometrial preparation increase operating time (39 versus 32 minutes and 37 versus 32 minutes, respectively) (Magos et al., 1991).

Concurrent Operative Procedures

TCRE may be combined with hysteroscopic myomectomy or polypectomy. In certain instances laparoscopy is necessary for sterilization or to treat co-existing pelvic pathology. Ewen and Sutton (1994) have suggested that patients with marked dysmenorrhea may benefit from combining TCRE with laparoscopic uterine nerve ablation (LUNA). It is also possible to treat ovarian pathology and endometriosis at the same time, bearing in mind that these other pathologies may lead to further pelvic surgery in which case TCRE will be deemed to have failed.

Histologic Examination of Resected Endometrium

All resected chips should be sent for examination. The histology report reflects the underlying pathology and whether or not the endometrium has been pharmacologically prepared, in which case it is usually reported as 'basal', 'inactive' or 'atrophic'.

The angle at which the endometrial chip is resected varies, making it difficult to comment on the relative proportions of endometrium and myometrium. Typically, chips are composed of 75% myometrium (range 10–100%) and adenomyosis is reported in up to 12% of cases (Magos et al., 1991).

Postoperative Recovery

Recovery is generally rapid and uneventful making TCRE ideally suited for day case surgery. If performed under local anesthesia and sedation patients are generally fit for discharge within a few hours.

Vaginal bleeding and discharge usually last for 2–4 weeks and gradually ease off. Increased discharge or bleeding may indicate infection. Return to normal domestic activity and work is rapid (Gannon et al., 1991; Dwyer et al., 1993; Pinion et al., 1994).

Effects on the Uterine Cavity

Hysteroscopy at three and 12 months following TCRE reveals marked fibrosis of the cavity with an overall reduction in volume; occasionally the cavity is completely obliterated. Biopsy of the uterine wall reveals histologic evidence of endometrium in up to 25% of amenorrheic women. This has implications for the use of estrogen replacement therapy post TCRE.

Ultrasonographic assessment shows no change in uterine volume, but a definite shrinkage of the uterine cavity, presumably due to fibrosis.

Operative Complications

The complication rate following TCRE is lower than following hysterectomy (Dicker et al., 1982). The operative and postoperative complication rates are usually less than 10%, the majority of complications being minor. However, the type of complication differs from those seen at laparotomy (Table 58.2). Large scale surveys have confirmed the safety of TCRE (MacDonald & Phipps, 1992).

Uterine Perforation

Uterine perforation is potentially the most serious complication of TCRE and is related to operator experience. Although 50% of perforations occur during the learning curve, the corollary is that the remainder occur when one is technically competent. This may reflect a more difficult caseload. The reported incidence varies from 1–3.7%. The myometrium is thinnest in the cornual region and paradoxically this is one of the more difficult areas to resect; extra care is therefore required in this region. Use of the rollerball in this area reduces the likelihood of perforation. The novice hysteroscopist should ensure that the

Table 58.2 Potential complications of TCRE.

Intraoperative	Postoperative	
	Short term	Long term
Uterine perforation	Infection	Recurrence of
Fluid overload	Hematometra	symptoms
Primary hemorrhage	Secondary hemorrhage	Pregnancy
Gas embolism	Cyclical pain	? Uterine malignancy
	Treatment failure	

endometrium is prepared and only operate on normal-sized uteri, using the rollerball to treat the ostia and fundus.

Perforation may occur at cervical dilatation, during electrosurgery or at retrieval of tissue. Clearly perforation with an active electrode is the most serious as there is a risk of damaging intra-abdominal structures such as bowel, bladder or major blood vessels. Such perforation should be managed by immediate laparotomy or laparoscopy, depending upon endoscopic experience. Perforation at other times can usually be managed expectantly, with observation and antibiotics. If there is concern about bleeding then it is usually possible to control this at operative laparoscopy. Perforation may not be recognized at the time, but an increase in fluid absorption, abdominal distention or collapse of the cavity should prompt a thorough inspection of the cavity. Visualization of intra-abdominal contents through the hysteroscope leaves no doubt. Developments in resectoscope technology may include incorporation of an ultrasound with or without a Doppler probe in the tip of the instrument, and this should lead to safer hysteroscopic surgery.

Fluid Overload

Glycine 1.5% is the irrigant fluid most used in hysteroscopic surgery. It is electrolyte free, but is also hypo-osmolar with respect to plasma. During electrosurgery, glycine is instilled into the uterine cavity at pressure to distend the cavity. Blood ves-

sels are opened when the resection is in progress and therefore some fluid is absorbed in virtually all cases of TCRE. Excessive absorption of glycine 1.5% can cause hyponatremia, hemolysis, hypertension, congestive cardiac failure and neurologic signs, and if untreated, death. Fluid overload complicates up to 4% of cases. The dilutional effects of glycine 1.5% absorption during TCRE have been well described (Baumann *et al.*, 1990; Boto *et al.*, 1990). Hematocrit and serum albumin concentration fall, but the fall in serum sodium concentration is more significant and is proportional to the volume of irrigant absorbed.

Fluid balance is measured throughout surgery. We suspend the bags of glycine from a spring weight, and collect the outflow from the uterus. The deficit is the difference between the two, allowing for leakage. The balance is measured at 5-minute intervals, but if absorption is high a continuous check is kept. New fluid monitoring systems give a running balance collating data on fluid instilled into the uterus and that returned from the patient. It is also possible to label glycine with ethanol and absorption can be measured by checking the expired breath ethanol concentration.

Fluid absorption is higher when the fallopian tubes are patent, the endometrium is unprepared and in patients having concurrent resection of fibroids.

With careful monitoring, fluid overload should be recognized and treated early (Table 58.3). Diuretics should be given and electrolytes and urine output should be appropriately monitored, thereby avoiding serious sequelae.

Table 58.3 Guidelines for the management of fluid absorption during hysteroscopic surgery

Volume absorbed (ml)	Effect	Action
<1000	Well tolerated by healthy patient	Continue surgery
1000–2000	Mild hyponatremia likely	Complete surgery as soon as possible
>2000	Severe hyponatremia and other biochemical disturbances likely	Stop surgery

Uterine Hemorrhage

Hemorrhage is uncommon at TCRE. The blended current seals many small vessels as they are cut and by not cutting deeply, the larger vessels in the myometrium are avoided. If bleeding is excessive, the bleeding points may be cauterized using electrocoagulation under direct vision. Failing this a 30 ml Foley balloon catheter, left *in situ* for 6–8 hours, can be used to tamponade the cavity. Pharmacologic preparation of the endometrium before surgery reduces uterine vascularity and hence the risk of hemorrhage. The average blood loss in our series of 525 cases was 9 ml and a Foley balloon was used on three occasions to control bleeding (O'Connor and Magos, 1996).

Gas Embolism

Gas embolism has been reported as a complication of both laser endometrial ablation (Baggish and Daniell, 1989) and endometrial resection (Wood and Roberts, 1990). Air embolism can occur when an open vein is exposed to air at a greater pressure than that in the vein, for example when the patient is placed in the Trendelenburg position and the heart is at a lower level than the operating site. The inflow and outflow sheaths should not be left in the uterus with the handle mechanism removed, as might occur when changing from loop electrode to rollerball, because this may promote air embolism. Wood and Roberts (1990) suggest the use of positive pressure ventilation rather than spontaneous breathing during anesthesia and avoiding the head down position during and after surgery may also help.

Irrigation systems that rely on gas pressure systems for irrigation should have air trapping valves.

Postoperative Complications and Considerations

Infection

Although infection is a rare complication following endometrial resection, we routinely administer prophylactic antibiotics, currently Augmentin (SmithKline Beecham, Worthing, UK) 1.2 g intravenously at induction. Endometritis and urinary tract infection complicate 2% of procedures. Immunosuppressed patients should have swabs taken in the week before surgery and be covered appropriately with antibiotics and antifungal agents.

Hematometra and Cyclical Pain

Hematometra formation following endometrial resection is an important cause of treatment failure. It occurs when islands of active endometrium are buried behind intrauterine adhesions. The presence of a hematometra is suspected when the patient complains of cyclical or constant pelvic pain some time following surgery. Ultrasound will typically show a fluid collection within the uterus. Treatment is by repeat resection, which may need to be carried out under laparoscopic or ultrasound guidance. The incidence can be reduced by attention to technique and by overdilating the cervix to Hegar 16 at the completion of surgery.

Cyclical abdominal pain in the absence of hematometra is one of the principal causes of treatment failure. Asherman described this phenomenon in his report on intrauterine synechiae (Asherman, 1950), and it is likely to be due to islands of endometrium becoming buried deep within the myometrium, resulting in adenomyosis. Treatment is difficult, and simple analgesics will often not suffice. LUNA may help, but has not been adequately validated. Ultimately hysterectomy may be necessary.

Pregnancy

Intrauterine and tubal pregnancy have been reported following endometrial resection. Goldberg (1994) has estimated the risk at 0.3%. The pregnancy outcome is variable with an increased early pregnancy loss. Uncomplicated term pregnancies have been reported (Maher and Hill, 1990), but there are isolated reports of fetal growth retardation and fetal abnormality (Whitelaw and Sutton, 1993).

Patients who have not been sterilized should be counselled carefully, and barrier methods of contraception advised. A small number of patients who are amenorrheic following endometrial resection and who have not been sterilized subsequently request sterilization for fear that the amenorrhea is due to pregnancy.

Uterine Malignancy

There is no reason to believe that endometrial resection or ablative techniques per se should result in an increased risk of uterine malignancy. It has been claimed that removal of the bulk of the endometrium may reduce the risk, but as endometrial cancer is principally a postmenopausal condition this is unlikely. Of greater concern is the possibility that a potential endometrial malignancy buried behind intrauterine adhesions might present at a later stage than if the cavity was patent. As yet this is a theoretic risk.

There are three case reports of endometrial cancer in association with endometrial resection in the literature and two further cases known to the author (Dwyer *et al.*, 1993; Copperman *et al.*, 1993; Horowitz *et al.*, 1995). Preoperative endometrial sampling will detect unsuspected cancer and identify those patients with atypical hyperplastic endometrium.

Long-term follow-up is needed to definitively answer this question, but the evidence to date is reassuring.

Hormone Replacement Therapy (HRT)

There are few reports in the literature on the use and safety of HRT following endometrial resection. A recent survey of our patients over 50 years of age revealed few problems in those women taking HRT. Most had either no bleeding or minimal loss on treatment, and were managed by their general practitioner. Combined estrogen/progesterone regimens should be used and prescribed according to manufacturer's instructions for the relief of symptoms and prophylaxis against osteoporosis and heart disease. Estrogen-only therapy should not be prescribed, even in those women who have been amenorrheic for years. Abnormal uterine bleeding on HRT should be managed as usual, with ultrasound and endometrial biopsy.

Endometrial resection has been used to reduce blood loss in women with heavy loss on HRT (Spaulding, 1994). In such cases hysteroscopic evaluation of the endometrium with biopsy should be carried out before surgery. Again, combined preparations should be used.

Results of Endometrial Resection

The reported results depend primarily upon the duration of follow-up and whether the results are reported by time from surgery or as an averaged figure. The outcome measure used is important as indices such as satisfaction with the procedure can be affected by external factors. Satisfaction, menstrual result and need for further surgery are the most useful outcomes to measure, with the need for further gynecologic surgery being the most robust measurement.

Menstrual Outcome

The majority of patients report an improvement with up to 97% reporting a reduction in menstrual flow following endometrial resection. The amenorrhea rate at one year is approximately 40% and this falls to 20% over five years (Figure 58.2). The effect on irregular or frequent periods is less satisfactory, resection will lighten the loss, but will not be curative unless amenorrhea is the outcome.

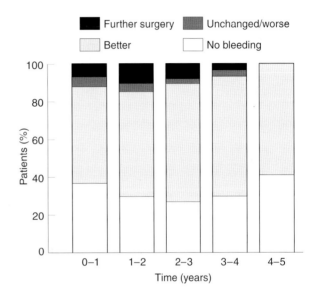

Figure 58.2 Effect of primary endometrial resection on menstrual flow in 525 women followed up for up to five years.

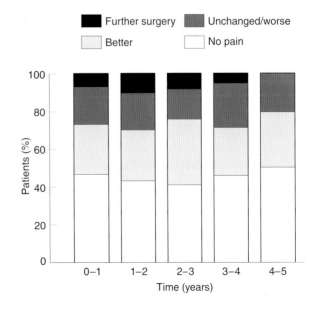

Figure 58.3 Effect of primary endometrial resection on menstrual pain in 525 women followed up for up to five years.

Interpretation of reported results is complicated by differences in technique, partial versus total resection, the use of postoperative suppressive therapy such as medroxyprogesterone acetate and the duration of follow-up. The effect on pain is similar with the majority reporting an improvement in symptoms (Figure 58.3).

If symptoms fail to improve it is usually possible to repeat the resection. Although not as successful as initial resection it is nonetheless a worthwhile procedure. Some patients will choose hysterectomy, especially if pain is a marked feature of their symptoms.

Objective measurement of menstrual loss in 25 patients showed a reduction to normal levels (< 80 ml per cycle) in 24 patients following endometrial resection (Figure 58.4). The results after partial TCRE were not as impressive, although the patients did report subjective improvement.

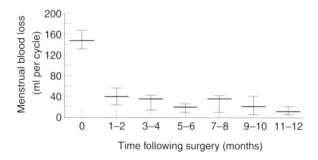

Figure 58.4 Actual menstrual blood loss following endometrial resection.

Further Gynecologic Surgery Following Endometrial Resection

We have used life table analysis to estimate the risk of further surgery following endometrial resection in 525 women followed up for up to five years. The cumulative possibility of undergoing further surgery is shown in Figure 58.5a–e. Only 8.8% of women underwent hysterectomy and most repeat surgery was done in the first three years. Very few women were on medication for recurrent menstrual problems over the course of the study, implying that those who were dissatisfied with the initial surgical procedure, chose further surgery for their complaint. Similar failure rates have been reported by Raiga *et al.* (1995) and Derman *et al.*, (1991).

Comparison of Ablative Techniques

Preliminary results of the MISTLETOE study (Minimally Invasive Surgical Techniques Laser EndoThermal Or Endoresection) (Royal College of Obstetrics and Gynaecology Audit Unit, 1994) suggest that visual techniques are superior to non-visual techniques of ablation, where failure rates of up to 56% were seen at one year. The failure rate at 12 months following combined resection and rollerball (15.1%) was lower than for resection (19.3%) or rollerball alone (20.7%) or laser abalation (32.2%); this is at the expense of a slightly higher complication rate (7.7% for resection/rollerball versus 5.5% for laser). It should be stressed that these are interim results and that significant data were missing when these figures were compiled.

Comparison with Hysterectomy

Four randomized trials have been reported to date comparing endometrial ablation with hysterectomy. Gannon *et al.* (1991), Dwyer *et al.* (1993), Pinion *et al.* (1994) and O'Connor *et al.* (1997) broadly report shorter operating time, reduced blood loss, reduced complications, shorter hospitalization and earlier return to normal activity and work for those patients treated with endometrial ablation compared to those treated with abdominal hysterectomy. A financial analysis of the Bristol trial showed significant savings to the health service, which were still apparent at three years follow up (Sculpher *et al.*, 1993).

The effects of both procedures on the use of general practitioner services and psychosocial parameters have been investigated in the Medical Research Council funded trial of endometrial resection and hysterectomy. These findings are confirmed by the MRC trial (O'Connor *et al.*, 1997). This trial includes vaginal and abdominal hysterectomy; as it is multicentered, the results are more generalizable.

Coulter (1994) has reported that the introduction of TCRE has had no effect on the hysterectomy rate in Oxford. Indeed, the total number of patients being treated surgically for menorrhagia has increased in this region. However, we know that the hysterectomy rate following TCRE in the Oxfordshire area is in the order of 20%, and it may be that the threshold for offering surgical treatment for menorrhagia has changed in this region. The randomized trials and the long-term reviews of TCRE show that it is a successful treatment and a genuine alternative to hysterectomy. It is possible that TCRE is being offered to women who would have been managed medically in the past, and therefore more women are having surgery for menorrhagia. This is a reflection on current practice rather than a criticism of TCRE.

Figure 58.5a Life table analysis: further surgery following primary and repeat endometrial resection.

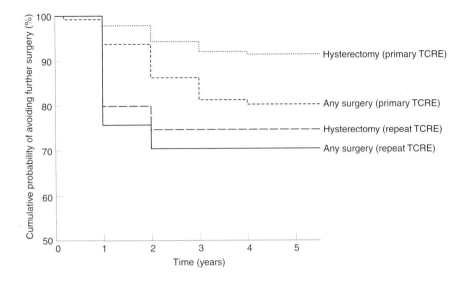

Figure 58.5b Life table analysis: further surgery following TCRE for dysfunctional uterine bleeding combined with hysteroscopic myomectomy.

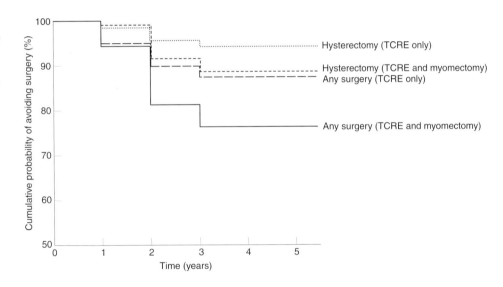

Figure 58.5c Life table analysis: further surgery according to uterine size.

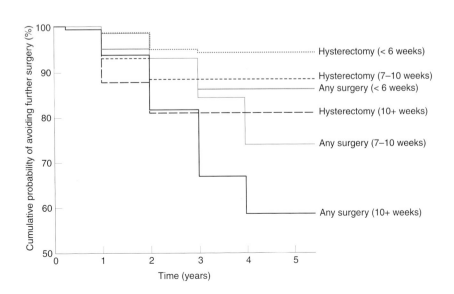

Figure 58.5d Life table analysis: further surgery according to endometrial preparation.

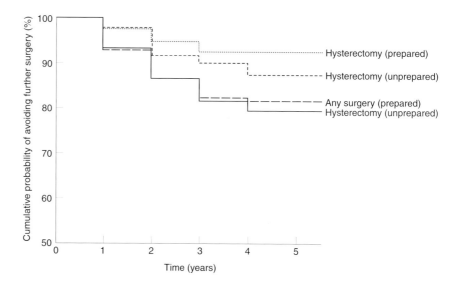

Figure 58.5e Life table analysis: further surgery according to age. (Reprinted by permission of *The New England Journal of Medicine*, from O'Connor *et al.* (1996) vol. **335**, pp. 151–156. Copyright (1996). Massachusetts Medical Society. All rights reserved.)

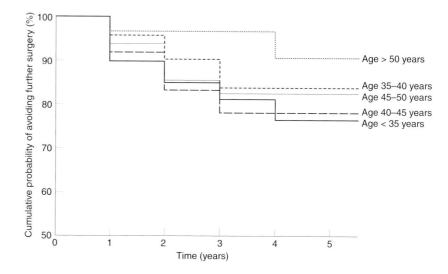

Conclusion

Endometrial resection is a cost-effective alternative to hysterectomy in the management of menorrhagia. Training, careful patient selection and counselling combined with correct technique are the keys to success. Long-term follow-up will be needed to determine long-term failure rates leading to additional therapeutic intervention (including surgery) in order to ascertain its true cost-effectiveness.

References

Amin HK, Neuwirth RS (1963) Operative hysteroscopy utilising dextran as distending medium. *Clinical Obstetrics and Gynecology* **26**: 277–284.

Asherman JG (1950) Traumatic intra-uterine adhesions. *Journal of Obstetrics and Gynaecology of the British Empire* **57**: 892–896.

Baggish MS, Daniell JF (1989) Catastrophic injury secondary to the use of coaxial gas-cooled fibres and artificial sapphire tips for intrauterine surgery. *Lasers in Surgery and Medicine* **9**: 581–584.

Baumann R, Magos A, Kays JDL, Turnbull AC (1990) Absorption of glycine irrigating fluid during transcervical resection of the endometrium. *British Medical Journal* **300**: 304–305.

Boto TCA, Fowler CG, Cockroft S, Djahanbakch O (1990) (letter) Absorption of irragating fluid during transcervical resection of the endometrium. *British Medical Journal* **300**: 748–749.

Brooks PG, Serden SP, Davos I (1991) Hormonal inhibition of the endometrium for resectoscopic endometrial ablation. *American Journal of Obstetrics and Gynecology* **161**: 1601–1608.

Copperman AB, DeCherney AH, Olive DL (1993) A case of endometrial cancer following endometrial ablation for dysfunctional uterine bleeding. *Obstetrics and Gynecology* **82**: 640–642.

Coulter A, Bradlow J, Agass M, Martin-Bates C, Tulloch A (1991) Outcomes of referrals to gynaecology outpatient clinics for menstrual problems: an audit of general practice records. *British Journal of Obstetrics and Gynaecology* **98**: 789–796.

Coulter A (1994) Trends in gynaecological surgery (letter). *Lancet* **344**: 1367.

DeCherney AH, Polan ML (1983) Hysteroscopic management of intrauterine lesions and intractable uterine bleeding. *Obstetrics and Gynecology* **61**: 392–397.

DeCherney AH, Diamond MP, Lavy G, Polan ML (1987) Endometrial ablation for intractable uterine bleeding: hysteroscopic resection. *Obstetrics and Gynecology* **70**: 668–670.

Derman SG, Rehnstrom J, Neuwirth RS (1991) The long term effectiveness of hysteroscopic treatment of menorrhagia and leiomyomas. *Obstetrics and Gynecology* **77**: 591–594.

Dicker RC, Greenspan JR, Strauss LT *et al.* (1982) Complications of abdominal and vaginal hysterectomy among women of reproductive age in the United States. *American Journal of Obstetrics and Gynecology* **144**: 841–848.

Dwyer N, Hutton J, Stirrat GM (1993) Randomised controlled trial comparing endometrial resection with abdominal hysterectomy for the surgical treatment of menorrhagia. *British Journal of Obstetrics and Gynaecology* **100**: 237–243.

Ewen SP, Sutton CJG (1994) A combined approach for painful heavy periods: laparoscopic laser uterine nerve ablation and endometrial resection. *Gynaecological Endoscopy* **3**: 167–168.

Gannon MJ, Holt EM, Fairbank J *et al.* (1991) A randomised trial comparing endometrial resection and abdominal hysterectomy for the treatment of menorrhagia. *British Medical Journal* **303**: 1362–1364.

Goldberg JM (1994) Intrauterine pregnancy following endometrial ablation. *Obstetrics and Gynecology* **83**: 836–837.

Hallez JP, Netter A, Cartier R (1987) Methodical intrauterine resection. *American Journal of Obstetrics and Gynecology* **156**: 1080–1084.

Horowitz IR, Copas PR, Aaronoff M, Spann CO, McGuire WP (1995) Endometrial adenocarcinoma following endometrial ablation for postmenopausal bleeding. *Gynecologic Oncology* **56**: 460–463.

Lockwood GM, Baumann R, Turnbull AC, Magos AL (1992) Extensive hysteroscopic surgery under local anaesthesia. *Gynaecological Endoscopy* **1**: 15–21.

MacDonald R, Phipps J (1992) Endometrial ablation: a safe procedure. *Gynaecological Endoscopy* **1**: 7–9.

Magos AL, Baumann R, Turnbull AC (1989a) Transcervical resection of endometrium in women with menorrhagia. *British Medical Journal* **298**: 1209–1212.

Magos AL, Baumann R, Cheung K, Turnbull AC (1989b) Intra-uterine surgery under intravenous sedation as an out-patient alternative to hysterectomy. *Lancet* **ii**: 925–926.

Magos AL, Baumann R, Lockwood GM, Turnbull AC (1991) Experience with the first 250 endometrial resections for menorrhagia. *Lancet* **337**: 1074–1078.

Maher PJ, Hill DJ (1990) Transcervical endometrial resection for abnormal uterine bleeding – report of 100 cases and review of the literature. *Australian and New Zealand Journal of Obstetrics and Gynaecology* **30**: 357–360.

O'Connor H, Magos A (1996) Endometrial resection for menorrhagia. Evaluation of the results at 5 years. *New England Journal of Medicine* **335**: 151–156.

O'Connor H, Broadbent JA, Magos A, McPherson K (1997) Medical Research Council randomized trial of endometrial resection versus hysterectomy in management of menorrhagia. *Lancet* **349**: 897–901.

Pinion SB, Parkin DE, Abramovich DR *et al.* (1994) Randomised trial of hysterectomy, endometrial laser ablation, and transcervical endometrial resection for dysfunctional uterine bleeding. *British Medical Journal* **309**: 979–983.

Raiga J, Mage MD, Bruhat MD *et al.* (1995) Factors affecting risk of failure after endometrial resection. *Journal of Gynecologic Surgery* **11**: 1–6.

Reid PC, Sharpe F (1988) Hysteroscopic Nd:YAG endometrial ablation: an *in vitro* and *in vivo* laser–tissue interaction study. *Abstract IIIrd European Congress on Hysteroscopy and Endoscopic Surgery, Amsterdam*. p. 70.

Royal College of Obstetrics and Gynaecology Audit Unit (1994) *MISTLETOE Update*, October.

Rutherford AJ, Glass MR, Wells M (1991) Patient selection for endometrial resection. *British Journal of Obstetrics and Gynaecology* **98**: 228–230.

Sculpher MJ, Stirling B, Dwyer N, Hutton J, Stirrat GM (1993) An economic evaluation of transcervical endometrial resection versus abdominal hysterectomy for the treatment of menorrhagia. *British Journal of Obstetrics and Gynaecology* **100**: 244–252.

Spaulding BB (1994) Endometrial ablation for refractory postmenopausal bleeding with continuous hormone replacement therapy. *Fertility and Sterility* **62**: 1181–1185.

Whitelaw N, Sutton C (1993) Nine years' experience of endoscopic surgery in a District General Hospital. In Sutton CJG (ed.) *New Surgical Techniques in Gynaecology*. Carnforth, Lancs: Parthenon Publishing.

Wood SM, Roberts PL (1990) Air embolism during transcervical resection of the endometrium. *British Medical Journal* **300**: 945.

59

Endometrial Electroablation

THIERRY G. VANCAILLIE

Royal Hospital for Women, Randwick, Sydney, NSW, Australia

Introduction

Although most gynecologists view electrodesiccation of the endometrium as 'new' and 'innovative', the actual history of this technique stretches back over half a century. In 1948, Baumann reported a success with the technique and this mode of therapy was extremely popular in Germany, Austria and the Netherlands (Bardenheuer, 1937; Baumann, 1948). This was despite the fact that the necessary technology was at that time virtually in its infancy. Surgeons in those days used a 5–8 mm steel ball electrode on a 20 cm long insulated shaft, employing the electrode in a blind fashion, using no anesthesia of any kind. Such a procedure would hardly be acceptable today! Despite these handicaps, Baumann, reporting on 387 cases treated in this manner over a period of ten years, experienced an astoundingly low failure and complication rate of only 3.4% (Table 59.1).

Economic and political change often result in dramatic shifts in therapeutic modalities, but nowhere is this influence more apparent than in the history of endometrial electrodesiccation. Born in a time of economic hardship and high-risk anesthesia and fostered during the wartime shortage of hospital beds, the technique foundered in the relative affluence of the 1950s because of the unjustified association with the use of X-rays or radium for 'menolysis', which were subsequently found to cause secondary malignancies. Furthermore the fashionable trend at that time was to extend the limits of invasive surgery. Proponents of electrodesiccation such as Baumann continued to defend the technique, but their views went unheeded. As the rise–fall–rise course of this modality appears to have been largely determined by extrinsic factors, the student of history may justifiably ask what shift in economic, political or social factors has produced the recent resurgence of interest in this form of therapy. Certainly the current economic climate plays a

Table 59.1 Complications and failures after electrocoagulation of the endometrium as reported by Baumann (1948).

Indication	Number	Early comp.	Late comp.	Early hyst.	Late hyst.	Repeat el.
Metrorrhagia	324	2	1	2	1	2
Myoma	58	3	0	0	2	0
Postmenopause	5	0	0	0	0	0
Total	387	5	1	2	3	2
%	100.0	1.3	0.26	0.52	0.78	0.52

Comp., complication; hyst., hysterectomy; el., electrocoagulation.

role, but I think the increasingly greater involvement of the patient in the decision-making process is probably the decisive factor, along with greater awareness on the part of both the physician and the patient concerning any possible undesirable secondary effects of clinical interventions. Although the original reports made no mention concerning possible secondary malignancy following electrodesiccation, and although conclusions of this sort are not hastily drawn, there has indeed been no reported carcinogenesis – leading the clinician to a cautious optimism.

In recent years, fueled by the potentially large market, a number of companies have funded the development of several technologies intended to simplify and therefore replace the current method. The three front runners are the hot water balloon from Gynecare (Johnson & Johnson, Somerville, New Jersey), the hot glycine balloon from Cavetherm (Walstrom, Lausanne, Switzerland) and the multi-electrode balloon from Valleylab (Boulder, Colorado). All devices have a mechanical component (i.e. the balloon), which brings the energy source (i.e. heat or electrical current) to the endomyometrium.

There is no doubt that to a certain extent, all these devices will work. Which one will be the winner, is unknown at this time. One thing is sure: the powerful engine of the companies promoting non-hysteroscopic ablation will return endometrial ablation into the limelight. Some predict that the balloon technologies will eliminate the need for the resectoscope. The armamentarium of the physician dealing with abnormal uterine bleeding increases, but this does not mean that one modality will eliminate the other. The mode of treatment shifts toward the least invasive technology. The results of this activity are a multiplication of different treatment modalities per patient and an increased awareness of the different modalities by the patient. The total number of hysteroscopic endometrial ablations may be reduced, but the modality will nevertheless subsist. Eventually the hysteroscopist will have to deal with a new category of patient, namely the one who failed to respond to a non-hysteroscopic method of reducing menstrual flow.

Patient Selection

Electrodesiccation is ideally suited for the treatment of excessive, rather than irregular bleeding; the surgery will reduce the amount of bleeding, but will not necessarily correct the erratic pattern of metrorrhagia. Endometrial carcinoma and other less common conditions, remain the purview of other therapeutic modalities. The ideal candidate for electrodesiccation is a multiparous woman with a uterus of normal size and heavy but regular bleeding in whom sterilization has already been accomplished by previous tubal ligation. Early reports on this technique pointed out that the greatest success was achieved with perimenopausal dysfunctional bleeding. Baumann reports that the greatest benefit is achieved in patients in their late forties. My personal experience tends to corroborate this statement.

Patients with organic lesions (i.e. submucous fibroids or polyps) represent another category in whom endometrial ablation may be indicated. Office hysteroscopy or hydrosonography readily identifies patients with intrauterine lesions who present with abnormal uterine bleeding. The question may be asked whether these patients should be offered endometrial ablation in addition to resection of the intrauterine lesion for treatment of the abnormal bleeding. For patients who have no further desire for fertility, this may represent a viable option. The rational for presenting this option is that patients may suffer from a combined organic and functional pathology, rather than from an organic pathology alone.

Reduction or complete elimination of menstrual bleeding is accompanied by certain beneficial side effects. Dysmenorrhea, which is induced by expulsion of blood clots, is usually diminished concomitant with a reduction in flow. A decline in premenstrual symptoms has been reported (Lefler, 1989; Vancaillie, 1989) and the incidence of pelvic inflammatory disease or its recurrence may be reduced, as well. An additional benefit of electrodesiccation is that this technique offers both the patients and the surgeon a physiologic indicator of its success. A successful procedure results in an obvious decrease in menstrual flow.

It is the experience of the author that long-term persistence of amenorrhea cannot be forecast with certainty at all. This fact should be made absolutely clear to the patient when she is counseled preoperatively to avoid subsequent disappointment and misunderstanding. If the objective of electrodesiccation is actually one of its beneficial side effects such as reduced premenstrual syndrome (PMS), the subject should be reviewed thoroughly with the patient. It should be clear to the physician and the patient that there may be some benefit, but that this benefit is unpredictable and most likely to be temporary.

Can endometrial ablation ever be a reliable alternative technique for sterilization? The answer depends upon whether amenorrhea will ever become a predictable outcome. Many factors play a role, most of them related to the armamentarium of the surgeon: experience, skill and training. With increasing experience, the surgeon will in the future become more adept at predicting which patient will become reliably amenorrheic. Implementation of additional techniques will hopefully enable the operator to ensure amenorrhea in a particular patient. The surgeon who has mastered only roller-ball ablation is unnecessarily restricted. Obviously a thorough knowledge and understanding of the endocrinology and pharmacology of the lower genital tract is imperative. It hardly need be mentioned that patients should be absolutely certain that they wish no future fertility and this decision is often heavily influenced by years of menstrual problems.

Patient Counseling

Expectations

Because of the variable outcome, it is essential that patients considering or intending to undergo electrodesiccation of the endometrium are counseled thoroughly to prevent subsequent misunderstanding and/or disappointment. Those patients with excessive menstrual flow will obtain relief from the procedure whether or not total amenorrhea is obtained. However, patients with other complaints, often multiple and minor, may be less enthusiastic about the outcome, if their prospects are not explained thoroughly and in detail before the surgery. Available information may be summarized for the patient as follows:

- Menstrual flow will be reduced in almost all (> 90%) cases.
- Post-surgical bleeding pattern is unpredictable.
- True dysmenorrhea will almost certainly be reduced in parallel with the reduction in menstrual flow; however, minor cramping similar to that of dysmenorrhea may persist, even if amenorrhea is obtained and there is no hematometra.
- Pelvic pain other than that of true dysmenorrhea (e.g. endometriosis), but which the patient has mistakenly thought to be dysmenorrhea, will remain unchanged.

Further examination and possible intervention (e.g. laparoscopy) may be needed to obtain a definitive diagnosis and/or relief. Persistence of pelvic pain is a major indication for subsequent pelvic surgery in women who undergo endometrial ablation.

PMS (Lefler, 1989) symptoms are relieved, in the author's experience only when total amenorrhea is obtained. Obviously, progesterone-influenced symptoms such as bloating and breast tenderness will remain relatively unrelieved. Psychosomatically, the patient may obtain relief from the 'vicious circle' of PMS symptoms when the physical signs of the menstrual cycle are eliminated. Some women with PMS feel better in anticipation of the surgery, perhaps as a result of their decision to take further control of their lives by finally 'doing something about it'.

Complications

Preoperative hormonal treatment may result in side effects such as hot flushes, but these are generally well tolerated in the patient who has received adequate counseling. The more serious complications are:

- Intravasation.
- Uterine perforation.
- Electrosurgical accidents.
- Excessive uterine bleeding.
- Infectious complications.
- Pregnancy.

INTRAVASATION

Intravasation always occurs! No control system exists that can totally eliminate this danger. The experienced hysteroscopist remains ever alert, because he or she never loses sight of this fact. Intravasation occurs because tissue and capillary pressures ($\leq$ 15 mm Hg) are less than the pressure needed to adequately distend the uterine cavity (35 mm Hg). Therefore there is always a pressure gradient toward the patient's vascular system. The goal of the surgeon and supporting operating room staff is, therefore, not elimination of intravasation, but its control within acceptable limits. Patients with normal metabolic functions should experience no difficulty with a fluid load of 1000 ml, and can tolerate even larger volumes. On the other hand, compromised patients such as those undergoing renal dialysis, will be unable to handle even a slight increase in vascular volume because of the resultant hyponatremia and hypokalemia. A brush-up course in electrolyte homeostasis would be helpful to the clinician, to assist in coping with the problems inherent in fluid overload. (Distension media are discussed in Chapter 53.) Only the main points will be mentioned here.

Dextran 70 and similar hyperosmolar media cause hemodilution, not by direct fluid overload, but by osmosis. Diuretics are of no effect because these macromolecules do not pass the renal filter. Therefore diuretics will worsen the fluid shift because of the increased loss of free water in the presence of continued osmotic pressure. One can only wait until the Dextran 70 is broken down by intravascular and hepatic enzymes and eliminated while monitoring vital signs.

Early in our experience we used Dextran 70 because this was the medium with which we had had the most experience, but it quickly became apparent that accidents resulting from intravasation were a major problem with this medium. The author's three most serious incidents occurred when Dextran 70 was being used as the distension medium. Delayed aspiration pneumonia occurring in one patient was undoubtedly a result of the patient's altered cognitive state due to hyponatremia. Careful monitoring of electrolytes can avoid this major complication. Two other patients with sickle cell trait suffered a hemolytic crisis.

Hypo-osmotic non-conductive media such as sorbitol (with or without mannitol) and glycine are current favorites. Preoperative serum electrolyte values should always be obtained to screen for borderline low values that can be corrected before surgery. Ingestion of a potassium-rich diet before operative hysteroscopy is also helpful, and should be routinely recommended. There are currently also iso-osmotic media based on mannitol. These media do cause fluid overload if absorbed, but no hypo-osmolarity.

When fluid overload does occur, diuresis can be initiated by use of a diuretic such as furosemide. Mannitol admixed with sorbitol will initiate diuresis by itself. All diuretics result in sodium and potassium loss and replacement should be considered at the time of diagnosis rather than waiting for values to drop further below normal. For example, an intravenous infusion of Ringer's lactate with added potassium (e.g. 4 meq 100 ml^{-1}) at a rate of 50 ml^{-1} can be started, replacing the glucose solution that was running before. Adding hypertonic saline to the intravenous infusion requires careful calculation of the sodium deficit. Consultation with a nephrologist is recommended. Remember that overcorrecting hyponatremia is as detrimental as hyponatremia itself. With a fluid overload of 1000 ml or over it is advisable to monitor serum electrolyte values until excess fluid has been filtered out. Note that at the time of suspicion of fluid overload, peripheral serum values may still be normal due to a latency period in the redistribution of fluids. Although an increased diuresis by the patient is welcome at this time, concomitant loss in sodium and potassium should also be anticipated. Electrolytes are considered stabilized when two series of determinations two hours apart show steady values.

A thorough understanding of the dynamics of electrolyte balance is essential in the immediate postoperative period. A patient may appear to be recovering well following a procedure and be discharged to go home two hours later. Upon arriving home, she may experience malaise and nausea or even become disoriented. Such an experience will leave the patient and her family with unpleasant recollections of the surgery at least. Moreover, more serious complications, such as aspiration pneumonia, can ensue, especially if the patient's state of consciousness is affected.

Fluid overload is less likely to occur if only a large contact electrode, such as the roller, is employed during the procedure because tissue is coagulated rather than cut, sealing rather than severing the vessels. However, if such a large contact electrode is used improperly it may slowly burn a path into the uterine wall, opening venous sinuses in the process.

To summarize, fluid balance must be monitored at all times and under all circumstances. A crude way to accomplish this is to recover the distension fluid using direct aspiration under low negative pressure, collecting the recovered fluid in containers of the same volume as the infusion bottles, thus enabling quick estimation and comparison of the volumes of fluid used and recuperated. Real-time measurement of fluid overload is achieved by commercially available equipment such as the AquaSens by Aquintel (Mountain View, California, USA).

UTERINE PERFORATION

This is the one complication that should never occur, as the endoscope is introduced under direct visual control. However, cervical dilatation preceding insertion of the resectoscope does sometimes result in perforation, which, of course, signals immediate termination of the procedure as a perforated uterus cannot hold the distension medium. Once the resectoscope is inserted into the endometrial cavity there should be no problem with outright perforation. Incomplete perforation remains a pitfall, however. Although it does not prevent retention of the medium and distension of the uterine cavity, the resultant increased intravasation into the vascular system is a hazard.

Perforation with the loop electrode results from improper handling of the resectoscope. The electrode should always, with few exceptions, be activated only when moved towards the optic. It is tempting to cut adhesions or a septum with a loop electrode while advancing the electrode towards the fundus. Invariably this will one day lead to inadvertent perforation at the fundus.

ELECTROSURGICAL ACCIDENTS

Fortunately, electrosurgical accidents rarely occur. Such misadventures are often the result of defective insulation and connectors and for this reason electrodes should be considered to be disposable items. If prolonged contact with any one place on the uterine wall for any extended period of time is avoided, burning through the wall of the uterus will not occur. However, thinner areas (such as the tubal ostia and uterotomy sites) can permit heat conduction to neighboring organs, with resulting injury. This heat conduction can result in necrosis and subsequent breakdown of the wall of the bladder or bowel. Particularly where there is direct and continuous contact, as in uterine–bladder or uterine–bowel adhesions. For this reason, desiccation at the level of the uterotubal junction and at uterotomy scars must be conducted with extreme care.

The most dangerous aspect of accidental electrical burns from large contact electrodes is that no symptoms will be noted until several days following the procedure. For this reason, patients should be instructed to report any symptoms such as hematuria, diarrhea, fever and pain. Any pain 24 hours following the procedure that requires pain medication other than mild analgesics such as aspirin should be carefully investigated.

Early reports mentioned fistula formation between the uterus and small bowel, which was treated by expectant management for up to nine weeks. These fistulas were most likely the result of transmural burns, which also affected the bowel. The role of a particular pathogen (i.e. tuberculosis) is unknown. In more recent times, there are only a few published reports of electrical injury to the bowel. Complications are not the favorite subject for publication so one may safely assume that more complications have occurred. These incidents, however, are anecdotal and rare.

The large contact electrodes are much less likely to burn through the uterine wall than the loop electrodes, the latter being designed for precisely that purpose, thus making large contact electrodes the preferred choice for the 'beginner'. Let us emphasize one more time that any electrode, but in particular the loop electrode, is moved only towards the optic and not advanced towards the fundus, when activated. When a loop electrode has perforated the uterus one should assume that injury of the bladder or bowel has

occurred. A laparoscopy should be performed to evaluate the bowel. A negative laparoscopy is not an absolute guarantee that there is no injury to the bowel or bladder. The patient should be told to remain in contact with the unit and to monitor temperature and other vital functions for at least ten days after the occurrence.

EXCESSIVE UTERINE BLEEDING

Excessive uterine bleeding rarely occurs, and is more likely to be the result of overenergetic cervical dilatation than electrodesiccation. If electrodesiccation is performed during an episode of heavy bleeding, uterine flow will be reduced significantly postoperatively. Indeed, in the 1930s and 1940s, procedures were performed during ongoing metrorrhagia for the purpose of successfully interrupting excessive bleeding. Postoperative bleeding should not exceed that of normal menstrual flow – an annoyingly vague concept, but one the patient understands quite well. Should postoperative bleeding exceed this, a potential problem should be suspected and investigated. Any lacerations of the cervix should be cauterized and repaired. If the bleeding seems to emanate from the uterine cavity itself, an intramuscular injection of ergotamin derivative (Methergin) or an intracervical injection of diluted synthetic vasopressin (Pitressin) should be administered. Branches of the uterine vessels can be injured through laceration of the uterine sidewall, whether electrosurgically or mechanically induced. Such injury is rare, however, if only large contact electrodes are used for intrauterine surgery. With the loop electrode, it is possible to sever larger vessels within the myometrium, especially if a myomectomy is performed before the endometrial ablation. In rare cases an intrauterine tamponade is performed with an inflatable balloon. A large Foley catheter will work well after the tip is cut off. The balloon is inflated until resistance is encountered. The pressure is maintained for a predetermined period of time. Personally, I order the balloon to be deflated to half its original volume after two hours. If no bleeding occurs after another two hours, the balloon is gently removed.

Intrauterine tamponade with a balloon will not be effective if a perforation has occurred at the same time. The inflated Foley catheter will obscure the external bleeding, but not prevent the escape of blood into the peritoneal cavity or broad ligament. Close observation of the patient is initially required. Should there be any doubt about the state of hemostasis, a laparotomy or laparoscopy, possibly followed by hysterectomy should be considered.

INFECTIOUS COMPLICATIONS

Acute Endomyometritis

Acute endomyometritis is better known as a puerperal condition. However, any intrauterine manipulation can theoretically facilitate this infection. The incidence is unknown. The clinical presentation is one of increased vaginal bleeding after a period of initial tapering off. There is not necessarily a high fever or severe pelvic pain and the discharge is not necessarily purulent. The clinical course is more one of 'failure to steadily improve'. Low-grade fever and increased leukocytosis are common findings, but not typical. A culture may be taken from the cervix or endometrial cavity, but more importantly, broad-spectrum antibiotics are started immediately.

Whether antibiotics should be administered prophylactically remains an open question. Most colleagues in the USA will order a standard regimen of preoperative antibiotics such as 1 g of a second generation cephalosporin intravenously before surgery.

Acute Pelvic Peritonitis and Tubo-ovarian Abscess

One case of tubo-ovarian abscess was presented to me several years ago during a scientific meeting, but I do not recall having seen this case or any other case published. However, theoretically, occlusion of the cervix for some reason within the first days postoperatively may lead to a hematometra, which may secondarily progress to pelvic peritonitis and tubo-ovarian abscess. The occurrence of this complication was also mentioned by Baumann (1948) in one of the earlier publications.

This type of infectious complication obviously differs from the peritonitis engendered by perforation of the uterus or a transmural burn of the uterus with subsequent bowel perforation. The occurrence of a bowel perforation is significantly more life-threatening and early surgical intervention should be encouraged. The presence of pelvic abscedation (the process of an infection progressing towards an abscess) should spur the physician to look for any form of bowel perforation, because early surgical intervention will make a distinct difference to the recovery and survival of the patient.

Chronic Endomyometritis

One of my patients recently underwent a hysterectomy approximately nine months after an endometrial ablation because of persistent, almost daily brownish discharge. There were no other physical or biochemical abnormalities. The pathology report of the specimen noted chronic inflammatory infiltrate with extensive giant cell reaction, no endometrium seen on the specimen'. During the months of battling with the patient's symptoms it was noted that the discharge did respond to treatment with short courses of antibiotics and hormones, but would invariably return. No long-term (longer than one month) periods of treatment were tried.

Hematometra

The occurrence of hematometra is well known and is the main reason why some colleagues recommend routine sounding of the uterus at the first postoperative visit. Whether this sounding prevents cervical occlusion is doubtful and I do not have any hard data on the incidence of hematometra. My clinical experience tells me that the condition can occur at any time after the procedure up to several years. One common denominator is that these patients all are amenorrheic for several months or years to start with. The hematometra becomes a problem at a time when the pain caused by the hematometra is no longer spontaneously linked to the uterus. In many cases an extensive work-up with scanning and barium enema is carried out before it is realized that one is dealing with a simple hematometra. Sounding of the uterus may be all that is needed to break up the synechia that holds up the flow of menses. In case of recurrence, a hysterectomy is the treatment of choice. Whether a repeat ablation is equally effective in treatment is unknown.

PREGNANCY

Pregnancy, either intrauterine or ectopic, can occur as a long-term complication. The estimated risk is approximately 1%. However, there are no reliable statistics for the occurrence of pregnancy, and this figure should be understood to apply only to experienced operators.

Endometrial Suppression

Preoperative endometrial suppression reduces the bulk of the endometrial tissue and makes surgery easier; furthermore, a suppressed endometrium is less likely to recover from a surgical insult, thus enhancing the effectiveness of endometrial electro-desiccation. It is difficult to recommend any one hormonal regimen above another; probably the regimen most familiar to the physician and most convenient for the patient is the one to recommend. We use a single intramuscular injection of leuprolide acetate depot (7.5 mg) during the luteal phase of the cycle, and 2–3 weeks before the date of surgery. Lupron Depot is effective for approximately six weeks, thus a single dose provides both pre- and postoperative endometrial suppression. Drawbacks of endometrial suppression are the delay it causes in scheduling the surgery and the cost of some of these drugs. Combining resection with desiccation may be one way of avoiding preoperative suppression. However, if a desiccation only technique is planned, then it is strongly advisable to treat the patient with hormonal suppression before the procedure.

Operative Technique

Room Set-up and Positioning of the Patient
(Figure 59.1)

The patient should be placed in the dorsal lithotomy position with the instrument table and scrub technician on one side, and the video monitor and fluid containers on the other. Ideally, a heating blanket should be available to keep the patient comfortable. Large volumes of fluid used for uterine distension will lower the patient's temperature significantly, depending upon the length of the surgery.

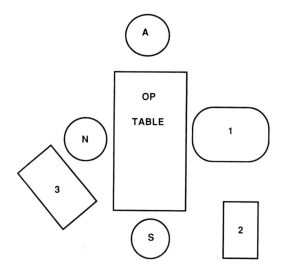

Figure 59.1 Room set-up. This diagram gives a schematic overview of the special arrangement of the operating room. (A, anesthesiologist; N, nurse; S, surgeon; 1, video cart; 2, in and outflow; 3, instrument table)

An excessive Trendelenburg position should be avoided because this changes the pressure gradient between the uterine cavity and the venous collection system, contributing to an increased risk of fluid overload.

Anesthesia

Virtually any form of anesthesia can be used for endometrial electrodesiccation. Note, however, that heat sensation is not blocked by local anesthesia and, additionally, patients may experience some pain under local anesthesia (i.e. paracervical block) when the surgeon operates in the cornual areas. The anesthesiologist should be instructed concerning the potential for fluid overload and the need to limit intravenous infusion.

Even when general anesthesia is used, a paracervical block is useful; its anesthetic effect will last some hours beyond the actual intervention, reducing the need for postoperative pain medication.

Vasoconstrictive Agents

If one anticipates using the cutting loop, it is helpful to administer a vasoconstrictor (e.g. synthetic vasopressin) in conjunction with local anesthesia. Vasoconstrictors prolong the effect of the local anesthetic agent. In addition, use of such a vasoconstrictive agent permits a virtually bloodless dilatation and curettage before electrodesiccation and when injected into the cervix the vasoconstrictor seems to make cervical dilatation easier. We find the use of vasoconstrictive agents extremely helpful, and use them for all hysteroscopic interventions except synechiolysis.

Cervical Dilatation

The operator must take great care in cervical dilatation. First, an obvious laceration or perforation automatically signals termination of the procedure; however, even more importantly, an unnoticed, perhaps incomplete perforation or laceration will almost certainly lead to rapid fluid overload owing to the injury of large venous sinuses. Many surgeons routinely employ laminaria preoperatively to assist in cervical dilatation. We do not use laminaria because we find they make it more difficult to distinguish the internal cervical os. Furthermore, a cervical dilatation of 10 mm is sufficient, and this can usually be achieved with any type of mechanical dilator.

Curettage

Following cervical dilation, a thorough suction curettage can be carried out to remove as much debris and endometrium as is possible. To encourage thorough curettage, it is helpful for the surgeon to set a time period (e.g. three minutes) for this procedure and then have someone actually time him or her, with a stopwatch, so he or she does not shorten this important step. If no endometrial sampling has been performed earlier, a specimen should be obtained at this point for histologic evaluation.

Selection of the Electrode

A variety of electrodes are now on the market, presenting the surgeon with the luxury (and burden) of making a choice. What constitutes an ideal electrode? Ideally, it would have no fixed form at all, but would rather adapt itself to whatever contour it encounters. Unfortunately, no such instrument exists at present. Given that one must make a very real choice among very real instruments, what factors are important, and what do we know about these factors?

SHAPE

My personal favorite is the ball-shaped electrode, because this shape seems best adapted to the irregularities one encounters. However, the effectiveness, electrophysically, of the various shapes of the electrodes has been investigated very little.

SIZE

The electrode must permit an adequate field of view for the endoscopist, and thus be relatively small.

TRANSMISSION OF ELECTRICAL ENERGY FROM THE AXIS TO THE ROTATING PART

This is an aspect of configuration that is very important for optimal transmission of the electrical energy from the electrode to the tissue. A loose connection will allow internal sparking between the axis and the bulk of the electrode. Sparking has two unwanted effects:

- First, it produces a significant amount of heat, leading to charring of tissue, which sticks to the electrode, thereby reducing its effectiveness.
- Second, sparking is a source of demodulation, which causes muscle twitching. These sudden jerky movements of the patient are in themselves harmless, but they make the surgeon lose control over the resectoscope. Injury to the patient may be the result of such jerky movements.

BUILD-UP OF CHAR ON THE ELECTRODE DURING SURGERY

Char is carbonized tissue and forms an electrical barrier between the electrode and the tissue. This increased resistance prevents in-depth desiccation of the endomyometrium. Charred tissue sticking to the electrode is to be avoided at all costs. The electrode is kept as clean as possible during the entire procedure.

The currently popular grooved ball end electrodes (e.g. Vaportrode (ACMI)) are not intended for desiccation, but for vaporization. They may be used for endometrial ablation, but the risk of perforation is definitely higher than with the regular ball electrodes because of the ability of the grooved electrodes to cut through tissue, rather than desiccate the tissue.

Selection of the Waveform and Power Settings
(Figures 59.2–59.5)

When a large electrode in contact with tissue is activated, desiccation occurs because the energy immediately spreads within a large volume of tissue. Early in this century, studies established that low power density electrical energy used over a relatively long period of time will cause deeper tissue destruction than an equivalent amount of energy delivered at a high power density. This is because rapid desiccation causes increased tissue impedance and a consequent decrease in current flow. Deep destruction (2 mm) would therefore be most effectively accomplished by using power of a continuous low density waveform ('cutting current' at e.g. 20–40 W). Tissue destruction is slow and therefore difficult for the surgeon to control. The process is more easily understood if the reader thinks of it as being divided into two phases: static and dynamic.

FIRST PHASE: INITIATION (see Figures 59.2, 59.3)

The operator presses the electrode gently into contact with the tissue and activates the current. A relatively large volume of tissue is being destroyed. The electrode should be held in one spot as long as required until blanching is observed around the electrode (less than one second).

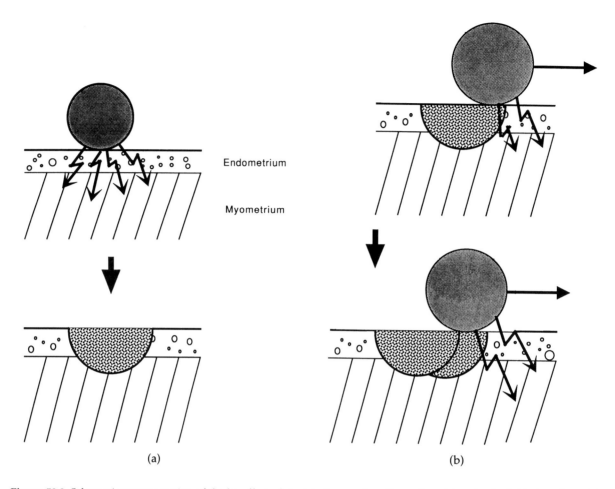

Endometrium

Myometrium

(a)   (b)

Figure 59.2 Schematic representation of the bioeffect of electrical current on the endometrium in the initiation phase (a) and dynamic phase (b).

SECOND PHASE: DYNAMIC (See Figures 59.4, 59.5)

When blanching has been observed all around the electrode, the operator can then move the electrode slowly towards the cervical canal. To determine at what speed the electrode should be moved, the operator must watch the zone of visible tissue destruction preceding the electrode. A relatively high level of power is required to pass through the desiccated tissue and coagulate tissue in front of it. Low-wattage 'desiccation' or 'blend' current best balances the need for surgical speed and required depth of tissue destruction. Different electrosurgical units vary in the amount of energy they provide. However, 40–60 W at 2000–5000 V will commonly provide sufficient energy to cause the desired level of destruction.

After the operator presses the electrode against the uterine wall and presses the control pedal, blanching should be visible around the electrode within one second. If the surgeon observes no visible effect, the connections are checked and if found intact the power setting is increased. On the other hand, rapid explosive action indicates that the power setting is too high. When the surgeon is sure the power setting is appropriate, the electrode is rolled slowly towards the optic. The operator should be able to see the desiccation zone preceding the electrode at all times. As the electrode progresses beyond the original, rather wide, area of desiccation, only the advancing edge of the electrode contacts as-yet-uncoagulated tissue – a rather small area, comparatively. The rest of the electrode is passing over already desiccated tissue where the current is impeded by the previous desiccation. This allows reduction in the time of exposure and therefore forward motion of the electrode. The most important aspect of the surgery is that the operator maintains a steady but slow pace in moving the electrode over the surface.

The Operation

There are different variations on how to perform an endometrial ablation with the resectoscope. There is

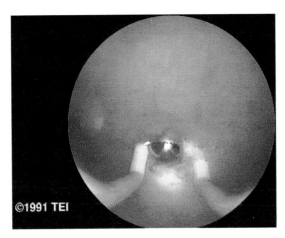

Figure 59.3 *In vivo* appearance of the 'initiation phase'. (Courtesy of Texas Endosurgery Institute.)

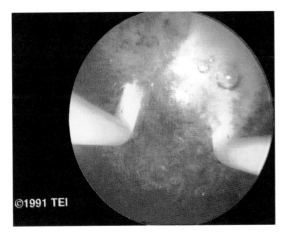

Figure 59.4 *In vivo* appearance of the desiccation effects preceding the electrode. (Courtesy of Texas Endosurgery Institute.)

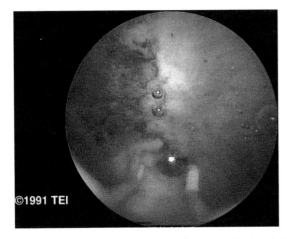

Figure 59.5 Aspect of the cavity after a single 'stroke' with the electrode. (Courtesy of Texas Endosurgery Institute.)

the roller ball only, the loop only and a combination of both. It appears that most physicians will start out with the roller ball only and then graduate to the roller ball plus loop. There is no doubt that roller ball ablation is easier and safer to learn than resection of tissue. Intrinsically it is unclear whether desiccation or resection is better in terms of reducing menstrual bleeding. The question may appear trivial, but is not. In-depth tissue destruction is fundamentally different from tissue resection.

Whether either modality is better than the other is an unanswered question and will remain unanswered for some time. Currently the majority of colleagues known to me combine both modalities. The roller ball is applied primarily to the cornua and the fundus whereas the walls of the uterus are resected, followed by an application of the roller ball to the cut surface. The reason for using the roller electrode after resection of the endomyometrium is primarily hemostasis. In addition, however, supplemental desiccation may have a positive impact on reducing menstrual flow.

The operation as currently performed, consists of three steps. (1) desiccation of fundus and ostia; (2) resection of endomyometrium; (3) desiccation of the cut surface. First desiccation of both cornual areas and the fundus with the roller electrode is performed. Electrodes are then exchanged and the walls of the uterine cavity are shaved with the loop electrode to remove the endomyometrium. The loop electrode is activated only when moved towards the internal cervical os. The current is switched on slightly before the electrode touches the tissue. This is exactly the opposite to the use of the roller electrode. The activated loop electrode is driven into the tissue to a depth predetermined by the operator. The loop is then pulled towards the internal cervical os in a continued smooth motion and remains activated until it exits the tissue to avoid it getting stuck within the uterine wall.

Resection of the uterine walls should be systematic. I favor starting on the right of the posterior wall and progressing clockwise. The electrodes are then exchanged again. Where desiccation is begun is unimportant, but once begun, desiccation should be pursued in a systematic fashion, and this sequence religiously followed, whether it is clockwise or counterclockwise. During the procedure, the surgeon should inspect both tubal ostia, note any visible uterotomy scars and look out for any unexpected pathology. The areas where complications are likely to arise are those that are technically most difficult to reach, namely areas of the fundus and tubal ostia. Rolling the electrode is often impossible in these areas; thus, the electrode must be placed in one spot, activated, retrieved, then relocated, activated again, and so on, until the entire fundus and adjacent cornual areas are coagulated. The operator must take care not to force the electrode into the tubal ostia.

It is important to locate the internal cervical os, because this represents the limit of desiccation. The operator should retrieve the resectoscope into the cervical canal, thus temporarily occluding the outflow and permitting visualization of the internal cervical os. It is not easy to determine the precise anatomic site and if laminaria have been used for dilatation, it is even more difficult. It is sometimes helpful to stain the mucosa of the uterus with methylene blue (a single drop diluted in 10–20 ml of physiologic solution and slowly instilled into the uterine cavity before dilatation). The operator can then use a 5 mm endoscope to perform a diagnostic hysteroscopy. The endometrium will be colored evenly blue, the endosalpinx will appear as dark blue spots, and the endocervix will appear as parallel blue lines.

To complete the ablation, the surgeon inspects the uterine cavity for any areas that appear untouched. Because the resection/desiccation significantly alters the appearance of the endometrial surface, this is not easy, thus emphasizing the need for a careful, systematic approach in the first place. Evaluation for adenomyosis is aided by the fact that the coagulated interface between the endometrium and myometrium presents as transverse grooves (Figure 59.6). This is because the cell-rich tissue of the endometrium conducts electricity better than the fibrous tissue of the myometrium, and will

therefore be more thoroughly destroyed. When the operator rolls the electrode over such an area, he will feel a 'bump', much as the driver of an automobile experiences when he drives over a 'speed bump'. The desiccation of the glandular tissue in such areas may be incomplete because endometrial glands reach deep into the myometrium, and resection may be indicated. It is probably an illusion to believe that adenomyosis can be resected completely.

Up until 1995, I instilled a suspension of tetracycline hydrochloride in Dextran 70 into the uterine cavity to enhance scarring. No clear benefit could be demonstrated. Since discontinuing tetracycline the results do not appear to have changed.

Follow-up

Vital signs, vaginal bleeding and diuresis must be monitored carefully during the immediate postoperative period. However, it is important to remember that bleeding and infection can arise several days following the surgery. It is therefore vital to keep in close contact with the patient for a period of ten days or more – an extremely important point, for instance, if one is treating a patient who lives some distance from the surgical clinic. A postoperative check should be scheduled within ten days. At that time, any delayed infection can be diagnosed and therapy begun. At 2–3 months following surgery, the patient should be checked a second time. Repeat ultrasonography can be performed at this visit to determine uterine measurements and to detect any hematometra. No intrauterine manipulation is performed, but pelvic examination should reveal a firm uterus that is slightly smaller than it was preoperatively.

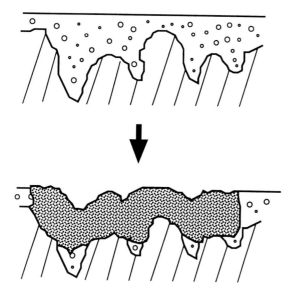

Figure 59.6 Graphic representation of the effect of an irregular interface between endometrium and myometrium.

Results

About 80% of patients will be pleased with the results of their operation. Because patient satisfaction is determined to a large extent by patient expectations, adequate preoperative counseling is of utmost importance. Results should be assessed in terms of reduction in menstrual flow, but because there is no accurate way to measure this, one must deal with total days of vaginal bleeding experienced by the patient per month. We define bleeding as follows:

- Amenorrhea – total absence of any cyclic vaginal bleeding.

Table 59.2 Results of roller-ball electrocoagulation of the endometrium (author's experience: follow-up > 9 months).

Series	0 d	<1/2 d	<2 d	>2 d	Re E.A.	Hyst.
A (n = 15)	*	10 (67)	1 (6)	4 (27)	1	1
B (n = 12)	1 (8)	4 (33)	3 (25)	4 (33)	1	2
C (n = 63)	17 (27)	24 (38)	16 (25)	6 (10)	0	0

Series A starts in June 1986, B in October 1988 and C in October 1989.
Numbers in parentheses are percentages.
Re E.A., repeat ablation; Hyst., hysterectomy; d, average number of days of menstrual bleeding per month.
*In series A the results of '0 d' and '< 1/2 d' are combined.

- Spotting – bleeding lasting less than half a day.
- Hypomenorrhea – bleeding lasting less than two days.

It is often difficult to obtain reliable data concerning bleeding because patients may not assess their own bleeding patterns reliably (e.g. if bleeding is sporadic, does not occur regularly or is so scant that it requires no protection). In the latter case, the patient may report complete amenorrhea when this is not really the case. The difference between scant bleeding for half a day or less and no bleeding at all generally matters very little to the patient, and my initial data also combined these two groups; however, in the interest of precision, I have, in my later data, separated these two groups. In Table 59.2, which shows the results of 90 patients treated between June 1986 and June 1991, series A represents the initial study, series B represents the intermediary period, and series C reports the results using the roller-ball electrode only with preoperative hormone treatment.

The observer will note that the results obtained in series A are superior to those in series B. This is because I capitulated to every surgeon's instinct to increase the speed of surgery by moving the electrode more rapidly, using an increased wattage. I later learned, through consultation with an electrical engineer, why precisely the reverse – low wattage and 'slow motion' surgery – were more effective in electrodesiccation. The temptation to increase speed is one every surgeon must confront and resist, in the face of everything he or she has learned previously, if optimal results are to be obtained in electrodesiccation of the endometrium.

The results presented in Table 59.2 were compiled in 1991 before publication of the first edition of this book. Meanwhile more than five years have gone by and the results have changed. The hysterectomy rate has passed the 10% mark, and slowly increases year after year. I refuse to predict at what level the reintervention curve will plateau. One of the issues still in debate is whether endometrial ablation can be repeated several times. Liberal use of repeat ablation will obviously affect the long-term hysterectomy rate. It should also be noted that hysterectomy is performed in many cases for other reasons (e.g. pelvic floor relaxation, pelvic pain, adnexal mass). Whether the patient consults a physician unfamiliar with endometrial ablation is also an important variable. However, the results within the first two-year time frame after endometrial ablation have not changed since publication of the first edition.

One patient in series B became pregnant. Her postoperative menstrual period lasted an average of five days.

Electrodesiccation as a technique for endometrial ablation is still in its evolution. I believe that further investigation and refinement of the three components involved in this technique – hormonal endometrial inhibition, thermal destruction and scar formation – will ultimately produce the optimal technique.

References

Baumann A (1948) Ueber die elektrokoagulation des Endometriums sowie der Zervikalschleimhaut. *Geburtshilfe fur Frauenheilkunde* **8**: 221.

Bardenheuer (1937) Elektrokoagulation der Uterusschleimhaut zur Behandlung klimakterischer Blutungen. *Zentralblatt fur Gynakologie* **209**: 16.

Lefler H Jr (1989) Premenstrual syndrome: improvement after laser ablation of the endometrium for menorrhagia. *Journal of Reproductive Medicine* **34**: 905.

Vancaillie T (1989) Electrodesiccation of the endometrium with the ball-end resectoscope. *Obstetrics and Gynecology* **74**: 425.

60

Nd:Yag Laser Ablation of the Endometrium

MILTON H. GOLDRATH* AND RAY GARRY[†]

*Sinai Hospital of Detroit, Michigan, USA
[†]Women's Endoscopic Laser Foundation, South Cleveland Hospital, Middlesbrough, UK

Until recently, women with normal uteri who did not respond to pharmacologic intervention for the treatment of menorrhagia were limited to one of the following two options:

- Hysterectomy.
- Continued cycles of heavy menstrual bleeding.

With the advent of hysteroscopic endometrial laser ablation (ELA) in 1979 (Goldrath *et al.*, 1981), women with menorrhagia refractory to or unable to tolerate other methods of therapy were offered an alternative to hysterectomy. ELA has also been employed in recent years to treat menorrhagic patients with moderate-sized fibroids (Goldrath, 1990a). Thus, the number of patients for whom this procedure is potentially beneficial is impossible to estimate.

The primary objective of ELA is to limit uterine bleeding or produce amenorrhea – in essence, Asherman's syndrome. Asherman (1948), identified uterine synechiae, usually resulting from post-abortal or postpartum uterine curettage, as the cause of amenorrhea and infertility in his patients.

It soon became apparent that any technique capable of reproducing Asherman's syndrome might be used to correct excessive uterine bleeding. Subsequently, a variety of chemical and physical methods were used for this purpose, the majority of which proved unsuccessful. Radium and cryocoagulation were both associated with limited success, but radium is no longer used and the cryocoagulation procedure described by Droegemueller *et al.* (1971a,b) was abandoned because of the potential for producing painful hematometra. DeCherney

and Polan (1983) have successfully destroyed the endometrium and produced amenorrhea through the use of a high-frequency coagulating current employing a modified urologic resectoscope. More recently, others have done the same using the so-called roller-ball technique (Townsend *et al.*, 1987; Vancaillie, 1989) with electrosurgery.

Photocoagulation of the Endometrium with the Nd:YAG Laser

The Nd:YAG (neodymium:yttrium-aluminum-garnet) laser is particularly well suited to photocoagulation of the endometrium as a result of its high power and transmission through optical fibers. Its deep tissue penetration (up to 4 mm beneath the surface) distinguishes it from carbon dioxide (CO_2), argon and potassium titanyl phosphate (KTP) lasers. Because of the danger to the surgeon's eye from backscatter after tissue impact, a protective filter over the eyepiece of the hysteroscope is essential or a video camera can be used.

Surgical Procedure

The human uterus is characterized by a relatively thick myometrium and thin endometrium, thus it is an ideal organ for laser surgery. The fact that only about 5% of the uterine thickness must be ablated in order to destroy the endometrium protects adjacent organs from thermal damage.

Ringer's lactate or physiologic saline are currently used to distend the uterus and have both proved to be excellent visualizing media. Gaseous distending media are useful for diagnostic purposes, but should *not* be used for extensive therapeutic hysteroscopic surgery because of the risk of fatal gas embolism.

The procedure is performed with the patient under general or spinal anesthesia. A continuous flow hysteroscope is used (Figures 60.1, 60.2). The fluid flows in by gravity only and is removed by low suction to provide a constant flow of fluid at low pressure. This is important not only for a clear operative field, but also to prevent excessive fluid absorption. Alternatively, a pressure-controlled pump can be used, as described in Chapter 53 (Figure 60.3).

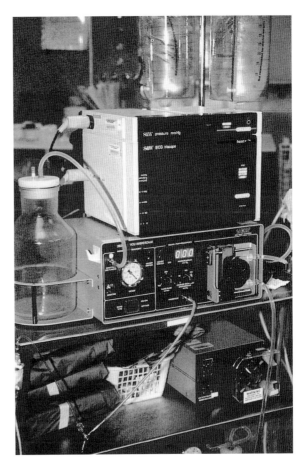

Figure 60.3 A uterine distension system using a Hamou Hysteromat.

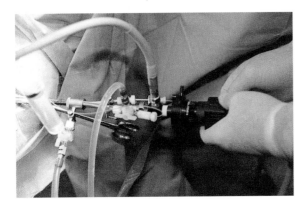

Figure 60.1 A Weck–Baggish hysteroscope with a laser fiber inserted in the left operating channel, a three-way tap with the fluid inflow and a catheter from the uterine cavity to a pressure transducer in the right channel, and a three-way tap for fluid outflow and syringe for channel flushing in the central channel.

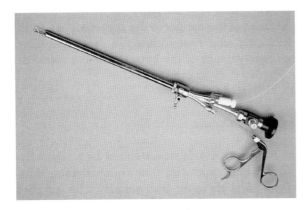

Figure 60.2 Flexible quartz fiber inserted down a channel of an operating hysteroscope.

Endometrial photovaporization and photocoagulation are performed under direct visualization using a power output of at least 50 W, continuous wave. The entire endometrial lining is treated, commencing in the cornual area (Figure 60.4) and extending across the fundus and down the anterior and posterior walls to the isthmus (Figure 60.5), terminating 4 cm from the external cervical os. To avoid treating the endocervix, the level of the internal os (4 cm) is marked on the sheath of the hysteroscope. Care is also taken to avoid perforation near the tubal ostia, the thinnest parts of the uterus.

The desired end-point is coagulation or charring of the entire endometrial surface (Figures 60.6, 60.7). This procedure takes 30–40 minutes in a normal-sized uterus and longer in a larger uterus. After up to 6 months, synechiae develop that are similar to those described by Asherman (Figures 60.8, 60.9).

The preoperative use of danazol or a gonadotiopin releasing hormone (GnRH) agonist greatly facilitates ablation of the endometrium. This pharmacologic manipulation decreases the thickness of the endometrial lining (Brooks *et al.*, 1991).

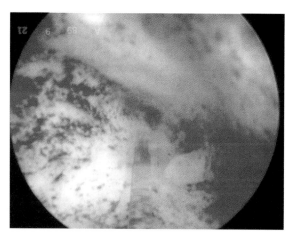

Figure 60.4 Laser quartz fiber applied close to the right tubal ostium before ablation.

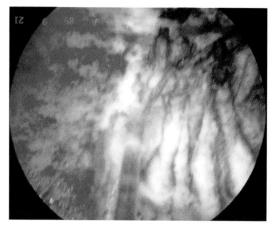

Figure 60.5 Laser quartz fiber 'dragging' a series .of parallel furrows across the fundus of the uterine cavity.

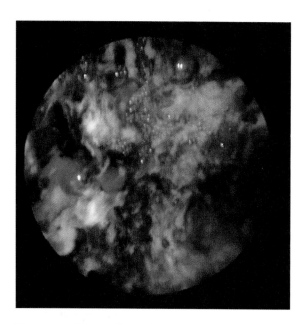

Figure 60.6 Tissue effects of endometrial ablation.

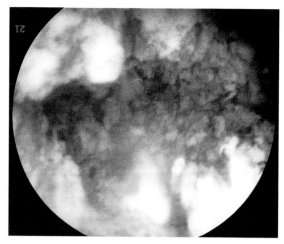

Figure 60.7 A completed ablation. All the endometrium has been removed with the Nd:YAG laser and the He–Ne aiming beam is seen glowing at the tip.

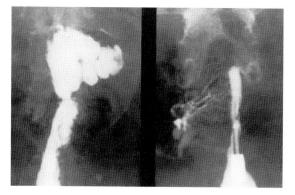

Figure 60.8 Hysterosalpingograms performed three months and one year after ELA. Note complete obliteration of cavity and intravasation of dye.

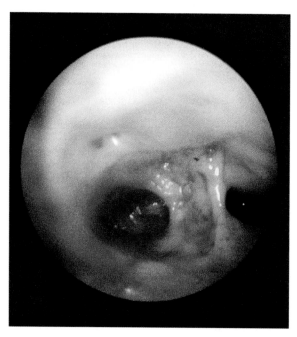

Figure 60.9 Synechiae ten months after laser ablation.

Hysteroscopic examination reveals a very thin atrophic endometrium with prominent telangiectases. It is interesting to note that this endometrium resembles that of a postmenopausal woman.

Clinical Experience in Detroit (USA) (Milton Goldrath)

To date, over 500 women have been operated upon in my department. The following is an analysis of 407 women aged 12–53 years who have undergone 427 hysteroscopic laser procedures for the treatment of menorrhagia in the 11 years ending January 1990. Over 60% of the patients ($n=274$) had fibroids, most of which were submucous, or adenomyosis. The criteria for patient selection included:

- Excessive and disabling bleeding.
- Inability or unwillingness to use other therapies.
- Future childbearing not desired.
- Dilatation and curettage (D and C) within six months of the surgical procedure to rule out adenocarcinoma of the endometrium or its precursors.

For the past eight years, patients have had preoperative hysteroscopic evaluation as well.

The procedure is usually performed on an outpatient basis, with the patients discharged 23 hours later. Although severe cramping typically occurs for the first two hours following surgery, it has recently been noted that the use of a bupivacaine hydrochloride 0.25% with epinephrine (adrenaline) 1 : 200 000 paracervical block on completion of the procedure greatly reduces the postoperative pain. The other postoperative symptoms resemble those associated with a D and C. All patients have varying degrees of serosanguineous discharge lasting for up to four weeks. None of the patients has become febrile.

Results

Table 60.1 summarizes the results of surgery. Overall, the results have been excellent in 379 procedures, 60% of which resulted in amenorrhea and the remainder resulted in a few days of spotting per cycle. Ten patients reported good results, meaning that they were satisfied with treatment and experienced what they considered to be normal menstrual flow. Of the 35 procedures that yielded poor results, 19 of the 22 which were repeated resulted in amenorrhea and three failed, necessitating hysterectomy.

Table 60.1 Results of ELA (Detroit).

Result	Number of procedures
Excellent	379
Good	10
Poor	35
Early failure	17
Late failure (1.5–8 years)	18

Of the remaining 13 failed patients, 12 underwent hysterectomy without retreatment and one has decided to 'put up' with her menorrhagia.

Among the patients 55 had clotting disorders, all of whom did well following surgery. Of these patients 22 were receiving warfarin therapy. It should be noted that patients receiving danazol while on warfarin therapy may have a very marked increase in prothrombin time. This could produce spontaneous retroperitoneal hemorrhage among other complications. It is therefore advisable to reduce the warfarin dose by 50% of the maintenance dose in these patients. Hysteroscopic laser ablation can be readily performed with the patient fully anticoagulated.

Of a total of 31 hysterectomies 18 were laser successes (i.e. no excessive bleeding) and 13 were laser failures (i.e. excessive bleeding). In two, laser use was abandoned because of the presence of large submucous myomas. In one patient cervical bleeding occurred ten days postoperatively necessitating hysterectomy. This latter complication deserves special comment. At the time, it was our practice to continue administering danazol for two weeks after the procedure. The patient was also taking warfarin. Ten days following surgery, excessive, uncontrollable bleeding occurred, necessitating hysterectomy. It has since been published that the dose of warfarin must be reduced in patients receiving danazol therapy. The two drugs may be administered concomitantly, but warfarin dosage should be reduced by 50%. Prothrombin times should be checked every three days. However, it should be restated that the use of danazol in these patients should be avoided by using GnRH agonists.

Of the 13 hysterectomies performed when ELA failed eight of the cases had adenomyosis. In view of the possibility that adenomyosis was associated with endometrial regeneration, it was decided to administer a single 150 mg dose of medroxyprogesterone acetate to patients with suspected adenomyosis or submucous fibroids on the day of surgery in an attempt to delay regeneration until some scarring had occurred. Of the patients treated with medroxyprogesterone acetate 69% became amenorrheic, compared with only 37% of those who did not receive treatment. This difference was highly significant. The remaining patients were hypomenorrheic.

Complications

Table 60.2 lists the complications associated with ELA. The major complication observed with this procedure has been fluid overload, which led to pulmonary edema in two cases. It should be noted that this problem occurred early on when a 'push' infusion method was used to distend the uterus. The use of a continuous flow technique with gravity feed of fluid into the uterus and actively controlled suction out of the uterus has largely avoided excessive absorption of distending medium.

Following surgery, profuse bleeding developed in 15 patients after release of the irrigating pressure. The bleeding was controlled by balloon tamponade using a Foley catheter inserted into the uterus (Goldrath, 1983).

One and three months after the procedure, all patients undergo a suction curettage; if a hematometra is found, suction curettage is performed weekly until the condition resolves. Routine suction curettage revealed 11 cases of postoperative hematometra. Experience had suggested that if a hematometra had not developed within three months following ELA, it would not develop subsequently. We have recently discovered nine cases of delayed hematometra. One developed nine years following laser therapy. Four patients with recurrent hematometra were treated by insertion of an intrauterine contraceptive device (IUD). One had a hysterectomy performed at the time of an operation for stress urinary incontinence. If a patient develops cyclic pain or other symptoms of hematometra, ultrasonic examination should be diagnostic.

Three patients had allergic reactions to danazol. The reaction was mild in two cases and therapy was continued. One patient had to discontinue treatment because of a severe allergic reaction.

Three patients had postoperative urinary tract infections related to intraoperative catheter drainage.

In one patient purulent endomyometritis developed approximately one week postoperatively. Although asymptomatic, she was hospitalized for two days and treated with intravenous antibiotics. The purulent discharge immediately stopped. She did not become febrile.

Laser ablation was not completed in one patient due to an instrument-related uterine perforation. The laser was not being used at the time. The patient returned to the hospital two months later, at which time the laser procedure was completed.

Clinical Experience in Princeton (USA), Middlesbrough (UK) and Farnborough (UK) (Ray Garry)

Table 60.3 lists the intraoperative and immediate postoperative results of a multicentre study of more than 1000 patients with menorrhagia treated with ELA (Garry et al., 1991). After the early learning phase the treatment time fell and the mean time to complete the ablation was 23 minutes (range 11–90). Almost all patients were discharged home within 24 hours and many went home on the day of surgery. Some complained of menstrual-like cramps for a few hours after ablation, but this was almost invariably relieved by simple analgesics and early postoperative pain was not a problem. A variable serosanguineous loss persists for up to six weeks after the

Table 60.2 Complications associated with ELA (Detroit).

Complication	Number of patients
Fluid overload (two with pulmonary edema)	6
Profuse bleeding (tamponade)	15
Urinary tract infection	3
Drug reaction	3
Uterine perforation	1
Cervical bleeding (hysterectomy)	1
Endomyometritis	1
Hematometra	20

Table 60.3 Operative details of multicenter study of ELA

	Princeton	Farnborough	Middlesbrough	Total
Number	342	359	318	1019
Operative time (min)	17 (11–27)	27 (17–90)	26 (11–90)	23
Mean fluid deficit (ml)	1500	1500	743 a 1416 b 289	1272

a, 115 cases with continuous flow non-pressure controlled pump.
b, 170 cases with pressure controlled variable flow rate pump.

ELA and during this time some women experience a heavy menstrual-like bleed attributed to shedding of the necrotic endometrium. In those in whom a simple continuous flow pump was used to distend the cavity the mean volume of normal saline absorbed was 1416 ml. In the 170 patients in whom the fluid was infused with a Hamou Hysteromat the mean volume absorbed was 289 ml, a reduction of 80%.

We have recently published the results of some 600 ELAs performed on 524 women with a mean follow-up time of 15 months (Garry et al., 1995). In this series no case of major operative morbidity occurred and there were no cases of primary or secondary hemorrhage, uterine perforation with the operating instrument or immediate laparotomy. A successful outcome was reported by 83.4% of patients, but a second ablation was required by 14.3% of the patients (Tables 60.4, 60.5). Success appeared to increase with increasing age and low fluid absorption. In contrast cavity length, operating time and duration of follow-up did not affect the success rate, although the hysterectomy rate did increase with increasing length of follow-up (Table 60.5).

We consider that it is essential to give preoperative medication to produce endometrial thinning before endometrial ablation. We have investigated several different regimens for this and found that both danazol and a GnRH agonist, goserelin (Zoladex Zeneca, Cheshire, UK) were effective in thinning the endometrium. However, goserelin appeared to be more effective and better tolerated than danazol resulting in a greater reduction in cavity length, a shorter operation, less fluid absorption and a higher rate of satisfactory menstrual reduction (Garry et al., 1996). Eight weeks of treatment resulted in slightly better operating conditions but more vasomotor side effects than four weeks of treatment; however, there was no difference in clinical outcome.

We have just completed a more detailed study on an enlarged series of 1000 ELAs followed up for up to 6.5 years (Phillips et al., 1997). This study reported the results in terms of survival curve analysis and proportional hazard regression to identify the predictors of having a hysterectomy after ELA. The survival curve analysis projected an overall hysterectomy rate of 21% at 6.5 years' follow-up. This more critical method of analysis again suggested that cavity length and operative time did not affect the risk of requiring a hysterectomy after ELA, but in apparent contradiction to the results of our previous analyses patient age and volume of fluid absorbed were also statistically insignificant clinically. The presence or absence of dysmenorrhea, premenstrual syndrome and the method of endometrial preparation did not significantly increase the risk of hysterectomy. In this study the only factor that clearly predisposed to subsequent hysterectomy was the need to have more than one ELA and the only factor that appeared to be associated with a reduced risk of hysterectomy was rather surprisingly the presence of intrauterine pathology such as fibroids and uterine polyps.

Table 60.4 Reported menstrual loss and frequency following ELA (multicenter study).

	Menstrual loss Number (%)	Menstrual frequency Number (%)
Amenorrhea	135 (28.9)	135 (28.9)
Reduced	309 (66.2)	172 (36.8)
Same	21 (4.5)	153 (32.8)
Increased	1 (0.2)	6 (1.3)
No response	1 (0.2)	1 (0.2)
Total	467 (100)	467 (100)

Note: This table excludes the 34 women who subsequently underwent hysterectomy.

Table 60.5 Outcome by age, length of follow-up, and operative data following ELA (Multicenter study).

Outcome	Number (%)	Mean age (years)	Mean length of follow-up (months)	Mean operation time (min)	Mean fluid balance (ml)	Mean uterine cavity length (cm)
Success	418 (83.4)	43.0*	14.7	25.1	559	8.1
Failure	83 (16.6)	40.2*	15.7	25.9	759	8.2
Amenorrhea †	135 (28.9)	45.0*	16.1*	24.3	462	8.1
Continuing menses †	332 (71.1)	41.8*	14.0*	25.6	638	8.1
Hysterectomy	34 (6.8)	39.7*	17.9‡	25.2	588	8.1
No hysterectomy	467 (93.2)	42.7*	14.6‡	26.5	667	7.9

*$P = 0.001$, t test.

†In this comparison, the 34 women who had a subsequent hysterectomy are excluded.

‡$P = 0.05$, t test

Complications

The principal short-term complications expected following ELA are:

- Uterine perforation with damage to bowel, bladder and blood vessels.
- Fluid overload with pulmonary edema and electrolyte disturbances.
- Intra- and postoperative hemorrhage.
- Infection (Garry, 1990).

The incidence of these complications in the 1015 patients reported by Garry *et al.* (1991) is shown in Table 60.6. The total short-term complication rate was extraordinarily low at only 1%. This was made up as follows:

- The uterus was perforated on three occasions, a rate of 0.3%. All occurred during insertion of the rigid hysteroscope. When this happened the procedure was discontinued, the patient was allowed home within 24 hours and in each case the treatment was successfully repeated within four weeks.
- No uterine perforation was caused by the laser, nor were there any cases of damage to bowel, bladder or other surrounding structure.
- None of the women had perioperative bleeding requiring active treatment or blood transfusion.
- None developed hematometra. Most of these women had uterine distension produced by simple non-pressure controlled pumps.
- Four women (0.4%) developed symptomatic pulmonary edema requiring management with postoperative intravenous diuretics. Each responded promptly and all left hospital within 6–48 hours. None of these cases required intensive care, but in other series severe fluid overload problems have been encountered.

- Significant postoperative pyrexia was noted in four women, but only one of these had proven pelvic inflammatory disease.

Summary of Complications

In summary, the relative thickness of the myometrium, the ease with which effective uterine tamponade can be produced to arrest hemorrhage, and the fact that endometrial destruction is produced by the Nd:YAG laser energy spreading from the quartz fiber placed superficially on the surface layers of the endometrium minimize the risk of serious complications. The large multicenter study reported above was associated with a very low early complication rate of only 1%. However, ELA, like any surgical procedure, is associated with the risk of severe complications. Three cases of uterine perforation and bowel damage have been reported (Perry *et al.*, 1990) attributed respectively to:

- An abnormally thin myometrium in a congenitally abnormal uterus.
- The use of laser power in excess of 90 W.
- Inexpert use of the laser in an inadequately supervised situation.

The inappropriate use of sapphire tips cooled by high-flow CO_2 or air under pressure has caused four deaths and an additional case of severe brain damage due to catastrophic gas embolism has also been reported (Baggish and Daniell, 1989). Significant intraoperative hemorrhage is unlikely, but major postoperative hemorrhage remains a possibility. Large amounts of necrotic tissue are produced by ELA and this can provide a focus for infection. The author recommends the use of a preoperative broad-spectrum antibiotic to reduce this risk.

The most common serious complication of ELA remains excessive intravasation of the distending medium into the systemic circulation with the risk of fluid overload, dilutional problems and pulmonary edema (Leake *et al.*, 1987). This complica-

Table 60.6 Complications in multicenter study (Garry *et al.*, 1991).

Complication	Princeton	Farnborough	Middlesbrough	Total
Pulmonary edema	2	2	0	4
Perforation with hysteroscope	1	2	0	3
Perforation with laser	0	0	0	0
Hemorrhage	0	0	0	0
Infection	0	2	2	4
Hematometra	0	0	0	0
Total	3	6	2	11 (1%)

tion, reported in Goldrath's original series, has been noted to a greater or lesser extent in almost every subsequent series. Careful monitoring at frequent intervals of infusion fluid inflow, outflow and deficit is essential. As described in more detail in Chapter 53, maintenance of a closed circuit, high flow, low pressure distension system with a continuously maintained clear outflow channel will minimize this risk. Using a pressure-controlled infusion system has been shown to reduce fluid absorption, and directly measuring the intrauterine pressure and adjusting flow rates appropriately has been shown to virtually eliminate the risk of excessive fluid absorption.

Discussion

ELA is a treatment for patients complaining of menorrhagia. Most women suffering from this complaint request relief of the symptom of heavy menstrual loss. They do not usually request amenorrhea or demand a hysterectomy. In fact, many women are delighted to be relieved of their symptoms and yet still retain their uterus. The distinction between absolute amenorrhea and profound oligomenorrhea appears to be of greater consequence to gynecologists than their patients. Goldrath's original clinical classification of outcome (1990a) into excellent (which includes both amenorrhea and oligomenorrhea), good (with continuing, but significantly reduced menstruation) and failure continues to seem relevant. It remains, however, the aim of most laser hysteroscopists to produce amenorrhea in every case and it is not yet clear why this is achieved in some cases and not others. The precise mechanism by which menstrual reduction is produced is not clear. It is certainly not due to the production of a complete Asherman's syndrome and in most cases a much reduced, but still patent cavity can be demonstrated at follow-up hysteroscopy. It is of particular interest that in many cases it takes 36 months to achieve the maximal reduction in menstrual flow. Many questions remain to be answered about how this technique works and about its long-term safety and effectiveness.

The endometrium is destroyed, the uterotubal junctions damaged and often occluded and considerable myometrial scarring is produced by ELA. These features all combine to reduce the chances of conception. Pregnancy, however, remains possible and three patients in the authors' total series of 1400 cases have become pregnant. It is important to counsel patients appropriately and to offer those at risk alternative contraceptive protection.

ELA requires a considerable amount of expensive equipment and questions have been raised about the cost-effectiveness of the procedure. No meaningful answers can be given until we know the long-term relapse and complication rates. Some facts are, however, already clear. Patients who have had an ELA spend less time in the operating room, less time in hospital, and less time off work or away from their family duties than those who have had a hysterectomy (Table 60.7). These savings in time can also lead to considerable financial savings for the hospital service. The magnitude of these savings will depend much more upon the number of cases dealt with than on the capital cost of the equipment. We have calculated that if a laser has a working life of seven years and 500 patients per year can be treated with it the cost per case of providing the laser is only about £22 (Table 60.8). The cost of theater consumables such as drapes, swabs and suture materials is 45% less for ELA than for hysterectomy. This saving alone, if continued for the life of the laser, is sufficient to pay for the equipment. We conclude that Nd:YAG lasers when used frequently in large and busy departments are cost-effective items and with a small cost per case the capital costs of buying the equipment are very quickly recovered. If the change from long-term inpatient hospital stay associated with hysterectomy to day case surgery permits closure of

Table 60.7 Operative details of ELA compared with hysterectomy.

	Hysterectomy	ELA
Time in theater (min)	88	44
Treatment time (min)	60	23
Mean hospital stay (days)	7	1
Mean convalescence (days)	56	10
Proportion with noted postoperative complication	45%	1%
Postoperative pain (< 24 hours)	94%	0%

Table 60.8 Costs of hysterectomy compared with ELA.

	Hysterectomy	ELA
Theater consumables	£ 58.09	£27.77
Laser depreciation		£21.42
Laser fiber costs		£9.60
Staff costs	£107.21	£74.07
Total theater costs	£165.30	£132.86
Ward costs	£800.00	£50.00
Total procedure costs	£965.30	£182.86

inpatient beds it is estimated that for every 500 patients treated with ELA rather than hysterectomy there could be a saving of £390 000. The financial benefits are even greater, if the savings associated with early return to work and reduced social benefit payments are included. In the short term, endometrial ablation is certainly very popular with the patients and with those who pay for their treatment. With an immediate morbidity of only 1% and a patient satisfaction rate in excess of 90% it is a technique worthy of further study. From a consideration of both the theoretic mode of action and the clinical evidence currently available, Nd:YAG laser ablation seems to be the safest of the ablative techniques now available. Well structured studies are, however, required to determine the long-term relapse rate, the effect of the procedure on various genital tract malignancies and the sustained safety and effectiveness of the procedure.

Conclusion

The data accumulated over the past 15 years suggest that ELA offers an alternative to hysterectomy in patients with menorrhagia who are not good candidates for other forms of conservative treatment. Our current experience in over 2000 patients indicates that this procedure can be safe and effective in trained hands and is usually associated with minimal perioperative morbidity and discomfort.

References

Asherman JG (1948) Amenorrhea traumatica (atretica). *Journal of Obstetrics and Gynecology* 55: 23–30.

Baggish MS, Baltoyannis P (1988) New techniques for laser ablation of the endometrium in high risk patients. *American Journal of Obstetrics and Gynecology* 159: 287–292.

Baggish MS, Daniell JF (1989) Death caused by air embolism associated with neodymium:yttrium-aluminum-garnet laser surgery and artificial sapphire tips. *American Journal of Obstetrics and Gynecology* 161: 877–878.

Bertrand JD (1989) Endometrial ablation using Nd-YAG laser for menorrhagia. In *Proceedings of the Second World Congress of Gynecologic Endoscopy, Clermont-Ferrand, France.*

Brooks MD, Philip G, Serden MD, Scott P, Davos I (1991) Hormonal inhibition of the endometrium for resectoscopic endometrial ablation. *American Journal of Obstetrics and Gynecology* 164: 1601–1608.

Daniell JF, Tosh R, Meisels S (1986) Photodynamic ablation of the endometrium with the Nd-YAG laser hysteroscopically as a treatment for menorrhagia. *Colposcopy and Gynecologic Laser Surgery* 2: 43–46.

Davis JA (1989) Hysteroscopic endometrial ablation with the neodymium-YAG laser. *British Journal of Obstetrics and Gynaecology* 96: 928–932.

DeCherney A, Polan ML (1983) Hysteroscopic management of intrauterine lesions and intractable uterine bleeding. *Obstetrics and Gynecology* 61: 392–397.

Donnez J, Nisolle M (1989) Laser hysteroscopy in uterine bleeding. Endometrial ablation and polypectomy. In Donnez J (ed.) *Laser Operative Laparoscopy and Hysteroscopy.* Leuven: Nauwelaerts Printing.

Droegemueller W, Makowski E, Macsalka R (1971a) Destruction of the endometrium by cryosurgery. *American Journal of Obstetrics and Gynecology* 110: 467–469.

Droegemueller W, Greer B, Makowski E (1971b) Cryosurgery in patients with dysfunctional uterine bleeding. *Obstetrics and Gynecology* 38: 256–258.

Gallinat A, Lueken RR, Moller CP (1989) The use of the Nd:YAG laser in gynecological endoscopy. In MBB-Medizintechnik GmbH (ed.) *Laser Brief 14.* Munich.

Garry R (1990) Safety of hysteroscopic surgery. *Lancet* 336: 1013–1014.

Garry R, Erian J, Grochmal S (1991) A multicentre collaborative study into the treatment of menorrhagia by Nd-YAG laser ablation of the endometrium. *British Journal of Obstetrics and Gynaecology* 98: 357–362.

Garry R, Shelley-Jones D, Mooney P, Phillips G (1995) Six hundred endometrial laser ablations. *Obstetrics and Gynecology* 85: 24–29.

Garry R, Khair A, Mooney P, Stuart M (1996) A comparison of goserelin and danazol as endometrial thinning agents prior to endometrial laser ablation. *British Journal of Obstetrics and Gynaecology* 103: 339–344.

Goldrath MH (1983) Uterine tamponade for the control of acute uterine bleeding. *American Journal of Obstetrics and Gynecology* 147: 869–872.

Goldrath MH (1990a) Use of danazol in hysteroscopic surgery for menorrhagia. *Journal of Reproductive Medicine* 35: 96.

Goldrath MH (1990b) Intrauterine laser surgery. In Keye WR (ed.) *Laser Surgery in Gynecology and Obstetrics*, 2nd edition. pp. 151–165. Chicago: Year Book Medical Publishers.

Goldrath MH, Fuller TA, Segal S (1981) Laser photo-vaporization of endometrium for the treatment of menorrhagia. *American Journal of Obstetrics and Gynecology* 140: 14–19.

Goulbourne IA, Macleod DAD (1981) Interaction between danazol and warfarin: case report. *British Journal of Obstetrics and Gynaecology* 88: 950–951.

Leake JF, Murphy AA, Zacur HA (1987) Noncardiogenic pulmonary edema: a complication of operative hysteroscopy. *Fertility and Sterility* 48: 497–499.

Loffer FD (1987) Hysteroscopic endometrial ablation with the Nd-YAG laser using a non-contact technique. *Obstetrics and Gynecology* 69: 679–682.

Lomano JM (1988) Photocoagulation of the endometrium with the Nd-YAG laser for the treatment of menorrhagia. *Journal of Reproductive Medicine* 31: 148–150.

Perry CP, Daniell JF, Gimpelson RJ (1990) Bowel injury from Nd-YAG endometrial ablation. *Journal of Gynecologic Surgery* 6: 199–203.

Phillips AG, Chien P, Garry R (1997) The risk of having a hysterectomy after endometrial laser ablation – analysis on 1000 consecutive cases. *American Journal of Obstetrics and Gynecology*. (In press).

Townsend DE, Richart RM, Paskowitz RA, Woolfork RE (1987) 'Rollerball' coagulation of the endometrium. *Obstetrics and Gynecology* **679**: 679–682.

Vancaillie TG (1989) Electrocoagulation of the endometrium with the ball-end resectoscope ('rollerball'). *Obstetrics and Gynecology* **74**: 425.

61

Endometrial Balloon Ablation

RICHARD W. DOVER

Royal Surrey County Hospital, Guildford, UK

Introduction

Menorrhagia sufficient to affect daily activities occurs in up to 25% of middle-aged women (Gath et al., 1987). However, this widespread problem, which has been responsible for an increasing number of hysterectomies over the last two decades (Coulter et al., 1991) is only associated with abnormal pathology in 50% of patients (Rees, 1989; Office of Population Censuses and Surveys, 1985). This, in addition to a complication rate of up to 42.8% associated with abdominal hysterectomy (Dicker et al., 1982), coupled with a steadily rising number of women who wish to retain their uterus, has led to the development of endometrial ablation (EA) as an alternative treatment for abnormal uterine bleeding.

Published figures concerning techniques in common use at the moment show that both hysteroscopic endometrial laser ablation (HELA) and transcervical resection of the endometrium (TCRE) are capable of achieving high levels of patient satisfaction when performed by experienced clinicans (Garry et al., 1991; Magos et al., 1991; O'Connor and Magos, 1996). The outcome is highly dependent upon the ability and technique of the surgeon, with more skill and experience giving better results, but more importantly fewer complications (Davis, 1989; Pyper and Haeri, 1991; Holt and Gilmer, 1995).

Until recently the long-term efficacy of EA has been unclear. However, recent data suggest that in experienced hands, 90% of women undergoing TCRE have not had a hysterectomy, and 80% have had no further gynecologic surgery during the first five postoperative years (O'Connor and Magos, 1996).

However, although EA has been shown to have long-term benefits, and avoids the high rates of morbidity associated with an abdominal hysterectomy, it does have a morbidity and complication rate of its own. Uterine perforation, fluid overload from the uterine irrigant, and hemorrhage have been estimated to occur in 1% of patients undergoing HELA (Garry et al., 1991), while perforation at the time of TCRE varies from 1–3.7% (Maher and Hill, 1990; Pyper and Haeri, 1991). It is of some interest that the incidence of perforation is related to the expertise of the surgeon, with one series reporting that 52% occurred during the first five cases of each individual's experience (MacDonald and Phipps, 1992).

The established therapeutic benefits of EA have led to many attempts to develop alternative, locally ablative techniques. These aspire to equal or exceed the efficacy of those currently available, while simultaneously aiming to eliminate the previously described complications. The intention is for them to be suitable for use by general gynecologists who have not undergone the lengthy periods of training necessary in order to achieve good outcomes and low complication rates with HELA and TCRE. Indeed, the only skills needed for successful use of one of these new techniques are those required to fit an intrauterine device (Vilos et al., 1996). This is in stark contrast to TCRE where the benefits of increasing surgical experience may still be apparent until at least 200 patients have been treated (Holt and Gilmer, 1995).

Three of these new therapies will be discussed

below, but it is important to appreciate that these procedures are comparatively recent innovations and that they do not have the wealth of published literature associated with HELA or TCRE, the techniques they are seeking to supersede. It is also important to be aware that the interpretation of patient outcomes following EA therapy is a confusing area. Many authors use differing terminology and this makes direct comparisons between alternative therapies difficult. In addition, many of the endpoints chosen are highly subjective and therefore difficult to assess accurately. An objective outcome measure is therefore desirable, with the most pertinent being the need for a second procedure or a hysterectomy. As mentioned earlier, one recent paper (O'Connor and Magos, 1996) has published results in this format. If one accepts that objective endpoints are more reliable, then papers not published in this style should perhaps be viewed with some caution.

The second issue of importance is that therapeutic failures can occur up to 36 months postoperatively, at which point a plateau is reached (O'Connor and Magos, 1996), and that almost 50% of those seeking further treatment do so 12 months after their original surgery (Holt and Gilmer, 1995). This implies that follow-up data for any period less than this is likely to show a higher success rate than that obtainable in the long term, and once again, some caution must be used in interpreting these results.

The Balloon Systems

Three of these techniques will be considered here. Although they are all variations on the basic idea of an inflatable balloon that conforms to the shape of the endometrial cavity, there are important differences between them:

- The VestaBlate (Valleylab, Boulder, CO, USA) balloon uses radiofrequency energy delivered to the endometrium via monopolar electrodes.
- The Cavaterm (Wallsten Medical SA, Morges, Switzerland) and the Thermal Balloon (Gynecare Inc., Menlo Park, CA, USA) rely on heated fluid to cause endometrial destruction.

Whatever differences may exist with regard to their mode of action, the preoperative assessment is common for all three procedures. In essence the aim is to select a group of patients with menorrhagia with structurally normal uteri who have no desire for further children or to undergo a hysterectomy. Cervical smears and endometrial biopsy should

exclude cellular abnormalities, while structural anomalies of the uterus such as leiomyomas or excessive cavity length are detected by ultrasound. As with EA, the procedures are not contraceptive and counselling needs to be given in this area. Patients about to undergo HELA or TCRE are usually treated with danazol or one of the gonadotropin releasing hormone (GnRH) analogs to thin their endometrium in order to aid the surgical procedure. However, pharmacologic endometrial suppression adds to the cost of the procedure and causes well documented, although transient, side effects. The balloon modalities deal with this aspect somewhat differently, and this will be mentioned in the section on each.

The other issue common to all three therapies is the use of heat, although as mentioned earlier, the source is different. All three modalities have undergone similar trials to assess their ability to destroy the endometrium. The extent of thermal spread has also been investigated, both *in vitro* and *in vivo*. Although none of the balloon systems caused significant thermal spread to adjacent viscera, only the manufacturers of Cavaterm and the Thermal Balloon have published their data.

The Thermal Balloon

The first of these new procedures to be considered is the Thermal Balloon Endometrial Ablation System (Gynecare Inc.). This consists of a 16 cm long by 3 mm diameter plastic catheter with a latex balloon attached to the distal end that houses a heating element and thermistor. The proximal end, which allows for inflation of the balloon, connects to a unit that monitors and controls preset intraballoon temperature, pressure and length of treatment.

Before insertion the system is tested for leaks, and the uterine cavity is then assessed hysteroscopically. The device is then inserted transcervically to reach the fundus. A solution of 5% dextrose is used to incrementally distend the balloon until a stable pressure is obtained. Initial work suggested this occurred at 70–80 mm Hg (Neuwirth *et al.*, 1994), but more recently clinicians have suggested that 160–170 mm Hg is optimal (Vilos *et al.*, 1996). Indeed, in this later study the first 15 patients were treated with pressures of 80–140 mm Hg, whereas the final 15 were treated with pressures of 150–180 mm Hg. When discussing their results the authors suggest that this may be a factor related to a poor outcome as their seven failures were all among the first 15 patients.

Once a stable intrauterine pressure has been

achieved the heater is activated and maintains the intraballoon solution at a temperature of 85 ± 5°C. Earlier work has suggested a treatment time of eight minutes (Neuwirth *et al.*, 1994; Singer *et al.*, 1994).

The patients treated more recently (Vilos *et al.*, 1996) have then been hysteroscoped immediately postoperatively. Uniform blanching has been noted over the fundus and anterior and sidewalls, with pink unblanched areas being seen near the ostia, especially if the uterus is arcuate, and on the posterior uterine wall. They summarized that this incomplete blanching was a result of uneven energy distribution within the balloon, and that it could perhaps be rectified by continual agitation of the balloon in order to improve the circulation. Unlike the Cavaterm, there is no mechanism to circulate the fluid automatically within the Thermal Balloon.

The first published data describing the therapeutic use of the Thermal Balloon is in relation to a multicenter trial involving 18 patients (Singer *et al.*, 1994). The follow-up ranges from 6–34 months (mean 17.5) during which seven of 18 (39%) reported light bleeding, and eight (44%) reported spotting or amenorrhea. A success rate of 83% is claimed, although it is notable that three patients underwent a second procedure – two hysterectomy and one TCRE, during this comparatively short follow-up. Of the failures, one had no identifiable endometrium at histological assessment, whereas the other two had varying amounts of normal endometrial tissue still present within the cavity.

The other published data relating to this device are also comparatively disappointing (Vilos *et al.*, 1996), even though the follow-up extends to only 12–18 months. Of the 30 patients undergoing the procedure seven (23%) were deemed to have experienced no improvement. These all underwent TCRE or hysterectomy. In addition, a further six patients, all of whom had improved to some degree, underwent further surgery. In total, therefore, 13/30 (43%) underwent a second procedure by 18 months. It is possible, as suggested earlier, that inadequate balloon distention may have contributed to seven of the treatment failures, and as a consequence of this, one may expect better results from the multicenter trial currently underway.

Studies are also in progress to assess the impact of endometrial preparation. In the more recent study nine women took a short course of danazol preoperatively, while the other procedures were performed at various times of the cycle. The results of the danazol-treated group are not given separately. This has significant implications since it is known that endometrial glandular elements may be present deep within the myometrium and that in order to destroy these areas, resection or ablation

should include the endometrium and up to 3 mm of myometrium (Reid and Sharp, 1992). The Thermal Balloon is capable of penetrating up to 5 mm into the myometrium (Neuwirth *et al.*, 1994) but this does not take account of the varying depth of the endometrium, which may be up to 7 mm deep in the secretory phase (Reid and Sharp, 1992). Endometrial suppression reduces the depth to 1.5–2.0 mm (Sutton and Ewen, 1994) and it is therefore possible that endometrial preparation may improve the outcome with this system.

Whatever the current concerns regarding the long-term efficacy of this procedure, one aspect is of major significance. The diameter of the system is only 3 mm and this has obvious implications regarding the ease of insertion. This technique has also been performed without general anesthesia, with 21 of the 30 procedures in the most recent trial being performed under neuroleptic anesthesia (Vilos *et al.*, 1996).

The narrow diameter of this system, compared to the other two balloon devices – the cervix needs to be dilated to Hegar 9 and 10 respectively to introduce the Cavaterm and Vestablate systems – is obviously an advantage when attempting to design a system for use as an outpatient. The eight-minute treatment cycle also compares favorably with the 15 minutes currently used by the Cavaterm, although it is longer than the four minutes needed by VestaBlate.

The Cavaterm System

The Cavaterm system (Wallsten Medical SA) also uses heated fluid to destroy the endometrium, but it differs significantly from the Thermal Balloon. It consists of two major components:

- A silicone balloon catheter and heating element (Figure 61.1).
- A central unit, which houses the power source and the pump to ensure continual circulation of the heated fluid.

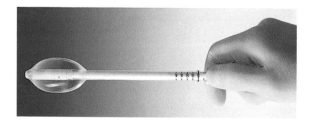

Figure 61.1 The Cavaterm balloon (Wallsten Medical SA, Morges, Switzerland).

There are three important points to note with regard to this system:

- The first is that the silicone balloon is adjustable and can thus be altered according to the length of cavity about to be treated.
- The second feature follows from the first. Ensuring an optimal fit of the balloon to the cavity reduces the chances of heat affecting the cervix, which may lead to stenosis or damage to the underlying major vessels. The shaft of the catheter is insulated in an attempt to eliminate the occurrence of high temperatures in the vagina and cervical canal, which have led to problems in the past with other ablative techniques (Phipps et al., 1990).
- Finally, an oscillating pump causes the liquid to vibrate, consequently activating a backvalve system within the catheter tip, which forces the liquid to circulate vigorously inside the balloon.

Adequate circulation ensures constant temperatures within the balloon and on its surface, and therefore a uniform degree of thermal damage. In the absence of circulation, temperature differences of up to 18°C have been noted within the balloon (Friberg et al., 1996a), and other workers have suggested that this may be a cause of unequal energy distribution within their systems (Vilos et al., 1996).

Before the procedure is performed the cervix is dilated to Hegar 9 in order to accept the 8 mm diameter catheter. Of the initial series of 44 patients, 29 had their procedure under general and 15 under spinal anaesthesia (Friberg et al., 1996b). After sounding the cavity to determine the balloon length, a curettage is performed. This mechanically prepares the endometrium, meaning that hormonal pre-treatment is not required, and the procedure can be performed at any phase of the menstrual cycle. In addition, a further histologic specimen is obtained.

After adjusting the balloon length to the sounded length, the Cavaterm catheter is then introduced to reach the fundus, and the balloon is filled with glycine until a pressure of 180–200 mm Hg is obtained. This level of pressure is thought to be important for two reasons, the first being that it ensures adequate contact between the balloon and endometrium. The second reason is that at this level of pressure, in excess of systolic blood pressure, there is a marked diminution in endometrial perfusion and consequently a reduction in heat loss from the system. This means that the therapeutic temperature can be reached more quickly, and maintained using less power.

Once the system is activated the therapeutic balloon surface temperature of 75°C is quickly reached, and then maintained for 15–30 minutes, after which the fluid is removed and the balloon is withdrawn. During manufacture the heating element is preset to a working temperature of 80°C, which yields a balloon surface temperature of 75°C. The element has a large surface area, minimizing the need for a high temperature. This temperature cannot be altered, thereby eliminating the possibility of boiling, which may lead to balloon expansion and possible rupture.

Apart from the initial in vivo and in vitro heating studies (Friberg et al., 1996b) this device has thus far been trialled in over 1000 patients, although published data are only available in relation to 44 (Friberg et al., 1996a). During this study the treatment time was set at 30 minutes. The follow-up time in this series is only 12 months, but the initial results are encouraging. Of the 44 patients, 38 had an improvement in their menstrual loss, with 12 being amenorrheic and 11 having minimal loss. None were postmenopausal on biochemical assessment. Three patients had not noticed any improvement, while three had undergone hysterectomy. Of these:

- One complained of continued heavy loss and histopathologic assessment revealed the presence of a 25 mm pedunculated fibroid. Interestingly the portion of the uterus accessible to the balloon had been totally destroyed.
- The second therapeutic failure was as the result of a uterine septum, which prevented adequate balloon coverage of the cavity.
- The third failure was the result of atypical hyperplasia being noted on the preoperative curettage, although at histologic assessment the endometrium had been completely destroyed.

The authors made the point that all three of these patients should have been excluded from the trial, since in keeping with the other balloon systems, cellular or structural abnormalities are contraindications to inclusion in these clinical trials.

The data on seven patients at 24 months have been presented and reveal that four patients are currently amenorrheic, although no mention is made about their status at 12 months.

After the initial series, the treatment time was reduced to 15 minutes, but follow-up on this group of 30 patients is very short, with only 14 having been followed for six months or longer. It should be noted that all of this group have had a reduction in their menstrual loss, although longer follow-up is obviously needed (Friberg, 1996).

The VestaBlate System

The final procedure to be considered is the VestaBlate system. In common with the previous devices it is based on the concept of an inflatable balloon, but in this instance rather than being a container for heated fluid, it acts as a carrier for monopolar electrodes.

The system is comprised of two components:

- The electrode balloon constructed of an expandable polymer that allows the balloon to conform to the shape of the uterine cavity as it is inflated (Figure 61.2).
- A hardware control component that connects to a standard electrosurgical generator, and controls the application of radiofrequency energy to the 12 monopolar electrodes located on the balloon.

Six electrodes are applied to each uterine surface, each containing its own thermistor, which is continually checked by the controller so that energy levels can be altered to maintain the desired temperature level.

Pre-clinical studies, in common with the previously described devices, did not reveal thermal spread to adjacent organs and demonstrated consistent thermal injury extending into the myometrium to a depth of 3±1 mm when the treatment protocol of temperature and time of 75°C and four minutes, respectively, were used.

Although long periods of endometrial suppression are not required with the VestaBlate system, it is the only one of the balloon systems to use pharmacologic methods to prepare the endometrium. Unless surgery can be scheduled for the early follicular phase, a withdrawal bleed is procured just before treatment by the use of either a short course of a progestogen or combined contraceptive pill.

The cervix is dilated to Hegar 10 and the treatment device is slowly inserted until the distal end is in contact with the fundus. To reduce the risk of perforation, the VestaBlate inserter has been designed with an atraumatic blunt-nosed sheath. Once this is adjacent to the fundus, the distal end is retracted to reveal the electrode balloon. The lumen of the instrument is patent, and used to test for unrecognized perforations before heating of the electrodes. A small volume (3–5 ml) of normal saline is injected through the lumen into the uterine cavity. Absence of resistance to this influx of fluid means that the uterine cavity must be carefully inspected to exclude a perforation.

The balloon is then maximally distended by the use of an air-filled syringe connected to the inflation port. The volume of air required is usually 10–15 ml and a constant pressure is maintained manually. In contrast to the other systems, the exact intrauterine pressure is not measured during the VestaBlate procedure.

Temperature and time of therapy are set at 75°C and four minutes, respectively, and the system is then activated. A warm-up period of 40–60 seconds is needed to reach the target tissue temperature, at which point the therapeutic phase begins. During this therapeutic phase, the thermistors sense the temperature at each electrode so that local energy levels can be adjusted to ensure that the temperature remains within a narrow range. At the end of four minutes the system automatically shuts off and the balloon can be removed.

This system is currently being trialed in an international therapeutic study, and although the data have yet to be published, they have recently been presented (Dover, 1996). To date 107 patients have been treated and 50 have been followed up for 12 months or longer. Based on their status at the most recent review, 81.3% are either amenorrheic or have had a marked decrease in their menstrual loss.

There have been eight documented treatment failures so far, and where factors have been identified, they appear to be similar to those noted by other workers using balloon systems, notably distortion of the uterine cavity by a submucous leiomyoma.

The need for the use of concrete endpoints in the presentation of results was discussed earlier. The VestaBlate group is the only one using a balloon system to have presented their data in an actuarial format. Comparison of their results with those dealing with the five-year follow-up of TCRE patients (O'Connor and Magos, 1996), reveals that they are on the same course. It must, however, be noted that the limit of review of the VestaBlate patients is 18

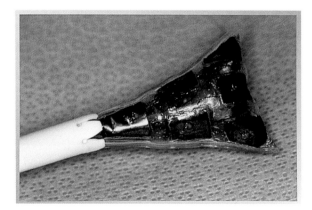

Figure 61.2 The VestaBlate™ electrode balloon (Valleylab, Boulder, CO, USA).

months, but that the TCRE data have shown that treatment failures may occur until 36 months. Caution is therefore needed when reviewing these initially promising results.

Conclusion

It appears that in the majority of cases good short-term therapeutic results can be achieved with the use of the balloon systems, but their long-term durability is as yet unproven. The numbers involved in the published and presented trials are small, and the length of follow-up is too short to demonstrate whether or not the results are equivalent to those achieved by TCRE or HELA.

The ease of use and apparent safety are encouraging aspects of these new modalities. All of the devices have been designed with simplicity in mind, and their use requires only basic skills that are well within the remit of all practising gynecologists. If the long-term outcomes are found to be satisfactory, then this ease of use may well be the pivotal factor in enabling many more women to gain access to this proven therapy.

There are some areas where improvements do need to be made, and these adjustments will become obvious with greater clinical experience with the therapies. The final treatment protocols have not yet been established in all cases and changes here, such as the role of pretreatment of the endometrium, may well improve efficacy.

The one area where all modalities need to improve is patient selection. The mode of action of all these devices is thermal damage to the adjacent endometrium. Any distortion of the cavity, whether from a leiomyoma or uterine septum will reduce the extent of balloon contact and leave a varying proportion of untreated endometrium. Identification and exclusion of patients with irregular endometrial cavities, an established cause of failure across all of the modalities, will mean that the therapies will not be performed on patients who can be expected to do badly and who would in all likelihood benefit more from an alternative treatment. This may be helped if all potential patients undergo a pretreatment hysteroscopy to exclude structural uterine anomalies, as the use of ultrasound alone, as in some protocols, appears to be insufficient for this purpose.

Based on initial experience there seems to be little in the way of serious complications developing following these new procedures. It should, however, be remembered that these complications occur infrequently and the numbers of patients who have received these therapies are small; perhaps the initially encouraging results reflect both the numbers involved, and the skill of the clinicians trialling these devices.

Undoubtedly there will be some clinicians who will be alarmed by the presence of atypical hyperplasia on one of the pretreatment specimens and will cite this, coupled with the lack of an operative histologic specimen as a reason not to use these techniques. The exception here is the Cavaterm system for which the preoperative curettage provides a histologic sample. It should, however, be remembered that of the currently used procedures only TCRE produces tissue for histologic assessment, as both HELA and rollerball coagulation destroy the endometrium *in utero*. It does, however, serve as a timely reminder of the need to obtain a good preoperative endometrial sample, which is as true for the present techniques as it is for balloon therapy.

Although the numbers and length of follow-up are small, it does seem that some observations can be drawn from the published trials with regard to the future. Further work with longer follow-up is undoubtedly necessary before the true benefits of these procedures are known, but on initial inspection they all appear to have some merit. As such it seems likely that ablative therapy based on an inflatable balloon system will be a treatment option for many women in the near future. This does not, however, mean the end of the currently practiced techniques. There are limitations to the balloon therapies that are unlikely to be overcome. Leiomyomas are common, and many women with menorrhagia will have a distorted uterine cavity and so be unsuitable for balloon therapy. These limitations have been recognized by the manufacturers, with cavity irregularities being both contraindications to inclusion in their trials, and responsible for some of their treatment failures. At the present time it would seem that TCRE or HELA are the only ablative options for these women and will consequently be in demand for the forseeable future.

References

Coulter A, Bradlow J, Agass M, Martin-Bates C, Tulloch A (1991) Outcomes of referrals to gynaecology outpatient clinics for menstrual problems: an audit of general practice records. *British Journal of Obstetrics and Gynaecology* **98**: 789–796.

Davis JA (1989) Hysteroscopic endometrial ablation with the Nd-YAG laser. *British Journal of Obstetrics and Gynaecology* **96**: 928–932.

Dicker RC, Greenspan JR, Strauss LT, Cowart MR, Scally MJ, Peterson HB (1982) Complications of abdominal and vaginal hysterectomy among women of reproductive age in the United States. *American Journal of Obstetrics and Gynecology* **144**: 841–848.

Dover R (1996) Thermoregulated radiofrequency endometrial ablation. Abstract. *British Society for Gynaecological Endoscopy*. London.

Friberg B (1995) A new technique for endometrial destruction by thermal coagulation; clinical results with 12–24 months follow-up. Abstract. *4th Congress European Society for Gynaecological Endoscopy*. Brussels.

Friberg B (1996) Cavaterm – A new technique for endometrial ablation by thermal coagulation. Abstract. *World Congress of Hysteroscopy*. Miami.

Friberg B, Wallsten H, Henriksson P *et al.* (1996a) A new, simple, safe and efficient device for the treatment of menorrhagia. *Journal of Gynecologic Techniques* **2**: 103–108.

Friberg B, Persson B, Willen R, Ahlgren M (1996b) Endometrial destruction by hyperthermia – a possible treatment of menorrhagia. *Acta Obstetricia et Gynecologica Scandinavica* **75**: 330–335.

Garry R, Erian J, Grochmal SA (1991) A multi-centre collaborative study into the treatment of menorrhagia by Nd-YAG laser ablation of the endometrium. *British Journal of Obstetrics and Gynaecology* **98**: 357–362.

Gath D, Osborn M, Bungay G *et al.* (1987) Psychiatric disorder and gynaecological symptoms in middle-aged women: a community survey. *British Medical Journal* (Clinical Research Edition) **294**: 213–218.

Holt EM, Gilmer MDG (1995) Endometrial resection. *Baillière's Clinical Obstetrics and Gynaecology* **9(2)**: 279–297.

Macdonald R, Phipps J (1992) Endometrial ablation: a safe procedure. *Gynaecological Endoscopy* **1(1)**: 7–9.

Maher PJ, Hill DJ (1990) Transcervical endometrial resection for abnormal uterine bleeding – report of 100 cases and review of the literature. *Australian and New Zealand Journal of Obstetrics and Gynaecology* **30(4)**: 357–360.

Magos AL, Baumann R, Lockwood GM, Turnbull AC (1991) Experience with the first 250 endometrial resections for menorrhagia. *Lancet* **337**: 1074–1078.

Neuwirth RS, Duran AA, Singer A, MacDonald R, Bolduc L (1994) The endometrial ablator: A new instrument. *Obstetrics and Gynecology* **83**: 792–796.

O'Connor H, Magos A (1996) Endometrial resection for the treatment of menorrhagia. *New England Journal of Medicine* **335**: 151–156.

Office of Population Censuses and Surveys (1985) *Hospital Inpatient Enquiry*. London: HMSO.

Phipps JH, Lewis BV, Roberts T *et al.* (1990) Treatment of functional menorrhagia with radiofrequency endometrial ablation. *Lancet* **335**: 374–376.

Pyper RJD, Haeri AD (1991) A review of 80 endometrial resections for menorrhagia. *British Journal of Obstetrics and Gynaecology* **98**: 1049–1054.

Rees MCP (1989) Heavy painful periods. *Baillière's Clinical Obstetrics and Gynaecology* **3**: 341–356.

Reid PC, Sharp F (1992) Hysteroscopic Nd-YAG endometrial ablation: an *in-vitro* and *in-vivo* laser tissue interaction study. Abstract. *III European Congress on Hysteroscopy and Endoscopic Surgery*. Amsterdam.

Singer A, Almanza R, Gutierrez A, Haber G, Bolduc L, Neuwirth R (1994) Preliminary clinical experience with a thermal balloon endometrial ablation method to treat menorrhagia. *Obstetrics and Gynecology* **83**: 733–735.

Sutton CJG, Ewen SP (1994) Thinning the endometrium prior to ablation: Is it worthwhile? *British Journal of Obstetrics and Gynaecology* **101**: 10–12.

Vilos GA, Vilos EC, Pendley L (1996) Endometrial ablation with a thermal balloon for the treatment of menorrhagia. *Journal of the American Association of Gynecologic Laparoscopists* **3(3)**: 383–387.

62

Photodynamic Therapy

Y. TADIR, B. TROMBERG AND M. W. BERNS

Beckman Laser Institute and Medical Clinic, University of California, Irvine, USA

Introduction

The use of laser in reproductive medicine is described in Chapter 7. Photodynamic therapy (PDT) is one example in which the principles of photomedicine (Parrish, 1982) can be applied to obtain selective tissue destruction in a non-surgical mode. The process typically involves systemic or topical administration of a photosensitizing drug. Although photosensitizers are generally retained in malignant tissue (Dougherty, 1984) these drugs also accumulate healthy tissue. When light of sufficient energy and appropriate wavelength interacts with the sensitizer, highly reactive oxygen intermediates are generated. These intermediates, primarily singlet oxygen, irreversibly oxidize essential cellular components. The resultant photodestruction of crucial cell organelles and vasculature ultimately causes tissue necrosis.

PDT may offer an optimal approach for treating lesions on:

- The external genital organs – genital warts and vulvar/vaginal intraepithelial neoplasia (VIN/VAIN) (Rettenmaier et al., 1984; Fehr et al., 1996a).
- The cervix – cervical intraepithelial neoplasia (CIN) (Muroya et al., 1996; Monk et al., 1997).
- The uterus – selective endometrial ablation for dysfunctional uterine bleeding (DUB) (Schneider et al., 1988; Bhatta et al., 1992; Yang et al., 1993a; Wyss et al., 1995).
- Intra-abdominal lesions such as endometriosis (Manyak et al., 1989) and ovarian cancer (Goff et al., 1994).

Several interrelated factors, including photosensitizer photophysical properties, optimal light and drug dose, and drug localization, determine the effectiveness of PDT.

Photosensitizers

The biophysical characteristics of various groups of photosensitizers are currently an area of intense research (Fisher et al., 1995). The better known among these groups are the porphyrins, a class of compounds that has been recognized since the beginning of the century (Von Tappeiner and Jesionek, 1903). The clinical effect of these photoactive substances is porphyria cutanea tarda, a cutaneous form of endogenous porphyrinopathy. These observations led to the development of exogenous porphyrins such as hematoporphyrin derivative (HPD). HPD is a mixture of porphyrins that tend to be selectively retained in tumors (Lipson et al., 1961). The purified fraction of HPD is primarily composed of a mixture of di-hematoporphyrin esters and ethers (DHE), and its use has allowed the therapeutic dose of HPD to be reduced by almost 50% (Richter et al., 1990). Additional modification to this compound has resulted in the development of a more potent photosensitizer, benzoporphyrin derivative monoacid ring A (BPD-MA), which is 10–70 times more phototoxic to various cell lines than HPD (Richter et al., 1987).

Another approach to PDT uses 5-aminolevulinic-acid (ALA), a precursor of protoporphyrin IX (Pp IX) in the heme biosynthetic pathway. Heme biosynthesis is essential to life and occurs in all aerobic cells. The slowest step in heme synthesis is the conversion of Pp IX to heme. Therefore, the exogenous administration of photodynamically inactive ALA induces the production and accumulation of Pp IX, which is a potent photosensitizer. Since only certain types of cells have a capacity to sensitize substantial amounts of Pp IX, the use of ALA in combination with appropriate light delivery systems can provide an additional element of selectivity in PDT (Kennedy and Pottier, 1992).

A growing number of second generation photosensitizers are being synthesized, which can be activated once exposed to light at wavelength over 650 nm. Some of these classes of compound include porphyrin and chlorine derivatives, purpurines, benzoporphyrins, phthalocyanines, and naphthalocyanines. Wavelength activation is important since tissue penetration is deeper with the longer wavelength, and this may define expected PDT effects and clinical indications.

Application Modes

Information on drug concentration and relative distribution in diseased and healthy tissue is of crucial importance in designing effective treatment protocols for selective photochemical therapeutic effects. Numerous studies have focused on the pharmacokinetics of photosensitizers in various experimental models, species, organs and application modes. Several groups are studying drug distribution in the uterus in order to develop a new treatment modality for dysfunctional uterine bleeding (Schneider et al., 1988). Drug distribution in rat uteri was studied following intravenous (IV), intraperitoneal (IP), and intrauterine (IU) administration of Photofrin (DHE, Quadra Logic Technologies, Vancouver, Canada) (Chapman et al., 1993). Extraction of Photofrin from uterine tissue was conducted according to a modified porphyrin fecal extraction technique (Lipson et al., 1961). Frozen sections were analyzed by fluorescence microscopy in order to characterize drug distribution in different uterine layers. Endometrial fluorescence was highest following topical administration (IU), and these levels remained elevated over time. In addition, myometrial and stromal drug uptake were minimized by IU application. Similar observations confirmed these effects for other drugs such as ALA and BPD (Petrucco et al., 1990; Wyss et al., 1994a; Steiner et al., 1996a). However, it is known that tissue fluorescence is not an accurate predictor of the expected PDT effects. PDT for endometrial ablation has been studied following systemic and topical application of photosensitizing agent in rats

and rabbits (Schneider et al., 1988; Petrucco et al., 1990; Bhatta et al., 1992; Yang et al., 1993a,b; Wyss et al., 1994a,b, 1995; Steiner et al., 1996a).

Another factor that plays a role in designing effective protocols is the pace of drug metabolism and concentration in the periphery, which may result in skin photosensitivity once exposed to sunlight. Topical application of photosensitizers may assist in reducing drug concentration and avoid skin photosensitivity. However, some photosensitizers (such as Photofrin) do not penetrate easily through mucous membrane barriers and penetration enhancing agents are used to improve PDT effects (Monk et al., 1997). Other photosensitizers such as BPD (Wyss et al., 1994a), or SnET2 (tin ethyl etiopurfurin) (Rocklin et al., 1996) have short half-life following systemic application (2–4 days) and this offers significant benefits when compared to first generation photosensitizers in which photosensitivity may still occur 4–6 weeks following IV administration. Information on photosensitizer distribution and PDT in primates (Van Vught et al., 1996) and human uteri (Fehr et al., 1996b), is minimal; however, several groups are actively involved in this field and it is expected that more information will be available in the near future. Information is available on photosensitization of the external (Fehr et al., 1996a) and internal genital tract (Lipson et al., 1961; Manyak et al., 1989) but clinical studies are still limited to anecdotal reports (Rettenmaier et al., 1984; Lobraico and Grossweiner, 1993; Korell et al., 1995).

Basic Physical Considerations for Light Application

Photosensitizers are more efficiently activated by blue light, but tissue penetrance at these short wavelengths is severely limited to a fraction of a millimeter, thus preventing PDT in deeper tissue layers. Since hemoglobin absorption diminishes at wavelengths longer than 600 nm, red light can be used to photosensitize tissue structures. For example, DHE and Pp IX red absorption maxima at 630–635 nm are significantly less intense than their corresponding 405 nm blue peaks (Figure 62.1). Newer compounds, such as SnET2, BPD or uterium Texaphyrin-LuTex (Texafrine; Pharmacyclics, Sunnyvale, California, USA), are designed to absorb light more readily further in the red spectral region. Deeper and more effective results are expected since the attenuation of light in tissue typically decreases with increasing wavelengths. Various light delivery systems will be discussed in relation to specific applications.

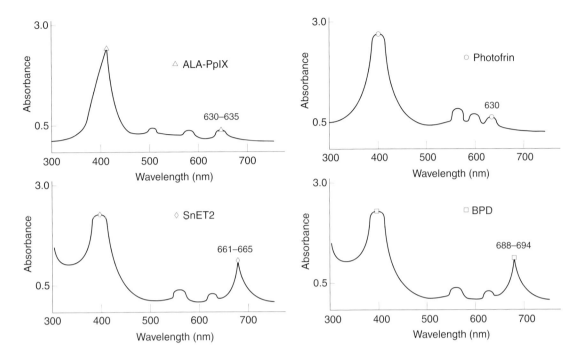

Figure 62.1 Absorption spectra of various photosensitizers.

Uterine PDT

Two main indications are the topic of research at several institutions involved in uterine PDT. These are:

- CIN
- Endometrial ablation for DUB.

CIN

In a preliminary study (Monk *et al.*, 1997), we determined the safety and efficacy of topically applied DHE in the PDT of CIN using fixed drug doses and application schedules, and a variable dose of 630 nm red light delivered by an argon pumped dye laser. Using a cervical cap, 2 ml of a 1% solution of DHE in a 4% 1,dodecylazacycloheptane-2-one (Azone; Whitby Research Inc., Richmond, Virginia, USA) and isopropyl alcohol vehicle were applied to the cervix 24 hours before PDT. An argon pumped dye laser providing light at 630 nm was then used to perform PDT. Light was coupled into a 400 μm silica fiberoptic terminating in a microlens, which focused the laser radiation onto a circular field of uniform light intensity perpendicular to the tissue. The entire ectocervix was treated in a single field including a margin of 3–5 mm of normal cervix. Using a constant power density (150 mW cm^{-2}). to avoid thermal injury, the PDT energy was gradu-

ally increased from 40 up to 140 J cm^{-2}. The maximal energy density was well tolerated with no patients experiencing local necrosis, sloughing or scarring. However, a mild vaginal discharge was noted in several patients, but systemic effects were absent. After 12 months of follow-up 68% are disease free. In a second study, ALA was topically applied in the same way and fluorescence microscopy revealed selective conversion to Pp IX and optimal CIN to normal tissue ratio at 1.5 hours after application. A PDT study for patients with CIN II–III is underway.

DUB

FLUORESCENCE DETECTION

The human endometrium, because of its cyclic rapid proliferation and neovascularization, is potentially well suited for PDT. Since endometrial thickness is dependent upon hormonal status, uterine light penetration can be modulated by manipulating hormone levels. Additionally, the thick myometrium, which surrounds the endometrial layer serves as a natural 'barrier', protecting pelvic organs from unwanted PDT effects.

Although questions and concerns remain, animal studies have thus far been informative. In studies on rat uteri, topical application of Photofrin yielded nearly identical fluorescence in the endometrial glands and stroma (Bhatta *et al.*, 1992). Yang *et al.*

(1993a) studied Pp IX fluorescence following topical administration of ALA in the mouse uterus. The endometrium became strongly fluorescent while the myometrium did not. Judd *et al.* (1992) studied fluorescence of the uterine layers following IV injection of ALA. Endometrial fluorescence peaked 2–3 hours after injection and the endometrial layer showed fluorescence levels five times higher than those of the myometrium.

Our group extensively studied various aspects of endometrial photosensitization and PDT in rats, rabbits (Wyss *et al.*, 1994a; 1994b; Steiner *et al.*, 1996a) and humans (Fehr *et al.*, 1996b). Various photosensitizers were administered and uteri removed for fluorescence microscopy at different time intervals following drug administration. In the case of topical application, only one uterine horn was photosensitized while the second horn served as a control. Low light level fluorescence imaging was performed with a slow scan, thermoelectrically-cooled charged coupled device (CCD) camera system coupled to an inverted fluorescence microscope. A special system was used to visualize bright field and fluorescence images of frozen sections. A 100 W mercury arc lamp filtered through a 405 nm bandpass filter provided excitation light. A dichroic filter was used to separate excitation from emission signals, and a 635 nm broad bandpass filter was used to isolate the fluorescence emission. Instrument control, image acquisition and processing were performed with a Macintosh computer.

The relative fluorescence of Photofrin, ALA, BPD and SnET2 in various animal models was determined, suggesting that selective endometrial PDT is feasible. ALA solution was instilled into the uterine cavity of 27 women before hysterectomy (Fehr *et al.*, 1996b). Fluorescence was first detected in the superficial endometrial glands 75 minutes after drug injection (Figure 62.2). In the endometrial gland

stumps fluorescence intensity peaked 4–8 hours after ALA instillation and was more than 48-times higher than in the underlying myometrium, suggesting that selective photodynamic destruction of the human endometrium may be possible 4–8 hours after intrauterine ALA instillation.

PDT EFFECTS

Similar animal models have served for studying the histologic effects on the endometrium following optimal drug dose and drug to light interval. The laser beam was transmitted into the uterine cavity via a fiber with a cylindrical diffusing tip. The Photofrin/Azone study revealed that Azone may enhance PDT selectivity by facilitating drug targeting to critical endometrial structures (Steiner *et al.*, 1995). Histologic studies in rats revealed PDT-induced endometrial destruction with marked atrophy after treatment with ALA (Steiner *et al.*, 1996a) and SnET2 (Rocklin *et al.*, 1996). In rabbits, persistent epithelial destruction with minimal regeneration following photosensitization with ALA and BPD was observed (Wyss *et al.*, 1994a, 1994b).

Since selective photochemical damage of the entire endometrium or even specific targets within the endometrium is feasible, we applied this unique modality to study mechanisms of regeneration. ALA was diluted to 200 mg ml⁻¹ dextran 70 and a volume of 1.2 ml was injected into the left uterine horn. Intrauterine illumination (wavelength 630 nm, light dose 40–80 J cm⁻²) was performed three hours after drug administration. Tissue morphology was evaluated by light and scanning electron microscopy 1, 3, 7 and 28 days after treatment. Regeneration of the endometrium following epithelial ablation by PDT was fully activated by 24 hours and was completed by 72

Figure 62.2 Fluorescence microscopic image of human endometrium sampled four hours after intrauterine ALA instillation. (A) shows an area at the endometrial–myometrial junction, the mark 'M' indicates where the myometrium is located. The endometrial gland stumps are highly fluorescent. (B) shows an area near the endometrial surface (S). The lumen of the uterine cavity is at the right edge of the picture. (Reprinted with permission from Fehr *et al.*, 1996b.)

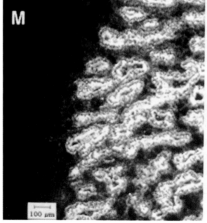
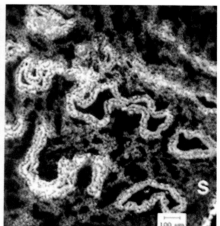

(a)   (b)

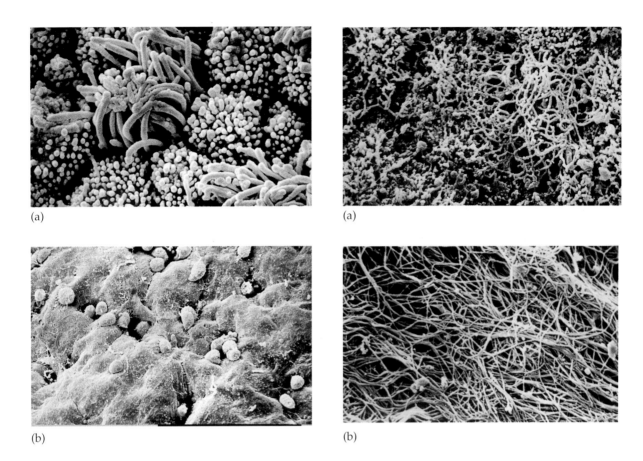

Figure 62.3 Scanning electronmicrographs (SEM) of (a) normal endometrium (control), and (b) 24-hours following PDT. Columnar epithelium after PDT is missing while cells migrate towards gland openings as part of the regeneration process.

Figure 62.4 Scanning electronmicrographs and treated endometrium one week (a) and four weeks (b) after PDT. (Reprinted with permission from Wyss *et al.*, 1994b.)

hours (Figure 62.3). Endometrial resurfacing occurred by proliferation, originating primarily in deeper regions of the glands. Findings from our morphologic follow-up support the origin of endometrial regeneration from mainly undifferentiated stem cells and residual glandular epithelium. By using a higher light dose and other drug combinations the endometrial surface was replaced by fibrous tissue (Figure 62.4).

REPRODUCTIVE PERFORMANCE FOLLOWING PDT

Some of the rat models were designed to evaluate the effect of PDT with Photofrin, Photofrin/Azone, ALA and BPD on embryo implantation (Steiner *et al.*, 1995, 1996a). Materials and methods were similar to the PDT histology research protocol. Functionality studies following mating with fertile males demonstrated a significant reduction in the number of implantations per treated uterine horns

when compared with controls. The mean number of implantations decreased systematically by increasing the interval between Photofrin administration and light application. Although the fluorescence pharmacokinetic studies suggested that both forms of topically-administered Photofrin were diffusely distributed throughout the endometrium at virtually the same rate, there productive performance study suggested that Azone may enhance PDT selectivity by facilitating drug targeting to critical endometrial structures. The same study with ALA (Yang *et al.*, 1993b) and BPD (Steiner *et al.*, 1996b) demonstrated a significant implantation failure in the treated uterine horns compared with various controls. The number of implantation sacs in the ALA-treated area was 0.4 ± 0.26 compared with 6.2 ± 1.39 in the untreated control side ($P <0.005$) and similar effects were noted with BPD. Reproductive performance studies were more sensitive than histology in defining PDT effects.

SOLVENTS FOR ENDOMETRIAL PHOTOSENSITIZATION

Instillation of low-viscosity solutions into the human uterine cavity may result in retrograde spillage and immediate passage through the fallopian tubes into the abdominal cavity. In our initial animal studies we mixed the photosensitizers with sterile water for injection. In order to decrease spillage and prolong the contact between the topically applied photosensitizer and the endometrial surface, a more viscous solution (32% dextrane, 70% dextrose; Hyskon, Pharmacia, Piscataway, New Jersey, USA) was tested. Hyskon is a viscid and hydrophilic branched polysaccharide fluid used for uterine distention during hysteroscopy. In all our endometrial studies since 1994 (Wyss *et al.*, 1994a) we have mixed the photosensitizers with Hyskon and demonstrated that it qualifies well as a new possible vehicle for PDT. Other viscous solutions and gel forms were tested in order to formulate the optimal compound dictated by uterine anatomy, histology and the chemical considerations (i.e. test solubility) of the drugs available.

BASIC OPTICAL CONSIDERATION FOR HUMAN ENDOMETRIAL PDT

The intensity of light propagating through tissue decreases exponentially with distance due to scattering and absorption. The penetration depth is defined as the distance corresponding to a decrease in the optical fluence rate by a factor of $1/e = 0.37$ ($e = 2.718$) (Judd *et al.*, 1992). The fluence rate measures the quantity of photons per second passing through a defined area (mW cm^{-2}). If, for example, the optical penetration depth for a given tissue is 3 mm, the fluence rate of photons at this depth is 37% of its rate at the surface. If the distance is doubled to 6 mm, the fluence rate is decreased by a factor $1/e^2$, that is, to approximately 10%. Since, the optical penetration depth is determined by absorption and scattering properties, it is a unique parameter that can be used to characterize a particular tissue.

Light in the wavelength region of 600–800 nm, which may be applied for endometrial ablation, will be reflected at an air–tissue interface by typically 30% (Svaasand *et al.*, 1989; Cilesiz and Welch, 1993). In other words, only 70% of the applied light will propagate into the tissue. Most of the photons that propagate into the endometrium will be scattered before they are absorbed. Scattering is caused by optical inhomogeneities, or more precisely, by refractive index discontinuities in cells and tissue. Although tissue scattering is predominately directed forwards, after a distance of about 1–2 mm, multiple scattering events produce nearly isotropic light distributions in most tissues.

Backscattered light in tissues enhances the optical fluence rate close to the surface. In a hollow organ such as the uterus, the surface fluence rate may be increased by a factor of 5–6 due to the additional reflection of light from the surrounding walls. Thus, in PDT of the endometrium, the fluence rate of the endometrial surface will generally be much higher than the incident unscattered light (Wyss *et al.*, 1995).

The fluence rate in the endometrium is therefore dependent upon the reflection conditions at the surface, the incident light, and the tissue scattering and absorption properties. Since the absorption and scattering coefficients typically decrease with increasing wavelength, longer wavelengths have greater tissue penetrance.

Endometrial optical properties (i.e., absorption and scattering coefficients) should be determined in order to optimize light dosimetry for uterine PDT. We have conducted optical property measurements on fresh uterine samples immediately after hysterectomy (Madsen *et al.*, 1994). Our results indicate that bulk tissue absorption and scattering coefficients are, respectively, in the ranges 0.19–0.52 cm^{-1} and 7.3–9.1 cm^{-1} at 630 nm. The corresponding values for the optical penetration depth are in the region of 2.59–5.11 mm. Although we have not observed substantial differences in light penetrance for human endometrium and myometrium, we continue to explore this possibility with additional measurements. The optical dose to the tissue is proportional to the incident light power per unit area and the exposure time. The tissue optical dose (J cm^{-2}) is defined as the product of the *in situ* fluence rate (W cm^{-2}) and the exposure time (seconds), and it decreases exponentially with depth. The optical dose at a given depth can be enhanced by increasing the incident optical power and/or prolonging the exposure time.

PDT is intended to induce photochemical changes at irradiation levels that do not cause thermal damage. In order to avoid hyperthermal effects, tissue temperature should be kept below 43–45°C. A temperature rise of 6–8°C above normal body temperature corresponds to an incident optical power density in the range of 100–200 mW cm^{-2} (Steiner *et al.*, 1996a). In order to achieve deep photodynamic effects with a power density limited to 100 mW cm^{-2}, the exposure time should be prolonged.

Another important factor is the photodegradation (bleaching) of the photosensitizer. In response to optical irradiation, photosensitizers tend to decompose. The concentration of the non-degraded sensitizer that can participate in the production of singlet oxygen, decreases continuously during irradiation (Moan, 1986; Svaasand and Potter, 1992). The efficiency of the singlet oxygen generation process is therefore maximal at the beginning of irradiation, and decreases to zero when the sensitizer has been completely degraded.

Bleaching will play an insignificant role in the deeper layers where the fluence has fallen off. In the case of endometrial destruction in the human, it is expected that bleaching will limit the 'overkill' in the upper layer of the endometrium and will have an insignificant effect on the depth of necrosis.

INTRAUTERINE LIGHT DIFFUSER

Light penetration depths at 630, 660 and 690 nm and the optimal configuration of intrauterine light diffusing fibers were determined in a theoretic model (Tromberg et al., 1996), and later confirmed in human uteri (Alfano et al., 1989) in order to design an optimal light intrauterine device. Postmenopausal uteri showed a significantly lower light penetration depth than premenopausal uteri. With insertion of a single central diffusing fiber, the fluence rate measured in the uterine wall at the most remote point of the cavity decreased to $1.1 \pm 0.4\%$ of that measured at closest proximity, whereas it decreased to only $40 \pm 9\%$ with three fibers. Distention of the uterine cavity with 2 ml of an optically clear fluid increased the fluence rate at the fundus between the fibers at a depth of 2 mm by a factor of four. It was concluded that in normal-sized uterine cavities, three diffusing fibers will deliver an optical dose above the photodynamic threshold at a depth of 4 mm, even at the most remote areas, in less than 15 minutes without causing thermal damage. For distorted and elongated cavities, either slight distention of the cavity or insertion of a fourth diffusing fiber is required.

Based on these studies we have designed an intrauterine light diffuser (Figure 62.5) for endometrial PDT (US Patent #5,478,339) and clinical trials using this device are in progress.

Fluorescence Diagnostics

Several groups have demonstrated that the fluorescence of endogenous chromophores may be useful for differentiating neoplastic and normal tissue in human breast (Alfano et al., 1989), bronchus (Hung et al., 1992), bladder (Kriegmair et al., 1995; Chang et al., 1996), and the gastrointestinal tract (Kapadia et al., 1990). In a recent study (Major et al., 1996), in vivo fluorescence detection of Pp IX could be used to identify intraperitoneal micrometastases of epithelial ovarian carcinoma after application of ALA. The area was illuminated with ultraviolet light, and the intensity of the fluorescence was concentration dependent. It was concluded that direct visualization of in vivo fluorescence after ALA application may improve the detection of intraperitoneal ovarian cancer micrometastases.

Spectroscopic techniques have also been investigated for improved detection of cervical neoplasia. An in vitro study of the gynecologic tract showed that the ratio of fluorescence intensities at 340 and 440 nm emission (at 300 nm excitation) and 383 and 460 nm emission (at 320 nm excitation) could be used to differentiate malignant and nonmalignant cervical, uterine and ovarian tissue with a

Figure 62.5 The intrauterine light diffuser for endometrial PDT (US Patent #5,478,339).

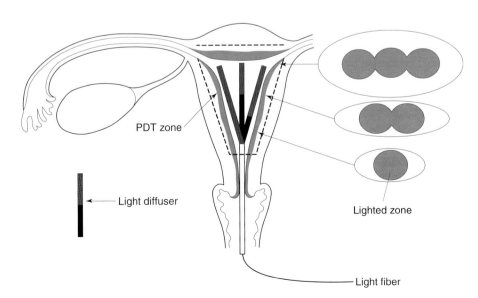

PDT zone

Light diffuser

Lighted zone

Light fiber

predictive value of 75–95% (Glassman *et al.*, 1992). Fluorescence excitation–emission matrices were obtained *in vitro* for cervical biopsies (Mahadevan *et al.*, 1993). Based on a sensitivity of 75%, positive predictive value of 86%, and specificity of 88% for spectroscopic identification of histologically proven abnormal specimens it was concluded that fluorescence spectroscopy may be useful in differentiating normal and abnormal tissue. These techniques can be integrated with endoscopes to improve diagnostic accuracy of neoplastic lesions or endometriotic implants.

Conclusion

Photomedicine of the female genital tract offers new diagnostic and therapeutic modalities based on the interaction of light with the reproductive organs. Preliminary human studies are in progress in several institutions. Different components of PDT such as choosing the preferred photosensitizer, testing the optimal dose, drug delivery mode, the interval between drug application and light treatment, light sources, light dose, and the use of specially designed delivery probes, are just a few examples of topics that are under development.

Data available suggest that PDT principles can be used to diagnose and treat various gynecologic diseases such as DUB, adenomyosis, endometriosis and ovarian cancer, and lesions on the vulva, vagina and uterine cervix. The ability to target specific lesions, and selectively ablate them with minimal or no damage to the healthy surrounding tissue, and the lack of thermal effects, which eliminates the need for any anesthesia, offer a promising combination for minimally invasive therapy.

References

Alfano RR, Pradhan A, Tang CG (1989) Optical spectroscopic diagnosis of cancer in normal and breast tissues. *Journal of the Optical Society of America B* **6**: 1015–1023.

Bhatta N, Anderson R, Flotte T, Schiff I, Hasan T, Nishioka NS (1992) Endometrial ablation by means of photodynamic therapy with Photofrin II. *American Journal of Obstetrics and Gynecology* **167**: 1856–1863.

Chapman JA, Tadir Y, Tromberg BJ *et al.* (1993) Effect of administration route and estrogen manipulation on endometrial uptake of Photofrin. *American Journal of Obstetrics and Gynecology* **168**: 685–692.

Chang SC, MacRobert AJ, Bown SG Biodistribution of protoporphyrin IX in rat urinary bladder after intravesical instillation of 5-aminolevulinic acid. *Journal of Urology* **155(5)**: 1744–1748.

Cilesiz IF, Welch AJ (1993) Light dosimetry: effects of dehydration and thermal damage on the optical properties of the human aorta. *Applied Optics* **32**: 477–487.

Dougherty TJ (1984) Photodynamic therapy (PDT) of malignant tumors. *CRC Critical Reviews in Oncology/Hematology* **2(2)**: 83–116.

Fehr MK, Madsen SJ, Svaasand, LO *et al.* (1995) Intrauterine light delivery for photodynamic therapy of the human endometrium. *Human Reproduction* **10**: 3067–3072.

Fehr KM, Chapman C, Krasieva T *et al.* (1996a) Selective photosensitization of vulvar condylomata acuminata following topical application of 5-aminolevulinic acid. *American Journal of Obstetrics and Gynecology* **174(3)**: 951–957.

Fehr KM, Wyss P, Tromberg B *et al.* (1996b) Photosensitization of the human endometrium using topically applied 5-aminolevulinic acid. *American Journal of Obstetrics and Gynecology* **175**: 1253–1259.

Fisher AMR, Murphee AL, Gomer CJ (1995) Clinical and preclinical photodynamic therapy. *Lasers in Surgery and Medicine* **17**: 2–31.

Glassman WS, Liu CH, Tang GC, Lubicz S, Alfano RR (1992) Ultraviolet excited fluorescence spectra from non-malignant and malignant tissues of the gynecological tract. *Lasers in Life Sciences* **5**: 49–58

Goff BA, Hermanto U, Rumbaugh J, Blake J, Bamberg M, Hasan T (1994) Photoimmunotherapy and biodistribution with an OC125–chlorin immunoconjugate in an *in vivo* murine ovarian cancer model. *British Journal of Cancer* **70**: 474–480.

Hung J, Lam S, LeRiche JC, Palcic B (1992) Autofluorescence of normal and malignant bronchial tissue. *Lasers in Surgery and Medicine* **11**: 99–105.

Judd MD, Bedwell J, MacRobert AJ (1992) Comparison of the distribution of phthalocyanine and ALA-induced porphyrin sensitizers within the rabbit uterus. *Lasers in Medical Science* **7**: 203–211.

Kapadia CR, Cutruzolla FW, O'Brien KM, Stetz ML, Enriquez R, Deckelbaum LI (1990) Laser-induced fluorescence spectroscopy of human colonic mucosa. *Gastroenterology* **99**: 150–157.

Kennedy JC, Pottier RH (1992) Endogenous protoporphyrin IX, a clinically useful photosensitizer for photodynamic therapy. *Journal of Photochemistry and Photobiology. B, Biology* **14**: 275–292.

Korell M, Untch M, Abels C *et al.* (1995) Use of photodynamic laser therapy in gynecology. *Gynakologisch-Geburtshilfliche Rundschau* **35(2)**: 90–97.

Kriegmair M, Stepp H, Steinbach P *et al.* (1995) Fluorescence cystoscopy following intravesical instillation of 5-aminolevulinic acid: a new procedure with high sensitivity for detection of hardly visible urothelial neoplasias. *Urologia Internationalis* **55**: 190–196.

Lipson RL, Baldes EJ, Olsen AM (1961) The use of derivative of hematoporphyrin in tumor detection. *Journal of the National Cancer Institute* **26**: 1–11.

Lobraico RV, Grossweiner LT (1993) Clinical experiences with photodynamic therapy for recurrent malignancies of the lower female genital tract. *Journal of Gynecologic Surgery* **9(1)**: 29–34.

Madsen SJ, Tromberg BJ, Wyss P, Svaasand LO, Haskell RC, Tadir Y (1994) The optical properties of human uterus at 630 nm. Advances in optical imaging and photon migration. *Optical Society of America, Topical Meeting March 21–23, Orlando, FL. Proceedings.*

Mahadevan A, Mitchell MF, Silva E, Thomsen S, Richards-Kortum RR (1993) Study of the fluorescence properties of normal and neoplastic human cervical tissue. *Lasers in Surgery and Medicine* **13**: 647–655.

Major A, Rose S, Chapman C *et al.* (1996) In vivo fluorescence detection of ovarian cancer in the NuTu-19 epithelial ovarian cancer animal model using 5-aminolevulinic acid (ALA). *Gynecologic Oncology* **66**: 122–132.

Manyak MJ, Nelson LM, Solomon D (1989) Photodynamic therapy of rabbit endometrium transplants: a model for treatment of endometriosis. *Fertility and Sterility* **52**: 140–145.

Moan J (1986) Effects of bleaching of porphyrin sensitizers during photodynamic therapy. *Cancer Letters* **33**: 45–53.

Monk B, Brewer B, Vannostrand K *et al.* (1997) Photodynamic therapy using topically applied dihematoporphyrin ether (DHE) in the treatment of cervical intraepithelial neoplasia (CIN). *Gynecologic Oncology* **64**: 70–75.

Muroya T, Suehiro Y, Umayahara K *et al.* (1996) Photodynamic therapy (PDT) for early cervical cancer. *Japanese Journal of Cancer and Chemotherapy* **23**: 47–56.

Parrish JA (1982) The scope of photomedicine. In Regan JD, Parrish JA (eds) *The Science of Photomedicine.* pp. 3. New York: Plenum Press.

Petrucco OM, Sathananden M, Petrucco MF *et al.* (1990) Ablation of endometriotic implants in rabbits by hematoporphyrin derivative photoradiation therapy using the gold vapor laser. *Lasers in Surgery and Medicine* **10**: 344–348.

Rettenmaier MA, Berman ML, Disaia PJ, Berns MW (1984) Gynecologic uses of photoradiation therapy. In Doiron DT, Gomer CJ (eds) *Porphyrin Localization and Treatment of Tumors.* p. 767. New York: Alan R Liss.

Richter AM, Kelly B, Chow J *et al.* (1987) Preliminary studies on a more effective phototoxic agent than hematoporphyrin. *Journal of the National Cancer Institute* **79**: 1327–1332.

Richter AM, Ceerruti-Sola S, Sternberg ED, Dolphin D, Levy JG (1990) Biodistribution of tritiated benzoporphyrin derivative (3H-BPDD-MA), a new potent photosensitizer, in normal and tumor-bearing mice. *Journal of Photochemistry and Photobiology. B, Biology* **5**: 231–244.

Rocklin GB, Kelly HG, Anderson SC, Edwards LE, Gimpelson RJ, Perez RE (1996) Photodynamic therapy of rat endometrium sensitized with Tin Etiopurpurin. *Journal of the American Association of Gynecologic Laparoscopists* **3**: 561–570.

Schneider D, Schellhas HF, Wessler TA *et al.* (1988). Endometrial ablation by DHE photoradiation therapy in estrogen treated ovariectomized rats. *Colposcopy and Gynecologic Laser Surgery* **4**: 73–77.

Steiner R, Tromberg BJ, Wyss P *et al.* (1995) Photodynamic destruction of rat endometrium using topically-administered Photofrin. *Human Reproduction* **10**: 227–233.

Steiner R, Tadir Y, Tromberg BJ *et al.* (1996a) Photosensitization of the rat endometrium following 5-aminolevulinic acid (ALA) induced photodynamic therapy. *Lasers in Surgery and Medicine* **18**: 301–308.

Steiner R, Tadir Y, Tromberg BJ *et al.* (1996b) Photodynamic therapy of the endometrium after topical intrauterine application of benzoporphyrin derivative mono acid and laser light. *Geburtshilfe and Frauenheilkunde* **56**: 1–7.

Svaasand LO (1984) Optical dosimetry for direct and interstitial photoradiation therapy of malignant tumors. In Doiron D, Gomer C (eds) *Porphyrin Localization and Treatment of Tumors.* pp. 91–114. New York: Alan R Liss.

Svaasand LO, Potter WR (1992) The implications of photobleaching for photodynamic therapy. In Henderson B, Dougherty TJ. (eds) *Photodynamic Therapy: Basic Principles and Clinical Aspects.* pp. 369–385. New York: Marcel Dekker

Svaasand LO, Gomer CJ, Profio AE (1989) Laser induced hyperthermia of ocular tumors. *Applied Optics* **28**: 2280–2287.

Tromberg BJ, Svaasand L, Wyss P *et al.* (1996) Light dosimetry for photodynamic destruction of the endometrium: mathematical model. *Physics and Biology* **40**: 1–15.

Van Vugt DA, Kizemien A, Roy BN *et al.* (1996) Photodynamic endometrial ablation in non-human primates. *Presented at the Xth Canadian Fertility and Andrology Society Meeting.*

Von Tappeiner H, Jesionek A (1903) Therapeutische Versuche mit fluoreszierenden Stoffen. *Muench Med Wochenschr* **50**: 2041–2051.

Wyss P, Tadir P, Tromberg BJ, Liaw L, Krasieva T, Berns MW (1994a) Benzo Porphyrin Derivative (BPD): a potent photosensitizer for photodynamic destruction of the rabbit endometrium. *Obstetrics and Gynecology* **84**: 409–414.

Wyss P, Tromberg BJ, Wyss MT *et al.* (1994b) Photodynamic destruction of endometrial tissue using topical 5-aminolevulinic acid (5-ALA) in rats and rabbits. *American Journal of Obstetrics and Gynecology* **171**: 1176–1183.

Wyss P, Svaasand L, Tadir L *et al.* (1995) Photomedicine of the endometrium: experimental concepts. *Human Reproduction* **10**: 221–226.

Yang JZ, van Vugt DA, Kennedy JC, Reid RL (1993a) Evidence of lasting functional destruction of rat endometrium after 5-aminolevulinic acid-induced photodynamic ablation: Prevention of implantation. *American Journal of Obstetrics and Gynecology* **68**: 995–1001.

Yang JZ, Van Vugt DA, Kennedy JC, Reid RL (1993b) Intrauterine 5-aminolevulinic acid induces selective fluorescence and photodynamic ablation of the rat endometrium. *Photochemistry and Photobiology* **57**: 803–807.

63

Microwave Endometrial Ablation

NICHOLAS C. SHARP*, IAN B. FELDBERG†, DAVID A. HODGSON*,
BRIAN BUTTERS‡ AND NIGEL CRONIN†

*Royal United Hospital, Combe Park, Bath, UK
†University of Bath, School of Physics, Bath, UK
‡Microsulis Ltd, Waterlooville, Hampshire, UK

Introduction

All techniques for endometrial ablation work on the basic principle of transfer of energy to or from the endometrium. To be effective, the transferred energy should destroy the regenerative capacity of the endometrium. The wide range of methods tried is testimony to the remarkable resilience of the endometrium and many techniques have been largely abandoned (ionizing radiation, chemical agents, cryosurgery, and radiofrequency ablation) due to poor results and lack of precision. Why then try and develop another technique?

The criteria for an ideal endometrial ablation technique are:

- Effective.
- Safe.
- Easy to learn.
- Quick to perform.
- Painless.
- Suitable for local anesthetic.
- Suitable for outpatient use.
- Portable.

Existing techniques have their own drawbacks and do not satisfy all the criteria for an ideal ablative procedure. This may be because all of these procedures try to adapt an existing technique or technology to the problem. If one considers that a thin atrophic endometrium can be achieved in preparation for any ablation procedure and that endometrial glandular elements will invariably be present deeper in the myometrium, an effective ablative procedure should set out to destroy tissue uniformly at a depth of at least 5 mm. The application of modern microwave technology has enabled us to develop a new treatment specifically for the purpose of endometrial ablation.

Physics of Microwave Energy

Microwaves, like all forms of electromagnetic energy, will penetrate into biologic tissue to a depth determined by the electrical properties of the tissue and the frequency of the electromagnetic wave. Figure 63.1 shows the 'penetration depth' in high water content tissue (uterine tissue) at varying frequencies.

A conventional microwave oven uses electromagnetic energy at a frequency around 2.45 GHz. At this frequency the plane wave penetration depth would be approximately 18 mm in tissue with a high water content. This corresponds to the depth at which the field amplitude is reduced to 10% of that at the surface of the tissue, therefore causing negligible heating in the tissue beyond this point. The plane wave penetration depth gives us an approximate guide to the resultant depth of necrosis at a particular electromagnetic frequency. Figure 63.1

Figure 63.1 Microwave penetration into tissue at differing frequencies.

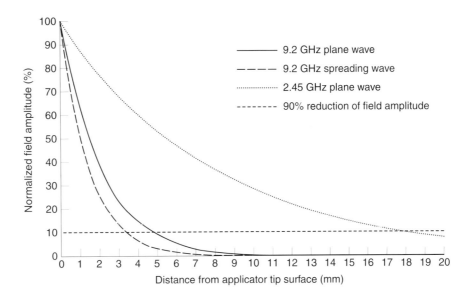

therefore shows that at around 9 GHz the plane wave penetration depth is closer to that required for the purposes of endometrial ablation.

To transmit energy at this frequency through the cervix into the uterine cavity, a dielectric filled circular waveguide has been chosen (Cronin, 1995). An air-filled waveguide would need to be almost 25 mm in diameter and the cervix can only be dilated to about 10 mm. The waveguide is therefore filled with a material that has a dielectric constant greater than that of air, which effectively reduces the wavelength of the propagating wave. By using this technique the overall diameter of the applicator has been reduced to 8.5 mm. The treatment frequency was chosen to be 9.2 GHz in order to propagate energy efficiently down the dielectric filled waveguide and produce the desired depth of penetration in uterine tissue.

To radiate energy into the uterine cavity efficiently an applicator tip was designed to produce semi-spherical heating patterns in tissue. This effectively spreads the microwave energy across the tip surface, causing a further reduction in field strength at distances removed from the applicator tip surface. Figure 63.1 shows that as a result of this factor the depth of microwave penetration will be closer to 3 mm.

The Microwave Endometrial Ablation (MEA) equipment began its development at the School of Physics, University of Bath in 1992 with early experimental trials in collaboration with the Department of Medical Physics and the Directorate of Gynaecology at the Royal United Hospital, Bath. Clinical trials commenced in October 1994. The MEA system (Figure 63.2) comprises a 9.2 GHz

Figure 63.2 MEA system.

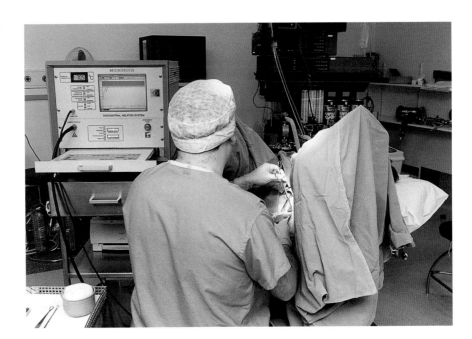

microwave generator, real-time thermometry graphics and system cables leading to the hand-held microwave applicator.

The generator status is controlled by an embedded computer system. A safety interlock prevents generator activation until the applicator thermocouple reading exceeds 30°C (i.e. warming up to body temperature) and is not in air but in close tissue contact. A thermocouple is also placed to record applicator shaft temperature, and both tip and shaft temperatures have safeguard warnings and cut offs.

The microwave energy enters the hand-held applicator and is guided to the tip where it is absorbed by adjacent endometrium. As shown using the simple spreading wave model in Figure 63.1, the semi-spherical field pattern emanating from the applicator tip surface will be reduced by 90% after approximately 3 mm. Beyond this zone of intense microwave heating, further tissue destruction occurs by conduction of thermal energy away from the heated region. The total depth of necrosis, therefore, depends upon the power level used and the length of time for which this power is applied. These parameters have been optimized in animal tissue, excised uteri, perfused excised uteri and finally *in vivo* before hysterectomy. In the latter experiment the specimens were stained with a vital tissue stain (nitroblue tetrazolium) (Kiernan, 1981), which stains viable tissue an intense blue while devitalized areas fail to stain and remain pale (Figure 63.3). Using the information obtained during these experimental trials it is now possible to achieve a depth of necrosis of 5–6 mm *in vivo*. The novel applicator (Figure 63.4) now provides the gynecologic surgeon with a new surgical tool, making it possible to deliver a very precise field of intense microwave energy to the uterine cavity.

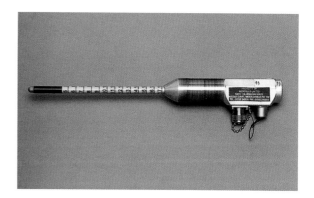

Figure 63.4 The microwave applicator – a new surgical tool.

Operative Technique

Under general anesthesia or local anesthesia using a four quadrant block technique (Ferry and Rankin, 1994a, 1994b) to the cervix, the uterine cavity is sounded, and the sounding checked against a centimeter rule. The cervix is dilated to Hegar 9 mm and the sounding with this dilator is also checked against the rule to ensure an identical measurement. The microwave applicator is then inserted until the tip rests against the fundus. The applicator is marked in centimeter graduations to check that the insertion is the same as the sounding. These simple precautions prevent the risk of inadvertent perforation. The applicator has a 'non-stick' fluoropolymer coating to permit easy passage through the cervix and to give the instrument a good 'feel' in the surgeon's hands.

After system checks are complete, taking a few moments, the applicator is energized. A thermocouple sensor at the applicator tip registers a temperature proportional to the tissue temperature in the microwave field. The indicated tissue temperature, which increases rapidly, is visualized on the system screen. This indicated temperature is slightly lower than the actual tissue temperature because the sensor is thermally heatsunk to the bulk of the applicator tip and it is lagged by the protective sheath.

During the initial temperature rise the applicator tip is moved slowly from side to side at the uterine fundus to ensure the fundal area is heated evenly and to make certain that the cornual areas are fully treated (Figure 63.5). By keeping the measured temperature within a therapeutic band visible on the system screen, the surgeon can apply the desired energy dose evenly to the endometrium. Once the fundal area has been treated the applicator is slowly withdrawn, continuing the side to side movements,

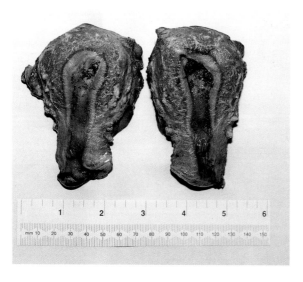

Figure 63.3 Vital tissue staining of uterus after microwave endometrial ablation.

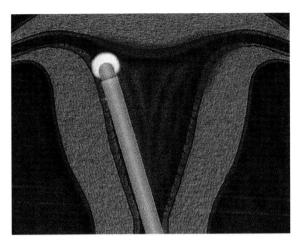

Figure 63.5 The microwave applicator treating the uterine fundus.

maintaining the temperature in the therapeutic band as far as possible (Figure 63.6). In an untreated area the temperature will be lower, so the applicator is held still in that region until it is heated, when the temperature will rise into the therapeutic band and the applicator can be moved again. In this way the entire uterine cavity is treated as the instrument is steadily withdrawn. A 35 mm solid black zone below the applicator tip alerts the surgeon on withdrawal of the applicator that the active tip is reaching the internal os. When this zone starts to appear at the external cervical os, the power is switched off to prevent endocervical heating and the instrument is withdrawn. The total treatment time is generally 2–3 minutes for an average-sized uterus. At the end

of a treatment the system can generate a printout, which shows the patient's treatment temperature profile for inclusion in the patient's notes (Figure 63.7). A record of each treatment is also stored in memory on the system's plug-in memory card.

Postoperatively most patients experience little or no discomfort. Two patients experienced severe pain unresponsive to opiates and were returned to theater from the recovery area; an intracervical local anesthetic block produced immediate relief. Most patients are treated as day cases, with an increasing number opting for local anesthesia. A few women have now been treated as outpatients in a colposcopy clinic setting. Diclofenac sodium suppositories are given routinely unless contraindicated. Patients are warned that a watery discharge is normal for up to three weeks post-operatively and will settle spontaneously.

Clinical Trial of Microwave Endometrial Ablation

All trial patients were evaluated in a dedicated research clinic. Each one had a transvaginal scan to assess the uterus, as well as endometrial sampling. Blood was taken for full blood count, thyroid function and gonadatropins. The patient's menstrual disorder was determined using a menstrual score questionnaire (Sharp *et al.*, 1995) as well as the severity of dysmenorrhea experienced by the patient. Preoperative endometrial thinning was arranged with subjects receiving either danazol

Figure 63.6 Picture of on-screen display.

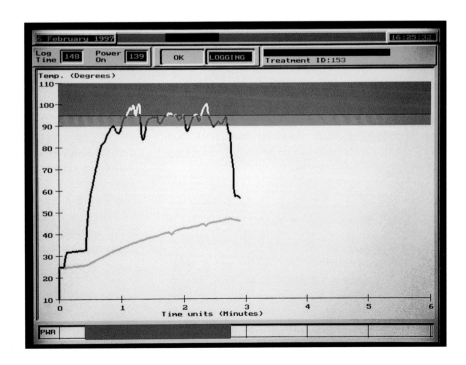

Figure 63.7 Copy of treatment profile printout.

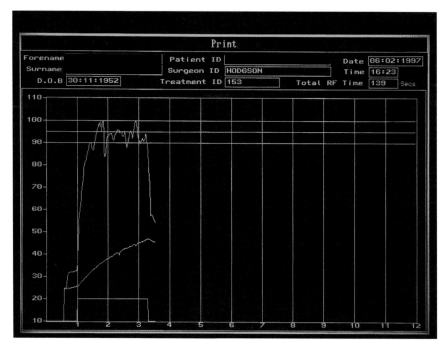

800 mg daily for at least four weeks, or goserelin (Zoladex, Zeneca, Cheshire, UK) 3.6 mg subcutaneously at least four weeks before admission. Immediately before ablation, all patients had a repeat vaginal ultrasound scan (usually in the operating theater) to assess endometrial thickness following pre-treatment.

Exclusion criteria were:

- Family incomplete.
- Submucous fibroids greater than 3 cm.
- Significant endometrial pathology or significant pelvic pathology.
- Previous uterine surgery, including failed resection.

Previous cesarean section is not a contraindication, but the region of the uterine scar was carefully scanned to ensure that there was no serious thinning of the myometrial tissues at that point, but only a few patients have had to be excluded for this reason.

Results

Over 180 women have now been treated with microwave endometrial ablation in Bath. Seven treated with 20 W of power had a poor outcome (only two patients improved), indicating that this low power level is ineffective. This group is excluded from subsequent data analysis.

Twenty six women were treated with 40 W and the remainder with 30 W. There was no significant difference in outcome between 30 W and 40 W treatments and the lower power setting is now the standard treatment.

The mean treatment time was 147 seconds. Approximately 35% of women treated were under 40 years of age, but there was no significant difference in outcome when this group was compared with the older age group and the data are presented for all ages.

Improvement in menstrual flow is shown in Figure 63.8. There is a good amenorrhea and overall satisfaction rate up to two years. Those women who did not have a satisfactory response were offered retreatment or hysterectomy. Their probability of not having further surgery is shown in Figure 63.9. The other major benefit of microwave endometrial ablation has been an improvement in dysmenorrhea for many women (Figure 63.10).

The initial high rate of 'no dysmenorrhea' at 64% shows signs of declining to just under 60% at two years, with a combined total of 77% having no or less dysmenorrhea at two years. Additional data are being accumulated to assess larger numbers over 2–3 years of follow-up and beyond.

Discussion

Although these are preliminary results for microwave endometrial ablation, they compare

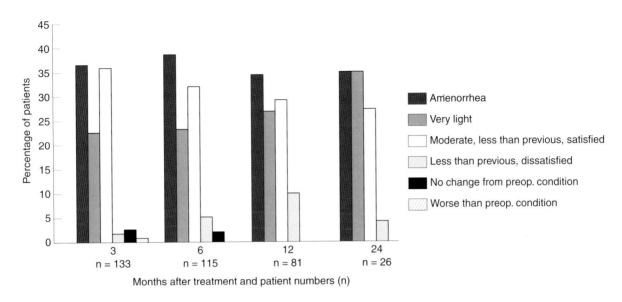

Figure 63.8 Histogram of periods assessment at 3, 6, 12 and 24 months.

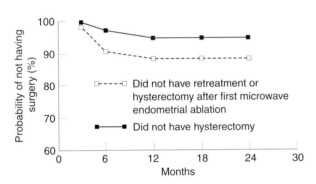

Figure 63.9 Probability of not having further surgery.

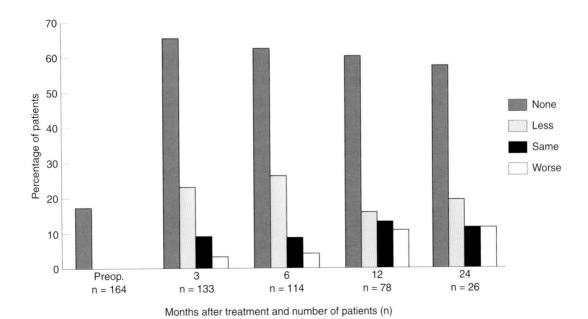

Figure 63.10 Dysmenorrhea assessment at 3, 6, 12 and 24 months.

very favorably with those reported for other techniques (Rankin and Steinberg, 1992; Pinion *et al.*, 1994; Garry *et al.*, 1995; Baggish and Sze, 1996; O'Connor and Magos, 1996; Unger and Meeks, 1996). During the course of this clinical trial some parameters were changed, and we now know that some of these women had a suboptimal treatment. Having optimized the treatment, it is expected that patients now being treated will have better outcomes, and even fewer should require re-treatment.

A good response to treatment is not dependent upon operator experience and is simply related to the technique. A few gynecologic surgeons from other centers have now been trained in the use of microwave endometrial ablation and more than 120 women have been treated at four other UK sites. Training consists of a 'hands on' experience at the Royal United Hospital, Bath, UK followed by a single supervised list at the trainee's own hospital. All trainees testify to the ease of use and rapid confidence in the technique and all are finding their initial results very similar to those reported here, indicating a minimal 'learning curve'.

Complications

There have been no intraoperative complications and no uterine perforations during microwave endometrial ablation. One patient with a stenosed cervix, largely due to a six-week exposure to goserelin, had a cervical perforation during attempted cervical dilatation, and the procedure had to be abandoned before microwave endometrial ablation. There is no post-operative bleeding. One patient was readmitted a few days after treatment with symptoms suggestive of endometritis, which settled rapidly with broad-spectrum antibiotics. Subsequent swab cultures were, however, negative.

Safety

The technique is inherently safe for a number of reasons:

- The physics is correct, with tissue penetration being strictly limited by the physical properties of the chosen microwave frequency.
- Uterine perfusion is unimportant. Thermal containment is not dependent upon blood flow, and initial research using unperfused and perfused hysterectomy specimens showed that uterine cavity temperatures near 100 °C failed to cause any temperature elevation at the serosa.
- Continuous thermometry gives the surgeon instantaneous information to guide applicator placement during treatment.
- The technique of steady applicator withdrawal after careful initial positioning prevents the risk of perforation during treatment.
- Power requirements are low – only 30 W.
- Energy requirements are low – a combination of low power and short treatment time. They are typically 1% of those that used to be required for radiofrequency ablation (Phipps *et al.*, 1990).
- Hysteroscopic fluids are not required.
- There is no risk of hemorrhage.

Summary

Returning to the criteria for an ideal endometrial ablation technique, microwave endometrial ablation fulfills most criteria well. It is safe, effective, very quick and easy to learn. There have been no adverse incidents during the experience in five centers with a two-year experience in the prime site (where the clinical trials took place).

Microwave endometrial ablation is virtually pain-free for most patients. The ease with which it is performed under local anesthesia and the short time required to complete the treatment makes it ideal for outpatient use. The applicators are autoclavable and soakable and therefore suitable for use in any outpatient treatment facility. It is expected that a hospital offering a colposcopy service would be able to adapt to incorporate microwave endometrial ablation into such a setting.

Microwave endometrial ablation produces results comparable to those of other existing techniques, but has a number of very real practical advantages, not least of which is the ease with which it can be learnt.

Acknowledgements

The authors gratefully acknowledge the collaborative effort of the other team members: Mr Martyn Evans and Dr Suzanne Smith of the Medical Physics Department, Royal United Hospital and Dr Lyn Hirschowitz, Consultant Histopathologist, Royal United Hospital.

References

Baggish MS, Sze E (1996) Endometrial ablation: A series of 568 patients treated over an 11 year period. *American Journal of Obstetrics and Gynecology* **174**: 904–913.

Cronin NJ (1995) *Microwave and Optical Waveguides.* IOP Publishing.

Ferry J, Rankin L (1994a) Low cost, patient acceptable, local analgesia approach to gynaecological outpatient surgery. A review of 817 consecutive procedures. *Australian and New Zealand Journal of Obstetrics and Gynaecology* **34**: 453–456.

Ferry J, Rankin L (1994b) Transcervical resection of the endometrium using intracervical block only. A review of 278 procedures. *Australian and New Zealand Journal of Obstetrics and Gynaecology* **34**: 457–467.

Garry R, Shelley–Jones D, Mooney P *et al.* (1995) Six hundred endometrial laser ablations. *Obstetrics and Gynecology* **85**: 24–29.

Kiernan JA (1981) *Histological and Histochemical Methods; Theory and Practice.* pp. 236–240. Oxford: Pergamon Press.

O'Connor H, Magos AL (1996) Endometrial resection for the treatment of menorrhagia. *New England Journal of Medicine* **335**: 151–156.

Phipps JH, Lewis BV, Roberts T *et al.* (1990) Treatment of functional menorrhagia by radiofrequency induced thermal endometrial ablation. *Lancet* **335**: 374–376.

Pinion SB, Parkin DE, Naji A *et al.* (1994) Randomised trial of hysterectomy, randomised endometrial ablation, and transcervical endometrial resection for dysfunctional uterine bleeding. *British Medical Journal* **309**: 979–983.

Rankin L, Steinberg LH (1992) Transcervical resection of the endometrium: A review of 400 consecutive patients. *British Journal of Obstetrics and Gynaecology* **99**: 911–914.

Sharp NC, Cronin N, Feldberg I *et al.* (1995) Microwaves for menorrhagia: A new fast technique for endometrial ablation. *Lancet* **346**: 1003–1004.

Unger JB, Meeks GR (1996) Hysterectomy after endometrial ablation. *American Journal of Obstetrics and Gynecology* **175**: 1432–1436.

Major Complications of Hysteroscopic Surgery – Avoidance and Management

64

Hazards and Dangers of Operative Hysteroscopy

BRUNO J. van HERENDAEL

Jan Palfijn General Hospital, Antwerp, Belgium and University of Varese, Varese, Italy

Operative hysteroscopy is a new and valuable technique in the treatment of non-malignant conditions of the uterine cavity. As the indications for endoscopic surgery become wider (Siegler and Valle, 1988) safety protocols become more important in the prevention of complications. This is particularly important since most complications tend to occur in the hands of inexperienced surgeons (Lindemann, 1975).

As with any other surgical technique, operative hysteroscopy requires an intensive training period. The operative field is new to gynecologists and requires a different approach compared to that of classical surgery (Martens, 1991; Slangen, 1991). It is therefore advisable that a surgeon starting hysteroscopic surgery should have performed at least 250 diagnostic procedures before embarking on operative work.

A further recommendation is that the surgery should be graded according to difficulty. The beginner should do approximately 50 minor surgical procedures, then 50 intermediate procedures and only start doing major hysteroscopic surgery after about 350 hysteroscopies.

The Safety Committee of the European Society of Hysteroscopy has issued a classification of the difficulty of hysteroscopic operative procedures. It seems reasonable to use such a classification to assess the progress of any trainee (Table 64.1).

Every uterine septum operation performed with the hysteroscope should have a full investigation including a laparoscopy before surgery to ascertain that the uterus is not bicornuate (Valle and Sciarra, 1986).

Table 64.1 Classification of operative difficulty.

Minor hysteroscopic surgery
  Endometrial biopsy
  Small polyps
  Non-embedded intrauterine contraceptive device
    (IUCD) (non-pregnant)
  Simple adhesions

Intermediate hysteroscopic surgery
  Cannulation of the fallopian tube
  Sterilization

Advanced hysteroscopic surgery
  Myomectomy*
  Large polyps
  Endometrial resection or ablation
  Resection of uterine septum*
  IUCD removal in pregnancy
  Extensive adhesiolysis*

*These procedures should probably be combined with either a laparoscopy or an ultrasound examination (Sugimoto *et al.*, 1984; Taylor *et al.*, 1984; van Herendael, 1988).

Complications of Hysteroscopic Surgery

Dilation of the Cervix

The use of rigid instruments may damage the cervical canal if appropriate care is not taken. The cervix can be lacerated by the tenaculum due to excessive traction during dilation (Siegler, 1983). Dilation itself can provoke bleeding. A certain amount of force is often necessary to dilate a cervical canal up to Hegar 9. Therefore the position taken with the direction of the force as well as a certain amount of patience should be taken into consideration. The use of Hegar dilators, increasing by half a size at a time is less traumatic. Some instruments such as the Pratt dilator seem to cause less trauma.

Pharmacologic cervical dilatation is useful in overcoming these problems. Laminaria stents are hygroscopic and distend by absorption of fluid over the course of a few hours. However, the laminaria tends to swell beyond the confines of the cervical canal and can therefore be difficult to remove and can introduce infection. Synthetic laminaria such as Lamicel (Cabot Medical Corporation, Langhorne, PA, USA) overcome this problem. The dilator consists of a polyvinyl core impregnated with less than 500 mg of sodium phosphate.

A better method of pharmacologic dilatation is the use of prostaglandins. The synthetic derivative of prostaglandin E_2 (sulprostone) is more effective at a lower dosage than prostaglandin $F_{2\alpha}$ and its maximum effect is reached within one hour. The route of administration is local by vaginal suppositories. The action is due to softening of the cervical stroma resulting in dilatation of the canal. This is enhanced by contractions of the myometrium induced by the drug. Doses of 125–250 mg given 1–2 hours before surgery produce sufficient cervical dilatation in 80% of women. Side effects reported include nausea, vomiting, hypertension and hypotension, and occasionally a cutaneous rash.

Hazards of Distension Media

Both carbon dioxide (CO_2) and liquid distension media are used in hysteroscopic surgery (Lindemann, 1983) and are comprehensively covered in Chapter 53.

Minor and intermediate hysteroscopic surgery can be performed using CO_2 gas with a specially adapted insufflator for hysteroscopy. Advanced hysteroscopic surgery is always performed using liquid distension, the one exception being removal of an IUCD in the gravid uterus where the distension medium of choice is still CO_2 under carefully controlled pressure.

Complications of CO_2 and other Gases

CO_2 is a soluble gas at body temperature since 57 ml of CO_2 per minute are absorbed in 100 ml of blood (Lindemann, 1972). There are no changes in P_{O_2} P_{CO_2} or pH if 100 ml of CO_2 are infused into the bloodstream per minute, but changes start to occur with more than 400 ml of CO_2 per minute. If 1000 ml are infused per minute an irreversible cardiac shock occurs due to acute CO_2 intoxication of the heart muscle.

This means that for operative hysteroscopy where the time used for the procedure is longer than for a classical diagnostic hysteroscopy it is mandatory to have a reliable and calibrated hysteroflator. The flow should not exceed 80 ml min^{-1}. The insufflation pressure should not exceed 200 mg Hg. The use of cervical cups is contraindicated as it prevents the outflow of gas through the cervical canal.

The use of hysteroflators equipped with the possibility of giving a boost of gas is dangerous and should not be used for hysteroscopy. These deliver a bolus of gas of 120 ml in ten seconds with the ability to repeat the bolus every minute; in doing so the blood buffer system could be overloaded. These hysteroflators should therefore not be used for operative procedures (Gallinat, 1978). Gas embolism is probably underdiagnosed due to the very high solubility of CO_2. It must, however, be assumed that because the intrauterine pressure rises above the diastolic blood pressure there must be frequent entry of gas into the venous circulation.

The physical properties of CO_2 are such that mixing with the blood and the mucus of the endocervix and the endometrium creates bubbles. Bubbles impair vision, but invariably disappear when the physical reaction of mixing ends. However, this can take a long time and CO_2 is less appropriate for hysteroscopic surgery since liquid distension media are safer and provide good visibility for the surgeon.

Air and other gases must never be used for uterine distension. Fatal air embolism has been recorded with both tubal persufflation and with hysteroscopy. Baggish and Daniell (1989) reported five fatal cases where air had accidentally been used to cool the sapphire tips of Nd:YAG laser fibers. Several other deaths have been reported throughout the world. All these women had sudden irreversible circulatory failure due to massive air embolism.

Anesthesiologists have been increasingly worried about so-called CO_2 emboli. Phil Brooks (personal communication) reports that at least three of the so-called CO_2 emboli were due to the absorption of room air, confirmed by gas analysis from samples of blood obtained by cardiac puncture. Therefore it is recommended to avoid self-retaining speculae during general anesthesia for operative hysteroscopy and to place the patients in a slight anti-Trendelenburg position. This procedure should reduce aspiration of air through opened vessels in the cervix by the negative pressure of the circulation.

Complications of Liquid Distension Media

Liquid distension media are absorbed and intravasated into the uterine vessels, especially if the latter are transected during operative hysteroscopy, which occurs particularly with resection. Transtubal intra-abdominal spillage occurs to a lesser extent. Although peritoneal absorption over a long period of time has been observed, aspiration of the spilled fluid by concomitant laparoscopy does not prevent complications.

High-viscosity Fluids

The fluid 32% dextran 70 in 10% dextrose (Hyskon) has excellent optical properties and does not conduct electricity. The risks are the same in hysteroscopy as with intravenous infusion and intraperitoneal instillation. The metabolism of intravascular dextran is dependent upon its molecular weight. Dextrans of molecular weight less than 50 000 are filtered through the kidney with little reabsorption. Larger molecules are metabolized by the reticuloendothelial system. Intravascular reabsorption has been linked to anaphylactic shock and noncardiogenic pulmonary edema.

The response to dextran is immediate in the case of anaphylactic shock due to the sensitization resulting from oral exposure to sugar beets and cross-reactivity with bacterial antigens such as streptococci, pneumococci and salmonella. The incidence of anaphylaxis is rare at 1 in 10 000 (Leake et al., 1987; McLucas, 1991). The so-called dextran-induced anaphylactic reaction (DIAR) is not predictable and does not depend upon the amount used. Witz et al. (1993) reported that several patients with DIAR were found to be negative when skin-tested late for allergy to dextran. Most authors attribute the edema to a direct toxic effect of dextran 70 on the pulmonary vasculature. This explanation is not accepted by all authorities as animal studies fail to show this direct pulmonary toxicity. Pulmonary edema is most likely due to an increased intravascular volume. High molecular weight dextrans are limited to the intravascular space. Because of their slow metabolization they significantly increase the plasma oncotic pressure. Fluid and electrolytes are drawn from the interstitial and third space into the intravascular compartment. Each gram of dextran 70 is capable of drawing 20–27 ml of water into the circulation.

Managing patients with dextran toxicity involves the treatment of fluid overload and of pulmonary edema. Basic treatment involves respiratory support and diuresis. The underlying problem of increased plasma oncotic pressure should be addressed. Because the molecular weight is over 50 000 dialysis is not effective in removing dextrans. Epinephrine (intratracheal and intravenous) and hydrocortisone may be necessary. Some advocate the administration of antihistamines.

OTHER SIDE EFFECTS OF DEXTRAN

Dextran 70 has been associated with coagulation disorders. Disseminated intravascular coagulation has been reported after Hyskon hysteroscopy. The antithrombotic effect of dextran is thought to be secondary to decreased platelet adhesiveness to the endothelium. Dextran may also alter fibrin clot structure making it more susceptible to lysis. It also reduces the activity of fibrinogen, clotting factors V, VIII and IX, and the factor VIII–von Willebrand complex.

Low-viscosity Fluids

A variety of symptoms associated with the absorption of large volumes of distension media are called 'post-TURP syndrome' by urologists. Patients with this syndrome present with bradycardia and hypertension followed by hypotension, nausea, vomiting, headache, visual disturbances, agitation, confusion and lethargy. These symptoms are the result of hypervolemia, dilutional hyponatremia and decreased osmolarity. If untreated the result may be seizures, coma, cardiovascular collapse and death.

GLYCINE 1.5%

Glycine is a non-essential, simple amino acid that is normally present in the circulation; mixed with water in a 1.5% solution it gives poor electrical conductivity and good visibility (Baumann et al., 1990). Intravascular absorption of large volumes may cause water intoxication with hypervolemia and hypernatremia. Due to oxidative deamination in the liver and the kidneys, glyoxylic acid and ammonia are formed. This may result in hyperconcentration of ammonia in the brain. High ammonia concentrations here alter the neural amino acid metabolism, resulting in the production of false inhibitory neurotransmitters in the retina in the ganglion and horizontal cells, decreasing visual acuity. Glyoxylic acid is metabolized to oxalate, the metabolic end-product, and is contraindicated in renal failure as it forms crystals in the urine.

Glycine in iso-osmotic concentration can lead to hemodilution and extracellular volume expansion with subsequent decrease of serum sodium. From the experiments of Donnez (personal communication) we know that it is possible to lose up to 1300 ml into the circulation without any adverse effect. It is therefore mandatory to monitor fluid input and output very carefully and to stop surgery when the deficit is over 1300 ml.

Glycine may get into the vascular space when large uterine vessels are transected during surgery. Serum sodium decreases as fluid enters the circulation. Sodium and its associated anions account for the majority of plasma osmolarity. A drop in serum sodium therefore reflects a drop in serum osmolarity. The osmotic activity of the glycine molecules initially helps to maintain the serum osmolarity. Glycine does not remain in the intravascular space – intravascular half-life is 85 minutes – it is absorbed intracellularly. This results in a surplus of free water. Hypo-osmolar hyponatremia results if this free water is not eliminated rapidly. Due to stress and the resulting release of antidiuretic hormone, diuresis is often delayed. The danger of this condition lies in the potential of hyponatremia causing irreversible brain damage. A rapid increase of intravascular free water will lead to decreased osmolarity and movement of water into the brain, causing cerebral edema. As the brain swells it may be injured by compression against the bony structures. Increased intracranial pressure may cause decreased blood flow and hence hypoxia. An increase of 5% in intracranial volume may lead to herniation. A 10% increase in volume is incompatible with life. Hyponatremia may be an independent factor as sodium influences cardiac and skeletal muscle, nerve impulses, membrane potentials and membrane permeability.

The treatment consists of removing the excess fluid and correcting the serum sodium level. Spontaneous evolution is not sufficient as patients with severe hyponatremia deteriorate rapidly. As the onset of severe symptoms is unpredictable the treatment should start immediately. If correction is too rapid, however, it may cause an injury to the brain called central pontine myelinolysis (CPM). This is a cerebral demyelinating lesion. Treatment methods are variable, but have to include intravenous saline and forced diuresis. Furosemide is the drug of choice to force diuresis: 20 mg intravenously are sufficient to initiate diuresis. If there is concomitant renal failure, larger doses will have to be used. Initially serum electrolytes should be monitored every four hours.

Mannitol and Sorbitol

Sorbitol and mannitol are six-carbon alditol isomers. Sorbitol is removed from the circulation and metabolized in the liver to fructose and glucose.

Mannitol is essentially inert. Only 6–10% of the absorbed mannitol is metabolized. The remainder is freely filtered by the kidney and excreted unchanged in the urine. With normal renal function, the half-life of mannitol in the plasma is 15 minutes. Mannitol therefore acts as an osmotic diuretic that should reduce the risk of water overload. Intravasation of large amounts can cause nausea, vomiting, headache and hyponatremia. It should not be used in patients with renal failure. The only severe complication known is fluid overload and water intoxication, the treatment of which is the same as described above (Wamsteker, 1991).

Mechanical Complications

Perforation

It is an accepted fact that perforations do occur when using dilators to dilate the cervix or when inserting the hysteroscope. Subsequently therapy is seldom necessary, but the patient should be carefully observed for several hours. A rising pulse and falling blood pressure usually indicates ongoing hemorrhage, in which case a laparoscopy should be performed to assess the bleeding. Usually the hemorrhage can be stopped by laparoscopic endocoagulation, diathermy or sutures, but occasionally it is necessary to perform a laparotomy or even a hysterectomy.

Instrumental Injuries

The more sophisticated the instrument the more essential it is that the surgeon knows its physical properties. Electric instruments have quite different physical properties to those of mechanical and laser instruments.

If the instrument or the heat generated by the instrument diffuses beyond the myometrium adherent bowel loops may be damaged. For this reason if a patient complains of increasing abdominal pain after surgery, a laparoscopy should be performed to check for bowel damage. A pelvic drain should be inserted and the patient kept under careful observation for signs of peritonitis.

Mechanical injury is circumscribed and mostly easy to detect with the laparoscope. If a perforation occurs during instrumentation, the operation must be terminated immediately. On no account must a laser or electric current be activated if perforation is suspected. This is certainly true if there is no clear vision of the operative field and the tissue to be treated. Most serious accidents have occurred when instruments have been without vision due to poor distension or to bleeding. The surgeon has to ascertain that there has been no major vessel injury and withdraws the hysteroscope only after removing the ancillary instruments (Haning *et al.*, 1980).

A possible complication is fluid overload due to massive absorption of the distension medium at the time of the perforation. The rate of fluid absorption is increased 20-fold. Sometimes collections of distension medium have been reported in the broad ligament, especially after perforations at the time of extensive adhesiolysis. These should be left undisturbed and will disappear over a period of time. Laparoscopic drainage should be performed only if the patient complains of pressure in the iliac fossa or persistent fever.

Injuries to the bowel – mostly colon or rectum (and very seldom the small bowel) – due to electric current are often not so obvious and require some expertise to be detected. If the perforation is performed by an experienced surgeon the current will not be activated at the time of the perforation in most cases. The injury will therefore be a thermal injury and sometimes it will take several days before the bowel perforates and the patient will present with a septic peritonitis. For this reason if perforation is suspected the patient should be kept under close observation in hospital for several days. If the current is activated during the perforation the results are more spectacular and require immediate intervention. There have been case reports of damage to the aorta, the external and internal iliac vessels, and the mesenteric and sacral vessels in these circumstances. Prompt intervention with emergency laparotomy and preferably the assistance of a vascular surgeon is necessary to save the life and limb of the patient.

PREOPERATIVE PREPARATION

Patients should have received some kind of bowel preparation. The easiest to perform is the one used by the radiologists to prepare the bowels for contrast radiography. The least expensive is a combination of an oral laxative the morning and the evening of the day preceding the hysteroscopy and an enema approximately two hours before the procedure.

ACTIVE AND PASSIVE RESECTOSCOPE

The procedure is best performed with a passive resectoscope (DeCherney *et al.*, 1987). The active resectoscope features a loop, a ball or a knife that protrudes in front of the instrument. This is useful for the urologist, but offers no advantage to the gynecologist. The automatic advancement of the loop can cause a perforation if the resectoscope is held too close to the uterine wall. The passive resectoscope automatically retracts the loop towards the end of the hysteroscope and requires an active movement from the fingers of the surgeon to move it outwards, thus reducing the danger of perforation.

When using a resectoscope the active phase should always be towards the lens so that the surgeon is able to control the section at all times. As long as the loop, the ball or the knife is not completely visible the current should not be activated.

HAZARDS OF ELECTROCAUTERY AND LASERS

Electricity has an effect beyond the visual field of the surgeon. Coagulation and devitalization occur up to 6 mm into the tissues. This has serious implications in the region of the uterine cornua where the safety margin before reaching the serosa is only approximately 8 mm (Neuwirth and Amin, 1976).

Inside the cavity the zona compacta of the myometrium, situated directly under the endometrium, is approximately 6–8 mm thick, and beneath this lies the vascular bed. Perforation of this layer causes intensive bleeding. Secondary bleeding one week or more after surgery has been reported due to the deep devitalization of the tissues after overzealous coagulation (DeCherney and Polan, 1983).

The most widely used laser for intrauterine surgery is the neodymium:yttrium-aluminum-garnet (Nd:YAG) laser (Goldrath *et al.*, 1981). All lasers used at hysteroscopy are fiber lasers. Some incidents have occurred where the fiber has perforated the uterus and the laser has been activated. As the fiber is then in the abdominal cavity out of the visual field of the surgeon the bowel and major vessels may be damaged. The power setting needed for intrauterine laser surgery is high, so damage can be extensive. If the surgeon recognizes the problem, a laparotomy should be performed to assess the damage as laparoscopy is not sufficient or reliable in these cases.

The Nd:YAG laser has a penetration of 6 mm into the tissues and therefore the surgeon needs to take the same precautions as when using electricity.

The argon or potassium titanyl phosphate (KTP) 532 lasers have a penetration of approximately 3 mm and require fewer precautions. The holmium:YAG laser seems to have even less penetration, approximately 1–2 mm, and this could be an advantage in some cases.

Laser procedures take much longer than electrosurgery; hence they increase the risk of fluid overload and should therefore only be used with continuous flow hysteroscopes or flexible hysteroscopes, which require less fluid. Flexible hysteroscopes, however, are more difficult for the beginner to use (Baggish and Baltoyannis, 1988).

There is one more pitfall in the tissue penetration. The endometrium is not a homogeneous layer and in adenomyosis crypts of endometrial tissue infiltrate the myometrium and facilitate conduction of both electricity and laser energy far deeper than would be expected in myometrium.

In an unpublished study on the follow-up of 70 patients after endometrial resection after 3, 6, 9 and 12 months, both with hysteroscopy and vaginal endosonography, we found lesions up to 3 mm from the serosa as measured by vaginal ultrasound in 3% of patients. The healing of the endometrial wound takes many months and hysteroscopically stabilization of scar tissue occurs only after nine months, thus explaining some of the delayed complications.

There is no evidence that hysteroscopic surgery causes displaced fragments of endometrium to seed and to produce endometriosis or encourages metastasis of endometrial carcinoma cells (Labastida *et al.*, 1991).

Anesthesia

Local Anesthesia

The main problems that may be encountered when using local anesthesia are anxiety, vasovagal reaction and pain. Most patients are understandably anxious when entering the hysteroscopy room. Not all patients are suitable for outpatient hysteroscopy and hysteroscopic surgery (Magos *et al.*, 1989). It is important to create a relaxed setting, which includes a gynecologic examination chair or couch, and above all, good communication between the surgeon and the patient.

Traction on the cervix itself and dilatation may cause a vasovagal reaction. The patient may feel unwell and have a slow pulse rate and a fall in blood pressure. Vagal reactions can be prevented by giving atropine 0.6 mg by intramuscular injection approximately 20 minutes before the procedure. Glaucoma is uncommon, but should be excluded before this drug is given. The patient has to be warned about blurred vision afterwards and it is advisable to ask patients to provide transport and an escort to take them home.

Pain results from dilatation of the cervix beyond Hegar 5–6 and also from overdilatation of the uterine cavity with CO_2. Pain can be diminished by preoperative administration of naproxen sodium 500 mg by rectal suppository two hours before the

Table 64.2 Recommended doses of commonly used anesthetics.

Local anesthetic	Maximum doses without vasoconstrictor	Maximum doses with vasoconstrictor
Lignocaine (1–2%) (Xylocaine)	200 mg	500 mg
Mepivacaine (1–2%) (Scandicaine, Carbocaine)	300 mg	500 mg
Prilocaine (1–2%) (Citanest)	400 mg	600 mg

Xylocaine, Scandicaine, Carbocaine and Citanest are manufactured by Astra, Sydney, Australia.

operation and/or by using a local anesthetic in a paracervical block.

The recommended doses of the commonly used anesthetics are shown in Table 64.2. The preparations are effective in 2–3 minutes and provide good pain relief for up to 30 minutes. The effect is prolonged threefold by combination with vasoconstrictive agents, but these are rarely necessary in office hysteroscopy where most procedures are of short duration.

COMPLICATIONS OF LOCAL ANESTHETICS

Provided the dosage is within accepted limits and care is taken to avoid an intravascular injection, complications are rare, although toxic reactions can occur. It is therefore imperative for the hysteroscopist to recognize and deal with them:

- An inhibiting effect on the conduction system of the heart may be caused by rapid absorption from the injection site, accidental intravascular injection or exceeding the maximum dose. The cardiac effect is manifest as bradycardia, cardiac arrest, shock or convulsions. The emergency treatment is atropine 0.5 mg IV immediately, intubation and oxygen at a rate of 4–6 l min⁻¹, adrenaline 0.5–1.0 ml IV of 1:1000 solution, and respiratory and cardiac resuscitation.
- An excitatory effect on the central nervous system may be caused by the same factors. The signs are drowsiness, tremor or convulsions and above all paresthesia of the tongue and the perioral area. The treatment is diazepam 10–20 mg IV immediately and respiratory support.
- Allergic reactions are mainly caused by hypersensitivity to the distension medium. Agitation, palpitations, pruritis, urticaria,

coughing, bronchospasm, shock and possibly convulsions occur after a very short period of time – usually within minutes. The emergency treatment is adrenaline 0.5 ml (1 : 1000) SC or IM, clemastine 2 mg (2 ml) IV, prednisolone 25 IV, aminophylline 240 mg (10 ml) slowly IV over several minutes, and supportive measures including IV fluids and oxygen.

General Anesthesia

General anesthesia should be administered with controlled positive pressure respiration and an endotracheal tube for all diagnostic and operative hysteroscopies and for combined laparoscopy and hysteroscopy. This is especially the case when CO_2 is used as the distension medium. CO_2 absorption leads to a raised plasma level of CO_2, especially if there is an associated hypoxia, as is often the case during the induction of the anesthesia. The blood pH falls and there is release of catecholamines, which in turn leads to vasoconstriction, raised central venous pressure and cardiac arrhythmias. The side effects of CO_2 absorption can usually be prevented by hyperventilation with 30% oxygen, although complications can occur if the patient has a metabolic acidemia even if there has been compensation.

Contraindications to Hysteroscopy

Absolute Contraindications

The one and only absolute contraindication is an inexperienced endoscopist. There is no area of gynecologic surgery that can result in such sudden and catastrophic disaster as a result of a lack of adequate supervised training.

Relative Contraindications

These are:

- Infection.
- Cardiorespiratory disease.
- Metabolic acidosis.
- Pregnancy.
- Uterine bleeding.
- Occult cervical malignancy.

Infection

Sometimes we have to perform an operation with an IUCD *in situ* in the nongravid uterus when we become aware that there is endometritis. It is then necessary to treat the patient for 48 hours with broad spectrum antibiotics (Salat-Baroux, 1984).

Cardiorespiratory Disease

As most of the operations are performed under general anesthesia there should be adequately controlled respiration with an endotracheal tube or a laryngeal mask. This should limit the risks. If CO_2 is used under local anesthesia or without anesthesia, cardiopulmonary disease is an absolute contraindication.

Metabolic Acidosis

This condition should be corrected before any surgery.

Pregnancy

If operative hysteroscopy must be performed in pregnancy it should be before the tenth week of gestation with a flow of 50 ml min^{-1} and a maximum pressure of 100 mm Hg. As the gestational sac does not adhere completely to the uterine cavity there should be no mechanical trauma and as the optic nerve does not function before the tenth week there should be no risk of damage to that nerve (Lindemann and Lueken, 1978).

Uterine Bleeding

This condition requires more experience in hysteroscopy or in practice with the hysteroscope, but is not a contraindication to surgery. The continuous flow hysteroscope allows good visibility, even in the presence of active bleeding.

Occult Cervical Malignancy

Operative hysteroscopy should not be performed in the presence of cervical or endometrial malignancy and if recognized during the procedure, the appropriate biopsies should be taken, the neoplasm should be staged according to the International Federation of Gynecology and Obstetrics (FIGO) criteria, the operative procedure should be discontinued and the patient's future treatment planned in the conventional manner.

References

Baggish MS, Baltoyannis P (1988) New techniques for laser ablation of the endometrium in high risk patients. *American Journal of Obstetrics and Gynecology* **159**: 287–292.

Baggish MS, Daniell JF (1989) Death caused by air embolism associated with Nd:YAG laser surgery and artificial sapphire tips. *American Journal of Obstetrics and Gynecology* **161**: 877–878.

Baumann R, Magos A, Kay JDS, Turnbull AC (1990) Absorption of glycine irrigating solution during transcervical resection of the endometrium. *British Medical Journal* **300**: 304–305.

DeCherney A, Polan MH (1983) Hysteroscopic management of intrauterine lesions and intractable uterine bleeding. *Obstetrics and Gynecology* **61**: 392–397.

DeCherney AH, Diamond MP, Lavy G, Polan ML (1987) Endometrial ablation for intractable uterine bleeding: hysteroscopic resection. *Obstetrics and Gynecology* **70**: 668–670.

Gallinat A (1978) Metromat – a new insufflation apparatus for hysteroscopy. *Endoscopy* **3**: 234.

Goldrath MH, Fuller T, Segal S (1981) Laser photovaporization of endometrium for treatment of menorrhagia. *American Journal of Obstetrics and Gynecology* **140**: 14–19.

Haning RV *et al.* (1980) Preservation of fertility by transcervical resection of a benign mesodermal uterine tumor with a resectoscope and glycine distension medium. *Fertility and Sterility* **39**: 209.

Labastida R, Montesinos M, Cararach M *et al.* (1991) Endometrial carcinoma and hysteroscopy. In van Herendael B, Slangen T, Martens P (eds) *Operative Endoscopy, Practical Aspects*. pp. 52–58. Antwerp: Gyntech.

Leake JF, Murphy AA, Zacur HA (1987) Non-cardiogenic pulmonary oedema: a complication of operative hysteroscopy. *Obstetrics and Gynecology* **48**: 497.

Lindemann HJ (1972) The use of CO_2 in the uterine cavity for hysteroscopy. *International Journal of Fertility* **17**: 221.

Lindemann HJ (1975) Komplikationen bei der CO_2 Hysteroskopie. *Archiv für Gynäkologie* 219.

Lindemann HJ (1983) The choice of distension medium in hysteroscopy. In Van der Pas H, van Herendael B, Van Lith D, Keith L (eds) *Hysteroscopy*. p. 83. Lancaster: MTP Press.

Lindemann HJ, Lueken RP (1978) Transcervical amniocentesis via hysteroscopy within the first three months of pregnancy. In Philips J (ed.) *Endoscopy in Gynecology*.

Downey, CA: American Association of Gynecologic Laparoscopists.

Magos A, Baumann R, Cheung K, Turnbull AC (1989) Intrauterine surgery under intravenous sedation as an out-patient alternative to hysterectomy (letter). *Lancet* **ii**: 925–926.

Martens P (1991) Basic notions for the endoscopic nurse. In van Herendael B, Slangen T, Martens P (eds) *Operative Endoscopy, Practical Aspects*. pp. 6–9. Antwerp: Gyntech.

McLucas B (1991) Hyskon complications in hysteroscopic surgery. *Obstetrical and Gynecological Survey* **46**: 196–200.

Neuwirth RS, Amin HK (1976) Excision of submucous fibroids with hysteroscopic control. *American Journal of Obstetrics and Gynecology* **126**: 95–97.

Salat-Baroux J (1984) Complications. In Hamou J (ed.) *Hysteroscopie et Microcolpohysteroscopie Atlas et Traité*. pp. 79–84. Palermo: COFESE.

Siegler AM (1983) Risks and complications of hysteroscopy. In Van der Pas H, van Herendael B, Van Lith D, Keith L (eds) *Hysteroscopy*. pp. 75–80. Lancaster: MTP Press.

Siegler AM, Valle RF (1988) Therapeutic hysteroscopic procedures. *Fertility and Sterility* **80**: 685.

Slangen T (1991) Adaption of a conventional operating theatre to a practical set-up for endoscopic surgery. In van Herendael B, Slangen T, Martens P (eds) *Operative Endoscopy, Practical Aspects*. pp. 19–21. Antwerp: Gyntech.

Sugimoto O, Ushiroyama T, Fukuda Y (1984) Diagnostic and therapeutic hysteroscopy for traumatic intrauterine adhesions. In Siegler AM, Lindemann HJ (eds) *Hysteroscopy, Principles and Practice*. pp. 58–62. Philadelphia: JB Lippincott.

Taylor PJ, Leader A, George RE (1984) Combined laparoscopy and hysteroscopy in the investigation of infertility. In Siegler AM, Lindemann J (eds) *Hysteroscopy, Principles and Practice*. pp. 207–210. Philadelphia: JB Lippincott.

Valle RE, Sciarra JJ (1986) Hysteroscopic treatment of the septate uterus. *Obstetrics and Gynecology* **67**: 253.

van Herendael BJ (1988) Hysteroscopy in infertility. *Pakistan Journal of Obstetrics and Gynaecology* **1**: 136–147.

Wamsteker K (1991) Fluid intravasation: risk and management. In van Herendael B, Slangen T, Martens P (eds) *Operative Endoscopy, Practical Aspects*. pp. 81–83. Antwerp: Gyntech.

Witz CA, Silverberg KM, Bburns WN, Schenken RS, Olive DC (1993) Complications associated with the absorption of hysteroscopic fluid media. *Fertility and Sterility* **60**: 745–756.

The Future

65

Fetal Surgery

JOSEPH P. BRUNER

Vanderbilt University Medical Center, Nashville, Tennessee, USA

Enthusiasm for the use of fetal endoscopy has waxed and waned since the first intrauterine procedure was performed during pregnancy more than 40 years ago (Westin, 1954). Initially, fetal endoscopy enjoyed a slow but steady growth in popularity as an increasing number of medical centers worldwide developed indications for direct examination of the fetus, fetal blood sampling and fetal tissue biopsy in families at risk (Rodeck, 1980; Rodeck and Nicolaides, 1983; Elias, 1983; Rodeck and Nicolaides, 1986; Romero *et al.*, 1986; Elias, 1987). In 1958, however, the first reported use of diagnostic ultrasound in clinical obstetrics and gynecology appeared in the literature (Donald *et al.*, 1958). With the introduction of real-time ultrasonography several years later, the collection of fetal fluid and tissue specimens by manipulation of fine needles under continuous ultrasonographic guidance became practical, and many of the more invasive endoscopic procedures became obsolete (Holzgreve and Golbus, 1984; Golbus *et al.*, 1989; Bakharev *et al.*, 1990; Buckshee *et al.*, 1991; Evans *et al.*, 1991; Lynch and Berkowitz, 1992; Holbrook *et al.*, 1993). During the late 1980s to the mid 1990s obstetric endoscopic procedures were rarely performed.

It now appears that the technical limits of ultrasound resolution are being reached. At the same time, the expanding role of minimally invasive approaches to the diagnosis and treatment of human illnesses has caused a resurgence of interest in fetal endoscopy. Instruments and techniques developed by general surgeons, gynecologists and other surgical subspecialists have been adapted and modified for obstetric use. Indeed, it sometimes seems that the introduction of innovative endoscopic therapies for specific fetal abnormalities is limited only by the rarity of the conditions suitable for such intervention. This chapter will provide an overview of current applications of fetal endoscopy.

Embryoscopy and Fetoscopy

The term embryo is correctly used to describe the developing child from conception to the end of the eighth menstrual week. The fetal period extends from week nine to delivery. In spite of this well-established terminology, 'embryoscopy' is commonly used to refer to intrauterine endoscopic procedures performed by the transcervical route. 'Fetoscopy', on the other hand, commonly identifies the transabdominal approach to fetal endoscopy. Recently, the terms 'needle embryofetoscopy' (NEF) (Reece *et al.*, 1994) and 'thin-gauge embryofetoscopy' (TGEF) (Quintero *et al.*, 1993a) have been introduced to describe the direct visualization of the embryo or fetus with thin-gauge needles and fiberoptic endoscopes passed transabdominally into the amniotic cavity.

Optical Systems Used in Fetal Endoscopy

Endoscopic fiberoptics employs bundles of long thin fibers aligned from one end of the instrument to the other. These fibers propagate captured light along their entire length with very little energy loss. The fibers can be engineered for maximal light transmission by manipulating such construction variables as fiber composition, the reflectance angle of captured light, and fiber length. The individual fibers are flexible and free to move except at the ends of the instrument where they are fixed. Fiberoptic endoscopes are therefore ideal for surgical situations that cannot be easily approached with rigid instruments. Since each individual fiber is self-contained, instruments can be custom made to the specific needs of each procedure. Within each device, some of the fibers transmit light from the light source, while the rest carry the optical image. Since more fibers generally translate into a clearer image, smaller fiber optic endoscopes usually have poorer image quality. The smallest instruments commonly used in fetoscopic procedures are 0.5 mm and 0.7 mm in diameter, with 3000 and 6000 fibers, respectively.

The image transmitted through the usual glass fiber is degraded by the variety of reflectance angles the light beam encounters. 'Solid lens systems' attempt to overcome this loss due to scattering by focusing the image onto a single plane. Solid rod lenses are not commonly used in fetal endoscopy.

'Multiple lens systems', the workhorses of laparoscopy, transmit light through a rigid hollow tube filled with air. The image is focused by a series of lenses arranged within the tube. The outer wall of these instruments carries the light fibers used to illuminate the field of view. Multiple lens systems have the advantages over other optical systems of a larger field of view for a given diameter, and more efficient light transmission. However, significant physical limitations restrict wide use of these instruments in early gestation – multiple lens system endoscopes are rigid and smaller diameter instruments have difficulty transmitting sufficient light to the target. The light carrying capacity of these systems is a function of area and is reduced to 25% by every reduction in diameter of 50%. Some of the size limitation has been overcome by the development of brighter light sources.

Embryoscopy

Early endoscopic efforts to visualize the products of conception used the natural entrance to the uterine cavity, the cervix. In these early procedures, the terminal objective lens of a contact hysteroscope was placed directly against the presenting fetal membranes, often without the need for maternal analge-

sia or cervical dilation. Hence, this technique came to be known as 'contact embryoscopy'. The first report of direct intrauterine observation of the fetus and fetal adnexa using this approach was by Westin (1954) at the Karolinska Institute in Sweden. A rigid 10 mm hysteroscope was inserted through the cervix of three women undergoing pregnancy termination at 16–20 weeks. In Venezuela embryoscopy was performed in 118 pregnant patients using rigid hysteroscopes 20–28 F (7 to 10 mm) in diameter (Agüero *et al.*, 1966). Most of the subjects were near term, however, and the most common indication for endoscopy was to observe the color of the amniotic fluid. Only one woman was studied in the first trimester of pregnancy, and one procedure was performed in the second trimester. Gallinat *et al.* (1978), attempted embryoscopy in women scheduled for abortion at 5–12 weeks, but only successfully visualized the embryo after 7 weeks. The first systematic study of fetuses in early pregnancy was reported by Dubuisson *et al.* (1979), who performed contact embryoscopy in 50 patients before termination of pregnancy at 8–12 weeks. Using a 6 mm contact hysteroscope, the fetal extremities were visualized in 41 cases. Using a similar technique, embryoscopy was performed in 30 women in whom fetal limb anomalies had previously been detected on ultrasonographic examination (Roume *et al.*, 1985). More than 50% of the extremity malformations were confirmed by transcervical endoscopic visualization of the fetus at 18–22 weeks' gestation.

Ghirardini (1991) was the first researcher to stress the importance of perforating the chorion to observe the human fetus more clearly through the transparent amnion. Without the aid of ultrasonography, an endoscope with an outer diameter of 4 mm and a length of 30 cm was inserted transcervically in 100 women at 8–13 weeks' gestation. The fetus was visualized in 75% of the cases, and all but two were followed immediately by pregnancy termination. In two women, pregnancy was continued to term and normal infants were delivered. An additional 62 procedures were performed at 7–12 weeks' gestation using a specially designed instrument 30 cm in length with a 2.7 mm outer diameter and a 70° viewing angle. No instances of amnion rupture, uterine perforation or postoperative infection were reported, although again all pregnancies were terminated after study.

Dumez (1988) provided the first report of first trimester embryoscopy in a large number of continuing pregnancies. Transcervical endoscopy was performed in more than 50 women, with a reported miscarriage rate of 7%.

The first contemporary description of embryoscopy was published by Cullen *et al.* (1990) at Yale

University. Using a modification of the technique developed by Dumez, embryoscopy was performed in the first trimester in 100 women scheduled for elective termination of pregnancy. Rigid fiberoptic endoscopes 30 cm in length with diameters ranging from 2–3.5 mm and a wide-angle 0° lens were used. With the patient in the dorsal lithotomy position, the vagina was cleansed with betadine. A sterile speculum was placed in the vagina, and the anterior cervix was grasped with a single tooth tenaculum. Using continuous ultrasonographic guidance, the endoscope was inserted through the uterine cervix. The chorionic membrane was punctured bluntly with the tip of the endoscope, allowing the yolk sac, vitelline vessels, and chorionic plate to be directly observed within the extracoelomic cavity. The embryo was visualized through the transparent amnion (Figure 65.1). Complete examination of the fetus included views of the head, face, dorsal and ventral surfaces, limbs and umbilical cord insertion. With experience, the length of time required to insert the endoscope and complete the examination was about two minutes. Chorionic perforation and visualization of the

embryo was accomplished in 96% of cases. The amnion was ruptured in five cases, all at gestational ages of 11 weeks or over, leading the authors to conclude that the ideal time for embryoscopy is at 7.5–11 menstrual weeks' gestation. Embryoscopy was performed in 12 women with complete or partial placenta previa, resulting in bleeding or placental separation in five.

In a follow-up study, 14 women scheduled for elective termination of pregnancy underwent transcervical endoscopic confirmation of congenital anomalies at 14–19 menstrual weeks' gestation. Unlike first trimester embryoscopy, in which amniotic entry was rare (5%), membrane rupture occurred in 79% of cases in the second trimester. The larger size of the fetus in the second trimester also made complete visualization of anatomy more difficult (Cullen *et al.*, 1991).

Overwhelming reluctance to perform embryoscopy in continuing pregnancies proved an insurmountable obstacle to the full development of this once promising technique. In one dramatic example of first trimester diagnosis, embryoscopy was used to identify cleft lip at 11 weeks' gestation in a fetus

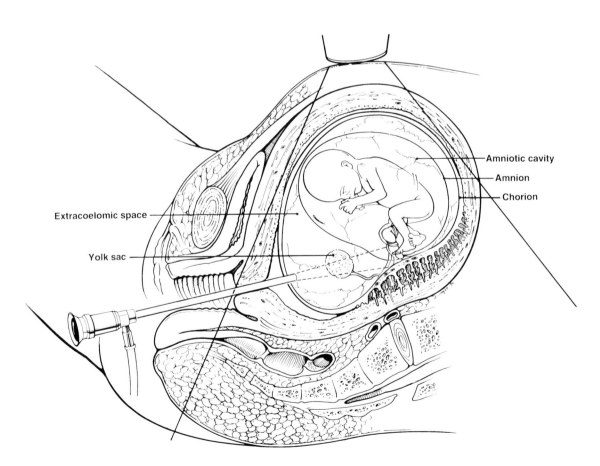

Figure 65.1 The tip of the endoscope is located within the extracoelomic cavity, allowing the fetus to be observed through the transparent amnion.

at risk for the Van der Woude's syndrome (Dommergues *et al.*, 1995). In another demonstration, fetal blood was successfully obtained from vessels in the chorionic plate or umbilical cord in five of eight attempted cases in pregnancies scheduled for termination at 8–12 weeks' gestation (Reece *et al.*, 1993). These potential applications of embryoscopy, however, never became widespread.

In a recent review of transcervical embryoscopy, Reece (1992) speculated about the potential role of this experimental procedure in modern obstetric care. Embryoscopy has been used for the first trimester diagnosis of structural fetal anomalies, and in experienced hands allows visualization of the fetus in 95% of cases with an average operating time of less than five minutes. The technique has been used to obtain fetal blood in the first trimester in a small number of cases, and may allow fetal tissue biopsy as well. Other benefits include the potential for expanding our current knowledge of human embryology and access to the developing embryo for possible stem cell or gene therapy.

Documented risks of embryoscopy include bleeding, infection and amnion rupture. Although the risks of bleeding and infection should be no greater than those of transcervical chorionic villous sampling (CVS), almost all reported cases have been performed in women undergoing termination of pregnancy. The only data available about risks in continuing pregnancies, obtained from a small number of unpublished cases, quotes a pregnancy loss rate of 7% (Dumez, 1988). The risk of amnion rupture increases dramatically with fusion of the membranes at the end of the first trimester (Cullen *et al.*, 1990; Cullen *et al.*, 1991; Reece, 1992). The risk of inadvertent amniotomy is minimized when embroscopy is performed at 7.5–11 weeks' gestation. Because of these limitations, transcervical embryoscopy has been largely replaced by transabdominal fetoscopy using thin-gauge endoscopes. One possible role that remains for embryoscopy is the confirmation of fetal structural anomalies identified by high resolution ultrasonography before pregnancy termination by suction curettage.

Fetoscopy

The transabdominal approach to direct visualization of the fetus was first used by Mandelbaum *et al.* (1967). Using a 16-gauge needle for illumination and a 14-gauge needle for observation, the maternal abdomen was entered percutaneously and the instruments advanced into the amniotic cavity without the aid of ultrasonographic guidance.

Although the instrumentation was crude by today's standards, and fetal viewing was limited by the narrow field of view, the fetus and placenta were directly observed and the first fetoscopic photographs were recorded. Although the procedure was confined to visualizing the fetus, the authors foresaw the day when hematologic testing and direct intravascular transfusion of the fetus would become possible.

Valenti (1972) used a modified pediatric cystoscope with an 18 F (6 mm) diameter to perform fetoscopy in 11 women undergoing abortion by hysterotomy at 14–18 weeks' gestation. Following preoperative localization of the placenta by ultrasonography, a laparotomy incision was made under general or regional anesthesia and the instrument was placed in utero. Skin biopsy specimens were successfully obtained from five fetuses, and 0.1–0.2 ml of pure fetal blood was aspirated from the abdominal cord insertion of three patients with a 27-gauge needle. After completion of the fetal biopsy procedures, the endoscope was removed and the insertion site secured uneventfully with a pursestring suture (Valenti, 1973). Using a similar technique, Scrimgeour (1976), who was the first to use the term 'fetoscopy', examined six fetuses at increased risk of myelomeningocele using a 2.2 mm endoscope. Direct visual inspection of the fetus was negative in three cases and normal babies were subsequently delivered at term. In one patient, a fetus with spina bifida was inadvertently impaled by the trocar on entry into the uterus. In a second case, fetoscopic examination of the fetus was considered to be normal, but an infant with myelomeningocele was delivered preterm. In a third patient, fetoscopy was negative, but the normal fetus miscarried 48 hours postoperatively after a large fetomaternal hemorrhage.

With major advances in both instrumentation and technique, successful outpatient percutaneous fetoscopy with local anesthesia was reported in 27 of 28 patients scheduled for therapeutic abortion at 15–20 weeks' gestation (Hobbins *et al.*, 1974). Using the well-known Needlescope (Dyonics, Woburn, Massachusetts, USA), a fiberoptic endoscope 15 cm in length and 1.7 mm in diameter, introduced through a 14-gauge needle with A-mode ultrasonographic guidance, fetal examination was performed and skin biopsies obtained. Only one procedure was abandoned because of bloody fluid after entering the uterus through an anterior placenta. In a further report, Hobbins and Mahoney (1974) aspirated blood from an additional eight women before therapeutic abortion at 15–20 weeks' gestation. Using a 27-gauge needle inserted under direct observation into a fetal vessel on the chorionic plate, 0.05–0.5 ml of blood was aspirated. However, pure fetal blood was obtained from only one sample. Using the same instrumentation, Rodeck and Campbell (1978) obtained pure fetal blood by sampling fetal vessels in the umbilical cord, rather than the chorionic plate. This technique proved so successful that it was subsequently used to perform direct intravascular fetal blood transfusions in two pregnancies complicated by rhesus isoimmunization (Rodeck *et al.*, 1981).

The classic approach to fetoscopy reached its zenith during the decade from the mid 1970s to the mid 1980s. The fourth meeting of the International Fetoscopy Group in 1982 reported almost 4000 procedures from 24 programs worldwide. Of these procedures 75% were performed for fetal blood sampling to test for fetal blood type, hemoglobinopathy, congenital infection, karyotype, coagulation disorder, metabolic disorder, genetic disorder, and blood cell deficiency. Direct visualization of the fetus was used to identify abnormal surface anatomy beyond the capabilities of ultrasonography available at the time. Fetal skin sampling was used for the prenatal diagnosis of a variety of hereditary skin disorders or clinical syndromes. Finally, fetal liver biopsy was performed to diagnose inherited metabolic disorders not detectable by other methods. Even at the height of its popularity, however, fetoscopy was beset with significant difficulties. The greatest of these was that the technique required a high level of operator expertise, thus limiting its application to a few diagnostic centers. Even in capable hands, the spontaneous abortion rate after fetoscopy was 6.8% for fetal blood sampling, and 7.7% overall. The rate of perinatal loss was 1.4% after fetal blood sampling, and 2.1% overall (International Fetoscopy Group, 1984).

In the 1980s the introduction of high resolution ultrasound imaging permitted noninvasive diagnosis of many congenital anomalies which had previously required fetoscopic confirmation. In addition, advances in molecular genetics made it possible to analyze DNA from amniotic fluid fibroblasts and chorionic villi to diagnose many genetic disorders. Finally, fetal blood sampling, skin biopsy, muscle and liver biopsy were all performed under direct ultrasonographic guidance. In 1985, Daffos *et al.* (1985) reported successfully obtaining fetal blood in more than 600 cases of cordocentesis performed solely with ultrasonographic guidance, and the era of classic fetoscopy came to an end.

TGEF and NEF

TGEF and NEF are competing terms for the same new endoscopic technique in which a thin flexible fiberoptic device is introduced transabdominally into the uterus through a small gauge needle. This procedure was first described in 15 women undergoing first trimester termination at 8–12 weeks' gestation (Pennehouat *et al.*, 1992). After administration of general anesthesia, a 21-gauge spinal needle 15 cm in length was placed transabdominally under direct ultrasonographic guidance into the amniotic cavity. A 0.5 mm flexible fiberoptic endoscope 50 cm in length, with a 55° field of vision and 1–20 mm depth of field was inserted through the needle sheath, connected to a xenon light source, and a video camera with monitor was attached to the eyepiece. Visualization of the ventral surface of the fetus was accomplished in every case in less than 15 minutes (mean duration five minutes, range 2–15 minutes).

Quintero *et al.* (1993a) coined the term 'thin-gauge embryofetoscopy' in a study of 28 women undergoing first- or second-trimester pregnancy termination from 7–20 weeks of gestation. A later report brought the total number of patients to 57, with a range of gestational ages from 5.5–20 weeks (Quintero *et al.*, 1993b). Fiberoptic endoscopes as small as 0.5 mm were delivered through a 21-gauge needle, although the examination was hampered by the shallow depth of field and the narrow field of vision. Most procedures were performed using a 0.7 mm endoscope placed through an 18- or 19-gauge needle specially designed for easy aspiration or irrigation with a blunt tip perforated with lateral holes and a hub with a checkflow-valve mechanism and side arm (Cook OB/GYN, Spencer, Indiana, USA). Before fusion of the amnion and chorion at 12–13 weeks' gestation, an attempt was made to guide the needle tip into the chorionic sac outside the amnion. Beyond this age, the needle was placed intraamniotically. After 16 weeks' gestation, fetal blood sampling was performed at the placental cord insertion site. TGEF was successful in 84% of subjects. The procedure could not be completed:

- In three patients at less than six weeks' gestation.
- In a patient with a severely retroverted uterus.
- In two obese women.
- In two pregnancies with turbid fluid due to open myelomeningocele and omphalocele, respectively.
- In one case with bloody fluid.

Extracoelomic placement of the needle could not be achieved in 35% of patients less than 12 weeks' gestation, and the amnion was entered inadvertently. Interestingly, the authors found direct visualization of the fetus after intraamniotic needle insertion to be superior to examination performed through the amniotic membrane with the needle in the extracoelomic space. In fact, a fetus with

Meckel–Gruber syndrome was successfully identified at 11 gestational weeks using the intra-amniotic approach (Quintero *et al.*, 1993a). All attempts at fetoscopic cordocentesis after 16 weeks' gestation were successful.

Transabdominal NEF was performed in 12 patients scheduled for first trimester abortion at 8–12 weeks as well as one continuing pregnancy (Reece *et al.*, 1994). A specially designed 16-gauge double-barrel instrument sheath equipped with a 0.8 mm fiberoptic endoscope and a 27-gauge needle was inserted transabdominally under ultrasonographic guidance into the amniotic cavity. Following examination of the fetus, the 27-gauge needle was directed into an umbilical vessel and a sample of fetal blood was aspirated. Inspection of fetal anatomy was completed in all cases, and fetal blood sampling was successful in all but three. The mean duration of the procedure was ten minutes. In a subsequent report, more than 20 cases of NEF were described, including one in which a suspected myelomeningocele was excluded by direct fetal examination at 15 weeks in a continuing pregnancy (Reece *et al.*, 1995). A normal full-term female infant was eventually delivered vaginally without complications. Hobbins *et al.* (1994) confirmed the diagnosis of Smith–Lemli–Opitz syndrome, type II, in an 11-week fetus with transvaginal ultrasonographic findings of a nuchal membrane and bilateral polydactyly. Using real-time ultrasonographic guidance with local anesthesia, an 18-gauge needle was inserted into the amniotic cavity, the stylet was removed, and a 0.75 mm flexible endoscope was placed through the lumen of the needle. The identification of polydactyly by direct visualization of the fetal hand confirmed the diagnosis in the at-risk fetus in less than 15 minutes.

The major roles of embryofetoscopy today are:

- Detection of small external structural anomalies that cannot be visualized easily even with transvaginal ultrasonographic imaging.
- Accurate description of embryologic development.

Although commercially available instruments are small enough to be passed through an amniocentesis needle, adding only a few minutes to the procedure, fetal fluid and tissue specimens are routinely obtained with fine needles under direct ultrasonographic rather than fetoscopic guidance. Fetoscopes are occasionally used as teaching aids during the evaluation of new percutaneous techniques (Evans *et al.*, 1994). Enormous potential exists for the development of first trimester cordocentesis and novel therapies such as stem cell transplantation and gene therapy.

Procedure-related risks of bleeding, infection, and amniotic fluid leakage have been minimized with the introduction of smaller endoscopes. Although the total number of patients studied is still too small to determine pregnancy loss rates with accuracy, it is reasonable to assume that risks are similar to those associated with transabdominal amniocentesis, which uses needles of the same caliber. The main limitations of fine NEF are the shallow depth of field (approximately 2–15 mm) and the narrow field of view (approximately 5 mm diameter at 1 cm). This results from a compromise between the number of optical versus light fibers that can be incorporated in ever-smaller endoscopes (currently 3000 fibers in a 0.5 mm flexible endoscope to 6000 fibers in a 0.7 mm instrument).

Early concerns about the possible teratogenic effects of thermal or light energy transmitted to the developing fetus have been largely allayed by appropriate laboratory studies and clinical surveillance of continuing pregnancies. Using an *in vitro* model, no temperature change could be elicited when using the endoscope for as long as 30 minutes (Quintero *et al.*, 1993b). Although teratogenic effects have been observed in chick embryos exposed to white light for prolonged periods (Aige-Gil and Murillo-Ferrol, 1992), no retinal damage could be detected when exposure time was limited to that more closely approximating the clinical situation (Quintero *et al.*, 1994a). Human infants born after performing transcervical embryoscopy in the first trimester manifested no apparent visual defects (Dumez and Daffos, 1990).

Fetoscopic Surgery

Improved instrumentation, a more complete understanding of the underlying pathophysiology of many fetal anomalies, and enhanced proficiency in endoscopic surgical techniques have fueled a proliferation of innovative approaches to fetal therapy over the past few years. While all these novel procedures share an imaginative application of fetoscopic techniques, it is useful for discussion purposes to differentiate procedures directed at the placenta and fetal adnexa from minimally invasive surgery of the fetus itself.

Endoscopic Surgery of the Placenta and Fetal Adnexa

The modern era of fetoscopic surgery began in 1990 when DeLia *et al.* (1990) at the University of Utah School of Medicine published a small case series announcing the use of the fetoscopic neodymium: yttrium-aluminum-garnet (Nd:YAG) laser for occlusion of placental vessels in ultrasonographically suspected cases of twin-to-twin transfusion syndrome (TTTS). TTTS is a serious complication of monochorionic twin pregnancies in which blood is shunted from one fetus (the donor) through placental vascular communications (chorioangiopagus) to the other fetus (the recipient). In some early reports, perinatal mortality in untreated cases was 100% (Weir et al., 1979). The theoretic basis of the novel application of fetoscopic laser technology in this disorder is that laser coagulation of interfetal vascular anastomoses on the placental surface of affected twins will prevent transfusion of the larger recipient twin by the smaller donor. After developing the surgical technique in a series of experiments in sheep and rhesus monkeys (DeLia et al., 1985; DeLia et al., 1989), the operation was performed in three women who developed acute polyhydramnios at 18.5, 22 and 22.5 weeks' gestation. Under general or regional anesthesia, a 10 cm laparotomy incision was created, followed by a stab wound through the uterine wall to the fetal membranes. A rigid fetoscope 25 cm in length was passed through a dual-channel oval cannula 3.85 × 2.9 mm in diameter into the amniotic cavity of the polyhydramniotic twin. After inserting the 400 μm Nd:YAG laser fiber into the operating channel of the endoscope, a video camera head was attached to the eyepiece. All vessels passing near the placental equator were identified, and the laser fiber was positioned 0.5–1.0 cm from the vessel and perpendicular to the vessel wall. Vessels were coagulated for 2–3 seconds over a length of 1 cm using a laser power output of 60 W. When all visible vessels had been coagulated, the fetoscope was removed and the stab wound was closed with a pursestring suture. The first two patients delivered at 27 and 34 weeks' gestation after premature rupture of the membranes and spontaneous labor, while the third patient developed severe preeclampsia at 29 weeks, requiring delivery. Four of the six infants survived. A later report brought the total number of patients evaluated for treatment to 35 (DeLia et al., 1995). Of the original 35 patients, five were excluded during preoperative examination, and four procedures were aborted shortly after uterine entry because the amniotic fluid was too bloody to allow adequate visualization of placental vessels, so 26 women underwent laser surgery. The 26 treated patients had a mean gestational age of 20.8 weeks (range 18–24 weeks). Six of these procedures were terminated prematurely because of excessive bleeding. Overall, 53% of treated fetuses survived, with a mean gestational age at delivery of 32.2 weeks (range 26–37 weeks), and a mean laser therapy-delivery interval of 11.7 weeks (range 6–17 weeks). Maternal operative morbidity was limited to one patient with upper gastrointestinal bleeding detected at the time of surgery, and complete wound dehiscence on the fifth postoperative day.

The largest series of patients treated for suspected TTTS with endoscopic laser photocoagulation of placental surface vessels was reported by Ville et al. (1995) at King's College, London. Using a rigid fetoscope 2 mm in diameter with a 75° field of view housed in a 2.7 mm cannula, placental anastomotic vessels were coagulated with a 400 μm Nd:YAG laser in 45 sets of twins. Technically, the procedure represented several major advances over that previously described, including a percutaneous approach under local anesthesia, aspiration and replacement of bloody fluid with Hartmann's solution, and treatment of the anterior placenta. Results, however, were remarkably similar to those achieved in the USA: the median gestational age at the time of surgery was 21 weeks (range 15–28 weeks); 53% of fetuses survived to delivery; the median gestational age at delivery was 35 weeks (range 25–40 weeks); and the median interval from surgery to delivery was 14 weeks (range 0–21 weeks).

Advocates of fetoscopic laser ablation of chorioangiopagus argue that theirs is the only therapy aimed specifically at the offending anastomotic vessels that make transfusion of blood from one twin to the other possible. As such, laser surgery of the placenta offers the opportunity for definitive treatment of this devastating obstetric complication. In spite of its application in a growing number of pregnancies, however, controversy continues to surround this innovative approach to the therapy of TTTS. First of all, antenatal diagnosis of TTTS is far from accurate. Bruner and Rosemond (1993) performed sequential cordocentesis in a series of patients with monochorionic diamniotic twin gestations, same fetal sex, a 'stuck twin' coexisting with a co-twin with subjective polyhydramnios, and fetal growth discordance over 20%. Even in this well-selected cohort, transfer of marked erythrocytes from the suspected donors to the suspected recipients could be documented in only 44% of cases. Since 'true' twin-to-twin transfusion may occur in less than 50% of those patients identified by currently accepted diagnostic criteria, concern exists about the application of endoscopic surgery in all suspected instances. For example, of the 30 patients DeLia et al. (1995) actually took to the operating room:

- Growth of one twin pair was concordant.
- 11 twin sets were within one week of each other.
- 13 twin pairs were only 2 weeks discordant.

- Only five twin pairs (16%) exhibited growth discordance of 3–4 weeks.

Similarly, some of the treated patients in the report from King's College (Ville *et al.*, 1995) were also concordant in growth. Furthermore, one of the pregnancies with suspected TTTS referred to DeLia *et al.* (1995) for evaluation underwent spontaneous resolution of abnormal ultrasonographic findings before arrival. Other misgivings center on the reported success rate of endoscopic surgery for TTTS of just over 50%. In the report from the UK (Ville *et al.*, 1995), for example, 42% of the donor fetuses died within 24 hours of endoscopy. In the series described from the USA (DeLia *et al.*, 1995), ten of the 30 cases in which the fetoscope was placed were terminated prematurely because of excessive bleeding or other complications. In contrast, Elliott *et al.* (1991) reported a survival rate of 79% among 17 cases of suspected TTTS managed only with aggressive decompression amniocentesis – a much less invasive approach than fetoscopic laser surgery that can be performed at any medical center. Elliott (1995) noted, in fact, that all women treated with laser surgery of placental vessels also underwent decompression of the polyhydramniotic sac of anywhere from 400–6500 ml, and suggested that the incidental amniocentesis may represent the source of any therapeutic benefit obtained from the operation. At the present time, no prospective randomized trial of fetoscopic laser occlusion of placental vessels versus serial decompression amniocentesis for the treatment of TTTS is planned. Until such a comparative study is undertaken, the least controversial role for fetoscopic laser surgery in this disorder is for very preterm fetuses with hydrops of one or both twins.

Twin reversed arterial perfusion sequence (TRAPS) is another unusual complication of monochorionic twin gestations in which the coexistence of artery-to-artery and vein-to-vein interfetal anastomoses leads to perfusion of a nonviable 'acardiac' twin by its anatomically normal co-twin. The added perfusion burden on the cardiovascular system of the normal 'pump' twin is the chief cause of increased morbidity and mortality for this fetus. Moore *et al.* (1990) studied the perinatal outcome in 49 twin pregnancies with TRAPS. The overall perinatal mortality of the 'pump' twin was 55%, but was greatest if the weight of the acardiac twin exceeded 70% that of the normal co-twin. Treatment of this ominous obstetric complication was revolutionized when Quintero *et al.* (1994b) successfully ligated the umbilical cord of an acardiac twin via transabdominal fetoscopy. At 19 weeks of gestation, the ultrasonographic measurement of the abdominal circumference of the acardiac twin was 156%

that of the normal co-twin. Under general anesthesia, two 12-gauge (28 mm) trocars were introduced percutaneously into the amniotic cavity using ultrasonographic guidance. A multi-lens endoscope 1.9 mm in diameter, 11 cm in length, and with a 5° field of view was inserted through one sheath and attached to a video camera with monitor. A 5 F (1.7 mm) semi-rigid automatic rat-tooth grasper was placed through the second port and used to pass two 1–0 polyglactin sutures around the umbilical cord of the acardiac fetus. The sutures were tied with a 19.5-gauge (1 mm) knot pusher, also inserted through the operating port. The suture ends were cut with a 5 F (1.7 mm) semi-rigid scissors. Cessation of blood flow through the ligated cord was confirmed with pulsed wave Doppler ultrasonography. The surviving infant delivered at 36 weeks' gestation after spontaneous rupture of membranes.

A second report of successful ligation of the umbilical cord of an acardiac fetus appeared shortly after (Willcourt *et al.*, 1995). At 24 weeks' gestation, the 'pump' twin developed nonimmune hydrops and cardiomegaly. Under general anesthesia, a paramedian laparotomy incision was created for uterine exposure. Under direct ultrasonographic guidance, a 10 mm viewing port and a 5 mm operating port were placed. Warm lactated Ringer's solution was used for continuous irrigation of the operating field. With direct endoscopic visualization, a 0 polydioxanone Endoloop suture (Ethicon, Somerville, New Jersey, USA) was passed through the operating port and two suture ligatures were placed around the umbilical cord of the acardiac twin. After removal of the instruments, the uterine incisions were closed with pursestring sutures. A liveborn infant was delivered by emergency cesarean section at 29 gestational weeks after the onset of preterm labor.

Endoscopic ligation of the umbilical cord of the acardiac fetus appears to be the most definitive and least morbid therapy currently available for the treatment of TRAPS. At the present time, the only controversy concerns timing of the procedure. Not enough cases have been performed to decide whether cord ligation should be performed prophylactically in every case of TRAPS, only in those cases in which the estimated size of the acardiac fetus exceeds 70% that of the normal fetus, or only when polyhydramnios, cardiomegaly, or nonimmune hydrops develops in the 'pump' twin.

DeLia *et al.* (1993) have suggested endoscopic laser photocoagulation of placental vessels for treatment of the acardiac twin in TRAPS and also for chorioangiomas associated with fetal compromise. To date, there are no reports that these procedures can be carried out successfully. There is some theoretic concern about the effects of laser surgery on the 'pump' twin in TRAPS, since one study of the same technique in TTTS resulted in death of the donor twin within 24 hours of surgery in 42% of reported cases (Ville *et al.*, 1995).

Endoscopic Surgery of the Fetus

The present generation has witnessed an astonishing array of stunning medical achievements that have changed the very way in which we think about human illness. Organ transplants, stem cell and gene therapy, the unraveling of the biochemical basis of mental illness, and victory over frightening new infectious organisms are just a few examples of sensational discoveries that have occurred in our lifetime. The public, however, never appears to lose its interest in new invasive fetal therapies. Virtually every revelation concerning a novel fetoscopic approach to a congenital malformation is greeted with headlines and cover stories. Minimally invasive fetal surgery is in every sense a new frontier awaiting development.

All endoscopic fetal surgery performed at this time must be considered experimental. Significant ethical issues involving disclosure of potential risks and benefits, case selection, and informed consent are therefore raised whenever an innovative fetal therapy is proposed. The International Fetal Medicine and Surgery Society has recommended guidelines for addressing ethical problems in investigational fetal therapy. The guidelines suggested are listed in Table 65.1. An earlier admonishment against innovative therapy in multiple gestation pregnancies has been relaxed so many times that it presently constitutes only a relative contraindication to treatment.

FETAL OBSTRUCTIVE UROPATHY

No fetal anomaly has been the target of as many innovative interventional therapies as congenital urethral obstruction. This is due primarily to the longstanding capability for ultrasonographic diagnosis of fetal urinary obstruction early in gestation. In addition, severe early obstruction usually leads to the development of lethal renal dysplasia (Bernstein, 1971) and pulmonary hypoplasia (Potter, 1946). Antenatal relief of the obstruction with restoration of amniotic fluid volume usually allows adequate pulmonary development and may decrease the severity of renal damage (Harrison *et al.*, 1982). *In utero* decompression of the urinary tract has been accomplished by continuous drainage of the fetal bladder into the amniotic cavity by placement of a double pigtail catheter or open cystotomy (Golbus *et al.*, 1982; Crombleholme *et al.*, 1988). The fine pigtail shunts currently in use, however, are notoriously prone to migration or obstruction, often requiring multiple reinsertion if placed during the midtrimester. Hysterotomy for open fetal surgery, on the other hand, is excessively morbid for the mother and associated with a high rate of fetal loss.

One innovative approach to fetal urethral obstruction early in the second trimester is creation of a cystotomy with an endoscopic argon laser probe (MacMahon *et al.*, 1992). Urethral obstruction was diagnosed ultrasonographically at 14 weeks' gestation because of the absence of amniotic fluid and megacystis. At 17.4 weeks, amnioinfusion of 200 ml of warmed sterile fluid was performed. A guide wire was placed through the amniocentesis needle and a 9 F (3 mm) sheath was introduced over the guide wire. A pediatric cystoscope was inserted through the sheath, and an argon laser probe was placed through the operating channel. Two small

Table 65.1 Guidelines for addressing ethical problems in experimental fetal therapy. (Adopted from Fletcher and Jonsen, 1991).

Only fetuses with a reasonable expectation of benefit from therapy should be considered for intervention

Lesions addressed should be isolated

A normal karyotype should be obtained

The mother and family should consent not only to treatment, but also to long-term perinatal and pediatric follow-up

A multidisciplinary team should develop a consensus plan for treatment and obtain approval from the appropriate Institutional Review Board

Experimental therapy should only be performed in a facility with immediate access to a tertiary care obstetric unit and neonatal intensive care unit

Both the parents and physicians should be free to request ethical or psychiatric consultation, if desired

---

openings were burned through the distended fetal abdomen resulting in the immediate release of large amounts of urine. Ultrasonographic surveillance documented a decompressed bladder and increased amniotic fluid. At 33 weeks' gestation, the bladder was again distended and the amniotic fluid volume decreased. The infant was delivered at 34 weeks with no respiratory distress, and the laser openings on the 'prune belly' of the newborn could not be found. Renal ultrasonography demonstrated only mild bilateral pelviceal dilation, and voiding cystourethrogram revealed bilateral vesicoureteric reflux and urethral obstruction. Although laser cystotomy proved successful in this single case report, the anticipated functional duration of the fistulous tract is unknown. Rapid healing of the cystotomy may require repetitive procedures to maintain decompression of the fetal urinary system.

An alternative approach to long-term bladder drainage has been performed by placing a wire mesh stent in fetal lambs (Estes et al., 1992). Time-dated pregnant ewes with surgically created urinary obstruction were placed under general anesthesia and laparotomy was performed to expose the pregnant uterus. A Veress needle was placed into the uterus and pneumometrium obtained by low-flow insufflation with carbon dioxide (CO_2) at a pressure of 3–5 cm H_2O. A 5 mm trocar was then inserted, and a 5 mm 0° endoscope was passed and attached to a xenon light source. Under direct endoscopic guidance, a second operating port was placed. A 16-gauge needle was then inserted into the distended fetal bladder under direct endoscopic guidance. After aspiration of urine, a 0.035 inch 'J' wire was passed into the bladder and the needle was removed. A Wallstent introducer (Schneider U.S. Stent, Inc., Minneapolis, Minnesota, USA) was passed over the guide wire into the bladder, and the wire mesh stent, 32 mm in length and 8 mm in diameter, was then deployed into the vesicoamniotic fistula. The pneumometrium was released, warmed Ringer's lactate with 1 g of penicillin was instilled, the instruments were removed, and pursestring sutures were used to close the uterine wounds.

The most innovative approach to the evaluation and treatment of fetal obstructive uropathy has been proposed by Quintero et al. (1995a). A fiberoptic endoscope was inserted through the lumen of the needle or trocar into the fetal bladder at the time of vesicocentesis or vesicoamniotic shunt placement, respectively. Direct visual examination of the fetal urethra, bladder neck, ureteral orifices and bladder mucosa was performed. Fetal cystoscopy was successful in 11 of 13 patients. The bladder mucosa appeared edematous or hemorrhagic in three cases. The ureteral orifices were adequately

visualized in nine of 11 fetuses, demonstrating dilation in five fetuses and ureteral webs in two others. A transurethral shunt was successfully placed in two of seven fetuses, while in an additional fetus urethral patency was achieved with urethral probing alone.

In another case (Quintero et al., 1995b) a fetus was evaluated ultrasonographically at 19 weeks' gestation and a distended bladder, dilated proximal urethra, bilateral hydroureters, bilateral pyelectasis, ascites, bilateral pleural effusions, and oligohydramnios were identified. Serial fine-needle vesicocentesis was performed to evaluate fetal renal function, and urine electrolyte, protein and osmolality determinations prognosticated a poor outcome. At the time of the first vesicocentesis procedure, a 0.7 mm fiberoptic endoscope was passed through the needle lumen into the fetal bladder and a diagnosis of posterior urethral valves was confirmed by direct observation. Although the fetus was judged to be a poor candidate for standard shunt placement, the parents consented to experimental endoscopic fulguration of the posterior urethral valves. At 22 weeks' gestation, under general anesthesia, a 10-gauge trocar was passed percutaneously into the fetal bladder using ultrasonographic guidance. A 2.5 mm steerable endoscope with a 1.3 mm operating channel was introduced and directed to the bladder neck. A soft-tip 0.025 inch wire guide was passed through the operating channel of the endoscope between the posterior urethral valves and into the amniotic cavity. The endoscope was advanced along the guide wire up to the valves, the guide was removed, and the valves were electrocoagulated with a 2 F (0.67 mm) ball-tip monopolar flexible electrode using 25 W of coagulating current. Frequent manual instillation of warmed lactated Ringer's solution through the operating channel of the endoscope aided in visualization of the operating field. Ultrasonographic follow-up demonstrated drainage of fluid through the patent urethra, resolution of the megacystis, thinning of the bladder wall, and resolution of the ascites and pleural effusions. Oligohydramnios persisted, however, and the 31-week newborn infant died of pulmonary hypoplasia. In the latest refinement of this technique, laser ablation of posterior urethral valves has now been accomplished by percutaneous fetal cystoscopy (Quintero, 1996).

CONGENITAL DIAPHRAGMATIC HERNIA (CDH)

After fetal obstructive uropathy, the developmental defect that has received the most attention from both the medical community and the general public is CDH. In babies that survive the newborn period, surgical repair is accomplished by removal of the herniated abdominal organs from the thorax and closure of the diaphragm. With modern surgical support, especially the recent introduction of extracorporeal membrane oxygenation (ECMO), neonatal survival approaches 50% (Harrison *et al.*, 1994). Severe pulmonary hypoplasia, however, results in neonatal mortality in many cases despite optimal postnatal therapy. At the present time, there is no consistently reliable means of discerning those fetuses likely to do well with standard therapy from those who will develop lethal pulmonary hypoplasia. Open fetal repair of CDH has been successfully performed in some instances, but like all surgical approaches using a hysterotomy incision, morbidity is common in both mother and fetus, usually as a result of intractable preterm labor. A review of unsuccessful cases of *in utero* correction of CDH has also led to the realization that when the fetal liver is incarcerated in the thorax, reduction will compromise umbilical blood flow and cause fetal death (Harrison *et al.*, 1993). Fetal therapy of CDH found itself at an impasse: if the fetal liver was positioned in the chest, *in utero* repair was unlikely to succeed; if the liver was not incarcerated, modern postnatal therapy was as likely to result in neonatal survival as antenatal correction.

While positioned thus at the crossroads of medical therapy, Hedrick *et al.* (1994a) reviewed 16 cases of congenital high airway obstruction (CHAOS) due to laryngeal atresia, tracheal stenosis, or rarely, subglottic stenosis. All cases were identified ultrasonographically by the presence of large echogenic lungs, flattened or inverted diaphragms, and dilated airways distal to the obstruction. These pathognomonic features of CHAOS develop because obstruction of lung fluid flow results in airway expansion. The authors noted that although only one infant survived the newborn period, the lungs, even in fatal cases, were histologically normal (Scurry *et al.*, 1989). Seizing upon this information, Hedrick *et al.* (1994b) proposed obstructing the flow of fluid from the lungs of fetuses with CDH in order to expand the airways and expel the abdominal contents from the chest, thus preventing pulmonary hypoplasia. This astonishing new concept was termed PLUG – 'plug the lung until it grows'. To test their hypothesis, a left-sided diaphragmatic hernia was created in 16 75-day-gestation fetal lambs (full term, 145 days). At 120 days the trachea was ligated in eight of the lambs. At 135–140 days, the fetuses were delivered and a tracheostomy performed. Newborns were ventilated for one hour and then killed. At autopsy, the abdominal viscera were reduced from the thorax of the lambs with a ligated trachea, while in the control lambs abdominal contents completely occupied the left chest. The

lungs of the ligated lambs had a higher dry weight, and at 60 minutes neonatal P_{O_2} was higher and P_{CO_2} lower. The authors concluded that 'plugging' the upper airway in the fetal lamb with a diaphragmatic hernia reduces the abdominal viscera from the chest, accelerates fetal lung growth, and improves oxygenation and ventilation after birth. Thus began a search for a reliable, reversible, and atraumatic technique of occluding the fetal trachea in CDH. Devices investigated in the fetal lamb CDH model included a foam-cuffed endotracheal tube, a foam-cuffed endotracheal tube modified with a magnetically controlled flow valve, and a tracheal insert constructed of a water-impermeable, expandable, polymeric foam placed by a translaryngeal approach (Bealer *et al.*, 1995).

Luks *et al.* (1994a) demonstrated the feasibility of *in utero* fetal tracheoscopy and esophagoscopy. Using a rigid 5 mm endoscope and a 3 mm steerable choledochoscope, the upper respiratory and gastrointestinal tracts were examined in six fetal lambs. The esophagus was visualized into the fetal stomach, and the trachea was visualized to the level of the right upper segment bronchus without apparent muscosal injury on retrograde examination. Building on this achievement, a number of researchers are laboring to develop an inflatable endotracheal balloon that can be inserted endoscopically in the fetus with CDH (Deprest *et al.*, 1996; Benachi *et al.*, 1996).

Using an alternative approach, VanderWall *et al.* (1996) have successfully placed a removable occlusive clip on the trachea of a human fetus with CDH. This procedure is performed through 3 mm, 4 mm, and 5.5 mm operating and viewing ports. Visualization during fetoscopically-guided dissection of the fetal trachea is aided by a specially designed irrigation device to remove blood and tissue debris from the operating field of view (Harrison, personal communication).

MYELOMENINGOCELE

As experience with fetoscopic approaches to the treatment of congenital fetal anomalies increases, and the true risks of minimally invasive fetal surgery become known, a fundamental shift is occurring with regard to the selection of suitable cases for fetoscopic surgery. Because of its prohibitively high morbidity and mortality, open fetal surgery was limited to the treatment of disorders likely to cause perinatal death without antenatal intervention. Today, the low morbidity and mortality of minimally invasive fetal surgery affords the possibility of treating not just lethal disorders, but also those anomalies likely to result in irreversible organ damage and a decreased quality of life.

The best current example of this new paradigm for fetoscopic surgery is antepartum treatment of fetal spina bifida. Myelomeningocele is one of the most common congenital malformations in humans, with an incidence of 0.5–2 per 1000 live births in the USA. Although the lesion is rarely lethal, affected infants may have varying degrees of somatosensory loss, neurogenic sphincter dysfunction of the bladder and bowel, hemiparesis and skeletal deformities. A study of 213 British children born with myelomeningocele from 1965–1992 reported a five-year survival of only 36% for open lesions, 60% for closed lesions, and 18% for lesions that were not classified (Althouse and Wald, 1980). Among those surviving with open unclassified lesions, 84% were severely handicapped, 10% were moderately handicapped, and only 6% had no handicap. Survivors with open lesions spent an average of more than six months in the hospital and had an average of six major surgical procedures during the first five years of life. With widespread maternal serum screening and the use of high-resolution ultrasonography, most cases of fetal myelomeningocele are now detectable in the mid-second trimester of pregnancy. The only management options currently available for affected pregnancies, however, are either termination or continuation of the pregnancy with neonatal therapy. This is partly due to the historic belief that the neurologic defects seen in children with myelomeningocele result from congenital myelodysplasia.

A growing body of experimental evidence suggests, however, that in addition to the developmental defects, much of the neurologic injury may be caused by prolonged exposure of the neural tube to amniotic fluid. In the first published animal study, intrauterine lumbar laminectomy (L3–L5) with displacement of the spinal cord from the central canal was performed in eight *Macaca mulatta* fetuses (Michejda, 1984). This condition was repaired in five animals, while the other three were left untreated. When the monkey infants were delivered by caesarean section near term, animals treated *in utero* were found to have developed normally. In contrast, the three control animals had paraplegia, incontinence and somatosensory loss. In a fetal rat model of surgically treated dysraphism, the spinal cord of each pup in the experimental group was intentionally exposed to amniotic fluid, but control fetal rats were subjected to the same procedure without directly exposing the spinal cord to the intrauterine environment (Heffez *et al.*, 1990). All fetal rats with open lesions were born with severe deformities and weakness of the hind limbs and tail, while control rats were normal at birth. Histologic studies of the exposed spinal cord revealed extensive erosion and necrosis, as seen in children with myelomeningocele. These findings were later confirmed in similar studies of fetal pigs (Heffez *et al.*, 1993) and lambs (Meuli *et al.*, 1995). Minimization of exposure of the spinal neural elements to amniotic fluid may diminish the severity of symptoms produced by myelomeningocele in humans, resulting in significant health benefits for the patient and family, and possible reduction of the long-term health care costs of affected infants. Accordingly, an animal model was developed in sheep for endoscopic intrauterine skin graft covering of surgically-induced defects (Copeland *et al.*, 1993).

Using the techniques developed in the animal model, Bruner (1996) and associates (Bruner *et al.*, 1996), repaired open spina bifida in two human fetuses. Under general anesthesia, a small split-thickness skin graft was obtained from the lateral aspect of the maternal thigh, following which a laparotomy incision was made. Real-time ultrasonography was used to determine fetal lie and the fetus was positioned in a cephalic, back-up presentation. Under direct ultrasonographic guidance, a needle was placed in the midline of the lower uterine segment, just above the bladder reflection, and a pressure transducer was attached to measure intrauterine pressure. A guide wire was inserted through the needle and used to place a 5 mm endoscopic port, through which an endoscopic camera was introduced. Two 3 mm operating ports were then placed through the anterior uterine wall, medial and inferior to the cornua, so that the endoscopic ports were triangulated around the fetal neural placode (Figure 65.2). Amniotic fluid was aspirated until the spinal lesion was clearly visible; the evacuated amniotic fluid was saved in a sterile warming container. Simultaneously, CO_2 was insufflated through a second port to maintain a constant intrauterine pressure. A 3 mm specially designed grasping forceps was used to situate the prepared, fitted maternal split-thickness skin graft into the crater of the neural placode. Finally, the skin graft and neural placode were covered with a fitted piece of Surgicel (Johnson and Johnson Medical Inc., Arlington, Texas, USA). Needles were inserted into two of the operating ports, and bovine thrombin was dripped liberally over the entire surface of the graft site, followed immediately by autologous maternal cryoprecipitate. The fetal spinal defect was thus completely obscured by a congealed layer of fibrin glue. The CO_2 was released while the preserved amniotic fluid was

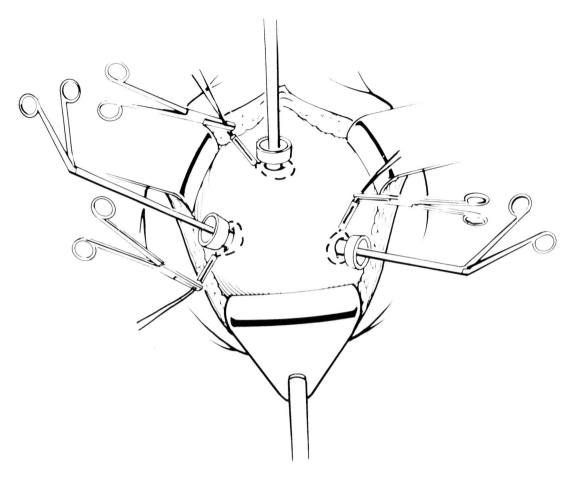

Figure 65.2 Using standard laparoscopic technique, the viewing and operating ports are triangulated around the intrauterine target and secured with pursestring sutures

put back into the uterine cavity. All endoscopic ports were removed and the entry points secured with pursestring sutures. The first fetus treated in this manner had an open myelomeningocele at the L4–S3 level diagnosed with ultrasonography, with mild ventriculomegaly, an Arnold–Chiari II malformation and no evidence of talipes. Endoscopic surgery was performed at 22.3 weeks, and scheduled cesarean delivery was performed after documentation of fetal lung maturity at 35.1 weeks. Definitive repair of the myelomeningocele was performed in the neonate, followed by ventriculoperitoneal shunt placement. This child is now 18 months old with only mild somatosensory deficit of the distal lower extremities. The second fetus treated endoscopically also had open myelomeningocele, in this case at the L3–S2 level, mild ventriculomegaly, an Arnold–Chiari II malformation and bilateral talipes. Endoscopic surgery was performed at 23.6 weeks. Unfortunately, the mother developed amnionitis a week later resulting in delivery of the fetus at 24.5 weeks. The newborn died in the delivery room from extreme prematurity.

CONGENITAL CYSTIC ADENOMATOID MALFORMATION (CCAM)

CCAM is the disordered cystic overgrowth of the terminal bronchioles of the lung at the expense of the alveoli. Stocker *et al.* (1977) proposed a classification of CCAM into three subtypes according to the size of the cysts:

- Type I has a few large cysts.
- Type II is multicystic.
- Type III consists of a noncystic lesion producing mediastinal shift.

Although most cases of CCAM are best treated surgically after birth, large lesions that displace the mediastinum and cause hydrops inevitably result in fetal demise. Adzick *et al.* (1993) have reviewed their experience with fetal therapy for cases of life-threatening CCAM:

- Three fetuses with a single predominant cyst were treated with placement of a thoraco-amniotic shunt. Two of the three survived after delivery with immediate neonatal resection and either high-frequency ventilation or extracorporeal membrane oxygenation (ECMO).

- Open fetal lobectomy was performed in an additional six cases with type III lesions. In four pregnancies, resection of the CCAM resulted in resolution of fetal hydrops, accelerated intrauterine lung growth and neonatal survival. In one case, *in utero* resection was followed by preterm labor and preeclampsia, requiring delivery of a nonviable fetus. In the last case, the fetus died unexpectedly after apparently successful resection of the tumor.

Although the success of open fetal surgery for the treatment of CCAM was greater than for any other indication for intrauterine surgery, morbidity and mortality were still high. Recently, however, a case of CCAM was successfully treated with an innovative fetoscopic laser procedure. A fetus was diagnosed ultrasonographically with a large type III lesion at 17 weeks' gestation. By 20 weeks, mediastinal shift and hydrops developed. Under general anesthesia with real-time ultrasonographic guidance, a 14-gauge needle was placed into the uterine cavity during the twenty-first gestational week. A 1.98 mm rigid endoscope was inserted through the needle lumen and used to guide the insertion of an 18-gauge needle into the fetal thorax. After the needle tip entered the fetal chest, it was guided, once again, with the aid of ultrasonography into the CCAM lesion. Amplitude-based color Doppler ultrasonography was used to avoid parenchymal vessels. When the needle was properly situated, a 400 μm Nd:YAG laser fiber was fed through the lumen. Using a power setting of 16 W, the lesion was photocoagulated under ultrasonographic guidance. Continued growth of the lesion necessitated a second procedure at 23 weeks. Preterm premature rupture of membranes occurred at 31 weeks, and vaginal delivery was achieved at 36 weeks' gestation. No ventilatory support was required in the neonate, who underwent resection of the tumor on the tenth day of life (Fortunato and Daniell, personal communication).

Complications of Minimally Invasive Fetal Surgery

Complications of all types of fetoscopic surgery include maternal pain, fetal movement during surgery, bleeding, infection, membrane rupture and preterm labor. Maternal pain for brief percutaneous procedures is usually relieved with local anesthesia and intravenous sedation. For longer, more extensive procedures general or regional anesthesia is often very effective. General anesthetic agents, many of which readily cross the placenta, also provide fetal anesthesia. Infection is usually addressed by the use of prophylactic antibiotics, administered systemically to the mother or added to the amniotic fluid. Although rupture of the membranes at the cervical os continues to defy attempts at occlusion of amniotic fluid leakage, in many instances the fluid leaks from the amnionic entry point in the uterine fundus. One case of a 'high leak' was treated by injecting a single autologous unit of platelets and one unit of cryoprecipitate into the amniotic cavity overlying the amnionic puncture site (Quintero *et al.*, 1996). Fluid leakage ceased on the second postoperative day. Finally, preterm labor is usually treated prophylactically by means of intravenous, subcutaneous or oral medications. One response to theoretic concerns about the effect of the endoscopic light source on the developing fetal eye was a proposal to perform 'night vision' fetoscopic surgery using an infrared light source and infrared video camera (Luks *et al.*, 1994b).

Table 65.2 Potential fetoscopic procedures.

Sacrococcygeal teratoma	Fetoscopic vascular occlusion by either: (1) Transcutaneous laser photocoagulation of vessels (2) Umbilical arterial catheterization and arterial embolization of vessels
Aqueductal stenosis	Laser ablation of stenotic lesion Third ventriculostomy
Tracheal atresia – stenosis – obstruction	Fetoscopic tracheoscopy Laser ablation of obstruction
Cleft lip – palate	Fetoscopic repair

The Future

Although fetoscopic approaches to complex developmental problems in the fetus are becoming increasingly sophisticated, minimally invasive fetal surgery is still in its infancy. Procedures that are theoretically possible or have been performed only in animals are listed in Table 65.2.

References

Adzick NS, Harrison MR, Flake AW *et al.* (1993) Fetal surgery for cystic adenomatoid malformation of the lung. *Journal of Pediatric Surgery* **28**: 806–812.

Agüero O, Aure M, López R (1966) Hysteroscopy in pregnant patients – a new diagnostic tool. *American Journal of Obstetrics and Gynecology* **94**: 925–928.

Aige-Gil V, Murillo-Ferrol N (1992) Effects of white light on the pineal gland of the chick embryo. *Histology and Histopathology* **7**: 1–6.

Althouse R, Wald N (1980) Survival and handicap of infants with spina bifida. *Archives of Disease in Childhood* **55**: 845–850.

Bakharev VA, Aivazyan AA, Karetnikova NA *et al.* (1990) Fetal skin biopsy in prenatal diagnosis of some genodermatoses. *Prenatal Diagnosis* **10**: 1–12.

Bealer JF, Skarsgard ED, Hedrick MH *et al.* (1995) The 'PLUG' odyssey: Adventures in experimental fetal tracheal occlusion. *Journal of Pediatric Surgery* **30**.

Benachi A, Dommergues M, Dumez Y, and Brunnelle F (1996) Endoscopic placement of an endotracheal balloon in fetal lambs with experimental diaphragmatic hernia. *International Fetal Medicine and Surgery Society, May 1996, Capri, Italy.*

Bernstein J (1971) The morphogenesis of renal parenchymal maldevelopment (renal dysplasia). *Pediatric Clinics of North America* **18**: 395–407.

Bruner J (1996) Endoscopic repair of fetal spina bifida *in utero. International Fetal Medicine and Surgery Society, May 1996, Capri, Italy.*

Bruner JP, Rosemond RL (1993) Twin-to-twin transfusion syndrome: A subset of the twin oligohydramnios–polyhydramnios sequence. *American Journal of Obstetrics and Gynecology* **169**: 925–930.

Bruner J, Tulipan N, Richards W (1996) Endoscopic repair of fetal spina bifida *in utero. American Journal of Obstetrics and Gynecology* **174**: 487.

Buckshee K, Parveen S, Mittal S *et al.* (1991) Percutaneous ultrasound-guided fetal skin biopsy: a new approach. *International Journal of Gynecology and Obstetrics* **34**: 267–270.

Copeland ML, Bruner JP, Richards WO *et al.* (1993) A model for *in utero* endoscopic treatment of myelomeningocele. *Neurosurgery* **33**: 542–545.

Crombleholme TM, Harrison MR, Langer JC *et al.* (1988) Early experience with open fetal surgery for congenital hydronephrosis. *Journal of Pediatric Surgery* **23**: 1114–1121.

Cullen MT, Green JJ, Reece EA, Hobbins JC (1990)

Embryoscopy: description and utility of a new technique. *American Journal of Obstetrics and Gynecology* **162**: 82–83.

Cullen MT, Whetham J, Viscarello RR *et al.* (1991) Transcervical endoscopic verification of congenital anomalies in the second trimester of pregnancy. *American Journal of Obstetrics and Gynecology* **165**: 95–97.

Daffos F, Capella-Pavlovsky M, Forestier F (1985) Fetal blood sampling during pregnancy with use of a needle guided by ultrasound: a study of 606 consecutive cases. *American Journal of Obstetrics and Gynecology* **153**: 655–660.

DeLia JE, Rogers JG, Dixon JA (1985) Treatment of placental vasculature with a neodymium:YAG laser via fetoscopy. *American Journal of Obstetrics and Gynecology* **151**: 1126–1127.

DeLia JE, Cukierski MA, Lundergan DK, Kochenour NK (1989) Neodymium:YAG laser occlusion of rhesus placental vasculature via fetoscopy. *American Journal of Obstetrics and Gynecology* **160**: 485–489.

DeLia JE, Cruikshank DP, Keye WR Jr (1990) Fetoscopic neodymium:YAG laser occlusion of placental vessels in severe twin–twin transfusion syndrome. *Obstetrics and Gynecology* **75**: 1046–1053.

DeLia JE, Kuhlmann RS, Cruikshank DP, O'Bee LR (1993) Current topic: placental surgery: a new frontier. *Placenta* **14**: 477–485.

DeLia JE, Kuhlmann RS, Harstad TW, Cruikshank DP (1995) Fetoscopic laser ablation of placental vessels in severe previable twin–twin transfusion syndrome. *American Journal of Obstetrics and Gynecology* **172**: 1202–1211.

Deprest J, Evrard V, Van Ballaer P *et al.* (1996) Fetoscopy – guided tracheoscopy for *in utero* tracheal obstruction in the fetal lamb with a detachable balloon. *International Fetal Medicine and Surgery Society, May 1996, Capri, Italy.*

Dommergues M, Lemerrer M, Couly G *et al.* (1995) Prenatal diagnosis of cleft lip at 11 menstrual weeks using embryoscopy in the van der Woude syndrome. *Prenatal Diagnosis* **15**: 378–381.

Donald I, MacVicar J, Brown TG (1958) Investigation of abdominal masses by pulsed ultrasound. *Lancet* **2**: 1188–1194.

Dubuisson JB, Barbot J, Henrion R (1979) L'embryoscopie de contact. *Journal de Gynécologie, Obstétrique et Biologie de la Reproduction* **8**: 39–41.

Dumez Y (1988) Embryoscopy and congenital malformations. *Proceedings of the International Congress on Chorionic Villus Sampling and Early Prenatal Diagnosis, May 1988, Athens, Greece.*

Dumez Y, Daffos F (1990) L'echographie interventionelle en medicine foetale. In Gillet P (ed.) *Echographie des Malformations Foetal.* pp. 407–408. Paris: Vigot.

Elias S (1983) Fetoscopy in prenatal diagnosis. *Clinics in Perinatology* **10**: 357–367.

Elias S (1987) Use of fetoscopy for the prenatal diagnosis of hereditary skin disorders. In Gedde-Dahl T, Wuepper KD (eds) *Prenatal Diagnosis of Heritable Skin Disease.* pp. 1–13. Basel: Karger.

Elliott JP (1995) Twin–twin transfusion syndrome. *New England Journal of Medicine* **333**: 387.

Elliott JP, Urig MA, Clewell WH (1991) Aggressive therapeutic amniocentesis for treatment of twin–twin transfusion syndrome. *Obstetrics and Gynecology* **77**: 537–540.

Estes JM, MacGillivary TE, Hedrick MH *et al.* (1992) Fetoscopic surgery for the treatment of congenital anomalies. *Journal of Pediatric Surgery* **27**: 950–954.

Evans MI, Greb A, Kunkel LM *et al.* (1991) In utero fetal muscle biopsy for the diagnosis of Duchenne muscular dystrophy. *American Journal of Obstetrics and Gynecology* **165**: 728–732.

Evans MI, Hoffman EP, Cadrin C *et al.* (1994) Fetal muscle biopsy: Collaborative experience with varied indications. *Obstetrics and Gynecology* **84**: 913–917.

Fletcher JC, Jonsen AR (1991) Ethical considerations in fetal treatment. In Harrison MR, Golbus MS, Filly RA (eds) *The Unborn Patient*, 2nd edn. p. 16. Philadelphia: WB Saunders.

Gallinat A, Lueken RP, Lindemann H-J (1978) A preliminary report about transcervical embryoscopy. *Endoscopy* **10**: 47–50.

Ghirardini G (1991) Embryoscopy: Old technique new for the 1990s? *American Journal of Obstetrics and Gynecology* **164**: 1361–1362.

Golbus MS, Harrison MR, Filly RA *et al.* (1982) In utero treatment of urinary tract obstruction. *American Journal of Obstetrics and Gynecology* **142**: 383–388.

Golbus MS, McGonigle KF, Goldberg JD *et al.* (1989) Fetal tissue sampling. The San Francisco experience with 190 pregnancies. *Western Journal of Medicine* **150**: 423–430.

Harrison MR, Nakayama DK, Noall R *et al.* (1982) Correction of congenital hydronephrosis in utero. II: decompression reverses the effects of obstruction on the fetal lung and urinary tract. *Journal of Pediatric Surgery* **17**: 965–974.

Harrison MR, Adzick NS, Flake AW *et al.* (1993) Correction of congenital diaphragmatic hernia in utero. VI. Hard-earned lessons. *Journal of Pediatric Surgery* **28**: 1411–1418.

Harrison MR, Adzick NS, Estes JM, Howell LJ (1994) A prospective study of the outcome of fetuses with congenital diaphragmatic hernia. *Journal of the American Medical Association* **271**: 382–384.

Hedrick MH, Ferro MM, Filly RA *et al.* (1994a) Congenital high airway obstruction syndrome (CHAOS): A potential for perinatal intervention. *Journal of Pediatric Surgery* **29**: 271–274.

Hedrick MH, Estes JM, Sullivan KM *et al.* (1994b) Plug the lung until it grows (PLUG): A new method to treat congenital diaphragmatic hernia in utero. *Journal of Pediatric Surgery* **29**: 612–617.

Heffez DS, Aryanpur J, Hutchins GM, Freeman JM (1990) The paralysis associated with myelomeningocele: Clinical and experimental data implicating a preventable spinal cord injury. *Neurosurgery* **26**: 987–992.

Heffez DS, Aryanpur J, Cuello-Rotellini NA *et al.* (1993) Intrauterine repair of experimental surgically created dysraphism. *Neurosurgery* **32**: 1005–1010.

Hobbins J, Mahoney ME (1974) In utero diagnosis of hemoglobinopathies. Technic for obtaining fetal blood. *New England Journal of Medicine* **290**: 1065–1067.

Hobbins J, Mahoney ME, Goldstein LA (1974) New method of intrauterine evaluation by the combined use of fetoscopy and ultrasound. *American Journal of Obstetrics and Gynecology* **118**: 1069–1072.

Hobbins J, Jones OW, Gottesfeld S, Persutte W (1994) Transvaginal ultrasonography and transabdominal embryoscopy in the first-trimester diagnosis of Smith–Lemli–Opitz syndrome, type II. *American Journal of Obstetrics and Gynecology* **171**: 546–549.

Holbrook KA, Smith LT, Elias S (1993) Prenatal diagnosis of genetic skin disease using fetal skin biopsy samples. *Archives of Dermatology* **129**: 1437–1454.

Holzgreve W, Golbus MS (1984) Prenatal diagnosis of ornithine transcarbamylase deficiency utilizing fetal liver biopsy. *American Journal of Human Genetics* **36**: 320–328.

International Fetoscopy Group (1984) Special report. The status of fetoscopy and fetal tissue sampling. *Prenatal Diagnosis* **4**: 79–81.

Luks FI, Deprest JA, Vandenberghe K *et al.* (1994a) Fetoscopy – guided fetal endoscopy in a sheep model. *Journal of the American College of Surgeons* **178**: 609–612.

Luks FI, Deprest JA, Peers KHE *et al.* (1994b) Infrared fetoscopy in the sheep. *Fetal Diagnosis and Therapy* 327–330.

Lynch L, Berkowitz RL (1992) Amniocentesis, skin biopsy, and umbilical cord blood sampling in the prenatal diagnosis of genetic diseases. In Reece EA, Hobbins J, Mahoney ME, Petrie RH (eds) *Medicine of the Fetus and Mother*. pp. 641–652. Philadelphia: JB Lippincott.

MacMahon RA, Renou PM, Shekelton PA, Paterson PJ (1992) In-utero cystotomy. *Lancet* **2**: 1234.

Mandelbaum B, Pontarelli DA, Brushenko A (1967) Amnioscopy for prenatal transfusion. *American Journal of Obstetrics and Gynecology* **98**: 1140–1144.

Meuli M, Meuli-Simmen C, Yingling CD *et al.* (1995) Creation of myelomeningocele in utero: A model of functional damage from spinal cord exposure in fetal sheep. *Journal of Pediatric Surgery* **30**: 1028–1033.

Michejda M (1984) Intrauterine treatment of spina bifida: Primate model. *Zeitschrift für Kinderchirurgie* **39**: 259–261.

Moore TR, Gale S, Benirschke K (1990) Perinatal outcome of forty-nine pregnancies complicated by acardiac twinning. *American Journal of Obstetrics and Gynecology* **163**: 907–912.

Pennehouat GH, Thebault Y, Ville Y *et al.* (1992) First-trimester transabdominal fetoscopy. *Lancet* **2**: 429.

Potter EL (1946) Bilateral renal agenesis. *Journal of Pediatrics* **29**: 68–76.

Quintero R (1996) In utero laser ablation of posterior urethral valves. *International Fetal Medicine and Surgery Society, May 1996, Capri, Italy*.

Quintero RA, Abuhamad A, Hobbins J, Mahoney ME (1993a) Transabdominal thin-gauge embryofetoscopy: A technique for early prenatal diagnosis and its use in the diagnosis of a case of Meckel–Gruber syndrome. *American Journal of Obstetrics and Gynecology* **168**: 1552–1557.

Quintero RA, Puder KS, Cotton DB (1993b) Embryoscopy and fetoscopy. *Obstetrics and Gynecology Clinics of North America* **20**: 563–581.

Quintero RA, Crossland WJ, Cotton DB (1994a) Effect of endoscopic white light on the developing visual pathway: A histologic, histochemical and behavioural study. *American Journal of Obstetrics and Gynecology* **171**: 1142–1148.

Quintero RA, Reich H, Puder KS *et al.* (1994b) Brief report: Umbilical cord ligation of an acardiac twin by fetoscopy at 19 weeks of gestation. *New England Journal of Medicine* **330**: 469–471.

Quintero RA, Johnson MP, Romero R *et al.* (1995a) *In-utero* percutaneous cystoscopy in the management of the fetal lower obstructive uropathy. *Lancet* **2**: 537–540.

Quintero RA, Hume R, Smith C *et al.* (1995b) Percutaneous fetal cystoscopy and endoscopic fulguration of posterior urethral valves. *American Journal of Obstetrics and Gynecology* **172**: 206–209.

Quintero RA, Romero R, Dzieczkowski J *et al.* (1996) Sealing of ruptured amniotic membranes with intra-amniotic platelet – cryoprecipitate plug. *Lancet* **2**: 1117.

Reece EA (1992) Embryoscopy: new developments in prenatal medicine. *Current Opinion in Obstetrics and Gynecology* **4**: 447–455.

Reece EA, Whetham J, Rotmensch S, Wiznitzer A (1993) Gaining access to the embryonic–fetal circulation via first-trimester endoscopy: A step into the future. *Obstetrics and Gynecology* **82**: 876–879.

Reece EA, Goldstein I, Chatwani A *et al.* (1994) Transabdominal needle embryofetoscopy: A new technique paving the way for early fetal therapy. *Obstetrics and Gynecology* **84**: 634–636.

Reece EA, Homko CJ, Wiznitzer A, Goldstein I (1995) Needle embryofetoscopy and early prenatal diagnosis. *Fetal Diagnosis and Therapy* **10**: 81–82.

Rodeck CH (1980) Fetoscopy guided by real-time ultrasound for pure fetal blood samples, fetal skin samples, and examination of the fetus *in utero*. *British Journal of Obstetrics and Gynecology* **87**: 449–456.

Rodeck CH, Campbell S (1978) Sampling pure fetal blood by fetoscopy in second trimester of pregnancy. *British Medical Journal* **2**: 728–730.

Rodeck CH, Nicolaides KH (1983) Fetoscopy and fetal tissue sampling. *British Medical Bulletin* **39**: 332–337.

Rodeck CH, Nicolaides KH (1986) Fetoscopy. *British Medical Bulletin* **42**: 296–300.

Rodeck CH, Holman CA, Karnicki J *et al.* (1981) Direct intravascular fetal blood transfusion by fetoscopy in severe rhesus isoimmunisation. *Lancet* **1**: 625–627.

Romero R, Hobbins J, Mahoney ME (1986) Fetal blood sampling and fetoscopy. In Milunsky A (ed.) *Genetic Disorders in the Fetus*. pp. 571–598. New York: Plenum.

Roume J, Aubry MC, Labbe F *et al.* (1985) Prenatal diagnosis of limb and digital abnormalities. Evaluation of the activity of the Port Royal University Clinic from 1979 to 1983. Apropos of 30 cases. *Journal de Genetique Humaine* **33**: 457–461.

Scurry J, Adamson T, Cussen L (1989) Fetal lung growth in laryngeal atresia and tracheal agenesis. *Australian Paediatric Journal* **25**: 47–51.

Scrimgeour JB (1976) Clinical experience with fetoscopy. In Kaback M, Valenti C (eds) *Intrauterine Fetal Visualization*. p. 150. New York: Elsevier.

Stocker JT, Madewell JE, Drake RM (1977) Congenital cystic adenomatoid malformation of the lung. Classification and morphologic spectrum. *Human Pathology* **8**: 155–171.

Valenti C (1972) Endoamnioscopy and fetal biopsy: A new technique. *American Journal of Obstetrics and Gynecology* **114**: 561–564.

Valenti C (1973) Antenatal detection of hemoglobinopathies. A preliminary report. *American Journal of Obstetrics and Gynecology* **115**: 851–853.

VanderWall K, Harrison MR, Bruch SR *et al.* (1996) Fetendo clip: endoscopic tracheal clip procedure in a human fetus. *International Fetal Medicine and Surgery Society, May 1996, Capri, Italy.*

Ville Y, Hyett J, Hecher K, Nicolaides K (1995) Preliminary experience with endoscopic laser surgery for severe twin–twin transfusion syndrome. *New England Journal of Medicine* **332**: 224–227.

Weir PE, Ratten VG, Beischer NA (1979) Acute polyhydramnios – a complication of monozygous twin pregnancy. *British Journal of Obstetrics and Gynaecology* **86**: 849–853.

Westin B (1954) Hysteroscopy in early pregnancy. *Lancet* **2**: 872.

Willcourt RJ, Naughton MJ, Knutzen VK, Fitzpatrick C (1995) Laparoscopic ligation of the umbilical cord of an acardiac fetus. *Journal of the American Association of Gynecologic Laparoscopists* **2**: 319–321.

66

Embryoscopy

YVES DUMEZ

Maternité Port Royal, Paris, France

Introduction

Over the past years, an objective of fetal medicine has been to offer early prenatal diagnosis. The possibility of first-trimester diagnosis encourages couples at risk of transmitting dominant or recessive disorders to attempt pregnancy. Chorionic villus sampling had made early diagnosis of karyotypic or metabolic disorders possible, and vaginal ultrasound imaging reveals some major morphologic abnormalities before 12 weeks gestation. Ten years ago, we developed the technique of embryoscopy for direct endoscopic visualization of the fetus at as early as nine menstrual weeks, when externally visible lesions cannot be diagnosed by any other means. Although any external malformation can theoretically be diagnosed by embryoscopy, this technique should be offered to patients with a high genetic risk for anomalies of the face and extremities. These anomalies may be either isolated or part of the phenotypic expression of a complex inherited syndrome. In selected cases, the risk of having a fetus affected by a limb or facial defect may reach 25–50%, thereby justifying early invasive prenatal diagnosis. Embryoscopy also has potential applications for fetal therapy, by opening access to the embryonic circulation at an early stage in development.

Technique

Principles

Embryoscopy consists of observing the embryo through the intact amniotic membrane via an endoscope introduced across the chorion into the extraembryonic coelom. The chorion is opaque and flimsy, while the amniotic membrane is transparent and strong. These anatomic features allow introduction of the endoscopic device across the chorion without damaging the amnion. Because of the relatively large size of the extraembryonic coelom, it is also possible to move the tip of the endoscope freely without tearing the amnion.

Embryoscopy should be performed after the major external features of the embryo's body have been established (i.e. after eight menstrual weeks), but before the extraembryonic coelom is obliterated by the growth of the amniotic cavity (i.e. before 11 menstrual weeks). Moreover, we believe that endoscopic lighting of the amniotic cavity should be avoided until the development of the embryo's eyelids has been completed (nine menstrual weeks) in order to prevent potential eye damage from excessive light exposure. As the maximal size of the extraembryonic coelom is also achieved at nine weeks, this is the ideal gestational age for performing embryoscopy.

Material

We use a rigid fiberoptic endoscope with a 0° wide-angle lens (Needlescope, Olympus, France), measuring 17 cm in length and 1.7 mm in diameter, which is introduced through a cannula (2 mm outer diameter).

The cannula is equipped with a side channel, allowing injection of normal saline while the endoscope is in place. Ultrasound guidance is achieved using a Combison 320, with a 5 MHz sector probe (Kretz, Vienna, Austria).

Methods

Embryoscopy is an outpatient procedure, performed by either a transcervical or transabdominal approach. Preoperative ultrasonic evaluation is required:

- To rule out a multiple pregnancy.
- To check the size of the embryo and extra-embryonic coelom.
- To confirm fetal vitality.

Intraoperative ultrasound is also needed.

- To guide the endoscope directly into the coelom.
- To avoid the trophoblast.
- To orient the tip of the device towards the part of the embryo to be viewed.

TRANSCERVICAL EMBRYOSCOPY

The technique originally described was transcervical, and this can be used unless the thickest part of the trophoblast is in direct contact with the internal cervical os. No anesthesia or sedation is required. The cervix is exposed by a single valve-weighted speculum and carefully cleaned. The endoscope within the cannula is then gently introduced under ultrasound guidance through the cervix and directed towards the lowest part of the ovum in contact with the chorion. The entire device is then briskly pushed forward to cross the chorion and enter the coelom. The smooth and relatively large tip of the endoscope may reach the amnion, but will not damage it. Direct visual inspection of the extraembryonic coelom confirms proper placement of the endoscope. If needed, the cannula can be flushed with 1–2 ml of normal saline to remove blood and particles. The tip of the endoscope is then brought in direct contact with the amniotic sac, through which the embryo can be observed. The initial inspection is made directly through the endoscope. A video camera is then attached to the endoscope, allowing the mother to view the embryo on a television monitor and to obtain a video tape recording when a malformation has been discovered. If the fetus is found to be normal, the duration of the procedure should be kept as short as possible to minimize the risk of miscarriage.

TRANSABDOMINAL EMBRYOSCOPY

A transabdominal approach can be used whenever the thickest trophoblastic area is not located on the anterior aspect of the uterus. After administering local anesthesia with 1% lidocaine solution, the cannula, containing a sharp trocar, is introduced into the coelom. The trocar is then removed and replaced by the endoscope. After confirming the integrity of the amniotic sac, the endoscopic tip is placed in contact with the transparent amniotic membrane and the remainder of the procedure is the same as for the transcervical approach.

Whichever route is used, the patient is discharged from the hospital the next morning after a follow-up ultrasound scan. Antibiotics are given following transcervical procedures. If indicated, termination of pregnancy is performed by suction and curettage.

Results

Normal Pregnancy

EXTRAEMBRYONIC COELOM AND YOLK SAC
(Figure 66.1)

Through the embryoscope, the extraembryonic coelom appears to be a clear space in which thin trabeculae may sometimes be observed. Numerous vessels run on the inner aspect of the chorion, which are easily identified by their red color. The embryo can be seen through the whitish amniotic sac that limits the coelom opposite the chorionic plate. The two vessels of the vitelline duct can be identified at the insertion of the amnion around the umbilical cord. The vitelline duct runs freely in the coelom and connects the yolk sac to the fetal circulation.

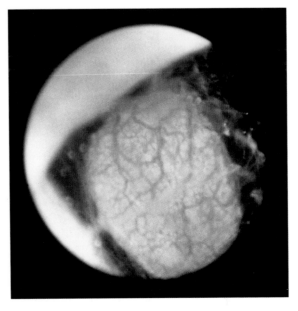

Figure 66.1 Yolk sac at nine weeks.

The yolk sac looks like a yellowish sphere with a rich vascular network connected to the vascular pedicle of the vitelline duct. Later in gestation, the vascular network of the yolk sac diminishes. By following the vitelline duct from the yolk sac, the cord insertion on the chorionic plate will be reached. At nine menstrual weeks, the umbilical cord adjacent to the chorionic plate is located within the coelom and outside the amniotic cavity. The umbilical vein appears deep blue while the umbilical arteries are bright red.

EMBRYO

After observing the coelom, the tip of the endoscope is moved into contact with the amnion. A nearly complete wide-angle view of the embryo can be obtained when crown–rump length does not exceed 35 mm. A detailed examination of the four extremities and the face can be performed within a few seconds of direct observation.

Embryonic extremities

When the endoscope is brought close to an embryonic hand or foot, the region studied occupies the whole visual field, and morphologic details can be studied with great accuracy. At nine weeks, the hands are found in a symmetric position in front of the embryonic face, with the radial borders directed cranially. Small spontaneous movements of the fingers, forearm and arm are often observed. The fingers can be visualized and easily counted, and the phalanges can also be clearly identified (Figure 66.2). The thumb has a typical two phalangeal appearance and is opposed to the other digits. The

size of the entire limb as well as the relative dimensions of each portion can be assessed. Both pre- and post-axial aspects of the hands and forearms can be observed in detail. Later in gestation, at ten weeks, the primary nail fields can also be identified. Earlier, at seven weeks, the fingers are normally fused at the distal end of the upper limb bud, but the outlines of all five future digits are clearly visible.

The feet have a different appearance. At nine weeks their plantar surfaces face each other and the tibial border of the leg is directed cranially. After visualizing the heel, however, it can be seen that the foot is oriented perpendicularly to the leg, forming a right angle in the region of the ankle. The toes can be clearly identified (Figure 66.3), and both their size and shape can be assessed. The pre- and post-axial borders of the leg can also be observed. Earlier in gestation, at seven weeks, the distal end of the hind limb bud has a grossly triangular shape, with the future toes still appearing as united rays.

Embryonic face

The face can be thoroughly analyzed (Figure 66.4). At nine weeks the eyes are located in the anterior aspect of the face, and the eyelids are fused, completely covering the eyes. The nose, nostrils, mouth and ears are well established and the upper lip is fused. The chin looks prominent. Earlier, at eight weeks, the eyelids have not been formed and deep blue eyes can be observed on the lateral aspect of the face. The eyes look like convex discs covered by a thin transparent membrane, which is the corneal ectoderm.

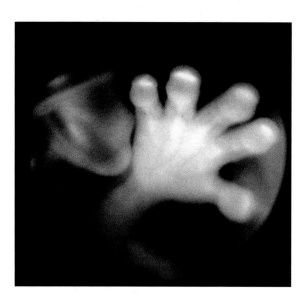

Figure 66.2 Hand at nine weeks.

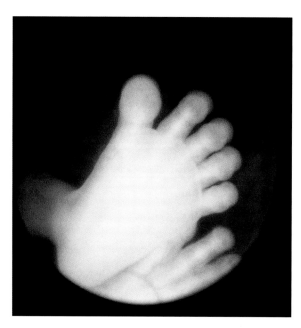

Figure 66.3 Foot at nine weeks.

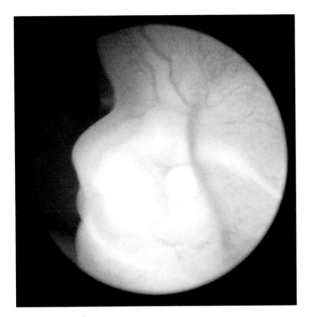

Figure 66.4 Face at nine weeks.

Embryonic abdomen and external genitalia

At nine weeks, the midgut is normally herniated into the embryonic insertion of the umbilical cord and the small intestine can be observed through the transparent wall of this physiologic umbilical hernia (Figure 66.5). At 11 weeks the hernia has usually, but not always, completely disappeared. When this has occurred, the abdominal wall is completely closed. At ten weeks, during the process of reduction of the physiologic hernia, a vestigial sac may persist adjacent to the umbilical cord.

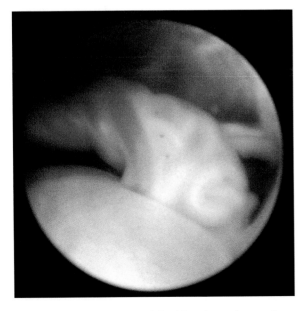

Figure 66.5 Physiologic umbilical hernia at nine weeks.

At 9–10 weeks the external genitalia are not yet differentiated and consist of a genital tubercle with two labioscrotal swellings. At this age, the embryonic sex cannot be phenotypically diagnosed.

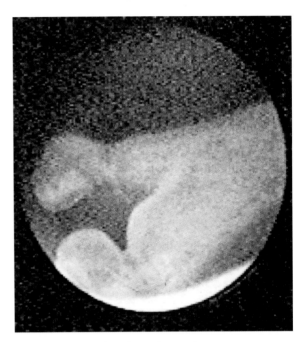

Figure 66.6 Ectrodactyly at nine weeks.

Skull and back

The shape of the skull is round and it is covered by thin skin through which subcutaneous blood vessels as well as the large sagittal suture can be seen. The neural tube is closed at nine weeks and this can be observed through the skin. Earlier in gestation, the neural tube is still open in its cranial and caudal regions.

Malformed Embryos

EXTREMITIES

The quality of embryoscopic imaging allows prenatal diagnosis of any foot or hand congenital defect at nine weeks.

Gross anomalies such as ectrodactyly (Figure 66.6), monodactyly and adactyly are obvious at first glance. However, because the expression of the disease may differ from one extremity to the other, the four extremities must always be studied. Hexadactyly is also easy to diagnose. The sixth digit is usually found on the ulnar border of the hand (Figure 66.7), but can also be located on the radial border.

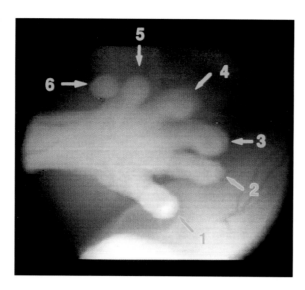

Figure 66.7 Polydactyly at nine weeks.

Syndactyly is slightly more difficult to diagnose. However, the appearance of the hand is globally abnormal. Part of the digits or all the digits are fused. The hand appears wide, but does not look flat like the distal end of the limb bud earlier in pregnancy.

More subtle anomalies can be diagnosed by embryoscopy such as hypoplasia of one digit, nail hypoplasia or a short phalanx.

FACE

The face may be slightly more difficult to observe than the extremities. A cleft lip can be unequivocally diagnosed based on a divided upper lip at nine weeks. Anophthalmy has not yet been diagnosed by embryoscopy, and the fusion of the eyelids is a potential limitation for such a diagnosis. Ear hypoplasia or aplasia can be diagnosed. However, in the absence of a well-defined malformation, facial dysmorphy cannot be demonstrated by embryoscopy.

Indications

In our opinion, prenatal diagnosis by embryoscopy should only be offered to patients with a high genetic risk of limb or face malformation. Genetic counseling is crucial to accurately identify the index case and to assess the risk of recurrence. Four types of indication should be considered:

- Isolated abnormalities of the extremities for which inheritance is likely to be dominant (e.g.

ectrodactyly, syndactyly, adactyly, acromesomelia).
- Isolated cleft lip with suspected dominant inheritance.
- Polymalformation syndromes that include anomalies of the face with probable inherited transmission. These include autosomal recessive diseases such as Carpenter's or Mohr syndromes, or syndromes with syndactyly and cleft lip. Autosomal dominant disorders include Nager's syndrome (radial ray agenesis and cleft lip) or EEC syndromes (ectodermic dysplasia and cleft lip).
- Polymalformation syndromes that include anomalies of the extremities with probable inherited transmission. These include recessive autosomal syndromes (e.g. Baller–Gerold, Saldino–Noonan, Bardet–Biedl, Rothmund–Thomson, Mekel, Quazi, Ellis–van Creveld, Smith–Lemli–Opitz) and X-linked disorders with hexadactyly such as the Golaby–Rosen syndrome.

Diagnostic Value and Obstetric Risk

Because of the small number of indicated cases, our experience with ongoing pregnancies is limited to 57 cases over a period of ten years. The diagnostic value of this technique, however, seems to be excellent. In our series all positive diagnoses were confirmed by postmortem examination, and no morphologic abnormality was missed. Six miscarriages occurred, all in procedures performed after ten menstrual weeks. Postnatal follow-up did not reveal any pediatric morbidity associated with the procedures.

Future Outlook

Embryoscopy may have considerable importance for future developments in fetal diagnosis and therapy. In the future, use of new very small optical fibers will make the procedure easier and safer and this will allow for new developments. This procedure might permit sampling of fetal blood or the yolk sac during the first trimester as well as injection of cells into the embryo. This latter approach has potential applications for early therapy of a variety of genetic disorders, including those involving the hematologic, metabolic or immune systems.

Conclusions

Embryoscopy permits prenatal diagnosis of facial and limb defects to as early as nine weeks. Although invasive, it is clinically useful use for couples with a high risk of having infants with severe disorders that cannot be diagnosed by any other means in the first trimester.

References

Cullen M, Reece A, Whetham J, Hobbins J (1990) Embryoscopy: description and utility of a new technique. *American Journal of Obstetrics and Gynecology* **162**: 82–86.

Cullen M, Whetham J, Viscarello R, Reece A, Sanchez-Ramos L, Hobbins J (1991a) Transcervical endoscopic verification of congenital anomalies in the second trimester of pregnancy. *American Journal of Obstetrics and Gynecology* **165**: 95–97.

Cullen M, Green J, Wethman J, Salafia C, Gabrielli S, Hobbins J (1991b) Transvaginal ultrasonographic detection of congenital malformations in the first trimester. *American Journal of Obstetrics and Gynecology* **163(2)**: 466–467.

Dumez Y, Dommergues M, Beuzard Y (1988) Study of a method for early first trimester fetal blood sampling and intravascular injection. *Symposium on Fetal Therapy and Development: Outlook for the 21st Century. November 27–30, 1988, Chicago, USA.*

Dumez Y, Oury JF, Dommergues M (1992) Diagnostic embryoscopy: 50 cases of early diagnosis. *International symposium from Gametes to Embryology. May 18–20, 1992, Milan.*

Dumez Y; Dommergues M, Gubler MC *et al.* (1994) Meckel Gruber syndrome: Prenatal diagnosis at 10 menstrual weeks using embryoscopy. *Prenatal Diagnosis* **14**: 141–144.

Gorlin R, Cohen M, Lewine S (1990) *Syndromes of the Head and Neck*, 3rd edition. Oxford: Oxford University Press.

Reece A, Rotmensch S, Whethman J, Cullen M, Hobbins J (1992) Embryoscopy: A closer look at first-trimester diagnosis and treatment. *American Journal of Obstetrics and Gynecology* **166**: 775–780.

Smith DW, (1982) *Recognizable Pattern of Human Malformation: Genetic, Embryologic, and Clinical Aspects.* Philadephia: WB Saunders Company.

Timor–Tritsch I, Monteagudo A, Peisner D (1992) High frequency transvaginal sonographic examination for the potential malformation assessment of the 9 week to 14 week fetus. *Journal of Clinical Ultrasound* **20**: 231–283.

67

Outpatient Local Anesthetic Laparoscopy

EDWARD J. SHAXTED

Three Shires Hospital, Northampton, UK

Ever since Ott first described optical inspection of the peritoneal cavity (he called it ventroscopy) in 1901, the technique has become more and more refined. Laparoscopy has now become a standard diagnostic tool of the gynecologist, and has been widely embraced by general surgeons and gynecologists for the performance of many surgical procedures. It allows a clear view of the pelvic organs and has become the main diagnostic instrument for diseases such as endometriosis, pelvic inflammatory disease and ectopic pregnancy. The laparoscope is also widely used in the management of infertility, and in some hands is considered useful in the management of intraperitoneal malignant disease (Childers *et al.*, 1992).

In recent years a wide range of gynecologic operations previously performed through abdominal incisions have come to be performed laparoscopically. Most female sterilizations in developed countries now involve the application of mechanical devices to occlude the fallopian tubes laparoscopically. There is a growing trend to treat ectopic pregnancies, ovarian cysts and other adnexal pathologies laparoscopically. In some hands other, more technically demanding operations such as hysterectomy, myomectomy and colposuspension can also be performed laparoscopically.

Almost all laparoscopies in UK are performed under general anesthesia. Many minor laparoscopic operations are, however, performed as a day case with the patient returning to their own home on the evening of their operation. It is unusual for patients who have major procedures performed laparoscopically to be discharged on the same day in UK. There is also a problem with training and accreditation in laparoscopic surgery in the UK. Although diagnostic and simple therapeutic laparoscopy is part of the routine training of all gynecologists, there are still relatively few senior gynecologists undertaking advanced laparoscopic procedures.

Despite the enthusiasm of a few gynecologists for performing laparoscopy under local anesthesia, and indeed the exaltations of some very well-known gynecologists about the advantages of local anesthesia (Gordon, 1984) local anesthetic techniques have never been popular with the majority of either patients or surgeons in the UK.

Anesthesia

The majority of laparoscopies are performed under general anesthesia with a degree of airway control. Previously this has often been thought to imply intubation (Chamberlain and Carron-Brown, 1978), but many laparoscopies are now performed without the patient being completely paralyzed and without intubation. Laryngeal masks are considered appropriate by many anesthesiologists.

Laparoscopy can be performed without general anesthesia using a combination of local anesthetic with or without (Khandala, 1984) a sedative technique. To perform laparoscopy without general anesthesia requires surgical skill and gentleness. It also requires appropriate patient selection and the confident use of local anesthetic agents.

Advantages of Local Anesthetic Laparoscopy

Clearly avoidance of general anesthesia avoids the inherent risks of general anesthesia. In the British Laparoscopy Survey (Chamberlain and Carron-Brown, 1978) two of the four deaths were due to the complications of general anesthesia. These risks should not be overemphasized, however, but many patients are more terrified of the anesthetic than they are of the operation. These patients may be unsuitable for local anesthetic techniques. If the investigation of pain is the primary indication for laparoscopy, then a local anesthetic technique has the advantage of allowing assessment with a cooperative patient. Some patients find real-time visualization of their own pelvis helpful and interesting.

Do not expect a local anesthetic technique to be quicker or cheaper. The additional time required to be gentle and kind and to achieve patient cooperation far exceeds the time taken by even the slowest anesthesiologist to give a general anesthetic. Recovery from the sedative technique must be considered, and if the operation is to be performed in the outpatient or office setting, there are unlikely to be recovery facilities.

Some authors insist that even with local anesthesia, the operation should take place in an operating theater (Gordon, 1984). Others are happy with the outpatient or office setting (Khandala, 1984; Childers et al., 1992). Certainly the major advantages of a local anesthetic technique are only seen when the procedure is performed outside the operating theater.

Local Anesthetic Laparoscopy

Patient Selection and Preparation

Clearly not all patients will be suitable to have a laparoscopy performed under local anesthetic. Laparoscopy under local anesthesia should not be considered if the patient has any fears about the procedure (Gordon, 1984). The patient must be prepared for some minor discomfort and it must be anticipated that the operation will be straightforward and without complications. The patient should not be excessively obese. In my view those patients who are most suitable for outpatient local anesthetic laparoscopy are those for whom laparoscopy is being performed for a specific diagnostic or therapeutic reason and for whom a prolonged and detailed searching examination of the entire peritoneal cavity will not be necessary. Minor

surgical procedures such as biopsy (Childers et al., 1992) aspiration of fluid (Childers et al., 1992) and female sterilization (Penfield, 1974; Khandala, 1984) can easily be performed under local anesthetic.

The patient should be starved and generally prepared in much the same way as if she was going to have a general anesthetic. Clearly the hospital concerned should have the facilities for general anesthesia and the facilities for dealing with any of the complications that can occur with laparoscopy. It might be considered appropriate to perform the operation in an operating theater fully equipped for general anesthesia, but certainly for diagnostic work this is not essential. While gaining experience of local anesthetic techniques, it is probably wise to start in the operating theater with an anesthetist present. With experience the need to convert from a local to a general anesthetic will be rare. Gordon quoted nine of 1200 in a personal series (1984). In my personal experience, conversion to general anesthesia is rare with the correct patient selection and appropriate technique.

Sedation and Local Anesthetic Techniques

Intravenous access should be obtained, usually by a cannula on the back of the hand. Intravenous sedation with a drug such as midazolam is generally helpful. A dose of 5–10 mg is usually sufficient. Midazolam has the added advantage of producing postoperative amnesia. An intravenous analgesic such as fentanyl may also be used in addition to the midazolam in a dose of 50–100 μg. Care must be taken, however, not to render the patient unconscious with an excessive dose. The precise dosage of sedative and analgesic should be titrated against the effect on the patient. The timing of administration of these drugs is imperative. They are relatively short acting and the operative procedure needs to be performed when the effects of the drugs are greatest. Staff should work quietly, efficiently and rapidly. They must be well trained and totally familiar with the technique, the equipment and the surroundings. They must be able to cope with any emergency that may arise. One member of the nursing staff should have no role other than to look after the patient. She should provide constant reassurance to the patient and must carefully observe her vital signs.

The anticipated abdominal wall puncture sites should be infiltrated with appropriate local anesthetic. I personally use bupivacaine 0.25% with adrenaline. Care should be taken to infiltrate all layers of the abdominal wall including, if possible, the peritoneum at the puncture sites. When sterilization is to be performed, the fallopian tube will need to be anesthetized before occlusion. This can be achieved by spraying the portion of the fallopian tube with a lignocaine spray or by injecting lignocaine into the tube transperitoneally, the former being easier. Instilling local anesthetic solution into the uterine cavity and through the fallopian tubes may have a similar effect. Dilute solutions of local anesthetic should be used; it is only too easy to give a toxic dose otherwise.

Maximal Local Anesthetic Doses

The following should be regarded as maximal doses of local anesthetic for the complete procedure:

- Bupivacaine – 2 mg kg^{-1} of body weight – for a 70 kg woman this is 140 mg or 28 ml of 0.5% Marcain.
- Lidocaine – 4 mg (plain) or 7 mg (with adrenaline) kg^{-1} of body weight – for a 70 kg woman at 3 mg kg^{-1} this is 210 mg plain lidocaine (or 42 ml of 0.5%); at 7 mg kg^{-1} this is 490 mg lidocaine with adrenaline (or 98 ml of 0.5%).

The Bladder

Catheterization of the patient can be avoided if the patient is asked to empty her bladder immediately before the operation. If there is any doubt about whether or not the bladder is empty, a simple transabdominal ultrasound scan will confirm this.

Patient Position

The patient should be placed comfortably in a modified Lloyd-Davies position, and after infiltrating the anterior lip of the cervix with a very small amount of local anesthetic agent, I grasp the cervix transversely with a single tooth tenaculum. Uterine manipulation will usually be required. This will call for the gentle insertion of some form of uterine manipulator through the cervix, so that the surgeon can antevert and retrovert the uterus at will. This can be a relatively uncomfortable part of the operation and I personally use a dilator that can be easily passed through the cervical canal without dilatation. Other authors avoid uterine manipulation and do not place the patient in any special position (Khandala, 1984).

The Pneumoperitoneum

A pneumoperitoneum should be obtained after passing a Veress needle at the usual site. If the patient is sufficiently cooperative she can be asked to tense her abdominal muscles and this aids passing the needle.

Carbon dioxide (CO_2) is usually used for insufflating the peritoneal cavity at general anesthetic laparoscopy, but some authors maintain that nitrous oxide causes less discomfort, and at least one has described the use of air in many patients without a problem (Khandala, 1984). It may prove difficult, however, to obtain a peritoneal insufflating machine with a connection for anything other than CO_2 cylinders. Ideally the gas should be prewarmed and pre-humidified before insufflation to reduce generalized peritoneal stimulation and discomfort from the gas.

The Laparoscope

The standard laparoscope used for most general anesthetic laparoscopies is a 10 mm 0° rod lens laparoscope. Such an instrument undoubtedly gives the best vision, but requires the passage of a relatively large trocar. Smaller laparoscopes are generally used for local anesthetic techniques.

Very adequate rod lens laparoscopes of 3–4 mm in diameter can be obtained and these produce a view that is only a slightly lower quality than that with a 10 mm laparoscope. Modern 5–7 mm laparoscopes are likely to be optically better than older 10 mm scopes.

Still smaller scopes are now available, several being available on the market with an external diameter of 1–2 mm. These scopes invariably have a fiber basis to their optics and while the optical resolution that can be obtained with them is good, it is not as high as that obtained with solid rod lenses. (Risquez et al., 1993). These small scopes are expensive and delicate and one of the big advantages in their use is that they encourage the surgeon to be gentle in handling both the instruments and the patient.

The system used by the author is an optical catheter (Figures 67.1, 67.2). The light source and camera system are statically mounted on the stand (Figure 67.3). An integral fiberoptic bundle carries both light fibers and imaging fibers to and from the box (Figure 67.4).

Many of the small fiberoptic scopes now available are designed to be passed down the Veress needle that has previously been used to create the pneumoperitoneum (Childers et al., 1992; Risquez et al., 1993). One of the problems with the use of minilaparoscopes is the need to avoid even the slightest contamination of the lens with blood or fluid. A single drop of blood will completely destroy the view down a 1.8 mm scope. Small scopes of this

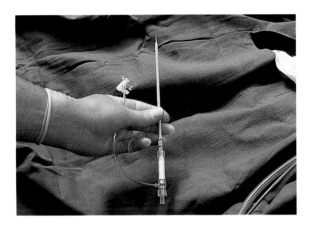

Figure 67.1 A modified Veress-type needle – the Adair needle (Medical Dynamics, Englewood, Colorado, USA) – which is used for insufflating the peritoneal cavity and as a cannula for the optical catheter laparoscope (Medical Dynamics, Englewood, Colorado, USA). Note the gas sealing valve at the proximal end.

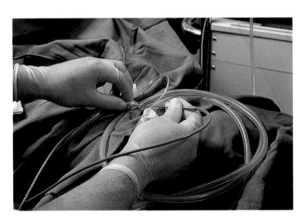

Figure 67.2 The optical catheter in use.

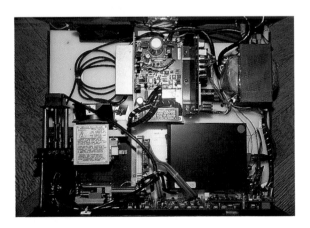

Figure 67.3 The camera and light source are both statically mounted in the case for maximal efficiency.

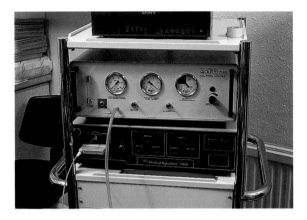

Figure 67.4 The equipment for using the optical catheter. Note that the light cable is integral with the optical viewing fibers.

nature will usually need a very high quality light source and light cable. Some may have their own inbuilt light source.

Video Equipment

Although eyeballing down the laparoscope is adequate for performing some operations, particularly diagnostic procedures, operations under local anesthetic have the advantage that the patient may wish to visualize the procedure in real-time. High-quality, lightweight video cameras attached to the scope give the opportunity not only for the surgeon and the patient to view the pelvis, but also for the findings to be recorded and viewed at a later date if necessary.

Monitoring

It is well to remember that even if the patient has not been anesthetized by a standard general anesthetic, intravenous midazolam and fentanyl have a strongly sedative effect and if given in excessive dosages can depress or even arrest respiration. In my view the minimum monitoring facility that should be considered is a pulse oximeter attached to the patient at all times. Facial oxygen might also be considered to be appropriate, but this can distress the patient and cause excessive anxiety. At the very least, however, facial oxygen should be available to be given if necessary. An ampoule of flumazenil drawn up and ready in case an excessive dose of midazolam has been inadvertently administered should also be available. Flumazenil rapidly reverses the effects of benzodiazepine agents such as midazolam. As the half-life of midazolam is longer than that of flumazenil, the effects of flumazenil will wear off first and the sedative effect of midazolam will return. Flumazenil should not be used routinely, but kept for emergency use.

Conclusion

Few gynecologists have wholeheartedly embraced local anesthetic outpatient laparoscopy. Some (Bhatt and Trivedi, 1981; Bhalerao, 1982; Khandala, 1984), however, have reported huge series of outpatient local anesthetic female sterilizations with few complications, and a high rate of patient acceptability. The growing trend towards shorter hospital stay and increased outpatient work requires us all to explore the benefits of outpatient laparoscopy under local anesthesia.

References

Bhalerao MN (1982) Laparoscopic sterilization: experience of 20 000 cases in rural areas. *Clinical Meeting of the Bombay Obstetrics and Gynaecological Society, Bombay, May 1.*

Bhatt RV, Trivedi GK (1981) Mortality in laparoscopic sterilization using fallope rings in rural camps in Gujarat. *First Asian Congress on Gynaecological Endoscopy, Bombay, February.*

Chamberlain GVP, Carron-Brown J (eds) (1978) *Gynaecological Laparoscopy*. London: Royal College of Obstetricians and Gynaecologists.

Childers JM, Hatch KD, Surwitt EA (1992) Office laparoscopy and biopsy for evaluation of patients with intraperitoneal carcinomatosis using a new optical catheter. *Gynecologic Oncology* **47**: 337–342.

Gordon AG (1984) Laparoscopy under local anaesthesia. *Journal of the Royal Society of Medicine* **77**: 540–541.

Khandala SD (1984) Development of a simplified laparoscopic sterilization technique. *Journal of Reproductive Medicine* **29**: 586–588.

Ott, D (1901) Illumination of the abdomen (ventroscopy). *J Akush Zhenksk Bolez* **15**: 1045.

Penfield JA (1974) Laparoscopic sterilization under local anaesthesia. In Phillips JM (ed.) *Gynaecological Laparoscopy: Principles and Techniques*. pp. 225–226. New York: Stratton International.

Risquez F, Pennehouat G, Fernandez R, Confino E, Rodriguez O (1993) Microlaparoscopy: a preliminary report. *Human Reproduction* **8**: 1701–1702.

68

Total Laparoscopic Hysterectomy Using Ultrasound Energy

CHARLES E. MILLER

The Center For Human Reproduction, Chicago, IL, USA

In 1989, Harry Reich performed the first laparoscopic hysterectomy (Reich *et al.*, 1989). Since this landmark in surgical history, multiple techniques have been described to enable hysterectomy to proceed at least in part via a laparoscopic route (Boike *et al.*, 1993; Bishop, 1993; Lyons, 1993; Angle *et al.*, 1994). Electrosurgical instrumentation, laser, vascular clips, and linear staplers and cutters have all been used. However, use of this instrumentation in laparoscopic surgery has not been without complication (Saye *et al.*, 1991; Reich 1992; Ata *et al.*, 1993; Ryder and Hulka 1993; Soderstrom, 1994; Tucker

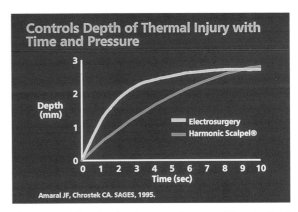

Figure 68.2 The depth of penetration noted in standard monopolar electrosurgery (30 W) is compared to a standard setting of the harmonic scalpel (level 3). Electrosurgery achieves maximum penetration within seconds and plateaus as tissue desiccates, as studied in porcine liver, stomach and skin tissues. In contrast, depth of penetration with the harmonic scalpel increases linearly with time when power and pressure are constant.

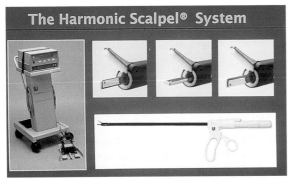

Figure 68.1 The harmonic scalpel. The generator converts electronic energy to mechanical motion. This enables the active blade of the LaparoSonic Coagulating Shears to vibrate 55 500 times per second. The active blade of the LaparoSonic Coagulating Shears can be rotated to three different positions. This enables varying tissue effect. This figure, and Figures 68.2–68.15, are reproduced with kind permission from Ethicon Endo-Surgery, Inc.

1995). Adverse events with electrosurgery have included stray current, insulation failure and capacitative coupling, while the linear stapler and cutter has been noted to misfire. Injury to the ureter has occurred, both with electrosurgery and with the linear stapler and cutter.

In contrast to the above, the ultrasonically activated scalpel (Harmonic Scalpel, Ethicon Endo-Surgery, Cincinnati, Ohio, USA) has proven to be a safe and effective tool in laparoscopic surgery (Amaral, 1993a) (Figure 68.1). When coagulating with the ultrasonically activated scalpel, both depth of penetration and lateral distribution of energy are far more gradual than in electrosurgery and therefore easier to control (Amaral and Chrostek, 1993) (Figures 68.2, 68.3).

The author's technique and experience with the use of an ultrasonically activated scapel in laparoscopic hysterectomy, more precisely the LaparoSonic Coagulating Shears, will now be presented.

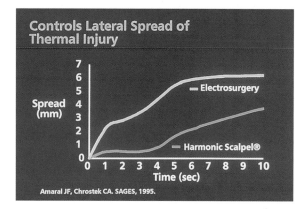

Figure 68.3 The lateral spread of coagulation noted in standard monopolar electrosurgery (30 W) is compared to a standard setting of the harmonic scalpel (level 3). The lateral spread of coagulation from the harmonic scalpel is much less than the tissue destruction with electrosurgery when compared in standard models (porcine liver, stomach and skin tissue) over time.

Ultrasonic Coagulation and Cutting Mechanics

Both electrosurgery and laser surgery cause hemostasis primarily via tissue desiccation with a resultant scab forming over the area. As blood and tissue is heated to far in excess of 100°C, however, tissue is destroyed and charring occurs. In contrast, an ultrasonically activated scalpel uses ultrasound energy to disrupt hydrogen bonds of protein moieties and thus denature the protein in tissue (Figure 68.4).

With the tip of the active blade of the unit vibrating 55 500 times per second in the longitudinal axis for 50–100 μm, blood vessels are accepted and sealed by a denatured protein coagulum. Vessels up to 5 mm in diameter can be coagulated in this fashion (Amaral, 1993a; Amaral and Chrostek, 1995) (Figure 68.5).

When necessary, secondary deep coagulation can be accomplished by heat generation resulting from the friction of the vibration of the blade on tissue. Char is still not noted, but greater desiccation will occur with heat generation. This desiccation effect

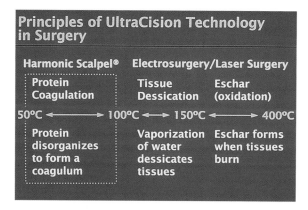

Figure 68.4 Electrosurgery and laser surgery cause hemostasis by raising temperatures far in excess of 100°C. Vaporization of cellular fluid occurs, thus leading to tissue desiccation. Ultimately, the eschar formed seals the vessel. In contrast, an ultrasonically activated scalpel is able to disrupt hydrogen bonds of protein moieties at temperatures less than 100°C. In doing so, small blood vessels are sealed by a denatured protein coagulum.

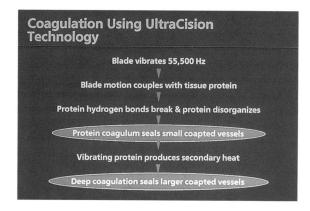

Figure 68.5 Small vessels are sealed by a protein coagulum at temperatures below 100°C. Larger vessels are coapted by heat generated over time due to the friction of the vibrating instrument on the tissue.

using an ultrasonically activated system, however, is far less and more gradual than with the use of electrosurgical techniques. Moreover, because temperature increase at the tissue is far lower than with electrosurgery, smoke production is greatly reduced. (Hambley *et al.*, 1988; Amaral, 1993a, 1993b, 1993c; Amaral and Chrostek, 1993; Ott, 1993; Markovecz *et al.*, 1994; Meltzer *et al.*, 1994; Amaral and Chrostek, 1995). Not only is visualization enhanced, but potential risk from smoke production is minimized (McCarus, 1996).

As tissue response is parallel to the direction of force of the energy, lateral tissue damage is minimized (Ott, 1993; Amaral and Chrostek, 1995) (Figure 68.6). This lateral tissue destruction is especially negligible when dissecting within the tissue plane. Furthermore, cutting may be enhanced by the cavitational effect (Figure 68.7). Due to a transient fluctuation in pressure generated at the blade tip, fluids vaporize at low temperatures; this, in turn leads to a separation of tissue planes similar to that occurring with dissection. Unlike hydrodissection, however, the tissue does not become edematous, which may have a deleterious effect on visualization. The ability to separate tissue planes with the cavitation effect is helpful for:

- Incising sidewall peritoneum to improve visualization of the ureters.
- Opening up the broad ligament for further dissection at the time of round ligament transection.
- Transection of the cervico-vesico-uterine peritoneum (creation of the bladder flap).
- Opening up of the broad ligament to skeletonize the uterine vessels (Amaral, 1993b).

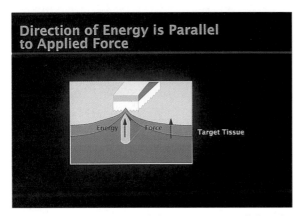

Figure 68.6 The direction of the energy is parallel to the applied force. Thus, lateral tissue damage is minimized.

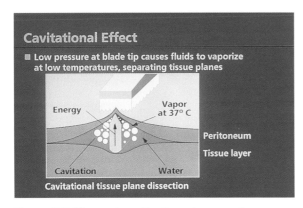

Figure 68.7 Ultrasonic vibration lowers the vapor pressure. As PV remains constant, this results in increased tissue volume. This expanding vapor opens tissue planes.

Instrumentation – LaparoSonic Coagulating Shears

The ultrasonically activated scalpel that proves to be the instrument of choice in the laparoscopic approach to hysterectomy is the LaparoSonic Coagulating Shears (see Figure 68.1). This particular instrument was designed to maximize the coagulation effect of large vessels and to allow coagulation of unsupported tissue. Studies in porcine models verified that vessels 5 mm in diameter could be coagulated and cut with this technology (Miller, 1996). The LaparoSonic Coagulating Shears consist of the 15 mm active blade, which vibrates at 55 500 times per second, and an inactive pad (Figure 68.8). As unsupported tissue is grasped between the active and inactive pads, coaptive coagulation is optimized. This multifunctional instrument can thus grasp, coapt, coagulate and cut tissue without instrument exchange (Amaral, 1993b).

The active blade has three different surfaces, which can be rotated into position using a thumb wheel on the hand piece (see Figure 68.1). Depending upon the surface of the blade, the tissue effect can be greater cutting with less coagulation or greater coagulation and less cutting (Figure 68.9; Robbins and Ferland, 1995). When the shear mode is used, the sharp side is against the inactive pad. In this position, the LaparoSonic Coagulating Shears function as hemostatic scissors – the coagulation effect is minimized (0.25–1 mm) while the cutting effect is maximized (Figure 68.10). In the blunt mode, the coagulation effect increases (0.75–1.75 mm) while cutting ability decreases (Figure 68.11). In this same position, the sharp surface will be directed outwards and it can therefore be used as an energized knife. Even greater coagulation effect (1.0–2.0 mm) can be gained when the active blade is

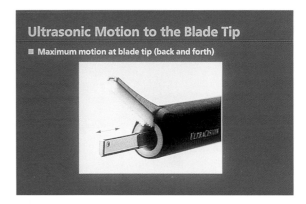

Figure 68.8 The LaparoSonic Coagulating Shears consists of the 15 mm active blade and an inactive pad. The active pad vibrates in a forward–backward direction 55 500 times per second.

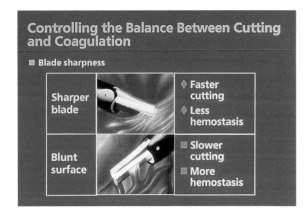

Figure 68.9 This illustration summarizes the ability to control the balance between cutting and coagulation with blade sharpness. A sharper blade provides more cutting and less hemostasis.

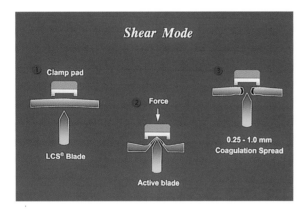

Figure 68.10 In the shear mode (the sharp side against the inactive pad) the coagulation effect of the LaparoSonic Coagulating Shears (LCS) is minimized (0.25–1 mm), while cutting is maximized.

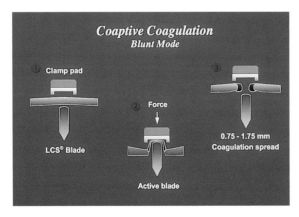

Figure 68.11 In the blunt mode, the coagulation effect of the LaparoSonic Coagulating Shears (LCS) increases (0.75–1.75 mm) while cutting ability decreases.

rotated 90° to the flat position. Along with the increased coagulation effect, there is greater lateral distribution of energy (Figure 68.12).

Cutting versus coagulation effect can be modified not only with the active blade position, but also by altering tissue tension, power setting and grip strength. At a power setting of one, the excursion of the blade is 50 μm, at three the blade moves 70 μm, and at the maximum level five, the distance traveled by the active blade is 100 μm. Coagulation and slower cutting occurs at lower power, while fastest cutting with minimal coagulation occurs at level five (Figure 68.13).

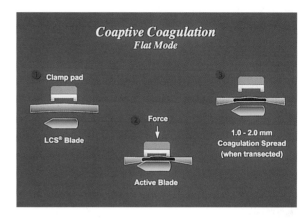

Figure 68.12 Even greater coagulation effect (1.0–2.0 mm) occurs with the active blade in the flat position. In this position, a greater lateral distribution of energy is noted with the LaparoSonic Coagulating Shears (LCS).

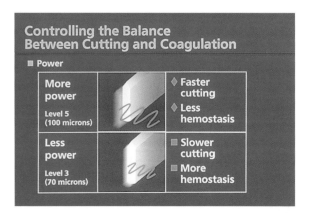

Figure 68.13 Cutting and coagulation can be modified by the power setting, which alters the blade excursion. At a power setting of one, the excursion of the blade is 50 μm, at three the blade moves 70 μm, and at the maximum level five, the distance traveled by the blade is 100 μm.

When tissue is placed on the greatest tension, cutting is maximized, while coagulation is minimized (Figure 68.14).

Likewise, when grip force is greatest, the fastest cutting and least coagulation are noted (Figure 68.15). Thus, maximum coagulation is noted with a blunt or flat blade position on a low power, minimizing tissue tension and grip force. On the other hand, greatest cutting occurs with strong grip force, a sharp blade, high power setting and with tissue on tension. As an example, coagulation and subsequent cutting of a large vessel (utero-ovarian ligament, infundibulopelvic ligament or uterine vessels) is initially performed using minimal tension, a light grip and a blunt blade at level three. Once coagulation has been initiated, cutting is performed by increasing tissue tension and grip force. In fact, to increase the coagulation effect, the vascular pedicle is coagulated at three adjacent sites

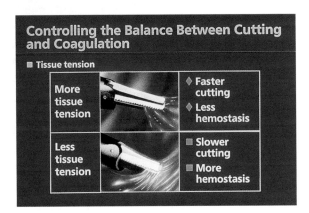

Figure 68.14 The amount of tension placed on the tissue determines whether a cutting or coagulation effect is noted. The more tension placed on the tissue, the greater the cutting effect.

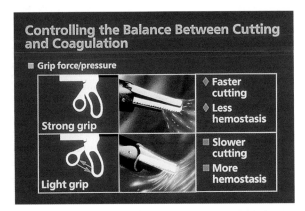

Figure 68.15 The force of the grip placed across tissue with the LaparoSonic Coagulating Shears determines the degree of cutting versus coagulation at the tissue site. When grip force is greatest, cutting is fastest and least coagulation is noted.

before cutting. On the other hand, cutting peritoneum over the broad ligament or bladder involves placing the tissue on tension using a firm grip and the sharp surface at a power level of five.

Results of the use of LaparoSonic Coagulating Shears in the Laparoscopic Approach to Hysterectomy

At the 1995 Annual Meeting of the American Association of Gynecologic Laparoscopists, the author presented 102 consecutive hysterectomies performed by a laparoscopic approach using the LaparoSonic Coagulating Shears (Miller, 1995). This discussion included laparoscopic assisted vaginal hysterectomy, laparoscopic hysterectomy with vaginal completion, and complete laparoscopic hysterectomy.

Only one patient during this study period required conversion to an open technique. This represents a conversion rate of less than 1%. This patient is in fact the only patient for whom a laparoscopic hysterectomy has been converted to an abdominal hysterectomy since the author began using the LaparoSonic Coagulating Shears 42 months ago.

As reported at the twenty-fourth International Congress of Gynecologic Endoscopy, few complications were noted among these 102 patients. One patient received one unit of autologous blood as ordered by her referring physician, although postoperative hemoglobin was normal before the transfusion. Minor complications consisted of one case of postoperative cuff cellulitis, which was treated with oral antibiotics on an outpatient basis, and one case of bleeding from the vaginal cuff, which was treated in the office with Monsel's solution.

Before the use of the LaparoSonic Coagulating Shears, the author noted a 10% conversion rate to open abdominal hysterectomy. As mentioned above, the present conversion rate using the LaparoSonic Coagulating Shears is negligible. The major impact with the use of the LaparoSonic Coagulating Shears on decreasing the need to proceed to abdominal hysterectomy is in the ability to treat the patient with a large myomatous uterus.

Special Consideration – the Large Myomatous Uterus

Before the LaparoSonic Coagulating Shears became available, the large bulky myomatous uterus was morcellated via a vaginal route using traditional techniques. However, at times, the fibroids were so large and subsequent visualization so poor, that it was virtually impossible to transect the lateral ligaments supporting the uterus. Moreover, the corpus of the uterus can be so enlarged that the uterus will not distend into the pelvis due to the bony structure of the pelvis.

The LaparoSonic Coagulating Shears are used to evacuate the large myoma or myomas from the uterus; thus, the uterus is reduced in size, allowing subsequent descensus and vaginal extraction. The fibroids remain in the cul-de-sac until the uterus has been removed. The fibroids are then retrieved and removed via the vagina.

Ideally, the uterine vessel pedicles are secured before evacuation of the fibroids. If this cannot be accomplished, a dilute synthetic vasopressin solution is used to control hemostasis. This synthetic vasopressin is infiltrated into the bed of the myoma.

The myoma or myomas are resected from the uterus using the LaparoSonic Coagulating Shears and a technique the author has previously described for laparoscopic myomectomy (Miller, 1996). The serosa and myometrium are incised to the level of the myoma using the LaparoSonic Coagulating Shears at level five with the sharp side out. Thus, the LaparoSonic Coagulating Shears perform as an activated knife (Figure 68.16). The LaparoSonic Coagulating Shears are then used to dissect out the myoma with blunt dissection (Figure 68.17). If particularly tenacious areas are noted between the myometrium and the fibroid, the LaparoSonic Coagulating Shears are activated to allow rapid dissection. With this technique, the author has performed laparoscopic hysterectomy in a woman with an 18-cm fibroid.

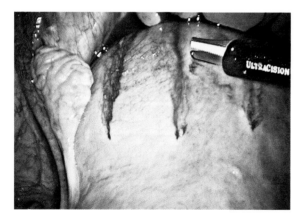

Figure 68.16 This uterus contains a 14-cm posterior wall myoma. With the sharp side facing away from the inactive pad, the LaparoSonic Coagulating Shears is used as an energized knife to cut through the serosa and myometrium to the level of the myoma.

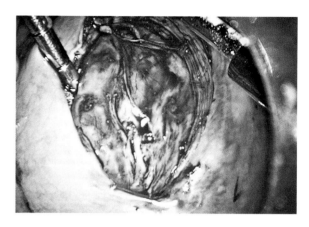

Figure 68.17 The myoma is then dissected out of the uterus with blunt dissection and sharp dissection. If further hemostasis is required, the blunt side is used against the inactive pad for increased coagulation.

Steps in Complete Laparoscopic Hysterectomy Using the LaparoSonic Coagulating Shears

The steps for complete laparoscopic hysterectomy using LaparoSonic Coagulating Shears are as follows:

1. Dissect out the ureters when necessary. Use the LaparoSonic Coagulating Shears in the shears position at level five. This provides the ability for opening up the peritoneum over the ureter with a minimum lateral distribution of energy.
2. Transect the round ligaments using the blunt or flat blade at level three. This enables a coagulation effect as the round ligament is transected.
3. Open up the cervico-vesico-uterine peritoneum with the shears mode at level five as this tissue is minimally vascular.
4. Mobilize the bladder off the cervix. Usually this can be performed without energy. If necessary, the shears at level five can be used.
5. Depending upon whether the ovaries remain or are removed, the utero-ovarian or infundibulopelvic ligament is initially coagulated and then transected. The blunt or flat blade is used at level three. In order to allow coagulation first, a light touch must be used and the area coagulated in three positions. Only then can hemostatic cutting occur (Figure 68.18).
6. The uterine vessels are now skeletonized by using the shears mode at level five as

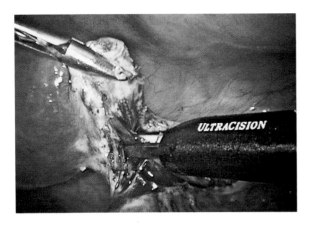

Figure 68.18 The LaparoSonic Coagulating Shears have been used to skeletonize the right infundibulopelvic ligament using a shears mode. Now the vessels are coagulated and cut with the LaparoSonic Coagulating Shears in the blunt or flat mode.

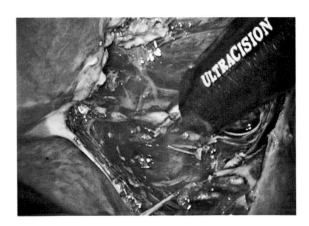

Figure 68.20 The right uterine vessels are now well visualized. The vessels are initially coagulated with the blunt or flat blade of the LaparoSonic Coagulating Shears at level three in three adjacent areas at level three.

concern with coagulation is minimal (Figure 68.19).

7. In a similar way to dealing with the utero-ovarian ligament or infundibulopelvic ligament, the uterine vessels are initially coagulated with the blunt or flat blade in three adjacent areas at level three and then transected. Care must be taken to maximize coagulation (Figure 68.20).

8. Cardinal ligaments are transected using the blunt or flat surface at level three.

9. The blunt position is now used to grasp, coagulate and cut across the uterosacral ligament at level three.

10. A sponge stick is now placed anterior to the cervix and the vagina is carefully entered.

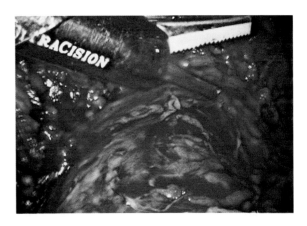

Figure 68.21 An anterior culdotomy incision is made at level five with the sharp side out (an activated knife) after a sponge stick has been placed in the vagina.

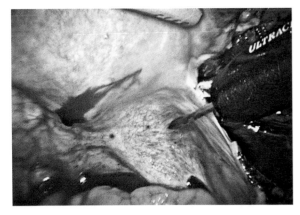

Figure 68.19 The posterior broad ligament is opened to begin skeletonization of the uterine vessels. A shears mode of the LaparoSonic Coagulating Shears at level five is used.

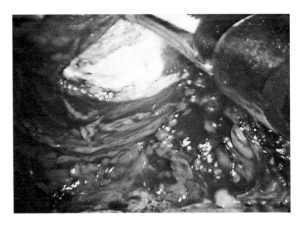

Figure 68.22 The cervix and uterus is now amputated from the apex of the vagina, utilizing the LaparoSonic Coagulating Shears.

11. An anterior culdotomy incision is made at level five using the sharp side to the outside (i.e. an activated knife) as the apex of the vagina is relatively vascular, and thus cutting with minimal coagulation (Figure 68.21).

12. The amputation of the cervix continues using the blunt mode at level 3–5 or as an energized knife at level five (Figure 68.22).

13. The specimen is removed through the vagina. The vaginal vault is then repaired via a laparoscopic route.

References

Amaral JF (1993a) Laparoscopic application of an ultrasonically activated scalpel. *GI Endoscopy Clinics of North America* **3**: 381–392.

Amaral JF (1993b) Comparison of the ultrasonically activated scalpel to electrosurgery and laser surgery for laparoscopic surgery. *Surgical Laparoscopy and Endoscopy* **7**: 141.

Amaral JF (1993c) The ultrasonically activated scalpel produces less tissue damage during seromyotomy than electrosurgery. *Surgical Laparoscopy and Endoscopy* **7**: 213.

Amaral JF, Chrostek C (1993) Sealing and cutting of blood vessels and hollow viscus with an ultrasonically activated shears. Presented at *American College of Surgeons, San Francisco, October 1993*.

Amaral JF, Chrostek C (1995) Depth of thermal injury: ultrasonically activated scalpel versus electrosurgery. *Surgical Laparoscopy and Endoscopy* **9**: 226.

Angle HS, Cohen SM, Midlebaugh D (1994) The initial Worcester experience with laparoscopic hysterectomy. *Journal of the American Association of Gynecologic Laparoscopists* **2**: 155–161.

Ata AH, Bellemore TJ, Meisel JA, Arambulo SM (1993) Distal thermal injury from monopolar electrosurgery. *Surgical Laparoscopy and Endoscopy* **3**: 323–327.

Bishop M (1993) Laparoscopic hysterectomy: how should it be done. *Surgical Laparoscopy and Endoscopy* **3**: 127.

Boike GM, Elfstrand EP, DelPriore G *et al.* (1993) Laparoscopically assisted vaginal hysterectomy in a university hospital: report of 82 cases and comparison with abdominal and vaginal hysterectomy. *American Journal of Obstetrics and Gynecology* **168**: 1690–1697.

Hambley R, Hebda PA, Abell E, Cohen BA, Jegasothy BV (1988) Wound healing of skin incisions produced by ultrasonically vibrating knife, scalpel, electrosurgery, and carbon dioxide laser. *Journal of Dermatology and Surgical Oncology* **14**: 1213–1217.

Lyons TL (1993) Laparoscopic supracervical hysterectomy – a comparison of morbidity and mortality results with laparoscopically assisted vaginal hysterectomy. *Journal of Reproductive Medicine* **38**: 763–767.

Markovecz, Chrostek CA, Amarel JF (1994) Surgical laparoscopic energy and lateral thermal damage. Presented at *The Society for Minimally Invasive Therapy, Berlin, October, 1994*.

McCarus SD (1996) Physiological mechanism of the ultrasonically activated harmonic scalpel. *Journal of the American Association of Gynecologic Laparoscopists* **3**: 601–608.

Meltzer RC, Hoenig DM, Chrostek CA, Amarel JF (1994) Porcine seromyotomies using an ultrasonically activated scalpel. *Surgical Laparoscopy and Endoscopy* **8**: 253.

Miller CE (1995) A follow up critical review of laparoscopic hysterectomy and laparoscopic assisted vaginal hysterectomy. Presented at *The Second World Symposium on Laparoscopic Hysterectomy, New Orleans, LA*.

Miller CE (1996) Laparoscopic myomectomy in the infertile patient. *Journal of the American Association of Gynecologic Laparoscopists* **4**: 522–529.

Ott D (1993) Smoke production and smoke reduction in endoscopic surgery. *Surgical Laparoscopy and Endoscopy* **1**: 230–232.

Reich H (1992) Laparoscopic bowel injury. *Surgical Laparoscopy and Endoscopy* **2**: 74–78.

Reich H., Decaprio J, McGlynn F (1989) Laparoscopic hysterectomy. *Journal of Gynecologic Surgery* **5**: 213–216.

Robbins ML, Ferland RJ (1995) Laparoscopic assisted vaginal hysterectomy using the Laparosonic Coagulating Shears™: a preliminary report. *Journal of the American Association of Gynecologic Laparoscopists* **2**: 339–343.

Ryder RM, Hulka JF (1993) Bladder and bowel injury after electrodesiccation with Kleppinger bipolar forceps: a clinicopathologic study. *Journal of Reproductive Medicine* **38**: 595–598.

Saye WB, Miller W, Hertzmann P (1991) Electrosurgical thermal injury: myth or misconception? *Surgical Laparoscopy and Endoscopy* **1**: 223–228.

Soderstrom RM (1994) Cutting your legal risks of electrosurgery. *OB/GYN Management* **6**: 19–32.

Tucker RD (1995) Laparoscopic electrosurgical injuries: survey results and their implications. *Surgical Laparoscopy and Endoscopy* **5**: 311–317.

69

Embolization of Myomas

BRUCE McLUCAS

100 UCLA Medical Plaza, Suite 310, Los Angeles, CA, USA

Introduction

Embolization of pelvic vessels has been used to treat acute pelvic hemorrhage and is now an established procedure within gynecology and obstetrics. Perhaps the longest history of efficacy is noted for hemorrhage associated with pelvic malignancy, when surgery is either impossible or must be postponed until radiation or further evaluation is necessary (Yamashita *et al.*, 1994). In treatment of postpartum hemorrhage, embolization has a success rate close to 100% (Greenwood *et al.*, 1987), compared to at the best a 50% success rate with either hypogastric artery ligation (Clark *et al.*, 1985) or uterine artery ligation (Fahmy, 1966). Several different occlusion techniques are available, including coils and permanent or temporary particles. The choice of occlusion method is determined by the nature of the disease and the desired function of the structure being embolized.

At the Hôpital Lariboisiere in Paris, France, Ravina and his co-workers followed patients who were initially referred for temporary measures before definitive surgery, either myomectomy or hysterectomy (Ravina *et al.*, 1995a). These patients were often able to avoid surgical intervention after initial embolization as the myomas shrank after arterial embolization. Ravina then began to study the effects of embolic therapy as an alternative to surgery. His initial work detailing the treatment of 16 patients was reported in 1995 in the *Lancet* (Ravina *et al.*, 1995b). Among others, our group at UCLA has been able to duplicate the results of the French (McLucas *et al.*, 1996).

Patient Characteristics

Patients who are candidates for embolization are also surgical candidates. All of our patients suffered from menorrhagia. Table 69.1 summarizes the details of the initial patients in our study group. Five women were perimenopausal or menopausal, the others were ovulatory. Eight of the patients had additional gynecologic problems – six with adhesions, two with endometriosis. All patients had multiple myomas documented on pelvic examination and ultrasound.

Every patient had previously undergone invasive procedures for control of symptoms including myomectomy (ten patients), myoma lysis (three patients), and endometrial ablation (five patients). All patients were screened by hysteroscopy to exclude a malignant cause for their symptoms. No patients were known to have conditions that would make them vulnerable to hemorrhage or ischemic or infectious complications of embolization such as coagulopathy, salpingitis, diabetes mellitus or other causes of vasculitis. All patients were offered hysterectomy as an alternative. The risks and benefits of the procedure were described both by a gynecologist and an interventional radiologist. At the time of writing, we are beginning to offer embolization to patients who desire fertility. However, the patients reported here were cautioned against future pregnancies until more could be learned about the long-term results of the procedure.

Table 69.1 Characteristics of patients undergoing uterine artery embolization.

Patient	Current Age	Prior Pregnancy	Menstrual Status	Gyne. History	Previous Procedures	Symptoms
1	55	$G_4P_4Ab_0$	Post-menop.	None	TCMR Cystectomy	Bleeding* and pelvic pain
2	47	$G_1P_1Ab_0$	Peri-menop.	Adhesions Hydrosalpinx	Laparoscopic myolysis	Pelvic pain
3	45	G_0	Pre-menop.	Adhesions	TCMR Adhesiolysis Abdom. myomectomy	Bleeding and pelvic pain
4	38	G_0	Pre-menop.	Adhesions	TCMR Cystectomy Endom. fulguration Adhesiolysis	Pelvic pain
5	53	$G_2P_2Ab_0$	Pre-menop.	None	Abdom. myomectomy	Bleeding and pelvic pain
6	55	$G_7P_2mAb_5$	Post-menop.	None	Abdom. myomectomy Endom. fulguration	Bleeding and pelvic pain*
7	27	G_0	Pre-menop.	Asherman's syndrome	TCMR Abdom. myomectomy L salp-oophorectomy	Pelvic pain
8	49	$G_3P_0Ab_3$ (mAb_2,tAb_1)	Peri-menop.	None	TCMR Endom. fulguration Laparoscopic myolysis	Bleeding and pelvic pain*
9	41	$G_3P_1mAb_2$	Pre-menop.	Adhesions	TCMR Adhesiolysis Cystectomy	Bleeding
10	32	$G_2P_0mAb_2$	Pre-menop.	Adhesions	TCMR Abdom. myomectomy Myolysis Endom. fulguration Adhesiolysis	Bleeding with anemia
11	32	G_0	Pre-menop.	Adhesions Endometriosis	Abdom. myomectomy TCMR Adhesiolysis Endom. fulguration	Bleeding and pelvic pain*

mAb, miscarriage.
Peri-menop., perimenopausal.
Pre-menop., premenopausal.
tAb, therapeutic abortion.
TCMR, transcervical myoma resection.
Endom., endometriosis.
Abdom., abdominal.
*dominant symptom.

Technique

The patient's right groin was prepared and draped and the right femoral artery was punctured under local anesthetic with a 4 or 5 F catheter and a glide catheter. The contralateral (left) common iliac, internal iliac, and anterior division were catheterized in sequence. Using digital subtraction arteriography, the uterine artery was selected. Five patients required use of a .018 Tracker microcatheter to enter the uterine artery; all catheterizations were aided by digital roadmapping. Once entered, the uterine artery was embolized with 500–700 μm polyvinyl alcohol particles (PVA), except one patient who received 300–500 μm PVA. The photographs show the left uterine artery outlined by contrast (Figure 69.1) and after embolization (Figure 69.2).

After stasis in the left uterine artery, a Waltman loop technique was used to enter the ipsilateral internal iliac artery in all but one patient. Similar subselective catheterization and free flow embolization was performed on the right side. The length of the procedure varied from 45–90 minutes (average

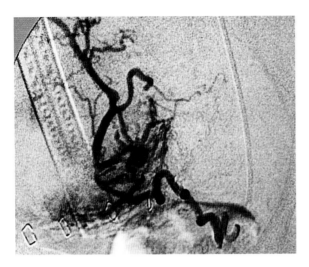

Figure 69.1 Dye injected through catheter inserted into right uterine artery reveals typical corkscrew appearance of myoma's blood supply.

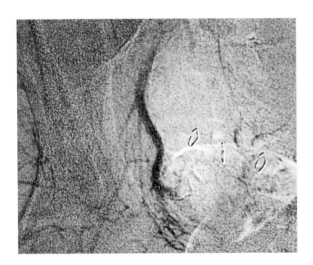

Figure 69.2 Following injection of polyvinyl alcohol no flow of contrast is seen beyond the tip of the catheter in the same artery.

75 minutes). After removal of the catheter and wire, hemostasis was obtained by direct compression for 15 minutes. Patients were confined to bed rest for six hours following embolization to prevent bleeding from the arterial site. No patient required overnight observation.

Analgesia

In the initial group of patients, an anesthesiologist provided general anesthesia for all except one patient who received conscious sedation (fentanyl and versed). Subsequent patients have all been managed by this latter method without difficulty. Five patients received 100 mg of lidocaine injected directly into the uterine artery for periprocedure analgesia. All patients received 30 mg of ketorolac in the post-anesthesia care unit, nine intravenously, and two intramuscularly. The total post-procedure analgesia and subsequent pain levels of patients were recorded.

Clinical follow-up

Measures of success were primarily the patients' responses to a questionnaire posted to them five months after embolization. Ultrasound examinations were performed at six weeks and six months following the embolization and included measurements of total uterine volume and myoma size, as well as Doppler flow studies of the uterine arteries pre- and post-procedure.

Results

Angiographic Findings

Hypervascular uterine masses with bilateral blood supplies were demonstrated in six patients, masses with unilateral blood supplies could be seen in two patients, and three patients showed diffuse vascularity without an obvious mass. One of the early patients with unilateral distortion of the blood supply underwent unilateral embolization; all of the other patients had bilateral procedures.

Clinical Results

No complications were encountered either in the procedure room or in the post-anesthesia suite. One patient has had incomplete follow-up.

Nine patients completed the questionnaires. Eight reported a decrease in menorrhagia and pain. The lack of response was seen in the patient who underwent unilateral embolization. One patient experienced post-procedure fever and leukocytosis to 22 000 three weeks after embolization. She was successfully treated with intravenous antibiotics and then returned to the hospital where a computed tomogram revealed a pelvic abscess – she then underwent a total abdominal hysterectomy, during which purulent material was seen.

Ultrasound Changes

All 11 patients underwent ultrasound examination before embolization, which demonstrated myomatous change. Nine patients had a follow-up ultrasound two months after embolization. One patient underwent an ultrasound examination where dimensions were not recorded, but for the other eight patients pre- and post-procedure dimensions were available. Before embolization, average uterine dimensions were 9.8 × 5.8 × 7.3 cm (calculated volume 224 + 99 cm³), whereas after the procedure the dimensions were 8.7 × 4.6 × 5.9 cm (calculated volume 127 + 48 cm³). The average reduction in uterine volume was 40%, with a range of 22–61%. Similar decreases in myoma volumes were observed. The sonograms of one patient before the procedure and six weeks and six months after the procedure are shown in Figure 69.3. The single patient who underwent unilateral embolization and did not obtain symptom relief nonetheless had a 34% reduction in uterine volume.

Morbidity

Among patients undergoing conscious sedation there were no observable intraoperative complaints of pain. In the recovery room following embolization, seven patients reported pain. Four rated the pain as mild, one described it as 'moderate cramping', and two recorded pain as severe. Four of the five women who received intra-arterial lidocaine during the procedure experienced pain, including all three women with moderate or severe pain. This injection practice is no longer part of the embolization protocol. Only two patients required intravenous morphine or hydromorphone in recovery, the rest were managed with oral ketorolac tromethamine. No patient required a patient-controlled anesthesia pump. All patients were discharged on the day of the procedure. Two patients experienced contraction-type pain 1–2 weeks after embolization, which was alleviated by oral medication alone. One patient complained of post-procedure fever – the patient who ultimately underwent hysterectomy. Seven patients stated they were satisfied with the procedure and would undergo it again if symptoms recurred.

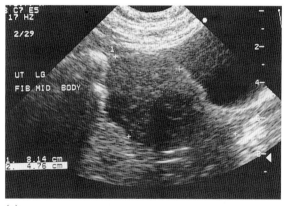

(a)

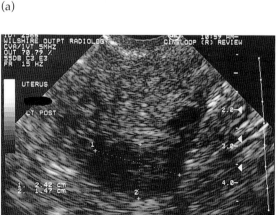

(b)

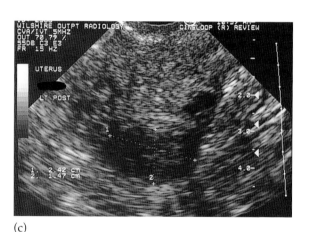

(c)

Figure 69.3 (a) Pre-operative sonogram showing an 8 cm myoma. (b) Six-week follow-up ultrasound of same myoma reveals shrinkage to 3.5 cm. (c) Six-month follow-up reveals further decrease to 2.4 cm. Patient is now symptom-free.

Discussion

Transcatheter embolization of uterine arteries is not a new procedure in either gynecology or obstetrics. Among others, we have urged physicians to consider this as an initial therapy for patients with acute bleeding (Vedantham *et al.*, 1997). Doppler ultrasound has demonstrated a decrease in uterine artery flow in patients with myomas who were treated with gonadotropin releasing hormone (GnRH) agonists (Matta *et al.*, 1988). The rationale for devascularization was therefore established. Initial work on embolization was performed by Ravina and his group in Paris, France. A multicenter study of 31 patients found that embolization significantly reduced blood loss when performed as an adjunct to surgical myomectomy (Ravina *et al.*, 1995a). Several patients who were treated with embolization so that they could donate autologous blood did not require surgery. This prompted Ravina to study the effect of embolization as an alternative to myomectomy or hysterectomy (Ravina *et al.*, 1995b). His group found that 88% of 16 patients with menorrhagia related to myomas demonstrated symptomatic improvement, and in 70% there was a recorded decrease in tumor volume.

All the patients in our study had failed to respond to both hormonal and surgical therapies, compared with only three of Ravina's population who had undergone previous myomectomy. The results we obtained supported Ravina's findings. Every patient undergoing embolization reported a decrease in menorrhagia, similar to the 88% reported by Ravina. Sonographic reductions in total uterine volume and individual myoma reductions were also consistent with Ravina's results. Ultrasound and clinical results did not necessarily match, however, since decrease in uterine volume did not predict the patient who failed to respond to embolization. The three patients who reported the best results did show very large reductions (>66%) in uterine size.

One difference between our group and Ravina's group was his choice of a smaller 300 μm PVA particle compared to our 500 μm range. Several of the differences between the results for our patients and Ravina's patients may be explained by this difference in particle size. The symptoms of 70% of the patients in Ravina's group completely resolved compared to complete resolution of symptoms in only 30% of our patients. However, the post-procedure pain experienced by Ravina's patients was greater, reflecting greater ischemia with smaller particles. The one patient who was embolized with 300 μm particles in our series had severe prolonged pain and the results of her embolization were no greater than those of the other patients embolized with the 500 μm PVA particles.

Our patient undergoing unilateral embolization represents the truth of pathologic studies demonstrating anastomoses between left and right uterine arteries in myomas (Sampson, 1912). Other studies have reported a failure to respond when only one artery was embolized (Rosenthal and Colapinto, 1985).

Antibiotic therapy before the procedure when the arterial bed is still open is now routine practice following abscess development in one patient without obvious predisposing factors. Fever after embolization is a commonly reported side effect (Gilbert *et al.*, 1992) so it is noteworthy that none of our patients complained of fever. Any report of delayed temperature elevation should therefore be vigorously evaluated.

Our initial procedures were performed under general anesthesia. However, as experience was gained, we changed to conscious sedation. No patients experienced discomfort during this method of analgesia. We speculate that the patients in whom intravenous lidocaine was used may have experienced a vasodilatation, which seeded particles more distally in the vascular bed, resulting in greater ischemia. Since the results did not improve with this technique, it has been abandoned.

Conclusion

Transcatheter embolization of the uterine arteries is a promising new method for the treatment of symptomatic myomas. Patients undergoing bilateral embolization can be informed of the likelihood of symptom relief as well as a reduction in uterine size and individual myoma dimensions. We have follow-up of over 18 months in many patients without any regrowth of myomas. Other studies have reported a 15% second surgery rate after myomectomy (Buttram and Reiter, 1981). It is possible that the embolization technique offers better overall results than myomectomy. Certainly the risks to the patient of the embolization are less than traditional myomectomy with its known morbidity of hemorrhage, adhesion formation and infection (Wallach, 1992).

Patients desiring fertility will be studied next for embolization. Ravina (personal communication, 1997) recently reported a follow-up of a larger group of patients, four of whom became pregnant and carried to term without complication; one of these patients delivered twins!

References

Buttram VC, Reiter RC (1981) Uterine leiomyomata: etiology, symptomatology, and management. *Fertility and Sterility* **36**: 433–445.

Clark SL, Phelan JP, Yeh S, Bruce SR, Paul RH (1985) Hypogastric artery ligation for obstetric hemorrhage. *Obstetrics and Gynecology* **66**: 353–356.

Fahmy K (1966) Ligation of the hypogastric and uterine arteries. *Australian and New Zealand Journal of Obstetrics and Gynaecology* **6**: 253–257.

Gilbert WM, Moore TR, Resnik R *et al.* (1992) Angiographic embolization in the management of hemorrhagic complications of pregnancy. *American Journal of Obstetrics and Gynecology* **166**: 493–497.

Greenwood CH, Glickman MG, Schwartz PE, Morse SS, Denny DF (1987) Obstetric and nonmalignant gynecologic bleeding: treatment with angiographic embolization. *Radiology* **164**: 155–159.

Matta WHM, Stabile I, Shaw RW, Campbell S (1988) Doppler assessment of uterine blood flow changes in patients with fibroids receiving the gonadotropin-releasing hormone agonist Buserelin. *Fertility and Sterility* **49**: 1083–1085.

McLucas B, Goodwin S, Vedantham S (1996) Embolic therapy for myomata. *Minimally Invasive Therapy and Allied Technologies* **5**: 336–338.

Ravina JH, Bouret JM, Fried D *et al.* (1995a) Value of pre-operative embolization of uterine fibroma: report of a multicenter series of 31 cases. *Contraception, Fertilité, Sexualité* **23**: 45–49.

Ravina JA, Herbreteau D, Ciraru-Vigneron N *et al.* (1995b) Arterial embolisation to treat uterine myomata. *Lancet* **346**: 671–672.

Rosenthal DM, Colapinto R (1985) Angiographic arterial embolization in the management of postoperative vaginal hemorrhage. *American Journal of Obstetrics and Gynecology* **151**: 227–231.

Sampson JA (1912) The blood supply of uterine myomata. *Surgery, Gynecology and Obstetrics* **XIV**: 215–234.

Vedantham S, Goodwin SC, McLucas B, Mohr G (1997) Uterine artery embolization: an underutilized method of controlling pelvic hemorrhage. *American Journal of Obstetrics and Gynecology* (In press).

Wallach EE Myomectomy (1992) In Thompson JD, Rock JA (eds) *Te Linde's Operative Gynecology*, 7th edn. pp. 647–662. Philadelphia: Lippincott.

Yamashita Y, Harada M, Yamamoto H *et al.* (1994) Transcatheter arterial embolization of obstetric and gynecological bleeding: efficacy and clinical outcome. *British Journal of Radiology* **67**: 530–534.

Directory of Manufacturers

DIANE MILES

Operating Department Superintendent, Mount Alvernia Hospital, Guildford, UK

Apple Medical Corporation
Insight Medical Ltd, ASMEC Centre, Eagle House, The Ring, Bracknell, Berks RG12 1HB, UK, Tel: +44 (0)1344 382086, Fax: +44 (0) 1344 382087;
Apple Medical Europe, 26–34 Avenue Croix St Martin, 03200 Vichy, France, Tel: +33 470 32 88 22, Fax: +33 470 32 87 83;
Apple Medical Corp, Bolton Office Park, 580 Main Street, Bolton, MA 01740, USA, Tel: +1 (508) 779 2926, Fax: +1 (508) 779 6927

Trocars and cannulas
Bipolar diathermy machines
Uterine manipulators
Ureter illumination systems
Single-use laparoscopic instruments
Rectal and vaginal probes
Rotating cone biopsy electrodes

Athrodax Surgical Ltd
Great Western Court, Ross on Wye, Herefordshire HR9 7XP, UK, Tel: +44 (0) 1989 566669, Fax: +44 (0) 1989 768140

Camera systems
Insufflators
Telescope demisting access
Trocars and cannulas
Bipolar diathermy machines
Pressure irrigation systems
Hysteroscopes – diagnostic
Hysteroscopes – therapeutic and accessories
Hysteroscopes – rectoscopes
Light source
Gas warmers
Laparoscopic instruments
Electrodiathermy machines
Endocoagulation system
Lateral vaginal retractor
Ultrasonic dissectors

Auto Suture Company UK
2 King's Ride Park, King's Ride, Ascot, Berks SL5 8BP, UK, Tel: +44 (0) 1344 277 21, Fax: +44 (0) 1344 874911;
United States Surgical Corporation, 150 Glover Avenue, Norwalk, Connecticut 06856, USA, Tel: +1 (203) 866 5050

Trocars and cannulas
Laparoscopic instruments
Single-use laparoscopic instruments
Laparoscopic stapling and suturing devices
Autosonix Ultrasonic Scalpel

Baxter Healthcare Ltd (UK)
Wallingford Road, Compton, Newbury, Berks RG20 7QW, UK, Tel: +44 (0) 1635 206421, Fax: +44 (0) 1635 206101

Irrigation fluids
Irrigation sets
Disposable suction systems

Cariad Technologies Ltd
Cornermount, Mount Park Road, Harrow on the Hill, Middlesex HA1 3LB, UK, Tel: +44 (0) 181 864 6072, Fax: +44 (0) 181 864 6072

CO_2 laser
Single-use laparoscopic instruments
Nd:YAG laser
Cryo surgical system
Laser fibers

Carl Zeiss
Carl Zeiss Strasse, PO Box 1380, D-7082 Oberkochen, Germany, Tel: +49 (0) 736 4200, Fax: +49 (0) 736 46808;
Carl Zeiss Inc, One Zeiss Drive, Thornwood, NY 10594, USA, Tel: +1 (914) 747 1800
Carl Zeiss Ltd, PO Box 78, Woodfield Road, Welwyn Garden City, Herts AL7 1LU, UK, Tel: +44 (0) 1707 871200, Fax: +44 (0) 1707 373210

Camera systems
CO_2 laser
Light source
Laparoscopic instruments
Single-use laparoscopic instruments
Colposcopes
Laser smoke evacuators

Circon ACMI/Cabot
UK agent: Cory Bros (Hospital Contracts) Co Ltd, 6 Bittacy Business Centre, Bittacy Hill, London NW7 1BA, UK, Tel: +44 (0) 181 349 1081, Fax: +44 (0) 181 349 1962

Camera systems
Insufflators
Trocars and cannulas
Pressure irrigation systems
Hysteroscopes – diagnostic
Hysteroscopes – therapeutic and accessories
Hysteroscopes – rectoscopes
Female sterilization MAS instruments
Light source
Laparoscopic instruments

Single-use laparoscopic instruments
Colposcopes

Coherent Inc
Coherent (UK) Ltd, Cambridge Science Park, Milton Road, Cambridge CB4 4RF, UK, Tel: +44 (0) 1223 424048, Fax: +44 (0) 1223 425902

CO_2 laser
Nd:YAG laser
Laser fibers

Conkin Surgical Instruments
PO Box 6707, Station A, Toronto, Ontario M5W 1X5, Canada, Tel: +1 (416) 922 9496, Fax: +1 (416) 922 3501;
UK agent: Endosafe Technologies, Suite 46, 32 The Calls, Leeds LS2 7EW, UK

Uterine manipulators

CONMED Corporation/Aspen Labs Surgical Systems
UK agents: Cory Bros (Hospital Contracts) Co Ltd, 6 Bittacy Business Centre, Bittacy Hill, London NW7 1BA, UK, Tel: +44 (0) 181 349 1081, Fax: +44 (0) 181 349 1962

Trocars and cannulas
Bipolar diathermy machines
Electrodiathermy machines
Argon beam coagulators

Cook (UK) Ltd
Monroe House, Letchworth, Herts SG6 1LN, UK, Tel: +44 (0) 1462 481 290, Fax: +44 (0) 1462 480 944;
William Cook Europe A/S, Sandet 6 DK-4632, Bjaeverskov, Denmark, Tel: +45 53 671133;
Cook Canada Inc, 111 Sandiford Drive, Stouffville, Ontario L4A 7X5, Canada, Tel: +1 (905) 640 7110

Insufflators
Trocars and cannulas
Laparoscopic instruments
Single-use laparoscopic instruments
Ureter illumination systems
IVF equipment

Cross Medical Ltd
1, The Chase Centre, 8, Chase Road, Park Royal, London NW10 6QD, UK, Tel: +44 (0) 181 453 0388, Fax: +44 (0) 181 453 0336

CO_2 laser
Pressure irrigation systems
Nd:YAG laser
Laser smoke evacuators
Laser fibers

D P Medical Systems Ltd
Sutton Business Centre, Restmor Way, Wallington, Surrey SM6 7AH, UK, Tel: +44 (0) 181 669 0011, Fax: +44 (0) 181 773 0929

Camera systems
Insufflators
Trocars and cannulators
Hysteroscopes – diagnostic
Hysteroscopes – therapeutic and accessories
Hysteroscopes – resectoscopes
Light source
Single-use laparoscopic instruments
Colposcopes

Diagnostic Sonar Ltd
Kirkton Campus, Livingston, West Lothian EH54 7BX, Scotland, Tel: +44 (0) 1506 411 877, Fax: +44 (0) 1506 412 410

Ultrasound scanner

Diomed Limited
The Jeffreys Building, Cowley Road, Cambridge CB4 4WS UK, Tel: +44 (0) 1223 421799, Fax: +44 (0) 1223 425011

Surgical diode lasers

Electroscope, Europe
Unit Q Floors Street, Floors Street Industrial Estate, Johnstone, PA68PE Scotland, Tel: +44 (0) 1505 329 500, Fax: +44 (0) 1505 336 733
Electroscope Inc, 4828 Sterling Drive, Boulder, CO 80301-2350, USA, Tel: +1 (800) 998 0986, +1 (303) 444 2600, Fax: +1 (303) 444 2693

Shielded monopolar electrosurgical electrodes
Active electrode monitoring system
Bipolar end point monitoring system

Elmed
60 West Fay Avenue, Addison, IL 60101-5106, USA, Tel: +1 (708) 543 2792, Fax: +1 (708) 543 2101

Camera systems
Insufflators
Trocars and cannulas
Bipolar diathermy machines
Pressure irrigation systems
Cold-coagulation system
Hysteroscopes – diagnostic
Hysteroscopes – therapeutic and accessories
Light source
Laparoscopic instruments
Electrodiathermy machines
Argon beam coagulators
Cryo surgical system
Uterine manipulators
Female sterilization MAS instruments
Lateral vaginal retractor
Colposcopes
Laser smoke evacuators

Eschmann Equipment
Peter Road, Lancing, West Sussex BN15 8TJ, UK, Tel: +44 (0) 903 753 322, Fax: +44 (0) 903 766 793

Bipolar diathermy machines
Electrodiathermy machines

Ethicon Endo-Surgery
(subsidary of Johnson & Johnson), Ethicon Ltd, Simpson Parkway, Kirkton Campus, Livingston EH54 7AT, Scotland, Tel: +44 (0) 131 453 5555, Fax: +44 (0) 1506 460714

Ethicon Endo-Surgery
4545 Creek Road, Cincinnati, OH 45242, USA, Tel: +1 (513) 786 7000, Fax: +1 (513) 786 7080;
Ethicon Endo-Surgery GmbH, Hummelsbuetteler, Steindamm 71, D-22851 Norderstedt, Germany

Trocars and cannulas
Laparoscopic instruments
Single-use laparoscopic instruments
Uterine manipulators
Harmonic scalpel

European Information Technology (UK) Ltd
240 Brox Road, Ottershaw, Surrey KT16 0RA, UK, Tel: +44 (0) 1932 874 642, Fax: +44 (0) 1932 873 655

Computerized patient records/notes and audit

Eurosurgical Ltd
Merrow Business Centre, Guildford GU4 7WA, UK, Tel: +44 (0) 1483 456007, Fax: +44 (0) 1483 456008;
Distributor: Coopersurgical, 15 Forest Parkway, Shelton, CT 06484, USA, Tel: +1 (203) 929 6321, Fax: +1 (203) 925 0135

Camera systems
Insufflators
Hysteroscopes – diagnostic
Hysteroscopes – therapeutic and accessories
Hysteroscopes – resectoscopes
Light source
Laparoscopic instruments
Cryo surgical system
Lateral vaginal retractor
Colposcopes
Uterine manipulators

Femcare Ltd
67 St Peter's Street, Nottingham NG7 3EN, UK, Tel: +44 (0) 115 9786322, Fax: +44 (0) 115 9420234

Trocars and cannulas
Female sterilization MAS instruments
Filshie clips

Fry Surgical Instrument
Unit 17, Goldsworth Park Trading Estate, Woking, Surrey GU21 3BA, UK, Tel: +44 (0) 1483 721 404, Fax: +44 (0) 1483 755 282

Camera systems
CO_2 lasers
Pressure irrigation systems
Laparoscopic instruments

Genesis Medical Ltd
7 Heathgate Place, Agincourt Road, London NW3 2NU, UK, Tel: +44 (0) 171 284 2824, Fax: +44 (0) 171 284 2675

Hysteroscopes – diagnostic
Hysteroscopes – therapeutic and accessories
Hysteroscopes – resectoscopes
Light source
Electrodiathermy machines
Cryo surgical system
Flexible hysteroscopes
Colposcopes

Johnson and Johnson Ltd
Ethicon Inc, US Route 22, Sommerville, NJ 08876, USA, Tel: +1 (908) 218 0707;
Johnson and Johnson Medical Ltd, Coronation Road, Ascot, Berks SL5 9EY, UK, Tel: +44 (0) 1344 871000, Fax: +44 (0) 1344 212 47

Interceed adhesion barrier
Haemostats – surgical
Absorbable haemostats
Surgical Nu-Knit
Absorbable haemostat spongostan
Gelatin sponge
Spongostan
Anal gelatine sponge
Instat
Collagen haemostat

Karl Storz GmbH & Co
UK agent: Rimmer Brothers, Aylesbury House, 18 Aylesbury Street, London, EC1R 0DD, UK, Tel: +44 (0) 171 251 6494, Fax: +44 (0) 171 253 7585;
Karl Storz GmbH & Co, Mittelstrasse 8, D78532 Tuttlingen, Germany, Tel: +49 7461 7080, Fax: +49 7461 708105

Camera systems
Insufflators
Telescope demisting access
Trocars and cannulas
Bipolar diathermy machines
Hysteroscopes – diagnostic
Hysteroscopes – therapeutic and accessories
Hysteroscopes – resectoscopes
Light source
Gas warmers
Laparoscopic instruments
Electrodiathermy machines
Uterine manipulators
Endometrial oblators
Flexible hysteroscopes
Ureter illumination systems
Endocoagulation system

Keymed (Medical and Industrial Equipment) Ltd
Keymed House, Stock Road, Southend-on-Sea, Essex SS2 5QH, UK, Tel: +44 (0) 1702 616333, Fax: +44 (0) 1702 465677;
Northern Office, Peel House, Ladywell East, Livingston EH54 6AG, Scotland

Camera systems
Insufflators
Trocars and cannulas
Pressure irrigation systems
Hysteroscopes – diagnostic
Hysteroscopes – therapeutic and accessories
Hysteroscopes – resectoscopes
Light source
Laparoscopic instruments
Flexible hysteroscopes
Colposcopes
Laparoscopic ultrasound
CCTV trolleys
Laparoscopes

Kontron Instruments Ltd
Blackmoor Lane, Croxley Business Park, Watford, Herts WD1 8XQ, UK, Tel: +44 (0) 1923 412214, Fax: +44 (0) 1923 412301

Camera systems
Nd:YAG laser
Laparoscopic ultrasound
Laser fibers

Laserscope
NWL Laser Technologie GmbH, Industriegebiet Dollnitz 12, 92690 Pressath, Germany, Tel: +49 9644 9203 0, Fax: +49 9644 9203 11;

Laserscope, Parc Technologie, 18 rue de Boid Chaland, 91090, Lisses, France, Tel: +33 1 60 86 20 49, Fax: +33 1 60 86 14 88;
Laserscope (UK) Ltd, Raglan House, Llatnarnam Park, Cwmbran, Gwent NP44 3AX, Wales, Tel: +44 (0) 1633 838081, Fax: +44 (0) 1633 838161;
Laserscope, 3052 Orchard Drive, San Jose, CA 95134, USA, Tel: +1 (408) 943 0636, Fax: +1 (408) 943 1051

CO_2 laser,
KTP/YAG laser
Nd:YAG laser
Micromanipulator enabling laser use from colposcope
Laparoscopic laser irrigation/aspiration systems
Photodynamic therapy devices

Litechnica Ltd
Kirby House, 122 Heston Road, Heston, Middlesex TW5 0QU, UK, Tel: +44 (0) 181 577 2450, Fax: +44 (0) 181 572 8292

Camera systems
Insufflators
CO_2 laser
KTP/YAG laser
Light source
Laparoscopic instruments
Nd:YAG laser
Argon beam coagulators
Laparoscopic ultrasound
Laser smoke evacuators
Laser fibers

Marlow Surgical Technologies Inc
1810 Joseph Lloyd Parkway, Willoughby, OH 44094, USA, Tel: +1 (800) 946 2453, Fax: +1 (216) 946 1997

Insufflators
Trocars and cannulas
Uterine manipulators
Laparoscopic instruments
Single-use laparoscopic instruments
CO_2 filters
Knot pushers
2 mm laparoscopic scope and instruments

Medical Dynamics
99 Inverness Drive East, Englewood, Colorado 80112, USA, Tel: +1 (303) 790 2990, Fax: +1 (303) 799 1378

Camera systems
Light source

Philips Medical Systems
Kelvin House, 63–75 Glenthorne Road, Hammersmith, London W6 0LJ, UK, Tel: +44 (0) 181 741 1666, Fax: +44 (0) 181 741 8716;
PO Box 10,000, Best DA 5680, The Netherlands, Tel: +31 40 762 710, Fax: +31 40 762 577;
Philips Medical Systems North America, 710 Bridgeport Avenue, Shelton, CT 06484, USA, Tel: +1 (203) 926 7475, Fax: +1 (203) 926 1272,

Mobile X-ray imaging systems

Richard Wolf UK Ltd
PO Box 47, Mitcham, Surrey, CR4 4TT, UK, Tel: +44 (0) 181 640 3054, Fax: +44 (0) 181 640 9709;
Richard Wolf GmbH, Postfach 1164/1165, D-75434 Knittlingen, Germany, Tel: +49 7043 350, Fax: +49 7043 35300;
Richard Wolf Medical Instruments,
353 Corporate Woods Parkway, Vernon Hills, IL 60061, USA, Tel: +1 847 913 1113, Fax: +1 847 913 1489

Camera systems
Insufflators
Telescope demisting access
Trocars and cannulas
Bipolar diathermy machines
Pressure irrigation systems
Hysteroscopes – diagnostic
Hysteroscopes – therapeutic and accessories
Hysteroscopes – resectoscopes
Uterine manipulators
Female sterilization MAS instruments
Endometrial oblators
Fexible hysteroscopes
Light source
Gas warmers
Laparoscopic instruments
Electrodiathermy machines
Laser smoke evacuators

Rocket of London Ltd
Imperial Way, Watford, Herts WD2 4XX, UK, Tel: +44 (0) 1923 239 791, Fax: +44 (0) 1923 230 212

Camera systems
Insufflators
Trocars and cannulas
Pressure irrigation systems
Cold coagulation systems
Light source
Gas warmers
Laparoscopic instruments
Single-use laparoscopic instruments
Uterine manipulators
Female sterilization MAS instruments
Ureter illumination systems

Sharplan
Sharplan Lasers (Europe) Ltd, 1st Floor, Merit House, Edgware Road, Colindale, London NW9 5AF, UK, Tel: +44 (0) 181 324 4200, Fax: +44 (0) 181 324 4222;
Sharplan GmbH, AM Lohmuhlbach 12A, Freising 85356, Germany, Tel: +1 49 8161 988 0, Fax: +1 49 8161 988010;
Sharplan Lasers Inc, 1 Pearl Court, Allendale, 07401 New Jersey, USA, Tel: +1 201 327 1666, Fax: +1 201 445 4048

Camera systems
CO_2 laser
KTP/YAG laser
Nd:YAG laser
Laparoscopic ultrasound
Laser smoke evacuators
Laser fibers

Smith and Nephew Healthcare Ltd (Incorporating: Acufex, Dyonics and Images products)
Smith and Nephew Richards Ltd, 6 The Techno Park, Newmarket Road, Cambridge CB5 8PB, UK, Tel: +44 (0) 1223 568100, Fax: +44 (0) 1223 568098;
Smith and Nephew PLC (Europe Offices), Temple Place, Victoria Embankment, London, WC2R 3BP, UK, Tel: +44 (0) 171 836 7922, Fax: +44 (0) 171 240 1343;
Smith and Nephew Endoscopy, 160 Dascomb Road, Andover, MA 01810, USA, Tel: +1 508 749 1000, Fax: +1 508 470 2227

Camera systems
Insufflators
Trocars and cannulas
Pressure irrigation systems
Hysteroscopes – diagnostic
Hysteroscopes – therapeutic and accessories
Hysteroscopes – resectoscopes
Light source
Laparoscopic instruments

Stryker Corporation
2725 Fairfield Road, PO Box 4085, Kalamazoo, MI 49003, USA, Tel: +1 (616) 385 2600, Fax: +1 (616) 385 1062;
Stryker SA, 19 Av de Belmont, 1820 Montreaux, Switzerland, Tel: +41 21 963 8701, Fax: +41 21 963 8700;
Stryker UK, Medway House, 5000 Newbury Business Park, London Road, Newbury, Berks RG14 2ST, UK, Tel: +44 (0) 1635 262400, Fax: +44 (0) 1635 580300

Camera systems
Insufflators
Trocars and cannulas
Hysteroscopes – diagnostic
Light source
Laparoscopic instruments
Single-use laparoscopic instruments

Sun Medical Inc
1179 Corporate Drive West, Suite 100, Arlington, TX 76006, USA, Tel: +1 (817) 633 1373, Fax: +1 (817) 640 1840

Laser smoke evacuators

Surgical Innovations Ltd
US distributors: Deknatel Snowden Pencer, 5175 South Royal Atlanta Drive, Tucker, GA 30084, USA, Tel: +1 (770) 496 0952, Fax: +1 (770) 934 8659;

Surgical Innovations Ltd, Clayton Park, Clayton Park, Clayton Wood Rise, Leeds LS16 6RF, UK, Tel: +44 (0) 113 230 7597, Fax: +44 (0) 113 230 7598

Insufflators
Telescope demisting access
Trocars and cannulas
Laparscopic instruments
Single-use laparoscopic instruments
Uterine manipulators
Endometrial oblators

United States Surgical Corporation
150 Glover Avenue, Norwalk, Connecticut 06856, USA, Tel: +1 (203) 866 5050

Trocars and cannulas
Laparoscopic instruments
Laparoscopic suturing and stapling devices
Retrieval bags
Autosonix Ultrasonic Scalpel

Valleylab Europe
Hoge Wei, Zaventum, Belgium, Tel: +32 2 722 0375, Fax: +32 2 725 1085;
Valleylab Inc, Pfizer Hospital Products Group, 5920 Longbow Drive, Boulder, CO 80301, USA, Tel: +1 (303) 530 2300, Fax: +1 (303) 530 6285;
Valleylab UK, Pfizer Hospital Products Group, 622 Western Avenue, Park Royal, London W3 0TF, UK, Tel: +44 (0) 181 896 7600, Fax: +44 (0) 181 896 7630

Trocars and cannulas
Bipolar diathermy machines
Light source
Single-use laparoscopic instruments
Electrodiathermy machines
Argon beam coagulators
Ultrasonic dissectors
Laser diathermy smoke evacuators
Endometrial ablation devices

Video South Medical Ltd
5 Kingsmead Square, Bath, Avon BA1 2AB, UK, Tel: +44 (0) 1225 461 985, Fax: +44 (0) 1225 444 425

Television links
Medical/surgical video conferencing

Walker Filtration Ltd
Spire Road, Glover East, Washington, Tyne and Wear NE37 3ES, UK, Tel: +44 (0) 191 417 7816, Fax: +44 (0) 191 415 3748

Laser smoke evacuators

Zeppelin Instruments Ltd
1 Godstow Road, Upper Wolvercote, Oxford, OX2 8AJ, UK, Tel: +44 (0) 1865 510111, Fax: +44 (0) 1865 514751

Camera systems
Trocars and cannulas
Pressure irrigation systems
Hysteroscopes – diagnostic
Light source
Laparoscopic instruments
Colposcopes

Zinnanti Surgical Instruments Inc
UK agent: Cory Bros (Hospital Contracts) Co Ltd, 6 Bittacy Business Centre, Bittacy Hill, London NW7 1BA, UK, Tel: +44 (0) 181 349 1081, Fax: +44 (0) 181 349 1962

Insufflators
Uterine manipulators
Light source
Laparoscopic instruments
Lateral vaginal retractor
Laser smoke evacuators

Index

Page numbers in **bold** refer to major discussions in the text, those in *italic* refer to figures or tables.

abdominal distension 43, 482
abdominal entry
adhesions/previous surgery **48–9**, *49*, 483
  bowel injury risk **482–4**, *483*
  CO_2 insufflation **46–7**, 482–3
  direct entry 290–1, 483
  incisions **57–8**
  ninth intercostal space 48, 57, 393
  problems 12–13
  technique *46*, **46**, **290–2**, **392–3**, 394
  verification of placement **47–8**, 490–1
  vessel injury 46, **51**, 296, **490–2**
abdominal scars 12, 13, 43, 172, 482
  laparoscope insertion **48–9**, *49*
  ninth intercostal space incision 48, 57
  vessel injury risk 489
abscess 12, 242
  see also tubo-ovarian abscess
Access to Health Records Act (1990) 10
Access to Medical Records Act (1988) 10
achondroplastic dwarfism 48
adenomyosis 262, 266, 360–1, *362*, 607
  post-endometrial transcervical resection (TCRE) 586
  see also rectovaginal septum adenomyotic nodule
adhesiolysis 58
  argon beam coagulator (ABC) 107, **109**
  complications 15, 66, **485**
  laser laparoscopy **75**
  tubal repair surgery 131–2, 133, *134*, 136
  see also adhesions; periadnexal adhesive disease; salpingo-ovariolysis
adhesions
  abdominal entry **48–9**, *49*, 483
  bowel injury risk 13
  distal tubal occlusion 129–30, **139–40**, 148

formation 142, 148, 398
  laparoscopy versus laparotomy **399**
  laser surgery **400**
  microsurgery **399–400**
  suture material 400
  ovum pickup impairment 139
  pelvic contents inspection 350–1
  postoperative re-formation **398–9**
  previous cesarean section 301
  second look laparoscopy **400**
  vaginal hysterectomy contraindications 300–1
  see also adhesiolysis; enterolysis; periadnexal adhesive disease; salpingo-ovariolysis
adhesions prevention **65–6**, 286, **398–402**
  adjuvants **400–2**
  barriers 364, 365, 395, 402
  endometriosis laser vaporization 364, 365
  post-enterolysis **394–5**
adnexal mass 477–8
  hysterectomy 301–2
    supracervical laparoscopic 308
  laparoscopic assessment *477*
  tissue extraction 111–12, 114
adnexectomy 469, *472*, *473*
adrenal vein 425
air embolism 642
Allen–Masters windows endometriosis 367, *367*
allergic reactions
  dextran 526, 643
  local anesthetics 646
5–aminolevulinic acid (ALA) 621, 622, 623, 624
ampicillin 242, 376
anatomic landmarks 490
anesthesia 32, **674**
  colposuspension 327
  diagnostic laparoscopy **45**
  endometrial electroablation 598

endometrial transcervical resection (TCRE) 583
  hysterectomy 296
  hysteroscopy **646–7**
  monitoring 11
  office laparoscopy 28
  problems **296**
  sterilization **161–2**, **170**
  uterine artery embolization 689
antibiotic prophylaxis 45, 54
  enterolysis 392
  hysteroscopic metroplasty 563
  large bowel endometriosis 376, 385
  myolysis 281
antibiotic treatment
  pelvic abscess 242
  tubo-ovarian abscess 244
anticoagulant prophylaxis 43, *44*
aortic lymph nodes 420
aortic lymphadenectomy *see* lymphadenectomy, aortic
aquadissection **58**, 142
  adhesiolysis 391, 393–4
  endometriosis 364, *365*, 385
  hysterectomy 303, 310
  ovarian surgery 216, 228
  rectovaginal septum adenomyotic nodule 358, 360
  tubo-ovarian abscess 243, 244
  ureter dissection 385, 494
argon beam coagulator (ABC) 23, **59**, **105–10**, *109*, 116
  animal investigations 106
  clinical use 107–10
    adhesiolysis 391, 394, 396
    early evaluation 107–8, *107*
  costs 109–10
  laparoscopic probe development 106, *106*
  laparoscopic technique 107
  method of action 105–6
argon laser 71, 72, **74**, 96

argon laser (*cont.*)
contact versus non-contact application
mode **99–102**
ovarian drilling **238**
ovarian endometrioma
photovaporization 227
periadnexal adhesiolysis 140
safety 645
tissue effects **98–9**, *100*
uterine nerve ablation 252
atracurium 45
atropine 162, 518, 646
atypical endometriosis 49, *49*
autologous blood donation 55, 385, 392

ball-shaped electrodes 95, *95*, *96*
basal body temperature chart 177
benign cystic teratoma 209
tissue extraction 112
transvaginal ultrasound 207, *207*
benign ovarian neoplasms 212
benzodiazepine 45
biomedical cart 26
biomedical technician 20
bipolar electrocautery 58–9, 116, 171
adhesiolysis 391
deep endometriosis 383
instruments 22, 23, 280
myolysis 280, 281, 282, *282*, 286
ovarian drilling **238**
ovarian endometrioma 381
safety 292
sterilization 14, **168–9**
bladder care 11, 45, 54, 676
bladder injury 13, **495–7**
deep infiltrative endometriosis 388
hysterectomy 294, **295**, 298
management 295, 497
prevention **495**, 497
recognition 298, 497
bleeding disorders 43
Bleier clip 167, *169*
borderline ovarian tumors 212, 213
laparoscopic diagnosis 215
bowel injury 12–13, 43, **66**, 173, 245,
481–7
abdominal entry *47*, **47–8**, **482–4**, *483*
secondary portals 484
adhesiolysis 394, **485**
electrosurgery 91–2, **294**, 378, **484–5**,
570
endometriosis
deep infiltrative 388, **485**
laser vaporization 367
monopolar electroexcision 378
rectovaginal 360
exiting abdomen **486**
hysterectomy 290, 291, **293–4**, 298
hysteroscopic surgery 15, 645
incidence 481
laser energy **485**
late diagnosis 394, **486–7**
management 483–4
medico-legal aspects 11, 484, 486
posterior colpotomy 485
postoperative detection **298**, **486–7**
predisposing factors 481, 482
preoperative factors **482**
prevention 43, 290, 291, **293–4**
procedure-related **484–5**
repair 13, 294, 378, 394, **483–4**, *484*
minimal access 48, 66
surgeons' training levels 482
transcervical sterilization 570
bowel preparation 43, 45, 54, 66, 266, **482**

enterolysis 392
hysteroscopy 645
information sheet *42*
laparoscopic radical hysterectomy 447
large bowel endometriosis 371, 376,
385
previous laparotomy scars 48
rectovaginal septum adenomyotic
nodule 358
tubal repair surgery 131
BPD-Ma 621
brachial plexus injury 11
Bret–Tomkins metroplasty 554, 555, *556*
bupivacaine 675
maximum dose 676
Burch colposuspension *see* retropubic
colposuspension
burden of proof 9

CA-125
assay 54
endometriosis 349
ovarian malignancy **213–14**, 468, 476
canal of Nuck endometriosis 367
capacitance coupling 89–91, **294**
carcinoembryonic antigen (CEA) 476
cardinal ligament 442, 450, *451*
cardiorespiratory disease 647
cart, laparoscopy 26, *26*, 27
catheterization 45, 54
post-colposuspension 329, *332*
Cavaterm system *616*, **616–17**
clinical trials 617
cefalexin 563
cefazolin 376, 563
cefotetan 54
cefoxitin 54, 242
Celio–Schauta operation **440–1**, 462
laparoscopic part 440–1
vaginal part 441
Celio–Schauta version 2 **441–4**
central pontine myelinosis 644
cerebral edema 15
cervical adenocarcinoma *in situ* **461**
cervical carcinoma
advanced cancer **462**
aortic lymphadenectomy 417, 418,
419, 420, 421, 422, 435, 461
indications 423, 424
early invasive adenocarcinoma **461**
fluorescence diagnostics 627–8
laparoscopic radical hysterectomy
438, **447–57**
lymph node involvement 420, 461, 462
management algorithm *439*, *449*, 457
microinvasive disease **460–1**
pelvic lymphadenectomy 407, 411,
414, 461
risk following supracervical
hysterectomy 312, *312*, 313
stage IB **461–2**
staging 414, 418, 419
cervical damage **641–2**
cervical dilation **641–2**
endometrial electroablation 598
pain 646
pharmacologic methods 642
trauma 641–2
cervical intraepithelial neoplasia (CIN)
459–60
photodynamic therapy 621, **623–5**
cervical plexus injury 11
cervical stenosis 266
Chlamydia trachomatis 130, 241, 242
chorioangiopagus 657

chromotubation
distal tubal patency assessment 131, 143
microsurgical tubal anastomosis 184
circulating nurse 20–1, 32, 34, 35, 56
responsibilities *33*, **33**
Clarke knot-pusher 60, *60*, 61
clavulanate 242
cleft lip 672
clindamycin 242
clinical trials 10
clip sterilization 159
failure rates 164
reversibility 178
clips 52, **61–2**
clomiphene citrate 233, 239
closure 52, 56
bowel injury **486–7**
large vessel damage 267–8, *268*
peritoneal cavity 297
CO_2 insufflation
abdominal entry **46–7**, 482–3
complications **642**
hysteroscopy 508, 516, *517*, 518, **525–6**
tubal occlusion 569
instrumentation **23**
out-patient procedures 508, 516, *517*,
676
sterilization 168
CO_2 laser 23, 26, **59–60**, 72, **73–4**, 96, 116,
117
adhesiolysis **75**, 140, 391, 395
CO_2 laser power density 74
ectopic pregnancy **76**
endometriosis vaporization **75**, 363,
364
myomectomy **76**
ovarian drilling **238**
ovarian endometrioma
photovaporization 227, 230
polycystic ovaries management 233,
238
rectovaginal septum adenomyotic
nodule 358, 360
safety 12, 73
smoke evacuation 73
terminal salpingostomy **75**
tissue effects 97, *97*, *98*
tubal repair surgery 131
ultrapulse mode 97
uterosacral ligament ablation **76**, *251*,
251, 253, 255, *256*
coagulation 116, 117
argon beam coagulator (ABC) 105,
106, 107
argon laser tissue effects 98, 99, *100*,
101
high-frequency (HF) surgical
equipment 94, *95*, **95**
forced coagulation 95, *96*
soft coagulation 95–6, *95*
spray coagulation *95*, 96
instruments 93
Nd:YAG laser tissue effects 97, *98*, **98**,
99, *100*, 101–2
ultrasonic scalpel 103, 680, *680*
see also LaparoSonic Coagulation
Shears
cold coagulation sterilization **169**
color Doppler ultrasound, ovary **207**
pre-operative tumor imaging **223**
colostomy 13, 43, 66, 378, 465
colposuspension **325–33**
anesthesia 327
closure 329
complications 15, **332**
extraperitoneal approach 328

patient position 327
postoperative care 329
results 332–3
retropubic (Burch) procedure **344–5**, *345*
retropubic space access 326, **327**
Retziusscopy approach 328
suture material 325
suturing 325, 326, **329**
technique **327–32**, *330, 331, 332*
transperitoneal approach 327–8
trials 327
common iliac lymphadenectomy **409–10**
common iliac vein injury 268
complications *12*, **52**, *122*, 485
aortic lymphadenectomy **432–3**
bowel *see* bowel injury
colposuspension **332**
embryoscopy 654
endometrial ablation 614
electroablation **594–7**
microwave **636**
Nd:YAG laser *608*, **608**, *610*, **610–11**
endometrial transcervical resection (TCRE) **584–7**
endometrioma **230**
endometriosis, deep infiltrative 388
endometriosis monopolar electroexcision **378**
enterolysis 394, 396
fetal endoscopic surgery **664**
genitourinary *see* bladder injury; ureter injury
hysterectomy **289–98**
laparoscopic assisted Doderlein 320
laparoscopic assisted vaginal 306, 315
laparoscopic radical 454
hysteroscopy 15, **641–7**
laparoscopy 41, **43**
local anesthesia **646–7**
myolysis **284–5**, *285*
myomectomy *276*, **278**
hysteroscopic Nd:YAG laser 537, 539
ovarian drilling **235–6**
ovarian surgery 218–19, **230**
pelvic lymphadenectomy **411–14**
personal damages claims 9, 11
postoperative recognition 52
presacral neurectomy **267–9**
rectovaginal septum adenomyotic nodule 360, *360*
sterilization 172, 173
mass procedures *163*, **163**
tissue extraction 114
tubo-ovarian abscess treatment 245
uterine nerve ablation 258
vessel injury *see* great vessel injury; vascular injury
computed tomography (CT)
ovarian lesions 208–9
tubo-ovarian abscess 241, 242
guided aspiration 244
congenital anomalies
distal tubal infertility 129
embryonic extremities 671, *672*
embryoscopic first trimester diagnosis 653, 654
congenital cystic adenomatoid malformation (CCAM) **663–4**
congenital diaphragmatic hernia **660–1**
congenital high airway obstruction (CHAOS) 661
consent **43**
enterolysis 392

medico-legal aspects 10
myolysis 281
new therapies 10
sterilization 172
supracervical laparoscopic hysterectomy 305
uterine nerve ablation 250
consent form 31
sterilization 172
contact quality monitors **89**
contraindications 48
diagnostic laparoscopy *43*, **43**, **45**
Corson needle 237, *237*
cost-effectiveness
argon beam coagulator (ABC) 109–10
myolysis 286
Nd:YAG endometrial ablation 611–12, *611*
counseling
sterilization **172**
uterine nerve ablation 250, 256
cryomyolysis 280
culdotomy 63
curettage 599
cutting 116, 117
argon laser 99, *100*, 101
CO_2 laser *97*, **97**, *98*
KTP laser 98
microneedletip electrodes 181
modalities for adhesiolysis 140
Nd:YAG laser 99, *100*, 101–2
ultrasonic scalpel 102–3, 680–1, *680, 681*
see also LaparoSonic Coagulation Shears
cystocele 336
cystoscopy 497
historical aspects 1–2, *2*
ovarian cyst 215
cytokeratins 361

danazol 261, 349, 357, 582
allergic reactions 608
pre-endometrial ablation 540, 605, 616, 634
pre-hysteroscopic myomectomy 535, 538
side effects 262, 535
day case surgery 674
deep epigastric vessel localization 57
Denonvilliers' fascia *see* rectovaginal septum
dermoid cyst 207
dextran distension medium **526**, 594, 595
complications 526, **643**
see also Hyskon
dextran-induced anaphylactic reaction (DIAR) 643
dextrose 5% solution distension medium 526
diagnostic laparoscopy **41–52**
abdominal insufflation 46–7
anesthesia 45
bleeding during trocar introduction 51
closure 52
confirmation of peritoneal entry 46–7
contraindications *43*, **43**, 45
historical aspects 3–4
incision 46
initial inspection 49
laparoscope insertion 48
lateral trocars placement 50–1, *50, 51*
patient preparation 45
position 45

postoperative care 52
previous laparotomy scars 48–9
suprapubic probe insertion 49–50
umbilical trocar insertion 48
diathermy *see* electrosurgery
diazepam 162
diclofenac 45
di-hematoporphyrin esters (DHE) 621, 623
distal fallopian tube
adhesions 129–30
anatomy **129**, **189**
laparoscopic evaluation 135–6, 137
pathology **129–30**
distal tubal infertility 129, 139
Boer–Meisel classification 135–6, *136*
fimbrioplasty **132**, 133, *134*, 141, **143**, **145**, 148
laparoscopic techniques **131–2**, **141**
results 133, *134, 135*, **144–6**
microsurgical principles 141–2
patency testing 131, 143
preoperative investigations 130, 141
referral for assisted procreation 135, 136
retrograde salpingoscopy (tuboscopy) **144**
salpingo-ovariolysis 141, **142–3**, **145**, 148
salpingoscopic assessment of epithelium **187–8**, *188*
salpingostomy (neosalpingostomy) **132–3**, 141, **143–4**, **145–6**, 148
transcervical salpingoscopy (falloposcopy) 144
treatment program 134–5
tubal repair contraindications 130–1
Tubal Scoring System 134, *135*, 136, *136*, 148
tubotubal anastomosis 141, **146–7**, 148
distal tubal patency assessment
chromotubation 131, 143
falloposcopy 194, 195, *195*
distal tubal phimosis (stenosis) 129, 139–40
fimbrioplasty **132**, 143
distension media, hysteroscopic **525–7**
hazards **642–4**
see also fluid overload
laser myolysis 535
metroplasty 556–7, 559, 560
monitoring of intake 535
tubal occlusion 569
doxycycline 242
Doyle technique (uterosacral ligament division) 249, **250**, 254, 261
dual image video
hysteroscopy/laparoscopy 28–9, *29*
duplex Doppler imaging, ovary **207–8**, *208*
duty of care 9
dye laser 74, 96
dysfunctional uterine bleeding 593
hysteroscopy *512*, **512–13**
laser endometrial ablation 70, **77**, **540–4**
dysmenorrhea
adenomyosis 262, 266
causes 265–6
diagnostic hysteroscopy **515**
Doyle technique (uterosacral ligament division) 250, 261
endometriosis 256, 257–8, 261
epidemiology 249
medical treatment 254, 261, 262

dysmenorrhea (*cont.*)
  presacral neurectomy 261, 262, 269
  uterine nerve ablation 249–58, 261
    results 253–4

ectopic pregnancy
  conservative treatment 15, 120, **150–6**
    exposure of tube 150
    failure rate 151–2, *152*
    fertility following 152, 153–6, *153,
      154*, *155*, *156*
    hemostasis 150, 151
    laser laparoscopy **76**
    persistence of trophoblast material
      111, 152
    salpingotomy 151
    selection criteria 151–3
    technical aspects 150–1
    therapeutic decision-making 155–6
    tissue extraction 111
  diagnosis **188–9**
  electrocautery versus laser treatment
    120, *121*
  following endometrial electroablation
    597
  following endometrial transcervical
    resection (TCRE) 586
  following sterilization 14, *171*, **171–2**
    electrosurgical transcervical 570
    mass procedures 164
  interstitial 151
  medical treatment 151, 152, 156, 188,
    189
  medico-legal aspects **15**
  recurrence risk 15, 153, *153*, *155*
  rupture 43, 151
  vaginal hysterectomy 302
ectrodactyly 671
El Mahgoub metroplasty 556
Electroshield monitoring system *91*, *92*
electrosurgery 11–12, **58–9**, **83–92**, 116
  adhesiolysis 140, 390, 391
  biophysical principles **84–5**
  clinical results 117–18, *117*, *118*
  cutting 84, **87–8**
  desiccation 84, 85, **87–8**
  ectopic pregnancy conservative
    treatment 151
  endometriosis excision **369–79**, 380,
    383
  fulguration 84, 85, **87**
  historical aspects 84
  hysterectomy 303
  myomectomy 273, 538
    hysteroscopic 538
  ovarian endometrioma 228
  polycystic ovaries management 233,
    234, 237, **237–8**
    adhesions formation 235, *235*, 239
  power density 85
  power formula 85
  rectovaginal septum adenomyotic
    nodule 358
  safety 11–12, 15, 41, 43, 84, 102, **292–3**,
    596, 645–6
    access through trocar cannulas
      89–91, *90*, *91*
    accidental burns 12, **88–9**, 89, *90*, *91*
    bowel injury **294**
    capacitance coupling 89–91, **294**
    contact quality monitors 89
    hysteroscopy **645–6**
    insulation failure 89, **294**
    intergated shielded instruments *91*,
      92

  isolated electrosurgical outputs 89
  urinary tract injury 295
sterilization 14, 159, 167, **168–9**
  ectopic pregnancy following *171*,
    172
  failure rate 171
  hysteroscopic transcervical 570
  reversibility 177, 178
tissue effects **93–6**, *94*, *95*, 117
  at different temperatures 84, *84*
tubal repair surgery 131
uterine nerve ablation **252–3**
see also bipolar electrocautery;
    monopolar electrocautery
electrosurgical generator **22–3**, 26
embryo
  abdomen 671, *671*
  external genitalia 671
  extremities 670, *670*, 671
  face 670, *671*, 672
  lasers in manipulation **78–9**
  skull 671
  use of tubal environment for growth
    188
embryoscopy 651, **652–4**, *653*, **668–73**
  chorion perforation 653
  complications 654
  diagnostic value 672
  embryonic abdomen 671, *671*
  embryonic external genitalia 671
  embryonic extremities 670, *670*, 671
  embryonic face 670, *671*, 672
  embryonic skull 671
  equipment 668
  extraembryonic celom 669–70
  fetal blood sampling 654
  first trimester diagnosis 653, 654
  indications 672, 673
  malformed embryos 671–2
  neural tube 671
  obstetric risk 672
  principles 668
  timing 668
  transabdominal technique **669**
  transcervical technique **669**
  yolk sac 669–70, *669*
endobag extraction *470*
endoclips 456
endometrial ablation
  balloon ablation **614–20**
    balloon systems 615
    Cavaterm system *616*, **616–17**
    monopolar electrodes (Vestablate
      system) *618*, **618–19**
    multi-electrode balloon 593
    patient selection 619
    therapeutic failure 615, 619
  complications 614
  electroablation *see* endometrial
    electroablation
  hysteroscopes 527
  hysteroscopic fluid absorption 528–9,
    529
  interstitial hyperthermia (ITT
    multifiber device) *547*, **547–50**
    clinical studies 547–8
    in vitro thermometric studies 547, 550
    results 548, *549*, 550
  microwave **630–6**
    animal experiments 632, *632*
    clinical trial 633–4
    complications 636
    equipment 631–2, *631*
    microwave applicator 632, *632*
    microwave energy penetration
      630–1, *631*

  results 634, *635*, 636
  safety 636
  technique 632–3, *633*
  treatment profile printout 633, *634*
Nd:YAG laser 77, **540–4**, **604–12**, 614
  clinical experience **607–11**, *608*,
    609
  complications 543, 608, *608*, 610–11,
    610
  cost-effectiveness 611–12, *611*
  fluid absorption 528–9, *529*
  hysteroscopes 527
  patient selection 542, 607
  postoperative pain 607, 608
  preoperative therapy 541, *541*, 542,
    605
  results 542–3, *542*, *543*, 607–8, *607*,
    609, *609*, 611
  safety 604
  technique 542, **604–7**, *605*, *606*
photodynamic therapy *see*
    endometrial photodynamic
    therapy
thermal balloon 593, **615–16**
  clinical trials 616
underwater rectoscope surgery 57
endometrial biopsy 518
  infertility evaluation 130
endometrial carcinoma **462**
  aortic lymphadenectomy 423, 435
  endometrial resection association 587
  hysteroscopic abdominal spill of fluid
    512–13, *513*
  pelvic lymphadenectomy 411, 414–15
  staging 414, 418, 419
endometrial electroablation **592–603**
  anesthesia 598
  complications 592, *592*, 594–7
    accidental burns 596
  electrode 599
  fluid balance monitoring 595
  follow-up 602
  operating room set-up 598
  patient position 598
  patient selection 593–4
  pregnancy following 597
  preoperative counseling 593, 594
  preoperative endometrial suppression
    597–8
  results 602–3
  secondary malignancy following 593
  technique **598–602**
    cervical dilatation 598
    curettage 599
    dynamic phase 600, *601*
    initiation phase 599, *601*
    operation **600–2**
    vasoconstrictive agents 598
    waveform/power setting selection
      599–600, *600*
endometrial hyperplasia 515
endometrial photodynamic therapy 621,
    622
  embryo implantation following **625**
  endometrial effects **624–5**
  fluorescence detection **623–4**, *624*
  intrauterine light diffuser 627, *627*
  optical aspects 626–7
  solvents 626
endometrial polyp 512, *512*, 515
endometrial polypectomy 518
endometrial suppression 616
  endometrial ablation 540, 541, *541*,
    542, **597–8**, 618, 634
  endometrial transcervical resection
    (TCRE) 582–3

laser hysteroscopic myomectomy 535, 538
endometrial transcervical resection (TCRE) 281, **581–90**, 614
  ablative techniques comparison 588
  anesthesia 583
  complications 584–7, *585*
    operative 584–6
    postoperative 586–7
  gynecologic surgery following 588, *589, 590*
  historical aspects 581–2
  hormone replacement therapy (HRT) following 587
  hysterectomy comparison 588
  postoperative recovery 583, *583*, 584
  pregnancy outcome 586
  preoperative endometrial suppression 582–3
  results 583–4, 587–8, *587*
  technique 582–3
    uterine distension 582
  treatment criteria 582, *582*
endometriomas *see* ovarian endometrioma
endometriosis 6, 49
  advanced disease **380–8**
    excisional equipment **380–1**
  anatomic distribution of lesions 349, *351*, **351–2**, *369*
  argon beam coagulator (ABC) 107, **108–9**
  bladder involvement **385**
  conservative laparoscopic treatment **118–19**
  deep infiltration 361–2, **381**, **383–5**, *384*
    complications 388, 485
  distal tubal infertility 129
  dysmenorrhea 256, 257–8, 261
  excision *119*, **119**
  hysterectomy
    contraindications to vaginal route 301
    laparoscopic assisted Doderlein 317
    with oophorectomy 266
    supracervical laparoscopic 308
  imaging 370
  implantation in laparoscopy scar 51, *51*
  laparoscopic appearances *352*, **352–5**, *353, 354, 355, 372–3, 373*, 380
  laparoscopic diagnosis **349–55**, 380
  laparotomy **387–8**
  large bowel **385–7**, *386, 387*, 388
    antibiotic prophylaxis 376
    bowel preparation 371, 376, 385
    cul-de-sac obliteration 377, 387
    rectal probe 385, *387*
    segmental bowel resection 377
  laser vaporization 70, *75*, 227, 228, *257*, **257–8**, **363–7**, *364, 365*, 383
    adhesions prevention 364, 365
    Allen–Masters windows 367, *367*
    bladder 365
    bowel preparation 367
    canal of Nuck 367
    colon 366–7
    cul-de-sac 366, *366*
    peritoneum 364–5
    postoperative adhesions prevention 364
    rectal/vaginal cavities identification 366, *366*
    residual carbon particles 365, *365*
    safety 363
    soft tissues 364–5

ureter/uterine vessels protection 366
  medical therapy 349, 357, 370
  monopolar electroexcision **369–79**
    advantages 370–1
    angiolysis 375
    bowel preparation 371
    complications 378
    cul-de-sac obliteration 377
    identification of lesions 372–3
    instrumentation 371–2, *372*
    large bowel 376–8, *376, 377*
    neurolysis 375
    ovaries 375–6
    patient position 371
    peritoneal resection 374, *374*
    postoperative adhesions 379
    postoperative care 378
    results 378–9
    technique **373–8**
    ureterolysis 375
    uterosacral ligament 374–5
  natural history 349
  pelvic contents inspection 350–1
  peritoneal defects 354, *354*
  photodynamic therapy 621
  physical signs 349, 370
  symptoms 369–70
  tissue extraction 111
  ureter involvement **385**
  see also rectovaginal septum adenomyotic nodule
endometritis 515, 647
  post-microwave endometrial ablation 636
  post-Nd:YAG laser hysteroscopic myomectomy 537
endomyometritis 608
  post-endometrial electroablation 597
endopelvic fascia 335, *335*
endoscopy team 30, *30*
endostapler 456
endotracheal intubation 45, 56, 674
enflurane 45
enterocele
  preoperative evaluation 336–7
  repair **334–46**
    technique **339–40**
enterolysis **390–6**
  bowel preparation 392
  complications 394, 396
  historical development 390
  methods 390–1
  operating room setup 392
  patient selection 391–2
  postoperative adhesion prevention **394–5**
  preoperative preparation 392
  results 395
  technique **393–4**
    abdominal entry **392–3**, 394
    secondary trocar placement 393
equipment **21–4**, 30–1, **55–6**
  embryoscopy **668**
  endometriosis excision 380–1
  hysterectomy 289–90
    supracervical laparoscopic 305
  laser hysteroscopic myomectomy **535**
  mass sterilization camp **161**
  microwave endometrial ablation 631–2, *631*
  out-patient procedures **676–7**, *677*
  ovarian surgery **216**
  postoperative nursing responsibilities **38**
  safety 482, 490

sterilization 290
  tubo-ovarian abscess management **242–3**
Er:YAG lasers 74
  embryo manipulation 79
estrogen receptors 361
ethical aspects
  clinical trials 10
  fetal endoscopic surgery *659*
exiting abdomen **297**, **486**
external iliac vessel damage *50*, 51
extraembryonic celom 669–70

facial defects 672
fallopian tube
  anatomy **129**, 189
  local anesthesia 675–6
  see also distal fallopian tube
falloposcopy **186–96**
  ectopic pregnancy diagnosis 189
  technique **194–5**
  tubal cannulation 187
  tubal epithelium assessment **187–8**
  tubal patency assessment 187, 194, 195, *195*
falope (Yoon) ring 159, 160, 167, *169, 170*
  applicators 168
  ectopic pregnancy following *171*, 172
  failure rate 164, 169
  technique **169**
Femcet system 569
fentanyl 45, 675, 677, 689
fertilization, use of tubal environment **188**
fetal blood sampling 654, 655
fetal endoscopic surgery **659–64**
  complications 664
  congenital cystic adenomatoid malformation (CCAM) 663–4
  congenital diaphragmatic hernia 660–1
  ethical aspects *659*
  fetal obstructive uropathy 659–60
  myelomeningocele 661–2, *663*
  potential procedures *664*
fetal endoscopy
  historical aspects 651
  optical systems 651–2
fetal obstructive uropathy **659–60**
fetal skin sampling 655
fetoscopic surgery **656–64**
  fetal adnexa 656–9
  placenta 656–9
  twin reversed arterial perfusion sequence (TRAPS) 658–9
  twin-to-twin transfusion syndrome (TTTS) 657–8
fetoscopy 651, **654–5**
  fetal blood sampling 654, 655
  fetal skin sampling 655
fibroids *see* myomas
Filshie clip 14, 159, 167, *169, 170*
  applicators 168
  ectopic pregnancy following *171*, 172
  failure rate 170
  migration 172
  technique **170**
fimbrioplasty **132**, 141, **143**
  results 133, *134*, **145**, 148
fine needle electrodes 94–5, *95, 96*, 181, 391
first-trimester diagnosis 653, 654, 668
Fitz–Hugh–Curtis syndrome 131
flash lamp dye lasers 74
fluid overload **643–4**, 645

fluid overload (*cont.*)
  endometrial ablation
    electroablation **594–5**
    Nd:YAG laser 543, 610–11
  endometrial transcervical resection
      (TCRE) *585*, **585**
  fluid balance monitoring 560–1, 585,
      595
  hysteroscopic metroplasty 559, 560–1
  management 595, 644
  prevention 57
fluorescence diagnostics **627–8**
fluorescent photosensitizers 70
fluoroscopic tubal cannulation **192**, *193*,
    194
follow-up sheet *36–7*
frozen sections
  nodal status 423
  ovarian mass 215
FSH serum levels 177

gamete manipulation **77**
gamete transfer to tube 188
gas embolism 610, 642
  endometrial transcervical resection
      (TCRE) **586**
gasless technique 168
general operating room accidents 41, 43
  medical-legal aspects **11–12**
genital warts 621
glycine distension medium **526–7**, 535,
    585, 595
  complications **643–4**
gonadotropin-releasing hormone
      (GnRH) analogues 55, 76, 113, 582
  endometriosis management 261–2,
      349, 357, 388
  myomas shrinkage 281, 285, 535, 538
  ovarian endometrioma management
      227, 230, 231
  pre-endometrial ablation 540, 541,
      541, 542, 605
  pre-Nd:YAG hysteroscopic
      submucous myomectomy 544,
      546–7
  side effects 262
goserelin 535, 634, 636
great vessel injury 13, 41, 48, **489–93**
  abdominal entry techniques **490–2**
  closure 267–8, *268*
  hysterectomy 296
  incidence 489
  management 296, 492
  pelvic lymphadenectomy 412
  presacral neurectomy 267–8, *268*
  recognition **492**
  retroperitoneal space anatomy **490**

Hasson cannula open approach 43
hemaclips 268, *268*
hematocolpometra 266
hematoma formation 12, 13, 296, 492
hematometra
  endometrial electroablation 597
  endometrial transcervical resection
      (TCRE) **586**
  Nd:YAG endometrial ablation 598,
      610
hematoporphyrin derivative (HPD) 621
hemorrhage *see* great vessel injury;
      vascular injury
hiatus hernia 43
high flow CO_2 insufflators **55**

high McCall vaginal vault suspension
    340, *341*
high-frequency (HF) surgical equipment
    93
  coagulation effects 94, *95*, **95**
    forced coagulation *95*, 96
    soft coagulation 95–6, *95*
    spray coagulation *95*, 96
  cutting effects 94, *94*
  monopolar versus bipolar technique
      96, *96*
  shape of electrode 94–5, *95*
historical aspects **1–6**
  electrosurgery 84
  endometrial transcervical resection
      (TCRE) 581–2
  fetal endoscopy 651
  hysteroscopy 2–3
  laparoscopic surgery 5–6
  laparoscopy 3–6
  ovarian cancer 468
  ovarian endometriomas 221–2
  pelvic pain procedures 261–2
  sterilization **167–8**
Ho:YAG laser
  embryo manipulation 78
  hysteroscopic myomectomy 538, 539
  safety 645
Ho:YSGG laser 79
hormone replacement therapy (HRT)
    587
Hulka Clemens clip 14, 159, 167, *169*
  applicators 168
  ectopic pregnancy following *171*, 172
  failure rate 170, 171
  migration 172
  technique **169–70**
hydrodissection *see* aquadissection
hydrosalpinx 130, 140
  distal tubal infertility 130
  referral for assisted procreation 136
  salpingostomy *132*, **132–3**, *133*, 143
hyperthermia electrode myolysis 280
hypogastric artery ligation 687
hyponatremia 585, 594, 595, 644
  correction 595, 644
hypothermia probe myolysis 280
Hyskon (dextran 70) **526**
  hysteroscopic tubal occlusion 569
  photosensitizer solvent 626
Hyskon pump *507*, **507**
hysterectomy, laparoscopic
  abdominal insufflation 290
  bowel perforation avoidance 290, 291
  complications
    anesthesia problems **296**
    avoidance **289–98**
    bowel injury **293–4**, **298**
    re-laparoscopy 297
    urinary tract injury **294–5**, **297–8**
    vascular injury 292, **295–6**, 297
  dissection modality safety **292–3**
  exiting peritoneal cavity 297
  historical development 5–6
  imaging systems 289–90
  LaparoSonic Coagulation Shears *see*
      LaparoSonic Coagulation
      Shears
  laser safety 293
  peritoneal cavity access **290–2**, 294
    direct entry 290–1
    first entry 290–1
    second entry 291–2
  postoperative care **297**
  staples **293**
  sterility 290

  sutures **293**
hysterectomy, laparoscopic assisted
      Doderlein **315–20**
  advantages 315–16
  classification 316, *316*
  complications 320
  indications 316
  patient preparation 316
  postoperative care 320
  results 320
  technique **316–20**
    laparoscopic component 316–18,
        317, *318*
    vaginal component 318–20, *319*
hysterectomy, laparoscopic assisted
      vaginal (LAVH) **300–7**
  adnexal mass 301–2
  benefits 306
  bladder dissection 304, *304*
  cervical carcinoma 460, 461
    ovarian conservation 461
  complications 15, 306, 315
  ectopic pregnancy 302
  endometriosis 301, 303
  laparoscopic pelvic inspection 300,
      301, 303
  pelvic adhesions 300–1
  pelvic inflammatory disease 302
  postoperative care 305–6
  previous cesarean section 301
  staging system 306, *306*
  technique **302–5**, *303*
    abdominal procedures 303–4
    vaginal procedures 304–5
    without salpingo-oophorectomy
        305
  uterine artery management 303–4, *304*
  uterine mobility 302, 303
  uterine myoma 302
  vaginal access 302, 303
  see also hysterectomy, laparoscopic
      assisted Doderlein
hysterectomy, laparoscopic radical
      447–57
  adnexa management 448, 450
  bleeding management 448, 451, 452,
      456
  bowel preparation 447
  cervical carcinoma stage IB 461
  complications 454
  indications 457
  instruments 448
  intraoperative dissemination of
      malignant cells 456
  large vessel bipolar coagulation 448,
      454
  limited procedure **453**
  lymphadenectomy **450**
  operating room set-up 448
  peritoneal cavity inspection 448
  peritoneal incision 448, 454
  preoperative work-up 447, 457
  radical hysterectomy **450–3**
    cardinal ligament section 452
    pararectal space dissection 451
    paravesical space dissection 450–1
    rectovaginal space dissection 451–2
    surgical anatomy 450, *451*
    ureter dissection 452–3
    vaginal procedure 453
    vesicouterine ligaments dissection
        453
  results 454, *455*, 456
  trocar entry sites 448
hysterectomy, laparoscopic vaginal
      radical **438–45**

Celio–Schauta operation 440–1,
Celio–Schauta version 2 **441–4**
indications 438–9
laparoscopic part 443–4, *443*, *444*
pelvic lymphadenectomy **439**
radical trachelectomy **445**
Schauta operation **440**
urological complications avoidance
441–2
vaginal part 444–5, *444*, *445*
hysterectomy, supracervical
laparoscopic **308–14**
cervical cancer risk following 312, *313*,
313
indications **308–9**
patient preparation 309
postoperative care 311
results 311–12, *312*, 313
technique 309–11
explorative laparoscopy 310
trocar placement 309, *310*
uterine vasculature management
310–11, *310*
tissue removal 311, *311*
hysterectomy, vaginal
adnexal mass 301–2
contraindications 289, **300–2**
ectopic pregnancy 302
endometriosis 301
limited vaginal access 302
minimal uterine mobility 302
pelvic adhesions 300–1
pelvic inflammatory disease 302
previous cesarean section 301
uterine myoma 302
hysterosalpingography 511
hysteroscopic metroplasty 563
infertility investigations 130, 141
intrauterine adhesions 513
intrauterine filling defects 513, *513*
microsurgical tubal anastomosis **177**
septate uterus 554
tubal debris displacement 186–7
tubal patency assessment 186–7, 194,
195, *195*
hysteroscopes 502, *503*, 516, *517*, **527–8**, *528*
tubal occlusion 568–9
hysteroscopic operating accessories *505*,
505–7, *506*
hysteroscopic pumps *507*, **507**, *508*, **528**,
535
hysteroscopic operating sheaths **503–5**,
504
dual operating 506, *507*
multichannel 504–5, *505*
resectoscope 505, 511
single cavity 504, *504*
hysteroscopy **28–9**
abdominal spill of distension fluid
512–13
adenomyosis 266
anesthesia **646–7**
cervical dilation problems 641–2
classification of operative difficulty *641*
complications **15**, **641–7**
contraindications **647**
diagnostic **511–24**
indications **512–16**
distension media 508, 516–17, **525–7**
hazards 642–4
documentation *519*, **519–21**
photography 520–1, *521*, 523
video 521
dual image video
hysteroscopy/laparoscopy
28–9, *29*

flexible **518**
fluid absorption 528, **529–32**
depth of penetration effects
531–2
intrauterine pressure effects 529–31,
530, *531*
reduction methods 528–9, *529*
fluid instillation 518, **528–9**
fluid overload 585, **594–5**, 598, 610–11
management *585*, 595
historical aspects **2–3**
infertility investigation 130, 141
infusion systems **527–9**
instrumentation **502–10**, 516
laparoscopic **57**
laser applications **76–7**
medico-legal aspects 15
metroplasty **556–66**
minor intrauterine procedures **518–19**
nursing responsibilities **35**, **38**
occult malignant disease 647
office **506–7**, **516–17**
operating theater **517–18**
outpatient unit **517**
in pregnancy 647
records 509
rigid **518**
septate uterus 554
technique 518, **518**
training **501–2**, 641, 647
tubal cannulation **191–2**
tubal occlusion **568–77**
tubal ostia visualization 568
uterine perforation 501
video endoscopy **521–3**, 524
camera 522–3, *523*
high-frequency interference 523
recording systems 522, 523
video printing 523

ileus 414, 482
iliac arteries 375
iliac veins 268, 292
iliac vessel damage 50, 51
iliococcygeus muscle 335
imaging 6
imipenem/cilastin 242
in vitro fertilization (IVF) **77–8**
incision 46, **57**
laparoscopic sterilization 168
lateral trocars placement 50, 51, 57
vessel injury 490
incisional hernia 52, 111, 297
incidence 486
prevention 486
incisional instruments *93*
high-frequency 94, *94*
infection
distal tubal infertility 130
endometrial electroablation **597**
endometrial transcervical resection
(TCRE) **586**
Nd:YAG endometrial ablation 608,
610
operative hysteroscopy 647
prevention 56
inferior epigastric vessel damage 12, 50,
51, 112
inferior epigastric vessels 292
inferior mesenteric artery 424–5
infertility
diagnostic hysteroscopy **513–15**
investigations 130, 141, 177
septate uterus 552–4, 566

information for patients 31, 32
bowel preparation *42*
endometrial electroablation 593, 594
enterolysis 391
myolysis 281
postoperative written instructions **38**
sterilization 172
mass procedures 160
infundibulopelvic ligament bulldog
clamps 57
instrument cart 508
instrument table 25
instrumental intrauterine manipulations
515
instruments *24*, **24**, 142
endometriosis monopolar
electroexcision 371–2, *372*
hysteroscopic tubal occlusion **568–9**
Ovabloc *572*, **572**, *573*, *574*
hysteroscopy **502–10**, 516, 517
laparoscopic radical hysterectomy 448
myomectomy **273**
postoperative nursing responsibilities
38
sterilization **168**
insulation failure 89, 294
interiliac lymphadenectomy *408*, **408–9**,
409
tissue extraction 409
interiliac trigone 263, *263*
interstitial hyperthermia endometrial
ablation 547, **547–50**
clinical studies 547–8
in vitro thermometric studies 547, 550
results 548, *549*, 550
intratubal devices 570–1, *571*
intrauterine adhesiolysis 518
intrauterine adhesions *516*
classification 513–14, *514*
hysteroscopic diagnosis 513, *514*
instrumental intrauterine
manipulations 515
intrauterine endosurgery 515–16
intrauterine focal coagulation 518
intrauterine light diffuser 627, *627*
intravenous pyelography 54, 495
intravenous urogram (IVU) 298
irrigation fluid
absorption 15
see also fluid overload
nursing responsibilities **35**, **38**
ischemic heart disease 43
isoflurane 45
isolated electrosurgical outputs **89**
isolation bags 112
isthmic plugs 186
isthmic-ampullary anastomosis 181
isthmic-isthmic anastomosis 181

Jones metroplasty 554, 555, *556*

ketorolac 689
knife-shaped electrodes 95, *95*
Koh Ultramicro Series 178, *179*
Krukenberg tumors 207
KTP (potassium titanyl phosphate) laser
23, 26, 71, 72, 96, 117
adhesiolysis 140, 391, 393, 394
endometriosis vaporization 363
hysteroscopic metroplasty 77
ovarian drilling **238**
ovarian endometrioma vaporization
227, 228, *228*, 229, 230
polycystic ovaries management 233

KTP (potassium titanyl phosphate) laser (*cont.*)
  safety 645
  tissue effects *97*, **98–9**
  uterine nerve ablation **251–2**, 253, 255–6, *255*, *256*

laminaria stents 598, 642
laparoscope **23–4**, 28
  insertion **48**
LaparoSonic Coagulation Shears *681*, **681–3**, *682*, *683*
  hysterectomy **683–6**
    large myomas resection 683, *684*
    results 683
    technique 684–6, *685*
laparotomy, deep endometriosis **387–8**
laryngeal mask airway 674
laser assisted hatching **78–9**
laser light **68–9**
laser nurse *33*, **33–4**
laser optical tweezers 77, 78
laser zona drilling (LZD) 78
lasers 6, **68–79**, **96–102**, 116
  adhesiolysis **75**, 140, 390, 391
  adhesions formation **400**
  clinical results 117–18, *117*, *118*
  complications 122
  delivery systems 71, **72–4**
  design **69**
  ectopic pregnancy conservative treatment 151
  emission wavelengths 97
  endometriosis vaporization **75**, *257*, **257–8**, **363–7**, 380, 383
  fetoscopic surgery 657
  fiber tips 99, *100*, 101–2, 252
  gamete/embryo micromanipulation **77–9**
  hysteroscopic metroplasty **560–1**, *561*
  hysteroscopy 509, **645–6**
    applications **76–7**
  instrumentation **23**, **26–7**
  laparoscopic applications **74–6**
  myomectomy **76**
  operating modes 69, *99*, **99–102**
  ovarian drilling **238**
  ovarian endometrioma photovaporization **227–9**
  ovarian surgery 216
  pelvic reconstruction **71–2**, *72*
  photodynamic therapy *see* photodynamic therapy
  physical principles **68–9**, *535*
  polycystic ovaries management 233
  power density of beam 69, 71, 73
  safety 12, 15, 33, **71**, 102, 293, **645–6**
  sapphire tips 99, *101*, 252, 391
  techniques **59–60**
  terminal salpingostomy **75**
  tissue interactions **69–71**, *70*, *97*, 117, *535*
    absorption 70
    experimental studies 96–7, *98*
    fluorescence 70
    heat production 70
    ionization 71
    photoablation 70–1
    photochemistry 70
    plasma formation 71
  uterine nerve ablation (LUNA) *251*, **251–2**, *252*, 253, *255*, **255–6**, *256*
  uterosacral ligament ablation 76
lateral trocars placement *50*, **50–1**, *51*, 57, 291–2, 393, 484

legal aid 11
leiomyoma *see* myoma
leuprolide acetate 55, 281, 598
levator ani muscle 334, **335–6**
light cables 676
  fetal endoscopy 651–2
  hysteroscopy **502–3**, *503*, 520
light source 22, 676–7
  hysteroscopy *503*, **503**, 520, *520*
  mass sterilization camp *161*, **161**
  safety 12
lignocaine 170, 676
  maximum dose 676
limb defects 671
Limitation Act (1980) 9
lithotomy position 11, 45, 56
  endometrial electrosurgery 371, 598
  hysterectomy 305, 316, 447
  myomectomy 273
  pelvic floor support procedures 327, 338
  presacral neurectomy 266
Lloyd Davies position 676
local anesthesia
  advantages 675
  dose *646*
  endometrial electroablation 598
  endometrial transcervical resection (TCRE) 583
  hysteroscopy **646**
    complications **646–7**
  mass sterilization procedures 161–2
  maximum dose 676
  out-patient laparoscopy **674–8**
    conversion to general anesthesia 675
    patient preparation 675
    sterilization 168, **170**, 675–6, 678
lumbar arteries 426
lumbar lymphatic nodal chain 424
LUNA (laser uterine nerve ablation) *251*, **251–2**, *255*, **255–6**, *256*
luteal cysts 223, *223*
lymph node sampling 418–19
lymphadenectomy, aortic 6, **417–35**, *422*
  cervical carcinoma 461
  complications 432–3
  elderly patients 423
  historical development
    laparoscopic procedure 421–3
    open operation 418
  indications 417, 418, **423–4**, 435
  laparoscopic radical hysterectomy 450
  obese patients 422–3
  ovarian cancer staging 476
  port-site recurrences **433–5**
  purpose 418, **419–21**
    curative treatment 420–1
    diagnosis 419
  radical systemic procedure 421
  surgical anatomy **424–6**, *425*
  survival advantage 422, 435
  technical issues 417
  technique **426–31**
    nodal tissue removal 429–31, *430*, *431*, *432*, *433*
    operating room setup 426–7
    patient position 426
    peritoneal incision 427, *427*, *428*
    planes of dissection 428–9, *428*, *429*, *430*
    trocar placement 426
lymphadenectomy, pelvic 6, **407–16**
  Celio–Schauta operation 441
  cervical carcinoma 461
  complications **412–14**, 416

    early postoperative 414
    late 414
    nerve injury 413
    ureteral injury 413
    vessel injury 412–13
  extraperitoneal approach 439
  indications 414–15
  laparoscopic radical hysterectomy **450**
  laparoscopic vaginal radical hysterectomy **439**, 443, *443*
  missing lymph nodes 413–14
  ovarian cancer staging 476
  with ovarian transposition **411**
  peritoneal healing 412, *412*
  results 412, 415
  technique **407–12**, **439**
    common iliac lymphadenectomy 409–10
    interiliac lymphadenectomy 408–9, *408*, *409*, 439
    parametrial lymphadenectomy 410–11
  tissue extraction 409
  transperitoneal approach 439
lymphedema 414
lymphocysts **464–5**
  pelvic lymphadenectomy 414
magnetic resonance imaging (MRI)
  cervical carcinoma 447
  ovarian endmetrioma **224**
  ovarian lesions 208, 209
  tubo-ovarian abscess 241
magnification/operating distance 350, *350*
Manhès Triton 150, 151
mannitol distension medium **644**
masking **56**
mass sterilization
  abnormalities follow-up 162
  anesthesia 161–2
  complications 163, *163*
  economic aspects 165
  ectopic pregnancy following 164
  failure rates 164
  information for patients 160
  mortality 163–4, *164*
  pneumoperitoneum 162, *162*
  postoperative care 162, *162*, *163*
  reversal 164
  selection of method 159
  sterilization camp **160–1**, *161*
    equipment 161
    preparations 160–1
    prerequisites 160
    problems 164–5
  surgical team 160
  tubal occlusion methods 159–60
  tubal occlusion procedure **162**
  viral infection transmission 163
medico-legal aspects 52
  bowel injury **484–5**, 486
  causes of action *10*
  clinical trials 10
  consent 10
  ectopic pregnancy 15
  entry into abdomen 12–13, 291
  general operating room accidents 11–12
  hysteroscopic surgery 15
  limitations periods 9
  minimally invasive surgery **9–16**
  records 10
  standard of care 9–10
  sterilization 13–15, **172–3**
    pregnant patient **173**
  ureter injury 15

menorrhagia 77, 581, 604, 607, 608, 611, 614, 687, 689, 691
   see also dysfunctional uterine bleeding
menstrual history taking 13
meperidine 162
mesenteric arteries 424–5
metabolic acidosis 647
metalloproteases 398
methotrexate 151, 152, 156, 189
methylcyanoacrylate tubal occlusion 188, 569
metoclopramide 45
metronidazole 47, 242
metroplasty
   abdominal methods **554–6**, *555*
   hysteroscopic **556–66**
     antibiotic prophylaxis 563
     comparison of methods *561*, 564
     complete uterine septum 561–3, *562, 563, 564*
     concomitant procedures 564, 566
     distension medium 556–7, 559, 560
     fiberoptic lasers 560–1, *561*
     laparoscopic/sonographic monitoring 557, 559
     postoperative management 563
     rectoscopic 558–60, *559, 560, 561*
     reproductive outcome 564
     results 564, *565*
     scissor technique 556–8, *557, 558, 561*
microneedle tip unipolar electrode 181
microsurgery
   applications 185
   equipment **178, 180–1**
   laparoscopic access **176–7**
   microinstrumentation 178, *179*
   postoperative adhesions **399–400**
   prerequisites of surgeon **181**
   principles **176**
     myomectomy 273
microsurgical tubal anastomosis **176–85**, 187
   equipment/instruments **178**
     microinstrumentation 178, *179*
   feasibility 177–8
   indications 178
   isthmic–ampullary anastomosis 181
   isthmic–isthmic anastomosis 181
   operating set-up 183
   patient selection 181
   pregnancy rates following 184, *185*
   preoperative work-up 177–8
   prerequisites of surgeon 181
   technique *182*, **183–4**
   tubo-cornual anastomosis 177, 178, 181
microsuturing 176, **178, 180, 181**
microwave applicator 632, *632*
Microwave Endometrial Ablation system 631, *631*
microwave energy **630–1**, *631*
   endometrial ablation *see* endometrial ablation, microwave
midazolam 675, 677
mini-laparoscope 676
minimally invasive surgery 83–4, *83*
   gynecological oncology 459
   medico-legal aspects **9–16**
   microsurgical principles 141–2
mirror-image operating skills 56
missing IUCD **515**
MISTLETOE study 588
monopolar electrocautery 116, 292
   adhesiolysis 140, 391
   coagulation current 58

cutting current 58
endometriosis electroexcision **369–79**
hysteroscopic transcervical sterilization 570
instruments 22, 23
myolysis 280
ovarian drilling *237*, **237**
polycystic ovaries 234
safety 292
   accidental burns 88–9
   sterilization 14, **168**, 171
morcellation procedures 113
morcellators 63, 64, 113, *113*, 277
mortality 41
   mass sterilization camps **163–4**, *164*
   sterilization **171**
mucinous cystadenoma 111–12
multiple staple applicator 62, 63, 121, 293
mycoplasma 130
myelomeningocele 661–2, *663*
myolysis 55, **280–7**
   antibiotic prophylaxis 281
   complications 284–5, *285*
   consent 281
   cost effectiveness 286
   patient selection 280–1
   postoperative adhesions 283, 285–6
   preoperative evaluation 281
   reoperation 284, *284*
   reproductive outcome 281, **283–4**, 286–7
   results **282–4**, *283*, 286
   second-look laparoscopy 283, *283*, 286
   technique **281–2**
   tissue extraction 281
myomas
   classification 534, *534*, 544
   diagnosis 281
   embolization *see* uterine artery embolization
   hysterectomy
     laparoscopic assisted Doderlein 317
     supracervical laparoscopic 308
     vaginal versus abdominal approach 302
   indications for treatment 280, 285
   intramural 534
   laparoscopic coagulation *see* myolysis
   medical treatment 285
   pedunculated 534, 536
   sarcomatous degeneration 281
   submucous 534, 593, 607
     classification 515, *515*, 544
     hysteroscopy 512, *512*, 514–15, *514*
   tissue extraction 63–4, 113
   transvaginal ultrasound 202, *202*, 205, *205*
myomectomy 6, 55, **272–8**, 285, 286
   adhesions
     postoperative 276, *276*, 278, 285
     prevention 65
   argon beam coagulator (ABC) 107, **109**
   complications 275–6, *276*, 278
   conversion to laparotomy 275, 277
   indications 272, 275, **276–8**
   instrumentation 273
   intramural myomas **537**
   laser hysteroscopic **534–9**
     complications 537, 539
     equipment 535
     postoperative management 537
     preoperative endometrial suppression 535, 538
     preoperative preparation 534–5
     results 537–8, *537*

     technique 536–7
   laser laparoscopic **76**
   location of myoma 277
   microsurgical principles 273
   myoma removal 272, **273**, *274*, 275, **277**
   pedunculated myomas 273, 286, *536*, **536**
   reproductive outcome 275–6, 278, *278*
   results 275–6
   sessile myomas 273, 286
   size limits for laparoscopic procedure 272
   submucous myomas *536*, **536**, **544–7**
   suprapubic trocar position 273
   sutures 273
   technique 272, **273–5**, *274*
   transcervical 281
   ultrasonic scalpel 121–2
   underwater rectoscope surgery 57
   uterine incision 272, 277
   uterine suture 273, 277, 278

naproxen sodium 646
Nd:YAG hysteroscopic myomectomy 76, **534–9**
   submucous myomas **544–7**
     fertility following 546
     gonadotropin-releasing hormone (GnRH) analogues therapy 544, 546–7
     results 545, *545*
     technique *536*, **536–7**, **544–5**
Nd:YAG laser 23, 26, 71, 72, **74**, 96, 117
   adhesiolysis 140, 391
   bare fiber 99, *100*, 101–2
   contact versus non-contact application mode **99–102**
   endometrial ablation *see* endometrial ablation, Nd:YAG laser
   fetoscopic surgery 657
   hysteroscopic applications 77
   hysteroscopic metroplasty 77, **560–1**, *561*
   hysteroscopic tubal occlusion 570
   hysteroscopy 509
     safety **645–6**
   myolysis 280, 281, 286
   ovarian drilling **238**
   polycystic ovaries management 233
   sapphire tips 99, *101*, 391
   sperm manipulation 78
   supracervical laparoscopic hysterectomy 310, 311
   tissue effects *97*, *98*, **98**, **99**, *100*
   uterine nerve ablation 252, 253
needle embryofetoscopy (NEF) 651, **655–6**
needles, microsuturing **178, 180**
negligence 9, 10–11, 13, 14
   sterilization procedures **172–3**
Neisseria gonorrhoeae 130, 241, 242
neostigmine 45
nerve injury **413**
neural tube 671
new techniques **54–66**
ninth intercostal space entry 48, 57, 393
nitrogen lasers 74
nitrous oxide insufflation
   out-patient procedures 676
   sterilization 168, 170
nitrous oxide/oxygen 45
non-steroidal anti-inflammatory drugs (NSAIDs) 254, 261, 262

nursing roles
    operative hysteroscopy **35**, **38**
    training **39**

obese patients 482, 675
    anticoagulant prophylaxis 43
    aortic lymphadenectomy 422–3
    complications 41
    large bowel injury 12
    pneumoperitoneum establishment 12,
        47, 162
    previous laparotomy scars 48
    retroperitoneal space anatomy 490
    sterilization morbidity 172, 173
    vessel injury risk 489
obliterated umbilical artery 50, *50*
office hysteroscopy **508–7**, **516–17**
    distending media 508, 516–17
    see also out-patient procedures
office laparoscopy 19, **27–8**
    operating room setup 27–8, *27*
    see also out-patient procedures
oophorectomy 15, 218, *218*, 469, *471*, *472*
    endometriosis 266
    ovarian endometrioma 381, *382*, *383*
operating room design 25, **25–7**
operating room nurse 20–1, **30–9**
operating room preparation *31*, **31–3**
operating room setup 19, 31, *31*, **56**
    aortic lymphadenectomy 426–7
    endometrial electroablation 598
    enterolysis 392
    hysterectomy
        laparoscopic radical 448
        supracervical laparoscopic *305*
    mass sterilization camp 160–1, *161*
    positioning of personnel **34–5**
    surgical team **20–1**, *21*
operating table 55, 142
optical catheter 47, *47*
optical trapping of sperm **78**
oral contraceptive pill 254, 261, 262
orogastric intubation 56
out-patient procedures **674–8**
    bladder care 676
    endometriosis monopolar
        electroexcision 378
    equipment 676–7, *677*
    hysteroscopy **517**
    laparopscope system 676–7, *677*
    monitoring 677
    patient position 676
    patient preparation 675
    patient selection 675
    pneumoperitoneum 676
    technique **675–6**
Ovabloc system **571–7**
    instrumentation 572, *572*, *573*, *574*
    patient selection 571–2
    pregnancy following plug removal
        577
    problems 575–6
        plug migration 576, *576*
    procedure 572–5, *575*
    radiographic follow-up 576, *576*
    results 576–7
ovarian arteries 424, 425
ovarian cancer **212–13**, **462–4**
    advanced disease **476–7**
    aortic lymphadenectomy 421
        indications 423–4
    clinical detection 214
    dissemination problems 212, 434–5, 467
    fluorescence diagnosis of metastases
        627

historical aspects 468
incidence *213*
laparoscopic diagnosis 215
lymph node spread 420, 463
management principles 468, **475**, 477
pelvic lymphadenectomy 411, 415
photodynamic therapy 621
port-site recurrences 434–5
risk factors *213*
screening 464
second-look procedures 463, 464, 467,
    468, **476–7**
serological markers 213–14
stage I **475–6**
staging 418
tissue extraction 114, 463
treatment experience *474*, **474–5**, *475*
tumor marker elevation 463–4
ultrasound screening **203–4**
ovarian cyst 212
    cystoscopy 215
    functional 469
    intraoperative diagnosis 469
    laparoscopic assessment **214–15**, *215*,
        477
    malignancy 206, 209, 212, 213, 462,
        474, *474*, *475*
        dissemination 434–5
    management **209**, 468, **475**, 477
    preoperative diagnosis 468, *468*
    spillage of contents 112, 218, 434–4335
    surgery 209, **215–17**, *216*, *217*, 469, *470*
        cyst lining destruction *in situ* 217
    tissue removal 63, 112, 114, 469
        adnexal bag 469, *470*
    transvaginal ultrasound 202, *202*, 203,
        204, 205, **205–7**, *206*, *207*, 209,
        210, **224**
        duplex Doppler imaging 208
        fine echoes 206, 209, 224
    treatment experience **469–75**, *473*
    ultrasound-guided aspiration 209, 214
        dissemination risk 214
    unilocular (simple) 205–6, 209, 212,
        213, 214
ovarian cystoscopy 215
    ovarian endometrioma **224–5**, *225*
ovarian endometrioma **221–31**, *222*, 351,
    357, 476
    classification 223
    fertility following treatment 230
    historical background 221–2
    laparoscopic excision **119–20**, *120*,
        225–7, *226*
        complications 230
        results **230–1**
        two-step procedure 227, *227*
    laparoscopic laser surgery 227–9
        adhesions prevention **229**
        results **230**
    laparotomy versus laparoscopic
        techniques 231
    luteal cysts association 223, *223*
    magnetic resonance imaging (MRI)
        224
    malignancy 381
    management techniques **381**, *382*, *383*
    monopolar electroexcision **375–6**
    ovarian cystoscopy **224–5**, *225*
    ovarian suppressive therapy 227, 230,
        231
    pain relief following treatment 230
    pathology 222–3, *223*
    postoperative adhesions 218, 230, 231
    transvaginal ultrasound **223–4**
        exclusion of malignancy 224

visual diagnosis 222
ovarian mass **467–78**
    computed tomography (CT) 208–9
    laparoscopic assessment *214*, **214–15**
    laparoscopic surgery **215–19**
    magnetic resonance imaging (MRI)
        208
    pre-laparoscopic assessment **213–14**
    pre-operative imaging **223–4**
    see also pelvic mass
ovarian remnant syndrome 393
ovarian reserve assessment 177
ovarian surgery **212–19**, *217*
    complications **218–19**
    equipment 216
    general principles 215–16
    peritoneal lavage 217, 218
    postoperative adhesions 217, 218
    preoperative imaging **201–10**
    suture of ovary *216*, 217, *217*
    technique 216–17, *216*
ovarian tissue extraction 111–12, 113,
    217
    adnexal bag 469, *470*
    ovarian cancer 114, 463
    ovarian cysts 63, 112, 114, 469
ovarian torsion **212**
    laparoscopic treatment **219**
ovarian transposition **411**
ovarian veins 425, 426
ovary
    laparoscopic inspection 49
    ultrasound **201–10**

papillary serous ovarian carcinoma 111
paracervical block 598, 607
paracolpos tumor 464
parametrial lymphadenectomy **410–11**
paravaginal suspension **343–4**, *344*
pelvic contents inspection **49**
    end of procedure underwater
        examination 65
    endometriosis diagnosis **350–1**
    hysterectomy 300, 301, 303, 310, 317,
        448
    ovarian mass assessment 214
    uterine nerve ablation 250
pelvic floor disorders 334, 346
    anterior compartment defects **336**
    middle compartment defects **337**
    multiple defects 334–5
    posterior compartment defects **336–7**
    symptomatology **337–8**
pelvic floor support anatomy *335*, **335–6**
pelvic floor support procedures **334–46**
    contraindications 338
    laparoscopic approach 338
    patient preparation 338
    postoperative care **345**
    preoperative evaluation 336–7
    suturing 338
    technique **338–40**
        enterocele repair 339–40
        paravaginal suspension 343–4, *344*
        pubocervical fascia repair 342–3
        rectovaginal septum repair 342–3
        retropubic colposuspension 344–5
        trocar placement 338
        vaginal vault suspension 340–2, *340*
    ureter identification/dissection 339,
        339
pelvic inflammatory disease 129, 241
    adhesions 139
    hysterectomy 302, 309

tubal infertility 130
  see also tubo-ovarian abscess
pelvic lymphadenectomy *see*
  lymphadenectomy, pelvic
pelvic malignancy
  ovarian transposition **411**
  pelvic lymphadenectomy **407–11**
  staging 407
pelvic mass
  management **209**
  ultrasound examination 202, *203*, **204**,
    224
pelvic nerve supply *264*, 265
pelvic organ injury 43
pelvic pain **261–70**
  ultrasound examination **203**
pelvic reconstructive surgery 6
  laser treatment **71–2**, *72*
pelvic vessel embolization 687
pelviperitonitis 597
periadnexal adhesive disease **139–40**
  causes 139
  cutting modalities 140
  instruments 141
  preoperative investigations 141
  surgical results 144–6, **144–6**, 148
  surgical techniques **141–4**
peritoneal cavity closure 297
peritoneal entry **46–7**, **290–2**, 294, 448,
    454
  confirmation **47–8**
photoablation 70–1
photodynamic therapy **621–8**
  cervical intraepithelial neoplasia
    (CIN) 621, **623**
  endometrial ablation *see* endometrial
    photodynamic therapy
  indications 623
  mode of action 621
  photosensitizers 621–2, *623*
photosensitizers 70, **621–2**
  application methods 622
  light activation 622, *623*
physiologic umbilical hernia 671, *671*
placental surgery **656–9**
plasminogen activator inhibitors 398,
    399
plastic plug tubal occlusion 188
pneumoperitoneum
  difficulty in establishment **12**
  enterolysis procedure 392
  induction technique **46–7**
  obese patients 12
  out-patient procedures 676
  sterilization 162, *162*, 168
polycystic ovaries **233–9**
  adhesion formation
    following laparoscopic treatment
      235, **235–6**, 239
    postoperative 233
  electrocautery versus laser treatment
    121, *121*, *122*
  hormonal changes following surgical
    treatment 236–7
  hormonal treatment 233
  management 239, *239*
  mechanism of action of surgical
    treatment **236**
  ovarian drilling **120–2**, 233, *233*, 234
    complications **235–6**
    methods **237–8**
    ovulation/pregnancy outcome *234*
    premature menopause/ovarian
      atrophy 236
  ovarian ultrasound 204, *204*
  ovarian wedge resection 120

polydactyly 671
porphyrin photosensitizer 621
port enlargers 112
port-site recurrences
  aortic lymphadenectomy **433–5**
  ovarian cancer 434–5
post-TURP syndrome 642
posterior colpotomy 111, 112, 275, 277
  bowel injury 485
posterior parietal peritoneum *425*
postoperative care 45
  complications recognition 52
  diagnostic laparoscopy **52**
  follow-up *36–7*, **38–9**
  hysterectomy **297**
  nursing responsibilities **38**
  written instructions **38**
postoperative pain relief 45
pregnancy
  following endometrial electroablation
    597
  following endometrial transcervical
    resection (TCRE) 586
  following microsurgical tubal
    anastomosis 184, *185*
  following Ovabloc plug removal 577
  following ovarian drilling *234*
  following tubal cannulation 187
  operative hysteroscopy during **647**
  sterilization failure 169, 170, **171**
    medico-legal aspects **13–15**, 172–3
  sterilization of pregnant patient **173**
premedication 161, 162
premenstrual syndrome (PMS) 593, 594
preoperative assessment 31, 32, **54**
preoperative nurses 31
preoperative preparation 31, 32, **45**, **54–5**
  starvation 45
presacral neurectomy 6, 249, 254, 261
  argon beam coagulator (ABC) 107, **108**
  bowel preparation 266
  complications 267–9
  dysmenorrhea 269
  efficacy of pain relief 269
  indications **262–3**
  laparoscopic procedure 262
  laparoscopic surgical skills 263, 269
  preoperative evaluation 266
  surgical anatomy *263*, **263–5**, *264*
  technique **266–7**
previous abdominal surgery *see*
  abdominal scars
progesterone receptors 361
prolapse of pelvic contents 334, 336
propofol 45
prostaglandin synthetase inhibitors 518
protoporphyrin IX 621, 622
  fluorescence diagnostics 627
proximal tubal occlusion
  isthmic plugs 186
  microsurgical tubo-cornual
    anastomosis 187
  tubal cannulation **186–7**
proximal tubal patency assessment **186**
  falloposcopy 194, 195, *195*
pseudomyxoma peritonei 112
pubocervical fascia 335, *335*
  repair technique **342–3**
pubococcygeus `sling' 335
pulmonary edema 15, 526, 598, 610

quinacrine tubal occlusion **569–70**

radical trachelectomy **445**, **462**

records
  circulating nurse responsibilities 35,
    35
  hysteroscopy 509, *519*, **519–21**
  medico-legal aspects 10
  Microwave Endometrial Ablation
    system 633, *634*
  sterilization failure 173
recovery room nurse 38
rectal probes 55–6, 142, 385, 426, 448
rectocele 336–7
rectoscope **509**, 527, 581
  active/passive 645
  endometrial ablation 540, 541, 543
  hysteroscopic metroplasty **558–60**,
    559, *560*
  myomectomy procedures 57
  safety **645**
rectovaginal septum adenomyotic
    nodule **357–62**
  complications 360, *360*
  histology *360*, **360–1**, *361*
  patient characteristics 357–8
  preoperative evaluation 358
  rectal wall infiltration 358, *358*
  surgical technique **358–60**, *359*
  symptoms 358
rectovaginal septum (Denonvilliers'
    fascia) 335, 336
  repair technique **342–3**
recurrent pregnancy loss
  diagnostic hysteroscopy 515
  septate uterus 552–3, 554, 566
renal artery 426
renal vein 424, 425, 426
retrograde salpingoscopy (tuboscopy)
    144
retroperitoneal space anatomy *425*
  vessel injury **490**
retropubic (Burch) colposuspension
    325–6
  technique **344–5**, *345*
retropubic space access 326, **327**

sacrocolpopexy **340–2**
sacrospinous vaginal fixation **340**, *342*
salpingectomy
  ectopic pregnancy 15
  tissue removal 112
salpingitis 139–40
salpingo-oophorectomy 218, 303
salpingo-ovariolysis 141, **142–3**
  laser versus electrosurgery or sharp
    dissection 117, *117*
  results **145**, 148
salpingostomy 75, *132*, **132–3**, *133*, *134*,
    135, *136*, 141, **143–4**
  laser versus electrosurgery or sharp
    dissection 117–18, *118*
  results *134*, *135*, *136*, **145–6**, 148
salpingotomy 15, 151
sapphire tips 99, *101*, 252, 391
Schauta radical vaginal hysterectomy
    440, 454, 461, 462
Schauta–Amreich operation 440
Schauta–Stoeckel operation 440
schistosomiasis 129
scissor dissection
  adhesiolysis 140, 391
  clinical results 117–18, *117*, *118*
  ectopic pregnancy conservative
    treatment 151
  endometriosis excision 380, 383
  hysteroscopic metroplasty **556–8**, *557*,
    558

scissor dissection (*cont.*)
   rectovaginal septum adenomyotic
     nodule 358
scissors **58**
scrub nurse 20
scrubbing **56**
sedation **675–6**, 689, 691
semen analysis 130, 141, 177
septate uterus **552–6**, 641
   anatomy 552, *553*
   embryology 552, *553*
   indications for surgery 552–4
   preoperative evaluation 554
   treatment methods 77, 554–6
seromyotomy *102*
shaving, preoperative 45, 54
shock, clinical 43
smoke evacuation 73
   instrumentation **23**
sodium chloride distension medium,
   0.9% **527**
sodium hyaluronidate 395
sorbitol distension medium **527**, 595
   complications **644**
speculum, historical aspects 1, *1*
sperm manipulation **78**
standard of care 9–10
Staphylococcus aureus 45
stapler, laparoscopic 62, 63, 121, 293
staples
   colposuspension 326–7
   hysterectomy **293**
   new techniques **61–3**
   safety 293
sterilization 159, **167–73**
   anesthesia **170**, 675–6, 678
   complications 172, 173
   counseling 172
   ectopic pregnancy following *171*,
     171–2
   electrocautery 14, **168–9**
   endometrial electroablation 593–4
   equipment 290
   failure 14, 169, 170, **171**, 172, 173
   historical aspects 167–8
   hysteroscopic *see* tubal occlusion,
     hysteroscopic
   instrumentation 168
   long-term problems 172
   mass population control *see* mass
     sterilization
   mechanical techniques 14, *169*, **169–70**
   medico-legal aspects **13–15**, **172–3**
   menstrual history taking 13
   mortality 171
   nitrous oxide pneumoperitoneum 168,
     170
   pregnancy exclusion 14
   pregnant patient **173**
   resterilization 14
   reversal 159, 172, 184–5
     see also microsurgical tubal
       anastomosis
   vaginal route 159
   see also tubal occlusion
sterilization camp *see* mass sterilization
stomach distension 482
stress incontinence 325, 326, 327, 337
suction irrigation
   enterolysis 393–4, *394*
   microsurgical tubal anastomosis 180
   ovarian endometrioma surgery 228,
     229
   see also aquadissection
sulbactam 242, 376
sulprostone 642

superior hypogastric plexus 265, *265*
superior mesenteric artery 424
suprapubic probe insertion **49–50**
surgeon's preference card 32
surgical assistant 20, 32, *32*, **35**, 56
   responsibilities *34*, **34**
   training 482
surgical barriers 65
surgical modality comparisons **116–23**
surgical team **20–1**, *21*, **34–5**, *35*
   mass sterilization 160
surgical techician 34, **35**
sutures 6, 52, 142
   adhesion formation 400
   colposuspension 325, 326, **329**
   hysterectomy **293**, 303
   large vessel injury repair 268
   microsurgical tubal anastomosis **178**,
     180, **181**
   myomectomy 273, 277, 278
   new techniques 60, **60–1**, *61*, *62*
syndactyly 672

telescope **23–4**
   office laparoscopy 28
thecoma 207
thermal tissue effects 84, *84*, *93*
thermal tubal occlusion **169**
   blind methods 569
thin patients
   complications 41
   large bowel injury 13
   pneumoperitoneum induction 47
   vessel injury 489
thin-gauge embryofetoscopy (TGEF)
   651, **655–6**
three-dimensional imaging 6
thromboembolism 43
ticarcillin 242
tiltable operating room tables 55
tissue extraction **111–14**
   delayed 112
   hysterectomy 305, 311, *311*
   interiliac lymphadenectomy 409
   isolation devices 112
   misplaced tissues 112
   myolysis 281
   myomectomy 272, **273**, *274*, **275**, **277**
   ovarian cancer 463
   ovarian cysts 217, 469, *470*
   port site enlargement 112
   port site recurrence prevention 435
   potential complications 114
   principles 111
   problems of tissue spillage 111–12
   techniques 63–4, 112–14
   tubal trophoblast 151
tissue metalloprotease inhibitors
   (TIMPS) 398
tissue retrieval bags 63, 64, 112, 469, *470*
titanium clips 391
training 9, 482, 674
   hysteroscopy **501–2**, 641, 647
   nursing roles **39**
   surgical assistant 482
transcervical myomectomy 281
transcervical resection of endometrium
   see endometrial transcervical
     resection (TCRE)
transcervical salpingoscopy
   (falloposcopy) 144
transcervical sterilization
   blind methods **569**
   hysteroscopic *see* tubal occlusion,
     hysteroscopic

transfer, postoperative 38
transvaginal ultrasound 54, 511
   ovarian cysts 202, *202*, 203, *204*, *205*,
     205–7, 209, 210
   ovarian mass **204–5**, 213, 214, **223**
   ovary 201, **204**
     color flow imaging **207**
     duplex Doppler imaging **207–8**, *208*
   resolution 201–2
   transabdominal ultrasound
     comparison 202–3, *202*
Trendelenburg's position 11, 43, 48, 56
   anesthetic problems 296
   aortic lymphadenectomy 426
   degrees of tilt 45, 55
   endometriosis monopolar
     electroexcision 371
   great vessel injury risk 490
   hysterectomy 294, 447
   hysteroscopy-associated fluid
     overload 598
   microsurgical tubal anastomosis 183
   myolysis 281
   pelvic floor support procedures 338
   sterilization 162, 168
   tiltable operating room tables 55
   tubo-ovarian abscess 243
trifluoropromazine hydrochloride 162
trocar sleeves 24, **56**
trocars 24
   disposable 483
   electrosurgical electrode access
     hazards 89–91, *90*, *91*
   microsurgical tubal anastomosis 180
   safety shields 483
   tissue extraction technique 112
   vessel injury 489
tubal anastomosis *see* microsurgical
     tubal anastomosis; tubotubal
     anastomosis
tubal cannulation **186–96**
   anatomical factors 189
   ectopic pregnancy 188, 189
   falloposcopy **194–5**
   fluoroscopy **192**, *193*, **194**
   hysteroscopic techniques **191–2**
   pregnancy rates following 187
   procedure **189–90**, *190*, *191*, **191**
   proximal tubal occlusion 186–7
tubal embryo transfer 188
tubal epithelium
   early embryo growth effects 188
   falloposcopic assessment **187–8**
tubal lavage 57
tubal occlusion 159
   hysteroscopic **568–77**
     distension medium 569
     instrumentation 568–9
     timing of procedure 568
     tubal ostia identfication/approach
       568–9
     see also Ovabloc system
   mass sterilization **159–65**
   methods **188**, 569–71
     electrocautery 14, **168–9**
     mechanical 14, *169*, **169–70**, 570–1,
       571
   reversal 159, 172, 184–5
   transcervical blind methods **569–70**
   see also sterilization
tubal patency assessment 131, 143, 184,
     186–7
tubal plugs 571, *571*
   Ovabloc system **571–7**
tubal repair surgery **131–7**
   adhesiolysis 131–2, 133, *134*, 136

contraindications 130–1
equipment 131
fimbrioplasty **132**, 133, *134*
patient preparation 131
results 133, *134, 135*
salpingoscopic assessment of
epithelium **187–8**, *188*
salpingostomy *132*, **132–3**, *133, 135, 136*
surgical techniques **131–2**
tubal status scoring 195
tuberculosis 129, 130, 162
tubocornual anastomosis 177, 178, 181
proximal tubal occlusion 187
tubo-ovarian abscess **241–5**, 309
antibiotic treatment 241, 242, 244
complications of laparotomy 241
diagnosis 241
laparoscopic treatment **242–4**, *243*
complications 245
equipment 242–3
postoperative care 244
preoperative management 242
technique 243–4
pelvic adhesive disease 241, 242
post-endometrial electroablation 597
radiological guided aspiration 244
surgical drainage 242
tuboscopy 136
tubotubal anastomosis 141, **146–7**
results 147, 148
technique 146–7
Tupla clip 167, *169*
twin reversed arterial perfusion
sequence (TRAPS) **658–9**
twin-to-twin transfusion syndrome
(TTTS) **657–8**

ultrasonic scalpel *102*, **102–3**, 116, *679*, **679–86**
coagulation/cutting mechanics 680–1, *680*
LaparoSonic Coagulation Shears *681*, **681–3**, *682, 683*
hysterectomy *see* LaparoSonic
Coagulation Shears
lateral distribution of energy 679–80, *680*
myomectomy 121–2
tissue effects 117
ultrasound
hysteroscopic metroplasty monitoring
557, 559
indications **203–4**
myolysis evaluation 281
ovarian mass assessment 213, 214, **223–4**
ovary **201–10**
equipment 201
technique **201–3**, *202*
tubo-ovarian abscess 241, 242
guided aspiration 244
see also transvaginal ultrasound
umbilical trocar insertion **48**
underwater surgery
adhesiolysis 391
end of procedure examination **64–5**
hysterectomy electrosurgery 294
ovarian endometrioma 229
rectoscope surgery 57
unipolar electrocautery *see* monopolar
electrocautery
ureter injury 173, **494–5**
deep infiltrative endometriosis 385, 388

endometriosis monopolar
electroexcision 375
hysterectomy 292, 293, 294–5, 297–8, 315, 320, 454
management 385, **495**
medico-legal aspects **15**
pelvic floor support procedures 339
pelvic lymphadenectomy **413**
prevention **294–5**, 339, 375, 385, **494–5**
recognition 297–8, **495**
uterosacral ligament division 253
ureteric obstruction 298
ureteric stents, transilluminating 295
uretero-neocystostomy 385
ureterolysis 385
ureters inspection 49
urinary incontinence 325, 326, 327, 337
urinary retention, postoperative 54
urinary tract injury 43
urodynamic tests 337
urogenital diaphragm 335
urological malignancy 411, 415
uterine artery embolization **687–91**
analgesia 689, 690
follow-up 689
patient selection 687, *688*
results 689–90, *690, 691*
technique 688–9, *689*
uterine bleeding
endometrial electroablation **596**
endometrial transcervical resection
(TCRE) **586**
Nd:YAG endometrial ablation 598, 610
uterine instrumental injuries **644–5**
uterine malignancy **462**
post-endometrial transcervical
resection (TCRE) 586–7
uterine manipulator **55**, 162, 168, 243, 251, 266, 281, 303, 316, *317*, 385
laparoscopic radical hysterectomy 447
microsurgical tubal anastomosis 180–1
out-patient procedures 676
uterine nerve ablation **249–58**
complications 15, 253, **258**
consent 250
electrosurgery **252–3**
laser procedure (LUNA) *251*, **251–2**, *255*, **255–6**, *256*
patient counseling 250, 256
preoperative pelvic inspection 250
results **253–4**, 255–6
uterine nerve supply **249–50**
uterine perforation 15, **644**
endometrial electroablation **595–6**
endometrial transcervical resection
(TCRE) **584–5**, 614
fluid overload 645
hysteroscopy 501
Nd:YAG endometrial ablation 608, 610, 614
uterine prolapse 336
uterine rupture 278, 286, 287
uterine septum *see* septate uterus
uterosacral ligament sensory nerve
fibers 249–50
uterosacral ligament transection
argon beam coagulator (ABC) 107
Doyle technique 249, **250**, 254
laser ablation **76**
see also uterine nerve ablation

vaginal intraepithelial neoplasia (VAIN)
621

vaginal probes **55–6**, 142, 448
vaginal vault prolapse 336–7
vaginal vault suspension *340*, **340–2**
high McCall vaginal vault suspension
340, *341*
sacrocolpopexy 340–2
sacrospinous vaginal fixation 340, *342*
vascular injury 13, 41, 43, 173, **489–93**
abdominal entry techniques 46, **51**, 296, **490–2**
aortic lymphadenectomy 433
hemorrhage management **296**
hysterectomy 292, **295–6**, 315
re-laparoscopy 297
incidence 489
pelvic lymphadenectomy 412, **412–13**
presacral neurectomy 267–8, *268*
prevention 292, 295
recognition **492**
repair **51**, 292, 295, 296
retroperitoneal space anatomy **490**
surgical errors 489–90
uterosacral ligament division 253
vasopressin 150, 151, 281, 282, 598
vasovagal reaction 646
Veress needle
injury 482
insertion technique 46, *46*, 393
placement confirmation **47–8**
VestaBlate system *618*, **618–19**
clinical trials 618–19
endometrial preparation 618
video camera 6, 20, 21, 22
hysteroscopy 507–8, **522–3**, *523*
out-patient procedures 677
video carts 32–3
video instrumentation **21–2**
video monitor 6, 21–2, 26, 30, 56, **523**
ceiling mounting 22, *22*
video printing **523**
video recording systems 522, **523**
video standards **521–2**
vimentin 361
viral infection transmission 163
volvulus 13
vulvar cancer 464
vulvar intraepithelial neoplasia (VIN)
621

wound infection prevention 45
written information
bowel preparation *42*
postoperative care **38**

XeCl laser 74
embryo manipulation 78

yolk sac 669–70, *669*
Yoon ring *see* falope ring

zona pellucida
laser assisted hatching **78–9**
laser manipulations 77, 78

Multimedia CD-ROM
Single User License Agreement

1. NOTICE. WE ARE WILLING TO LICENSE THE MULTI-MEDIA PROGRAM PRODUCT TITLED "CD-ROM TO ACCOMPANY ENDOSCOPIC SURGERY FOR GYNECOL-OGISTS, 2ND EDITION" ("MULTIMEDIA PROGRAM") TO YOU ONLY ON THE CONDITION THAT YOU ACCEPT ALL OF THE TERMS CONTAINED IN THIS LICENSE AGREEMENT. PLEASE READ THIS LICENSE AGREEMENT CAREFULLY BEFORE OPENING THE SEALED DISK PACKAGE. BY OPENING THAT PACKAGE YOU AGREE TO BE BOUND BY THE TERMS OF THIS AGREEMENT. IF YOU DO NOT AGREE TO THESE TERMS WE ARE UNWILLING TO LICENSE THE MULTIMEDIA PROGRAM TO YOU, AND YOU SHOULD NOT OPEN THE DISK PACKAGE. IN SUCH CASE, PROMPTLY RETURN THE UNOPENED DISK PACKAGE AND ALL OTHER MATER-IAL IN THIS PACKAGE, ALONG WITH PROOF OF PAY-MENT, TO THE AUTHORIZED DEALER FROM WHOM YOU OBTAINED IT FOR A FULL REFUND OF THE PRICE YOU PAID.

2. **Ownership and License.** This is a license agreement and NOT an agreement for sale. It permits you to use one copy of the MULTIMEDIA PROGRAM on a single computer. The MULTIMEDIA PROGRAM and its contents are owned by us or our licensors, and are protected by U.S. and international copyright laws. Your rights to use the MULTIMEDIA PRO-GRAM are specified in this Agreement, and we retain all rights not expressly granted to you in this Agreement.

   - You may use one copy of the MULTIMEDIA PROGRAM on a single computer.

   - After you have installed the MULTIMEDIA PROGRAM on your computer, you may use the MULTIMEDIA PROGRAM on a different computer only if you first delete the files installed by the installation program from the first computer.

   - You may not copy any portion of the MULTIMEDIA PROGRAM to your computer hard disk or any other media other than printing out or downloading nonsubstantial portions of the text and images in the MULTIMEDIA PRO-GRAM for your own internal informational use.

   - You may not copy any of the documentation or other printed materials accompanying the MULTIMEDIA PROGRAM.

   Neither concurrent use on two or more computers nor use in a local area network or other network is permitted without separate autho-rization and the payment of additional license fees.

3. **Transfer and Other Restrictions.** You may not rent, lend, or lease this MULTIMEDIA PROGRAM. Save as permitted by law, you may not and you may not permit others to (a) dis-assemble, decompile, or otherwise derive source code from the software included in the MULTIMEDIA PROGRAM (the "Software"), (b) reverse engineer the Software, (c) modify or prepare derivative works of the MULTIMEDIA PROGRAM, (d) use the Software in an on-line system, or (e) use the MULTIMEDIA PROGRAM in any manner that infringes on the intellectual property or other rights of another party.

   However, you may transfer this license to use the MULTI-MEDIA PROGRAM to another party on a permanent basis by transferring this copy of the License Agreement, the MULTI-MEDIA PROGRAM, and all documentation. Such transfer of possession terminates your license from us. Such other party shall be licensed under the terms of this Agreement upon its

acceptance of this Agreement by its initial use of the MULTI-MEDIA PROGRAM. If you transfer the MULTIMEDIA PRO-GRAM, you must remove the installation files from your hard disk and you may not retain any copies of those files for your own use.

4. **Limited Warranty and Limitation of Liability.** For a period of sixty (60) days from the date you acquired the MULTI-MEDIA PROGRAM from us or our authorized dealer, we warrant that the media containing the MULTIMEDIA PRO-GRAM will be free from defects that prevent you from installing the MULTIMEDIA PROGRAM on your computer. If the disk fails to conform to this warranty, you may, as your sole and exclusive remedy, obtain a replacement free of charge if you return the defective disk to us with a dated proof of purchase. Otherwise the MULTIMEDIA PRO-GRAM is licensed to you on an "AS IS" basis without any warranty of any nature.

   WE DO NOT WARRANT THAT THE MULTIMEDIA PRO-GRAM WILL MEET YOUR REQUIREMENTS OR THAT ITS OPERATION WILL BE UNINTERRUPTED OR ERROR-FREE. THE EXPRESS TERMS OF THIS AGREEMENT ARE IN LIEU OF ALL WARRANTIES, CONDITIONS, UNDER-TAKINGS, TERMS AND OBLIGATIONS IMPLIED BY STATUTE, COMMON LAW, TRADE USAGE, COURSE OF DEALING OR OTHERWISE ALL OF WHICH ARE HEREBY EXCLUDED TO THE FULLEST EXTENT PERMITTED BY LAW, INCLUDING THE IMPLIED WARRANTIES OF SAT-ISFACTORY QUALITY AND FITNESS FOR A PARTICULAR PURPOSE.

   WE SHALL NOT BE LIABLE FOR ANY DAMAGE OR LOSS OF ANY KIND (EXCEPT PERSONAL INJURY OR DEATH RESULTING FROM OUR NEGLIGENCE) ARIS-ING OUT OF OR RESULTING FROM YOUR POSSESSION OR USE OF THE MULTIMEDIA PROGRAM (INCLUDING DATA LOSS OR CORRUPTION), REGARDLESS OF WHETHER SUCH LIABILITY IS BASED IN TORT, CON-TRACT OR OTHERWISE AND INCLUDING, BUT NOT LIMITED TO, ACTUAL, SPECIAL, INDIRECT, INCIDEN-TAL OR CONSEQUENTIAL DAMAGES. IF THE FOREGO-ING LIMITATION IS HELD TO BE UNENFORCEABLE, OUR MAXIMUM LIABILITY TO YOU SHALL NOT EXCEED THE AMOUNT OF THE LICENSE FEE PAID BY YOU FOR THE MULTIMEDIA PROGRAM. THE REM-EDIES AVAILABLE TO YOU AGAINST US AND THE LICENSORS OF MATERIALS INCLUDED IN THE MULTI-MEDIA PROGRAM ARE EXCLUSIVE.

5. **Termination.** This license and your right to use this MULTI-MEDIA PROGRAM automatically terminate if you fail to comply with any provisions of this Agreement, destroy the copy of the MULTIMEDIA PROGRAM in your possession, or voluntarily return the MULTIMEDIA PROGRAM to us. Upon termination you will destroy all copies of the MULTIMEDIA PROGRAM and documentation.

6. **Miscellaneous Provisions.** This Agreement will be gov-erned by and construed in accordance with English law and you hereby submit to the non-exclusive jurisdiction of the English Courts. This is the entire agreement between us relating to the MULTIMEDIA PROGRAM, and supersedes any prior purchase order, communications, advertising or representations concerning the contents of this package. No change or modification of this Agreement will be valid unless it is in writing and is signed by us.